DEWHURST'S
TEXTBOOK OF OBSTETRICS AND GYNAECOLOGY FOR POSTGRADUATES

This book is the fourth edition of
Integrated Obstetrics and Gynaecology for Postgraduates
Edited by Sir John Dewhurst

DEWHURST'S TEXTBOOK OF OBSTETRICS AND GYNAECOLOGY FOR POSTGRADUATES

EDITED BY

C.R. WHITFIELD
MD, FRCOG, FRCP

Regius Professor of Midwifery, University of Glasgow
Consultant Obstetrician and Gynaecologist
Queen Mother's Hospital and
Western Infirmary, Glasgow

FOURTH EDITION

BLACKWELL SCIENTIFIC PUBLICATIONS

OXFORD LONDON EDINBURGH
BOSTON PALO ALTO MELBOURNE

© 1972, 1976, 1981, 1986 by
Blackwell Scientific Publications
Editorial offices:
Osney Mead, Oxford, OX2 0EL
8 John Street, London, WC1N 2ES
23 Ainslie Place, Edinburgh, EH3 6AJ
3 Cambridge Center, Suite 208
   Cambridge, Massachusetts 02142, USA
667 Lytton Avenue, Palo Alto
   California 94301, USA
107 Barry Street, Carlton
   Victoria 3053, Australia

First published 1972
Second edition 1976
Third edition 1981
Fourth edition 1986
Reprinted 1987, 1988

Spanish edition 1978

Printed and bound in Great Britain by
Butler & Tanner Ltd, Frome and London

DISTRIBUTORS

USA
   Year Book Medical Publishers
   200 North LaSalle Street
   Chicago, Illinois 60601
   (*Orders*: Tel. 312-726-9733)

Canada
   The C.V. Mosby Company
   5240 Finch Avenue East
   Scarborough, Ontario
   (*Orders*: Tel. 416-298-1588)

Australia
   Blackwell Scientific Publications
   (Australia) Pty Ltd
   107 Barry Street
   Carlton, Victoria 3053
   (*Orders*: Tel. 03-347-0300)

British Library
Cataloguing in Publication Data

Dewhurst's textbook of obstetrics and gynaecology for
   postgraduates.—4th ed.
   1. Gynaecology
   I. Dewhurst, *Sir* C. John   II. Whitfield, C.R.
   III. Integrated obstetrics and gynaecology for
   postgraduates
   618   RG101

ISBN 0-632-01369-9

CONTENTS

LIST OF
CONTRIBUTORS

J. M. BEAZLEY   MD FRCOG
Professor of Obstetrics and Gynaecology
Royal Liverpool Hospital
University of Liverpool

G. V. P. CHAMBERLAIN   MD FRCS FRCOG
Professor of Obstetrics and Gynaecology
St George's Hospital Medical School, London

F. COCKBURN   MD FRCP (Ed & Glas) DCH
Professor of Child Health
Royal Hospital for Sick Children, Glasgow

D. A. DAVEY   MB BS PhD FRCOG
Professor of Obstetrics and Gynaecology
Director of Reproductive Medicine Research Unit
University of Cape Town
South Africa

SIR JOHN DEWHURST   FRCS(Ed) FRCOG
DSc MD FRCSI FRCOG(SA) FACOG FRACOG
Emeritus Professor of Obstetrics and Gynaecology
Queen Charlotte's Hospital for Women London

P. W. HOWIE   MD FRCOG
Professor of Obstetrics and Gynaecology
Ninewells Hospital, Dundee

K. R. PEEL   MB ChB FRCS(Ed) FRCOG
Consultant Gynaecological Surgeon
The General Infirmary at Leeds
Honourary Consultant Gynaecologist
Cookridge Hospital, Leeds
Senior Clinical Lecturer in Obstetrics and
Gynaecology, University of Leeds

J. W. K. RITCHIE   MD FRCOG FRCS(C)
Professor of Obstetrics and Gynaecology
University of Toronto
Director of Obstetric Perinatology
Mount Sinai Hospital, Toronto
Canada

J. S. SCOTT   MD FRCS(Ed) FRCOG
Professor of Obstetrics and Gynaecology
University of Leeds

R. P. SHEARMAN   MD FRCOG FRACOG
Professor of Obstetrics and Gynaecology
University of Sydney
Head of Obstetrics and Gynaecology
King George V Memorial Hospital
Royal Prince Alfred Hospital
Australia

D. W. WARRELL   MD FRCOG
Consultant-in-charge
Department of Gynaecological Urology
St Mary's Hospital, Manchester

C. R. WHITFIELD   MD FRCOG FRCP(Glas)
Regius Professor of Midwifery
University of Glasgow

PREFACE TO
FOURTH EDITION

It has been a great privilege and considerable responsibility to follow Sir John Dewhurst as Editor of the textbook which he launched in 1972 and which, in its first three editions, has become established as a main reading source for many obstetricians and gynaecologists in training, and as a useful reference book for the established specialist. Happily, Sir John remains in the team of contributors, writing several chapters dealing with matters in which he is an acknowledged expert and renowned teacher. We are delighted that he has also agreed that his name should be given to the new title: that is our public tribute to him.

Our objective remains to provide a coherent and advanced account of obstetrics and gynaecology, of the related physiology and pathology on a knowledge of which clinical expertise must be built, and of the common ground shared with other closely associated specialties. As stated by Sir John in his preface to the first edition, some basic knowledge is assumed, and the text is not so much 'on how things are done, but on how correct treatment is chosen, what advantages one choice has over another, what complications are to be expected, etc'. Practical matters, including history taking and physical examination and also operative techniques, should be learned in outpatient clinics and at the bedside and in the labour wards and operating theatres. Reinforcement of this practical experience by reference to detailed descriptions of operative procedures (in obstetrics, gynaecology and relevant general surgery) in specialized textbooks is essential complementary reading for the trainee. Likewise, those training to be subspecialists must read extensively in the journals and textbooks dealing with their particular fields—gynaecological oncology or urology, fetal medicine or reproductive endocrinology and infertility.

Inevitably, as new knowledge is gained and new developments are made at an ever increasing pace, there must be substantial revision from one edition to another. Although we remain conscious of the need to remove outdated material, to minimize overlap and repetition between chapters, and to keep cost within an acceptable limit, some lengthening of the text has been unavoidable. New chapters have been added and others reorganized, and, while thanking retiring authors who have contributed so effectively to previous editions, we welcome several newcomers to the team. Their expertise reflects the need for those with very specialized knowledge to remain involved in teaching the great majority of obstetrician–gynaecologists who will practise as generalists, as well as in training a small number of intending subspecialists. Thus, Dr Knox Ritchie, formerly Senior Lecturer in Fetal Medicine in Belfast and now directing an obstetrical perinatology service in Toronto, brings to the team his experience in managing the high risk fetus and of operative obstetrics. The chapters by Professor Peter Howie of Dundee, by way of Glasgow and Edinburgh, include those on the coagulation and fibrinolytic systems and their disorders and on the puerperium, in which fields he has made important contributions. In taking over from Sir Rustam Feroze responsibility for the chapters dealing with gynaecological cancer, Mr Roger Peel draws on his experience of providing a referral service in Leeds, while Dr David Warrell of Manchester has taken over two chapters that reflect his particular knowledge of urological problems in obstetrics and gynaecology. Finally, because many obstetricians, especially in developing countries, must still practise without close paediatric support, a chapter on neonatal care has been provided by my academic partner at the Queen Mother's Hospital, Professor Forrester Cockburn.

I am of course most grateful to those who have so willingly updated their chapters from the preceding edition, some of them readily accepting additional commitments. Thus, Professor Shearman continues to be responsible for the chapters that relate to the broad field of reproductive endocrinology, now including those on contraception and infertility; besides taking over the chapter on hypertensive disorders occurring in pregnancy, Professor Davey extends his contribution on normal pregnancy to include a section on obstetric care in undeveloped and developing communities; immunological disorders in pregnancy now have their own chapter, written by Professor Scott; Professor Beazley adds the third stage to his chapters on normal and abnormal labour; Professor Chamberlain adds a new chapter on the increasingly important topic of prepregnancy care and another that brings together well established and more recent methods for gynaecological diagnosis. The features and particular problems of multiple pregnancy also now have their own chapter, while the minor symptoms of pregnancy (so named by men) have, in the interests of space, been excluded from the chapter on miscellaneous disorders in pregnancy which is now given over almost entirely to the important TORCH and fetal alcohol syndromes and to the new potential threat posed by AIDS. Special thanks are due to Sir John Dewhurst, Sir Rustam Feroze and Mr David Morris for generously allowing considerable material from their earlier contributions to be used by others

in preparing the corresponding chapters this time; and I have made use of the experience of my colleagues who provide a referral service for prenatal diagnosis (particularly Drs Whittle, McNay and Gilmore) for a new chapter on detection of the abnormal fetus. We are grateful to many others who have permitted us to use their already published illustrations, acknowledged in each case, and have helped in other ways. The unstinting support of my hospital colleagues, senior and junior, was indispensable in reducing other demands upon my time; and it is a great pleasure to record special thanks to my secretary, Mrs Helen Mackenzie, without whose patience and diligence my own chapters and the editorial task could not have been completed. I am also indebted to Blackwell Scientific Publications, particularly Mr Nigel Palmer and Ms Jane Starling, who also showed considerable patience and provided much useful advice.

C. R. Whitfield
Glasgow, 1986

PREFACE TO
FIRST EDITION

Our purpose in writing this book has been to produce a comprehensive account of what the specialist in training in obstetrics and gynaecology must know. Unfortunately for him, he must now know a great deal, not only about his own subject, but about certain aspects of closely allied specialities such as endocrinology, biochemistry, cytogenetics, psychiatry, etc. Accordingly we have tried to offer the postgraduate student not only an advanced textbook in obstetrics and gynaecology but one which integrates the relevant aspects of other subjects which nowadays impinge more and more on the clinical field.

To achieve this aim within, we hope, a reasonable compass we have assumed some basic knowledge which the reader will have assimilated throughout his medical training, and we have taken matters on from there. Fundamental facts not in question are stated as briefly as is compatible with accuracy and clarity, and discussion is then devoted to more advanced aspects. We acknowledge that it is not possible even in this way to provide all the detail some readers may wish, so an appropriate bibliography is provided with each chapter. Wherever possible we have tried to give a positive opinion and our reasons for holding it, but to discuss nonetheless other important views; this we believe to be more helpful than a complete account of all possible opinions which may be held. We have chosen moreover to lay emphasis on fundamental aspects of the natural and the disease processes which are discussed; we believe concentration on these basic physiological and pathological features to be important to the proper training of a specialist. Clinical matters are, of course, dealt with in detail too, whenever theoretical discussion of them is rewarding. There are, however, some clinical aspects which cannot, at specialist level, be considered in theory with real benefit, examples of these are *how* to palpate a pregnant woman's abdomen and *how* to apply obstetric forceps. In general these matters are considered very briefly or perhaps not at all;

this is not a book on *how* things are done, but on how correct treatment is chosen, what advantages one choice has over another, what complications are to be expected, etc. Practical matters, we believe, are better learnt in practice and with occasional reference to specialized textbooks devoted solely to them.

A word may be helpful about the manner in which the book is set out. We would willingly have followed the advice given to Alice when about to testify at the trial of the Knave of Hearts in Wonderland, 'Begin at the beginning, keep on until you come to the end and then stop'. But this advice is difficult to follow when attempting to find the beginning of complex subjects such as those to which this book is devoted. Does the beginning lie with fertilization; or with the events which lead up to it; or with the genital organs upon the correct function of which any pregnancy must depend; or does it lie somewhere else? And which direction must we follow then? The disorders of reproduction do not lie in a separate compartment from genital tract disease, but each is clearly associated with the other for at last part of a woman's life. Although we have attempted to integrate obstetrics with gynaecology and with their associated specialities, some separation is essential in writing about them, and the plan we have followed is broadly this—we begin with the female child *in utero*, follow her through childhood to puberty, through adolescence to maturity, through pregnancy to motherhood, through her reproductive years to the climacteric and into old age. Some events have had to be taken out of order, however, although reiteration has been avoided by indicating to the reader where in the book are to be found other sections dealing with different aspects of any subject under consideration.

We hope that our efforts will provide a coherent, integrated account of the field we have attempted to cover which will be to the satisfaction of our readers.

Sir John Dewhurst, 1972

CHAPTER 1
NORMAL AND ABNORMAL DEVELOPMENT OF THE GENITAL ORGANS

SIR JOHN DEWHURST

An understanding of the manner in which the genital organs develop in the early embryo is clearly important for the gynaecologist. But it is also necessary to appreciate the reason why these organs develop differently in the two sexes. This chapter will open, therefore, with a brief outline of sexual differentiation which will be discussed more fully in Chapters 2 and 3.

Sexual development depends initially on the arrangement of the sex chromosome. Normal men have an XY sex chromosome arrangement and normal women an XX one. Sometimes, however, individuals are born with additional sex chromosomes and are XXY, XYY, XXYY, XXX, XXXX, etc., and others with a single X only; still others have different arrangements which need not concern us here but which are dealt with in greater detail later. Normally if a Y chromosome is present with one or more X chromosomes, testes will form in the early embryo and if two or more X chromosomes are present without a Y, ovaries form. If a single X chromosome is present alone, normal definitive gonadal tissue does not form and the gonads are represented by whitish streaks of tissue. It is likely that the effect of the Y chromosome in promoting testicular differentiation is concerned with a substance known as H–Y antigen which is thought to be the gene product of the male determining genes on the Y chromosome (Wachtel 1979).

The relationship between the differentiated gonad and the development of the other genital organs is, in summary, this. If testes form in the early embryo, that individual will develop male genital organs. If testes do not form, the individual will develop female genital organs whether ovaries are present or not. It may be concluded that the arrangement of the sex chromosomes normally determines the nature of the gonad, which in turn determines the differentiation of the other genital organs.

We will now turn our attention to how the genital organs develop.

THE DEVELOPMENT OF THE GENITAL ORGANS

Most embryological accounts agree on the principles of genital tract development as a whole, although different views are held on the development of the vagina.

The genital organs and those of the urinary tract

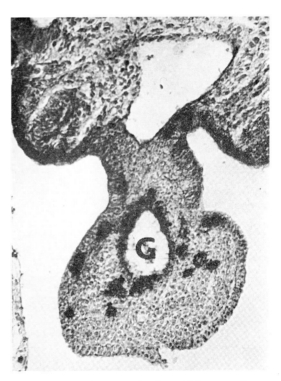

Fig. 1.1. Section of a 3.5 mm (28 days old) human embryo stained with alkaline phosphatase. The picture shows the primitive gut marked 'G' above which is the root of the mesentery. Above this again on either side is the intermediate mesoderm in which the genital organs develop. Germ cells are stained black and seen on either side of the primitive gut. (By courtesy of Dr Jan E. Jirasek, Dr Joe Leigh Simpson and Academic Press Inc.)

arise in the intermediate mesoderm on either side of the root of the mesentery, beneath the epithelium of the coelom (Fig. 1.1). The pronephros, a few transient excretory tubules in the cervical region, appears first but quickly degenerates. The duct which begins in association with the pronephros persists and extends caudally to open at the cloaca, connecting as it does so with some of the tubules of the mesonephros shortly to appear. The duct is called the mesonephric (Wolffian) duct. The mesonephros itself, the second primitive kidney, develops as a swelling bulging into the dorsal wall of the coelom of the thoracic and upper lumbar regions. The mesonephros in the male persists in part as the excretory portion of the male genital system; in the female a few vestiges only survive (Fig. 1.2). The genital ridge in which the gonad of each sex is to develop is visible as a swelling on the medial aspect of the mesonephros; the paramesonephric (Müllerian) duct, from which much of the female genital tract will develop,

forms as an ingrowth of coelomic epithelium on its lateral aspect (10 mm C.R. length; 5–6 weeks). The ingrowth forms a groove and then a tube and sinks below the surface.

DEVELOPMENT OF THE UTERUS AND FALLOPIAN TUBES

The two paramesonephric (Müllerian) ducts then extend caudally until they reach the urogenital sinus, at about 9 weeks; the blind ends project into the posterior wall of the sinus as the Müllerian tubercle (Fig. 1.3). At the beginning of the third month the Müllerian and Wolffian ducts and mesonephric tubules are all present and capable of development (Fig. 1.2[a]). From this point onwards in the female there is degeneration of the Wolffian system and marked growth of the Müllerian system (Fig. 1.2[b]). In the male the opposite occurs (Fig. 1.2[c]). The lower ends of the Müllerian ducts come together in the mid-line

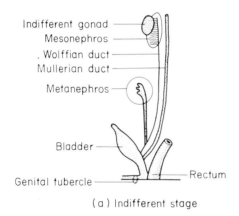

Indifferent gonad
Mesonephros
Wolffian duct
Mullerian duct
Metanephros

Bladder

Genital tubercle — Rectum

(a) Indifferent stage

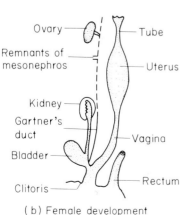

Ovary — Tube
Remnants of mesonephros
Kidney
Gartner's duct — Uterus
Bladder — Vagina
Clitoris — Rectum

(b) Female development

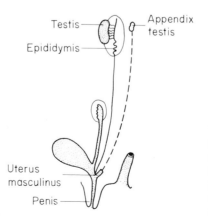

Testis — Appendix testis
Epididymis

Uterus masculinus
Penis

(c) Male development

Fig. 1.2. Diagrammatic representation of genital tract development. (a) Indifferent stage. (b) Female development. (c) Male development. (By courtesy of Ballière Tindall.)

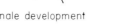

and fuse and develop into the uterus and cervix; the cephalic ends of the duct remain separate to form the Fallopian tubes. The thick muscular walls of the uterus and cervix develop from proliferation of mesenchyme around the fused portions of the ducts.

DEVELOPMENT OF THE VAGINA

There is difference of opinion about the precise events in vaginal development. At the point where the paramesonephric ducts protrude their solid tips into the dorsal wall of the urogenital sinus as the Müllerian tubercle (30 mm stage; 9 weeks; Fig. 1.3) there is a marked growth of tissue from which the vagina will ultimately form. Koff (1933) describes the formation of paired sinovaginal bulbs as posterior evaginations of the urogenital sinus; there is also stratification of the cells lining that part of the sinus, and this obliterates the Müllerian tubercle. The sinovaginal bulbs, which become solidified by further epithelial proliferation, fuse with the lower end of the Müllerian ducts to form the vaginal plate (Fig. 1.4[a]). This plate quickly grows in all dimensions, greatly increasing the distance between the cervix and the urogenital sinus. Later, the central cells of this plate break down to form the vaginal lumen (Fig. 1.4[b]).

According to Koff, approximately the upper four-fifths of the vagina is formed by the Müllerian ducts

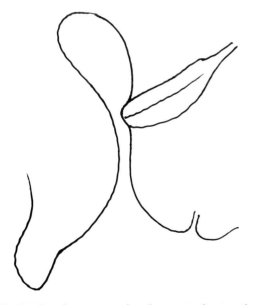

Fig. 1.3. Paired paramesonephric ducts protruding into the urogenital sinus as the Müllerian tubercle at 9 weeks of intrauterine life.

and the lower fifth from the urogenital sinus by the growth of the sinovaginal bulbs. He regards the hymen as being totally derived from the sinus epithelium. Vilas (1932) and Bulmer (1957) and others hold a different view. They believe that the sinus upgrowth extends up to the cervix, displacing the Müllerian component completely, the vagina being thus derived wholly from the endoderm of the urogenital sinus. It seems certain that some of the vagina is formed from the urogenital sinus, but it is not certain whether the Müllerian component is involved or not. See also Chapter 3 page 26.

THE DEVELOPMENT OF THE EXTERNAL GENITALIA

The primitive cloaca becomes divided by a transverse septum into an anterior urogenital portion and a posterior rectal portion. The urogenital portion of the cloacal membrane breaks down shortly after division is complete (15 mm C.R. length). The urogenital sinus develops further into three portions (Fig. 1.5). There is an external, expanded, phallic part, a deeper, narrow, pelvic part between it and the region of the Müllerian tubercle, and a vesico-urethral part connected superiorly to the allantois. Externally in this region the genital tubercle forms a conical projection around the anterior part of the cloacal membrane. Two pairs of swellings, a medial pair (the genital folds) and a lateral pair (genital swellings) are then formed by proliferation of mesoderm round the end of the urogenital sinus. Development up to this time (50 mm C.R. length; 10 weeks) is the same in the male and the female. Differentiation then occurs. The bladder and urethra form from the vesico-urethral portion of the urogenital sinus and the vestibule from the pelvic and phallic portions (Fig. 1.5). The genital tubercle enlarges only slightly and becomes the clitoris. The genital folds become the labia minora and the genital swellings enlarge to become the labia majora. In the male greater enlargement of the genital tubercle forms the penis. The genital folds fuse over a deep groove formed between them to become the penile part of the male urethra. The genital swellings enlarge, fuse and form the scrotum.

The final stage of the development of the clitoris or penis and the formation of the anterior surface of the bladder and the anterior abdominal wall up to the umbilicus is the result of growth of mesoderm extending ventrally round the body wall on each side to unite in the mid-line anteriorly.

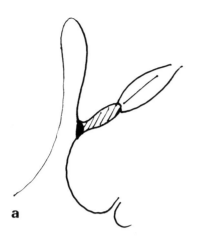 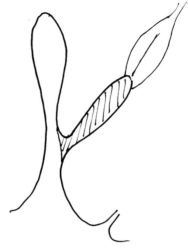

a

Fig. 1.4(a). On the left the earliest development of the vaginal plate is seen. The sino vaginal bulbs with which the lower portion of the Müllerian ducts fuse are indicated in black and the developing vaginal plate is hatched. On the right further development of the vaginal plate is shown displacing the lower end of the Müllerian ducts cranially.

DEVELOPMENT OF THE GONADS

The primitive gonad is first evident in embryos of 5.5–7.5 mm C.R. length (5 weeks). According to Gillman (1948) the gonad is of triple origin from the coelomic epithelium of the genital ridge, the underlying mesoderm and the primitive germ cells which come from an extragenital source (see below).

The gonad forms as a bulge on the medial aspect of the mesonephric ridge. Its histological appearances are alike in the early stages, whether it is to be testis or ovary. There is a proliferation of cells in and beneath the coelomic epithelium of the genital ridge. By 5 or 6 weeks these cells are seen spreading as ill-defined cords (sex cords) into the ridge, breaking up the mesenchyme into loose strands. Primitive germ cells are distinguishable as much larger structures, lying at first between the cords and then within them.

The differentiation of the testes is evident at about 7 weeks by the disappearance of germ cells from the peripheral zone and gradual differentiation of remaining cells into fibroblasts and later into the tunica albuginea. The deeper parts of the sex cords give rise to the rete testis, the seminiferous and straight tubules. The first indication that the gonad will become an ovary is failure of these testicular changes to appear. The primitive ovary passes first into the stage of differentiation and growth, and later into that of follicle formation. The sex cords below the coelomic epithelium develop extensively, with many primitive germ cells evident in this active cellular zone (Fig. 1.6). The epithelial cells in this area are known as pregranulosa cells. The active growth phase then follows, involving the pregranulosa cells and the

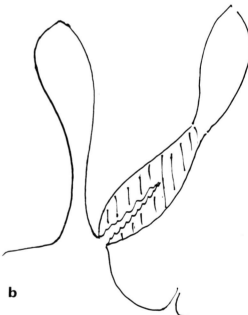

b

Fig. 1.4(b). The central cells of the vaginal plate are breaking down to form the vaginal lumen.

germ cells, which are now much reduced in size (14–16 weeks). This proliferation greatly enlarges the bulk of the gonad. The next stage (20 weeks onwards) shows the primitive germ cells (now known as oocytes) becoming surrounded by a ring of pregranulosa cells; stromal cells, developed from the ovarian mesenchyme, later surround the pregranulosa cells, now known as granulosa cells, and follicle

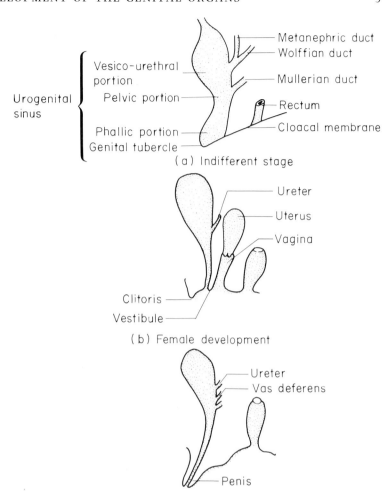

(a) Indifferent stage

(b) Female development

(c) Male development

Fig. 1.5. Diagrammatic representation of lower genital tract development. (a) Indifferent stage. (b) Female development. (c) Male development. (By courtesy of Ballière Tindall.)

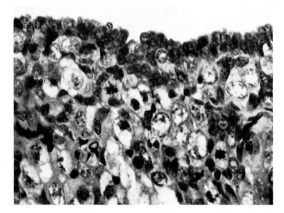

Fig. 1.6. Detail of immature ovary showing small epithelial cells (pregranulosa cells) and larger germ cells. (By courtesy of Dr J. Pryse-Davies.)

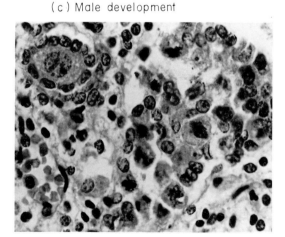

Fig. 1.7. A later ovary (31 weeks) showing a well formed primary follicle (top left) and a germ cell (centre right) which is not yet completely surrounded by granulosa cells.

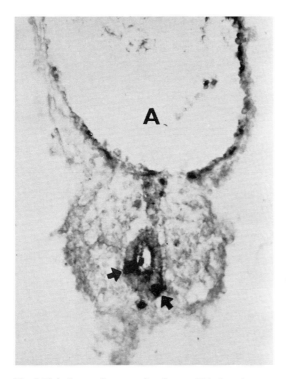

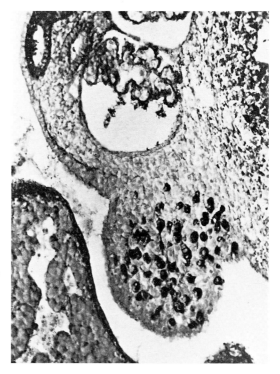

Fig. 1.8(a). Germ cells arrowed and stained black with alkaline phosphatase in the alantois of a human embryo 17–19 days old. 'A' indicates the amniotic vesicle.

Fig. 1.8(c). The indifferent gonad in a 9 mm human embryo (38 days old). The darkly stained primitive germ cells are clearly seen. (Figs. 1.8(a), (b), and (c) by kind permission as for Fig. 1.1.)

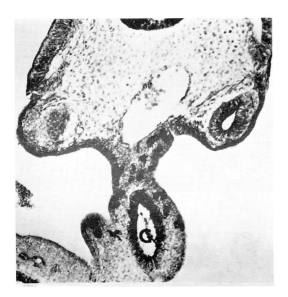

Fig. 1.8(b). Germ cells migrating to the genital ridge area in a 4 mm human embryo (see also Fig. 1.1).

formation is complete (Fig. 1.7). An interesting feature of the formation of follicles and the development of stroma is the disintegration of those oocytes which do not succeed in encircling themselves with a capsule of pregranulosa cells.

It is now generally accepted that the germ cells arise in the endoderm before the formation of the mesoderm of the lateral plate and somite formation (Pinkerton *et al.* 1961). Pinkerton and his colleagues described germ cells as migrating along the endoderm of the yolk sac, into the gut, through the mesenchyme at the root of the mesentery and into the primitive gonad (Fig. 1.8 [a], [b] and [c] and Fig. 1.1). Rapid proliferation of germ cells follows, until they become surrounded by granulosa cells as described above and become oocytes. Mitotic division, by which the germ cells have been increasing in numbers, then ceases and they enter the first stage of meiosis.

The number of oocytes is greatest some time during pregnancy, and thereafter declines. Baker (1963) found that the total population of germ cells rose

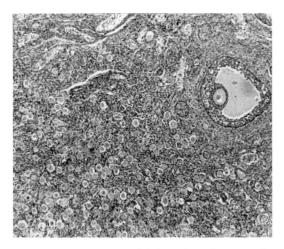

Fig. 1.9. Numerous primary follicles and one showing early development in the ovary of a child stillborn at 38 weeks.

from some 600 000 at 2 months to a peak of almost 7 000 000 at 5 months. At birth the number had fallen to 2 000 000, of which half were atretic. After 28 weeks or so of intrauterine life an increasing degree of follicle development is evident in the ovary. Follicles at various stages of development, and of various sizes, are seen (Pryse-Davies & Dewhurst 1971, de Sa 1975) (Figs. 1.9, 1.10). Simpson (1976) gives an excellent account of these events.

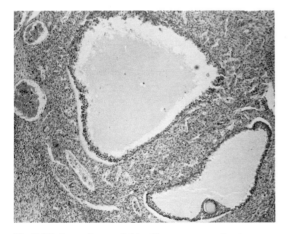

Fig. 1.10. Ovary from a child stillborn at 41 weeks showing a mature Graafian follicle, and a cystic follicle. (By courtesy of the Editor of *Journal of Pathology and Bacteriology*.)

GENITAL TRACT MALFORMATIONS

Numerous malformations of the genital tract have been described, some of little clinical significance, others of considerable importance. Perhaps it is not surprising that many gynaecologists try to explain malformations in terms of variation of the normal development just described. It is doubtful if there is any merit in this since malformations are by definition abnormal and many curious malformations may be seen for which variations of the normal development do not offer a convincing explanation.

Uterine anomalies

ABSENCE OF THE UTERUS

The uterus may be absent or of such rudimentary development as to be incapable of function of any kind. This type of anomaly is usually found when the vagina is absent also, the case presenting is one of primary amenorrhoea (*see* Chapter 6). Absence of the uterus may be associated with the development of the lower part of the vagina, which then ends blindly. This combination of features should suggest a diagnosis of androgen insensitivity (testicular feminization) (*see* Chapter 3). The absence of pubic hair in a patient with androgen insensitivity will be the physical sign which should suggest this diagnosis. However, similar development of the lower vagina only, and absence of the uterus, may occasionally be found in XX patients with ovaries. No treatment is of course possible for the uterine abnormality as such; it must be stressed however, that if the diagnosis is androgen insensitivity, testicular removal may be indicated on account of the increased risk of malignant change in the testes. Whether the patient is XY or XX, however, attention to psychological aspects of the case may be almost the most important facet of management.

FUSION ANOMALIES

Fusion anomalies of various kinds are not uncommon (Fig. 1.11) and may present clinically either in association with pregnancy or in other ways. The lesser degrees of fusion defects are quite common, the cornual parts of the uterus remaining separate, giving the organ a heart-shaped appearance. It is doubtful if such a minor degree of fusion defect *per se* gives rise to clinical symptoms or signs. The presence of a septum extending over some or all of the uterine cavity, however, is likely to give rise to clinical

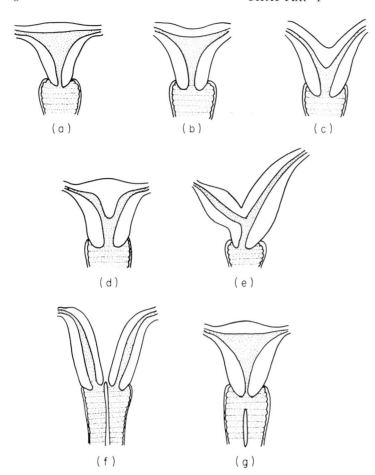

Fig. 1.11. Various fusion abnormalities of the uterus and vagina. (a) Normal appearance. (b) Arcuate fundus with little effect on the shape of the cavity. (c) Bicornuate uterus. (d) Subseptate uterus with normal outline. (e) Rudimentary horn. (f) Uterus didelphys. (g) Normal uterus with partial vaginal septum.

features. Such a septate or subseptate uterus may be of normal external appearance or of arcuate outline. Clinically, this state of affairs may come to light as a case of repeated unsuccessful pregnancy (*see* Chapter 14); a second likely method of presentation is as repeated transverse lie of the fetus in late pregnancy, since it tends to lie with the head in one cornu and the breech in the other (*see* Chapter 27).

In more extreme forms of failure of fusion the clinical features may be less, rather than more, marked. Two almost separate uterine cavities with one cervix are probably less likely to be associated with repeated abnormal lies than the lesser degrees of fusion defect mentioned above. Complete duplication of the uterus and cervix (uterus didelphys) if associated with any clinical fault at all might present as obstruction to descent of the head in late pregnancy or labour by the non-pregnant horn.

Rudimentary development of one horn may give rise to a very serious situation if a pregnancy is implanted there. Rupture of the horn with profound bleeding may occur as the pregnancy increases in size. The clinical picture will, in some ways, resemble that of a ruptured ectopic pregnancy, with the difference that the amenorrhoea would probably be measured in months rather than weeks; shock may be profound. A poorly developed or rudimentary horn may give rise to dysmenorrhoea and pelvic pain if there is any obstruction to communication between the horn and the main uterine cavity or the vagina. Surgical removal is then indicated.

Vaginal anomalies

ABSENCE OF THE VAGINA

Absence of the vagina is generally associated with absence of the uterus, as indicated above. Rarely, the uterus may be present and the vagina, or a large part of it, absent.

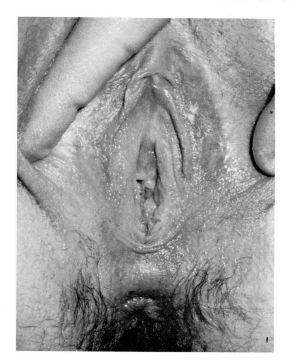

Fig. 1.12. Vulval appearances in a case of absence of the vagina.

In the more common circumstances of absence of both vagina and uterus the patient will probably present about 16 or so years of age with primary amenorrhoea. Secondary sexual characteristics will be present, since the ovaries are normally developed. This combination of normal secondary sexual development and primary amenorrhoea suggests an anatomical cause, such as an imperforate or absent vagina, for the failure to menstruate. Inspection of the vulva, abdominal examination and rectal examination will be required to exclude the presence of any retained blood in a part of the upper genital tract.

Vulval development is normal apart from the absence of a patent vaginal introitus (Fig. 1.12).

The presumptive diagnosis of absence of the vagina can generally be made without difficulty at the first examination. A very short vagina arising in androgen insensitivity may be mistaken for simple absence, so in every case of apparent vaginal absence a buccal smear, at least, should be performed and, if possible, a chromosome analysis. If the buccal smear is chromatin negative and the chromosome analysis confirms XY sex chromosomes, the case takes on an entirely different aspect (see Chapter 6).

An ultrasound scan of the renal areas should be undertaken to determine the presence or absence of two normal kidney echoes; if the scan is not normal an intravenous pyelogram is desirable in view of the frequent association of the renal tract anomalies which may have a bearing on treatment (Fig. 1.13). Should the ultrasound scan be normal, however, an intravenous pyelogram can probably be dispensed with. If there is any suggestion that there is a functioning uterus present an ultrasound pelvic scan will usually confirm or refute this: if doubt remains laparoscopy is employed. If laparoscopy is employed in any apparent case of vaginal absence to avoid the possibility of error a scan or an intravenous pyelogram should first be performed since there would be a real risk of injury of a pelvic kidney with the laparoscope if the organ were in this position.

Once the diagnosis is certain, consideration must be given to the construction of an artificial vagina. Rarely, one sees patients in whom this is unnecessary, since attempted intercourse has so indented the perineal area that enjoyable coitus for both wife and

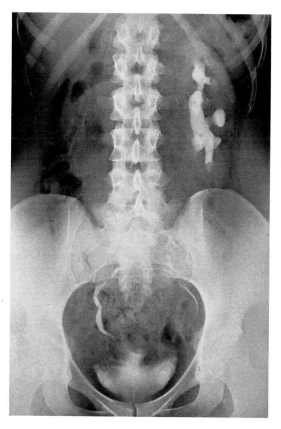

Fig. 1.13. An intravenous pyelogram in a patient with absence of the vagina, showing a single kidney and a gross abnormality of the course of the ureter.

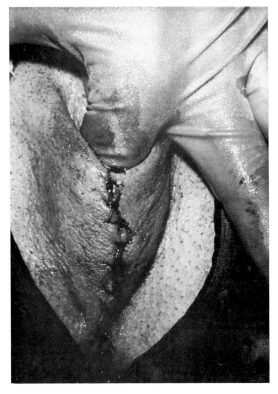

Fig. 1.14. A vagina constructed by the Williams vulvovaginoplasty method.

husband has been experienced. Such cases are, of course, exceptional. Their existence, however, indicates the possibility of non-surgical treatment by intermittent pressure with vaginal dilators referred to below.

The timing and nature of any surgical procedure required to construct an artificial vagina require some discussion. The technique introduced by McIndoe and Read (McIndoe & Bannister 1938) was the one most commonly used until some years ago. In this procedure a cavity is created between the bladder and bowel at the site which the natural vagina would occupy; this cavity is then lined by a split-skin graft taken from the thigh and applied on a plastic mould. The anatomical result in successful cases can be remarkably good.

There are, none the less, difficulties and disadvantages to this technique (Jackson 1965). The postoperative period is painful and sometimes protracted; the graft does not always take well and granulations can form over part of the cavity, giving rise to some discharge; pressure necrosis between the mould and

the urethra, bladder or rectum can lead to fistula formation. A further, and greater, disadvantage is the tendency for the vagina to contract unless a dilator is worn or the vagina is used for intercourse regularly. The ideal timing of the procedure, therefore, is some 6 months or so before marriage, so that the woman can wear a dilator throughout this time to prevent contraction, which thereafter can be prevented through natural intercourse; a longer interval may lead to irregular use of a dilator, when contraction can occur very rapidly. It is, moreover, a great psychological disadvantage for a girl who knows she has such an abnormality. Her relationship with young men is certain to be influenced.

The operation of vulvovaginoplasty introduced by Williams (1964) has obvious psychological advantages in this respect, since it can be performed on 17- or 18-year-old unmarried girls without the risk of significant contraction if regular intercourse is not indulged in for some time. Williams's account should be consulted for the details of this unusual technique, when it will be evident that the operative procedure is simple, quick and relatively comfortable for the patient. Functionally, the results seem good. The only apparent disadvantage is the unusual angle of the vagina (Fig. 1.14), which may displease a purist surgeon. The angle may, however, lead to a maximum of clitoral stimulation at intercourse and may account for good functional results. Feroze *et al.* (1975) have reviewed these two forms of surgical approach to the construction of an artificial vagina. The comparison favours the Williams procedure from several points of view but particularly from those of its surgical simplicity and freedom from complications. Morris (1973), however, suggests that with good patient cooperation intermittent pressure with graduated vaginal dilators, as suggested many years ago by Frank, can give such good results that surgical treatment may be unnecessary. The patient commences by pressing the tip of the glass dilator firmly on to the perineum at the region of the fourchette for 10–15 minutes twice a day at first; gradually, as the area becomes indented, more and more of the dilator can be 'inserted' and then a larger one may be used. My own recent experience with patients managed in this way suggests that in well-adjusted well-motivated patients such good results are possible that this should be the first line of approach (Dewhurst 1980). In a more recent series 12 out of 15 patients obtained a satisfactory vagina by this method. Ingram (1981) has constructed an ingenious bicycle stool seat which allows the patient to wear a small dilator beneath her underclothes which keeps up pressure for as long as she sits on the stool. A recent review by Smith (1983) compares the results of various procedures in the USA.

HAEMATOCOLPOS

An imperforate membrane may exist at the lower end of the vagina; this is loosely referred to as an imperforate hymen, although the hymen can usually be distinguished separately (Fig. 1.15). The condition is seldom recognized clinically until puberty, when retention of menstrual flow gives rise to the clinical features of haematocolpos; rarely, the case may present in the newborn as hydrocolpos (*see* page 41). The features of haematocolpos are, predominantly, three: abdominal pain; amenorrhoea; and interference with micturition. The patient is usually aged about 14 or 15 years, but may be much older. A clear history may be given of regular lower abdominal pain for some months past, but irregular pain is more common. The patient may be brought to hospital as an acute emergency if urinary retention develops. The examination will reveal a lower ab-

dominal swelling if there is urinary retention; *per rectum* a large, bulging mass in the vagina may be appreciated (Fig. 1.16). Vulval inspection will reveal the imperforate membrane, which may or may not be bluish in colour depending upon its thickness. Diagnosis may be more difficult if the vagina is imperforate over some distance in its lower part or if there is obstruction in one half of a septate vagina (Dewhurst 1976, 1980).

Treatment is usually very simple, since all that is required is incision of the membrane and the release of the retained blood. Redundant portions of the membrane may then be snipped away, but nothing more should be done at that time. Fluid will drain away naturally over some days. Examination a few weeks later is desirable to ensure that no pelvic mass

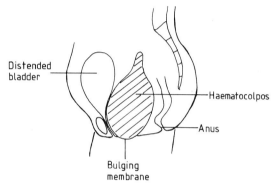

Fig. 1.16(a). Diagrammatic view of haematocolpos. Note how the blood collecting in the vagina presses against the urethra and bladder base ultimately causing retention of urine.

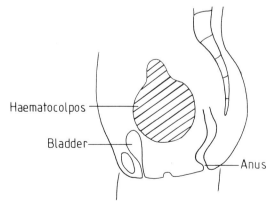

Fig. 1.16(b). Haematocolpos associated with absence of the lower portion of the vagina. Note that the retained blood is now above the bladder base and retention of urine unlikely.

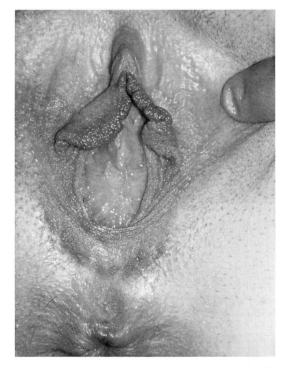

Fig. 1.15. An imperforate membrane occluding the vaginal introitus in a case of haematocolpos. Note the hymen clearly visible immediately distal to the membrane.

remains which might suggest the condition of haematosalpinx. In fact, haematosalpinx is most uncommon except in cases of very long standing, or in
association with retention of blood in a fragment of
upper vagina. On those rare occasions when a haematosalpinx is discovered, laparotomy is desirable,
the distended tube being removed or preserved, as
seems best. Haematometra scarcely seems to be a
realistic clinical entity, the thick uterine walls permitting comparatively little blood to collect therein.
The subsequent menstrual history and fertility of
patients who are successfully treated for haematocolpos is probably not significantly different from that of
normal women.

When the obstruction is more extensive than a
thin membrane and a length of vagina is absent,
diagnosis and management is less straightforward
and the ultimate interference with fertility may be
greater.

The combination of absence of most of the lower
vagina in association with a functioning uterus
presents a difficult problem. The upper fragment of
vagina will collect menstrual blood and a clinical picture, similar in many ways to haematocolpos will be
seen. Urinary obstruction is rare however since the
retained blood lies above the level of the bladder base
(Fig. 1. 16[a] and [b]). Diagnosis, however, is more difficult and it may not be at all certain how much of
the vagina is absent, nor how extensive the dissection
requires to be to release the retained fluid. An ultrasound scan may be helpful in determining this difficult point (Bennett & Dewhurst, 1983). Rectal examination may reveal a bulging swelling at a high
level but if doubt remains, the abdomen should be
opened to establish for certain the precise state of
affairs.

Treatment is difficult. If a dissection upwards is
made as in the McIndoe–Read technique, the blood
can be released, but its discharge for some time later
may interfere with the application of the mould and
the 'take' of the skin graft in the artificial vagina. The
approach advocated by Jeffcoate (1969) has been to
open into the fragment of upper vagina, the walls of
this portion, now stretched and greatly extended,
should then be brought down and stitched to the
introital area, so lining the new vagina with its own
skin and obviating the risk of contraction (advancement of the vagina). In my experience, however, the
upper fragment retracts upwards resulting in a narrow area of constriction some way up the vagina.
Dewhurst (1976, 1980) and Beazley (1974) discuss
these difficult cases more fully.

Mention must be made of the finding of endometriosis in the pelvis even in teenage girls in association
with high vaginal obstruction of this kind. Complete
drainage of the retained blood with local excision of
the lesions of endometriosis has prevented spread in
several personal cases of this rare condition.

VAGINAL SEPTA

A vaginal septum extending throughout all or part of
the vagina is not uncommon. Such a septum lies in
the sagittal plane in the mid-line, although if one side
of the vagina has been habitually used for coitus the
septum may have become displaced laterally to such
an extent that it may not be obvious that one is
present. The condition may be found in association
with a completely double uterus and cervix, or with
a single uterus only. In obstetrics the septum may be
important if a fetus presenting by the breech enters
the vagina astride it, when serious tearing may
occur. For this reason it is wise to arrange division of
the vaginal septum as a formal surgical procedure
whenever one is discovered during pregnancy. The
septum may occasionally be associated with dyspareunia, when similar management will be indicated.

Vulval anomalies

Doubt about the sex of a child due to faults in the
development of the external genitalia is discussed
fully in Chapter 3. Rarely, anomalies in the development of bowel or bladder may give rise to considerable abnormality in the appearance of the vulva. The
anus may open immediately adjacent to the vagina
or just within it (Fig. 1.17). Bladder exstrophy will

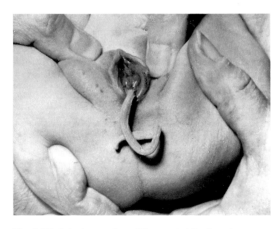

Fig. 1.17. Ectopic opening of the anus at the fourchette.

give rise to a bifid clitoris and anterior displacement of the vagina, in addition to the bladder deformity itself. These unusual cases are more fully discussed by Stephens (1963) and Dewhurst (1980).

Gonadal anomalies

Gonadal development may be markedly interfered with in certain patients with sex chromosome abnormalities.

These conditions are discussed in detail in Chapter 3.

Wolffian duct anomalies

Remnants of the lower part of the Wolffian duct system may be evident as vaginal cysts, or remnants of the upper part as thin-walled cysts lying within the layers of the broad ligament (parovarian cysts). It is doubtful whether the vaginal cyst *per se* calls for surgical removal, although removal is usually undertaken. Cysts situated at the upper end of the vagina may be found to burrow deeply into the region of the broad ligament and base of the bladder, and should be approached surgically with considerable caution. A palpable, and probably parovarian, cyst will require surgical exploration, since its precise nature will be unknown until the abdomen is opened. Such cysts normally shell out easily from the broad ligament.

Renal tract anomalies

The association between congenital malformations of the genital tract and those of the renal tract has already been mentioned. Whenever a malformation of the genital organs of any significant degree presents in clinical practice some investigation to confirm or refute a renal tract anomaly will be wise. An ultrasound scan can be arranged without any upset to the patient and will probably be sufficient in the first instance. If a fault is suspected an intravenous pyelogram may be performed. Lesions such as absence of one kidney, a double renal element on one or both sides, a double ureter, a pelvic kidney (Fig. 1.13), etc., may not call for immediate treatment but may do so later; moreover, it is as well to be aware of such anomalies if the abdomen is to be opened for exploration or treatment of the genital tract lesion itself. The author recently saw a patient with a single pelvic kidney which, at laparoscopy, had been thought to be haematocolpos and drainage had been proposed.

ECTOPIC URETER

One abnormality which can apparently present with gynaecological symptoms is the ectopic ureter (Fig. 1.18). A ureter opening abnormally is usually an additional one, although sometimes a single one may be ectopic. The commonest site of the opening is the vestibule, followed closely by the urethra and then the vagina; other sites are less common. The main symptom is uncontrollable wetness. The amount of moisture appearing at the vulva may, however, be small and is sometimes mistaken for a vaginal discharge. This confusion, together with difficulties in confirming the diagnosis of an ectopic ureter even when this is suspected, may lead to many patients being investigated for years before the condition is recognized.

Diagnosis can sometimes be easy, but is usually not so. The orifice at the vestibule may be clearly visible, but more often careful search is necessary to locate it, if it can be seen at all. Cystoscopy and urethroscopy may be necessary to establish, if nothing else, whether normal ureteric openings exist in the bladder. Radiological study is often helpful by

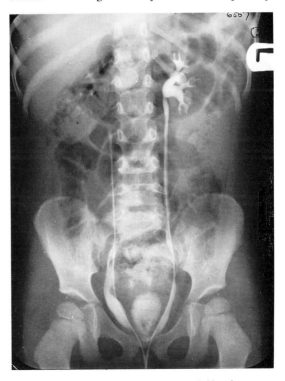

Fig. 1.18. An intravenous pyelogram in a child with an imperforate vagina. Both ureters open ectopically into the posterior urethra.

indicating a double element on one or both sides. The intravenous injection of indigocarmine, although theoretically likely to be useful, is often of little value, since concentration in the affected part of the kidney is often too poor to show up the opening well. Treatment will generally involve the urological surgeon rather than the gynaecologist. Partial nephrectomy and ureterectomy may be indicated or reimplantation of the ectopic ureter into the bladder.

Finally, mention may be made of the curious condition of ectopic ureterocele. This cystic malformation of an ectopic ureter may prolapse through the urethra and present at the vulva as an obvious swelling. The ureterocele may then quickly retract and by the time the patient is examined may have disappeared (Kasby & Parsons 1980).

REFERENCES

BAKER T. G. (1963) *Proc. Roy. Soc.*, **158**, 417.

BEAZLEY J. M. (1974) In *Clinics in Obstetrics and Gynaecology* (Dewhurst C. J. ed.), vol. 1 no. 3, p. 571. Saunders, Philadelphia.

BENNETT M. J. & DEWHURST Sir J. (1983) *Ped. Adol. Gynec.*, **1**, 25.

BULMER D. (1957) *J. Anat.*, **91**, 490.

DE SA D. J. (1975) *Arch. Dis. Childh.* **50**, 45.

DEWHURST C. J. (1972) *The Transactions of The College of Medicine of South Africa* **16**, 39–53.

DEWHURST C. J. (1976) In *Recent Advances in Obstetrics and Gynaecology* (Stallworthy J. & Bourne G. eds.). Churchill Livingstone, London.

DEWHURST SIR JOHN (1980) *Practical Pediatric and Adolescent Gynecology*. Marcel Dekker Inc., New York.

FEROZE R. M., DEWHURST C. J. & WELPLY G. A. C. (1975) *Brit. J. Obstet. Gynaec.*, **82**, 536.

GILLMAN J. (1948) *Contributions to Embryology, No. 210*, Vol. 32 p. 83. Carnegie Institute of Washington, Publication 575.

INGRAM J. M. (1981) *Amer. J. Obstet. Gynec.*, **140**, 867.

JACKSON I. (1965) *J. Obstet. Gynaec. Brit. Cwlth.*, **72**, 336.

JEFFCOATE T. N. E. (1969) *J. Obstet. Gynaec. Brit. Cwlth.* **76**, 961.

KASBY C. B. & PARSONS K. F. (1980) *Brit. J. Obstet. Gynaec.*, **87**, 1178.

KOFF A. K. (1933) *Contributions to Embryology, No. 140*, Vol. 24, p. 61. Carnegie Institute of Washington, Publication 443.

McINDOE A. H. & BANNISTER J. B. (1938) *J. Obstet. Gynaec. Brit. Emp.*, **45**, 490.

MORRIS J. M. (1973) Personal communication.

PINKERTON J. H. M., McKAY D. G., ADAMS E. C. & HERTIG A. H. (1961) *Obstet. Gynec., N.Y.*, **18**, 152.

PRYSE-DAVIES J. & DEWHURST C. J. (1971) *J. Path.*, **103**, 5.

SIMPSON J. L. (1976) *Disorders of Sexual Differentiation*. Academic Press, New York.

SMITH M. R. (1983) *Amer. J. Obstet. Gynec.*, **146**, 488.

STEPHENS F. D. (1963) *Congenital Malformations of the Rectum, Anus and Genito-urinary Tracts*, p. 4. Churchill Livingstone, Edinburgh and London.

VILAS E. (1932) *Z. Anat. Entwickl. Gesch.*, **98**, 263.

WACHTEL S. S. (1979) *Obstet. and Gynec. N.Y.*, **54**, 671.

WILLIAMS E. A. (1964) *J. Obstet. Gynaec. Brit. Cwlth.*, **71**, 511.

CHAPTER 2
CYTOGENETICS FOR GYNAECOLOGISTS

SIR JOHN DEWHURST

The increasing importance of chromosomal analysis in clinical practice indicates that an understanding of some aspects of cytogenetics is essential for clinicians. Such an account now follows. For more detailed consideration see Simpson (1976, 1982), Dewhurst (1981), de là Chapelle (1982), Maraschio and Fraccaro (1982).

GENERAL CONSIDERATIONS

The normal diploid number of chromosomes in the human is 46: 22 pairs of autosomes and an X and Y sex chromosome in normal males, the same number of autosomes and 2 X sex chromosomes in normal females. It is now widely realized that numerous individuals exist with a chromosomal fault of one kind or another. These faults may be broadly divided into:
1 abnormalities of chromosome number;
2 abnormalities of chromosome structure (Fig. 2.1).

Anomalies of number			Anomalies of structure
	45 (monosomy)	47 (trisomy)	
Autosomes	LETHAL	D E G (Down's syndrome)	Translocations
Sex chromosomes	Many abort ——— Some 45, X survive	47, XXX 47, XYY 47, XXY	Deletions

Fig. 2.1. Commoner chromosome abnormalities.

Abnormalities of chromosome number

Individuals exist whose chromosome number is more than 46, when it is generally 47 (trisomy) but is rarely 48 or even 49; others have a chromosome number less than 46, when it is always 45 (mono-somy). A variation on the theme of abnormal chromosome number is the mosaic individual whose body is composed of cells of different chromosomal complement derived from the same zygote; there may be two cell lines (such as 45,X/46,XX), three (45, X/46,XX/47,XXX) or even more. Mosaicism is not infrequently found when an abnormal chromosome is present as well, as we will see later.

Excluding mosaicism, abnormalities of chromosome number arise as a result of non-disjunction occurring during meiosis (Fig. 2.2[a]). Instead of each of the sex chromosomes entering a daughter cell during, for example, spermatogenesis, two enter one secondary spermatocyte and none enters the other; oogenesis may be similarly affected (Fig. 2.2[b]). The result, following fertilization, is indicated in these two figures. If non-disjunction affects more than one division of gametogenesis more bizarre chromosome abnormalities may result (Figs. 2.3[a] and [b]). Mosaicism arises by one of two mechanisms affecting the very early divisions of the zygote—non-disjunction or anaphase lag (Fig. 2.4[a] and [b]). Autosomal faults may arise by similar mechanisms.

Loss of a sex chromosome is lethal to the zygote if the X is lost and only a Y remains; loss of one of two XXs or of the Y with an X remaining is likely to result in abortion, although a small percentage of such embryos are born alive, as examples of gonadal dysgenesis (see later and p. 64). Possession of an extra sex chromosome is less likely to cause abortion of the zygote; trisomy of the sex chromosomes is compatible with normal mental and physical development and even with fertility. There is an increased risk of mental sub-normality, however, if an extra chromosome is present, especially if there are 48 chromosomes or more. The clinical picture associated with sex chromosome mosaicsm is variable and is likely to depend on the proportion of normal to abnormal cells and the distribution of these in the early embryo. This is discusseed further below.

If the autosomes are affected by non-disjunction,

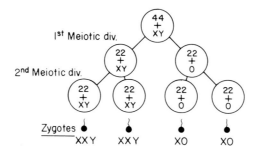

Fig. 2.2(a). Non-disjunction affecting the first division of spermatogenesis

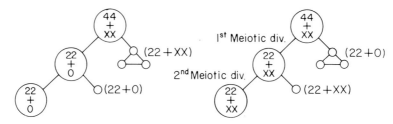

Fig. 2.2(b). Non-disjunction affecting the first division of oogenesis. (Both figures by courtesy of Ballière-Tindall.)

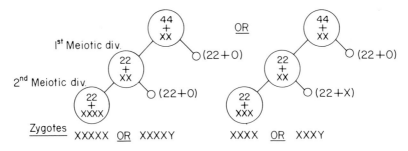

Fig. 2.3(a). Non-disjunction affecting both divisions of oogenesis.

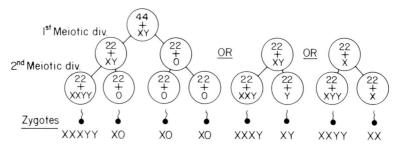

Fig. 2.3(b). Non-disjunction affecting both divisions of spermatogenesis. (Both figures by courtesy of Ballière-Tindall.)

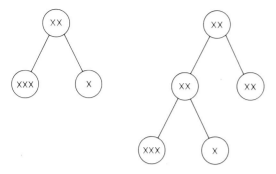

Fig. 2.4(a). Non-disjunction affecting early divisions of the zygote. (By courtesy of the Editor of *The British Journal of Obstetrics and Gynaecology*.)

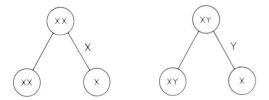

Fig. 2.4(b). Anaphase lag affecting the early division of the zygote. (By courtesy of the Editor of *The British Journal of Obstetrics and Gynaecology*.)

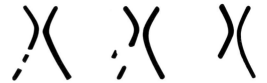

Fig. 2.5. Diagrammatic representation of chromosome deletion.

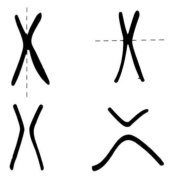

Fig. 2.6. Isochromosome formations. On the left is shown a normal vertical division of a chromosome at metaphase, on the right transverse division resulting in a chromosome representing the two short arms and another, the two long arms. (By courtesy of the Editor of *The British Journal of Obstetrics and Gynaecology*.)

loss of one of the pair is lethal and the zygote is aborted; an extra autosome is compatible with the birth of a child which is abnormal in various possible ways shortly to be mentioned.

Abnormalities of chromosomal structure

Abnormalities of chromosomal structure can be broadly divided into two groups:
(a) chromosome deletions,
(b) chromosome translocations.

DELETIONS

If breakage of a chromosome occurs during division, a portion may be lost and the resulting chromosome will be deficient in part of its long or short arm (Fig. 2.5). Occasionally breakage during division results in the ends of the long and short arms becoming adherent to each other and a ring chromosome forms; such a ring always indicates that some material has been lost although we cannot say how much nor which part. A deletion may also result from what is called isochromosome formation (Fig. 2.6). Here transverse

instead of vertical division occurs, leaving two chromosomes which are not identical; one represents the two short arms, one the two long arms. It is important to realize that if the former is involved in fertilization the genetic material carried on the long arm will be missing and vice versa. The clinical picture associated with an abnormal sex chromosome usually resembles that of gonadal dysgenesis. As mentioned above, a chromosome deletion and mosaicism often coexist.

TRANSLOCATIONS

The complex problem of chromosome translocations will, for simplicity, be summarized briefly. Two forms exist:

1 the Robertsonian translocation or centric fusion in which two chromosomes adhere to each other at the centromere (Fig. 2.7); the actual chromosome number will then be 45 but one chromosome will represent the two which have been joined together;
2 the reciprocal translocation in which a portion of one chromosome is exchanged with a portion of

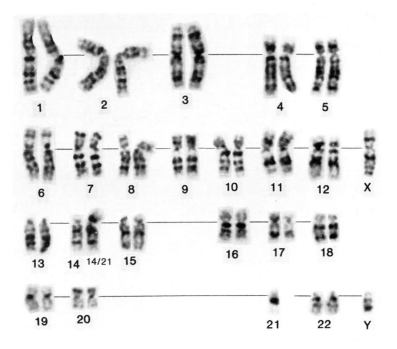

Fig. 2.7. Centric fusion affecting chromosomes 14 and 21. Note the absence of the second 21 chromosome from its normal position and the abnormal shape and size of the second chromosome in group 14. (We are grateful to Dr David Hughes for supplying this figure.)

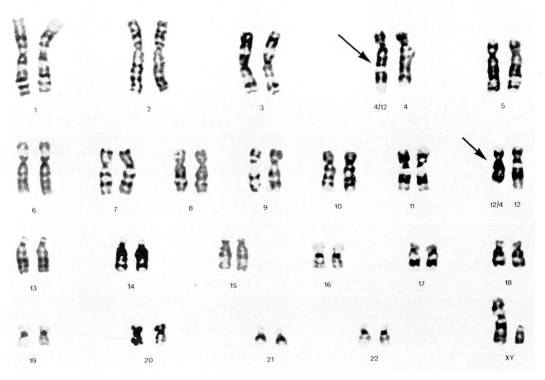

Fig. 2.8. Reciprocal translocation between chromosomes 4 and 12 demonstrated by the banding pattern technique. (By courtesy of Dr Mary Lucas and the Editor of *The British Journal of Hospital Medicine*.)

another (Fig. 2.8) so that two abnormal chromosomes exist although the number is 46.

Individuals with a translocation may be entirely normal if they have neither more nor less chromosome material than usual (balanced translocation). The risk, however, is that during gametogenesis, when chromosomes pair up and exchange genetic material prior to reduction division, the gamete may gain or lose genetic material (unbalanced translocation) and the resulting zygote will also have more or less chromosome material than is normal. An abnormal child or an abortion, respectively, may result. The clinical aspects of this are discussed more fully below.

TECHNICAL CONSIDERATIONS

Chromosome behaviour may be studied in several ways. Those most applicable to gynaecological practice are:

1 buccal smear examination for the presence of nuclear chromatin (Barr body) or F body fluorescence;
2 chromosome analysis of lymphocyte culture of peripheral blood;
3 chromosome analysis following fibroblast culture of skin, gonad or amniotic fluid.

Buccal smear examination

Buccal smear examination for nuclear chromatin can give only indirect information about a possible sex chromosome abnormality and none at all about a possible autosomal abnormality.

The buccal smear should be taken with a metal spatula from inside the cheek. Better results are obtained if the mouth is washed out first. The material obtained is then smeared directly onto a clean glass slide and fixed at once in a mixture of equal parts of 95% alcohol and ether. Slides should be left fixing for an hour at least before staining and examining. Examination of a buccal smear from normal females will show the presence in many nuclei of a densely staining triangular mass (the Barr body) some 0.8–1 μm in size (chromatin positive) which can be seen lying at the periphery of the nucleus. This body is formed from the second X chromosome which condenses into the hetero-chromatic mass. Males and 45,X females have no second X chromosome so no Barr body is visible (chromatin negative).

Patients with a 47,XXY karyotype (Klinefelter's syndrome) will have such a Barr body in their nuclei whilst females with a 47,XXX karyotype will have two masses present in some of their cells and 48,XXXX females three Barr bodies. Variations in Barr body size and percentage may occur in patients with abnormal chromosomes or mosaicism, but these are difficult to recognize. Barr body studies give such imprecise results that they are seldom employed now with chromosome analysis much more readily available.

Chromosome analysis

In clinical practice chromosome analysis is usually carried out following lymphocyte culture of a sample of peripheral blood. A venous sample of 2–3 ml of blood is preferred but if this amount cannot be obtained, as when the patient is a small child, micro techniques can be employed on quantities such as 0.2–0.4 ml. Venous samples are usually placed directly into heparin and set up in culture on the same day on which they are taken. They are incubated for two to three days, the cells are harvested and chromosome preparations are made. If the patient can attend the laboratory undertaking the culture, this will give the best results of all; if she cannot, the blood should be taken into suitable containers with anticoagulant supplied by the laboratory, and transported to it as quickly as possible without being exposed to extremes of temperature. In the case of very small quantities of blood, samples are inoculated directly into the culture bottle containing the medium and incubated soon afterwards.

In chromosome analysis it is customary for the chromosomes in some 30 cells to be counted, full analysis being undertaken in only 8–12 cells. The count on the 30 cells may reveal 46 chromosomes in all. It is not uncommon, however, for one cell or more to be found to have 45 or 47 chromosomes. These cells must then be analysed carefully to determine whether the apparent fault is due to some technical accident such as loss or fragmentation during culture or whether there is a possibility of mosaicism being present. If mosaicism is suspected, a larger number of cells is usually studied. These may show the presence of two cell lines with a different chromosome number, the same chromosome being absent or an extra one being present in all amodal cells. It is often possible to detect mosaicism in this way although sometimes it may be necessary to examine other tissues before a second cell line is revealed.

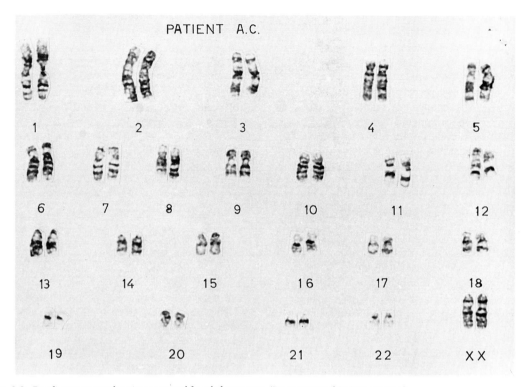

Fig. 2.9. Banding patterns showing a normal female karyotype. (By courtesy of Dr Mary Lucas.)

Mosaicism can never be disproved since we clearly cannot examine all the tissues of any individual patient.

The analysis is undertaken by looking carefully at the chromosomes spread on a slide, photographing the spread, cutting out the individual chromosomes and pairing up each with its opposite number. With conventional techniques such as have been used for many years it is not possible to identify every individual pair of chromosomes. In particular, chromosomes of the 6–12 group (Group C) resemble the pair of X chromosomes closely and until more recently only special techniques could identify one of the X chromosomes. The Y chromosome can generally be recognized by conventional techniques since it is a small acrocentric chromosome similar to numbers 21–22 (Group G) but distinguishable from these by certain features such as the more parallel direction of the long arms. For several years now it has been possible to identify the Y chromosome with certainty by staining the preparation with quinacrin hydrochloride and viewing slides under special illumination. The ends of the long arms of the Y chromosome can then be seen to fluoresce if the technique is properly applied. Similar fluorescence can be demonstrated on buccal smear (F body fluorescence) but the technique is not easy and is open to misinterpretation. It is now possible to identify each individual pair of chromosomes by special stains (Fig. 2.9) since a particular banding pattern is characteristic of each pair of chromosomes. The techniques are, of course, more difficult and more time-consuming and may not be necessary in all cases in which a routine chromosome analysis seems indicated. In certain circumstances, however, notably that of reciprocal translocation, positive identification of the portions of the chromosomes which have been reciprocally exchanged can be carried out (Fig. 2.8).

Fibroblast culture
Many tissues of the body (skin, amniotic fluid, rectus sheath, gonad, etc.) may be used for culture and chromosome analysis but it must be realized that it is always the fibroblasts that grow. Such culture requires to be maintained for much longer than do peripheral blood cultures, and sub-cultures from the original one may be required. Analysis may not be possible for two to three weeks or even longer. It is possible that during the growth process a particular

cell line, if more than one is present, may be selectively favoured by the culture and analysis of the cells obtained may not, therefore, be precisely representative of the karyotype of the original tissue.

Fibroblast culture is used in purely clinical practice in certain cases of suspected mosaicism which cannot be confirmed by lymphocyte culture of peripheral blood, in cases of exceptional cytogenic interest such as true hermaphroditism and on amniotic fluid for the antenatal detection of fetal abnormalities (*see* p. 317).

CLINICAL APPLICATION

Chromosome analysis has several important applications to obstetrical and gynaecological practice. Some of the conditions in which it is indicated are considered elsewhere in this book. These include suspected cases of:

1 gonadal dysgenesis (p. 64);
2 androgen insensitivity (testicular feminization) (p. 35);
3 congenital absence of the vagina (p. 8);
4 virilization at puberty (p. 84);
5 ambiguous sexual development (p. 26).

These conditions will not be reconsidered here. Other applications of chromosome analysis to clinical practice which will now be dealt with more fully include:

6 47,XXX females;
7 47,XXY males;
8 recurrent abortions;
9 malformed infants;
10 antenatal detection of genetic abnormalities.

47,XXX FEMALES

Most patients with this karyotype are normal women who may be fertile; if they are fertile it is extremely likely that their offspring will be chromosomally normal (Barr *et al.* 1969). Some patients with this karyotype, however, may develop secondary amenorrhoea or a premature menopause. They may also present with mental subnormality since the risk of this is raised in patients with more than 46 chromosomes and considerably raised in those with more than 47. Beyond the possible association of secondary amenorrhoea with mental subnormality no other clinical feature will suggest this particular diagnosis.

47,XXY MALES (KLINEFELTER'S SYNDROME)

Most patients with this syndrome have microtestes and aspermia; some have eunuchoid proportions of their limbs and a smaller number still (perhaps 15%) have gynaecomastia. Outwardly in many there may be little fault to draw attention to the possible diagnosis. Such men are, however, infertile and they may be discovered if a buccal smear is carried out on a man with aspermia or marked oligospermia who may then be found to be chromatin positive. Subsequent chromosome analysis will disclose this karyotype and further investigation will be unnecessary since no treatment will be of any avail.

RECURRENT ABORTIONS AND CONGENITAL MALFORMATIONS

These conditions will be considered together since they have much in common cytogenetically.

What has already been said must first be re-emphasized. If a zygote possesses only a single X sex chromosome, it is likely to abort; if it has only a single autosome of a pair, it is certain to abort. If a zygote is trisomic for the sex chromosomes (XXY or XXX), the pregnancy may continue to term and the child will have the appropriate clinical features of these syndromes outlined above; if the zygote is trisomic for an autosome, the child will have several congenital abnormalities, the nature depending upon the chromosomes involved. Trisomy for chromosomes no. 21 is Down's syndrome, the features of which do not require elaboration; trisomy 13 is characterized by low birth weight, microcephalus, cleft lip and palate, micropthalmos with narrow palpable fissure and often supernumerary digits; trisomy 18 is associated with a prominent occiput, micrognathos, a curious hand deformity with flexed 3rd and 4th metacarpals and the index finger deviated to the ulnar side over the 3rd digit, and 'rocker-bottom' feet; also common are central nervous system lesions.

In certain circumstances there can be said to be an increased risk of loss of genetic material, and so of abortion, or an increased risk of extra genetic material and thus of a congenitally malformed child. These risks are raised as follows:

1 increasing maternal age;
2 a previous child affected by a chromosome abnormality;
3 a balanced translocation in one parent.

Increasing maternal age

It is known that an older mother has a greater risk of having a child with a trisomic abnormality. The risk figures for Down's syndrome quoted to older mothers at Queen Charlotte's Hospital are: age 35, 1 in 450; age 36, 1 in 275; age 37, 1 in 210; age 38, 1 in 170; age 39, 1 in 130; age 40, 1 in 100; age 41, 1 in 80; age 42, 1 in 60; age 43, 1 in 45; age 44, 1 in 30; age 45, 1 in 25.

Previously affected child

The fact that a mother has previously given birth to a child with a known chromosomal abnormality probably increases the risk of her having another similarly affected. The extent to which the risk is raised is uncertain but in the case of Down's syndrome, for example, it is customary to quote a subsequent risk of 1 in 100 unless the patient or her husband has a translocation, now about to be described, in which case the risk will be higher.

Translocations

If either parent has a translocation, the risk of abortion or of a malformed child is increased. Again Down's syndrome may be used by way of illustration. The usual variety of Down's syndrome is simple trisomy 21 (Fig. 2.10) and neither parent has a chromosome abnormality. Translocation Down's syndrome may arise, however, if one parent has a translocation involving chromosome number 21, the most common variety being a 14–21 translocation

(Fig. 2.7). The parent will not be abnormal as the translocation is balanced. During gametogenesis, however, chromosomes pair up normally, exchange genetic material and then divide, one to each daughter cell. When this happens in a patient with a 14–21 translocation and, of course, also a normal no. 21 chromosome, the distribution of the chromosome 21 material during gametogenesis may be normal or abnormal. For example, the sperm or ovum may receive two 21 chromosomes (the normal one and that translocated to the number 14) or neither; after fertilization in the former instance the conceptus will be trisomic for 21 and will be an example of translocation Down's syndrome (Fig. 2.11), or in the latter instance, monosomic and will be aborted. The risks of this happening have been computed variously but if the mother is the carrier the risk quoted is about 1 in 10 or perhaps higher, whilst if the father is the carrier the risk is perhaps no greater than 1 in 25–50.

Other centric fusions may carry an even greater risk. A translocation between both 21 chromosomes in the father, for example, can only mean that his sperm will have this abnormal chromosome representing two 21s or neither; in the former instance his child will have Down's syndrome, in the latter abortion will occur; there is no other possibility.

Reciprocal translocations carry a high risk of abortion or malformation. Our knowledge of the karyotype of a patient believed to have a reciprocal translocation can now be much more exact than formerly

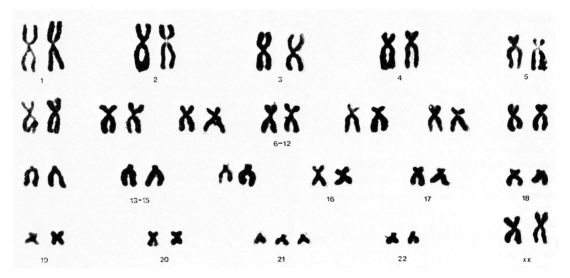

Fig. 2.10. Karyotype of patient with trisomy 21 Down's syndrome. (By courtesy of Dr Mary Lucas and the Editor of *The British Journal of Hospital Medicine*.)

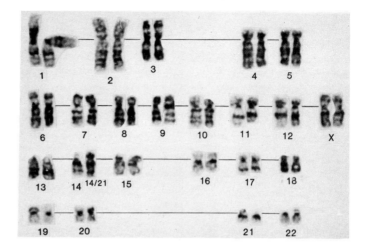

Fig. 2.11. Karyotype of a patient with translocation Down's syndrome. Note that there are two 21 chromosomes in the normal position and, in addition, a third 21 translocated onto chromosome 14. (We are grateful to Dr David Hughes for supplying this figure.)

if the banding pattern techniques described above are used (Fig. 2.8). The risk of the offspring of such a parent being abnormal is probably of the order of 1–4 so amniocentesis in a subsequent pregnancy to allow chromosome analysis of cultured cells, to determine if the fetus is abnormal or not, is usually undertaken.

Practical implications

There are several practical implications to all this. If a patient has had repeated abortions, the reason may lie in her karyotype or her husband's if either has a translocation. Lucas *et al.* (1972) estimated that in patients with two or more spontaneous abortions with or without an abnormal child the risk of discovering a chromosomal abnormality in one of other parent may be one in 26 pregnancies using older techniques and perhaps even higher using banding techniques; lower percentages are usually quoted, however. Chromosome analysis of parents may be indicated if no other fault can be found. Similarly, if a couple have had a child known to have a chromosomal fault, examination of the parents may disclose one to be a carrier with an increased likelihood of another affected child. Sometimes a history is obtained of a Down's syndrome child being born to a near relative of the father or mother. If such a relative's child had a regular trisomy 21 abnormality the risk that the patient will bear a child with Down's syndrome is no greater than in any other mother of her age. The precise karyotype of the relative's child is often unknown, however and if this child had been

a translocation Down's syndrome the patient who is attending you or her husband may be a translocation carrier too. The karyotype of the pregnant woman or of the husband, depending upon whose relative bore the abnormal child should then be established to exclude a balanced translocation. It is important to stress, however, that many congenital malformations (spina bifida and anencephaly are examples) do not have their origin in chromosomal abnormalities. If it is suspected that an abnormal child may have a chromosome fault, chromosome analysis should be arranged at once. If the child dies within hours of birth, as it well may, a piece of skin should be snipped off with sterile precautions, placed in sterile saline and forwarded at once to the cytogenetic laboratory; alternatively, a sample of cardiac blood may be obtained, placed in heparin and similarly sent off immediately.

It must be emphasized, too, that consideration of the problem of a couple with an abnormal baby should be undertaken before a subsequent pregnancy in order that decisions may be taken carefully and at leisure and not in haste when another pregnancy has already begun.

PRENATAL DIAGNOSIS OF GENETIC ABNORMALITY

The investigation during the early antenatal period of the possibility of a fetal genetic abnormality is nowadays commonly undertaken when an increased risk is believed to exist. The abnormalities which can be recognized at this time are not all chromosomal; in addition to the trisomy and translocations already referred to, it is possible to recognize fetal neural tube defects and a variety of inborn errors of metabolism. Amniotic fluid is obtained by amniocentesis between the 14th and 16th week of pregnancy having first identified the position of the placenta by ultrasonic scan; this not only permits the placenta to be avoided but excludes the possibility of more than one fetus being present. If a chromosomal abnormality or inherited metabolic disorder is suspected, the fibroblasts are cultured as described above and either the chromosomes are analysed, in the former case, or the presence or absence of the specific enzyme in question is established in these fibroblasts in the latter circumstances. A possible fetal neural tube defect is sought by measurement of the level of alphafetoprotein present in the maternal blood or amniotic fluid in the presence of such a defect a considerably raised alphafetoprotein level is usually found. The amniotic fluid is taken about week 16 of pregnancy since in any case involving fibroblast culture the fibroblasts may take two or three weeks to grow and be analysed; if growth is poor, a second sample may need to be taken so the patient may be approaching 20 weeks when the result is available. Any later therefore may be too late to undertake therapeutic abortion. The need for a second sample is variable but may arise in some 5% or so of cases.

The risk of a spontaneous abortion following amniocentesis at about 16 weeks has been the subject of a study by the Medical Research Council (1978). This suggested an abortion risk associated with amniocentesis of 1 to 1.5%; premature rupture of membranes and respiratory difficulty at birth was also noted (*see also* p. 317). It follows, therefore, that only high-risk cases are suitable for such investigation; these will include the patient who has had a previous child affected by a trisomy abnormality, an older mother, a parent known to have a balanced translocation, a patient with a previous child affected by a sex-linked abnormality (in which only the sex of the fetus is established, not whether it is affected or not), and a previous child affected by a known metabolic disorder capable of antenatal detection. When and how the possibility of the increased fetal risk of trisomy is broached with the older mother is an important matter for consideration. Some obstetricians tend to recommend the procedure at a certain age (often 37 to 38, but sometimes earlier). Others adopt what seems to be the more suitable approach of indicating to the patient of 35 years or more what the risk of her bearing a child with Down's syndrome might be and what the risk is of performing amniocentesis: the patient and her husband (who should if possible be counselled at the same time) can then decide for themselves whether they wish amniocentesis or not. The view is sometimes expressed that unless the patient will accept therapeutic abortion, the amniocentesis is pointless: however against this may be the view of some patients that although they would not accept the abortion of their fetus with an abnormality, they wish to know this in order that they can prepare for the event and not be confronted with the news of the malformation when the child is born. The whole area of genetic counselling and antenatal diagnosis of fetal abnormalities is a delicate but exceedingly important one.

The whole subject of the antenatal diagnosis of fetal defects has been well reviewed by Brock (1982) and is described in Chapter 22.

REFERENCES

BARR M.L., SERGOVICH F.R., CARR D.H. & SHAVER E.L. (1969) *Can. med. Ass. J.,*. **101**, 247–258.

BROCK D.J.H. (1982) *Early Diagnosis of Fetal Defects,* Churchill Livingstone, Edinburgh.

DE LA CHAPPELLE, A. (1982) In Crosignani P.G. & Rubin B.L. (eds) *Genetic Control of Gamete Production and Function,* pp 33–48. Academic Press, London.

DEWHURST J., (1981) Chromosomal aspects of reproductive failure. *J. Obstet. Gynec.,* **1**, 235–246.

DEWHURST C.J. & LUCAS M. (1973) *Brit. J. Hosp. Med.,* **10**, 735.

HARVEY D. (1973) *Brit. J. Hosp. Med.,* **10**, 591.

LUCAS M., WALLACE I. & HIRSCHHORN, K. (1972) *J. Obstet. Gynaec. Brit. Cwlth.,* **79**, 1119–1127.

MARASCHIO P. & FRACCARO M. (1982) *Genetic Control of Gemete Production and Function* (eds. Crosignani P.G. & Rubin B.L.). pp 275–285, Academic Press, London.

Medical Research Council (1978) *Brit. J. Obstet. Gynaec.,* **85** (Supplement 2).

SIMPSON J.L. (1976) *Disorders of Sexual Differentiation,* pp 1–50. Academic Press, New York.

SIMPSON J.L. (1982) In *Genetic Control of Gamete Production and Function* (eds. Crosignani P.G. & Rubin B.L.) pp 199–228. Academic Press, London.

CHAPTER 3
INTERSEXUALITY

SIR JOHN DEWHURST

There are several reasons for abnormal sexual development and several ways, in clinical practice, in which it may present. Though a complex subject, work in recent years has considerably clarified it and our understanding of some of the intricacies is greater than it was only a comparatively few years ago.

A knowledge of normal sexual differentiation is essential before we can understand how sexual differentiation occurs abnormally so this chapter will begin with a somewhat more detailed account of normal sexual differentiation, amplifying that given in outline in Chapter 1.

NORMAL SEXUAL DIFFERENTIATION

Three factors determine an individual's sexual development. These are: the effect of the sex chromosomes on the differentiation of the gonad; the proper functioning of the differentiated testes (ovaries are not important here); and the response of the end organs to testicular activity.

THE EFFECT OF THE SEX CHROMOSOMES ON THE DIFFERENTIATION OF THE GONAD

Sex chromosomes have only one function to perform in sexual development and that is to determine the differentiation of the undifferentiated gonad. If a Y chromosome is present in association with one or more X chromosomes, the undifferentiated gonad will become a testis. If the Y chromosome is present with more than one X chromosome, differentiation of that testis during intrauterine life will still be normal, although the subsequent development of the testis at and after puberty may be imperfect.

If two or more X chromosomes are present without a Y, the undifferentiated gonad will develop as an ovary. Unlike the subsequent development of the testis when two X chromosomes are present with a Y, subsequent development of the ovary at puberty when more than two X chromosomes are present, is likely to be normal.

It has been disclosed in the last few years (Wachtel 1979 and 1981, Wachtel & Koo 1982) that the probable mechanism by which the Y chromosome promotes testicular differentiation is by the production of a substance known as H-Y antigen which is thought to be the product of testis-determining genes on the Y chromosome. This H-Y antigen is a plasma membrane protein widely distributed in the animal kingdom. It has been given this name because it was first recognized as a result of histocompatibility studies using laboratory mice where it was found that female mice rejected the grafts from males, presumably as a result of an antigen present on the Y chromosome. H-Y antigen was first recognized in the human when it was discovered that rare phenotypic males who, nonetheless, have an apparent female (46,XX) karyotype, were found to be H-Y antigen positive; the presence of the antigen, it was thought, had caused the differentiation of the testes despite the fact that no Y chromosome was present. Similar findings were demonstrated in 46,XX true hermaphrodites who possessed both ovarian and testicular tissue who were also H-Y antigen positive. There is still much more to be learned about this interesting matter and what is learned will undoubtedly be of considerable scientific interest. At the moment let it suffice to say that although it is probable that H-Y antigen is closely related to testicular differentiation, the circumstances in which this happens have not been fully clarified. Moreover, in clinical practice the demonstration of the presence or absence of H-Y antigen does not apppear to be an important matter in the management of patients. Testing for H-Y antigen is difficult and the investigation can be undertaken at only a few centres at the time of writing. Bono and Fellous (1981) have described the technique of testing.

RELATIONSHIP BETWEEN THE FUNCTION OF
THE TESTIS AND GENITAL TRACT
DEVELOPMENT

When testes develop and function normally in an
early embryo, that embryo will develop as a male.
Should testes be absent, however, or if they do not
function normally, the embryo will become female
whether ovaries are present or not. It should be realized that male development is concerned with having
testes and female development with not having testes.

Testes carry out their intrauterine function by producing two substances, testosterone and anti-
Müllerian hormone.

The testosterone gives rise to the development of
the external genitalia and of the Wolffian system
whilst the anti-Mullerian hormone inhibits the development of Müllerian structures which are always
present and capable of development. Anti-Müllerian
hormone has recently been isolated (Picard and Josso
1984); it is a glycoprotein produced by the sertoli
cells (Josso *et al.* 1977, Josso *et al.* 1980). Anti-
Müllerian hormone has a unilateral action so that
each testis appears to produce the hormone which
results in regression of the Müllerian structures on its
own side. The sensitivity of Müllerian structures to
anti-Müllerian hormone is present only during the first
eight weeks of gestation.

END ORGAN SENSITIVITY TO ANDROGEN

The manner in which testosterone produced by the
developing testis is utilized to bring about masculinization has recently been clarified. To utilize testosterone effectively the external genital organs must convert testosterone to dihydrotestosterone through the
action of 5-alpha-reductase (Josso 1981, Liao *et al.*
1972). Wolffian structures, on the other hand, are
capable of utilizing testosterone directly and are,
therefore, independent of 5-alpha-reductase activity.
5-alpha-reductase activity is therefore essential to
normal development of the external genitalia and 5-
alpha-reductase deficiency will lead to intersexuality
in a manner shortly to be described. For effective
utilization of both testosterone and 5-alpha-reductase
it is necessary for these substances to be bound to
receptors in the cytoplasm of the cells and ineffective
binding of testosterone also leads to abnormal sexual
differentiation in the disorder known as androgen insensitivity. This also will be described below.

ABNORMAL SEXUAL DEVELOPMENT

It will be evident therefore that sexual development
may be abnormal in the following circumstances:

1   There may be a sex chromosome abnormality interfering with testicular differentiation; the only common one is 45,X/46,XY mosaicism giving rise to one
of the forms of gonadal dysgenesis.
2   Testes may be incapable of producing testosterone
either because of a complete failure of testicular differentiation (anatomical testicular failure) or a biosynthetic defect of testosterone production (enzymatic
testicular failure).
3   The end organs may be incapable of utilizing testosterone because of 5-alpha-reductase deficiency or
because of failure to bind testosterone effectively (androgen insensitivity).
4   The production of anti-Müllerian hormone may be
deficient leading to the growth of Müllerian structures
in an otherwise normal, or near normal, male.
5   In a genetic female (46,XX) masculinization of
the external genitalia may result from congenital
adrenal hyperplasia in the fetus or from androgen
stimulation from some other source.
6   Rarely, in a genetic female testicular differentiating genes capable of producing H-Y antigen may be
present on the X chromosome or on an autosome
leading to testicular differentiation (46,XX males).
7   True hermaphroditism (the presence of testicular
tissue and ovarian tissue in the same individual) may
be present; such patients are most commonly genetic
females (46,XX), sometimes mosaics and, least commonly, genetic male (46,XY).

These various conditions will be dealt with more
fully in the following sections but, before this is done,
the approach to the intersexual patient in clinical
practice must first be discussed.

Presentation in clinical practice

We will now consider the practical aspects of the
investigation and management of an intersexual
patient who presents in clinical practice. Here the list
of causes given above may, with benefit, be much
simplified, at least initially, to allow the important
issues to be more clearly seen.

An individual with ambiguous genitalia will be
either:

1   A masculinized female due to congenital adrenal
hyperplasia or to androgen stimulation from some
other source.

2 An under-masculinized male for one of the reasons discussed above.

3 A true hermaphrodite.

We will presently consider these various conditions which may cause intersexuality, but first important generalizations must be made.

It will be immediately evident that in this simplified classification the masculinized female has been placed first. The reason is a simple one: if the patient is a masculinized female due to congenital adrenal hyperplasia she may be unable to retain salt and water in the body and may die within a few weeks of birth from salt loss and dehydration. Congenital adrenal hyperplasia, therefore, is a condition which threatens the patient's life and it must be confirmed or excluded at the outset.

The second important generalization concerns the age at presentation. If, as is usually the case, the patient presents at birth with sexual ambiguity it is important that full investigation be undertaken at once in order that the more appropriate choice of the sex of rearing can be made at the earliest possible moment. There are two reasons for this. One is that if the child has congenital adrenal hyperplasia she may die within a short time unless correctly treated. The other reason is that whatever the diagnosis the orientation of the child to the chosen sex of rearing will be better if that child is placed in that gender role as soon as possible after birth and is allowed to grow up in it without further doubts about gender being expressed. If a wise decision is not made soon after birth, and the child is placed in the gender role later found to be wrong, an attempt to change this sex of rearing may result in considerable psychological confusion—confusion which is not seen if the sex of rearing is correctly chosen at birth and adhered to.

The third generalization to be made is that only thorough investigation can establish the correct diagnosis which cannot be determined by a superficial examination of the external genitalia.

The last generalization concerns the management of the patient who presents some years after birth. Such patients who have lived in a gender role for a time may have become well orientated to it and it may be wiser not to attempt to change that role even though it is later established that the original diagnosis of sex had been incorrect.

Patients presenting in the neonatal period

The first diagnosis to be confirmed or refuted is congenital adrenal hyperplasia. It must be admitted that if a probable testis can with certainty be palpated the likelihood of congenital adrenal hyperplasia is very small, but it should still be formally exclude by the investigations now to be described.

CONGENITAL ADRENAL HYPERPLASIA

This is a disorder in which the affected fetus suffers from one of several possible enzyme defects which interfere with the metabolism of cortisol and aldosterone. The commonest enzyme defect is 21-hydroxylase

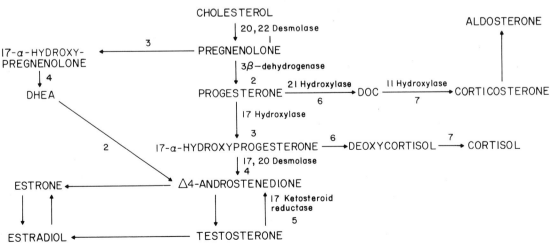

Fig. 3.1. Diagram of the enzyme steps necessary to convert cholesterol through its various intermediate stages to aldosterone, cortisol and testosterone. Note that 3-β-dehydrogenase (labelled 2) is active at two places as are 17-hydroxylase (labelled 3), 17,20-desmolase (labelled 4), 21-hydroxylase (labelled 6) and 11-hydroxylase (labelled 7).

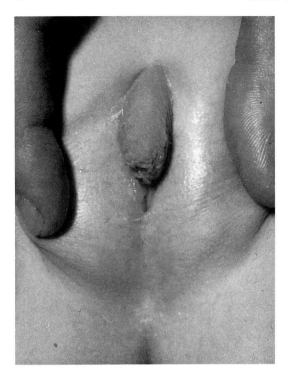

Fig. 3.2. The external genitalia of a child with congenital adrenal hyperplasia. Note the clitoral enlargement and the excessive fusion of labial folds which have resulted in only a single opening on the perineum.

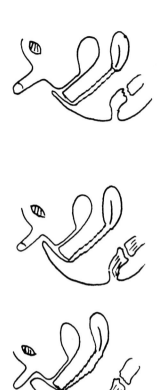

Fig. 3.3. Diagrammatic representation of clitoral enlargement and excessive fusion of labial folds to show the different thickness of the folds, the narrowing of the vagina in the most marked cases, and variations in the point at which the urogenital sinus opens.

deficiency which interferes with the conversion of 17-alpha-hydroxyprogesterone to desoxycortisol and with the conversion of progesterone to desoxy-corticosterone (Fig. 3.1). Two other less common defects are 3-beta-hydroxysteroid dehydrogenase deficiency and 11-beta-hydroxylase deficiency (New & Levine 1981). In the most common form, 21-hydroxylase deficiency, which will now be described, affected female fetuses demonstrate enlargement of the clitoris and excessive fusion of the genital folds which obscure the vagina and urethra (Fig. 3.2), forming in the process an artificial uro-genital sinus which has a single opening at some point on the perineum, usually near the base of the clitoris, sometimes along its ventral surface and rarely at the tip. Thickening and rugosity of labia majora are evident and they bear some resemblance to a scrotum. There is much variation in the thickness of fused labial folds and in extreme cases they are very thick indeed with narrowing of the lower part of the vagina (Fig. 3.3). The uterus, fallopian tubes and vagina, however, are always present and the vagina opens at some point in the urogenital sinus; in the more severe cases, how-

ever, it may be difficult to identify the opening precisely.

The underlying explanation of the masculinization is that lack of cortisol results in failure to inhibit ACTH production by the pituitary. ACTH is therefore produced in large quantities and overstimulates the adrenal which produces androgens in large amounts which masculinize the genitalia.

In some patients a dangerous salt-losing syndrome may arise because of the associated aldosterone deficiency; the child may die of wasting and vomiting within the first few weeks of life, perhaps before the true nature of the condition is appreciated, but such deaths have been known even though the child was in hospital under investigation.

Investigation of a suspected case of congenital adrenal hyperplasia should include the following:

1   Chromosome analysis to establish the karyotype (buccal smear examination is insufficiently precise to be reliable).
2   Measurement of androgen levels in urine by assay of urinary 17-oxosteroids.
3   Assay of 17-hydroxyprogesterone in the blood. Since a 21-hydroxylase deficiency prevents the further metabolism of 17-hydroxyprogesterone to desoxycortisol the former builds up in the body and considerably raised levels are found. If this assay is not available increased pregnanetriol excretion in the urine may be helpful, pregnanetriol being the excretion product of 17-hydroxyprogesterone.
4   Examination of electrolytes to check the possibility of a dangerous salt-losing syndrome; if the salt-losing state is present sodium and chlorides may be low and potassium raised.

Brook (1981) gives an excellent account of the investigation and diagnosis of this condition.

The immediate management of such a child should always be undertaken by or in cooperation with a paediatrician. Cortisol or one of its related substances must be given to suppress excess ACTH secretion. If the patient is a salt loser this salt loss must be very carefully controlled since if uncontrolled the outcome may be fatal.

The immediate management of any salt loss is concerned with establishing a normal blood volume at the earliest opportunity by saline infusion combined with the administration of mineralocorticoid hormones (desoxycorticosterone or aldosterone). Brook (1981) again gives an admirable account of this aspect of the patient's care.

Once the disorder has been brought under control, attention can be paid to surgical correction of the external genitalia. It must be emphasized that such patients are genetic females and potentially fertile and must be brought up in the female role regardless of the degree of masculinization of the external genitalia which can always be corrected.

Two corrective procedures need to be considered: reduction in size of the clitoris and division of the fused labial folds to expose the urethra and vagina beneath. A clitoral reduction is best undertaken in the neonatal period before the child is discharged from hospital; by so doing the visible evidence of maleness is removed, the parents can more readily regard their child as female and there is no risk of a third party seeing masculinized genitalia and reporting the child's doubtful sex. The division of the fused labial folds, however, is better left until later and, in

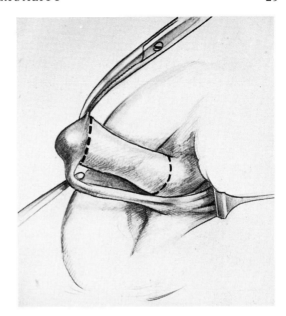

Fig. 3.4. Showing the identification of the corpora cavernosa which are excised following preservation of the nerve and blood supply to the glans.

many instances where the folds are thick, until after puberty.

The clitoris may be reduced in size by amputation which gives a good cosmetic result (Dewhurst 1981) and is compatible with normal coitus and orgasm. An attempt to preserve the sensitive glans with its nerve and blood supply is desirable however and the technique described by Allan (Dewhurst 1981) is to be preferred.

Briefly, the skin and subcutaneous tissues are stripped away from the body of the clitoris, the blood supply entering from the ventral surface and the nerve supply running in the anterior sheath of the corpora cavernosa being carefully preserved. The corpora cavernosa are then excised (Fig. 3.4) and the glans stitched back in place. A good cosmetic result is obtained (Fig. 3.5) and a good functional result likely. Operations which seek to bend the clitoris ventrally and bury it so as to render it unobtrusive are not recommended as they lead to painful erections later whilst with a large clitoris they give a poor cosmetic result.

The division of the fused labial folds is simple if they are thin (Fig. 3.6), when it may be performed at almost any age. It is the author's view that operations on the fused folds performed in childhood often give an indifferent result and need to be repeated later when, in view of the previous operation, they are

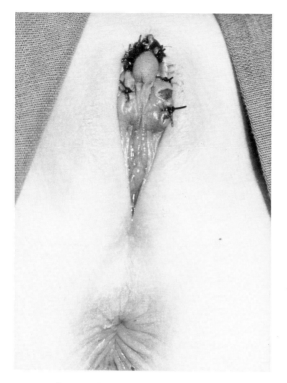

more difficult. The author favours performance of the procedure for the first time soon after the age of puberty. If the folds are very thick and especially if the vagina is narrowed, more elaborate procedures which bring extra skin to the introital ring are required (Dewhurst & Gordon 1969)

Careful supervision by a paediatrician of a child with congenital adrenal hyperplasia is essential throughout childhood. A recent review of subsequent menstrual and fertility patterns (Grant *et al.* 1983) indicates that the menarche is often delayed by up to two years. Good hormone control of the disease usually leads to an earlier menarche (Jones & Verkauf 1971, Klingensmith *et al.* 1977) and less menstrual irregularity, but in some cases, despite meticulous control, oligomenorrhoea or even amenorrhoea occur. Fertility is probably reduced to some extent, although a number of successful pregnancies have been reported in salt-losing (Andersen *et al.* 1983) and non-salt-losing (Porter & de Swiet 1983) patients.

Fig. 3.5. The immediate post-operative result after reduction in size of the clitoris by the Allan technique in the patient seen in Figure 2.

OTHER SOURCES OF MASCULINIZATION IN GENETIC FEMALES

Other sources of masculinization in genetic females are nowadays few. In former times masculinization was not infrequently reported following treatment of the patient's mother during pregnancy with a pro-

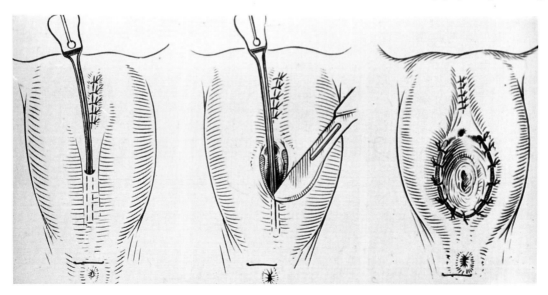

Fig. 3.6. Diagrammatic representation of division of fused labial folds. (By courtesy of Dr R. R. Gordon and Messrs Baillière-Tindall.)

gestogen (Wilkins 1960, Overzier 1963), methyltestosterone (Dewhurst & Gordon 1969), rarely progesterone alone (Hayles & Nolan 1958) or oestrogen and progesterone in combination (Wilkins *et al.* 1958). The progestogens now in clinical use possess little androgenic activity so such cases are a rarity. More recently, masculinization of the genitalia of the female fetus has been reported when the mother has become pregnant whilst under treatment with Danazol which has some androgenic activity (Peress *et al.* 1982). Masculinization has also been reported (Dewhurst 1981) when the mother was affected by Cushing's syndrome during pregnancy.

It may be mentioned that the features of the masculinized genetic female from other androgen sources are not likely to be significantly different from those seen in congenital adrenal hyperplasia so far as the degree of masculinization at birth is concerned (Fig. 3.7). There will, however, be no other metabolic defect and no salt-losing syndrome nor will the condition be progressive.

In the management of such a case congenital adrenal hyperplasia must first be excluded by the tests described above after which an attempt should be made to identify the source of androgen. If this can be determined further investigation is not required. The infant must be reared in her correct female role and her surgical treatment carried out as for congenital adrenal hyperplasia. If no source of androgen can be identified consideration must be given to the possibility of the child being a 46,XX true hermaphrodite (see later). Should the degree of external masculinization be considerable it will be wise to consider operation to permit gonadal biopsy; if masculinization is mild this step can probably be omitted.

Rarely no obvious androgen source can be detected to explain the masculinization of the external genitalia of a genetic female fetus (Dewhurst 1963, Jones 1981).

MALE INTERSEXES AND TRUE HERMAPHRODITES

Once masculinization of a genetic female from congenital adrenal hyperplasia or other androgen source has been excluded, which can usually be done within the first week of life, a distinction must be made between an undermasculinized male and a true hermaphrodite with ovarian and testicular tissue.

This distinction can be made for certain only by laparotomy and gonadal biopsy. Laparoscopic biopsy is not an adequate procedure for establishing the nature of a gonad in an intersex child. The organ may be an ovotestis and unless a representative biopsy is taken along the length of the gland this fact may be missed.

It must be stressed at this point, however, that the biopsy of the gonad is not undertaken to determine what the sex of rearing should be; this decision is principally made on the suitability of the external genitalia for sexual life in the one or other gender role. It is necessary to know the nature of the gonad however so that if gonadal tissue is present which is inappropriate to the chosen gender role, as it always will be in a true hermaphrodite and in a male intersex being brought up as a female, that gonadal tissue can be removed.

The various conditions present under the general heading of male intersexuality and true hermaphroditism will now be considered in more detail.

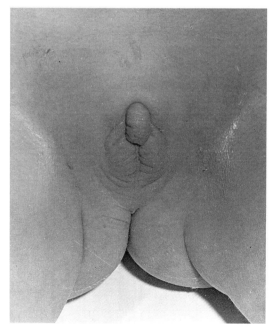

Fig. 3.7. Considerable masculinization of the external genitalia of a female child whose mother was treated with methyl testosterone in early pregnancy.

INTERSEXUALITY IN GENETIC MALES

1   *Faults in androgen production*

Anatomical testicular failure. Failure of normal testicular differentiation and development may be the result of chromosome mosaicism affecting the sex chromosomes or possibly associated with an abnormal chromosome such as an isochromosome (Simpson 1976), but usually the sex chromosomes appear to be normally male and the condition is sometimes referred to as pure gonadal dysgenesis. Clinically such cases show variable features depending upon how much testicular differentiation is present. Since differentiation is often poor most patients have mild masculinization or none at all and the uterus, tubes and vagina are generally present (Dewhurst 1980). The presence of the uterus in this condition contrasts with the other forms of XY female shortly to be described.

Management in this group is concerned with reconstruction of the external genitalia in the manner already described, should this be required, and removal of the streak or rudimentary gonad in view of their raised cancer potential. The degree of masculinization of such patients is often minimal and if it is limited to a minor degree of clitoral enlargement with little or no fusion of genital folds, surgery need not be undertaken.

The risk of malignancy in the rudimentary testes is probably of the order of 30% or so at some time in the patient's life (Dewhurst *et al.* 1971) and gonadal removal during childhood will be wise. Around the age of puberty replacement oestrogen and progestogen therapy can be started to produce secondary sexual development and menstruation.

Enzymatic testicular failure. Several metabolic steps are necessary for the complete formation of testosterone from cholesterol (Fig. 3.1). Faults have been reported at each stage of the process (Forrest 1981). Clinical features as a result are somewhat varied, but since such enzyme defects are generally incomplete there is external genital ambiguity of varying degrees; the uterus, tubes and upper vagina are absent, since the production of anti-Müllerian hormone by the testes is normal.

The decision on the sex of rearing will depend upon the degree of masculinization of the external genitalia, as already indicated, but the female role will often be chosen (Fig. 3.8). Surgical management is as already described. The identification of the precise enzyme defect can be difficult but may be approached by HCG stimulation of the gonads with measurement of DHEA, androstenedione and testosterone in an attempt to determine where the enzyme block occurs. Forrest (1981) may be consulted for further information.

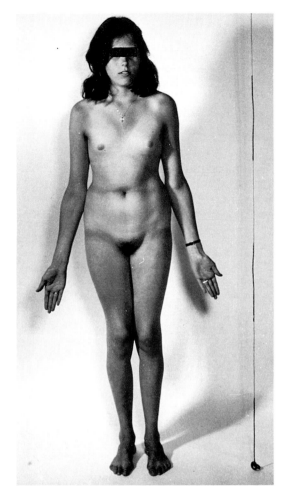

Fig. 3.8. A patient with enzymatic testicular failure believed to be due to 17-ketosteroid-reductase deficiency. (By kind permission of Marcel Dekker & Co.)

2   End organ insensitivity

5-Alpha-reductase deficiency. It has already been indicated that for normal masculinization of the external genitalia to occur testosterone must be converted to dihydrotestosterone by 5-alpha-reductase activity, although Wolffian structures can respond directly to testosterone. In the presence of 5-alpha-reductase deficiency a male fetus will have poor masculinization of external genitalia but the uterus, tubes and upper vagina will be absent since anti-Müllerian hormone production will be normal. As a rule the degree of genital masculinization is small or, at the best, moderate and most children are placed initially in the female role (Fig. 3.9). At puberty, however, the testes produce increasing amounts of testosterone and there

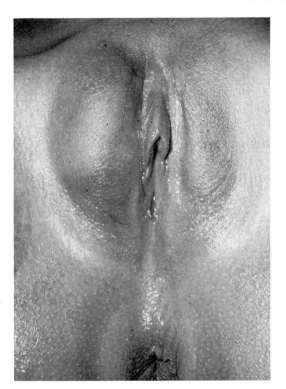

Fig. 3.9. The external genitalia of a 10-year-old 46 XY child with 5-alpha-reductase deficiency. (By courtesy of the Editor of *Pediatric and Adolescent Gynecology* and Marcel Dekker & Co.)

is greater virilization, perhaps to such an extent that the patient may wish to change the gender role from female to male. Penis size tends to remain barely adequate however and the female gender role will often be the better one for such patients. Imperato-McGinley *et al.* (1979), Savage *et al.* (1980) and Dewhurst *et al.* (1983) have described the condition. It is a familial disorder due to an autosomal recessive abnormality so that evidence of other similarly affected members of the family is often present to assist diagnosis. If there is no such history, precise diagnosis may be attempted by HCG stimulation of the genitalia for three days with measurement of testosterone and dihydrotestosterone at the beginning and end of the test. It must be stressed, however, that such testing is not important to the decision on the sex of rearing which depends upon the degree of masculinization of external genitalia.

Androgen insensitivity. This syndrome is seen only in the newborn if the enzyme defect giving rise to it is

partial. It is described below where patients presenting in later life are considered. When present in partial form and presenting at birth as ambiguous sex the principles of management are those already outlined for 5-alpha-reductase deficiency.

TRUE HERMAPHRODITES

True hermaphrodites are rare in Europe and in the United States of America. In some countries, however, notably the Southern part of the African continent, they appear to be much more common.

They present with varying degrees of sexual ambiguity (Fig. 3.10[a] and [b]), maleness preponderating in some patients, femaleness in others. In the majority the uterus and vagina are present.

The karyotype in most true hermaphrodites is that of an apparently normal female (46,XX) which occurred in 58% of 172 cases reviewed by Van Niekerk (1974, 1981). The next most frequent karyotype was 46,XX/XY which appeared in 13% followed by 46,XY (11%), 46,XY/47,XXY (6%) and 45,X/46,XY (4%); other mosaics occurred in 6%.

It has been possible to date to estimate the H-Y antigen status of only a few true hermaphrodites. Van Niekerk reports that in his own patients whose karyotype was 46 XX there was reduced expression of H-Y antigen in somatic tissues such as blood, skin and fascia when compared with 46 XY males, although the antigen could be detected. The ovotestes however showed testicular H-Y positive portion and an ovarian H-Y negative portion. Wachtel and Koo (1982) may be consulted for further details in this important area.

The distribution of the gonads is interesting. The commonest combination is for an ovotestis to be present on one side and an ovary on the other with a testis on one side and an ovary being almost as frequent. Ovotestes may be bilateral or combined with a testis.

The diagnosis of true hermaphroditism can be made as already indicated only by gonadal biopsy and the demonstration that ovarian and testicular tissue are both present. Sex of rearing, however, is determined on the functional capability of the external genitalia after which inappropriate organs are removed. In some cases it may be possible to identify the ovarian and testicular portions of an ovotestis for certain and to remove only that part which is unwanted. If this is not possible both must be removed and, if the patient then requires to be brought up in a gender role for which there is no appropriate gon-

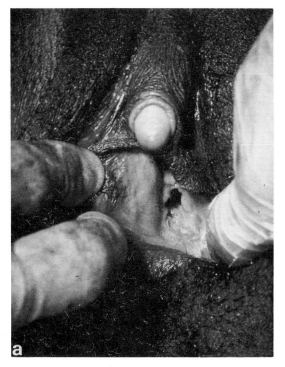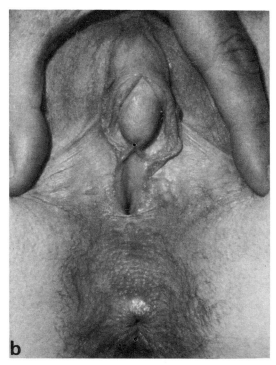

Fig. 3.10. External genitalia in two true hermaphrodites. In (a) there is a considerable degree of clitoral enlargement behind which it is possible to identify the urethra (not shown in the figure) and the vagina which is illustrated. In (b) there is an equivalent amount of clitoral enlargement, but the excessive fusion of labial folds has led to only a single perineal opening and it is not possible to identify the urethra and vagina separately.

adal tissue, replacement hormone therapy at puberty will be required.

Patients presenting after infancy

Doubt about an individual's sex may arise for the first time some years after birth, generally around puberty, some heterosexual feature becoming evident or a pre-existing minor one more pronounced. Sometimes an older patient is seen whose intersexual state had been recognized at birth but not investigated.

The investigation of such patients follows the general pattern outlined in the earlier part of this chapter and is different in only minor respects; if, for example, a patient is seen with late onset congenital adrenal hyperplasia about the time of puberty the likelihood of a salt-losing syndrome is minimal and investigation of this aspect of the case need not be intensive.

Management is, however, different in one particular and very important respect. The patient, of necessity, will have lived in one or other sex for some time and may have become so well adjusted that no attempt should be made to change this gender role. This aspect of the matter is best illustrated by 46,XY patients with androgen insensitivity to be discussed in a moment. Such patients have no masculinization of the external genitalia whatever and in most instances are well developed, very attractive phenotypic females. To suggest that they change to the male role because they have a male karyotype and intra-abdominal testes would be both ludicrous and the height of folly.

The intersexual condition most likely to be evident for the first time at or after puberty but which may sometimes be encountered earlier in childhood is the condition of androgen insensitivity which will now be considered further.

ANDROGEN INSENSITIVITY

The disorder of androgen insensitivity was formerly known as that of testicular feminization. It will be evident, however, from what has already been said in this chapter that there are several mechanisms by which a patient who has testes may be feminized, so this term is no longer appropriate. Since the basis of the condition is insensitivity to androgen this term is the more satisfactory. The clinical picture of complete androgen insensitivity is remarkably uniform although it now seems probable that two distinct mechanisms of insensitivity are present.

Most patients with androgen insensitivity present for the first time after puberty when despite normal breast development there is primary amenorrhoea. Further clinical examination will reveal absent or very scanty pubic and axillary hair, a normal vulva (Fig. 3.11), but a short, blind vagina with no cervix palpable. If a laparoscopy or laparotomy is performed the uterus will be found to be absent and probably only rudiments of fallopian tube present; testes are generally to be found either within the abdomen, in the groins or, occasionally, in the labia. Examination of the karyotype will disclose a normal 46,XY male pattern.

Endocrine investigation reveals testosterone levels to be within the normal male range (Southren et al. 1964, Tremblay et al. 1972). Oestrogen levels are generally within the range where normal male and normal female values overlap (Jeffcoate et al. 1968).

LH values are generally elevated due, it is believed, to the insensitivity of the hypothalamus and pituitary to testosterone (Zarate et al. 1974). FSH levels are more variable but are ususally within the normal male range or slightly raised.

There appear to be two aetiological mechanisms for this syndrome (Migeon et al. 1981). One group of observers (Keenan et al. 1974) identified faulty androgen receptor binding in the cytoplasm whilst another (Amrheim et al. 1976) showed receptor binding to be normal in some patients with an identical syndrome and it must be concluded that the fault in this group occurs after that step is complete. It is seldom difficult to make the clinical diagnosis of androgen insensitivity in a complete syndrome. Rarely, minor variations occur such as the presence of scanty or even moderate pubic hair, but axillary hair is seldom if ever present. The vagina may be somewhat longer in some patients, especially those who have had repeated intercourse. The combination of the clinical features and the male karyotype is usually sufficient for a confident diagnosis so that demonstration of the presence of testes can be combined with their removal if the time for this is ripe.

Although most patients present some time after puberty because of primary amenorrhoea the condition is occasionally seen in the child when a testis is found to occupy a hernial sac or when the presence of the full-blown syndrome in an older sister leads to examination of a younger one when the male karyotype is revealed.

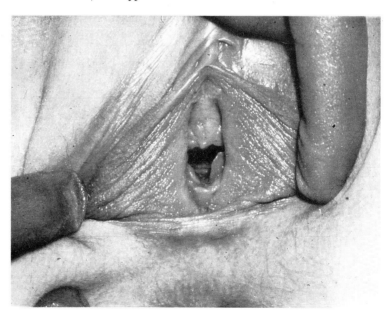

Fig. 3.11. The external genitalia of a patient with androgen insensitivity.

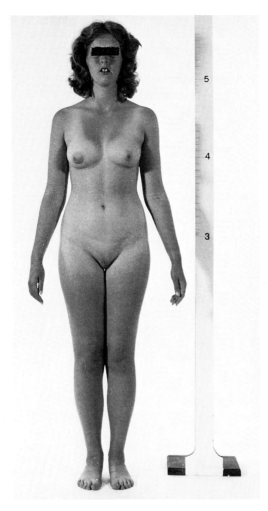

Fig. 3.12. The external appearance of a 46,XY individual with androgen insensitivity. Note the excellent breast development and complete absence of pubic hair.

The management of the patient with androgen insensitivity depends upon the age at which the patient is seen. If seen after puberty, with breast development complete (Fig. 3.12), the management to be considered is whether or not the testes should be removed. It seems likely that they have a raised cancer potential which is probably of the order of 5% or so at some time (Jones & Scott 1971). Many would regard this as sufficiently high to call for gonadectomy and have usually advised this treatment. It is probably unwise to let the patient know of the presence of the male karyotype and testes and it may be better to refer to 'gonads' or even to 'abnormal ovaries' which need to be removed because they may be a

danger in later life. If gonadectomy is carried out, replacement hormone therapy with oestrogen should be undertaken. This need not be cyclical since the uterus is absent (Dewhurst 1980).

If the patient is seen for the first time in childhood, and it can be confidently stated that feminization will occur at puberty, nothing need be done until after that time. If however there are heterosexual features present it is likely that masculinization may occur to some extent at puberty which would have a profound psychological effect upon a patient being brought up in the female role. In these circumstances gonadectomy in childhood will be wise followed by replacement hormone therapy at the appropriate time (Fig. 3.13).

Surgery is seldom necessary to elongate the vagina. Should elongation be required these cases respond well to graduated dilatation using Frank's method (*see* page 10); if this is unsatisfactory surgical elongation using amnion on a solid mould to promote epithelialization will probably be best.

The disorder of androgen insensitivity is inherited

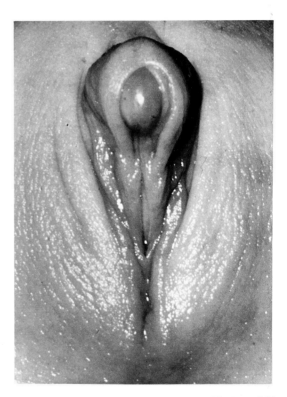

Fig. 3.13. External genitalia of a seven-year-old 46,XY child with a degree of masculinization. (By kind permission of Marcel Dekker & Co.)

as either an X-linked recessive, or sex limited autosomal dominant gene (Simpson *et al.* 1976).

Other disorders encountered in the older patient

When the disorders already discussed as presenting at birth are seen in later life, certain differences in clinical features and the management must be emphasized.

The patient with congenital adrenal hyperplasia who has been reared as a female is unlikely to have significant masculinization of the external genitalia (Fig. 3.14), so reconstructive surgery is less commonly necessary. Secondary sexual development is apt to be poor or absent (Fig. 3.15) but once the diagnosis has been made and the condition controlled by cortisol spontaneous secondary sexual development should follow soon afterwards. If however a serious error has been made at birth because of an extreme degree of masculinization the child being placed in the male role, management depends entirely upon the orientation of the patient to the male sex. If this is good and the phallus is of a size judged

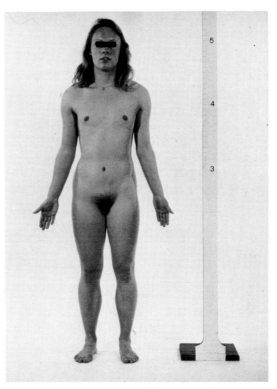

Fig. 3.15. External appearance of the patient whose genitalia are illustrated in Fig. 3.14.

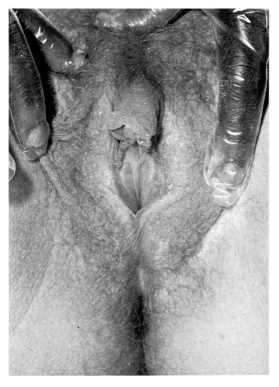

Fig. 3.14. External genital appearances of a 46,XX individual with congenital adrenal hyperplasia seen for the first time at the age of 16.

suitable for intercourse it may be wiser to allow the patient to continue in that gender role. It should be remembered however that if cortisol is used to inhibit the excessive ACTH activity the apparent male will probably begin to menstruate so total hysterectomy and oophorectomy will need to be performed, testosterone administered and, if judged appropriate, testicular prostheses inserted.

Patients with 5-alpha-reductase deficiency placed in the female role, but otherwise untreated, are likely to have a male-type puberty and may wish to change sex. An extremely difficult decision must then be made since, as already indicated, the phallic size is seldom really sufficient for coitus (Savage 1983). Many patients wish to change their gender role nonetheless and this important psychological aspect of management must be fully assessed in deciding what to do for the best.

Menstruation and/or breast development may occur at puberty in a true hermaphrodite who has been thought to be male (Gordon *et al.* 1960). In such a case the adjustment to masculinity is likely to be good so mastectomy and hysterectomy with removal of the ovary will be indicated.

Two other conditions require brief mention although it is unlikely that they will be encountered by the gynaecologist.

Phenotypic males are rarely found to have a 46 XX karyotype (Court-Brown *et al.* 1964, de la Chapelle *et al.* 1964, Therkelsen 1964). Wachtel and Bard (1981) refer to more than 80 cases reported in the literature. Those who have been appropriately examined have been shown to be H-Y antigen positive. There is little clinical ambiguity in this group, the external genitalia being generally normal although under-development of the penis and hypospadias have been mentioned several times. Cryptorchidism has also been reported (de la Chapelle 1972).

Isolated deficiency of Müllerian inhibitor has also been reported on rare occasions. Such cases do not present clinically as examples of doubtful sex until some unrelated surgical procedure reveals the surprising presence of Müllerian structures in an otherwise normal or near-normal man. Brook (1981) has briefly described the disorder.

REFERENCES

ANDERSEN M., ANDREASEN E., JEST P. & LARSEN S. (1983) *Pediat. adol. Gynec*, **1**, 47.

AMRHEIM J. A., MEYER W.J. III, JONES H. W. JR. MIGEON, C. J. (1976) *Proc. Acad. Sci. U.S.A.*, **73**, 891.

BONO R. & FELLOUS M. (1981) In Josso, N. (ed) *The Intersex Child*. p. 29. Karger, Basel.

BROOK C. G. D. (1981) In Josso, N. (ed) *The Intersex Child, Pediatric Adolescent Endocrinology*, **8**, 100, Karger, Basel.

DE LA CHAPELLE A., HORTLING H., NIEMI M. & WENNSTROM J. (1964) *Acta med scand.*, **suppl 412**, 25.

DE LA CHAPELLE A. (1972) Amer. J. hum. Genet., **24**, 75.

COURT-BROWN W. M., HARNDEN D.G., JACOBS P.A., MACLEAN N. & MANTLE D.J. (1964). Medical Research Council, Special Report Series No. 305, HMSO, London.

DEWHURST C.J. (1963) *Gynaecological Disorders of Infants and Children*, p. 77. Cassell and Co. Ltd., London.

DEWHURST SIR J. (1980) *Practical Pediatric and Adolescent Gynecology*, p. 168. Marcel Dekker Inc., New York.

DEWHURST SIR J. (1981) In Hawkins D.F. (ed) *Gynaecological Therapeutics*, p. 26. Baillière Tindall, London.

DEWHURST C.J. & GORDON R.R. (1969) *The Intersexual Disorders*, pp. 82–83. Baillière Tindall & Cassell, London.

DEWHURST C.J., FERREIRA H.P. & GILLETT P.G. (1971) *J. Obstet. Gynaec. Brit. Cwlth.*, **78**, 1077.

DEWHURST SIR J., CHAPMAN M., MURAM D. & DONNISON B. (1983) *Pediat. adol. Gynec.*, **i**, 85.

FORREST M.G. (1981). In Josso N. (ed) *The Intersex Child*, p. 133. Karger, Basel.

GORDON R.R., O'GORMAN F.P.J., DEWHURST C.J. & BLANK C.E. (1960) *Lancet*, **ii**, 736.

GRANT D., MURAM D. & DEWHURST SIR J. (1983) *Pediat. adol. Gynec.*, **i**, 97.

HAYLES A.B. & NOLAN R.B. (1958) *Proc. Mayo Clin.*, **33**, 200.

IMPERATO-MCGINLEY J., PETERSON R.E., GAUTIER T. & STRULA E. (1979) *New Engl. J. Med.*, **300**, 1233.

JONES H.W. & SCOTT W.W. (1971) *Hermaphroditism, genital anomalies and related endocrine disorders*, 2e, Williams and Wilkins, Baltimore.

JONES H.W. JR. & VERKAUF B.S. (1971) *Amer. J. Obstet. Gynec.*, **109**, 292.

JONES H.W. (1981) In *The Intersex Child* (ed. Josso N.) p. 65–79, Karger, Basel.

JEFFCOATE S.L., BROOKS R.V. & PRUNTY F.T. (1968) *Brit. med. J.*, **1**, 208.

JOSSO N. (ed) (1981) In *The Intersex Child. Pediatric and Adolescent Gynecology*, **8**, 1, Karger, Basel.

JOSSO N., PICARD J.Y. & TRAN D. (1977) *Recent Progr. Hormone Res.*, **33**, 117.

JOSSO N., PICARD J.Y. & TRAN D. (1980) In Steinberger and Steinberger (eds) *Testicular Development, Structure and Function*, p. 21. Raven Press, New York.

KEENAN B.S., MEYER W.J. III, HADJIAN A.J., JONES H.W. JR. & MIGEON C.J. (1974) *J. clin. Endocr.*, **38**, 1143.

KLINGENSMITH G.J., JONES H.W. JR. & BLIZZARD R.M. (1977) *J. Pediat.*, **90**, 996.

LIAO S., LIANG T. & TYMOCZKO J.L. (1972) *J. steroid Biochem.*, **3**, 401.

MIGEON C.J., BROWN T.R & FICHMAN K.R. (1981) In Josso N. (ed) *The Intersex Child*, p. 171. Karger, Basel.

NEW M.I. & LEVINE L.S. (1981). In Josso N. (ed) *The Intersex Child*, p. 51. Karger, Basel.

OVERZIER C. (ed) (1963). In *Intersexuality*, p. 387. Academic Press, London.

PICARD J.Y. & JOSSO N. (1984) Purification of testicular anti-Müllerian hormone allowing direct visualisation of the pure glycoprotein and determination of yield and purification factor. *J. molec. cell. Endocr.*, **34**, 23.

PORTER R.J. & DE SWIET M. (1983) *Pediat. adol. Gynec.*, **1**, 39.

PERESS M.R., KREUTNER A.K., MATHUR R.S. & WILLIAMSON H.O. (1982) *Amer. J. Obstet. Gynec.*, **142**, 708.

SAVAGE M.E. (1983) Personal communication.

SAVAGE M.E., PREECE M.A., JEFFCOATE S.L., RANSLEY P.G., RUMSBY G., MANSFIELD M.D. & WILLIAMS D.I. (1980) *Clin. Endocr.*, **12**, 397.

SIMPSON J.L. (1976) *Disorders of Sexual Differentiation*, p. 199. Academic Press, New York.

SIMPSON J.L., SUMMITT R.L., MERKATZ I.R. & GERMAN J. (1976) *Gynec. Invest.* **7**, 37.

SOUTHREN A.L., SHARMA D.C., ROSS H., SHERMAN D.H. & GORDON G. (1964). *Bull. N.Y. Acad. Med.*, **40**, 86.

THERKELSEN A.J. (1964). *Cytogenics* **3**, 207.

TREMBLAY R. R., FOLEY, T. P. JR., CORVOL P., PARK I. J., KOW-ARSKI A., BLIZZARD R. M., JONES H. W. JR. & MIGEON C. J. (1972) *Acta endocr. Copenhagen*, **70**, 331.

VAN NIEKERK W. A. (1974) *True Hermaphroditism: Clinical Morphologic and Cytogenic Aspects.* Harper and Row, Hagerstown, Maryland.

VAN NIEKERK W. A. (1981) True Hermaphroditism. In: Josso N. (ed.) *The Intersex Child*, p. 80. Karger, Basel.

WACHTEL S. S. (1979) *Obstet. Gynec.*, **54**, 671.

WACHTEL S. S. (1981) *Contemp. Obstet. Gynaec.*, **17**, 137.

WACHTEL S. S. & BARD J. (1981) In Josso N. (ed.), *The Intersex Child*, p. 116. Karger, Basel.

WACHTEL S. S. & KOO G. C. (1982) In Austin, C. R. & Edwards R. G. (eds.), *Mechanisms of Sex Differentiation in Animals and Man.* Academic Press, London.

WILKINS L. (1960) *J. Amer. med. Ass.*, **172**, 1028.

WILKINS L., JONES H. W. JR., HOLMAN G. H. & STEMPFIELD R. S. (1958) *J. clin. Endocr.*, **18**, 559.

ZARATE A., CANALES E. S., SORIA J. & CARBALLO O. (1974) Studies on LH and FSH releasing mechanisms in testicular feminisation syndrome. *Amer. J. Obstet. Gynec.*, **119**, 971.

CHAPTER 4
GYNAECOLOGICAL DISORDERS IN CHILDHOOD AND ADOLESCENCE

SIR JOHN DEWHURST

Gynaecological disorders are not common during childhood, but to say this is not to say that they are unimportant. Because the conditions which affect the child are comparatively rare, a gynaecologist may never have encountered a particular disorder before he or she is called upon to treat it. Examination and investigation moreover are more difficult in children. The parents are frequently deeply alarmed by a disease of the sexual organs which they fear will have serious repercussions in later life. Finally, the gynaecological disorders which do affect the child tend not to be the same disorders in miniature as affect the adult, but are special ones seldom seen at other times. A knowledge of some of these conditions and an approach to management are, therefore, important for the specialist gynaecologist. Around puberty a variety of disorders may present which, whilst seldom serious, are particularly distressing to patients and parents alike so that correct and gentle management is of the essence. At a later stage of adolescence the disorders encountered become more and more those seen in the adult, but nonetheless the emotional immaturity of the patient is always an important factor which must be fully appreciated in management.

Endocrinology, anatomy and physiology

The endocrinology of the childhood years will first be discussed briefly so that some of the disorders encountered may be understood more fully. The subject has been reviewed by Pennington (1974) and Dewhurst (1984). During the first week or two of life, a child enjoys a certain amount of passive oestrogenic stimulation which has passed across the placenta from the mother. This time is characterized by transient, but distinct, clinical features. Some growth of the breasts occurs then in most babies born at term, and the enlargement can sometimes be quite considerable and may be accompanied by a discharge of fluid from the nipple. A clear or mucoid vaginal discharge is evident in most female babies also (Fig. 4.1);

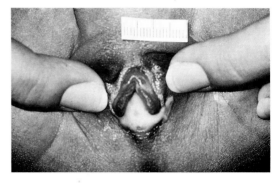

Fig. 4.1. A quantity of vaginal discharge seen at the vulva of a newborn child.

moistening of the genitalia is noticeable which will not be evident for most of the rest of childhood. This discharge may be blood-stained, a form of withdrawal bleeding occurring because oestrogen levels in the baby gradually fall and are no longer able to sustain the endometrium. The amount of bleeding is seldom sufficient to cause concern, but may alarm the attendants if they are unaware of its nature. Ten to fifteen per cent of babies may have a blood-stained loss of this kind during the first few weeks or so of life. After this neonatal period of passive hormone stimulation there follows a number of years when the genital organs receive little stimulus from the sex hormones. Oestrogens, gonadotrophins and adrenal hormones may be found in the child's urine during this time, but in small amounts only. The pelvic organs suffer from an oestrogen deficiency which is responsible for some of the clinical conditions shortly to be described. Gradual increase in hormone secretion during childhood leads ultimately to the commencement of secondary sexual development, growth spurt and menstruation.

A child's genital organs reflect this hormone background. The uterus at birth is somewhat larger than it will be for some years. Uterine hypertrophy has taken place under the influence of maternal oestrogens, but very soon the uterus becomes smaller and shows the characteristics of the unstimulated uterus of the child. It is straight in form, without fundal hypertrophy and the cervix is relatively longer than in the adult; the ratio of cervix to body of the uterus in the first week of life may be 1:1; later, when this hypertrophy has disappeared, the ratio of cervix to body becomes 2:1; at puberty, when the uterus has developed as a result of the child's own oestrogenic stimulation, this ratio will again be 1:1; as further oestrogenic stimulation affects the uterus in the few years after puberty the fundus increases still more in size and the cervix/body of uterus ratio becomes 1:2. The changes in the ovary during intrauterine life are dealt with in Chapter 1. At birth, and during the first few weeks of life, more cystic follicles may be seen than is the case later. Limited follicle development continues throughout childhood, however, reducing still further the number of ova present at puberty.

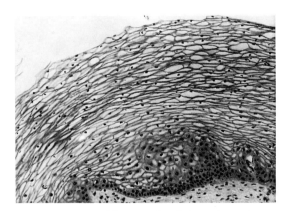

Fig. 4.2(a). Section of the vaginal epithelium of a newborn baby (compare b).

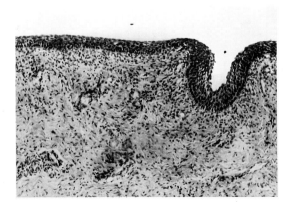

Fig. 4.2(b). Section of vaginal wall of an infant dying after the neonatal period.

The changes that occur in the vagina have the most significance, so far as clinical disorders are concerned. The vagina at birth is lined by squamous epithelium which is many layers thick (Fig. 4.2[a]), the cells being rich in glycogen. Within 2 or 3 weeks, however, most of the superficial layers become exfoliated and the vagina is lined by stratified squamous epithelium a few cells thick only (Fig. 4.2[b]). The reaction of the vagina, which in the newborn child is acid, with a pH of less than 5, soon rises (pH 7) due to oestrogen deprivation. It is lack of this protective acid secretion which makes the vagina of the child so susceptible to infections by low-grade organisms that cause the vaginitis shortly to be described.

CLINICAL DISORDERS

Most of the gynaecological disorders of childhood may conveniently be discussed in three groups, Group I, disorders of the newborn period. Group II, disorders of the years of oestrogen deficiency between this time and puberty. Group III, pubertal disorders.

Group I
Neonatal disorders

Some of the transient clinical manifestations of the early neonatal period have already been described. In addition to these, however, various congenital malformations involving the genital tract may call for investigation and treatment. These have been reviewed by Dewhurst (1968, 1980). The intersexual disorders form one important group which is discussed in Chapter 3. Another group of congenital malformations is that in which the bowel opens into the upper or lower genital tract. Surgical treatment of some kind is generally necessary at a comparatively early stage and a surgical opinion should always be requested quickly. Consultation between a gynaecologist and a paediatric surgeon will be an advantage in such cases. In one malformation, that of a congenital imperforate membrane occluding the lower vagina, mistakes in diagnosis may arise if the doctor is unaware of the disorder or does not elicit the physical signs correctly. This condition is called hydrocolpos.

HYDROCOLPOS

The lower part of the vagina is occluded by an imperforate membrane usually situated immediately

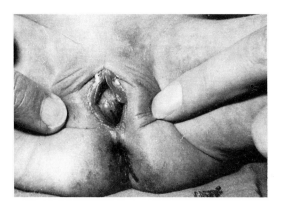

Fig. 4.3. Bulging vaginal membrane in a child with hydrocolpos.

above the hymen (Fig. 4.3). Above this obstruction the vagina becomes distended to a varying amount by watery, or usually milky, fluid, which probably collects there as a result of the passive hormone stimulation already mentioned, to which the fetus *in utero* in late pregnancy is always subjected. The quantity of fluid which collects may vary from a few millilitres to many ounces, so modifying the clinical features of the condition. If a large quantity of fluid is present there may be retention of urine, abdominal pain and a lower abdominal swelling which sometimes assumes large proportions. Inspection of the vulva usually reveals a bulging membrane, and the diagnosis can readily be made. Difficulties in diagnosis may occur if the abdominal swelling is thought so large that hydrocolpos is not seriously considered (Fig. 4.4), or if the obstruction at the lower end of the vagina is more extensive than a simple membrane. In the latter case no bulge will be evident, but rectal examination should disclose a swelling at

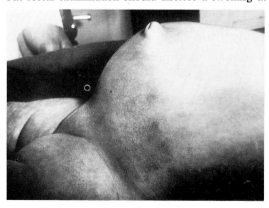

Fig. 4.4. Enormous abdominal swelling in an 8-day-old child with hydrocolpos.

a higher level. Correct diagnosis permits the condition to be treated properly by simple incision of the membrane and release of the retained fluid. It must be emphasized, however, that there are several cases on record in which laparotomy, or even hysterectomy, has been performed without the correct diagnosis being made; in one such case the child died (Joseph *et al.* 1966).

An interesting aspect of this condition is the origin of the fluid. It has already been suggested that the fluid accumulates as a result of passive hormone stimulation. Study of histological sections of the vagina and cervix from children stillborn or dying in the neonatal period indicates that considerable desquamation and outpouring of the fluid may be seen (Pryse-Davies & Dewhurst 1971). If there is vaginal obstruction but only a small volume of fluid collects, symptoms may not arise until the amount is increased by the menstrual flow about puberty; the case then presents as haemotocolpos (*see* p. 11). If a much greater quantity of fluid collects in the vagina at birth, clinical features will be evident very soon and treatment will be called for. Most cases of hydrocolpos become manifest during the first week or so of life, or not until they present as haemotocolpos at puberty. A further interesting aspect of the condition, as with genital tract malformations in general, is the association with anomalies of the renal tract so urinary tract investigation will usually be wise.

Group II
Disorders of the low oestrogen years

The commonest gynaecological disorder of childhood, vulvovaginitis, occurs during these years. There are several possible aetiological factors concerned but the most important are the ease with which infection may be introduced into the child's vagina and the lack of protective acid secretion during this time. Many cases of childhood vulvovaginitis are due to infection with organisms of low virulence rather than to specific pathogenic ones. Gonorrhoea was, at one time, a common cause of this condition, but is now fortunately seen much less often. The usual bacteriological finding in a case of vulvovaginitis is a mixed bacterial flora, no specific organism preponderating; specific organisms are sometimes found, but this is seldom the case by the time the patient is seen by the gynaecologist, although it may be more common at an earlier stage in the illness. Sore throats, scarlet fever and other exanthemata have sometimes been noted in cases of vulvovaginitis, and in some of these haemolytic streptococci have been isolated. *Tricho-monas vaginalis* infestations in children are not common, although they may be seen more frequently in the child near to puberty. Similarly, infestations with *Candida albicans* are rare and when they are found predisposing factors are present, such as diabetes or treatment with a broad-spectrum antibiotic. A foreign body in the vagina of a little girl will undoubtedly give rise to discharge and vulval soreness. In these circumstances the discharge is usually blood-stained and foul-smelling. In the presence of these features examination under anaesthesia is necessary to exclude a foreign body, but in the absence of them it is unlikely to be indicated; foreign bodies are comparatively rare findings in children presenting with vaginal discharge, and vulval soreness and examination under anaesthesia has been undertaken too often in the past. A further cause worthy of mention is a threadworm infestation which sometimes gives rise to this condition.

Although the presence of a vaginal discharge and vulval soreness is common to all cases, the degree of annoyance or discomfort caused is variable. If the vulva is sore, the child is likely to complain of pain on micturition. It is important to establish if a vaginal discharge is a prominent feature or whether the soreness is the main one, discharge being only slight or absent (see lichen sclerosus). Inquiry as to how often, and in what manner, the vulva is cleansed will also be helpful; imperfect vulval hygiene is sometimes evident and is certain to aggravate the irritation.

Examination can usually be performed without upset to the parent or child. Simple inspection of the vulva will show whether there is considerable soreness or not (Fig. 4.5). The vulva is usually reddened and may be swollen, and gentle separation of the labia will reveal a small amount of discharge present. If none can be seen, a rectal examination may permit a small amount of the discharge to be 'milked down' to the introitus. Bacteriological studies are not always helpful in cases of vulvovaginitis in childhood. If useful results are to be obtained, however, it is necessary to provide suitable samples for examination; a swab hastily taken from the region of the introitus will not give reliable information. With gentleness, however, a small amount of discharge may be taken with a platinum loop from within the lower vagina itself, and a smear made on a slide, which can then be examined. It should be possible to obtain a small amount of discharge also with a pipette, and some of this discharge may be added at once to a transport medium, cultured, and the remainder put directly on

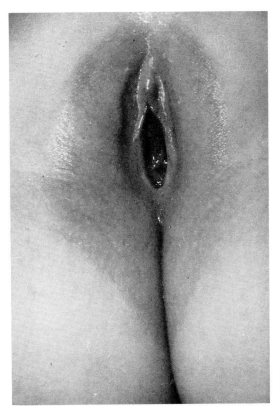

Fig. 4.5. Vulval soreness secondary to a vaginal discharge.

to a slide for examination for *Trichomonas vaginalis* or *Candida albicans*. Threadworm ova may also be recognized in this way.

Treatment with an appropriate antibiotic will be helpful if a specific organism has been isolated, but as has already been said, such cases are uncommon. For non-specific vaginitis the application of an oestrogen cream to the vulva each night for about 2 weeks is often most helpful, since it increases the natural vaginal protection and allows the infection to be overcome; because the soreness is relieved, the morale of the patient and parents is greatly improved. It is wise also to give some instruction to parents and child in elementary hygiene of the vulva. The vulva should be bathed daily at least, perhaps more often. Antiseptics should not be added to the water used, since they usually make matters worse. Bubble baths too are best avoided since it may be difficult to rinse these bubbles out of the skin folds of the vulva unless a shower is taken afterwards. After cleansing, drying with a soft towel should be undertaken. If soap or detergent used to wash the child's underclothes is not completely removed by rinsing, this may maintain a vulval irritation. Clothing the child unwisely in unsuitable thick undergarments in warm weather may increase vulval moisture and, again, aggravate the symptoms.

If the discharge is gonococcal, advice from a venereologist should be sought, since other members of the family may need examination and treatment as well. *Trichomonas* and *Candida* infestations in children respond well to oral therapy; Metronidozole may be used against *Trichomonas* in doses of 200 mg three times daily for 10 days; a smaller dose for a younger child—say 100 mg for a child under 12 years—may be necessary. For *Candida albicans*, nystatin may be given as an oral suspension or as a tablet; one tablet (500 000 units) three times daily for a week may be taken by an older child; for a younger one a suspension in doses of 2–4 ml (200 000–400 000 units) three times daily may be preferable. Threadworm infestations usually respond well to a piperazine preparation such as Antipar or Thiabendazole. Childhood vulvovaginitis and the clinician's approach to it in practical terms have been thoroughly considered by Huffman (1977) and Dewhurst (1980).

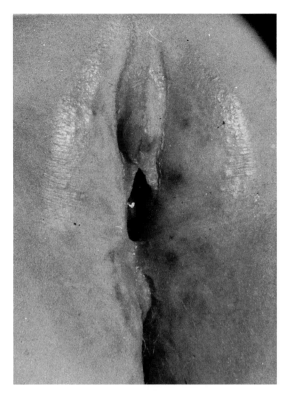

Fig. 4.6. Lichen sclerosus of the vulva in a four-year-old child showing typical features.

HYPOPLASTIC VULVAL DYSTROPHY (LICHEN SCLEROSUS)

Vulval soreness is not always secondary to a vaginal discharge. A generalized skin disease such as eczema or lichen sclerosus may be to blame. Lichen sclerosus can be present anywhere on the body surface, but has a special tendency to affect the genital area, where it is best termed hypoplastic dystrophy (see page 711). Discrete, white, flattened papules may be seen in the early stages; later, these coalesce to form larger plaques (Fig. 4.6). The histological appearances are hyperkeratosis of the epidermis itself, flattening of the rete pegs, and disappearance of elastic fibres from the superficial layers of the dermis where the collagen shows a hyaline change. In the deeper layers a zone of round-cell infiltration is seen. In many cases the degree of irritation is less severe than would be expected from the appearance of the skin, but itching can be marked, especially if any secondary infection is present. For treatment of acute cases, careful attention to vulval hygiene is desirable in all instances. Cleansing with 1% cetrimide may be helpful and is less painful than soap and water. Aureomycin cream may be useful if the lesion is infected. It is still uncertain to what extent disappearance of

the lesion may be expected around the time of puberty. Barclay *et al.* (1966) reviewing the literature at the time concluded that spontaneous resolution was common but not invariable. Kauffman and Gardner (1980) hold a similar view but believe that improvement cannot be linked to a specific event such as the menarche. Dewhurst (1983) reviews six patients who were followed into or through puberty.

LABIAL ADHESIONS

This is a simple condition not uncommon in young girls, and is sometimes seen even in older ones, in which the labia minora become adherent to each other, usually from behind, forwards, leaving a tiny opening through which urine is passed. The line of adhesion is quite thin and almost translucent in early cases (Fig. 4.7) but becomes firmer and thicker as time goes by. The importance of the condition is concerned with the fact that it may be mistaken for absence of the vagina; this may result in inaccurate and disturbing advice being given to the parents, who already may be greatly distressed by the condition.

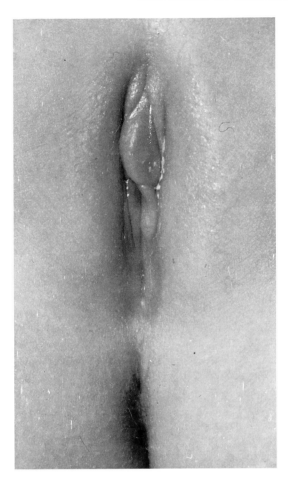

Fig. 4.7. Labial adhesions in a three-year-old child. Note the vertical translucent line in the centre where the labia minora are stuck to each other.

The aetiology is unknown but is thought to be concerned with the low oestrogen values of early childhood as the adhesions seldom persist after the pubertal period (Dewhurst 1984) and can be encouraged to separate spontaneously by local oestrogen therapy (see below); moreover, a similar condition sometimes occurs in very old ladies. Such labial adhesions are not congenital in origin but may develop quite soon after the neonatal period.

Simple treatment is all that is required. The adhesions can be separated with a fine probe or oestrogen cream may be applied by the child's mother to the line of the adhesions each night; the adhesions then usually separate spontaneously in some 10–14 days (Dewhurst 1980, Capraro & Greenberg 1972). Aribarg (1975) has shown that oestrogen cream has a specific effect which simple creams do not. It may be advisable to warn the mother that the adhesions may re-form, suggesting that she looks for early signs of it from time to time; if they seem to be re-forming they can easily be drawn apart and simple cream applied. If they repeatedly re-form it is best not to distress the child by repeated treatment but to await spontaneous separation at puberty.

Group III
Puberty and its disorders

PHYSIOLOGICAL CONSIDERATIONS

A general account only of the physiology of puberty and menstruation will be given here, the endocrine control of menstruation under normal and abnormal conditions being examined in greater detail in Chapter 5 (p. 55).

Hormonal changes
The hormone control of menstruation begins in the hypothalamus with the production of releasing hormones which pass down the pituitary portal system to the anterior pituitary where FSH is produced. This stimulates the development of many Graafian follicles in the ovary, one of which ovulates as a result of a pronounced LH surge at the appropriate stage of follicle development. During any single cycle one Graafian follicle alone achieves full development and ovulates; rarely, two and, more rarely still, more than two follicles ovulate. For the production of the meagre return of one ovum per month many follicles commence development and undergo follicle atresia once an ovum is shed by one of them. This abortive development occurs to a considerable extent even during childhood, evidence of it being visible in the ovaries at any age before the menarche. Such development can be explained by the recognition of gonadotrophic excretion throughout childhood indicating gonadotrophin production even during these early days (Grumbach et al. 1974, Sizonenko & Paunier 1975, Kantero et al. 1975). Gradually we are learning more of the important subject of gonadotrophin production during childhood and of the relationship of FSH to LH during this period. Detailed considerations by Faiman and Winter (1974). Grumbach et al. (1974), Hafez and Peluso (1976) and Dewhurst (1984) may be consulted by the reader wishing to look further into this interesting problem. The degree of ovarian activity in childhood, however, probably accounts for the gradual increase in oestrogen pro-

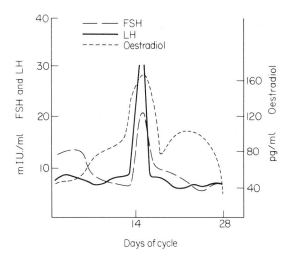

Fig. 4.8. FSH, LH and oestradiol levels in blood during a normal menstrual cycle. The height of the LH peak is open to much variation.

duction and excretion as the child grows older, resulting first in secondary sexual development and later in a uterine response and menstruation.

The developing Graafian follicle produces oestrogens; after ovulation the corpus luteum produces oestrogens and progesterone. These hormones have an important interrelationship with hypothalamic releasing hormones, and so indirectly with FSH and LH, which may be summarized as follows. At the time of menstruation in response to falling levels of oestrogen and progesterone there is further production of FSH. This stimulates early follicle maturation. As oestrogen levels rise, however, further FSH production is prevented by the inhibitory feed-back mechanism and FSH levels fall. Still greater oestrogen production acts directly to stimulate a surge of LH and, to a lesser extent, FSH and ovulation occurs. This surge of LH and FSH is quickly shut down as a result of the sharp fall in oestrogen production which accompanies ovulation. The steroidal output from the corpus luteum rises again quickly and is maintained until towards the end of the cycle when a fall causes menstruation and the cycle goes round again (Fig. 4.8).

Ovarian changes
As a result of stimulation by the pituitary gonadotrophins many follicles in the ovary commence maturation each month. In the primary follicle the ovum is surrounded by a single layer of granulosa cells. These cells multiply quickly, many layers being pro-

duced. During multiplication the cells secrete a fluid, liquor folliculi, which gradually distends the developing follicle to form a central, fluid-filled cavity. The layers of granulosa cells surrounding the cavity are then called the membrana granulosa. There is a localized proliferation of granulosa cells at one point, the discus proligerus, or cumulus oophorus, which contains the ovum within its depths. The stromal cells outside the granulosa layer become formed in a layer of spindle cells, the theca interna, whilst outside this, in turn, is a zone of flattened cells, the theca externa (Fig. 4.9).

Gradual increase in the size of the Graafian follicle occurs. At the same time, the follicle makes its way towards the periphery of the ovary, the discus proligerus always facing the surface; this progress is evidently facilitated by the formation of a cone-shaped development of theca interna cells which form at the same point.

Ovulation occurs at full follicle maturation, the ovum being discharged into, or very close to, the ostium of the Fallopian tube, which by normal tubal motility has been approximated to the ovary at the appropriate time. At ovulation the ovum has

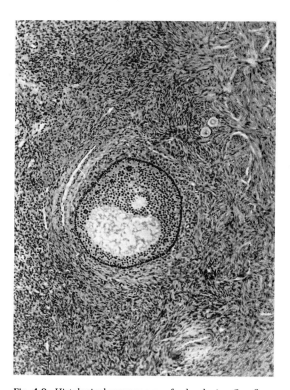

Fig. 4.9. Histological appearances of a developing Graafian follicle.

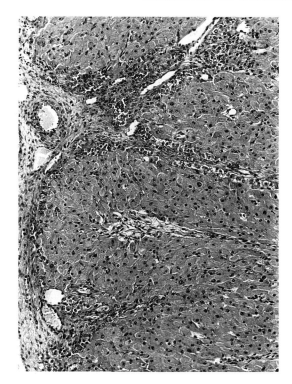

Fig. 4.10. Histological appearances of a well-formed corpus luteum.

undergone the first stage of meiotic division (maturation division) reducing the number of chromosomes from 46 to 23 and casting off the first polar body. The second maturation division occurs after fertilization. At the time the ovum is surrounded by a pale-staining zone, the zone pellucida, and outside this area is a ring of granulosa cells, the corona radiata.

The ruptured follicle collapses over a small quantity of blood and fluid left within and is transformed into the corpus luteum. The granulosa cells and the theca interna cells increase in size and take on a swollen appearance as a result of the process of luteinization; during this process, fluid, rich in carotene, is deposited within the cell cytoplasm, giving the corpus luteum an increasingly yellow colour as development proceeds. The cells of the corpus luteum become thrown into folds as they collapse into the empty cavity, giving it a characteristic appearance histologically (Fig. 4.10).

Activity of the corpus luteum continues for some 10 days, when degenerative changes commence if there has not been fertilization of the ovum. This coincides with a fall in oestrogen and progesterone

production, until the endometrium cannot be maintained and menstruation occurs.

It is probable that many early menstrual cycles are anovulatory, the developing follicles producing oestrogens which bring about the proliferation changes in the endometrium shortly to be described; when the follicle finally degenerates, oestrogen levels fall and anovular withdrawal haemorrhage results; early cycles are, therefore, frequently irregular both in interval and duration of flow (see below). At a still earlier stage in the pubertal years the slow rise in the secretion of oestrogen by increasing follicular activity produces the secondary sexual development shortly to be described.

Uterine changes

The changes occurring in the uterus as a result of the ovarian activity described above are most important ones. Immediately following menstruation the endometrium is thin; glands are narrow and straight and are lined by cuboidal epithelium; the stroma is compact. The action of oestrogen on this thin uterine lining is to produce growth of all the elements present. Glands become longer but remain straight; the epithelial lining becomes tall and columnar, the nuclei occupying a basal position (Fig. 4.11). The stromal cells increase in number and become more loosely packed together, the whole stroma being vascular and abundant. This is the stage of proliferation.

Following ovulation and the addition of progesterone activity to the oestrogen effect described, the secretory phase of development occurs. The glands become more tortuous and corkscrew-like. The epithelial lining demonstrates a series of changes during which the nuclei become displaced from their basal position towards the centre of the cell by the formation of subnuclear vacuoles (Fig. 4.12). These are usually readily recognizable as clear areas deep to the nucleus. The gland lumina are seen to contain more secretion as the days go by, until maximum secretion is achieved about day 25 of a 28-day cycle; this secretion is rich in glycogen (Fig. 4.13). Stromal cells become further increased in size and are loosely arranged, giving the stroma an oedematous appearance which may begin to resemble the decidua of early pregnancy. The arterioles of the endometrium, which are spiralling outwards towards the cavity from the arteries in the basal area, become more and more coiled.

With regression in the corpus luteum the levels of oestrogen and progesterone in the blood fall, and the maintenance of the endometrium is withdrawn.

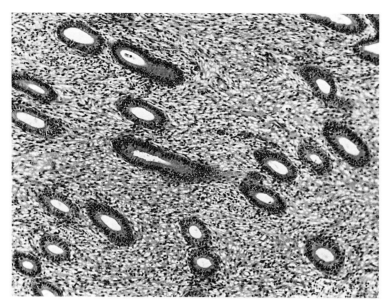

Fig. 4.11. Endometrium in
the proliferative phase.

Shrinkage occurs and there is constriction of the
spiral arteries, stasis, necrosis and bleeding. The
endometrium, with the exception of the deeper basal
zone which retains an effective blood supply, breaks
down and is cast off as menstrual flow.

The changes in cervical mucus during the ovarian
cycle are equally important to the occurrence of a
pregnancy. The cervical mucus in the days immediately following menstruation is thick, opaque and
of small amount only. Increased secretion of mucus

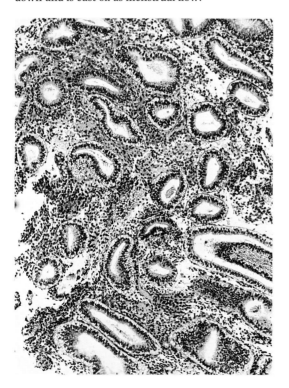

Fig. 4.12. Endometrium in the early secretory phase.

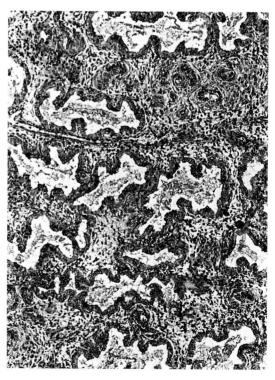

Fig. 4.13. Endometrium in the late secretory phase.

occurs during the proliferative phase, the peak corresponding with that of oestrogen production shortly before ovulation. At this point the cervical mucus is not only much greater in amount but is thin and watery and allows the passage of spermatozoa with great facility. A property of the mucus demonstrable with increasing oestrogen secretion and maximal about the time of ovulation is that of spinnbarkeit; this refers to the property of being able to be drawn out in long threads. A further property exhibited to its greatest extent at the time of ovulation is arborization; that is, fern-like formation visible when a drop of mucus is placed on a glass-slide, allowed to dry and examined under a microscope.

During the secretory phase of the cycle there is a return to the viscid, thicker mucus of the time immediately following the end of menstruation.

Hormone cytology of the vagina

The vaginal epithelium is the most accessible end-organ reflecting the hormonal turmoil of the menstrual cycle. Provided that they are interpreted with care by an experienced cytologist, smears from the vaginal fornix will help to form a general impression of hormonal activity. Clear changes in cytology are to be seen throughout the normal menstrual cycle, so that for maximum information serial smears are needed.

The vaginal epithelium during reproductive life is made up of four discernible types of cell (Fig. 4.14). Basal cells are firmly attached to the basement membrane and do not exfoliate, but parabasal cells, intermediate cells and superficial cells may be seen in different circumstances. When oestrogen levels are low there will be preponderance of parabasal cells staining blue with Papanicolau's stain. With greater oestrogen activity there is increase in the number of superficial cells, which stain pink at high oestrogen levels. The nucleus of these cells is pyknotic. Progesterone dominance gives a smear containing a large percentage of intermediate cells which may stain either pink or blue with Papanicolau's stain.

In essence, therefore, throughout one menstrual cycle postmenstrual smears show a relatively high proportion to intermediate cells; with progressive follicular maturation there is a rapid increase in cornified superficial cells. At the time of ovulation the smear shows few leucocytes, whilst the squames are large, separate and have small pyknotic nuclei. After ovulation the leucocyte population increases rapidly, the squames become folded and grouped in clumps, while the number of intermediate cells increases.

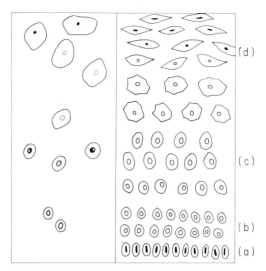

(a) Basal layer (not seen in smears).
(b) Parabasal layer.
(c) Intermediate squames.
(d) Superficial squames.

Fig. 4.14. Diagram of vaginal epithelial cell types. On the right the cells are represented in their normal orientation; on the left they are seen in vaginal smears.

Later in the luteal phase there is progressive cytolysis.

To attempt more objective assessment the maturation index, eosinophilic index and cornification index have been evolved by various workers. The maturation index relates to the percentage of parabasal, intermediate and superficial cells present, the eosinophilic index to the percentage of pink-staining cells, and the cornification index to the percentage of squamous cells with pyknotic nuclei, omitting from the count, in this instance, parabasal cells.

CLINICAL FEATURES

The first sign of pubertal development is usually breast growth (Tanner 1962). Growth in height occurs about the same time. Breast growth is usually seen first between the ages of 8 and 13 years, with an average around 11 years. Pubic hair development usually follows next, and later the appearance of axillary hair; this in turn is followed by the first menstrual period. Variations in this pattern are frequent, however, and anxiety on this account is needless (Marshall & Tanner 1969, Dewhurst 1984b). The most common variation is the appearance of menstruation before axillary hair, perhaps even before pubic hair or pubic hair growth may occur before

breast growth. It is worthy of mention that breast
growth is not uncommonly unequal during the early
stages, the breasts becoming equal in size as growth
proceeds Dewhurst (1984).

The age of the menarche has been investigated in
great detail by workers in many countries. The onset
of menstruation is influenced by several factors especially nutrition and environment. Largely as a result
of the improvement in the standard of living the age
of menarche has been declining throughout the 20th
century, girls now reaching the menarche approximately one year sooner than did their mothers. This
trend, however, appears to have stopped in parts of
Europe (Bruntland & Walloe 1973, Tanner 1973),
although it is still continuing in countries where economic improvements are still taking place. The whole
subject of growth and secondary sexual development
at puberty has been well reviewed by Marshall
(1981) who indicates that in developed European
countries and in the USA 95% of girls were menstruating for the first time between the ages of 11–
15 years, most of the remainder doing so between
10–11 and 15–16. Dewhurst (1984) has stressed
the variations that occur during puberty pointing out
that of two girls of the same age one may be menstruating and one may not have begun her secondary
sexual development, yet both could be normal.

PRECOCIOUS SEXUAL DEVELOPMENT

Sexual development must be considered precocious if
there is breast and pubic hair growth before the age
of 8 years or menstrual periods before the age of 10
years (Fig. 4.15).

The most common cause of this finding is the
premature release of the gonadotrophins from the
anterior pituitary without any organic lesion being
present—the so-called constitutional precocious
puberty (*see* Dewhurst 1984 for review). Here, the
signs of puberty usually appear in their correct order
and the bone-age and the child's height are several
years in advance of the chronological age. Gonadotrophins are detectable in blood and urine. There
should, of course, be no abdominal or pelvic swelling
palpable, although in some cases retention cysts of
follicular type may form in the ovaries and may reach
a considerable size. These, however, are the result of
the premature ovarian stimulation and are not the
cause of the abnormality. The next most common
cause of precocious sexual development is, again, the
premature release of gonadotrophin by the pituitary,
this time stimulated by the presence of some intra-

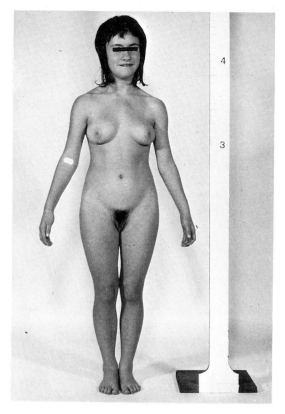

Fig. 4.15. A child aged 7 years with constitutional
precocious puberty. (By permission of Marcel Dekker and
Co.)

cranial lesion, such as meningitis, encephalitis, a
cerebral tumour, a third ventricle hamartoma or Albright's syndrome. In this last condition cystic
changes in bone (polyostotic fibrous dysplasia) are
combined with precocious puberty and café au lait
spots on the child's skin (Fig. 4.16). This syndrome
must always be remembered, as vaginal bleeding
may be the first sign of precocious puberty. X-ray of
the long bones and skull for the characteristic cystic
bony changes is important.

Less common than any of these lesions is premature sexual development due to a feminizing tumour
of the ovary (*see* Chapter 48). Here, the various landmarks of puberty may not appear in their usual order
and vaginal bleeding may be out of all proportion to
the degree of breast development. FSH and LH will be
detectable in blood or urine and their presence does
not indicate a hypothalamic/pituitary cause for the
condition. The presence of a pelvic tumour (Fig. 4.17)
will be the most significant feature pointing to this
diagnosis and will call for laparotomy; what has been

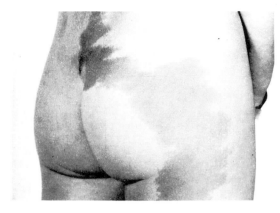

Fig. 4.16. Precocious puberty due to Albright's syndrome.

said already, however, about the possibility of a large follicular cyst in a case of constitutional precocious puberty should be remembered, and if such a lesion be found at operation, ovarian tissue must be conserved. A feminizing tumour if present is best treated by oophorectomy, as most are benign. Constitutional precocious puberty formerly treated with medroxyprogesterone acetate 100–200 mg intramuscularly every two to four weeks is now believed to respond better to treatment with cyproterone acetate in doses of 70–150 mg/m² daily by mouth. This suppresses menstruation, and breast growth is likely to regress. It is still uncertain whether there is any deceleration of bone growth.

Three other examples of premature sexual development must be mentioned. Premature thelarche (Fig.

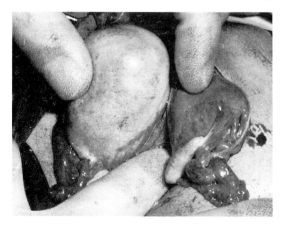

Fig. 4.17. Granulosa cell tumour of the left ovary causing precocious secondary sexual development and menstruation. Note that the uterus to the right of the picture is somewhat enlarged under the influence of oestrogen but the right ovary is normal.

4.18) is a condition in which breast growth is the only sign of precocious development, and premature pubarche a condition in which pubic hair growth is the only sign of sexual development. The conditions may represent unusual sensitivity of end-organs to the usual low level of hormones in the blood during childhood. In neither case is treatment required beyond simple explanation once careful examination and appropriate investigation have been carried out. The breast enlargement may be unilateral and is sometimes transient, as it was in the case shown in Fig. 4.18. The breasts began to decrease in size again after 6 months.

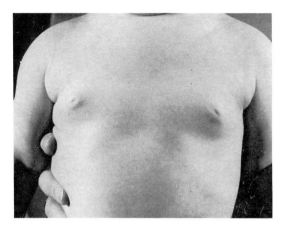

Fig. 4.18. Premature thelarche.

A third variety of an isolated feature of sexual precocity is premature menarche in which a prepubertal child without any evidence of secondary sexual development 'menstruates' at fairly regular intervals (Heller *et al.* 1979). Usually the precocity ceases after a time and the child passes through normal puberty at the normal time (Muram *et al.* 1983).

EXCESSIVE MENSTRUAL BLEEDING

In considering this symptom it must again be emphasized that early menstrual cycles seldom occur so regularly as in later life. The interval between periods, their duration and the amount of loss are often variable for some months or longer in most girls. Such variation is within physiological limits, and investigation and treatment are unnecessary. Occasionally, however, periods occur more frequently or are more heavy, the parents are alarmed and take their daughter to see a doctor.

The mother and child should then be questioned closely to determine the amount of loss, in order to decide if there is real cause for anxiety or not. A general examination is necessary to exclude any important associated abnormality but a pelvic examination can seldom be carried out in full. Inspection of the vulva, and bimanual rectal examination are nearly always possible and are often helpful in excluding a gross lesion. Examination of the blood should be undertaken in case any significant anaemia is present. Dickens (1974) stresses the need to keep in mind possible complications of early pregnancy even in young girls whose virtue may not seem to be in question. She mentions also the complications of irregular oral contraceptive pill taking as another possible cause.

In the treatment of mild cases it may be sufficient to give firm reassurance to mother and child that such episodes are not uncommon and are usually transient. The patient may be given a small calendar on which to keep a record of the days of future bleeding which may help to indicate that little is, in fact, wrong. Iron and dietary advice may be useful. In more severe cases admission to hospital may be necessary. This allows the severity of the condition to be assessed more accurately, and permits more intensive treatment of anaemia, should this be necessary. Heavy bleeding can generally be controlled by a progestogen such as norethisterone (Primolut N) 5 mg three times a day which should stop the bleeding within a few days. The drug should be continued for a further 3 weeks and then stopped to permit withdrawal haemorrhage to occur. Two or three courses are advisable, after which the treatment may be stopped to see if regularity will be resumed. Curettage may be required in protracted cases as may more complete blood studies in view of the possible association of a blood-coagulation defect (Claessens & Cowell 1981). Only in very exceptional cases indeed is more surgery to be contemplated. Excessive puberty bleeding is usually a self-limiting disease; any delaying tactics are therefore likely to be helpful by allowing spontaneous recovery to take place (Dewhurst 1984). Southam and Richert (1966) stressed the possibly more serious nature of adolescent menorrhagia in those few cases which do not respond quickly to treatment. They noted frequent recurrences, especially in patients whose excessive bleeding did not settle down within four years. The most serious consequence was hysterectomy which was required in four patients aged 20–23 for continuous bleeding and in another four for endometrial carcinoma at the ages of 23, 29, 30 and 33 years. Fraser and Baird (1972) also emphasized the need for more

careful and longer follow-up in the more protracted cases of adolescent excessive bleeding.

DYSMENORRHOEA

Not only are early menstrual cycles irregular, but they are frequently anovular. Anovular menstruation seldom causes pain, so that a girl's first few periods will probably be pain-free. Dysmenorrhoea becomes more common later when regular ovulation is established. Dysmenorrhoea during the first few cycles may suggest it to be due more to the incorrect attitude of the girl and her parents towards menstruation than to painful contraction of the uterine muscle. In such cases it may be manifest when interviewing the parents that the girl has been influenced by hearing graphic accounts of her mother's suffering, which not surprisingly may affect her own. It may not be easy to undo the harm done in this kind of case, but a simple explanation of the physiology of menstruation given sympathetically should help. Exercise should be encouraged and the patient should join in games at school whenever she can. Codeine or aspirin may be helpful in providing a more traditional remedy as well. Simple measures of this kind should be used for a while. In more severe cases success has been reported with the prostaglandin synthetase inhibitors (Jacubowicz & Wood 1978) whilst in older girls, the use of the 'Pill' to inhibit ovulation and to allow painless menstruation has obvious advantages. Simple dilatation of the cervix under general anaesthesia may be effective, at least for a time, if a progestogen is not favoured.

Other childhood disorders

GENITAL TRACT TUMOURS

Embryonal Rhabdomyosarcoma (sarcoma botryoides)
Tumours during childhood are, fortunately, uncommon. The most serious is the embryonal rhabdomyosarcoma (botryoid sarcoma), which is often grape-like (as its name suggests) but at other times may look like a simple polyp (Fig. 4.19). Histological features are varied; the stroma is myxomatous and contains fusiform cells singly or in groups; pleomorphism is usually marked; two distinguishing features are the presence of rhabdomyoblasts (large cells with vacuolated eosinophilic cytoplasm) and muscle fibres showing cross-striations.

In the early stages the tumour spreads extensively in the subepithelial tissues of the vagina or cervix

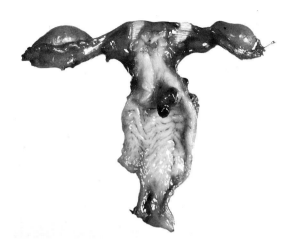

Fig. 4.19. Botryoid sarcoma of the cervix presenting as a cervical polyp in a 5-month-old child. Treatment was by extended hysterectomy and total vaginectomy.

whilst retaining a covering of epithelium, giving it a polyp-like appearance. Progress of the disease may be rapid and the outcome fatal unless early and vigorous treatment is undertaken, but in more and more cases nowadays good results are being obtained. Delay in treatment may arise because of the similarity of early lesions to simple polypi, and only when they have been removed and have recurred and been removed again is their nature apparent. It must be emphasized that, rare though botryoid sarcoma is, simple polypi in childhood are rarer still.

The outlook for these tumours is now more favourable than formerly since they have been shown to be sensitive to chemotherapy. Triple chemotherapy with vincristine actinomycin D and cyclophosphamide has been used in several of the author's own patients and combined with radiotherapy for a pre-operative period of 6 months. Extended hysterectomy and vaginectomy was then performed and, if at all possible, exenteration avoided. A further year of chemotherapy was then undertaken. More recently the radiotherapy has been omitted because if its affect upon the growing pelvic bones and sometimes the surgery too has been unncessary because of the good response to chemotherapy. Much more favourable results are being obtained by this kind of approach (Dewhurst 1983).

Carcinoma of the vagina and cervix

This is very rare indeed during childhood and nearly all examples reported have been adenocarcinomata. The presenting feature has always been vaginal

bleeding, subsequent investigation leading to the discovery of a tumour. During the last 15 years an increase in clear cell adenocarcinoma of the vagina and cervix has been identified in girls whose mothers were treated by diethylstilboestrol (DES) during pregnancy. Many children and adolescents so exposed will be affected by benign vaginal adenosis (Chapter 49, p. 764) and their cervices will show extensions of columnar epithelium onto the ectocervix and even onto the fornices; protruberant pseudo polyp formations may be seen, or the vaginal vault may be deformed by ridges almost obscuring the cervix from view. The alarming nature of the changes which may be evident to some degree in 90% or more of exposed girls is now considered to be a less serious matter than was at one time supposed. The benign lesions of adenosis show evidence of healing by squamous metaplasia as the patient gets older, whilst the chances of a clear cell adenocarcinoma making its appearance are considered to be of the order of 0.4–1.4 per 1000. Herbst recommends vaginoscopy to determine the extent of adenosis and to identify suspicious lesions once the patient has begun to menstruate or has reached the age of 14 years. Anaesthesia will be required in the younger patients but not necessarily later. A careful chart of the extent of vaginal lesions should be constructed, colposcopy should be employed and a cervical smear taken: at subsequent examinations at yearly intervals (or less in certain more affected patients) the investigation may be repeated and the degree to which healing has occurred may be noted. For further details Hurst & Bern (1981) may be consulted.

Ovarian cysts and tumours

These have been reported not infrequently during childhood. Certain tumours tend to be seen more often than in later life. The commonest ovarian tumour of the child and adolescent is the teratoma, which is usually found in the form of the well-known dermoid cyst. Simple cysts of follicular type may be found especially in the new-born and very young baby; dysgerminomata appear to be relatively more common than in the adult. In a review of 81 cases from Finland and Sweden (Lindfors 1971) 17 tumours were benign teratoma and 13 malignant teratoma; there were 11 dysgerminomas, also noted by others as more common in childhood, and 8 granulosa cell tumours. Breen and Maxson (1977) reported that one-third of ovarian masses in children were cysts of existing follicles and two-thirds were new growths: of the new growths 65–70%, were benign and 30–35% malignant.

Clinically, the presenting feature is more often torsion than is the case in older patients; sometimes, operation for undiagnosed abdominal pain has led to the tumour's discovery. In Lindfors' series pain was the main presenting symptom in more than half the cases and was far more common than the next most frequent feature of abdominal distension (18%); torsion was present in 23% of cases. This author stresses the value of plain X-rays in detecting teratomatous calcification, so helping to establish the correct diagnosis. When there is a palpable swelling present other conditions must be considered in the differential diagnosis such as Wilm's tumour, mesenteric cysts, enlarged spleen, distended bladder and hydrocolpos. Operation is required and the tumour must be dealt with in the most appropriate manner. Cysts which are clearly benign must be removed by ovarian cystectomy, and not by oophorectomy. It should be recalled that the common cyst, the dermoid, is often bilateral, and ovarian conservation is most important.

Solid ovarian tumours may be benign (fibroma) or malignant (teratoma, carcinoma or dysgerminoma). A solid, well-defined tumour likely to be benign should be dealt with by oophorectomy in the first instance; subsequent treatment may be considered in the light of the report on a frozen section or later histology. The dysgerminomata are not of a high degree of malignancy and are relatively radiosensitive, two characteristics which suggest that unilateral removal may be sufficient here too. The child may then be left with a chance of fertility; if a recurrence were detected later, radiotherapy could be employed.

REFERENCES

ARIBARG A. (1975) *Brit. J. Obstet. Gynaec.*, **82**, 424.

BARCLAY D.L., MACEY H.B. & REED R.J. (1966) *Obstet. Gynec., N.Y.*, **27**, 637.

BREEN J.L. & MAXSON W.S. (1977) *Clin. Obstet. Gynaec.*, **20**, 607.

BRUNTLAND G.H. & WALLOE L. (1973) *Nature*, **241**, 478.

CAPRARO V.J. & GREENBERG H. (1972) *Obstet. Gynec., N.Y.*, **39**, 65.

CLAESSENS E.A. & COWELL C.A. (1981) *The Pediatric Clinics of North America*, **28**, 369.

DALLEY V.M., DEWHURST C.J. & FLOOD C.M. (1971) *J. Obstet. Gynaec. Brit. Cwlth*, **78**, 1133.

DEWHURST C.J. (1969) *J. Obstet. Gynaec. Brit. Cwlth.*, **76**, 831.

DEWHURST SIR JOHN (1980) *Practical Pediatric and Adolescent Gynecology*. Marcel Dekker Inc., New York.

DEWHURST SIR JOHN (1983) *Ped. Adol. Gynec.*, **2**, 149.

DEWHURST SIR JOHN (1984) *Female Puberty and Its Abnormalities*, Chapter 5.

DICKENS A. (1974) In *Clinics in Obstetrics and Gynaeclogy* (Dewhurst C.J. ed.), Vol. 1, no. 3, p. 649.

FAIMAN C. & WINTER J.S.D. (1974) In *The Control of the Onset of Puberty* (Grumbach M.M., Grave G.D. & Mayer F.E. eds.), p. 32. John Wiley & Sons, New York.

FRASER I.S. & BAIRD D.T. (1972) *J. Obstet. Gynaec. Brit. Cwlth.*, **79**, 1009.

GRUMBACH M.M., GRAVE G.D. & MAYER F.E. (eds) (1974) *The Control of the Onset of Puberty*. John Wiley & Sons, New York.

HAFEZ E.S.E. & PELUSO J.J. (1976) In *Sexual Maturity: physiological and clinical parameters*. Ann Arbor Science Publishers Inc., Michigan.

HARRIS G.W. & JACOBSOHN D. (1952) *Proc. roy. Soc. B.*, **139**, 263.

HELLER M.E., DEWHURST SIR JOHN & GRANT D.B. (1979) *Arch. Dis. Childh.*, **54**, 472.

HERBST A.L. & BERN H.A. (eds) (1981) *Pregnancy*, Thieme-Stratton Inc., New York.

HUFFMAN J.W. (1977) *Clin. Obstet. Gynaec.*, **20** (No. 3), 581.

JACUBOWICZ D.L. & WOOD C. (1978) *Aust. N.Z. J. Obstet. Gynaec.*, **18**, 135.

JOSEPH M.K., NAYAR B.G. & KANNANKUTTY M. (1966) *Brit. med. J.*, **i**, 89.

KANTERO R.L., WIDE L. & WIDHOLM O. (1975) *Acta Endocr.*, **78**, 11.

KAUFMAN R.H. & GARDNER H.L. (1980) *Benign Diseases of the Vulva and Vagina*, pp. 178–191. G.K. Hall, Boston.

LEGIER J.F. (1961) *J. Urol.*, **86**, 583.

LINDFORS O. (1971) *Ann. Chir. Gynaec. Fenn.*, **60**, suppl. 177.

MARSHALL W.A. & TANNER J.M. (1969) *Arch. Dis. Childh.*, **44**, 291.

MURAM D., DEWHURST SIR JOHN & GRANT D.B. (1983) *Arch. Dis. Childh.*, **58**, 142.

PENNINGTON G.W. (1974) In *Clinics in Obstetrics and Gynaecology* (Dewhurst C.J. ed.), Vol. 1, no. 3, p. 509.

PRYSE-DAVIES J. & DEWHURST C.J. (1971) *J. Path.*, **103**, 5.

SIZONENKO P.C. & PAUNIER L. (1975) *J. clin. Endocr. Metab.*, **41**, 894.

SOUTHAN A.L. & RICHERT R.M. (1966) *Amer. J. Obstet. Gynec.*, **94**, 637.

TANNER J.M. (1962) *Growth at Adolescence*. Blackwell Scientific Publications, Oxford.

TANNER J.M. (1973) *Nature*, **243**, 95.

CHAPTER 5
CONTROL OF OVARIAN FUNCTION

RODNEY P. SHEARMAN

While there continues to be much perturbation in physiological literature about ovarian functions since the last edition, little of this has immediate clinical significance.

Puberty and the pineal gland

During the last 100 years there has been a progressive reduction in the age of menarche (Tanner 1968). For example, in Norway the age of the menarche in the 1850s was 17 years, dropping to 13.5 years in the mid 1950s. There are now data indicating that this progressive reduction can no longer be demonstrated; the age of menarche appears to have stabilized (Tanner 1973).

There is very suggestive evidence in many experimental animals and inferential evidence in the human that coordination of puberty may be under the control of the pineal gland (Wurtman & Anton-Tay 1969). Described by Wurtman as a 'neuro endocrine transducer', the input to the pineal is neural and its output hormonal. Major afferent pathways are sight and possibly smell. Its effects are transmitted to the hypothalamus by a group of specific indoles-melatonin, 5-hydroxytryptophol, serotonin and 5-methoxy-tryptophol. The first two compounds appear to have a specific inhibiting effect on luteinising hormone (LH) while the latter inhibit follicle stimulating hormone (FSH) (Editorial Comment 1974).

The physiological interactions between melatonin, LH concentrations and puberty have been nicely delineated by Waldhauser et al. (1984). They confirm the substantial diurnal variation in melatonin levels and showed that 'night time melatonin levels declined progressively from the early years of life throughout pre-puberty and puberty, thereafter remaining relatively constant during adolescence and young adulthood. Nocturnal LH concentrations are inversely related to serum melatonin, being low in pre-puberty and rising continuously during sexual maturation until adult levels are attained'.

Gonadotrophin releasing factor

The hypothalamus produces a series of specific releasing and inhibiting factors effecting production of specific pituitary hormones. A single releasing factor is responsible for synthesis and release of LH and FSH. Gonadotrophin releasing factor (GnRF) was characterized in 1971 (Schally et al. 1971) and is a deca-peptide. Judd (1984) discusses in detail the relationships between the hypothalamus and the pituitary.

GnRF has been identified in the median eminence and the arcuate nucleus. Its release is probably mediated by dopamine responding to afferent neural and hormonal pathways.

The major hormonal controls in the human female are oestradiol and progesterone. These hormones exercise both negative and positive feedback. As an example of the latter, increased levels of circulating GnRF are found at mid-cycle in normally cycling women.

GnRF will cause both synthesis and release of FSH and LH, assuming there are any stores of the two gonadotrophins within the pituitary. For example, if an acute bolus of GnRF is given to a patient with hypogonadotrophic hypogonadism (see Chapter 6) there is no response of FSH and LH. However, if a pulsed infusion is given, following a lag during which synthesis occurs, LH and FSH release will occur.

Prolactin inhibitory factor (PIF)

Although prolactin release can be induced by a bolus of thyrotrophic releasing factor (TRF) there is no very good evidence that this is an important mechanism of normal physiological control. Unlike the other pituitary trophic hormones prolactin is under chronic inhibition by PIF, and dopamine is almost certainly this physiological inhibitor.

Prolactin

The physiological role of prolactin in ovarian control is still unclear. It is a single chain polypeptide weighing about 20 000 daltons. The complete amino acid sequence has been reported by Shome and Parlow (1977).

Secretion in normal individuals is pulsatile with a superimposed diurnal rhythm. There are no major changes during the normal menstrual cycle and it is generally believed that prolactin in the human, unlike many other animals, has no effect on ovarian activity. The possibility that it may exert a 'permissive' effect on steroid secretion by the human Graafian follicle cannot be ruled out (McNatty et al. 1974).

There is, so far, only one clear-cut relationship between prolactin secretion and ovarian control. In those patients where prolactin secretion is increased pathologically, either by drugs such as phenothiazines or a prolactin-secreting pituitary tumour, there is often inhibition of the hypothalamic release of GnRF with subsequent secondary amenorrhoea. Specific inhibition of abnormal prolactin production by a dopamine agonist such as bromocriptine is usually followed by restoration of spontaneous ovulation (see Chapter 7).

THE GONADOTROPHINS

Follicle stimulating hormone (FSH)

Probably the most graphic description of the action of pure FSH is Greep's (1959), '. . . . it will not lead to stimulation of the uterus: the ovaries will exhibit many mature but not cystic follicles and no follicles that are in pre-ovulatory swelling; the preparation will not produce any trace of luteinization or thecal swelling in the hypophysectomized female rat nor any enlargement of the prostate in males'.

More recently, studying biologically pure human FSH extracted from urine, Petrusz et al. (1970) while supporting most of Greep's statements, do indicate that the human material does have some slight but definite effect on uterine weight and vaginal cornification, indicating that FSH alone may have a minor effect on steroid production.

The physiological obsession with the action of 'pure' FSH is clinically of little importance since there are no known circumstances where the human female produces FSH alone without associated LH release. However, in a unique female with a high level of LH antibodies we could elicit no steroid response after large amounts of FSH (Healy et al. 1978).

Dizerega and his colleagues (1983) have isolated a follicular protein in the human female that inhibits the action of FSH on the follicle. This may play a role in the selection of the dominant follicle that is selected to proceed to ovulation.

Luteinizing hormone (LH)

Like FSH, LH is a glycoprotein and its structure, partially clarified by Li (1961), has been documented further by the Birmingham group (Butt 1967). LH consists of two non-identical sub-units (α and β) different from each other in amino-acid composition, carbohydrate content and electrophoretic mobility (Holcomb et al. 1968).

Greep (1961) has pointed out that while LH administered alone has no detectable effect in the immature animal, in the adult animal many of its effects can be seen with the naked eye: superovulation, luteinization, and the effects of promoted steroidogenesis on the genital tract. For all of these effects prior priming with FSH is essential.

For obvious reasons there is little known of the effect of LH on human ovarian steroidogenesis in vivo. Even the somewhat coarse index of its effect on the lifespan of the corpus luteum is uncertain. Short (1964) reviews the evidence of others, and provides much of his own, that the lifespan of the ovine corpus luteum is unaffected by either LH or hCG. Moor and Rowson (1964) provide evidence that hysterectomy in the sheep before the thirteenth day of a 16-day cycle will prolong the life of the corpus luteum, and because of this a uterine 'luteolysin' has been postulated. The weight of evidence suggests that the endometrium produces this 'luteolysin' in the sheep, cow and some small laboratory animals. There is now a consensus that this luteolysin is prostaglandin $F_{2\alpha}$.

The situation in the human is still confused. While there is no evidence in the human for a uterine luteolysin as found in other animals, and while infusion of $PGF_{2\alpha}$ directly into the uterine cavity during the luteal phase of the cycle has no effect on hormonal production from the corpus luteum (Lyneham et al. 1975), injection of $PGF_{2\alpha}$ directly into the corpus luteum of the human does produce transient luteolysis (Korda et al. 1975). The true role of prostaglandins in human luteolysis, if they have such a role, will await further studies of the levels of this substance in the corpus luteum throughout the luteal phase of the normal cycle.

It would be an abuse of the Queen's English to say that controversy rages about the role of LH on the lifespan of the corpus luteum, but argument certainly continues. While Knobil (1973) produced good evidence that LH was necessary for maintenance of the primate corpus luteum, more recently Baumaceda et al. (1983) have produced cogent evidence that it is not. However there is general agreement that both LH and human chorionic gonadotrophin (hCG) will increase the synthesis of all steroids from the corpus luteum (Savard et al. 1965, Baumaceda et al. 1983).

The mechanisms by which LH increases steroidogenesis have been documented by Savard (1967, 1973). LH has a site-specific effect on the concentration of cyclic AMP (adenosine-3', 5'–monophosphate) in luteal tissue. In tissue slices of corpus luteum exposed to LH, increased concentration of cyclic AMP precedes by 15 to 120 minutes any significant increase in steroid synthesis. Cyclic AMP is very firmly established as the 'second messenger' in the steroidogenic cells of the ovary.

OVARIAN STEROIDOGENESIS

Accepting that LH promotes ovarian steroidogenesis, exclusive attention should not be focused on the follicle and corpus luteum as the sole sites of response. Savard et al. (1965) on the basis of in vitro findings discuss three separate steroidogenic compartments in the ovary, all of which are responsive to LH stimulation after prior or concurrent exposure to FSH. These are as follows:

1 The stroma, which may synthesize androstenedione, dehydroepiandrosterone, testosterone and small quantities of oestradiol and progesterone. This role of the stroma has been amplified by Mattingly and Huang (1969).
2 The follicle, synthesizing mainly oestradiol with trace amounts of progesterone and androgens.
3 The corpus luteum, producing progesterone as the dominant hormone, but significant quantities of oestradiol also.

There are very few data on the changes in steroidogenesis coincidental with cellular changes during the human menstrual cycle. Short (1962, 1964) has taken advantage of the large amount of follicular and luteal fluid present in the mare ovary to study steroid production in vivo. On the basis of his results he puts forward the 'two cell theory' which 'postulates that the theca interna cells have all the enzyme systems

necessary for the synthesis of oestradiol-17β from cholesterol, whereas the granulosal cells have only a weak 17-hydroxylase ability and little or no 17-desmolase activity'. Short suggests that the synthetic potential of the granulosal cells is not evident in the follicular phase because of its avascularity. After ovulation with a rapid in-growth of blood vessels, the capacity of the lutein-transformed granulosa becomes dominant. He concludes that in the mare, changes in steroid secretion so clearly evident after ovulation are 'a direct result of the change in cell type', the thecal cells of the follicle producing oestrogens and androstenedione, the granulosal-derived luteal cells producing predominantly progesterone.

Savard (1964) and Pearlman (1964) emphasize the species variability in production of steroids by the corpus luteum. In vitro, the human corpus luteum produces significant quantities of oestrogen, while the urinary excretion pattern and plasma levels of oestrogens in the luteal phase of the cycle indicate that this also occurs in vivo. It may be relevant that whereas in the mare, studied by Short, the thecal cells almost entirely disappear after ovulation, in the human they remain prominent as the theca lutein cells.

Ryan and Petro (1966) have studied the steroidal potential of human granulosal and thecal cells in vitro. They conclude that in the human the differences are quantitative rather than qualitative. McNatty et al. (1979) have shown that in the human, granulosal cell secretions accumulate preferentially in the intrafollicular fluid, whereas the majority of secretion from the thecal cells is secreted directly into blood.

There are many adequate reviews of ovarian steroid biogenesis and metabolism (Brooksbank 1964, Dorfman et al. 1963, Goldzieher 1964, Ryan & Smith 1965) and these have been summarized by Shearman and Cox (1966).

The main pathways are shown in Fig. 5.1. The Δ^4 (A) pathway hitherto considered dominant has ample support from the Δ^5 (B) steps (Ryan & Smith 1961, Smith & Ryan 1962). Kase (1964) has suggested that the Δ^5 pathway may be characteristic of all non-luteinized tissue.

While it should be noted that all oestrogens appear to be produced from androgenic precursors (Chapter 8), it must be emphasized that steroids occurring as part of a biosynthetic pathway may not be secreted in appreciable amounts.

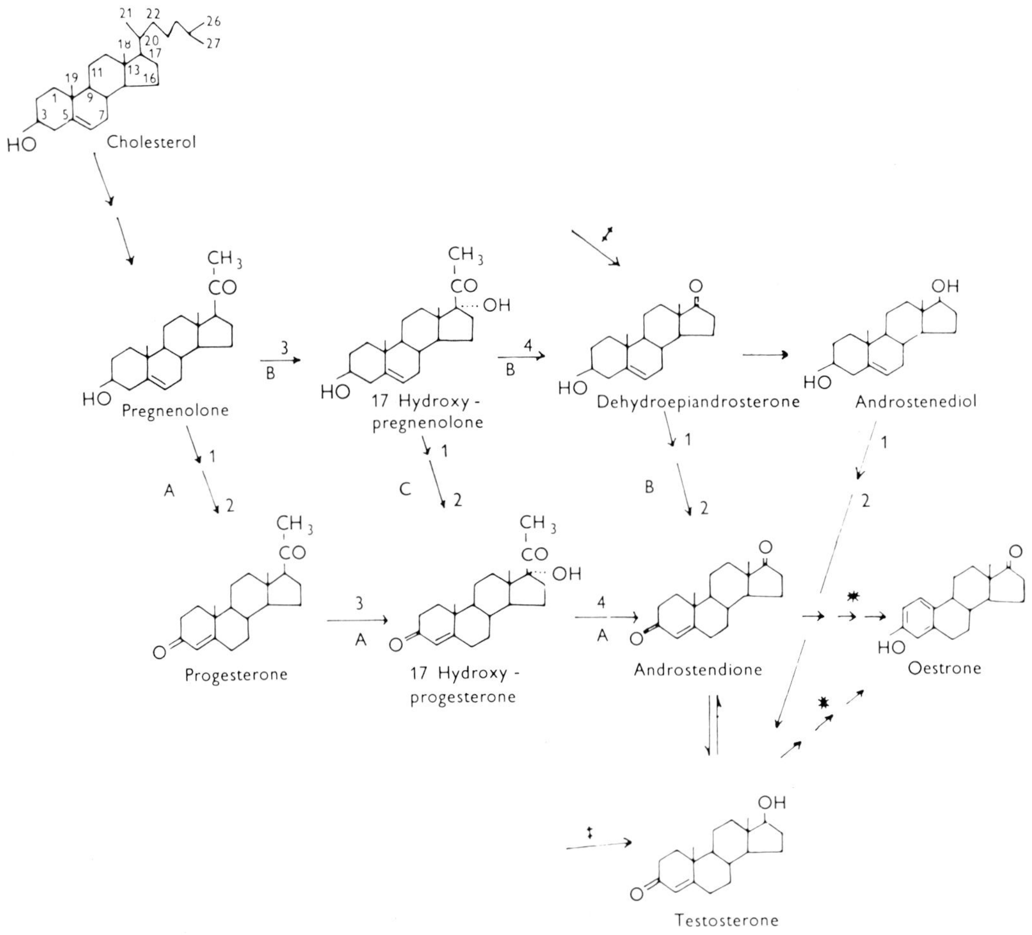

Fig. 5.1. Some pathways of ovarian steroidogenesis. (From Shearman & Cox (1966), by courtesy of the Editor of *Obstetrical and Gynaecological Survey*.)

SECRETION AND EXCRETION PATTERNS OF GONADOTROPHINS AND OVARIAN STEROIDS IN OVULATORY CYCLES

Gonadotrophins

For obvious reasons there are virtually no data on the pituitary content of gonadotrophins in the human during the menstrual cycle. Using prostatic weight in the hypophysectomized rat as the endpoint, McArthur (1965) has long held that there is a peak of LH excretion at mid-cycle and that it is detectable at all other times of the cycle. Using the more sensitive ovarian ascorbic acid depletion test, Fukushima *et al.* (1964), and Rosemberg and Keller (1965) have

also found a mid-cycle peak in LH excretion. Similar results have been reported by Wide and Gemzell (1962) and Mishell (1966) using an immunological method. In plasma, Yokata *et al.* (1965) have found clear evidence of a mid-cycle increase in LH levels. Using a radioimmunoassay for LH, which is more sensitive than methods hitherto developed, Bagshawe *et al.* (1966) described mid-cycle peaks of LH in both serum and urine and their findings in plasma have been confirmed by Odell *et al.* (1967) and Neill *et al.* (1967). When seen in global terms throughout the menstrual cycle, LH release appears to be fairly stable, apart from the single mid-cycle peak. This however is not the physiological situation. Throughout the cycle there is a pulsatile release of LH, at a frequency of approximately one pulse every hour. The neologism 'circhoral' has been provided for this pulsatile pattern (Knobil 1974).

Using radioimmunoassay Faiman and Ryan (1967) found two peaks of FSH, one early in the proliferative phase and the second occurring concurrently with the LH peak see at about mid-cycle. The results of concurrent radioimmunoassay of FSH and LH in urine and plasma throughout the menstrual cycle are shown in Fig. 5.2 (Stevens 1969).

Although still called the 'mid-cycle peak' of LH, this peak, in fact, occurs about 36 hours before ovulation. A very close analysis of the detailed interactions of LH, FSH, oestradiol, progesterone and 17-hydroxyprogesterone during this critical mid-cycle phase has been described by Haff et al. (1983).

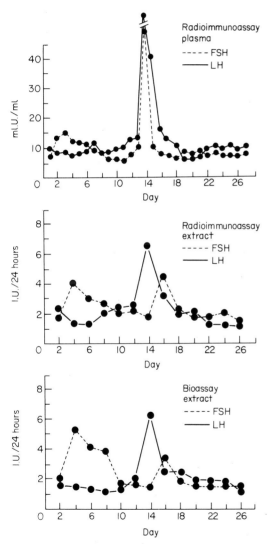

Fig. 5.2. FSH and LH patterns in plasma and urinary extract by radioimmunoassay and in urinary extract by bioassay during the menstrual cycle. (From Stevens 1969 by courtesy of the Editor of the *Journal of Clinical Endocrinology and Metabolism*.)

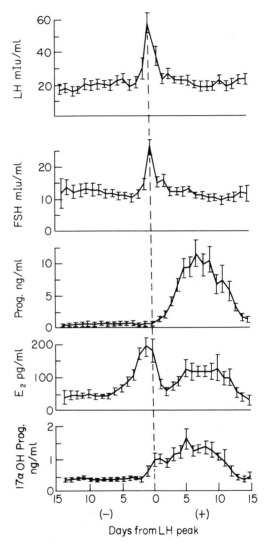

Fig. 5.3. Mean values of LH, FSH, progesterone (Prog.), oestradiol (E_2), and 17-hydroxyprogesterone (17αOH Prog.) in daily serum samples of 9 women during ovulatory menstrual cycles. Data from different cycles combined with the use of the day of the mid-cycle LH peak as the reference day (Day 0). The vertical bars represent one standard error of the mean. (From Thorneycroft et al. 1971 by courtesy of the Editor of the *American Journal of Obstetrics and Gynecology*.)

Ovarian steroids

Development of specific radioimmunoassay has allowed precise documentation of the plasma levels of
oestradiol and progesterone throughout the menstrual cycle. Oestradiol shows a characteristic biphasic pattern with a high peak at about the time of
ovulation and a secondary peak corresponding to
function of the corpus luteum. Progesterone levels
are low (less than 3.18 nmol/l) throughout the follicular phase. There is a very slight increase immediately before ovulation and a rapid rise corresponding to development of the corpus luteum followed by
a further fall before menstruation begins. A plateau
of progesterone is reached in the middle of the luteal

phase. The pattern of these steroids, related to gonadotrophin levels throughout the menstrual cycle, is
shown in Fig. 5.3.

For research purposes and increasingly in clinical
practice, plasma assays have largely replaced those
in urine. Nevertheless urinary assays are still employed in clinical practice. The excretion patterns of
the three classical oestrogens and pregnanediol are
fully documented following the early work of Brown
(1955a, b) and Klopper (1957). Oestrogen excretion
patterns have been fully reviewed by Brown *et al.*
(1959) and Brown and Matthew (1962). The mean
and normal range values for oestrogens (oestrone,
oestradiol and oestriol) obtained from a study of sixteen women are shown in Fig. 5.4. Typically, the

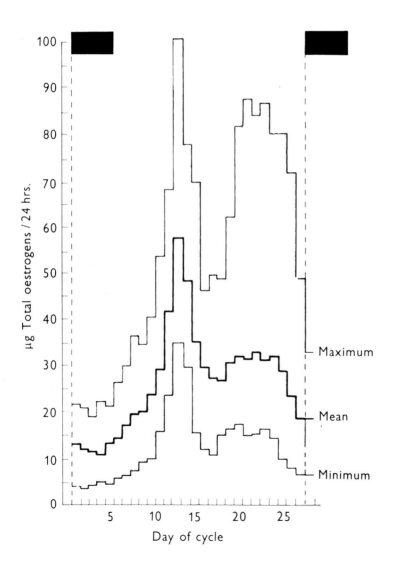

Fig. 5.4. Mean and range
of urinary excretion of total
oestrogens during the
normal menstrual cycle.
(From Brown *et al.* (1959)
by courtesy of the Editor of
*Journal of Obstetrics and
Gynaecology of the British
Commonwealth.*)

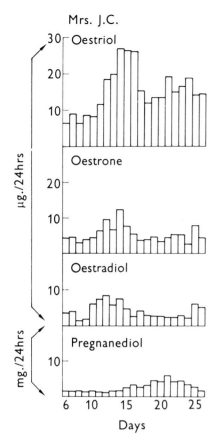

Fig. 5.5. Excretion of oestrogens and pregnanediol during the normal menstrual cycle. (From Shearman (1969), by courtesy of Charles C. Thomas, Publisher.)

pattern is biphasic. During the first 2 or 3 days of menstruation oestrogen excretion is low. In a 28-day cycle there is then a fairly rapid rise to a well-defined peak at mid-cycle, usually termed the *ovulation peak*. This is followed by a fall in oestrogen excretion and then a second, broader rise known as the luteal maximum. In the last few days of the cycle there is a decrease in oestrogen excretion, and menstruation follows.

It has been believed that in the non-pregnant individual, urinary oestriol is derived only from secreted oestrone and/or oestradiol, although it is now well established that oestriol in pregnancy is predominantly derived from non-oestrogenic precursors produced by the fetus. Work by Barlow and Logan (1967) suggests that at least in the luteal phase, precursors of urinary oestriol other than oestrone and/or oestradiol may be involved.

In contrast, the excretion pattern of pregnanediol is uniphasic. During the follicular phase excretion is usually less than 3.12 μmol/24 h. Shortly after ovulation the levels increase, reaching a maximum midway through the luteal phase and then declining before menstruation. The results in Fig. 5.5 are typical of those seen in a spontaneous ovulatory cycle.

The pattern on conceptual cycles is different. Brown (1956) produced data on the pattern of oestrogen excretion in the conceptual cycle of a woman ovulating spontaneously. A further increase beyond the luteal maximum is already obvious before the first missed period. If ovulation is physiologically induced in anovulatory females, an identical pattern can be produced.

It should be emphasized that although there is a qualitative similarity in excretion patterns from one woman to another, quantitatively there are large interpersonal differences. A clear picture may be obtained only by serial assays.

REFERENCES

BAGSHAWE K. D., WILDE C. E. & ORR A. H. (1966) *Lancet*, i, 1118.

BARLOW J. J. & LOGAN C. M. (1967) *Amer. J. Obstet. Gynec.*, **98**, 687.

BAUMACEDA J. D., BORGHI M. R., COY D. H., SCHALLY A. V. & AJCH R. H. (1983) *J. clin. Endocrin.*, **57**, 866.

BROOKSBANK B. W. L. (1964) *Clin. Obstet. Gynec.*, 7 (No. 4), 1120.

BROWN J. B. (1955a) *Lancet*, ii, 320.

BROWN J. B. (1955b) *Mem. Soc. Endocr.*, **3**, 1.

BROWN J. B., KELLER R. & MATTHEW G. D. (1959) *J. Obstet. Gynaec. Brit. Cwlth.*, **66**, 177.

BROWN J. B. & MATTHEW G. D. (1962) *Recent Progr. Hormone Res.*, **18**, 337.

BUTT W. R. (1967) In *Recent Research on Gonadotrophic Hormones* (Bell E. T. & LORAINE J. A. eds), p. 129. Churchill Livingstone, Edinburgh and London.

DIZEREGA G. S., CAMPEAU J. D., MAKAMURA R. M., UGITA E. L., LOBO R. & MARRS R. P. (1983) *J. clin. Endocrin.* **57**, 838.

DORFMAN R. K., FORCHIELLI E. & GUT M. (1963) *Recent Progr. Hormone Res.*, **19**, 251.

EDITORIAL COMMENT (1974) *Lancet*, ii, 1235.

FAIMAN C. & RYAN R. J. (1967) *J. clin. Endocr.* **27**, 1711.

FUKUSHIMA M., STEVENS V. C., GANTT C. L. & VORYS N. (1964) *J. clin. Endocr.* **24**, 205.

FUKUSHIMA M., STEVENS V. C., GANTT C. L. & VORYS N. (1964) *J. clin. Endocr.* **24**, 205.

GOLDZIEHER J. W. (1964) *Clin Obstet. Gynaec.*, 7 (No. 4), 1160.

GREEP R. O. (1959) *Recent Progr. Hormone Res.*, **15**, 139.

GREEP R. O. (1961) In *Sex and Internal Secretions* (Young W. C. ed.), p. 240. Williams & Wilkins, Baltimore.

HAFF J. D., QUIGLEY M. E. & YEN S. S. C. (1983) *J. clin. Endocr.*, **57**, 792.

HEALY D. L., FRASER I. S., LEE V. W. K., SHEARMAN R. P. & BURGHER H. G. (1978) *J. clin. Endocr.*, **47**, 823.

HOLCOMB G. N., LAMKIN W. M., JAMES S. A., WADE J. & WARD D. N. (1968) *Endocrinology*, **83**, 1293.

JUDD S. J. (1984) In *Clinical Reproductive Endocrinology* (Shearman R. P. ed), Churchill Livingstone, London. In press.

KLOPPER A. K. (1957) *J. Obstet. Gynaec. Brit. Cwlth.*, **64**, 504.

KNOBIL E. (1973) *Biol. of Reprod.*, **8**, 246.

KNOBIL E. (1974) *Recent Progr. Hormone Res.*, **30**, 1.

KORDA A. R., SHUTT D. R., SMITH I. D., SHEARMAN R. P. & LYNEHAM R. C. (1975) *Prostaglandins*, **9**, 443.

LI C. H. (1961) In *Human Pituitary Gonadotrophins* (Albert A. ed.), p. 364. Charles C. Thomas, Springfield, Illinois.

LYNEHAM R. C., KORDA A. R., SHUTT D. A., SMITH I. D., & SHEARMAN R. P. (1975) *Prostaglandins*, **9**, 431.

McARTHUR J. W. (1965) In *Human Ovulation* (Keffer C. S. ed.), p. 94. Churchill Livingstone, London.

McNATTY K. P., SAWERS R. S. & McNEILLY A. S. (1974) *Nature*, **250**, 653.

MATTINGLY R. F. & HUANG W. Y. (1969) *Amer. J. Obstet. Gynec.*, **103**, 679.

MISHELL D. P. (1966) *Amer. J. Obstet. Gynec.*, **95**, 747.

MOOR R. M. & ROWSON L. E. A. (1964) *Nature*, **291**, 522.

NEILL J. D., JOHANSSON E. D. B., DATTA J. K. & KNOBIL E. (1967) *J. clin. Endocr.*, **27**, 1167.

ODELL W. D., ROSS G. T. & PLAYFORD P. L. (1967) *J. clin. Invest.*, **46**, 248.

PEARLMAN W. H. (1964) *Recent Progr. Hormone Res.*, **20**, 338.

PETRUSZ P., ROBYN C. & DICSFULUSY E. (1970) *Acta Endocr.*, **60**, 454.

ROSEMBERG E. & KELLER P. J. (1965) *J. clin. Endocr.*, **25**, 1262.

RYAN K. J. & PETRO Z. (1966) *J. clin. Endocr.*, **26**, 46.

RYAN K. J. & SMITH O. W. (1961) *J. biol. Chem.*, **236**, 2207.

RYAN K. J. & SMITH O. W. (1965) *Recent Progr. Hormone Res.*, **21**, 367.

SAVARD K. (1964) *Recent Progr. Hormone Res.*, **20**, 334.

SAVARD K. (1967) In *Recent Research on Gonadotrophic Hormones* (Bell E. T. & Loraine J. A. eds.), p. 170. Churchill Livingstone, Edinburgh and London.

SAVARD K. (1973) *Biol. of Reprod.*, **8**, 183.

SAVARD K., MARSH J. M. & RICE B. F. (1965) *Recent Progr. Hormone Res.*, **21**, 285.

SCHALLY A. V., ARIMURA A., BABA Y., NAIR R. M. G., MATSUO H., REDDING T. W., DEBELJUK L. & WHITE W. F. (1971) *Biochem. Biophys. Res. Com.*, **43**, 393.

SHEARMAN R. P. (1969) *Induction of Ovulation.* Charles C. Thomas, Springfield.

SHEARMAN R. P. & COX R. I. (1966) *Obstet. gynec. Surv.*, **21**, 1.

SHOME B. & PARLOW A. F. (1977) *J. clin. Endocr.*, **45**, 1112.

SHORT R. V. (1962) *J. Endocr.*, **24**, 59.

SHORT R. V. (1964) *Recent Progr. Hormone Res.*, **20**, 303.

SMITH O. W. & RYAN K. J. (1962) *Amer. J. Obstet. Gynec.*, **84**, 141.

STEVENS V. C. (1969) *J. clin. Endocr.*, **29**, 904.

TANNER J. M. (1968) *Sci. Amer.* **218**, 21.

TANNER J. M. (1973) *Nature*, **243**, 95.

WALDHAUSER F., WEISZENBACHER G., FRISCH H., ZEITLHUBER V., WALDHAUSER M. & WURTMAN R. J. (1984) *Lancet*, **i**, 362.

WIDE L. & GEMZELL C. (1962) *Acta endocr.*, **39**, 539.

WURTMAN R. J. & ANTON-TAY F. (1969) *Recent Progr. Hormone Res.*, **25**, 493.

YOKATA N., IGARASHI M. & MATSUMOTO S. (1965) *Endocr. Jap.*, **12**, 92.

CHAPTER 6
PRIMARY AMENORRHOEA

RODNEY P. SHEARMAN

The differential diagnosis of primary amenorrhoea has long been an interesting intellectual exercise which has become more fascinating with the unfolding knowledge of genetic and hormonal influences on phenotypic development. With proper management it should be possible for all of these patients to lead a normal life, although many will be infertile.

The normal menarche requires an integration of hypothalamus, pituitary, ovary and uterus, and a patent effluent canal for menstrual bleeding. Aberrations in any of these may result in failure of sexual maturation or absence of menarche. It is now apparent that many, if not the majority, of abnormalities responsible for primary amenorrhoea are determined *in utero*, some of them prior to conception. It is very rare indeed that a precise reason cannot be found for primary amenorrhoea.

A working knowledge of the endocrinology of sexual differentiation *in utero* is necessary for a true understanding of many of the problems of primary amenorrhoea. Details will be found in Chapter 3. In summary, the important concepts of sexual differentiation are that:

1 XX is usually needed for normal ovarian development and maintenance. Ovarian development including germ cell migration will occur in the presence of a single X, but is almost invariably followed by rapid disappearance of these follicles, two X chromosomes normally being required for follicular maintenance.
2 The H-Y antigen probably evokes the testis as long as there are specific receptors. However, it will not by itself induce germ cell colonization of the gonads.
3 In the absence of a gonad, female development is the neutral or asexual norm.
4 The Sertoli cells of the testes produce anti-Müllerian factor (AMF). The male intersex lacking AMF will have a uterus, tubes and vagina.
5 Fetal testosterone evokes Wolffian structures but has no effect on Müllerian ducts.

6 Fetal testosterone will virilize the cloaca if it is bound to the target cells and can be converted to dihydrotestosterone (DHT).
7 A relative deficiency of 5α reductase will impair the cloacal response to testosterone, but it will not affect Wolffian evocation, the latter being dependent on testosterone without need of conversion.
8 Abnormal or ectopic androgen stimuli, depending on timing and biological potency, may cause variable or even almost complete masculinization of the female cloaca but never affect Müllerian development in chromosomal or gonadal females.

THE CLINICAL PROBLEM

There is difference of opinion about the age at which primary amenorrhoea should be investigated. Eighteen years is an age often suggested, and this may be reasonable in the patient who has developed normal secondary sexual characteristics and in whom cryptomenorrhoea has been excluded. However, those with primary amenorrhoea and sexual infantilism should be investigated at the age of 15 or 16, or even earlier if there are stigmata suggestive of Turner's syndrome or virilism.

A classification of the causes of primary amenorrhoea is shown in Table 6.1. A full discussion of each of these is inappropriate in a general text, but will be found in Shearman (1985).

In the majority of individuals wiith primary amenorrhoea it is possible to arrive at a fairly firm provisional diagnosis from the history and the results of physical examination. It is only in a minority that there is a need to go beyond fairly simple out-patient investigations.

The most important initial distinction is whether the patient is sexually infantile or whether there is evidence of secondary sexual characteristics. The importance of this distinction should be clear. A girl of 15 or 16 who has no secondary sexual characteris-

Table 6.1. Classification of primary amenorrhoea.

Hypergonadotrophic hypogonadism
1 Chromosomally incompetent ovarian failure includes
   classic Turner, all other X deletions and 45X/46XY
2 Chromosomally competent ovarian failure 46XX 46XX
      (i) True agenesis
      (ii) Premature ovarian failure (radiation chemo-
           therapy, autoimmune)
      (iii) Galactosaemia
      46XY

Hypogonadotrophic hypogonadism
1 Reversible
      Physiological delay
      Weight loss/anorexia nervosa/heavy exercise
      Primary hypothyroidism
2 Irreversible
      (i) Congenital
          Isolated GnRF deficiency (with or without anosmia)
          Partial or total hypopituitarism
          Congenital CNS defects
      (ii) Aquired
          Hyperprolactinaemia (no tumour)
          Pituitary adenoma
             a Prolactinoma
             b Mixed activity (a + acromegaly or Cushing's)
             c Producing gonadotrophins
             d Inert
          Empty Sella
          Craniopharygioma
          Other intracranial tumours
          Trauma (including surgery)

Eugonadal
1 Anatomical
      Uterovaginal agenesis
      Imperforate hymen (including transverse septum)
2 Polycystic ovaries
3 Testicular feminization
4 Noonan's syndrome

Virilism
1 Adrenal hyperplasia
2 Tumour (adrenal, ovary)
3 5-α-reductase deficiency
4 Partial adrogen receptor complex deficiency
5 Absent anti-Müllerian factor
6 True hermaphrodite

tics obviously has not been exposed to any form of stimulation from gonadal hormones. Individuals with sexual infantilism can be further divided into those in whom there is idiopathic delay of sexual development and those in whom there is pathological sexual infantilism, the cause of which may lie in the hypothalamic pituitary area or in the gonad.

Idiopathic delay and precocious puberty are two ends of a fairly wide frequency distribution curve. Girls with idiopathic delay may not commence sexual maturation until the age of 15 or 16. Differentiation of this condition from pathological sexual infantilism may require observation for a year or more. Closely related is the obese young girl with delayed menstruation and puberty, frequently mislabelled Fröhlich's syndrome. Most young girls who show this triad have no detectable pathological lesion, and spontaneous remission will occur in the majority.

The majority of patients with sexual infantilism due to congenital hypothalamic pituitary disturbances, such as Lorain–Lévi syndrome or Laurence–Moon–Biedl syndrome, will have been recognized clinically before the age of puberty, and its absence is only another incident in a long history. Lorain-type dwarfism is usually manifest by the third or fourth year with evidence of growth retardation and unfolds with evidence of persistently juvenile features, hypogonadism, hypothyroidism and sometimes hypoadrenocorticism. Although there is no doubt about the homogeneity of the Laurence–Moon–Biedl syndrome, the classical features of retinitis pigmentosa, polydactylism or syndactylism, and mental retardation will be evident in infancy.

Most girls with sexual infantilism who are seen by the gynaecologist appear to be quite well in every way except for the infantilism. The patient's height is important. If she is less than 4 ft 10 in (147 cm) tall, it is very likely that one or other of the chromosomal abnormalities leading to gonadal dygenesis will be present. Much less frequently, the diagnosis will be panhypopituitarism, or craniopharyngioma. Because of the possibility of the latter lesion, a skull X-ray is mandatory in these patients. Less frequently, a diagnosis of partial or total hypopituitarism will be reached. In many pituitary dwarves lacking endogenous growth hormone, puberty will occur but as a rule will be later than normal (sexual dwarves). In others the sexual infantilism will persist (asexual dwarfism).

If in addition to being short the patient has a web neck, increased carrying angle or perhaps even a congenital cardiac lesion, then it requires only modest clinical skill to suspect a diagnosis of Turner's syndrome (Fig. 6.1). This will be confirmed by finding a karyotype of 45,X or less frequently mosaics such as 45,X/46,XX. Although most mosaics are sexually infantile with a female phenotype, some may have menstruated, while others (X/XY) may show variable degrees of virilism. This last group is probably better

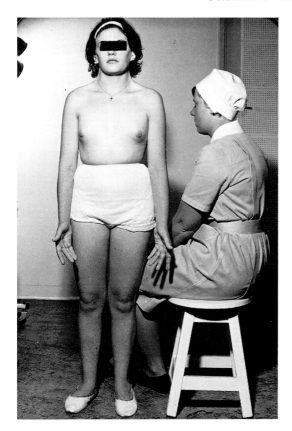

Fig. 6.1. Turner's syndrome. Height 4 ft 10 in. Note webbed neck and widely spaced nipples. Oestrogens have caused breast growth.

classified under the heading of mixed gonadal dysgenesis. Knowledge of the exact karyotype is essential for proper clinical management as surgical excision of streaks or dysgenetic gonads will be necessary in girls with XY or X/XY mosaicism (see below). Laparotomy or laparoscopy should only be considered when there is disparity between clinical findings, especially phenotype, and laboratory investigations.

For the taller patient with sexual infantilism the diagnosis usually lies between true gonadal agenesis and hypogonadotrophic hypogonadism. This important distinction cannot be made on purely clinical grounds. A karyotype of 46,XX will be found most commonly and the distinction between hypogonadotrophic hypogonadism and 46,XX true gonadal agenesis (chromosomally competent ovarian failure) will be made only by assay of FSH and LH which will be high in the latter and low or normal in the former. Gonadal biopsy is not needed in this group. If the karyotype is 46,XY (another variant of chromoso-

mally competent ovarian failure), gonadotrophins will be high and excision of the streaks essential (see below).

This group of patients should always have their sense of smell tested, as some of them may belong to the 'olfacto-genital' syndrome (Belaisch et al. 1965, Mroueh & Kase 1968, Teter 1967), also sometimes known in its familial form as Kallmann's syndrome (Kallmann et al. 1944). Sixteen cases of the author's own have shown anosmia, sexual infantilism, normal or above normal height and absent of or scanty sexual hair. The familial type of this condition is fully discussed by Santen and Paulsen (1973).

Delay in menstruation in a patient who has reached puberty is a different problem. An initial and simple distinction is to note whether the changes of puberty have been feminizing or masculinizing. If the patient has some female secondary characteristics, then obviously she has been exposed to some endogenous sex steroid stimulation. This statement is valid only if one can be certain that this sexual maturation has not been induced by the prolonged administration of exogenous steroids in an unwise attempt to induce vaginal bleeding before a proper diagnosis has been made. Far too frequently a patient in her late teens or early twenties will present with 'secondary amenorrhoea'. On careful questioning it is found that all of the patient's periods have been induced by hormone therapy given intermittently over many years, and that neither the patient, nor her mother, can recall whether the secondary sexual characteristics preceded or followed this treatment.

In a patient with normal female habitus, some local abnormality within the genital tract should be excluded forthwith. There may be an imperforate hymen or undeveloped vagina with cryptomenorrhoea. The uterus and vagina may be congenitally absent, in which case ovarian function is usually normal (Brown et al. 1959). These patients with Müllerian agenesis should have an intravenous pyelogram as 30% of them have major abnormalities of the renal tract including solitary kidney (Shearman & Roberts 1982). If it is found that the patient has a blind vagina without any evidence of a uterus, even though she may otherwise be quite feminine, the most likely diagnosis is the syndrome of testicular feminization. The testes may be palpable in the inguinal region, while axillary and pubic hair is usually scanty or absent. The karyotype in this condition is 46,XY and since the condition is familial, 'sisters' with the same problem may present.

If the patient has no local genital abnormality, and

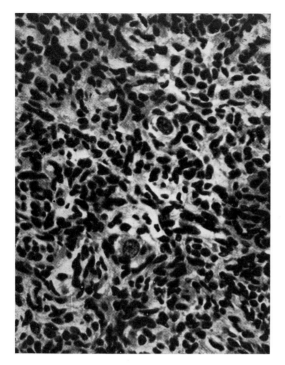

Fig. 6.2. Biopsy of ovarian tissue from true hermaphrodite. (From Shearman *et al.* 1964, by courtesy of the Editor of *Journal of Obstetrics and Gynaecology of the British Commonwealth.*)

While both true hermaphroditism and virilizing ovarian tumour are extremely rare, each must, nevertheless, be considered as a possible diagnosis in any apparent female who presents at puberty with virilism. Figs. 6.2 and 6.3 show biopsies from the gonads of a patient known to be a true hermaphrodite at the age of 4 years. The testis was left *in situ* and at the age of 13 the patient suddenly developed a masculinizing puberty, having been brought up as a female. The abdominal testis was removed and the early virilism regressed rapidly.

These individuals bearing testes, will of course have normal male levels of plasma testosterone.

Short of virilism, primary amenorrhoea may be the presenting symptom in some girls who, having had a female type of onset of puberty, develop severe acne and hirsutism. Mild postpubertal adrenal hyperplasia should be considered in this instance. Rarely, the diagnosis will prove to be prepubertal polycystic ovaries (Teter 1967). These patients show the expected high levels of LH and high LH/FSH ratio and the diagnosis can be confirmed by laparoscopy. It is important to be certain that the polycystic ovaries are

if some female secondary sexual characteristics have developed spontaneously, it is possible to await, with some degree of confidence, the onset of spontaneous menstruation. This may be delayed until the age of 19 or 20.

Primary amenorrhoea may occur in an apparent female who shows virilizing changes at puberty. This may be due to mild congenital adrenal hyperplasia that has not been detected previously, or the postpubertal form of adrenal hyperplasia. The steroidal aberrations are the same as those found in congenital adrenal hyperplasia presenting in children (Brooks *et al.* 1960). Such a diagnosis may be confirmed by finding a normal female karyotype, increase in serum 17-hydroxyprogesterone or if urinary steroids are still used, an increase in 17-oxosteroids, and pregnanetriol. An adrenal tumour may be excluded by the ability of dexamethasone to suppress these levels (*see* Chapter 8).

Apart from testicular feminism, there is a wide spectrum of XY females in whom primary amenorrhoea may occur. These are described in more detail in Chapter 3 dealing with intersexuality.

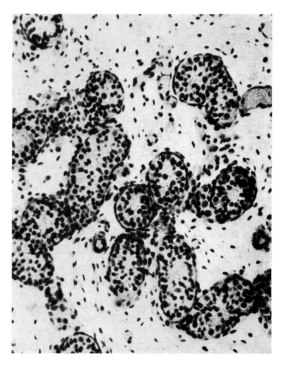

Fig. 6.3. Biopsy from testis removed from a true hermaphrodite during infancy. (From Shearman *et al.* 1964, by courtesy of the Editor of *Journal of Obstetrics and Gynaecology of the British Commonwealth.*)

'primary' and not secondary to adrenal hyperplasia, as they sometimes may be. The latter could be excluded by finding normal levels of 17-hydroxyprogesterone in plasma.

TREATMENT

The aim of treatment should be to attain the maximum physiological function of which the individual patient is capable. This may be complete fertility; it may be the prospect of fertility; often it will end with attainment of functional sexual maturation but irrevocable infertility. Only very rarely, if ever, will it be necessary to settle for anything less. No attempt should ever be made to treat these patients until a firm diagnosis is reached.

Turner's syndrome and gonadal agenesis

The only treatment for these patients is to achieve sexual maturation with exogenous steroids. An initial

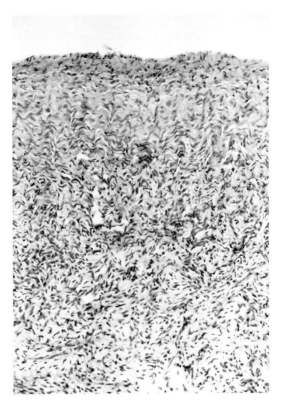

Fig. 6.5. Section from streak gonad on the contralateral side to that shown in Fig. 6.4.

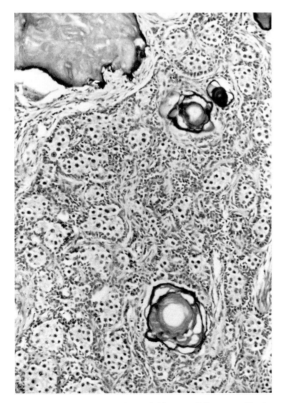

Fig. 6.4. Dysgerminoma (gonadoblastoma) from a patient with a mixed gonadal dysgenesis.

dose of 0.01 mg of ethinyloestradiol twice daily for 3 weeks in every month will cause primary breast-bud development if it is given for several months, but only rarely will withdrawal bleeding occur. Then definitive treatment with a larger amount of oestrogen and an added progestin is started and continued cyclically for an indefinite time. While the cheapest way to do this would be to use an ordinary oral contraceptive, the growing concern about the long-term metabolic effects of this regime probably renders this undesirable. Recognizing that many of the long-term sequelae of oral contraceptives relate not only to the dose of oestrogen but also to the amount of progestin and in particular the specific progestational effect on high density lipo-protein cholesterol, it might be preferable to use a 'tailor-made' pill containing 30 or 50 μg of ethinyloestradiol together with 5 mg of medroxyprogesterone acetate given for 21 days and repeated again after a week's gap. Many people use oestrogens alone, but the addition of a progestin for 10 days each month gives much better cycle control and appears to cause better breast development. It is also unequivocally clear that prolonged use of unopposed oestrogens in these girls can cause the early development of endometrial malignancy so that the addition of a progestin for at least 10 days in each treatment cycle is mandatory for this reason alone. Laparotomy should be considered only when there is discrepancy between the clinical findings and the laboratory data.

Patients with XY karyotype or XY mosaicism should have the area of the gonadal streak removed to prevent the risk of development of a dysgenetic tumour (Teter & Boczkowski 1967).

Although virilism is usual, a similar problem may arise in the non-virilized chromosomal intersex. Figure 6.4 shows a gonadoblastoma removed from a non-virilized but sexually infantile patient of normal height whose chromosomes showed X/XY mosaicism. The gonadal streak from the contralateral side is shown in Fig. 6.5. Because of the frequency of this complication (see Chapter 3) it is preferable to perform laparotomy on all XY or X/XY mosaics and perform bilateral adnexectomy.

Gonadal causes with or without virilism

Definitive treatment aims to achieve transformation to a potentially sexually competent adult; this means the surgical removal of sources of inappropriate hormonal stimulus (usually testicular tissue) and reconstruction of the external genitals along female lines. This should be done before the age of 4 years.

The testes should be removed from patients with the testicular feminizing syndrome because of the risk of development of a malignant gonadal tumour. The degree of risk is not known with certainty, but Jones (1958) states that the incidence of malignant degeneration is 'not above 5%'. These testes produce normal quantities of oestrogens and testosterone. The problem of target cell response is discussed in Chapter 3. If the testes are removed before puberty, breast development will not occur, but surgery should be considered after sexual maturation.

Disorders of hypothalamus and pituitary gland

Pituitary dwarfs with an isolated deficiency in human growth hormone (hGH) will undergo spontaneous puberty. Those who have panhypopituitarism from a craniopharyngioma or other causes should be treated initially with hGH, made sexually mature with gonadal steroids, and then treated with human pituitary or human menopausal gonadotrophin to induce ovulation when pregnancy is desired. Ateliotic asexual dwarves will require the same treatment.

With the exception of the need for hGH, the same treatment is used for those with hypogonadotrophic hypogonadism with or without anosmia. An alternative to intramuscular injections of pituitary gonadotrophins is to use pulsed administration of GnRF either by the subcutaneous or intravenous route. This is dealt with more fully in Chapter 7.

Adrenal hyperplasia

If this condition presents at the time of puberty, it is treated specifically with corticosteroids. In the rare event that ovulation does not follow, clomiphene is the additional treatment of choice. Unlike those cases diagnosed in infancy, the external genitals of the patients discussed here are usually normal.

Gynaetresia

Cryptomenorrhoea obviously requires treatment as soon as the diagnosis is made. This presents no difficulty in patients with a simple imperforate hymen, but when there is total absence of the vagina with haematometra above it, there may be great difficulty in retaining reproductive potential. However, this may not be impossible (Jeffcoate 1969).

Congenital absence of the uterus, vagina and most of the Fallopian tubes (the Mayer–Rokitansky–Kuster–Hauser syndrome) is usually the commonest single cause of primary amenorrhoea in any large series of patients (Reindollar et al. 1981, Shearman & Roberts 1982). Surgical reconstruction in this group is now rarely indicated, much better results being obtained by the use of graduated glass dilators.

Delayed menarche

Clearly, this diagnosis may be made only in retrospect. The onset of puberty in these patients is usually late, but provided that some secondary female characteristsic have developed spontaneously and progressively, and provided that all other causes have been excluded, no treatment should be offered. Spontaneous resolution will occur, but sometimes not until the age of 20.

CONCLUSIONS

Abnormalities in the normal progression of factors responsible for sexual differentiation in utero are the commonest causes of primary amenorrhoea. The factors responsible for normal differentiation should be understood for a rational approach to the clinical problem of primary amenorrhoea, and these are discussed in Chapter 3.

With suitable investigation a precise diagnosis can usually be reached, and it is possible to treat these patients on rational and physiological principles. All should be able to lead normal, sexually mature lives, but the prospect of fertility may be possible for a minority only. It may well be that for those women with gonadal agenesis and a normal uterus, ovum donation, *in vitro* fertilization and embryo transfer will become an appropriate and acceptable treatment for their infertility (*see* Chapter 40).

REFERENCES

BELAISCH J., MUSSET R. & NETTER A. (1965) *Ann. Endocr.* (Paris), **26**, 267.

BROOKS R.V., MATTINGLY D., MILLS I.H. & PRUNTY F.T.G. (1960) *Brit. med. J.*, **i**, 1294.

BROWN J.B., KELLAR R. & MATTHEW G.D. (1959) *J. Obstet. Gynaec. Brit. Cwlth.*, **66**, 177.

FORD C.E. (1963) In *Intersexuality* (Overzier C. ed.), p. 86. Academic Press, London and New York.

JEFFCOATE T.N.A. (1969) *J. Obstet. Gynaec. Brit. Cwlth.*, **76**, 961.

JONES H.W. (1958) In *Hermaphroditism, Genital Anomalies and Related Disorders* (Jones H.W. & Scott W.W. eds), p. 172. Williams & Wilkins, Baltimore.

KALLMANN F.H., SCHOENFELD W.A. & BARRERA S.W. (1944) *Amer. J. ment. Defic.*, **48**, 203.

MROUEH A. & KASE N. (1968) *Amer. J. Obstet. Gynec.*, **100**, 525.

PHILIP J., SELE V., TROLLE D. & MILLER B. (1965) *Fertil. Steril.*, **17**, 795.

REINDOLLAR R.H., BYRD J.R. & McDONOUGH P.G. (1981) *Amer. J. Obstet. Gynec.*, **140**, 371.

RIMION D.C., MERIMEE T.J., RABINOWITZ D. & McKUSICK V.A. (1968) *Recent Progr. Hormone Res.*, **24**, 365.

SANTEN R.J. & PAULSEN C.A. (1973) *J. clin. Endocr, Metab.*, **36**, 47.

SHEARMAN R.P. (1969) *Induction of Ovulation.* Charles C. Thomas, Springfield.

SHEARMAN R.P. (1985) *Clinical Reproductive Endocrinology,* p. 481. Churchill Livingstone, London.

SHEARMAN R.P., SINGH S., LEE C.W.G., HUDSON B. & ILBERY P.L.T. (1964) *J. Obstet. Gynaec. Brit. Cwlth.*, **71**, 627.

SHEARMAN R.P. & ROBERTS J. (1982) *Clin. Reprod. Fertil.*, **1**, 117.

TETER J. (1967) In *Proceedings of the Vth World Congress of Gynaecology and Obstetrics* (Wood E.C. ed.), p. 272. Butterworth, Sydney.

TETER J. & BOCZKOWSKI K. (1967) *Cancer* (New York), **20**, 1301.

CHAPTER 7
SECONDARY AMENORRHOEA

RODNEY P. SHEARMAN

In this chapter the term secondary amenorrhoea is applied to women of reproductive age who have secondary absence of menstruation for 12 months not due to pregnancy, lactation, or hysterectomy. Premature menopause is defined here as secondary ovarian failure before the age of 35 years.

Not all women who menstruate ovulate, and not all amenorrhoeic women are anovulatory. It is essential that precise diagnosis precedes any attempt to treat these patients. It is unlikely that those with major organic disease such as Cushing's disease or virilizing ovarian tumours will have their lesion undiagnosed, but with the increasing availability of powerful therapeutic weapons to treat amenorrhoeic women, such a possibility cannot be ignored. In the substantial group of women who are apparently well apart from amenorrhoea and infertility, treatment that is initiated before a correct diagnosis has been reached may be unnecessary, imprecise or potentially dangerous.

CLINICAL INVESTIGATION

Most truisms become blunted with frequent repetition. It is a truism to say that an adequate history is essential if an accurate diagnosis is to be reached. Although the spontaneous history given by the patient is of great value, specific questioning will usually be necessary to elicit relevant information in the large group of women who feel and look perfectly well. Is the amenorrhoea, for example, truly secondary? It is not uncommon to be presented with a patient who complains of secondary amenorrhoea only to determine that all menstrual bleeding has been induced with exogenous steroids and she has, in fact, primary amenorrhoea, a very different problem from secondary amenorrhoea and not relevant to this chapter. Any factors operative at the time of onset of amenorrhoea must be elicited specifically. If the amenorrhoea followed pregnancy, the patient should be asked whether curettage was performed for

secondary postpartum haemorrhage or repeat curettage for spontaneous or induced abortion. When this history is given, *amenorrhoea traumatica* (Asherman's syndrome) is a far more likely diagnosis than pituitary failure (Asherman 1950, Foix *et al.* 1966). If the patient gives a history of a large postpartum haemorrhage and failure of lactation, Sheehan's syndrome should certainly be considered. However, with the advent of better obstetric care and adequate blood replacement this now appears to be exceptionally rare in developed countries.

Weight change, at or near the onset of secondary amenorrhoea, is common. While many standard texts draw attention to related obesity, the association is far more frequently one of weight loss. Although it is usually recognized that the young girl with true *anorexia nervosa* has secondary amenorrhoea, it is not so widely recognized that lesser degrees of voluntary weight loss are very frequently associated with suppression of menstruation. The commonest history is that of a mildly overweight teenager who goes on to a 'crash diet'. The onset of amenorrhoea is usually abrupt, as a rule precedes significant weight loss, and it often persists even when the lost weight is regained.

A more modern variant of weight loss amenorrhoea is 'joggers' amenorrhoea. This is seen frequently in women training for marathon racing, in ballet dancers, and in those in heavy training for swimming and other forms of athletics (Frisch *et al.* 1981). The problem here seems to be not so much as absolute change in weight but a redistribution between the proportion of body fat mass and body muscle mass. There is also some evidence that the amenorrhoea may be mediated by exercise related changes in β-endorphins.

Secondary amenorrhoea will often occur abruptly with a major environmental stress and is seen not infrequently in migrants, in young women when they leave home, or in university students around the time of examinations.

Pharmacological causes of amenorrhoea are appearing more commonly. The most frequent syndrome seen clinically these days is the development of amenorrhoea after treatment with oral contraceptives (Shearman 1966a, Shearman & Fraser 1977). Although there must be a high index of suspicion that this association is causal, absolute proof that it is so has not yet been obtained (Vessey *et al.* 1978). Other drugs that may be related causally are phenothiazines, tricyclic antidepressants, reserpine and digoxin. The mechanism in these patients is pharmacological induction of hyperprolactinaemia.

The only clinical clue to premature ovarian failure may be the presence of hot flushes about which the patient should be questioned specifically. Any change in hair growth should be noted and she should be asked about acne. Progressive hirsutism associated with amenorrhoea would suggest adrenal disease, polycystic ovaries or, less frequently, virilizing ovarian tumours.

A history of breast secretion is highly significant. True but inappropriate galactorrhoea (Fig. 7.1) may persist after childbirth and breast feeding but far more frequently there is no temporal relationship to pregnancy. In these circumstances an otherwise asymptomatic pituitary tumour is very frequently present (Shearman & Fraser 1977). This statement is true irrespective of the apparent clinical association at the time these symptoms begin. Because of this it seems reasonable to abandon the confusion of names such as Chiari–Frommel, Forbes–Albright and others, no matter how appealing they may be on emotional or other grounds. It is clinically and scientifically more

acceptable to group these patients together as secondary amenorrhoea with inappropriate lactation.

Physical examination should be meticulous and include clinical assessment of thyroid status, hair growth patterns, the presence or absence of galactorrhoea and, of course, adequate vaginal examination which in some unmarried women with secondary amenorrhoea is better performed under anaesthesia. In women with secondary amenorrhoea the uterine size bears no relationship to the diagnosis or the prognosis, unless, of course, she is pregnant. Uterine hypoplasia as a *cause* of secondary amenorrhoea does not exist. The uterus is oestrogen-dependent and if oestrogen production is low, as it very frequently is in these women, the uterus will inevitably be smaller than normal.

Other rare causes of secondary amenorrhoea such as endometrial tuberculosis, pseudocyesis and lymphocytic-adenohypophysitis are discussed in Shearman (1985).

FURTHER INVESTIGATIONS

Those factors that cause the patient concern should be the key in determining what further investigations are needed. If there is any suspicion of organic disease it is mandatory to undertake the fullest investigation necessary to reach a precise diagnosis. In the clinically well woman who is concerned only with the reason for the amenorrhoea but not with her future fertility, investigation need be directed only to the exclusion of otherwise asymptomatic organic

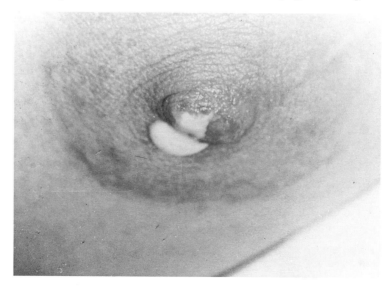

Fig. 7.1. True galactorrhoea in a nulliparous patient.

disease. Almost without exception the only problem here is an otherwise asymptomatic pituitary tumour or asymptomatic hypothyroidism.

The mandatory investigations in these women are X-ray of the skull and pituitary fossa, assay of prolactin and thyroid stimulating hormone (TSH). It is exceptionally rare for a pituitary tumour to cause secondary amenorrhoea without associated hyperprolactinaemia. It should be borne in mind that acromegaly may present with amenorrhoea and galactorrhoea but in most cases the pituitary tumour will be evident on X-ray. If the prolactin levels, X-ray of the skull and pituitary fossa and TSH (see below) are normal, then no other investigation is warranted in this otherwise healthy woman. If, however, she is worried by actual or potential infertility, investigations additional to those already mentioned are needed. Their only purpose is to decide whether or not she is suitable for the definitive treatment of ovulation induction.

If the patient is married, the decision to undertake these further investigations should rest with her and her husband. In unmarried women it is completely reasonable to assess the possibility of inducing ovulation so that a prognosis may be given. Specific treatment should not be undertaken, however, until pregnancy is desired.

Seminal analysis of the married patient's husband should be compatible with potential fertility. Apart from the basic investigations mentioned above, it is then necessary to determine if there are ova within the ovaries, as it is only in these circumstances that induction of ovulation is possible. Other and unrelated causes of infertility must also be excluded.

Although ovarian biopsy will provide absolute proof that ova are present, this is unnecessarily invasive and usually meddlesome. It is very disappointing to see a patient with remedial anovulation whose tubal status has been compromised by an unnecessary surgical assault on the ovaries.

An outline of the main investigations usually employed in the author's unit is shown in Fig. 7.2. These involve both anatomical and hormonal assessment. Any anatomical factor that may preclude pregnancy even if ovulation is induced must be determined, so tubal patency should be tested either by hysterosalpingography or laparoscopy.

Apart from assay of the pituitary hormones already mentioned, it is important to determine gonadotrophin levels in these patients. Radioimmunoassay of luteinizing hormone (LH) and follicle stimulating hormone (FSH) is the best method and in routine clinical practice two or three estimations of these hormones will be adequate to determine whether levels are low, normal or substantially increased. Apart from those few women with panhypopituitarism, it is uncommon to find low levels of LH and FSH in women with secondary amenorrhoea. If very high levels are found, this is strong evidence of a premature menopause, or far less likely, the resistant ovary syndrome.

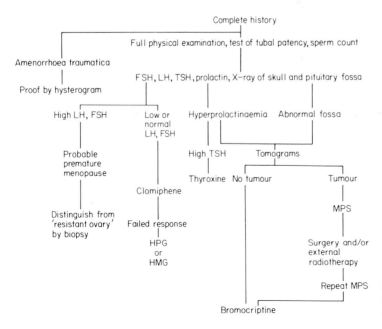

Fig. 7.2. Flow chart for investigation of secondary amenorrhoea.

Prolactin assays are mandatory to screen for the presence of pituitary tumour and will also have a major role in the selection of appropriate treatment. It is important to remember that stress, particularly including vaginal examination, will increase levels of prolactin. It is often practical to take blood for prolactin assays before examining these patients. It should also be emphasized that otherwise asymptomatic hypothyroidism can rarely present with hyperprolactinaemia with or without galactorrhoea and amenorrhoea. It is for this reason that TSH assays are needed. Thyrotrophin releasing factor (TRF), as well as increasing TSH levels, will also increase the secretion of prolactin. As will be discussed below, the appropriate treatment for these very few women is thyroxine.

The true place of multiple pituitary stimulation (MPS) (Mortimer et al. 1973) is now becoming clearer. This is a complex investigation that generates a very large number of radioimmunoassays and a substantial cost. Basal levels of growth hormone, cortisol, TSH, prolactin, LH and FSH are assessed and then measured further after a bolus injection of insulin (0.1 unit/kg body weight), gonadotrophin-releasing factor (GnRF, $100 \mu g$), and TRF ($200 \mu g$). Typical results in a patient with hyperprolactinaemia and pituitary tumour are shown in Table 7.1. Research needs apart, the only justification in clinical practice for this procedure seems to be in a patient who has a pituitary tumour.

It might be noted that the results in Table 7.1 show a normal capacity in these patients to release gonadotrophins. The old idea that amenorrhoea with pituitary tumours is due to compression of the pituitary is not tenable. Hyperprolactinaemia in its own right will induce secondary amenorrhoea.

X-rays of the pituitary fossa need to be viewed with a great deal of care. A large tumour will show ballooning of the fossa with erosion of the floor and/or clinoid processes, while with small tumours the only abnormality frequently seen is doubling or blistering of the floor of the fossa. Older invasive methods to outline more clearly the pituitary fossa and its environment such as arteriography and pneumoencephalography have been superseded by high resolution CT scanning. It might be noted that a better delineation of the pituitary region is obtained with coronal reconstruction of CT scans than with axial reconstruction. Even very small tumours (microadenomata) will be detected with this technique, usually using an iodine medium given intravenously for tumour enhancement. There is no satisfactory method, hormonally, of being certain whether a tumour is present or not (Editorial Comment 1980).

It should be recognized that although most women with a pituitary tumour and hyperprolacinaemia have an uncomplicated prolactinoma, mixed tumours producing acromegaly and hyperprolactinaemia, Cushing's syndrome and hyperprolactinaemia or destructive lesions such as craniopharyngioma may also be present. It is a great error to assume that a woman with a pituitary tumour and high prolactins has only a prolactinoma (Shearman 1983).

Premature ovarian failure

If very high levels of gonadotrophins are found in association with low urinary oestrogens the patient

Table 7.1. Results of multiple pituitary stimulation from a patient with a functioning pituitary tumour.

Time (min)	Insulin hypoglycaemia			TRF stimulation		GRF stimulation	
	Glucose (mmol/l)	Plasma cortisol (nmol/l)	HGH (ng/ml)	TSH (μu/ml)	Prolactin (ng/ml)	LH (mu/ml)	FSH (mu/ml)
0	4.9	520	1	2	245	13	10
10	2.3		2				
20	0.9		10				
30				25	250	86	25
45	1.9		13				
60	2.8	780	13	12	235	61	25
90	3.8	740	4	7		51	22
120	4.7		1	4	240	45	20
150	4.3		1				
180	4.4		1				

will almost certainly be suffering from a premature menopause; much more rarely she will have the resistant ovary syndrome (Dewhurst *et al.* 1975), and here the final court of appeal is ovarian biopsy, which is preferably done by open laparotomy. This is almost the only indication for ovarian biopsy in women with secondary amenorrhoea.

If premature menopause is proven, chromosomal studies are justifiable, although this will not affect patient management. Some of these women will have mosaicism (45,X/46,XX) while others will be triple X females (47,XXX). Tissue antibody screening should be done against the thyroid, gastric parietal cells, adrenal cortex and ovary. It is not only of academic importance that an auto-immune basis needs to be established if it is present. These women are at special risk of developing true pernicious anaemia, hypothyroidism and, less frequently, auto-immune Addison's disease, and the gynaecologist can be alerted to this possibility by finding antibodies against the appropriate target cells.

The clinical and pathological spectrum of hypergonadotrophic ovarian failure is discussed by Russell *et al.* 1982. Due to the increasingly common survival of girls and women with lymphoma and some forms of leukaemia after treatment with combined radiotherapy/chemotherapy, hypergonadotrophic amenorrhoea after this treatment is being seen more frequently.

Hypothalamic amenorrhoea

These patients will have normal or low normal levels of LH and FSH, normal levels of prolactin and TSH, normal X-rays of the skull and pituitary fossa.

Polycystic ovaries

While many of these women will have the classical Stein–Leventhal syndrome of oligomenorrhoea, obesity, hirsutism and infertility, a substantial group will have secondary amenorrhoea unassociated with hirsutism or obesity. This diagnosis would be highly suspect if persistently high levels of LH were found and a high LH/FSH ratio was present. If necessary, the diagnosis may be confirmed by laparoscopy.

TREATMENT

If anovulation proves to be secondary to other organic disease such as Cushing's disease, virilizing or other functioning ovarian tumours, or adrenal tumour, then obviously the primary treatment must be directed to the primary cause. These problems will not be discussed further in this chapter. The overwhelming majority of women with secondary amenorrhoea seen by gynaecologists are clinically well and normal on physical examination. It is to this group that the remainder of the chapter will be devoted.

Surgery

The only gynaecological surgery relevant to this chapter is bilateral ovarian wedge resection, and treatment of intrauterine adhesions. Although considered by many gynaecologists to be of historical interest only, the author believes that wedge resection has a very real place in the management of some patients with proven polycystic ovaries.

Although the treatment of first choice would be clomiphene (see below), a minority of these patients will not ovulate in response to clomiphene and bilateral ovarian wedge resection should be seriously considered as a suitable alternative to the only other remaining treatment, the use of human gonadotrophins. Particularly in a country such as Australia where many women live in geographic isolation and are not able to have regular medical supervision, this operation in suitably selected patients yields very good and usually permanent results. If bilateral ovarian wedge resection is undertaken, about one-third of the ovarian mass on each side should be resected and meticulous attention should be given to haemostasis to avoid subsequent peritubal adhesions. An early and useful clinical prognostic sign is the onset of vaginal bleeding within two to four days after operation. The majority of patients who subsequently reestablish regular ovulatory menstruation have this type of bleeding. Those who do not have this 'withdrawal' bleeding are much less likely to be cured by the surgical procedure.

Asherman's syndrome

The standard treatment for this syndrome has been to break down intrauterine adhesions, usually done blindly under anaesthesia with a uterine sound. An IUD, such as a Lippes loop, has been inserted after the procedure to keep the uterine walls apart and many workers have then used oestrogens in order to increase the chances of endometrial proliferation from the undamaged basalis.

This approach is certainly successful in re-establishing menstrual bleeding and pregnancy will frequently follow. However, there is an exceptionally high incidence of morbid pregnancy mainly related to pathological adherence of the placenta (Jewelewicz et al. 1975). The reproductive future of these patients may not, however, be unrelievedly gloomy. March et al. (1978) described division of intrauterine adhesions under direct vision using an operating hysteroscope followed by treatment with oral oestrogens and a synthetic progestin. Ninety-eight per cent of these patients had restortation of normal spontaneous menstruation, while seven of ten patients who wished to conceive did so and had uncomplicated pregnancies. This gratifying improvement in results needs to be confirmed.

Hyperprolactinaemia and pituitary tumour

There is not yet a consensus about the place of surgery in the treatment of pituitary tumours of all types. There is general agreement that intracranial surgery is indicated in women with craniopharyngoima or Cushing's syndrome and it may have a place in those women with hyperprolactinaemia and acromegaly, although Bromocriptine treatment is successful in a substantial number of these women. Until relatively recently there seemed to be general agreement that a prolactinoma with an extension outside the pituitary fossa should be treated surgically. While this surgery was very rarely curative (in the sense that menstrual function was restored and prolactin levels returned to normal) there was a very real fear that if pregnancy occurred in these women, rapid enlargement due to the high oestrogen levels of pregnancy might lead to abrupt enlargement of the tumour or even pituitary apoplexy. With the more recent evidence that even large tumours will show rapid reduction in size during treatment with bromocriptine and that it may be safely used in pregnancy there is much more of a move towards medical control of the uncomplicated prolactinoma (Hammond et al. 1983, Konopka et al. 1983).

A clearer picture is also emerging of the role of surgery in microadenometa. Although high cure rates may be obtained after transphenoidal excision of these tumours, not all neurosurgical units can achieve these results. In addition it is now quite clear that recurrence of tumour may occur after apparently complete initial surgical removal. With the evidence that enlargement of microadenometa to a significant degree is uncommon, and that when

it does occur it can be controlled as a rule with bromocriptine, it is probably fair to say that the neurosurgeons are losing this particular race.

Although radiation was widely used initially in the treatment of these lesions on the assumption that it would reduce possible growth rate at a later stage and particular during pregnancy, there now is agreement that there is little place for radiotherapy in the treatment of prolactinomas because of the very high incidence of panhypopituitarism several years after this treatment.

MEDICAL TREATMENT

Thyroxine

Gynaecologists have traditionally, if rather illogically, treated many women suffering from secondary amenorrhoea with thyroxine or other thyroid extracts. It is now clear that there has been some scientific merit in this treatment, at least for a small minority of the women so treated. About 4% of our own patients with hyperprolactinaemia are shown to have elevated levels of TSH. While many of these women will have evidence of hypothyroidism as indicated by assays of tri-iodothyronine and thyroxine, some of the levels are only marginally low. Provided the increase in TSH is confirmed then treatment with thyroxine will cause restoration of both TSH and prolactin to normal, and will be followed by regular ovulatory menstruation. It should be stressed that in the absence of proven hypothyroidism, thyroxine treatment has no place in the management of secondary amenorrhoea.

Gonadotrophin-releasing factor (GnRF)

If GnRF is given in high doses or very frequently by injection, 'down regulation' of the pituitary occurs and there is further depression of LH and FSH. However, given by pulsed intravenous or subcutaneous administration, there is now very good evidence that GnRF is a highly satisfactory treatment for women with hypogonadotrophic hypogonadism or hypothalamic secondary amenorrhoea who wish to ovulate and conceive (Hammond et al. 1979, Ory 1983, Pepperell 1983). It should be noted that the pumps to administer this drug are very expensive and that in many countries it is not approved for the purpose of induction of ovulation. At the time of writing, this treatment should therefore be regarded as a research approach.

Gonadal steroids

There is some evidence that a minority of women with hypothalamic amenorrhoea will begin to ovulate after a series of induced bleedings with gonadal steroids, presumably as a placebo effect. Since, however, one of the commonest clinical associations in patients presenting with amenorrhoea is 'post pill amenorrhoea' it seems quixotic to use this approach. However, there may possibly be a role for steroidal treatment of this type in women with the resistant ovary syndrome. Brosens et al. (1979) describe a very small number of patients with the resistant ovary syndrome who had hormone replacement therapy with cycloprogynova* on the assumption that they had premature menopause. Following this treatment, spontaneous pregnancy and ovulation ensued and six similar cases have been published in the literature. There are not yet sufficient data to show that this treatment is genuinely therapeutic and, if it is, what proportion of successes could be expected but it is an approach worth bearing in mind for this extremely rare clinical condition. The author has tried this in three patients, without success.

Bromocriptine

Although the pharmaceutical industry is sometimes accused of developing drugs in search of a disease, this allegation cannot be cast at bromocriptine. It is one of the nicer coincidences of human physiology and developmental pharmacology that a drug specifically suppressing prolactin secretion was developed concurrently with the proof that prolactin did exist, after all, as a separate discrete hormone in the human. An exhaustive discussion of these subjects will be found in Crosignani and Robyn (1977).

Within the context of this chapter bromocriptine is the treatment of choice for those amenorrhoeic women with hyperprolactinaemia in whom there is no indication for surgery, or when surgery/radiotherapy has been unsuccessful.

The only commonly observed side-effects with bromocriptine therapy are nausea, occasionally with vomiting, and, less frequently, postural hypotension. Headaches are sometimes described. In the author's experience, almost all women develop tolerance to these side effects as treatment continues and only one patient has withdrawn from treatment because of the severity of vomiting.

The very substantial advantage of this treatment is that it is specific in suppressing prolactin secretion. This then allows normal spontaneous cyclic release of FSH and LH and for this reason the incidence of multiple pregnancies following bromocriptine treatment is no different from that seen in the normal population. Although it is not yet possible to give an absolutely clear bill of health for teratogenicity, the incidence of abnormality in babies that were conceived as a result of this treatment is, to date, no different from that seen in other populations.

The initial dose is 1.25 mg given for seven days last thing at night with food when in bed. This regime will certainly reduce the incidence of nausea and postural hypotension. After this first week, the dose is increased to 1.25 mg twice daily with food and then to the usual definitive dose of 2.5 mg twice daily. Measurement of prolactin secretion is vital to assess response. If after two to three weeks on the final dosage already mentioned, prolactin levels are still above the normal range for the laboratory concerned, the dosage should be increased further. In practice this is seldom necessary.

Although prolactin levels are usually suppressed very promptly, ovulation does not usually return until three to six weeks after prolactin levels have been shown to be normal.

Very rarely doses even greater than 20 mg a day will still not suppress prolactin levels to normal. In a small number of these women where pregnancy is desired, addition of gonadotrophins to the therapeutic regime may be necessary.

Even when pregnancy is induced successfully, prolonged follow-up of these patients is mandatory. The author's results of follow-up (Rowe et al. 1979) show that all of the patients who have been treated with bromocriptine have had recurrence of hyperprolactinaemia after delivery and breast feeding have been completed. Although this recurrence is usual, there is some evidence that prolonged suppression with bromocriptine may have continuing effects after treatment is withdrawn (Eversman et al. 1979).

Pituitary tumours have been found at follow-up in some of our very long-term patients who had no such evidence when first seen. For this reason assay of prolactin after terminating breast feeding, and repeat cone views of the pituitary fossa, if indicated, are mandatory.

Other dopaminergic drugs will certainly appear in the future and information is now available on an additional synthetic ergot derivative, lisuride (de Cecco et al. 1979).

---

* Oestradiol valerate 1 mg for 21 days, with norgestrel 0.5 mg for the last 10 of these days.

Bromocriptine is now being used more widely in the long-term management of these patients even when conception is not desired. Substantial osteoporosis occurs more rapidly in hyperprolactinaemic amenorrhoeic women than it does in women with normoprolactinaemic amenorrhoea including a normal menopause (Schlechte *et al.* 1983). Long-term bromocriptine treatment is a rational alternative in these women to the use of oestrogens and progestins such as would be used in a normal post-menopausal patient.

Clomiphene citrate

Clomiphene is an anti-oestrogen that acts predominantly on the hypothalamus. Where successful its action is by increasing the secretion of FSH and LH. While the best results are obtained in women who have relatively high levels of endogenous oestrogens, it works sufficiently well in those patients with very low oestrogen secretion to make this the treatment of first choice in women with normoprolactinaemic amenorrhoea not due to a premature menopause.

True side effects with clomiphene are usually of a minor nature. A substantial minority of women will experience hot flushes which are like those of the menopause and are explained by the antioestrogenic action of the drug. Transient blurring of vision may be noted and very rarely there will be loss of scalp hair. In 7% of treatment cycles ovarian enlargement, usually asymptomatic, will occur and for this reason the patient must have a vaginal examination between each treatment course.

If ovarian enlargement is detected on vaginal examination, no further treatment should be given until complete regression occurs which usually takes two to three weeks. Provided these precautions are taken and the dosage schedule described here is not exceeded, serious side effects will be extremely rare.

When pregnancy occurs there is no increase in the risk of abortion and the only specific complication is an increase in the incidence of multiple birth. About one in ten conceptions due to clomiphene treatment will be multiple. While, overwhelmingly, these are twin pregnancies, in the author's unit there have been two triplet pregnancies. For practical purposes the main consideration is the increased incidence of twinning which should be explained to the patient and her partner before the treatment begins.

When ovulation occurs it is usually 7–12 days after starting a course of treatment. The initial dosage is 50 mg daily for five days. Basal body temperature is recorded throughout. If by day 30 menstruation does not occur and the patient is not pregnant, 100 mg are given daily in a divided dose for five days. If after a further 30 days menstruation does not occur and the patient is not pregnant, 50 mg are given three times daily for five days. If there is no response to 150 mg daily for five days some women will respond to higher doses up to 250 mg daily for five days but responses to higher dose levels have not been seen. If, however, ovulation is induced by any of these courses, clomiphene continues at that dose level, each new course starting on day five of the cycle until the patient conceives or withdraws from treatment. As already indicated, vaginal examination is mandatory between treatment courses where there has been some response.

Some patients previously suffering from amenorrhoea will have anovulatory bleeding with clomiphene. In these women there may be justification for using human chorionic gonadotrophin to act as an 'LH surge', the usual dose being 5000 international units given eight or nine days after the first day's treatment with clomiphene. The pregnancy rate is disappointing with this combined treatment.

It has been known for many years that there is a relatively wide discrepancy between the rate of 'apparent ovulation' and pregnancy. Various factors have been described that may contribute to this disparity such as luteinization of ovarian stroma, luteinization of unruptured follicles, defects in corpus luteum function and ovum entrapment. Since clomiphene is an anti-oestrogen it is not surprising that it has substantial effects on cervical mucin. It has been suggested that part of the low pregnancy rate may be attributed to poor penetrability of the cervical mucus and because of this some investigators recommend starting treatment on day two of the menstrual cycle rather than day five. However, there are no hard data that can explain this dilemma.

Human gonadotrophins

These preparations should be used only if there is evidence that they will succeed in inducing ovulation and if alternative treatments such as clomiphene or bromocriptine have been used, where indicated, and have failed to produce ovulation. Two main types of preparation are available throughout the world. One is extracted from the urine of postmenopausal women (HMG), the second is extracted from human pituitaries at the time of autopsy (HPG). Each of these preparations is equally effective and each contains a mixture of FSH and LH. While human menopausal gonadotrophins are most widely used, in several countries including Australia, Sweden and New Zealand, pituitary gonadotrophins have been employed for many years.

The theoretical basis of treatment is disarmingly simple. Follicular maturation is induced with daily injections of HMG or HPG and the ovulation is induced with HCG. While cumulative conception rates of up to 91% can be expected (Dor *et al.* 1980), in practice the treatment is complicated, often difficult and sometimes dangerous.

Since the material used is homologous, true side effects in the usual pharmacological sense are exceptionally rare. The author has had one patient who developed antibodies against LH during treatment which precluded further use of these drugs (Healy *et al.* 1978).

The major difficulties relate to problems in control of dosage, clinically reflected in a high incidence of multiple pregnancies and the development of the 'hyperstimulation syndrome'. The incidence of multiple pregnancy varies widely in published series from a high of about 60% down to a relatively low figure of about 20%. In the Australian series, about 20% of conceptions are multiple and while most of these are twins, 3% are triplets. Obviously maternal and fetal problems increase substantially if there is a multiple pregnancy, particularly with higher multiples. There is some evidence that the incidence of ectopic pregnancy may be increased in these patients (McBain *et al.* 1980).

Hyperstimulation syndrome can be a grave complication of treatment given to a previously healthy woman. The best classification of this complication remains that of the Israeli group (Rabau *et al.* 1967). In very severe cases there will be gross ovarian enlargement, ascites, hydrothorax and haemo-concentration of such a degree that arterial thromboses have been described.

Nobody can yet claim to have developed an infallible method of reducing the incidence of multiple pregnancies to that seen in women conceiving after spontaneous ovulation, nor of avoiding completely the risk of some degree of hyperstimulation. The various methods of control that have been utilized to minimize these complications have been discussed in detail elsewhere (Shearman 1978). Most people using human gonadotrophins now believe that some method of control based on the endocrinological response of the patient is essential and gives far better control than those methods based on purely clinical

assessment, such as ovarian size and the amount and quality of cervical mucus. In Australia it is customary to monitor the patient's urinary oestrogen response or, alternatively, plasma oestradiol levels during the administration of HPG, changing the dose if necessary during a course of treatment. When urinary or plasma oestrogens reach a level which is known to be compatible with ovulation, ovulation is induced by giving a single dose of chorionic gonadotrophin (3000–5000 units) and the supporting doses of 1000–1500 units of chorionic gonadotrophin at intervals of four to seven days in the luteal phase. The major problems of hyperstimulation appear to occur most frequently if the inducing dose of chorionic gonadotrophin is given when urinary or plasma levels of oestrogens are substantially higher than those seen during physiological ovulation. It is probable, but by no means certain, that a high rate of multiple conception and particularly multiple pregnancies beyond twins can be reduced by the same means. This method of control has recently been reassessed and examined by Biggs *et al.* (1978).

There is no doubt that this method of control presents many problems. It is very tedious for the patient, imposes a heavy burden on laboratory facilities and excludes patients who by reason of geography cannot reach a suitably equipped laboratory every day or arrange to have the appropriate sample of biological fluid sent to such a laboratory almost every day. Despite these difficulties, control of this type has the overwhelming advantage of safety.

Twenty years ago Shearman (1966b) discussed this problem in some detail and said at that time, 'Whichever treatment is used, the patient and her husband should be fully appraised of the problems and potential dangers. The final decision to be treated or not should be left to them. Although induction of ovulation is in a sense life-giving, it is not life-saving. The inherent problems in this type of treatment should be examined with this in mind.' Nothing has happened in the last decade to suggest to the writer that he should change this view.

REFERENCES

ASHERMAN J. G. (1950) *J. Obstet. Gynaec. Brit. Cwlth.*, **57**, 892.
BERGH T., MILLIUS S. J. & WIDE L. (1978) *Brit. med J.*, **i**, 875.
BIGGS J. S. G., HENNESSEY J. & JONES I. (1978) *Obstet. and Gynec. N.Y.*, **51**, 10.
BROSENS I. A., KONICKX P. H. & VLAEMYNCK G. (1979) *Infertility*, **2**, 219.

DE CECCO L., VENTURINI P.L., RAGNI N., ROSSATO P., MAGANZA C., GAGGERO G. & HOROWSKI R. (1979) *Brit. J. Obstet. Gynaec.*, **86**, 905.

CROSIGNANI P.G. & ROBYN C. (1977) *Prolactin and Human Reproduction.* Academic Press, London.

DEWHURST C.J., DE KOOS E.B. & FERREIRA H.P. (1975) *Brit. J. Obstet. Gynaec.*, **82**, 341.

DOR J., ITZKOWIC D.J., MASHIACH S., LUNENFELD B. & SERR D.M. (1980) *Amer. J. Obstet. Gynec.*, **136**, 102.

EDITORIAL COMMENT (1980) *Lancet*, **i**, 517.

EVERSMAN T., FAHLBUSCH R., FJOSK H.K. & VON WERDER K. (1979) *Acta Endocr. (Kbh.)*, **92**, 413.

FOIX A., BRUNO R.O., DAVISON T. & LEMA B. (1966) *Amer. J. Obstet. Gynec.*, **96**, 1027.

FRISCH R.E., GOTZ-WELBERGEN A.V., MCARTHUR J.W., ALBRIGHT T., WITSCHI J., BULLEN B., BIRMHOLT J., REED R.B. & HERMANN H. (1981) *J. Amer. med. Ass.* **246**, 1559.

HAMMOND C.B., WIEBE R.H., HANEY A.F. & YANCY S.G. (1979) *Amer. J. Obstet. Gynec.*, **135**, 924.

HAMMOND C.B., HANEY A.F., LAND M.R., VAN DER MERWE J.V., ORY S.J. & WIEBE R.H. (1983) *Amer. J. Obstet. Gynec.* **147**, 148.

HEALY D.L., FRASER I.S., LEE V.W.K., SHEARMAN R.P. & BURGER H.G. (1978) *J. clin. Endocr.*, **47**, 823.

JEWELEWICZ R., KHALAF S., NEUWIRTH R.S. & VAN DE WIELE R.L. (1975) *Obstet. and Gynec. N.Y.*, **47**, 701.

JEWELEWICZ R. & VAN DE WIELE R.L. (1980) *Amer. J. Obstet. Gynec.*, **136**, 339.

KONOPKA P., RAYMOND J.P., MERCENON R.E. & SEMEZE J. (1983) *Amer. J. Obstet. Gynec.*, **146**, 935.

MCBAIN J.C., EVANS J.H., PEPPERELL R.J., ROBINSON H.P., SMITH M.A. & BROWN J.B. (1980) *Brit. J. Obstet. Gynaec.*, **87**, 5.

MARCH C.M., ISRAEL R. & MARCH A.D. (1978) *Amer. J. Obstet. Gynec.*, **130**, 653.

MORTIMER C.H., BESSER G.M., MCNEILLY A.S., TURNBRIDGE W.M.G., GOMEZ-PAN A. & HALL R. (1973) *Clin. Endocr.*, **2**, 317.

ORY S.J. (1983) *Fertil. and Steril.*, **39**, 577.

PEPPERELL R.J. (1983) *Fertil. and Steril.*, **40**, 1.

RABAU E., SERR D.M., MASCHIACH S., INSLER V., SALOMY M. & LUNENFELD B. (1967) *Brit. med J.*, **4**, 446.

ROWE T.C., SHEARMAN R.P. & FRASER I.S. (1979) *Obstet. and Gynec. N.Y.*, **54**, 535.

RUSSELL P., BANNANTYNE P., SHEARMAN R.P., FRASER I.S. & CORBETT P. (1982) *Int. J. Gynec. Path.*, **1**, 185.

SCHLECHTE J.A., SHERMAN B. & MARTIN R. (1983) *J. clin. Endocr.*, **56**, 1120.

SHEARMAN R.P. (1966a) *Lancet*, **ii**, 1110.

SHEARMAN R.P. (1966b) *Aust. Ann. Med.*, **15**, 266.

SHEARMAN R.P. (1978) *Mod. Med. Aust.*, July, 33.

SHEARMAN R.P. (1983) in *Progress in Gynaecology.*, (Studd J. ed) **3**, 257.

SHEARMAN R.P. (1985) *Clinical Reproductive Endocrinology.* Churchill Livingstone, London.

SHEARMAN R.P. & FRASER I.S. (1977) *Lancet*, **i**, 1195.

VESSEY M.P., WRIGHT N.H., MCPERSON K. & WIGGINS P. (1978) *Brit. med. J.*, **i**, 265.

CHAPTER 8
HIRSUTISM AND VIRILISM

RODNEY P. SHEARMAN

It is easier to define virilism than hirsutism. Although one may define hirsutism as 'excessive growth of hair in an abnormal position on the body' there are immediate difficulties in trying to quantitate the word excessive. Initially, it appears reasonable to apply the word excessive, in this context, to a degree of hair-growth that worries the patient. It must be admitted that some women will become obsessed with a degree of hirsutism that would escape all but the most careful scrutiny, but if the patient is worried she is not to be dismissed lightly.

Hirsutism is very commonly present without any evidence of virilism; virilism is very rarely, if ever, present (apart from the neonate) without evidence of hirsutism. Virilism is defined here as one or more of the following: clitoral hypertrophy; breast atrophy; male-type baldness and deepening of the voice. It is usual to include amenorrhoea in this spectrum but it has been deliberately excluded here, both because amenorrhoea unassociated with actual or potential virilism is common, and because some grave cases of virilism may present with ovulatory or menstrual function still intact.

A great deal of progress has been made in unravelling the endocrinological intricacies of hirsutism; a comprehensive and good review will be found in Hammerstein *et al.* (1980). The last decade has also seen some improved prospects for the treatment of this vexing condition.

THE BIOCHEMISTRY OF HIRSUTISM AND VIRILISM

Hirsutism may be the outcome of excessive androgen stimulation or excessive end-organ response. Virilism is invariably due to excessive androgenic stimulation. Although the prime mover may be as disparate as the hypothalamus, the pituitary, or even bronchogenic carcinoma, the final source of production in the non-pregnant individual will always be steroidogenic tissue, either the adrenal cortex or the gonad. It is fortunate, and embryologically understandable, that the ovary and the adrenal cortex share many common steps in biosynthesis.

Figure 8.1 shows a skeletal outline of some of the more important pathways of adrenocortical biosynthesis. Aldosterone is excluded as it is not relevant to the present topic. It will be noted: that in the synthesis of cortisol from progesterone, sequential hydroxylation at C_{17}, C_{21} and C_{11} occurs, steps of considerable importance in the genesis of congenital adrenal hyperplasia; that androstenedione is produced from 17-hydroxyprogesterone; and that oestrogens are produced from androgenic precursors.

The last two statements are equally valid for the ovary, but as the ovary possesses neither 21- nor 11-hydroxylases, the first is not applicable.

It should also be noted that alternate pathways occur both physiologically and pathologically. An important alternate pathway is present in ovary and/or adrenal in either circumstance (Fig. 8.2). Conversion of androgens of weak biological activity, such as androstenedione or dehydro-epianodrosterone (DHEA), to the strongest androgen, testosterone, may occur either in abnormal ovarian or adrenal tissue, particularly the former, or by conversion elsewhere in the body (Fig. 8.3). The chemical similarity but different biological potency of three of these androgens should be stressed (Fig. 8.4). Although the hair follicle and the sebaceous glands can respond to testosterone, most of the androgenic activity of testosterone in these tissues occurs after conversion to dihydrotestosterone by a 5α reductase.

It has also been recognized that a minority of women with hyperprolactinaemia will have greasy skin, acne and sometimes hirsutism, probably due to the direct action of prolactin on the production of adrenal androgens (Parker *et al.* 1978).

It is necessary to have a grasp of the significance of some hormone assays that are used in assessing

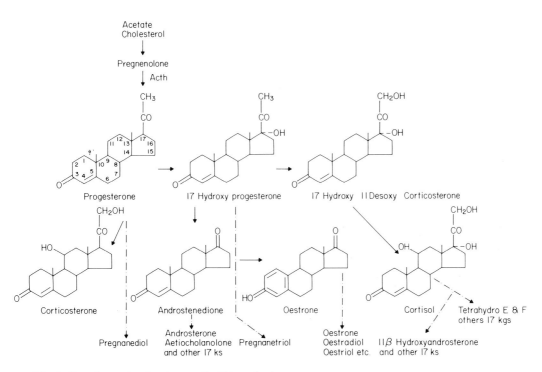

Fig. 8.1. Outline of some steps in adrenocortical biosynthesis.

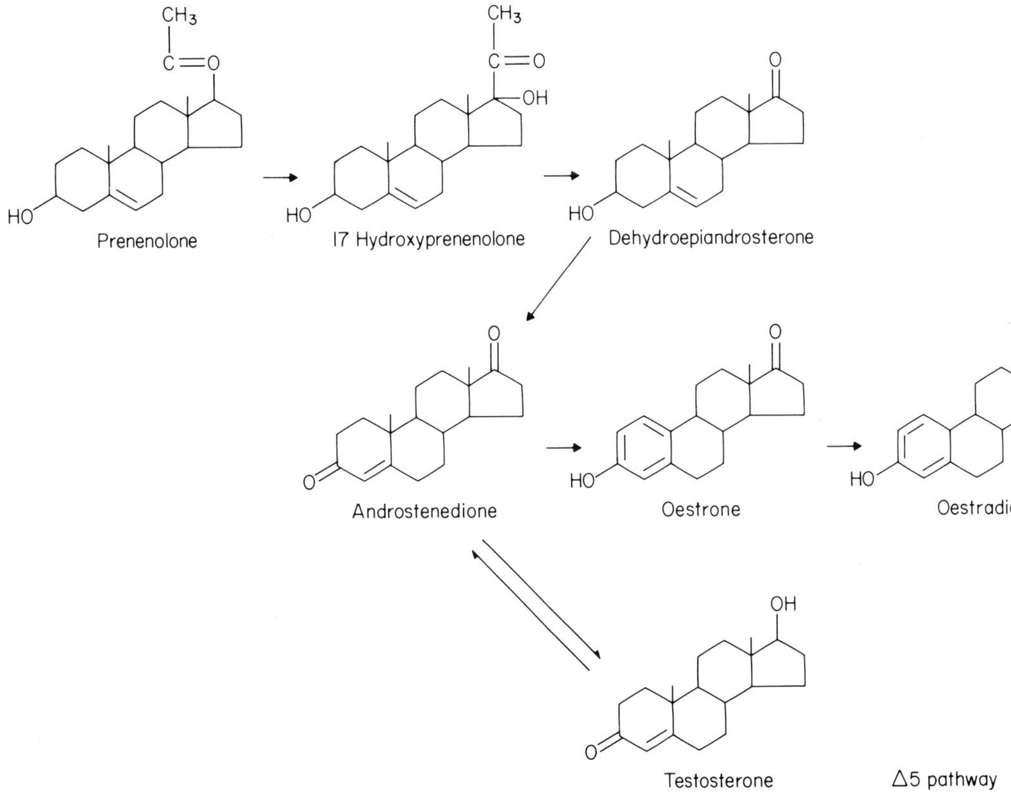

Fig. 8.2. An alternate pathway of steroid biosynthesis.

the clinical problems to be discussed in this chapter. Some, or all, of the following may be employed.

1   Prolactin, LH and FSH. (Discussed fully elsewhere in this book.)
2   Cortisol and ACTH.
3   Testosterone.
4   17-hydroxyprogesterone and dehydroepiandrosterone sulphate.

Cortisol and ACTH

Cortisol may be measured by radioimmunoassay in plasma and, very usefully, as urinary-free cortisol in urine. It should be recognized that plasma assays measure, with routine methods, total plasma cortisol and not the biologically effective component which is unbound to corticosteroid-binding globulin (CBG). Normally, there is a significant circardian rhythm— high levels in the morning, low levels at night. The diurnal variation is lost in Cushing's syndrome and depressive states. Radioimmunoassay for ACTH is very helpful in the differential diagnosis of Cushing's syndrome.

Probably the most sensitive method of assessing tissue exposure to biologically active cortisol is to measure urinary-free cortisol over a 24-hour period. This is an extremely useful method in screening patients suspected of having Cushing's syndrome.

Testosterone

Testosterone is most conveniently measured by radioimmunoassay in plasma. As with cortisol, routine measurements reflect total levels of testosterone, both free and that majority bound to sex hormone-binding globulin. As will be discussed below, there is good evidence that increases in free testosterone will be found in most women with 'idiopathic' hirsutism even where total testosterone levels are normal (Paulson *et al.* 1977). However, the assay methods for free testosterone are very tedious and are not available in many centres. Although assay of dihydrotestosterone is sometimes of interest and indeed important in some intersexes, in the majority of patients with hirsutism this assay is of little clinical use.

17-hydroxyprogesterone and dehydroepiandrosterone sulphate (DHAS)

Examination of Figs. 8.1 and 8.2 will show where these steroids fit into the pathway of synthesis. 17-hydroxyprogesterone is produced by both the ovary and the adrenal cortex. Its particular value is in patients where adrenal hyperplasia is suspected as plasma levels will always be increased. This is discussed more fully in Chapter 3. Dehydroepiandrosterone is secreted by the adrenal in conjugated form as the sulphate and is a uniquely adrenal steroid. Substantial increases in DHAS, therefore, point very strongly to an adrenal cause for hirsutism, recollecting, as will be discussed below, that the majority of women with polycystic ovaries also have some secondary adrenal involvement.

THE CLINICAL PROBLEMS

The individual syndromes producing hirsutism or virilism will be discussed initially. A clinical approach to the investigation and differential diagnosis of the hirsute patient will then be presented.

The features of the various syndromes are most conveniently considered under the following headings.

1   Congenital causes.
2   Iatrogenic virilization.
3   Masculinizing tumours of the ovary.
4   Adrenal hyperplasia.
5   Tumours of the adrenal cortex.
6   Cushing's syndrome.
7   Stein–Leventhal syndrome (polycystic ovaries).
8   'Idiopathic' hirsutism.
9   Acromegaly.
10 Hirsutism during pregnancy.

1   CONGENITAL CAUSES

For the most part, these have been considered in Chapter 3. Congenital adrenal hyperplasia has been discussed in that chapter and will be mentioned briefly in (4) below. Very rare congenital anomalies associated with hirsutism such as *hypertrichosis lanuginosa* and the Cornelia de Lang syndrome may need to be considered (Muller 1969).

2   IATROGENIC VIRILIZATION

This may occur during treatment with androgens. There are no absolute indications to use androgens in women, and in most women virilized in this way this unfortunate complication is unnecessary and

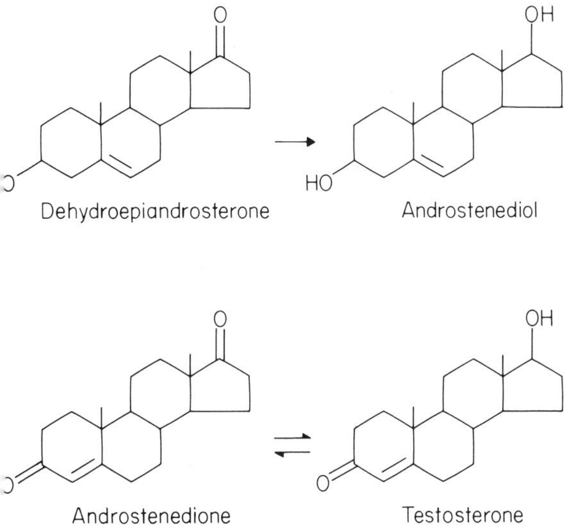

Fig. 8.3. Interconversion of some androgens.

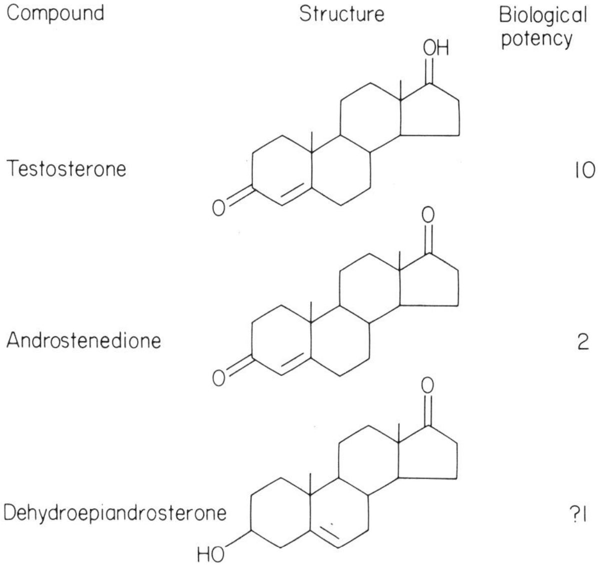

Fig. 8.4. The chemical similarity, but biological disparity of three androgens.

avoidable. With the exception of its use in some women with disseminated breast carcinoma, testosterone has little valid place in the treatment of women. If used for any of the more arguable reasons (endometriosis, frigidity, premenstrual tension) the dose should not exceed 150–200mg of methyltestosterone by mouth in any one month. In susceptible women even this amount will cause acne, or even early hirsutes.

Danazol is now widely used in the treatment of endometriosis and in a minority of women will cause acne and hirsutism.

It should be recognized that Dilantin can cause acne and hirsutism in some susceptible women. It is also worth noting that drugs that increase prolactin secretion, and in clinical practice the commonest group are the phenothiazines, may also be associated with skin changes due to the effect of the hyperprolactinaemia on the adrenal cortex.

3 MASCULINIZING TUMOURS OF THE OVARY

The pathology of ovarian tumours has long been a field of conflict among morbid anatomists. With functioning tumours of the ovary it may be impossible to correlate structure with function. Although the classical arrhenoblastoma is clearly masculinizing, virilism may also occur with granulosal tumours, thecomas, luteomas, hilus-cell tumours or adrenal-rest tumours. Although usually endocrinologically inert, pseudomucinous cystadenomata, Brenner and Krukenberg tumours may rarely cause virilism. The problem is fully discussed by Prunty (1967).

It is doubtful whether the endocrine changes attributable to the dysgerminoma or gonadoblastoma are truly causal. Where virilism does occur it is more reasonably explained on chromosomal and other intrauterine influences (Chapter 3).

Virilizing ovarian tumours may present at any age. The clinical picture is usually one of initial defeminization (amenorrhoea and breast atrophy) with concurrent, or rapidly following, hirsutism and virilism (Fig. 8.5). The changes in personality may be striking, and have been well documented by Elliott and Heseltine (1967).

Clinically, the presence of palpable ovarian pathology would suggest such a diagnosis. These tumours, particularly hilus-cell tumours, are often so small that they are not palpable, in which case hormonal investigations are of considerable assistance.

An ovarian cause for hirsutism/virilism should be highly suspect if there is a substantial increase in plasma testosterone. If normal levels of 17-hydroxyprogesterone and DHAS are found, this would firmly increase the suspicion.

If significant ovarian enlargement cannot be felt on clinical examination, or if obesity makes such an examination difficult, ultrasonography will often

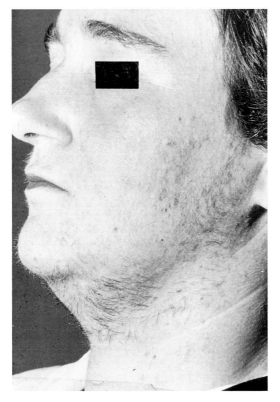

Fig. 8.5. Patient with arrhenoblastoma. (From Elliot & Heseltine 1967, by courtesy of the editor of *Australian and New Zealand Journal of Obstetrics and Gynaecology.*)

prove a helpful investigation, but the final court of appeal may be laparotomy.

4 ADRENAL HYPERPLASIA

Although this condition has been discussed more fully in Chapter 3, it must be referred to briefly here. The more severe forms will usually cross the obstetrician's path when a child is born with equivocal external genitals. If salt loss does not dictate early treatment, there may be progressive virilism with very early growth of pubic hair.

Occasionally, adrenal hyperplasia may not become obvious until after puberty. In these cases, hirsutism and oligomenorrhoea progressing to amenorrhoea are usual, but normal ovulatory menstruation may persist in a minority of women. The biochemical disturbance in these patients is essentially similar to that seen in infants with congenital hyperplasia (Brooks *et al.* 1960). In the most common form where there is a 21-hydroxylase deficiency, 17-hydroxyprogester-

one and DHAS will be increased in plasma. If urinary assays are used, 17-oxosteroids are always increased. While plasma testosterone will usually be increased, the increase is far smaller than that seen in patients with hirsutism associated with ovarian causes.

In patients presenting after puberty, a distinction will need to be made between adrenal tumour and adrenal hyperplasia and this can usually be done by a formal dexamethasone suppression test. Suppression tests should be done and interpreted properly. After two days for basal study, dexamethasone is given at a dose of 0.5 mg four times daily for two days and then 2 mg four times daily for four days. In the presence of adrenal hyperplasia there will be a very prompt fall in 17-hydroxyprogesterone and urinary 17-oxosteroids. With adrenal tumour, although there may be some fall, complete suppression does not occur. It should be noted that DHAS has an extremely long plasma half-life, and it is an inappropriate steroid to examine during a dexamethasone suppression test.

Jones and Klingensmith (1985) have provided an excellent historical and clinical review of this fascinating problem.

5 TUMOURS OF THE ADRENAL CORTEX

These tumours may produce a wide variety of clinical features: primary aldosteronism, Cushing's syndrome, virilization in women or gynaecomastia in men. The endocrine disturbances may be related to the area of the cortex from which the tumour arises. Aldosterone is secreted by the glomerulosa, and tumours of this area will cause hypertension and potassium loss (Conn & Louis 1956). Pure tumours of the fascicular zone will secrete excessive amounts of cortisol and corticosterone, causing Cushing's syndrome. Neoplasia of the reticularis will produce a clinical picture that varies with the age and sex of the patient and the relative amounts of androgen and oestrogen secreted. Very frequently there is considerable overlap in the clinical picture produced, particularly in the two last-mentioned groups. Some patients with Cushing's syndrome will present with virilization, whereas in others this may be minimal.

Virilizing tumours may occur at any age. In children the onset is usually with growth of axillary and pubic hair, development of acne, clitoral enlargement and deepening voice. In the adult the clinical picture may be identical with that of virilizing ovarian tumours or adrenal hyperplasia. Occasionally, ovulatory menstruation may persist, but amenorrhoea is the general rule.

These virilizing tumours are associated with very large increases of plasma 17-hydroxyprogesterone and DHAS. With adrenal carcinoma the increases are even greater. While testosterone is increased it is usually not nearly as high as the levels found in women with primary ovarian pathology. It should be emphasized, again, that if a dexamethasone suppression is done there may be partial suppression of these increased steroids but not to the same degree that is seen with adrenal hyperplasia.

6 CUSHING'S SYNDROME

When this syndrome was first described in 1932, Cushing ascribed it to pituitary dysfunction. In 1943 Albright pointed out that overactivity of the adrenal cortex, whether from hyperplasia or tumour, was an invariable feature of this syndrome. It is now recognized that the changes in secretion of ACTH are a fundamental problem in Cushing's syndrome related to adrenal hyperplasia and this is obviously of significance in determining the correct treatment.

The symptoms and signs of Cushing's syndrome in its classical form are well known, but the spectacular combination of obesity, moon face, cutaneous striae, subcutaneous ecchymoses, osteoporosis, hyperglycaemia, hirsutism and amenorrhoea is rarely seen in any one patient, and often some of the 'classical' manifestations may be absent. The disease is more common in women, and may be difficult to recognize in its early states.

The essence of Cushing's syndrome is overproduction of cortisol, and final diagnosis will depend on confirming this overproduction. Apart from the unusual patient with episodic Cushing's syndrome, this presents no difficulty. Urinary-free cortisol will be substantially above the normal range. In addition, the normal diurnal variation in plasma cortisol and ACTH will be lost as is the ability to suppress the morning peak of ACTH and cortisol with dexamethasone given at midnight. A useful routine is to take plasma for cortisol and ACTH examination at 8 am and midnight. Immediately after the midnight sample of blood is taken 2 mg of dexamethasone should be given and the assays repeated the following morning. If increased urinary-free cortisol is associated with loss of diurnal rhythm and inability to suppress the morning peak, then the diagnosis is almost assured. X-ray of the skull and pituitary fossa is mandatory since, in the majority of cases, the primary disturb-

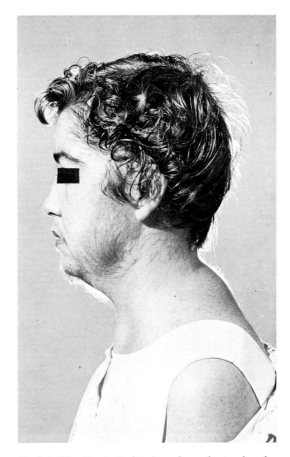

Fig. 8.6. Hirsutism in Cushing's syndrome due to adrenal carcinoma.

ance is in the hypothalamus/pituitary. However, the disease may be due to neoplasm which in some patients may be malignant (Fig. 8.6). Whole body CT scanning can be invaluable in locating adrenal tumours.

7 STEIN–LEVENTHAL SYNDROME (POLYCYSTIC OVARIES)

It is now 40 years since Stein and Leventhal first described this baffling syndrome. The classical picture is of an obese, hirsute, infertile female with oligomenorrhoea and bilaterally enlarged polycystic ovaries. It is now apparent that obesity is not common, and that while hirsutism is customary, it is by no means universal. It may, however, be impressive (Fig. 8.7). Clitoral enlargement is uncommon, but may occur.

The enlarged ovaries may be difficult to feel on examination, even under anaesthesia, and additional

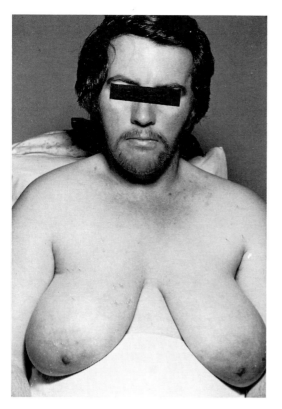

Fig. 8.7. Extensive hirsutism associated with polycystic ovaries. (From Shearman 1969, by courtesy of Charles C. Thomas, Publisher.)

help by laparoscopy is frequently needed. Occasionally, the ovaries, although polycystic, may not be enlarged. The macroscopic appearance is typical, but microscopic examination of the ovarian tissue reveals no unique feature.

The most constant endocrinological change is an absolute increase in levels of LH and a high LH/FSH ratio. Plasma testosterone is frequently slightly above the normal range. 17-hydroxyprogesterone will be normal but DHAS is usually increased, although not to the level seen in adrenal hyperplasia. This DHAS is coming from the adrenal cortex. This should not be surprising as the evidence that the adrenal cortex is secondarily involved in the majority of patients with polycystic ovaries, although old, is still incontrovertible (Shearman 1961, Shearman & Cox 1965). Hypothalamic pituitary function in this syndrome has been fully discussed by Rebar et al. (1976). About 10% of these patients will have elevated levels of prolactin.

8 'IDIOPATHIC' HIRSUTISM

This classification remains a convenient categorization of these women with hirsutism who lack completely any evidence of organic disease. While it seems indisputable that there are some women whose hair follicles are excessively responsive to a normal androgenic stimulus, there is now very good evidence that many of these women, while having normal reproductive function and normal urinary oxosteroids do have increased levels of plasma testosterone (Abraham & Chakmakjian 1974, Casey et al. 1966) and, in particular, plasma-free testosterone levels (Paulson et al. 1977). The excessive androgens may come from either the adrenal or the ovary, or both (Casey 1975).

9 ACROMEGALY

This is an uncommon disease, and it is even less common for hirsutism to be the presenting, or even the main, symptom. However, it may be, and the alert clinician will suspect the condition if these is associated atypical arthropathy, carpal tunnel syndrome and growth of extremities. Most women with acromegaly will have amenorrhoea and, as is discussed in Chapter 7, 50% will have hyperprolactinaemia. Assessment of hGH as part of a multiple pituitary stimulation or in response to stimulation with pancreatic tumour derived hGH releasing factor will help to establish the diagnosis. For screening purposes the most satisfactory assay is of somatomedin.

10 HIRSUTISM DURING PREGNANCY

It is unusual for hirsutes to develop for the first time during pregnancy, but there are many well-documented cases (Sohval 1965). Very rarely this may be due to the first manifestation of a genuinely coincidental cause such as an arrhenoblastoma (Brentnall 1945). Sometimes this may be due to an androluteoma which is an hCG-dependent tumour (Zander et al. 1978). More commonly, no such intercurrent pathology is found. This problem has been discussed by Fayez et al. (1974) and reviewed fully by Novak et al. (1970).

Clinical approach to differential diagnosis

There is no uniformly satisfactory method of grading the degree of hirsutism present. Efforts to quantitate this precisely by weighing shaved hair at regular intervals or by measuring hair shaft diameter are not ideal and certainly not very useful in routine clinical practice. Of the various methods of clinical assessment, probably the old one based on a differential scoring system produced by Ferriman and Gallwey (1961) remains the best.

One popular misconception should be dismissed forthwith. It is often stated that provided there is no interference with menstrual function, hirsutism must be either familial or idiopathic. Although it is usually correct, this belief is wrong sufficiently often to make it essential to look further into the problem of the woman with excessive hair growth, even in the presence of normal ovulatory menstruation, or even in those who have been recently pregnant.

Figure 8.6 shows a florid example of this problem. This woman's presenting symptom was hirsutism. She had, when first seen, completely normal ovulatory cycles. She also had carcinomatosis from an adrenal carcinoma producing Cushing's syndrome.

It is not meant as a placebo to say that a full history and examination are mandatory. The gynaecologist who restricts his field of vision to the subumbilical area will deservedly flounder.

The history itself may suggest adrenal hyperplasia, the appearance Cushing's syndrome (Figs. 8.6 and 8.8), or even acromegaly. Often, in fact usually, clinical suspicion may be directed along a certain line, but confirmation will require extensive assessment of the patient's hormonal environment which may be beyond the capacity of many hospitals.

It should be re-emphasized that hirsutism must be investigated, irrespective of the patient's menstrual cycle.

In the majority of hirsute women seen with normal periods, plasma testosterone will be only very slightly increased or at the upper limit of normal. Appropriate investigations will confirm normal ovulation and in the vast majority of women in this category 17-hydroxyprogesterone and DHAS will also be normal. In most of these women free levels of plasma testosterone will be increased if this assay is available.

If, on the other hand, the patient has oligomenorrhoea or amenorrhoea, the plasma testosterone levels are in the high normal range or slightly increased, LH/FSH ratios are high, 17-hydroxyprogesterone is normal and DHAS increased, then polycystic ovarian disease (the Stein–Leventhal syndrome) should be considered. This may be confirmed by laparoscopy.

Gross virilism associated with higher levels of testosterone will suggest that there is an inappropriate gonad or a virilizing ovarian tumour. Plasma levels of 17-hydroxyprogesterone and DHAS will usually be normal. Virilism with a lesser increase of testosterone, higher levels of 17-hydroxyprogesterone and DHAS point very firmly to a virilizing cause arising in the adrenal. Where Cushing's syndrome is suspected, assay of urinary-free cortisol, plasma cortisol and ACTH as outlined above will usually define the problem.

Acromegaly should be a constant phantom in the mind of the clinician who sees this type of patient. Like most phantoms, proof of existence is more difficult than initial suspicion, but without the latter proof will never be forthcoming.

TREATMENT

Treatment here, as in any other branch of medicine, if it is to be rational, must be based on a proper diagnosis of cause, and an equally proper knowledge of the natural history of the causal condition. Where there is serious underlying pathology, treatment must be directed at this cause, and the results may be singularly rewarding both for the patient and her medical advisors (Figs 8.8 and 8.9).

This treatment may involve hypophysectomy for Cushing's syndrome due to hyperplasia, or acromegaly; removal of adrenal or ovarian tumours; or corticosteroids for virilizing adrenal hyperplasia. Here the treatment is life-saving and a cure of hirsutism and associated infertility a bonus issue.

Numerically, the largest group will be those lacking serious pathology: those with the Stein–Leventhal syndrome or 'idiopathic' hirsutism.

The simultaneous treatment of hirsutism and infertility in patients with polycystic ovaries is mutually incompatible. In the writer's experience, wedge resection has no effect on any hirsutism present, a failing shared by clomiphene, although either approach has a place in the treatment of infertility.

Ovarian inhibition

There is no doubt that many women with either idiopathic hirsutism or excessive hair-growth associated with polycystic ovaries will have substantial improvement after long-term treatment with oral contraceptives. It should be recognized that of the oral contraceptives available, those containing norgestrel suppress sex hormone-binding globulin levels more severely than those containing norethisterone

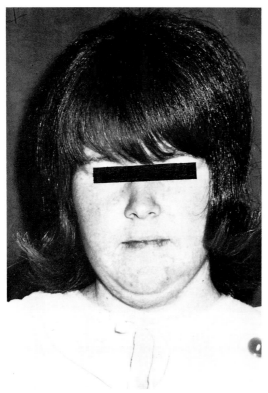

Fig. 8.8. Cushing's syndrome from adrenal hyperplasia before treatment.

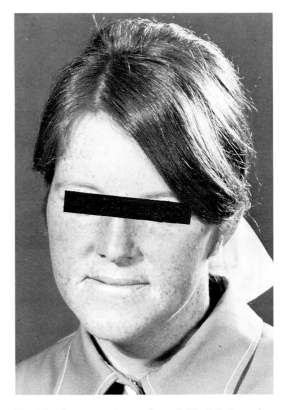

Fig. 8.9. The same patient as shown in Fig. 8.8, 6 months after bilateral adrenalectomy, maintained on cortisone acetate, 25mg twice daily and 9α fluorohydrocortisone, 0.1 mg daily. She has since developed Nelson's syndrome.

or one of its precursors. The corollary of this is that there is a relatively greater increase in plasma-free testosterone if oral contraceptives containing norgestrel are used. In general terms, a preparation containing 50 micrograms of ethinyl oestradiol and norethisterone or one of the related progestins is a reasonable first line of treatment. The patient should be warned that if she has acne, there may be very rapid improvement in this, but that it will be a matter of months before changes in hirsutism can be determined.

Wiebe and Morris (1984) have demonstrated that both ovarian and adrenal androgens may be reduced to some extent by this treatment in women with 'idiopathic' hirsutism or polycystic ovaries. However, it should be stressed that this treatment by itself is very rarely effective in causing regression of mature hirsutism.

Corticosteroids

Not everyone would be prepared to use corticosteroid therapy on a long-term basis for a condition that is

non-life-threatening like 'idiopathic' hirsutism. However, there can be no doubt that simultaneous adrenal and ovarian suppression causes a much greater reduction in testosterone production rate than does suppression of either structure alone (Casey 1975). If this approach is to be used, an oral contraceptive of the type outlined above should be employed together with Dexamethasone in a dose of 0.25 mg or 0.5 mg given last thing at night in a single dose.

Cyproterone acetate

This compound is an anti-androgen that inhibits testosterone binding to the cytoplasmic receptor. It has a very long half-life, and if used alone there is usually disruption of the menstrual cycle. More importantly, if pregnancy should occur, there is a grave danger of interfering with sexual differentiation of a male fetus.

The most commonly employed regime is the 'reversed sequential' method, originally developed by

Hammerstein (1980). In this regime between 30 and 50 μg of ethinyl oestradiol are given each day from the fifth to the twenty-fourth day of the cycle and cyproterone acetate is given in a dose of 100 mg daily from the fifth to the fourteenth day of the cycle. Withdrawal bleeding is often delayed for six to seven days after the last tablets are taken. Because of this we prefer to have a 21-day treatment cycle with a seven-day gap, ethinyl oestradiol being taken as above for 21 days and 100 mg of cyproterone acetate for the first 10 days of each treatment cycle (Fraser et al. 1983). Long term therapy for 12 or sometimes 24 months is usually needed and while this drug does not cause complete remission in all patients, in about 70% of women there is a very substantial improvement. It should be noted that cyproterone is not readily available in many countries.

Spironolactone

It was noted some years age that men being treated with spironolactone often develop gynaecomastia. This drug inhibits cytochrome P450, an enzyme required for androgen biosynthesis (Menard et al. 1979) and, like cyproterone acetate, is also a competitive inhibitor of androgen action in target cells (Corvol et al. 1975). Its usefulness in an initial small study by Boiselle and Tremblay (1979) has been confirmed in larger studies by Shapiro and Evron (1980) and Cumming et al. (1982). The author's practice is to use 50 mg twice daily every day except for the first four days of the menstrual cycle. It should be remembered that since this compound interferes with androgen binding it could, theoretically, interfere with sexual differentiation of the male fetus. It should therefore not be used during pregnancy and if a patient is exposed to the risk of pregnancy an oral contraceptive of the type outlined earlier in this chapter should be used in addition.

Cosmetic management

This should not be ignored but cannot be expected to cure the problem. Depilatory creams are often associated with skin hypersensitivity and, if the patient can be persuaded to do so, shaving is probably the best local approach followed by the use of bleaches which will cause regrowth to be initially less noticeable.

Finally, it should be emphasized to any patient who is to undergo medical treatment for hirsutism that with an androgen inhibitor good results will occur in 70–80% but that long term treatment will be essential.

REFERENCES

ABRAHAM G. E. & CHAKMAKJIAN Z. H. (1974) Obstet. and Gynec. N.Y., 44, 171.

BOISELLE A. & TREMBLAY R. R. (1979) Fertil. and Steril., 32, 276.

BRENTNALL C. P. (1945) J. Obstet. Gynaec. Brit. Cwlth., 52, 235.

BROOKS R. V., MATTINGLEY D., MILLS I. H. & PRUNTY F. T. G. (1960) Brit. med. J., i, 1294.

CASEY J. H. (1975) Clin. Endocr., 4, 313.

CASEY J. H., BURGER H. G., KENT J. R., KELLIE A. G., MOXHAM A., NABARRO J. & NABARRO J. D. N. (1966) J. clin. Endocr., 26, 1370.

CONN J. W. & LOUIS L. H. (1956) Ann. intern. Med., 44, 1.

CORVOL P., MICHAUD A., MENARD J., FREIFELD M. & MAHOUDEAU J. (1975) Endocrinology 97, 52.

CUMMING D. C., YANG J. C., REBAR R. W. & JYEN S. S. C. (1982) J. Amer. med. Assoc., 247, 1295.

ELLIOTT P. & HESELTINE M. (1967) Aust. N.Z. J. Obset. Gynaec., 7, 194.

FAYEZ J. A., BUNCH T. R. & MILLER G. L. (1974) Obstet. Gynec. N.Y., 44, 511.

FERRIMAN D. & GALLWEY J. D. (1961) J. clin. Endocr., 21, 1440.

FRASER I. S., SHEARMAN R. P., ALLEN J. K. & McCARRON G. (1983) Aust. N.Z. J. Obstet. Gynaec., 23, 93.

JONES H. W. & KLINGENSMITH G. J. (1985) In Clinical Reproductive Endocrinology (Shearman R. P. ed.). Churchill Livingstone, London.

HAMMERSTEIN J. (1980) In Androgenization in Women (Hammerstein, Lachnit-Fixson, Neumann & Plewig eds.), pp. 21, 221. Excerpta Medica, Amsterdam.

HAMMERSTEIN J., LACHNIT-FIXSON U., NEUMANN F. & PLEWIG G. (1980) In Androgenization in Women. Excerpta Medica, Amsterdam.

MENARD R. H., GUENTHER T. M., KON H., GILLETTE J. R. (1979) J. biol. Chem., 254, 1726.

MULLER S. A. (1969) Amer. J. Med., 46, 803.

NOVAK D. J., LAUCHLAN S. C., McCAWLEY J. C. & FAIMAN C. (1970) Amer. J. Med., 49, 281.

PARKER L. N., CHANG S. & ODELL W. D. (1978) Clin. Endocr., 8, 1.

PAULSON J. D., KELLER D. W., WIEST W. G. & WARREN J. C. (1977) Amer. J. Obstet. Gynec., 128, 851.

PRUNTY F. T. G. (1967) J. Endocr., 38, 85.

REBAR R., JUDD H. L., YEN S. S. C., RAKOFF J., VANDENBERG G. & NAFTOLIN F. (1976) J. clin. Invest., 57, 1320.

SHAPIRO G. & EVRON S. (1980) J. clin. Endocr., 51, 429.

SHEARMAN R. P. (1961) Aust. N.Z. J. Obstet. Gynaec., 1, 24.

SHEARMAN R. P. & COX R. I. (1965) *Amer. J. Obstet. Gynec.*, **92**, 747.

SOHVAL A. R. (1965) In *Medical, Surgical and Gynecological Complications of Pregnancy*, 2e. Williams and Wilkins, Baltimore.

WIEBE R. H. & MORRIS C. V. (1984) *Obstet. and Gynec.*, **63**, 12.

ZANDER J., MICKAN H., HOLZMANN K. & LOHE K. J. (1978) *Amer. J. Obstet. Gynec.*, **130**, 170.

CHAPTER 9
FERTILIZATION, IMPLANTATION AND
EARLY DEVELOPMENT OF THE EMBRYO

G. V. P. CHAMBERLAIN

In this chapter a number of important events are examined. These include fertilization and implantation of the zygote; the early development of the embryo will be briefly considered, with special reference to the importance of early embryonic development in obstetric practice. Detailed discussion of all these is not possible in the space available; the following reference is recommended for further reading: *Reproduction and the Fetus*—Findlay (1984)

Germ-cell maturation

Primordial germ cells appear in the yolk sac after about 25 days' gestation and migrate via the ventral duct mesentery to the primary gonadal folds. At the end of a month there may be over a thousand in the area of the future gonad.

At $7\frac{1}{2}$ weeks the testis is recognizable, at which time multiplication by mitosis ends and the germ cells enter upon a long-resting premeiotic phase. The central cells of tubules degenerate. Much later the attached cells will divide to form spermatogonia, whose successive redivisions produce the primary spermatocyte, the secondary spermatocyte and spermatids. The latter mature to spermatozoa by a series of at least six recognizable stages (Clermont 1963). In man the division of spermatogonia to mature spermatozoa (Fig. 9.1) occupies a period of not less than 64 days. The process of spermatogenesis occupies a longer time than mitosis and is under the control of local factors which are as yet ill-understood. These stimulate maturation in waves of activity. The tubules are apparently controlled by FSH and the Leydig cells by ICSH. The microanatomy of the mature spermatozoon is reviewed by Gould (1980). Human and gorilla sperm alone among primates are characterized by great pleomorphism. (See also Cohen & Hendry 1978.)

In the future female, mitosis continues during migration of germ cells to the primary gonadal folds and up to 2 months' gestational age (Baker & O 1976).

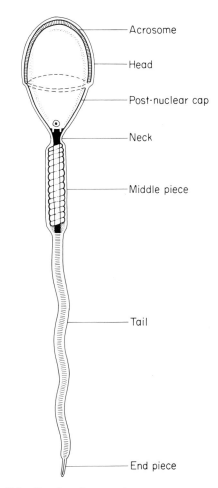

Fig. 9.1. Drawing of a spermatozoon.

Meiosis then begins under the influence of meiosis-inducing substances derived from the rete cords with polarization of chromosomes which are clumped at one edge of the nucleus; then follows the zygotene stage with homologous pairs of chromosomes lying parallel to each other; by 4 months the first pachytene oocytes can be detected. In the human female at

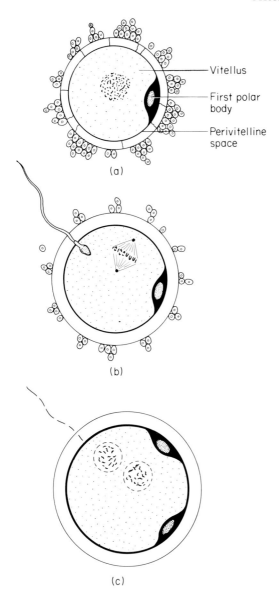

Vitellus

First polar
body

Perivitelline
space

(a)

(b)

(c)

Fig. 9.2. (a) Secondary oocyte and first polar body
formation following the first stage of meiosis.
(b) Penetration of the sperm stimulating the second
meiotic division of the oocyte. (c) The seond polar body
has formed; male and female pronuclei have formed prior
to fusion. (Redrawn from Llewellyn-Jones, *Fundamentals of
Obstetrics and Gynaecology.* Faber & Faber, London.)

5 months there are nearly seven million eggs present.
Many of these have entered the diplotene stage, the
chromosome pairs beginning to split but remaining
together at various points (chiasmata) where genetic
exchange is thought to occur. Meiosis is arrested by

a meiosis-preventing substance secreted by the granulosa cells of the follicle (Byskova 1978) and the oocytes rest until just before ovulation. Rest is a mis-
nomer as growth and much metabolic activity
continue (Moor & Warnes 1979).

Pre-ovulation follows removal of the intrafollicular
inhibiting substances under gonadotrophin, steroid
and possibly intrafollicular influences as it can occur
in tissue culture (Moor & Warnes 1979). The cell
passes from rest to the first metaphase, remaining
there for 12 hours before passing through the first
anaphase with elimination of the first polar body (Fig.
9.2[a]). It then enters the second metaphase, which
is followed after some time by fertilization. With fertilization is associated the production of the second
polar body, and the ovum (now having reached its
final stage) joins the male gamete to form the zygote.

Fertilization

Despite a vast amount of literature the processes of
capacitation and acrosome reaction in spermatozoa
are poorly understood. Capacitation involves the removal of epididymal and seminal proteins which coat
sperm surfaces. Some are highly immunogenic and
at least one inhibits fertilization (Brackett 1978). Hy-
aluronidase is liberated by the acrosome as the sperm
passes through the cumulus, and proof that the acrosome reaction is complete in the human is the ability of the sperm to penetrate the zona pellucida of
human eggs, pellucida binding sites being species
specific and penetration occurring by production of
the enzyme acrosin (Whittingham 1979). Following
entry of a sperm into the egg, there spreads from the
entry site over the zona pellucida a reaction which
prevents the passage of further sperms. This prevents
polyspermia and the risk of polyploidy.

The number of sperms reaching the oviduct is related directly to the number inseminated and study
of the distribution of sperms in the human female
genital tract has shown that they can reach the oviduct within 5 minutes of coitus though very few can
be found in the uterus (Settlage *et al.* 1973). It may
be that some constituent of seminal plasma increases
solubility of cervical muscus and that prostaglandin
E_2 in seminal fluid speeds the transport through the
uterus. Of clinical significance also are the survival
time and effects of ageing of spermatozoa which have
been reviewed by van der Vliet and Hafez (1974).
The ability to produce a viable embryo is probably
lost before the ability to fertilize, whilst motility and
metabolic activity persist slightly longer than either.

The survival time is related to the region in which the sperm is located: after 35 minutes in the acid vagina they are much less active and can no longer penetrate cervical mucus and do not survive in the vagina for more than 10–12 hours. In the cervical mucus at the time of ovulation the mean survival time is 1–3 days whilst in the oviduct a figure of 40–50 hours is guessed at. The ovum too is subject to ageing which has been implicated as a possible cause of early pregnancy wastage.

Following entry of the sperm, its post-nuclear cap disappears and the head detaches from the tail. The head, possibly with the mid-piece still attached, re-organizes in the centre of the ovum and becomes larger, exhibiting many nucleoli and showing distinct chromatin material. Entry of the sperm, as noted, triggers off the second maturation division of the ovum (Fig. 9.2[b] and [c]), following which the chromosomes of ovum and sperm fuse. Much of the recent information has been derived in studies of extracorporeal fertilization (Edwards *et al.* 1980, Evans *et al.* 1980, Whittingham 1979) to which the reader is referred.

Following fusion the nucleoli disappear and there ensues a brief period of rest, which is succeeded by much chemical activity. A first cleavage division occurs within 24 hours of fertilization and divisions follow roughly every 22 hours, successive ones occurring at right-angles. Divisions are normally into equal halves. The factors controlling early development have been summarized by Adamson and Gardner (1979).

Implantation

A progesterone-dominated environment is essential for subsequent implantation and there is increasing evidence that substances passing from conceptus to mother before implantation may prolong luteal functions (Heap *et al.* 1979). During this time the fertilized ovum is being transported along the Fallopian tube by a mixture of ciliary action and peristalsis, passing the isthmus at 72–120 hours when of the 16–50-cell size. Until this time there has been little alteration in overall size, and the cell mass (likened to a mulberry) is known as a morula (Fig. 9.3). Within the centre of this mass there soon develops a space filled with fluid known as the blastocyst cavity (Fig. 9.4[a]). The surrounding sphere of cells forms the trophoblast. The inner aspect of the trophoblast is at one pole thickened by the inner cell mass. Only in humans is tubal pregnancy seen suggesting a more robust blastocyst

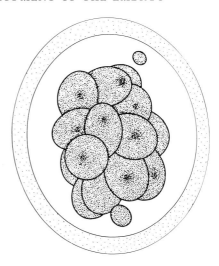

Fig. 9.3. Diagrammatic representation of the morula stage.

or a better tubal environment than in other animals. The size of the ovum now rapidly increases to about 300 μm and the zona pellucida becomes extremely thin. The zona may possibly be dissolved by endometrial enzymes or by enzymes from the blastocyst and either or both of these may be under ovarian steroid control.

The inner cell mass will form the embryo, yolk sac and amniotic cavity, whilst the trophoblast forms the placenta, chorion and extra-embryonic mesoderm. The change from morula to blastocyst is seen in the first 24 hours after entry of the fertilized ovum into the uterus, which normally occurs at $3\frac{1}{2}$–5 days after fertilization. Shortly thereafter the amniotic cavity appears in the inner cell mass (Fig. 9.4[b]) and erosion of the endometrium by the trophoblast usually begins in an area between the mouths of two decidual glands. Decidual glycogen is concentrated in the area of implantation, possibly in response to the presence of trophoblast. The mechanisms of endometrial preparedness are considered by James and Pasqualin (1979). Maternal cells and glycogen are both absorbed as embryotrophe. Regeneration of maternal epithelium at the implantation site is rapid and the trophoblast is fully embedded by the eighth or ninth day after ovulation. The embryonic pole with the inner cell mass penetrates first, and most deeply, into the decidua.

Early chorionic development

When the blastocyst imbeds at 7 days syncytiotrophoblast and cytotrophoblast are defined, and lacunar

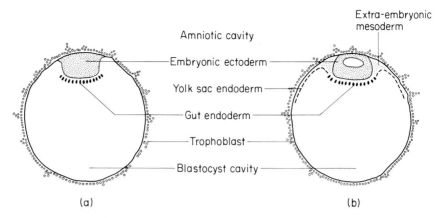

Fig. 9.4.   Drawing of the formation of the inner cell mass and amniotic cavity.

spaces appear in the syncytium in the next 48 hours. Two or three days after this these advance into the surrounding tissues as early villi, each of which consists of cytotrophoblast surrounded by syncytium. The lacunar clefts soon become filled with maternal blood from eroded maternal capillaries, and a slow circulation of this is evident by 12 days (Fig. 9.5).

Mesodermal cores become evident in the villi by the thirteenth day (Fig. 9.6), fetal blood vessels appearing subsequently and a fetal placental circulation being established when the heart starts to beat at 21–22 days. At 16–17 days the surface of the blastocyst is covered by branching villi which are best developed at the embryonic pole where the placenta will finally be established; the chorion here is known as chorion frondosum, in contrast to the smooth chorion (chorion laeve) covering the remainder of the embryonic sphere. At 4 weeks spiral arteries of the

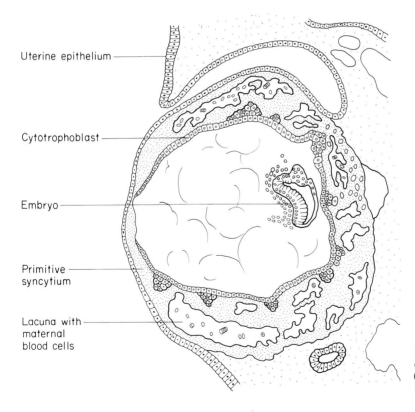

Fig. 9.5.   Drawing of the early development of the trophoblast. (Redrawn from Hamilton-Boyd & Mossman, Human Embryology.)

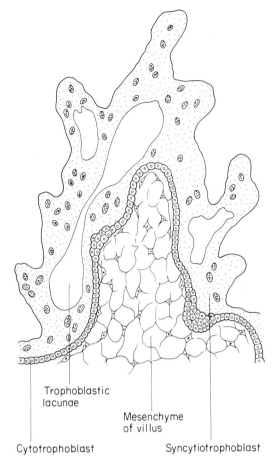

Trophoblastic
lacunae

Mesenchyme
of villus

Cytotrophoblast   Syncytiotrophoblast

Fig. 9.6. More definitive development of chorionic villi with entry of mesodermal cores.

endometrium, which in the progestational phase exhibit to-and-fro looping and marked dilatation, become eroded, with an increased rate of flow in the intervillous space.

The definitive number of stem villi is apparently established by 12 weeks' gestation. Placental growth thereafter continues until term, and possibly beyond, by a continuing increase in size of stem villi with sprouting and branching of their growing ends. This branching and rebranching causes the villi to fill the expanding lacunar space, which itself expands by virtue of coincident uterine growth in the area of placental attachment. We can now speak of this as the intervillous space, in which a brisk circulation has been established by about 5–6 weeks.

FETAL VESSELS IN THE PLACENTA

Main branches of the umbilical arteries and veins can be seen running together on the fetal surface of the placental chorion outside the transparent amnion. From these main branches at the chorionic surface paired branches are given off at intervals which enter the stalk of a primary villus, following its ramifications to reach the terminal villi. Up to 200 of these fetal units have been described in the mature placenta, though more recent writers suggest that between 60 and 80 may be a more usual number. Each primary stem villus, with all its ramifications, forms one fetal unit, but these fetal units are grouped together by incomplete septa which, arising from maternal tissues, divide the maternal aspect of the placenta into the somewhat indistinct lobulations known as cotyledons. Each cotyledon must include more than one fetal unit, as there are normally some 30 cotyledons. Each cotyledon may be supplied by its own spiral artery (Rushton 1973).

THE INTERVILLOUS SPACE

This develops as the lacunar spaces of the early trophoblast expand and fuse, an arterial in-flow to the spaces being developed after the fourth week of gestation by erosion of spiral arteries. From the way in which the space develops it is unlikely that preformed and static channels exist for maternal blood flow. On the maternal aspect the intervillous space is enclosed by a layer of basal cytotrophoblast fused with decidua and interrupted by ridges and septa, the largest of which separate the placental cotyledons. Maternal spiral artery in-flow and venous out-flow openings are distributed throughout the basal plate. The circulation within the space must be comparatively brisk, though variable, whilst the nature of the flow would lead one to expect that the composition of intervillous blood would not be uniform. Intervillous circulation has been studied by Indian ink injection studies in monkeys and in isolated human uteri, and by angiography. Some 60–80 spiral arterial in-flows are evident in the mature placenta, which are fewer than the number of arterial openings which can be demonstrated histologically. Thus, even when the uterus is at rest, some arterial in-flow sites may be temporarily out of action. This will be referred to later when discussing alteration in flow during uterine activity.

Though the quantitative aspects of the intervillous circulation are still speculative, and even the size of the space is uncertain, it is known that maternal arterial blood enters through the spiral arteries in the basal plate as forceful jets, each about 1 mm in diameter, and that venous drainage also occurs through openings scattered haphazardly in this plate. Crawford (1962) emphasized that the area immediately above an arterial in-flow is relatively free of villi, forming an intracotyledonary space, a concept confirmed by Freese et al. (1966). The latter suggested that such an arrangement would permit a constant unobstructed in-flow of maternal blood at sufficiently hydrostatic pressure to facilitate exchange of substances between maternal and fetal blood. An increase in size of the functioning vessels in the last trimester has been described. The entering blood jet (Borell jet) enters at a pressure 60–70 mmHg above the resting intervillous space pressure (10–15 mmHg) and is directed towards the chorionic plate.

Losing momentum, the blood flow is further impeded by the villi and is displaced from the centre of the cotyledon by the entry of the succeeding jet, so producing a doughnut shape on injection studies. As it spreads laterally the blood percolates progressively more slowly between villi, and finally leaves the intervillous space by the venous openings in the basal plate. Villi near these out-flows will be surrounded by poorly oxygenated blood and those near the chorionic plate by well-oxygenated blood. This has been termed a multivillous flow system. The mixed flow in the intervillous space accounts for the variable results which have been obtained in analysing that blood. During uterine relaxation the pressure in the space approximates to the intra-amniotic pressure (Martin 1965), while the pressure in the pelvic veins is slightly, but significantly, lower. Earlier authors demonstrated considerable variations in intra-amniotic resting pressure and found that the intervillous space pressure could actually be lower (Hellman et al. 1957). Injection studies have demonstrated that as uterine contractions become stronger the amount of contrast medium entering the intervillous space is reduced proportionally. In monkeys the in-flow will cease when contractions exceed 35 mmHg. It will be recalled that individual spiral arteries can be shut off from time to time even during uterine relaxation.

The volume of the space is important in considering the speed of blood flow, but it may not be constant. Moreover, in the normal full-term placenta the parenchymatous tissues which are involved in exchange of gases or metabolites are thought to account for 79% of its volume, and the intervillous space occupies between 37.5 and 42.5% of the par-

enchyma from the twenty-eighth week to term (Aherne & Dunnill 1966).

EARLY FETAL DEVELOPMENT

The early development of the fetus is considered in outline; for details standard works should be consulted (Williams & Warwick 1980). Of particular interest to gynaecologists is the mechanism of sex determination and development (Bercu & Schulman 1980, Short 1979; see also Chapter 1).

The development of the human fetus in utero is usually described in three stages. The first is from fertilization to implantation of the ovum. The changes of this period have been further elucidated by the studies of ova fertilized in vitro (Edwards et al. 1980). The second stage continues until the end of the eighth week, by which time the development of nearly all the major organs has begun. The third stage, from the eighth week until the end of pregnancy, constitutes largely one of organ growth.

At the end of the first week following fertilization the amniotic cavity is just making its appearance between the ectoderm and the covering of trophoblast. The embryo itself at this point is a disc composed of two layers, ectoderm and endoderm. The formation of the third embryonic layer, the mesoderm (Fig. 9.7[a]), is evident at this time; the mesoderm becomes divided into two zones, the embryonic mesoderm between the ectoderm and endoderm of the embryonic disc (Fig. 9.6[c]) and the extra-embryonic mesoderm which begins to fill the blastocyst cavity and leads to the formation of the primitive yolk sac (Fig. 9.7[b]). A further change in the extra-embryonic mesoderm is the coalescence of numerous spaces which form the extra-embryonic coelom dividing the mesoderm into two layers: an outer layer lining the trophoblast and called the somatopleure, and an inner one lining the embryonic area and yolk sac known as the splanchnopleure.

Rapid development now takes place in the region of the embryonic disc. Initially, the ectoderm proliferates on its posterior surface, causing the primitive streak to bulge into the amniotic cavity. The disc itself expands into a pear-shaped mass by marked development of mesoderm in the area. A groove appears throughout the length of the primitive streak, ending in the primitive pit situated anteriorly. The head process of the embryo develops from mesodermal growth anterior to the primitive pit. Further development of the head process coincides with shrinking of the primitive streak as the whole embryonic axis lengthens.

Further changes follow very quickly. In an embryo which is 3 weeks old an extension of the extra-embryonic coelom has been formed within the lateral plate, to give rise to the true coelom of the embryo. A little later, part of this is again separated off as the pericardial cavity. The heart begins pulsations. Blood vessels containing corpuscles are evident. Closure of the neural tube begins. The pronephros becomes evident and its duct begins to grow towards the cloaca. Still further development is evident in the 4-week-old embryo. Paired limb buds are evident. Abundant blood is seen in the yolk sac and circulating through the blood vessels and heart. The mesonephros and metanephros are forming. The neural tube becomes completely closed and early brain development is evident.

By 5 weeks the embryo is beginning to look more recognizably human, due largely to changes in the formation of the face. Important developments take place in the eye, with the formation of the lens and

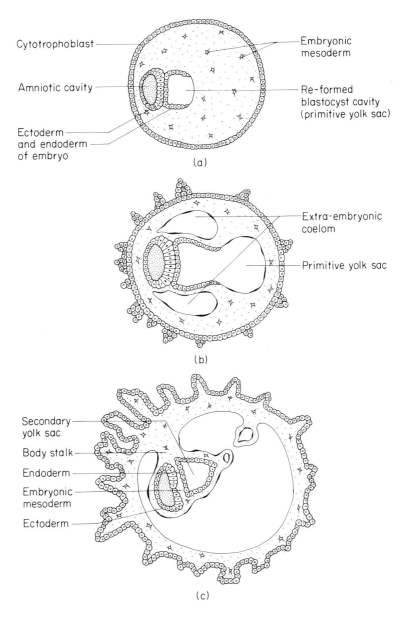

Fig. 9.7. The formation of the mesoderm, extra-embryonic coelom and yolk sac. (Redrawn from Llewellyn-Jones, *Fundamentals of Obstetrics and Gynaecology*. Faber & Faber, London.)

choroid fissure. The genital ridges may be seen by this time, and complete formation of the mesonephros has taken place. So rapid are these changes that by the end of the first 2 months the fetus looks clearly human in form. Almost every organ has been laid down, although development is not complete,. The sex of the fetus cannot be determined from the external genitalia at this time, differentiation usually occurring during the period 8–12 weeks, although not until later is it easy to recognize a male from a female. During this early period of rapid formation and development of primordial organs drugs such as thalidomide and diseases such as rubella can have an extremely important effect upon fetal development and can result in devastating fetal abnormalities (*see* p. 111).

Fetal circulation

A mass of cells, becoming so large that the inner units can no longer diffuse metabolic materials with the extracellular fluid, requires an internal transportation system. The human embryo reaches that stage by about 20 days. After this, a full vascular system

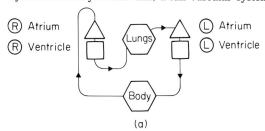

(a)

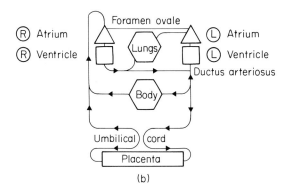

(b)

Fig. 9.8. The bypass mechanisms in the fetal circulation. (a) Shows the flow pattern of blood through the adult circulation and cardiopulmonary unit. (b) Shows the fetal situation with the added low resistance and high flow zone of the placenta and the two channels to bypass the non-functioning fetal lungs.

is evolved to carry fetal blood to the trophoblastic surface and return it to the central body. In both fetus and adult, high blood flow is maintained to homeostatic organs while flow to other areas of the body varies with needs. The fetal and adult cardiovascular systems differ because of the alterations in homeostatic mechanisms at each phase, the placenta acting instead of the adult lung or kidney in oxygenation or catabolite excretion (Fig. 9.8).

Blood returning from the placenta is shunted along the ductus venosus directly to the inferior vena cava, so avoiding the liver. Approaching the heart, the larger portion of the blood passes from the inferior vena cava to the left atrium through the foramen ovale, without entry to the right heart (Fig. 9.9). A lesser quantity of blood from the umbilical circulation is not diverted by the crista dividens and mixes in the right atrium with the deoxygenated blood from the head of the fetus. In fact, there is very little mixing of the two streams in the right heart. Most of the blood returning from the placenta passes straight to the left atrium, for in the fetus that chamber is beneath the rest of the heart and blood is diverted by the crista straight from the inferior vena cava. This simplification of ideas on fetal haemodynamics can be shown by measuring oxygen-saturation levels in superior or inferior vena cava and comparing them with the left atrial levels, and has been confirmed by injecting ^{131}I-labelled albumin into inferior or superior vena cava in turn. The first leads rapidly to a very high increase in scintillation counts in the carotid loop, the latter making no immediate change (Dawes 1968).

The blood with a higher oxygen saturation is pumped to the left ventricle and so to the aorta, from where the relatively big carotid arteries direct a larger share to the cerebral circulation. The lesser portion of oxygenated blood which actually entered the right atrium mixes with relatively deoxygenated blood from the superior vena cava and the coronary sinus, passing to the right ventricle and so to the pulmonary trunk. Pressures in the pulmonary circulation are higher than in the aorta, so most of this blood is diverted along the ductus arteriosus to join the aorta below the exit of the carotid arteries, less than 10% of the cardiac output passing through the pulmonary vessels. The blood which circulates to the fetal viscera, comes mostly from that which has circulated through the head and arms, together with a lesser quantity from the left ventricle. It passes down the aorta and about two-thirds of it is pumped along the umbilical arteries to the placenta, with a little going down the femoral arteries to the legs.

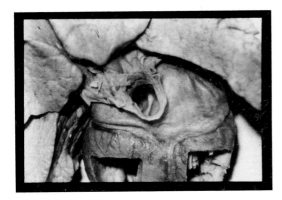
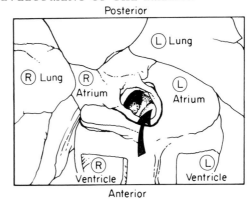

Fig. 9.9. The underside of the fetal heart with the inferior vena cava removed. The crista is clearly shown and it can be appreciated how this deflects most of the blood coming from below into the left atrium (arrow).

The circulation in the placenta has a low resistance, and must be sustained by high flow rates. Blood pressures drop sharply in the placenta, so that while umbilical artery pressures may be approximately 60 mmHg, those in the vein are only 10 mmHg. The effects of the flow of blood down a long vessel with numerous changing curves in the umbilical cord might be important, but most resistance to flow seems to occur in the cotyledonal vessels, while the pressure inside the villus vessels themselves is less than that of the intervillus space.

In early pregnancy more of the blood volume is outside the body (in placenta and cord) than inside but once body weight exceeds that of the placenta, at about 16 weeks, the ratio is reversed. Umbilical blood flow increases proportionally with fetal growth at a level of about 100 ml/kg a minute. Alterations in flow may be due to variations in placental vascular resistance in early pregnancy, but later on are related to fetal arterial blood pressure, which by term often reaches 75/55 mmHg. Return of blood from the placenta is by *vis à tergo*, although it has been suggested that pulsations of the umbilical arteries wrapped in a spiral fashion around the vein may help to milk the blood along.

Mild hypoxia causes a rise of fetal arterial pressure, and since there is usually no alteration of the placental vascular resistance, flow rates would increase; severe hypoxia, however, can slightly increase placental vascular resistance and so might reduce blood returned to the body. Since there seems to be no sympathetic enervation of the umbilical vessels after they have emerged from the fetal body, this effect is probably a reflection of increased catecholamine release by the fetal adrenal glands. Under these conditions a relatively large volume of the fetal blood stays in the placental vessels, possibly exposing a greater amount of blood to the exchange of gases. It has yet to be proved that this is an advantageous response of the fetus, for the catecholamines also increase metabolic rates and so increase the usage of oxygen by the fetus, so that although there may be more blood in the region, it might be exposed to oxygen exchange for a shorter time.

Much remains to be learned about the fetal circulation and its responses. Those wishing to learn more about the interim position should consult Dawes (1968).

Thanks are due to Mr E. D Morris, a previous contributor, for allowing much of his material to be used in this chapter.

REFERENCES

ADAMSON E. D. & GARDNER R. L. (1979) *Brit. med. Bull.*, **35**, 113.

AHERNE W. & DUNNILL M. S. (1966) *Brit. med. Bull.*, **22**, 5.

BAKER T. G. & O W-S. (1976) *Clin. Obstet. Gynec.*, **3**, 3.

BERCU B. B. & SCHULMAN J. D. (1980) *Obstet. gynec. Surv.*, **35**, 1.

BRACKETT B. G. (1978) In *Methods in Mammalian Reproduction*, p. 333. Academic Press, London.

BYSKOVA G. (1978) *Ann. Biol. anim.*, **18**, 327.

CLERMONT Y. (1963) *Amer. J. Anat.*, **112**, 35.

COHEN J. & HENDRY W. F. (eds) (1979) *Spermatozoa, Antibodies & Infertility*. Blackwell Scientific Publications, Oxford.

CRAWFORD J. M. (1962) *Amer. J Obstet. Gynec.*, **84**, 1543.

DAWES G. S. (1968) *Foetal and Neonatal Physiology*, Ch. 2. Year Book Medical Publishers, Chicago.

EDWARDS R. G., STEPTOE P. C., FOWLER R. E. & BAILLIE J. (1980) *Brit. J. Obstet. Gynec.*, **87**, 742.

EVANS M. I., MUKHERJEE A. B. & SCHULMAN J. D. (1980) *Obstet. gynec. Surv.*, **35**, 71.

FINDLAY A. L. (1984) *Reproduction and the Fetus.* Edward Arnold, London.

FREESE U. E., RANNIGER K. & KAPLAN A. (1966) *Amer. J. Obstet. Gynec.*, **94**, 361.

GOULD K. G. (1980) *Int. Rev. Cytol.*, **63**, 323.

HEAP R. B., FLINT A. P. & GADSBY J. E. (1979) *Brit. med. Bull.*, **35**, 97.

HELLMAN L. M., TRICOMIT V. M. & GUPTA O. (1957) *Amer. J. Obstet. Gynec.*, **74**, 1018.

JAMES V. H. T. & PASQUALINI J. R. (eds) (1979) *J. Steroid. Biochem.*, **11**(1c), 695.

MARTIN C. B. (1965) *Anesthesiology*, **26**, 447.

MOOR R. M. & WARNES G. M. (1979) *Brit. med. Bull.*, **35**, 99.

RUSHTON D. I. (1973) *Brit. med. J.*, **i**, 344.

SETTLAGE D. S. F., MOTOSHIMA M. & TREDWAY D. R. (1973) *Fertil. and Steril.*, **24**, 655.

SHORT R. V. (1979) *Brit. med. Bull.*, **335**, 121.

VAN DER VLIET W. L. & HAFEZ E. S. E. (1974) *Amer. J. Obstet. Gynec.*, **118**, 1006.

WHITTINGHAM D. G. (1979) *Brit. med. Bull.*, **35**, 105.

WILLIAMS P. L. & WARWICK R. (1980) *Gray's Anatomy*, 36e. Churchill Livingstone, Edinburgh.

CHAPTER 10
THE FETUS, PLACENTA AND AMNIOTIC FLUID

G. V. P. CHAMBERLAIN

From implantation to delivery the human fetus lives for 38 weeks in the uterus, an encapsulated organism shut off from the external world, dependent upon the umbilical and placental circulation. The fetus and placenta become a body compartment of the mother, the composition of fetal tissues being kept constant by the transfer function of the placenta, while the fetal homeostatic organs do exist, by and large it is only the placenta that communicates with the environment (the milieu extérieur) (Fig. 10.1). Virtually all fetal intake and output occurs across the placental membrane which separates the fetal and maternal milieu intérieur. Only via the maternal extracellular

fluid compartment can the external environment be reached, for the fetal organs of homeostasis mostly communicate with the amniotic cavity, which is a closed-off zone. At the placenta, the fetal and maternal circulations are close but are kept separate; it is important to remember the dual development and functional anatomy of the placenta, for any activity may be considered from the fetal or maternal side, depending on what is being measured.

Alterations in the ability of the placenta to handle the exchange of gases, fluids or nutrients lead to deprivation of the fetus, and are considered to be placental insufficiency; this is a clinical concept, but

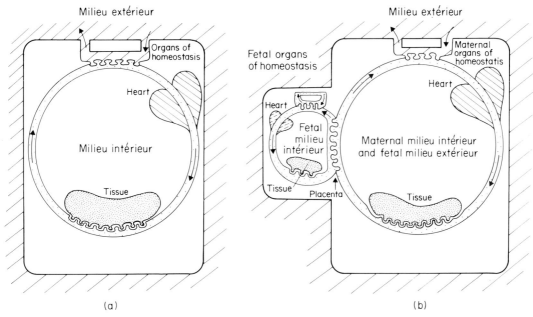

Fig. 10.1. A diagrammatic representation of the body compartments. (a) Shows the nonpregnant adult whose blood equilibrates with the tissues through the extracellular compartment and is restored to normality at the homeostatic organs in communication with the milieu extérieur.

(b) Represents the fetal situation. Although it has its own milieu extérieur in the amniotic sac, this is completely closed off and its milieu extérieur is really that of the mother; the fetus has its own homeostatic organs, but the most effective homeostasis must take place across the placenta.

many efforts are being made to measure it qualitatively. As well as its function as an exchange station, the placenta is a metabolic organ which provides a wide variety of hormones and enzymes. The two activities (regulation of exchange and hormone production) may be independent of each other, but it is the second activity of the placenta that is usually investigated when placental function tests are performed. There may be a relationship between the efficiency of the organ in each of these functions, but if there is, it is probably a complex and altering one and there is no justification to extrapolate automatically from one to the other. While weak correlations exist between the various placental activities and between them and the clinical state of the fetus, it is probable that many of the measures of placental hormones and enzymes in the maternal milieu are assuming the same thing and do not really give different indications of fetal prognosis.

THE FETUS IN PREGNANCY

The fetus grows in the uterus from a single fertilized cell into a complex organism, increasing its weight about six billion times. The rate of growth is the product of the rate of multiplication of cells and growth of the cells themselves. Since the former is mostly under genetic control, it is the latter which is often responsible for variations in the body size in a given species. The rate of growth of a cell depends on the availability of nutrients. In the fetus this depends upon the maternal blood arriving at the placenta. Except in extreme conditions of starvation, the concentration of nutrients in the maternal blood is the same in most women, and so the availability of foodstuffs to the fetal cells depends upon the blood flow to the maternal side of the placenta and the transfer of nutrients across the placenta membranes to the fetus.

In the first 12 weeks of pregnancy the developing embryo does not have a full placental system. For the first few days it is suspended in the secretion of the Fallopian tube and then in endometrial fluid. After implantation in the decidua as a blastocyst, all exchange of gases, foodstuffs and waste products takes place with the surrounding pool of blood and degenerating cells. Figure 10.2, showing the rate of growth of the fetus in the uterus, indicates that there is not an overall linear relationship between growth and maturity. By about 12 weeks, when the fetus weighs about 30 g, the placental system is evolved; thence there is an acceleration of growth rate followed by a flattening in the latter weeks.

The data shown in Fig. 10.2 are derived from two sources: weight of hysterotomy specimens in early pregnancy and birth weights in later pregnancy. The former can be accurately and reproducibly obtained but the latter are less accurate as the time from birth to the time of weighing may be many hours, and the weight of various impedimenta may be included (such as umbilical cord clips, forceps and maybe

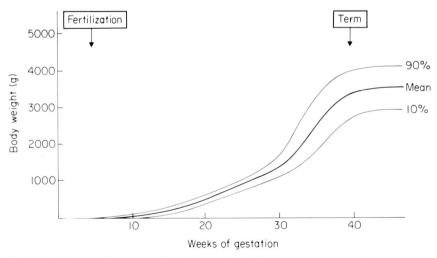

Fig. 10.2. Mean growth-gestation chart of human fetus. This is a composite chart from hysterotomy specimens in early pregnancy and from birth weights in the second half. The lighter lines indicate the 10th and 90th percentiles of the range of weights at any given gestation.

nappies in some cases). Further, it must be remembered that the delivery of many babies before term is for some pathological reason; induction of labour may be performed because of a hypertensive problem or the mother may go into spontaneous labour, producing a small baby because of an inefficient placenta. Hence the groups of weights in later pregnancy are a less reliable reflection of normality, even when careful screening has been done to exclude all known abnormalities of pregnancy and allowance has been made for the parity of the mother and sex of the infant.

Variations within these groups can be defined by one of two mathematical methods. The mean curve of weight at birth is established for any gestation and curves at one or two standard deviations above and below that mean for each week of gestation are derived and by joining them the outer lines are drawn. Babies outside the second standard deviation are considered to be significantly large or small for dates. This method is used by pathologists. The other technique involves the plotting of the weights on a percentage notation when weights above the 90th or below the 10th percentile are considered to be outside normal range. Such a method of measurement is commonly used by paediatricians when following babies' progress into childhood. If the distribution of babies' weights at any given maturity was random, then two standard deviations on either side of the mean contain about 95% of the population, while the tenth and ninetieth percentile method includes only 80% of all the babies. There is, however, usually a bias towards the lower weights, when the percentile method is more useful in practice. Using either of these methods, two groups of babies can be demonstrated a group of those that are larger, and a group that are smaller, than the expected gestation weight. Into the first group fall babies born to mothers with diabetes or prediabetes. Into the latter group fall the babies with congenital abnormalities following chromosomal abnormality, e.g. Trisomy 21 and Turner's syndrome, those with intrauterine infections (such as the chronic rubella syndrome or toxoplasmosis), and those who mothers are suffering from conditions known to affect placental exchange (hypertension and pre-eclampsia). Also in this group are babies born after multiple pregnancies and, sometimes, babies born to mothers who live at high altitudes. After all these recognizable groups have been identified, there is still a group of babies small for dates for no obvious reason.

It has long been understood that there are variations in intrauterine growth rate, but until recently, growth-retarded infants have been confused with premature babies. This is due partly to the birthweight definition of prematurity (2.5 kg or less) being used as the only criterion. The use of weight-gestation charts has differentiated these two groups: the baby born before its time, which is small but of the correct size for its gestation and the baby which may be born at any time in pregnancy but which is small for its period of gestation. The small-for-dates (or growth-retarded) babies undoubtedly result from chronic malnutrition while in the uterus.

These growth-retarded babies appear long and thin with relatively large heads, as the head circumference and baby length are less retarded than body weight. They show a lack of subcutaneous fat and many organs such as the liver, the lungs and the heart are smaller relative to total body weight than are those of the truly premature infant. Neurological development is mature and the brain weight is relatively greater in relation to birth weight, and so the ratio between liver and brain, which normally is 1:3, may be as high as 1:6. The reduction in organ size is due to reduction in individual cell mass rather than cell number, and is common to both the intrauterine small-for-dates fetus and the post-natal baby suffering from malnutrition.

The nutritional block to the fetus might be either in the blood supply to the placental bed, in the placenta itself or in the fetal vessels leading from the placental mass. Experimental work in which the uterine arteries of pregnant animals were banded has shown various degrees of fetal growth retardation, the fetuses in the parts of the oviduct furthest from the residual blood supply being most affected. This effect might be an exaggeration of the normal constraint mechanisms of fetal growth in the latter weeks of pregnancy. The blood supply to the uterus, in total and, separately, that component passing to the placental bed, is sensitive to alterations in oestrogen and progesterone balance. Since much of the oestrogen in late pregnancy is the result of fetal metabolism, this implies a certain coarse fetal control over its own environment.

The effects of reduced blood supply may be seen further in certain pathological conditions when the lumen of blood vessels on the maternal side of the placenta is diminished. Thrombotic occlusion of the arteries of the placental bed in pre-eclampsia has been shown, and this is a condition well known to be associated with chronically malnourished babies. Alterations in the structure of the placental membrane are often seen in conditions associated with such babies (e.g. 'syncytial knotting'). The fetal circulation may be impaired by endothelial cushions found in the vessels on the fetal side of the placentas of growth-retarded babies, and these obstructions may affect the fetal circulation just as the thrombotic conditions can affect the maternal blood flow. Preeclampsia is a well-known clinical state associated with small-for-dates babies, but fetal pathological conditions are only diagnosed after delivery of the placenta. Many growth-retarded babies are not so flagged by any obvious clinical state of the mother, who may have a good reproductive background.

Fetal distress may be divided into two phases: the chronic and the acute. The former is long-term malnutrition of the fetus in pregnancy, the latter the shorter reflection of this in labour, when the stress of uterine contractions is added to the chronic lack of transfer, causing the fetus to show the classical signs associated with clinical fetal distress. If exchange has been good until labour starts, the fetus can stand the extra stresses well. It is as though one wished to borrow money from the bank. To raise a debt when the account is in reasonable balance can be done easily. If, however, there is a chronic overdraft already, it is much harder to deal with acute debts as they arise.

Growth-retarded fetuses have a greatly increased risk of hypoxia during labour. The National Birthday Trust Perinatal Mortality Survey (Butler 1965) showed these babies to have a threehold risk of asphyxia during delivery and massive pulmonary haemorrhage in the neonatal period. They can also be shown to have a high risk of neonatal hypoxia. By recognizing chronic intrauterine malnutrition during pregnancy, more stringent monitoring can be used in labour to produce a less affected infant. The identification of these fetuses is by a mixture of clinical and other estimates, and an increasing proportion of antenatal care is now being devoted to the recognition of this group of babies in the uterus.

THE PLACENTA

The placenta, an apposition or fusion of the fetal membranes with the uterine mucosa for physiological exchange, has been investigated by gross anatomy, injection techniques, large-tissue sections, histochemistry, histology, electron-microscopy and enzyme digestion, as well as by placental perfusion. Some confusion has arisen because each different approach may involve its own vocabulary. Even with a single method of study there are revealed wide discrepancies between different areas and even between contiguous areas of the same placenta. Finally, it may be difficult to distinguish between normal ageing processes and pathological change. Indeed, no pathological change has been described which has not also been reported in normal placentas (Bernirschke & Driscoll 1967). It is probable that the composition of the placenta, as well as its size, could alter during development. Whilst the well-being of the fetus must, of course, demand sufficient healthy placental tissue to allow transfer or synthesis of substances needed for fetal homeostasis, growth and differentiation, one cannot correlate every functional change with convincing morphological change. The Grosser (1927) classification of placental types was based upon the number of tissue layers which intervened between fetal and maternal blood in different species. In the haemochorial placentas of man and monkey all the layers are of fetal origin. They comprise syncytiotrophoblast, the connective tissue of the villi and the fetal capillary wall. This classification does not tell us anything about the functional efficiency of any placental type which can vary from one area to another and can be modified by such diverse factors as high altitude, anoxia, hypertension, endotoxin and ageing. Placental growth continues until term, and perhaps beyond, with the formation of new villi and with no general senescence or decrease in efficiency (Crawford 1962).

In a normal mature placenta dilated capillaries occupy most of the cross-sectional area of villi, less than 5% of villi being small with contracted vessels and a fibrous stroma. Light- and electron-microscopy reveal that in the normal human placenta cytotrophoblast cells persist to term, though they may be so flattened between the triple-layered basement membrane and the syncytiotrophoblast that they do not necessarily form a complete layer. Nuclei of the syncytium are smaller and more electron-dense than those of the cytotrophoblast. The cytoplasm is also more highly differentiated and the surface of the syncytium is covered with microvilli. At term the number of these falls, evidence of pinocytosis, lessens and fetal vessels approach the villous surface. Thinning of syncytium, reduction in the number of cytotrophoblast cells, increased stromal fibrosis, fibrin deposition, infarction and fetal endarteritis have been described as normal ageing processes in villi. It was stressed by Amoroso (1961) that fetal capillaries are always covered with a layer of cytotrophoblast as well as by syncytium, however thin the former may become. In areas where the capillary lies close to the surface of the villi and the syncytium has become very thin, passive filtration is possibly facilitated. Such areas are known as vasculosyncytial membranes, but are not common in the normal placenta. In other areas the syncytium is relatively thick, contains many nuclei and a considerable amount of alkaline phosphatase, which suggests involvement in active transfer. These are known as syncytial knots.

A close relation has been demonstrated between placental and birth weights and chorionic villous area (Aherne & Dunnill 1966). Gross changes (e.g. accessory lobes, circumvallate placenta, and even placenta accreta) are comparatively unimportant. The overall size or weight of a placenta is only a very crude guide to its functional capacity, except for the very small placenta, which often proves inadequate, possibly because it produces a high fetal peripheral vascular resistance. Placento-fetal weight ratios are a crude measurement and, moreover, depend on a meticulous, reproducible method of preparation of the placenta before it is weighed. Calcification of the placenta on the other hand, seems comparatively unimportant (Tindall & Scott 1965). A reduction of villous surface area in pre-eclampsia has been confirmed by Aherne and Dunnill (1966). However, it is probable that reduction of intervillous blood flow will not only decrease concentration gradients from maternal to fetal blood but might also interfere with the function of placental tissue itself, as this depends for its nourishment upon maternal, and not fetal, blood. This, of course, need not produce structural changes, though there is experimental evidence that placental size can be limited by uterine blood supply.

Experiments involving high-altitude sheep suggested that chronic hypoxia can result in a placenta which permits oxygen to diffuse more easily. This could result from an increased functional area or involve alterations in thickness and composition of trophoblast, or be caused by opening-up and formation of extra capillaries. The experiments of Metcalfe et al. (1962) showed that the placenta became larger in relation to fetal size, whilst the incidence of twinning in high altitudes lessens (Lichty et al. 1957). Immunological factors may also alter placental size and function. Placental ultrastructure has been reviewed by Steven and Samuel (1979).

PLACENTAL FUNCTION

Many functions may be attributed to the placenta:
Transport
Respiratory
Nutrient production
Hormone, steroid and protein production
Excretory
The barrier function, probably a myth
These cannot be discussed without reference to cental transport mechanisms. (See also Longo 1972.)

Transport mechanisms

Various mechanisms are involved in the transport of substances across the placenta:
1   Simple diffusion.
2   Facilitated diffusion.
3   Active transport.
4   Special processes.

In most cases the passage may be in either direction. A most important placental function is to allow the loss of heat by the fetus.

SIMPLE DIFFUSION

Molecules of a substance in solution pass from a region of higher to one of lower concentration until the concentrations in the two areas become equal. The driving force is the thermal agitation of the molecules and no additional energy is needed. Two main groups of substances have been thought to be involved:
1   Substances concerned with the maintenance of biochemical homeostasis (water, electrolytes, oxygen, carbon dioxide).
2   The majority of foreign substances (with the important exception of antimetabolites).

The quantity of a substance transferred in unit time follows Fick's equation. This will be considered in more detail when oxygen transfer is discussed (p. 106); it will suffice here to say that the constant K for a substance other than oxygen is determined by its molecular size (compounds of molecular weight below 600 passing easily whilst those of molecular weight above 1000 pass hardly at all), its spatial configuration (the l-isomer passing more readily than the d-isomer), the degree of ionization (unionized molecules passing more freely), its lipid solubility (lipid-soluble drugs being favoured) and the partition coefficient for the substance between maternal and fetal blood. With increasing knowledge it is likely that the only substances to remain in this group will be the gases.

FACILITATED DIFFUSION

Transfer between compartments occurs more quickly than in simple diffusion, though there is no difference in the equilibrium eventually attained. Carrier systems are thought to be involved. The process is concerned mainly with substances involved in fetal nutrition such as natural sugars and most water-soluble vitamins.

ACTIVE TRANSPORT

Here it is postulated that placental work is involved, because the concentrations reached on the fetal side cannot be explained by the physical laws of diffusion. Antimetabolites, inorganic ions, endogenous substrates and amino acids (where again selective transfer of the l-isomer is most marked) are substances which make up this group.

SPECIAL PROCESSES

These involve substances of immunologic, but not pharmacologic, importance. Two mechanisms are included under this heading:
1 *Pinocytosis*. This is a process whereby tiny droplets of plasma are engulfed by a villus and discharged into the fetal circulation at a relatively slow rate.
2 *Leakage*. Minute breaks in a placental villus have been implicated as a route of transfer to intact blood cells to the fetus from the maternal circulation. It has been demonstrated by the injection into the mother of red blood cells of abnormal shape and their subsequent recovery from the fetus.

The outer layer of the endothelial cells may on occasions and in some species be separated by a gap of $12.5\,\mu$m (Boyd *et al.* 1976).

In transfer of IgG in the middle trimester it is thought that special receptors on the trophoblast allow selective transfer over such smaller molecules as albumin (Gitlin & Gitlin 1973). With increasing knowledge therefore the complexity of the processes involved is emphasized.

Nitrogen probably reaches the fetus entirely by the transfer of amino acids through the placental membrane. Branched chain neutral essential amino acids and basic amino acids are transported readily across the placental membrane (Young & McFadyen 1973).

Respiratory function

OXYGEN TRANSFER

An adequate supply of oxygen is needed for the transfer to the fetus of enough oxygen to satisfy fetal needs at a tension that enables the interior of fetal cells to receive sufficient oxygen that allows cell activity to continue. Intracellular Po_2 in adult cells of 1–6 mmHg, in fetal myocardium of 3 mm and a critical Po_2 for mitochondria of less than 1mmHg have been reported (Forster 1973). It had previously been suggested that the critical oxygen tension in capillary blood must be 15 mmHg or above to allow adequate penetration of cells. Oxygen is rapidly utilized and, with the possible exception of fetal myoglobin in the heart, there is no means of storing it so that the supply of the gas cannot be disturbed, even temporarily, without serious metabolic consequences to the fetus. It has been suggested that if oxygen supply to the fetus is adequate, the supply of other substances will also prove sufficient—but intrauterine growth retardation can occur in the absence of hypoxia.

As oxygen is a substance that is transferred by diffusion, its passage through the placenta will occur according to a modified form of Fick's equation. The quantity of oxygen transferred in unit time (Qt) will be proportional to the effective area available for gas exchange (A), and will depend on the size of the gradient between the mean oxygen tension of maternal blood in the intervillous space and the mean oxygen tension in fetal placental blood:

$$Po_2(m) - Po_2(f)$$

Transfer of the gas will be inversely related to the distance that separates fetal and maternal blood (d). The equation is completed by inclusion of the constant K, which relates to the physical properties of the intervening tissues and the nature of the substance being transferred. In the case of oxygen it is a comparatively small figure. The equation may now be written:

$$Qt = [Po_2(m) - Po(f)]K$$

Oxygen transfer is facilitated by a high-pressure gradient, a small diffusion distance, freely permeable intervening tissues and a large available area of exchange.

To understand the quantitative aspects of oxygen transfer, more would need to be known about the extent to which trophoblast acted as a barrier to diffusion. We would also have to measure oxygen tension and saturation in umbilical venous, umbilical arterial, uterine arterial and uterine venous blood, as well as knowing the umbilical and uterine blood flows. It is obvious that many of these facts are not obtainable at present. During life the area of exchange cannot be measured, and measurement of villous surface area even *in vitro* is difficult and time-consuming. The area available for diffusion could be greater than the villous surface if the additional surface provided by microvilli is included, or, alternatively, could be less than the villous surface area if the limiting factor is the surface area of the fetal capillary bed. The distance will vary in different regions of the same placenta. It could be increased by local fibrin deposition, by formation of syncytial knots and possibly by the presence near the villi of a layer of relatively stagnant blood. The distance would lessen in areas of temporary or permanent thinning of trophoblast or where dilated fetal capillaries bulge the villus surface. Evidence has been adduced of reversible thinning in response to hypoxia. The average distance involved has been estimated as 3.5–6.5 mm, which is 5–10 times that in the lung. Despite this, Adamson (1965) has presented evidence suggesting that the efficiency of the placenta is very similar to that of the lung, though its reserve of function is less.

It has been suggested that Qt, $Po_2(m)$ and $Po_2(f)$ are measurable or calculable. Were this so, then the expression could be rewritten:

$$KA/d = Qt/[Po_2(m) - Po_2(f)] = D$$

a value which has been named the diffusing capacity of a given placenta. Diffusing capacity has been shown to increase under high-altitude conditions (Metcalfe *et al.* 1962).

The relation between the rates of blood flow on maternal and fetal sides of the placenta is important. If they are not matched at each point of diffusion exchange, gas exchange becomes less efficient. It is known that shunts exist on both maternal and fetal sides of the placenta that would reduce efficiency. Theoretically it would be expected that a countercurrent blood flow might prove the most efficient but in the absence of preformed, static, maternal vessels in the human this cannot exist. These and other factors are discussed by Forster (1973).

Maternal oxygen tension: $Po_2(m)$

Despite the hyperventilation of pregnancy, maternal arterial blood has a mean oxygen tension of only 97.1 mmHg (88.8–109.6) during pregnancy, which is similar to the range in the non-pregnant state, though Pco_2 has fallen from 40 mmHg to between 31 and 33 mmHg. This represents a pH change of 0.06 pH unit.

Arterial blood reaching the uterus has three functions. One portion supplies the needs of the myometrium; estimates suggest that 25% of the blood may be so utilized. The remaining blood, which enters the intervillous space, subserves two functions. Firstly it supplies the oxygen needs of the placenta itself. At term the oxygen requirements of this very active organ have been estimated as 10 ml/kg a minute, compared with 5 ml/kg a minute for the fetus itself. Up to a third of the intervillous space flow could, therefore, be taken up in supplying placental needs. Secondly, the remaining intervillous blood supplies the fetal needs.

During pregnancy it is probable that the relative needs of myometrium, placenta and fetus will vary, and consequently the proportions of uterine blood supply involved in each function will also vary. Uterine contractions, hypo- and hypertensive states, regional block analgesia, general anaesthesia and drugs given to inhibit or stimulate labour may all cause changes in the relative and absolute amounts of these vital flow rates (Greiss 1973). In experimental situations maternal hypoxia and hyperoxia, maternal aortic occlusion and fetal death have had little effect on maternal uterine blood flow (Meschia & Battaglia 1973), suggesting that hormonal factors may be more important. Maternal alkalosis, however, has produced fetal hypoxia and acidosis, a relevant point when considering various methods of psychoprophylaxis or of anaesthesia for Caesarean section which could give rise to alkalosis by overbreathing (Dawes 1968).

The anatomy of the intervillous space makes it obvious that the blood within it is not likely to be of uniform composition and it is, therefore, unlikely that sampling will produce consistent readings or ones from which $Po_2(m)$ would be calculated.

If over a given short time fetal and placental oxygen needs remain steady, a quicker flow through the intervillous space would result in decreased maternal arteriovenous oxygen difference. This would, in turn, produce a higher $Po_2(m)$ so favouring materno-fetal transfer. Although it has been calculated that the intervillous space occupies 37.5–42.5% of the parenchymatous volume of the placenta (which is 79% of its total volume), it is not known whether this is the size in life nor is it certain that the size in constant.

There is evidence that maternal anaemia can be compensated for by an increased rate of flow, as can the chronic hypoxia of high-altitude conditions.

Fetal oxygen tension: Po$_2$(f)

The defects of studying cord blood oxygen levels have already been stressed. As on the maternal side, alterations of fetal blood flow in the placenta will have a profound effect upon Po$_2$(f). It was shown by Dawes (1962) that the placenta provides the maximum peripheral resistance in the fetus, and that the steadily increasing fetal blood-flow rates of pregnancy are initially the result of the opening-up of new vessels, but during later pregnancy are related to an increasing fetal blood pressure; the larger the fetus the higher the blood pressure which has to be maintained. For a fetus of 3.3 kg requiring 5 ml of oxygen/kg a minute, cord blood flows of between 165 and 330 ml/min would be necessary (Bartels *et al.* 1962). These, in turn, demand a cardiac output of about 118 ml/kg a minute. It was shown by Metcalfe *et al.* (1962) that up to a fifth of the fetal blood reaching the placenta is shunted from arterial to venous side without entering into gaseous exchange. It has been claimed that arteriovenous communications occur at all levels in villi, and it is known that fetal blood can continue to flow in cotyledons which are temporarily deprived of maternal arterial in-flow. Hypoxia can in part be countered by an increase of fetal blood pressure and of fetal placental flow. The placental perfusion experiments of Panigel (1962) suggest that fetal placental vessels dilate in response to carbon dioxide and constrict in response to oxygen so that part of the control of flow, and hence Po$_2$(f), may be peripheral. During hypoxia the umbilical blood flow is maintained by the response of fetal pulmonary blood vessels to asphyxia. This causes intense constriction, so diminishing the already small pulmonary blood flow and diverting the blood to the aorta and umbilical circulation.

Consideration of Po$_2$(m) − Po$_2$(f) gradient demands close examination of fetal and maternal perfusion ratios. In long-term sheep catheterization experiments Battaglia (1967) found a Po$_2$ gradient of 40 mmHg between maternal arterial blood entering the intervillous space and fetal reduced blood entering the villi. Further, the blood in the uterine vein and that in the umbilical vein had an identical Po$_2$. Umbilical venous blood has an oxygen saturation of between 70 and 80% at a Po$_2$ of 30–40mmHg. It must be remembered, however, that umbilical arterial blood is more representative of the arterial supply to fetal tissue, and this is normally 50–60% saturated with a Po$_2$ of 20–25 mmHg. Despite this low Po$_2$ the oxygen supply to tissues is usually adequate.

BLOOD PROPERTIES INVOLVED IN GAS EXCHANGE

Oxygen is slightly soluble in plasma, but the amount carried in solution is normally small, being of the order of 0.3 ml/100 ml of blood. The quantity so carried will depend on oxygen tension and upon the solubility coefficients of oxygen in plasma and in the substance of the red blood cell, respectively. The bulk of oxygen is transported as oxyhaemoglobin. The quantity carried will depend on the number of grams of haemoglobin per 100 ml of blood. Each gram when fully saturated carries 1.34 ml of oxygen at standard temperature and pressure, a conversion factor being necessary for other temperatures and pressures. If the percentage saturation of a given blood is plotted against oxygen tension, the result is the oxygen dissociation curve for that blood. For haemoglobin F and haemoglobin A this is an S-shaped curve. Its shape and position will be altered by changes in Pco$_2$ and pH (the Bohr effect). As the blood becomes more acid it gives up oxygen.

Maternal blood in the intervillous space acquires fixed acid and carbon dioxide from the fetus. These liberate oxygen, which is the more avidly taken up by fetal blood because it has surrendered both fixed and volatile acid. This double effect is probably extremely important in oxygen transfer, and may increase the effective Po$_2$ difference by at least 12 mmHg.

In vitro, fetal and maternal blood exhibit different dissociation curves, the Po$_2$ required to produce half-saturation being much lower in fetal than in maternal blood. The difference is closely related to the percentage of haemoglobin F in the fetal whole blood, yet it is known that in concentrated solution haemoglobin A and haemoglobin F produce identical curves. Further, when blood was tested which contained 69% haemoglobin F as a congenital abnormality a normal adult curve was obtained. Thus factors other than the difference in haemoglobin structures must be responsible for the fetal/maternal blood differences. It has been suggested that the difference may be related to a lower pH within the fetal red cell, to absence of carbonic anhydrase within the fetal red cell (similar curves can be obtained from adult blood when this enzyme is destroyed), or from increasing cell thickness during fetal life.

It is known that fetal cord blood has a haemoglobin content of 16–17 g/dl; this provides an oxygen capacity up to 23 ml% compared with 15–16 ml% provided by the haemoglobin of 11 or 12 g/dl present in the mother. This would favour oxygen uptake by fetal blood. More recent work has, however, suggested that the high haemoglobin levels of cord blood are, to a large extent, an expression of a response to stresses during a delivery. It is known that in the human there is a comparatively small increase in haemoglobin concentration between 22 weeks and term. In animals there is a wide scatter of results for fetal blood oxygen capacity. In the rhesus monkey, rabbits and goats there is no great difference at term between maternal and fetal oxygen capacity, while in the rat the haemoglobin content is actually lower than that of the mother. Cases of severe fetal anaemia of unknown origin have been reported in live lambs of normal weight or age, and it is known that the human fetus in cases of rhesus incompatibility can survive at least to the thirty-fourth week with a haemoglobin as low as 4 g/dl. Furthermore, intraperitoneal transfusion with adult blood permits survival and further growth of the fetus, even though at delivery 98% of the haemoglobin detected is adult. These points have been summarized by Dawes (1967).

If it is accepted that the pH of the fetus is 7.24 whilst the maternal pH is 7.42, the result would be that the relevant parts of the two dissociation curves would become superimposed, so minimizing the differences between them. This point has become less relevant since the demonstration that the difference in pH across the placenta in an unstressed preparation lies between 0.02 and 0.05 of a pH unit.

To summarize, by maintaining adequate flows within the fetus it is possible to provide sufficient oxygen despite the low oxygen tension. The perfusion rate on the maternal side of the placenta is also important. The pulmonary changes of pregnancy in the mother have an insignificant effect on her arterial oxygen saturation, whilst the differences between fetal and maternal blood in oxygen content and capacity are less important than was formerly believed. Finally, the Bohr effect is of the utmost importance in maintaining adequate oxygen transfer.

CARBON DIOXIDE TRANSFER

This gas diffuses through a wet membrane 20–30 times as fast as oxygen and, therefore, it passes much more rapidly across the placenta. Carbon dioxide carriage in blood involves three mechanisms.

1 A small amount, probably less than 7%, is transported as carbaminohaemoglobin; this fraction, however, provides 20% or more of the carbon dioxide exchanged. Formation of carbaminohaemoglobin re-quires reduced haemoglobin. At a Pco_2 over 10 mmHg this mechanism is saturated.

2 An even smaller amount is present in simple solution.

3 The bulk of carbon dioxide is carried as bicarbonate in plasma. Dissolved carbon dioxide is in equilibrium with a minute amount which combines with water, producing carbonic acid (H_2CO_3). When this dissociates to form HCO_3^- and H^+ the latter ion is removed by a hydrogen acceptor within the erythrocyte. The bicarbonate ion now diffuses into the plasma, whilst an equivalent amount of Cl^- ion enters the cell (Hamburger shift). This chain of reactions can continue until some 90% of the carbon dioxide is eventually transported as HCO_3^-, over two-thirds of which is accommodated in the plasma. As oxyhaemoglobin is less able to accept hydrogen than reduced haemoglobin, it follows that when blood becomes oxygenated carbon dioxide will be given off (Haldane effect). At the placenta the taking up of oxygen by fetal blood helps displace CO_2 from that blood; whilst simultaneous reduction of maternal blood facilitates the uptake of CO_2 by that blood.

Transfer of inert gases is of importance for studying placental diffusion as they are not produced or consumed by the placenta, have no chemical interaction with tissues and are carried in solution only. Carbon monoxide (which is normally produced and catabolized in the body), because of its high affinity for haemoglobin, has been of particular interest as a means of roughly assessing placental diffusing capacity in women and also with reference to the levels produced in smokers—whose smaller babies could result from a shift to the left of effective oxygen equilibrium by the presence of fetal HbCO at a level exceeding that of the mother.

Nutrient function

A liberal supply of carbohydrate is essential for fetal energy production, since a fetus derives its energy almost completely from this source. Moreover, with the exception of sucrose and lactose all dietary carbohydrates are broken down to glucose on complete hydrolysis, so a brief consideration of the transport of this material across the placenta is appropriate.

All the supply of glucose is obtained by passage across the placenta. It has already been mentioned that the process by which glucose is transferred is facilitated diffusion. Rapid transfer is evident after glucose loading of the mother (Fig. 10.3). Paterson et al.

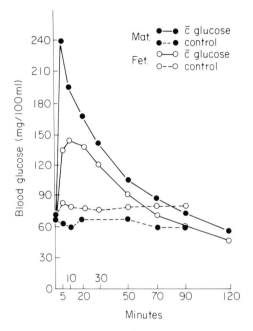

Fig. 10.3. Rapid transfer of glucose from mother to fetus following maternal glucose loading. (By courtesy of Coltart *et al.* 1969.)

(1968) applied the technique of fetal blood sampling to the study of glucose transfer and demonstrated very rapid passage across the placenta; this was confirmed by Coltart *et al.* (1969). In this respect it appears that there is little passage of insulin from the mother to fetus and a variable response in the fetal production of insulin following the glucose loading of the mother.

Placental glucogen was at one time thought to be a source of glucose for the fetus, the amount present providing a ready store of energy for fetal activity. This is now considered unlikely. A very important relationship exists between the glycogen stores of the fetus and its ability to withstand hypoxia.

Although the fetus obtains its energy almost exclusively from the metabolism of carbohydrate, lipids of growth and development must be deposited in significant qualities through fetal life. These lipids will be transported across the placenta, or at any rate built up from other substances so transported. The direct transport of triglycerides and fatty acids from the mother to fetus has been demonstrated in animals; from the fact that adipose tissue of the newborn contains essential fatty acids, direct transport in the human seems a probability (Bagdade & Hirsch 1966). On the other hand, fetal tissues are able to synthesize

triglycerides and fatty acids from early pregnancy onwards. Which mechanism is the more important during pregnancy is uncertain; it is suggested that direct transport from mother to the fetus is probably the more common in early pregnancy, synthesis in the fetus becoming increasingly evident later in fetal life. Cholesterol is capable of direct transport across the placenta from mother to fetus in the experimental animal. However, fetal synthesis is the more important process, accounting for the majority of fetal cholesterol which can be synthesized in most tissues (Myant 1970). No direct passage of more complex lipids such as glycolipids or phospholipids has been demonstrated. These substances are quickly synthesized within the fetus.

Protein transfer is for the most part achieved by the breakdown to amino acids on the material side of the trophoblast, followed by active transport. Here, pinocytosis is the process chiefly involved. Direct transfer may be achieved in the case of a few proteins.

In general, it may be said that in many instances transfer of nutrient materials across the placenta is a fairly rapid process, perhaps occupying only a few minutes in substances transported by simple and facilitated diffusion; in the case of active transport, duration of 30 min to 1 h, or less, is likely to be involved.

Hormone production

This extremely important placental function is considered in detail in Chapter 11.

The barrier function

In early years a good deal of attention was paid to the barrier function of the placenta. The placenta was thought to protect the fetus from a number of noxious substances which might be circulating in the mother if she had, say, an infectious disease or if she had been injected with a drug of some particular kind. We now believe that this barrier function is largely illusory. Many substances cross the placental barrier by physical diffusion or by an active transport system, so much so that in practice almost any drug ingested by or injected into the mother will be found within the fetus within a fairly short time. A high molecular weight has been thought to inhibit passage across the placenta, but this does not interfere with transmission to the fetus except to impose a brief time-lag on the process.

That certain common infections can pass across the alleged placental barrier and affect the fetus *in utero* has been known for many years. One of the most famous of all obstetricians, Mauriceau, is said to have been born pockmarked. The occurrence of congenital syphilis has also been known for many years. It is to modern obstetrics, however, that we have to look for the most dramatic examples of the devastating effects of disease and drugs on the fetus *in utero*.

The effects on the fetus of rubella contracted by the mother in early pregnancy are now well known, and are referred to in more detail in Chapter 23, as are the effects of other viral infections. The percentage of affected children has varied considerably in reported series, suggesting that the teratogenic affect of rubella will vary from one epidemic to another, and probably between epidemic and sporadic forms of the disease. It seems probable, however, that most deformities of the fetus follow an attack of rubella during the first 12 weeks of pregnancy when organogenesis is at its height; occasionally, abnormalities may follow the disease at a slightly later period. If the mother contracts rubella during the first 12 weeks of pregnancy, the chances of her giving birth to a seriously affected child may be somewhere between 15 and 50%. No other diseases have shown such devastating effects as rubella; indeed, it is by no means certain that any are teratogenic, although it has been suggested that mumps, infective hepatitis and influenza may act in a similar way.

A number of acute infections predispose to abortion and fetal death as a result of the toxaemia and pyrexia which are usually present, but teratogenic effects are absent. Chickenpox is known to affect the fetus if contracted by the mother in late pregnancy, leading to congenital or neonatal chickenpox.

The pregnant woman is apparently more liable to infection by poliomyelitis, and the disease is more dangerous if she is infected. It would appear not to be teratogenic, but the virus passing across the placenta may infect the fetus, so fetal wastage as abortion, stillbirth or neonatal death may result. Studies of Salk vaccine and orally administered, live, attenuated vaccine in pregnancy have shown no apparent fetal adverse effects, and one or other should be used if the risk of poliomyelitis is considerable.

The parasitic condition of toxoplasmosis deserves mention. This is an infestation by the parasite *Toxoplasma gondii* which may be virtually asymptomatic in the mother, but its effects on the fetus may be very grave. The parasite may pass across to the fetus during the parasitaemic phase and may give rise to serious abnormalities such as choroidoretinitis, hydrocephalus, cerebral calcification, jaundice, hepatosplenomegaly and convulsions. In some communities the disease is a significant cause of abortion, and perhaps should be more often considered in this country. Since the disease is only dangerous during its parasitaemic stage a person who has given birth to a child affected by toxoplasmosis need not concern herself in the future about a recurrence.

The appalling deformities caused by thalidomide administered in early pregnancy should make all obstetricians acutely aware of the risks of prescribing drugs in early pregnancy and in the case of some drugs, in late pregnancy also. Whilst with no other drug has such a close relationship to fetal deformity been established as with thalidomide, several have had the finger of suspicion pointed at them. It is difficult to know whether a particular drug can be held responsible for occasional defects, and an extremely cautious approach to prescribing in early pregnancy is necessary if further calamities are to be avoided (Stirrat & Beard 1973).

Some drugs, even when administered in late pregnancy, may pass to the fetus with harmful effects. Examples are a fetal goitre caused by potassium iodide or thiouracil treatment, fetal haemorrhage and death following dicoumarol treatment (heparin appears safe in this respect), and inhibition of bone growth with teeth discoloration following tetracycline therapy. Other antibiotics may also exert undesirable effects (Charles 1979). With transferable drugs we should perhaps be more interested in the effects of the drug on the fetus than in the actual blood levels reached in the fetus.

All things considered, the circumstances in which the placenta can really be regarded as a barrier are so few that this so-called function can be disregarded.

AMNIOTIC FLUID

Since the fetus lives surrounded by amniotic fluid, the idea has grown that examination of this milieu exterieur might give information about its metabolism, a similar philosophy to the classical physiologist's examination of expired air or of urine in the adult extrauterine human. It must be remembered, however, that amniotic fluid contains only a part of excretion products of the fetus, and that the vast majority of exchange takes place across the placenta. Amniotic fluid in late pregnancy, however, is largely made by the fetus and contains many products of its metabolism, but to those investigating the fetus the

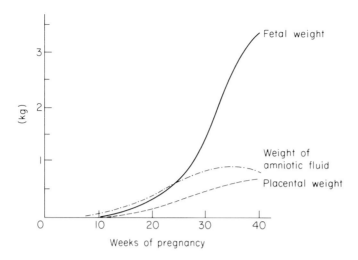

Fig. 10.4. The weight of amniotic fluid, fetus and placenta throughout pregnancy. (Redrawn from Hytten 1980.)

amniotic fluid is like the rubbish pit of an excavated site to the archaeologist. Both provide fragments of evidence about happenings from several episodes in the past history; they are often mixed up, and the time-relations require careful sifting.

The volume of amniotic fluid is used by clinicians as an estimate of the fetal state. Studies have shown the fluid volume to increase up to about 37 weeks' gestation in the normal patient and to diminish after this. However, measurements are increasingly difficult in the second half of pregnancy and Fig. 10.4 is a proportional illustration of the means of readings which are widely scattered and may vary, for example, from 500 to 1500 g in the last weeks. When patients with pre-eclampsia or essential hypertension are tested, they show a similar pattern but a decline in volume may occur earlier, possibly indicating a failing placental function early in pregnancy. Clinical surveys using girth as the measure of uterine content (Elder *et al.* 1970) have shown a significant correlation between liquor status and the production of a dysmature baby, particularly in the presence of essential hypertension.

Fetal urine becomes an increasingly important component of the amniotic fluid, and so content of the fluid may reflect fetal renal functions. Estimating the osmolality by the depression of freezing point is a guide to the electrolytes present in the amniotic fluid. The osmolality of liquor declines in an almost linear fashion in the second half of normal pregnancy, veering towards values in fetal urine rather than those of either maternal or fetal plasma. Deviations from this pattern are associated with an increased fetal death rate, but correlations are not yet

significant and readings may be more useful in the assessment of fetal maturity; if levels of 245 mmol/kg or below are obtained, it is probably that the fetus is beyond 38 weeks' gestation. Creatinine concentrations stay at a constant low level until the last few weeks of pregnancy when there is an abrupt increase, so that by 38 weeks the concentration is 1.5 mg% or more although in rhesus isoimmunization higher levels can occur earlier in pregnancy. This change may indicate fetal physiological maturity, and alterations in the rate of increase of concentration might be indicative of poor renal function and thus of poor fetal metabolism.

The acid-base state of liquor has been investigated in both chronic and acute deterioration in the fetal state. As pregnancy advances, the amniotic fluid pH drops with a rising $P\text{CO}_2$ and a falling bicarbonate. There is a very wide variation of normal levels in pregnancy and in labour. As in blood estimations, $P\text{O}_2$ in amniotic fluid has a poor correlation with the fetal state; large amounts of fixed acids, high $P\text{CO}_2$ levels and a low pH are found in the fluid of those with hypoxic fetal distress, but the correlations have not been significant.

It is the chronic diseases and conditions which will be best diagnosed from liquor investigations. The scanning of amniotic fluid in rhesus-affected pregnancies has led to assessment of the degree of affect on the baby. This is discussed in Chapter 18. The cellular content of the amniotic fluid increasingly comes from the fetus as pregnancy proceeds. These cells are hard to obtain before 16 weeks of gestation, but once present they can be used for the investigation of chromosomal abnormalities. After cell culture,

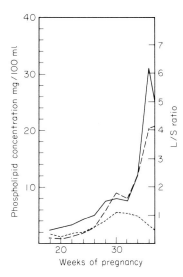

Fig. 10.5. The relationship in the amniotic fluid of lecithin and sphingomyelin and the alteration in the L/S ratio as pregnancy advances (redrawn from Gluck 1971).
——— L/S ratio; – – – – Lecithin; - - - - - Sphingomyelin.

the fetal sex and certain chromosomally labelled conditions (such as Down's syndrome) can be determined. Unfortunately, very few diseases are chromosomally flagged in a manner that present methods can detect, so that the use of this technique is limited. It takes 2–4 weeks to culture cells, and pregnancy is often well advanced by the time a diagnosis is made by this method; if termination of pregnancy is to be recommended on karyometric grounds, a patient is often well into the mid-trimester before this can be done.

In consequence, the technique of chorionic villus biopsy may be more attractive despite their higher risk of abortion for they allow examination of fetal cells so much earlier, at 8–10 weeks of gestation.

Maturity of the lung is related to its secretion of the phospholipids lecithin and sphingomyelin. These surfactant substances lower the surface tension of lung fluid so that alveoli can be opened more easily when the newborn baby breathes. Lecithin accumulates in the amniotic fluid more than does sphingomyelin so a ratio of these increases as maturity advances (Fig. 10.5). An L/S ratio of 2:1 is rarely associated with respiratory distress in the baby. Such lung maturity, as measured by this index seems to be reached by 33–34 weeks but maturation delay is found in severe diabetes, renal disease and indentical twins. Occasional acceleration of maturity occurs in pre-eclampsia and care should be taken to obtain a

blood-free sample of amniotic fluid for this can affect results. Assuming that surfactant activity is a result of fetal adrenal maturity. Liggins (1972) suggested that increased surfactant might be produced if women who were at risk of producing premature babies were given corticosteroids. This seems to be so.

All the methods discussed so far of examining the amniotic fluid have involved broaching the amniotic cavity. Whilst in mid or late pregnancy this is a safe procedure after the placenta has been localized, once the cervix permits, transcervical amnioscopy would leave the cavity intact. A tapered amnioscope is introduced through the vagina and manoeuvred through the cervix of the patient. With a good light source, a view is usually obtained through the amniotic sac of the liquor in front of the fetal presenting part. The colour and content of the fluid, including meconium flecks, can be seen. The major use for amnioscopy used to be in patients who had reached term by their gestational dates, and showed no signs of labour. Unfortunately, it has been shown that the use of amnioscopy alone has not caused any significant reduction in perinatal mortality rates in prolonged pregnancy and its use in the United Kingdom has been greatly reduced.

In its place, estimations of the volume of amniotic fluid have become important. Too much and too little (polyhydramnios and oligohydramnios respectively) can be recognized in their extremes clinically. More subtle changes can be found by ultrasound, and the diameter of the largest pocket of amniotic fluid can be measured. If less than 2cm, fetal growth is poor and well-being is suspect. If the largest pool is more than 8cm across, polyhydramnios is diagnosed and again the fetus is considered at higher risk. Ultrasound measurements allow the volume of amniotic fluid to be measured fairly accurately. Interpretation of the measurements is a clinical matter.

Thanks are due to Mr E. D. Morris, a previous contributor, for allowing much of his material to be used in this chapter.

REFERENCES

ADAMSONS K. (1965) *Birth Defects*, Series 1, No. **1**, p. 27.
AHERNE W. & DUNNILL M. S. (1966) *Brit. med. Bull.*, **22**, 5.
AMORSO E. C. (1961) *Brit. med. Bull.*, **17**, 81.
BAGDADE J. D. & HIRSCH J. (1966) *Proc. Soc. exp. Biol. Med.*, **122**, 616.
BARTELS H., MOLL W. & METCALFE J. (1952) *Amer. J. Obstet. Gynec.*, **84**, 1714.

BATTAGLIA F. C. (1967) *Modern Trends in Obstetrics*, 4e., p. 284. Butterworths, London.

BENIRSCHKE K. & DRISCOLL S. D. (1967) *The Pathology of the Human Placenta*. Springer, New York.

CHARLES D. (1979) *Obstet. & Gynec. Annual*, p. 19 (Wynn R. M. ed.) Appleton Century Crofts, New York.

BOYD R. D., HAWORTH C., STACEY T. & WARD R. (1976) *J. Physiol. (Lond.)*, **254**, 169.

BUTLER N. R. (1965) *Medicine*, **19**, 74.

COLTART T. M., BEARD R. W., TURNER R. C. & OAKLEY N. W. (1969) *Brit. med. J.*, **4**, 17.

CRAWFORD J. M. (1962) *Amer. J. Obstet. Gynec.*, **84**, 1543.

DAWES G. S. (1962) *Amer. J. Obstet. Gynec.*, **84**, 1634.

DAWES G. S. (1967) *Sci. Basis Med. Ann. Rev.*, p. 74.

DAWES G. S. (1968) *Foetal and Neonatal Physiology*, Ch. 2. Year Book Medical Publishers, Chicago.

ELDER M. G., BURTON E. R., GORDON H., HAWKINS D. F. & McCLURE BROWN J. D. (1970) *J. Obstet. Gynaec. Brit. Cwlth.*, **77**, 48.

FORSTER R. E. (1973) In *Foetal and Neonatal Physiology*, p. 223. Proc. Sir Joseph Barcroft Centenary Symposium. Cambridge Univ. Press.

GITLIN J. D. & GITLIN D. (1973) *Pediat. Res.*, **7**, 290.

GLUCK L. (1971) *Hosp. Pract.*, **6**, 45.

GREISS F. C. JR. (1973) *Obstet. & Gynec. Annual* (Wynn R. M. ed.), p. 55. Appleton Century Crofts, New York.

GROSSER O. (1927) *Funihartwicklung, Einhantbildung und Placentation des Menschen und der Säugetier*. Bergnaun, Munich.

LICHTY J. A., TING R. T., BRUNS P. D. & DYER E. (1957) *Amer. J. Dis. Child.*, **93**, 666.

LIGGINS G. C. & HOWIE M. B. (1972) *Pediatrics*, **50**, 515.

LONGO L. D. (1972) In *Pathophysiology of Gestation, vol II, Fetal Placental Disorders* (Assali N. S. ed.). Academic Press, London.

MESCHIA G. & BATTAGLIA F. C. (1973) In *Foetal & Neonatal Physiology*, p. 272. Proc. Sir Joseph Barcroft Centenary Symposium. Cambridge Univ. Press.

METCALFE J. MESCHIA G., HELLEGERS A. E., PRYSTOWSKY H., HUCKABEE W. E. & BARRON D. H. (1962) *Q.J. exp. Physiol.*, **47**, 74.

MYANT N. B. (1970) *Scientific Foundations of Obstetrics & Gynaecology*, p. 354 (Philip, Barnes & Newton eds.). Heinemann, London.

PANIGEL M. (1962) *Amer. J. Obstet. Gynec.*, **84**, 1664.

PATERSON P., PAGE D., TAFT P., PHILLIPS L. & WOOD C. (1968) *J. Obstet. Gynaec. Brit. Cwlth.*, **75**, 917.

STEVEN D. & SAMUEL C. (1979) In *Placental Transfer* (Chamberlain G. V. P. & Wilkinson A. eds.). Pitman Medical Publications, Tunbridge Wells.

STIRRAT G. M. & BEARD R. W. (1973) *Prescribers Journal*, **13**, 135.

TINDALL V. R. & SCOTT J. S. (1965) *J. Obstet. Gynaec. Brit. Cwlth.*, **72**, 356.

YOUNG M. & McFADYEN I. (1973) *J. Physiol.*, **235**, 409.

CHAPTER 11
ENDOCRINE CHANGES DURING PREGNANCY

RODNEY P SHEARMAN

Until relatively recently, it was believed that the endocrine changes in pregnancy did not become manifest until after implantation of the blastocyst. From that time until the delivery of the placenta, there is a progressive and profound modification of the woman's hormonal environment. Much of this is immediately due to direct endocrine activity of the placenta and fetus; some of it is a secondary effect of the feto-placental hormones on the maternal endocrine glands.

Although considerable progress has been made in unravelling the hormonal interrelationships of the mother–placenta–fetus, there are still large areas of ignorance. Since it is not possible to study pregnancy in the absence of the placenta, this denied to the investigator a classical method of understanding its hormonal function. Once considered endocrinologically inert, it is now clear that the human fetus is very active hormonally and this gave rise to the concept of the feto-placental unit.

Two further developments have now become apparent. Firstly, even the pre-implantation blastocyst is endocrinologically active; secondly, the fetus itself throughout pregnancy plays an important and probably autonomous role in the regulation both of its own development and perhaps in the initiation of spontaneous labour.

PEPTIDE HORMONES OF THE PLACENTA

Substances to be discussed here are human chorionic gonadotrophin (hCG) and human placental lactogen (hPL), with some discussion on the now resolving question of whether or not the human placenta produces one or more thyrotrophic hormones.

Human chorionic gonadotrophin (hCG)

The first of the human pregnancy-specific hormones to be isolated, hCG is a glycoprotein consisting of α and β sub-units. The former is common to thyroid-stimulating hormone (TSH), luteinizing hormone (LH) and follicle-stimulating hormone (FSH). The β sub-unit on the other hand shares structural and more importantly, immunological characteristics only with the β sub-unit of LH, but there is a terminal peptide sequence of about 30 amino acids that makes the β sub-unit unique (Morgan et al. 1973) but not perhaps to trophoblast alone (see later). hCG is secreted from the trophoblast before implantation and well before the first missed period (Mishell et al. 1974). Peak levels of hCG are detected between 11 and 14 weeks of gestation both in fetal serum and amniotic fluid (Clements et al. 1976). In the mother, precise and specific quantitative data are now available. Earlier immunological results that measured the total molecule of hCG had shown a secondary rise in the third trimester. Using a specific radioimmunoassay for β-hCG, Braunstein et al. (1976) have confirmed that the original bioassays were correct after all. hCG rises rapidly in early pregnancy, reaching a peak between days 56 and 68. There is then a relatively rapid drop to 18 weeks and levels remain more or less constant until after delivery. Spellacy et al. (1975) could not confirm earlier reports that hCG levels at term were related to fetal sex.

It may be all very well to know something of the structure of hCG, a little of its pharmacodynamics and even a fraction of its pharmacology, but it would be far more comforting to know what this hormone does in normal pregnancy. Obviously, it is not just there to provide the clinician with a convenient pregnancy test. Almost certainly hCG rescues the corpus luteum of pregnancy from its otherwise inevitable dissolution during menstrual bleeding. Although specific binding sites for hCG in the corpus luteum cannot be demonstrated after the 6th week of pregnancy, very specific binding can be shown in the corpus luteum during the normal cycle (Ashitaka & Koide 1974). Specific binding to the testis has also been demonstrated (Catt et al. 1972). Because fetal pituitary LH does not begin to rise before the 12th week (Clements *et al.* 1976; and also see below) it is now accepted that hCG is the prime mover in the induction of fetal testosterone secretion from the Leydig cells which makes the newborn baby boy so obviously male.

It is really quite extraordinary that so little should be known about the physiological roles of hCG. Its action in the early stimulation of Leydig cells is both crucial and clear. It has substantial activity as a luteinizing hormone. Having said this, one runs into the sands from a rapidly receding tide, and nothing is known of its control. For the mechanically or quantitatively minded it is very odd to consider the pattern of hCG secretion when compared with, for example, hPL or SP$_1$. These are all produced by the trophoblast and the last two increase hand in hand with placental weight. hCG breaks all the rules by retiring into relative obscurity after the eighteenth week when all the other indices of placental hormone production go from strength to strength. It would be nice to believe that hCG had something to do with the control of steroid synthesis from the placenta (something must control it after all) but there is no good evidence that it does. While many clinicians believe that hCG is responsible, at least in part, for 'morning sickness' both because of the natural history of this affliction in a temporal sense and its greater frequency in the two classic conditions where pathologically high levels of hCG are found (multiple pregnancy and hydatidiform mole), this is empiricism at its best. A conclusion based on observation and experience will show an association. It does not constitute proof.

The elusive hormone has achieved a minor triumph in a study of pathophysiology. While it was previously believed that the placenta produced a true and unique thyrotrophic hormone clinically evident in some women and men with trophoblastic tumours, it is now known that this action is due to pathologically high levels of hCG.

The trophoblastic uniqueness of hCG has been challenged by work from the laboratories of the National Institues of Health in the United States of America (Chen *et al.* 1976). The C-terminal peptide group, referred to earlier and thought to be peculiar to trophoblastic hCG has been found in body fluid of postmenopausal women, one man with Klinefelter's syndrome and in extracts from human pituitaries. However, Yoshimoto *et al.* (1979) have indicated that this material does not possess the carbohydrate component of placental hCG and therefore would have

little or no bioactivity *in vivo*. The trophoblastic uniqueness of hCG is, therefore, not its ability to synthesize hCG but its ability to glycosylate it.

While it is possible that hCG may play some role in the early regulation of the fetal zone of the human adrenal cortex (Séron-Ferré *et al.* 1978), it now seems evident that fetal ACTH and cortico-trophin-like intermediate lobe peptide (CLIP) are the trophic hormones in later pregnancy (Gray & Abramovich 1980).

It has also been shown that the fetus is capable of synthesizing the α and β sub-units of hCG in the kidney, while low, but consistent rates of α sub-unit synthesis occur in the liver (McGregor *et al.* 1983). It has been suggested that this fetal hCG has a role as a thyrotrophic hormone early in pregnancy while in anencephalic fetuses, in the absence of their own TSH, this may continue well into the second trimester.

Human placental lactogen (hPL)

Also known as human chorionic sommato-mammotrophin (hCS) the presence of this hormone was forecast by Ehrhardt in 1936. Following the precedent set by human growth hormone and prolactin, Schneider *et al.* (1975) have shown that while the traditional small molecule of hPL is dominant in body fluids, 'big' hPL is probably the active hormone secreted by the placenta. Although this observation explains the paradox of immunological heterogeneity of hPL that had been described in earlier papers and is of some importance for the fundamental physiologist, the actual or potential clinical physiologist should not feel unduly disadvantaged. As Gertrude Stein said in her famous latter-day trisagion 'a rose is a rose is a rose' (Brinnin 1960) whether it be large, middle-sized or small.

The trophoblastic origin of hPL was confirmed by Grumbach and Kaplan in 1964. Unlike hCG there is a close correlation between placental weight and hPL production throughout pregnancy. The normal levels in maternal venous blood throughout pregnancy are shown in Fig. 11.1. Total secretion rate at term is about 0.5 g/100 g of placental tissue in 24 hours (Josimovich 1977).

Earlier studies had indicated that hypoglycaemia or hyperglycaemia had no effect on hPL production (and this is still probably true in the physiological state), but pharmacological changes do alter serum hPL levels in late pregnancy, with hypoglycaemia increasing levels and hyperglycaemia causing a decrease (Josimovich 1977).

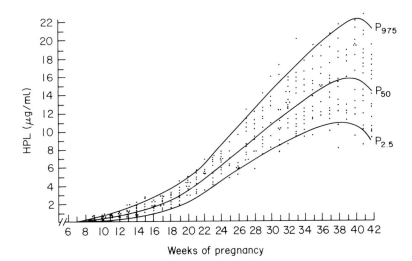

Fig. 11.1 hPL concentrations in 263 normal pregnancies. (Reproduced from Ylikorkala (1973) by courtesy of the Editor of *Acta Obstetrics et Gynaecologica Scandinavia*.)

Chemically and biologically, hPL has much in common with hGH and, to a lesser extent, prolactin.

Although negligible quantities of hPL are found in fetal serum, amniotic fluid levels increase *pari passu* with those seen in maternal blood.

Josimovich (1977) and Josimovich and Archer (1977) discuss the possible physiological roles of hPL. They may be summarized as follows:

1 It is lactogenic and will cause milk production in rhesus monkeys after pre-treatment with oestrogens and progestins. In this sense it is almost certainly complementary to the changes in maternal prolactin to be discussed below.

2 Since hPL inhibits maternal hGH, the former is probably the prime mover in lypolysis, nitrogen retention, hyperinsulinism and peripheral resistance to insulin, all of which are observed in normal human pregnancy.

3 It is not luteotrophic in humans, despite adequate evidence of this activity in rodents.

4 It may exert some control over progesterone synthesis.

Placental thyrotrophins

As already mentioned, the chorionic and molar thyrotrophins appear not to be unique hormones. There is now very good evidence that the pregnancy thyrotrophin is, in fact, hCG (Kenimer *et al.* 1975).

Other placental proteins

A review of these new placental proteins will be found in Grudzinskas *et al.* (1984).

RELAXIN

Although this hormone was first isolated in the guinea pig many years ago, interest in the human has been rekindled during the last decade. There is now unequivocal evidence for the presence of this hormone throughout human pregnancy, the site of origin being the corpus luteum (Quagliarello *et al.* 1979). Levels are highest during the first trimester, followed by a decline in the second and third trimesters when levels are relatively stable. There is good evidence that relaxin secretion can also be induced in the non-pregnant corpus luteum by administration of human chorionic gonadotrophin (Quagliarello *et al.* 1980). More recent immunohistochemical studies have shown that relaxin can be found in the placental syncytiotrophoblast, decidua and corpus luteum during pregnancy (Yki-Järvinen *et al.* 1983). The same workers have also confirmed the presence of relaxin in the corpus luteum and secretory endometrium of the normal non-pregnant woman without the need for prior administration of hCG. The origin and role of this endometrial relaxin remains to be determined.

The amino acid sequence of human relaxin derived from a genomic clone has been described by Hudson *et al.* (1983). Commercial production of relaxin using recombinant DNA technology is now feasible. Although there is only a 50% homology between porcine relaxin and human relaxin, the former will certainly induce ripening of the human cervix without uterine contractility (MacLennan *et al.* 1980; Evans *et al.* 1983). An outline of the established and speculative roles of relaxin in mammals is shown in Table 11.1.

Table 11.1. Possible biological roles of relaxin in mammals.

Established in some species

   Relaxation of pelvic ligaments near parturition
   Uterine stromal remodelling during pregnancy
   Inhibition of myometrial activity during pregnancy
   Cervical ripening and facilitation of parturition
   Mammary growth during pregnancy
   Enhancement of sperm mobility

Speculative

   Facilitation of follicle rupture at ovulation
   Facilitation of blastocyst implantation
   Fetal growth factor
   Facilitation of fetal membrane rupture
   Factor influencing skin collagen metabolism and collagen
   disorders

STEROID HORMONES OF THE PLACENTA

Progesterone

While the maternal ovary contributes some progesterone in the very earliest stages of pregnancy, after this the placental contribution dominates, and there is no doubt that the placenta is the source of virtually all the progesterone produced during pregnancy. However, there is clear evidence for some progesterone secretion by the corpus luteum throughout the whole of pregnancy. In addition to progesterone, two other biologically active progesterones (20α- and 20β-hydroxypregn-4-ene-3-one) are secreted in much lower quantities.

The placenta is able to synthesize progesterone from the same precursors as those discussed in Chapter 5 (Jaffe 1967). Unlike oestrogens, progesterone production is only very slightly affected by the fetal circulation (Cassmer 1959). These feto-placental relationships have been fully reviewed by Solomon et al. (1967).

Although some progress has been made in determining the control of progesterone secretion in the ovary, there is very little known of the controlling mechanism(s) in pregnancy. Certainly it is independent of maternal pituitary control (Fotherby 1964), and no negative feedback mechanism can be demonstrated.

The metabolic effects of progesterone and its activity on the uterus have been fully reviewed by Fotherby (1964) and Hytten and Leitch (1964). Progesterone probably antagonizes the action of aldosterone on the renal tubule, but this action is compensated by the increased secretion of aldosterone seen in pregnancy. In large amounts progesterone has a slight catabolic action and there is suggestive evidence that fat deposition may be increased.

The effects of progesterone on the uterus are complex and ill-understood. It is probable that progesterone effects the membrane potential of myometrial fibres, thereby reducing the excitability of the uterus. The effect of progesterone on the protein and collagen content of the uterus remains unresolved. It appears to increase the activity of alkaline phosphatase and succinate dehydrogenase in the uterus.

It is widely believed (but objective evidence for the belief is scanty) that the high levels of progesterone in pregnancy reduce smooth muscle tone in the ureter, colon and stomach. It is of interest that large doses of progesterone induce overbreathing with a reduction in alveolar and arterial Pco_2; changes normally observed in pregnancy.

Levels of progesterone and its metabolites in biological fluids

Progesterone levels in blood during pregnancy have been documented by Eton and Short (1960) and Yannone et al. (1968), showing a progressive increase throughout gestation. Although the presence of urinary progesterone has been indicated in pregnancy (Ismael & Harkness 1966), there are no adequate data on excretion patterns in normal or abnormal pregnancy.

Urinary pregnanediol levels have for many years been used as a means of assessing changes in progesterone production. The limitations of such an approach need to be clearly recognized. Although there is general recognition of the poor correlation between the excretion of urinary pregnanediol and either progesterone secretion or blood progesterone levels, for both historical and technical reasons pregnanediol assays have been widely used in endocrinological studies for many years. Adequate data using reliable methods are well documented. Using the same method, Shearman (1959) and Klopper and Billewicz (1963) produced very similar findings. Their results, together with those of Eton and Short for progesterone in blood, are shown in Fig. 11.2.

Csapo (1970) has long been a champion of the 'progesterone block' theory of the onset of labour. Although there is very good evidence that this is operative in many animals (vide infra), suggestions

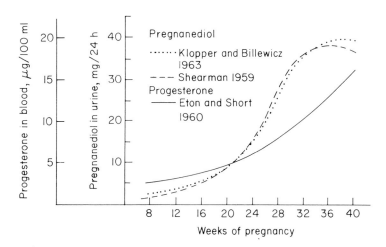

Fig. 11.2 Urinary pregnanediol excretion and blood progesterone levels during pregnancy. (Reproduced from Hytten & Leitch (1964), Blackwell Scientific Publications Ltd.)

that the same changes occur in the human (Turnbull et al. 1974) have not been confirmed (Dawood & Kelmkamp, 1977).

Oestrogens

In the last two decades there has been a large amount of data collected on the interrelationships of the maternal, fetal and placental contributions to oestrogen synthesis in pregnancy. Much of this has been reviewed extensively during this time (Bolte, 1967, Cassmer 1959, Diczfalusy et al. 1961, Frandsen 1963).

Although more than 25 different oestrogens have been isolated from human pregnancy urine, to simplify a complex problem only the three 'classical oestrogens' (oestrone, oestradiol and oestriol) will be discussed here.

The metabolism of oestrogens in the non-pregnant female is discussed in Chapters 5 and 8 where it will have been noted that the biologically actively secreted steroids, oestrone and oestradiol, are derived from androgenic precursors. Oestriol is predominantly a metabolite of these, but is secreted as such in small quantities by active steroidogenic tissue (Barlow & Logan 1966). It is also usually accepted that a hallmark of 'secreted' as distinct from 'metabolized' oestrogen in the non-pregnant state, is that they are unconjugated. Conjugation under these circumstances is usually accepted as part of the biological inactivation and metabolism of the secreted parent hormone.

The picture in pregnancy is different, involving a complex of maternal and fetal precursors, the fetal contribution being very dependent on the fetal

adrenal and liver, and an intact feto-placental circulation.

In the non-pregnant individual the proportions of oestriol:oestrone:oestradiol in urine varies, but approximates 3:2:1. As indicated above, most of the oestriol is derived from the metabolism of oestrone/oestradiol. In late pregnancy the urinary proportion of the three steroids is radically different, 30:2:1. There is clear evidence for secretion of oestriol by the placenta during pregnancy from predominantly fetal precursors, and of oestradiol from predominantly maternal precursors (Fig. 11.3).

Studies, both in vitro and in vivo, indicate that there is increasing ability of the placenta to convert maternal dehydro-epiandrosterone sulphate (DHAS) to oestradiol during pregnancy, conversion rates increasing from about 5% at 16 weeks' gestation to 40% at term (Siiteri & MacDonald 1966). Fetal DHAS also contributes to placental oestradiol production.

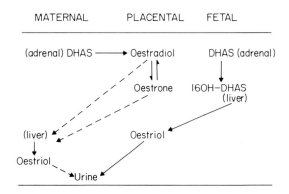

Fig. 11.3. Outline of oestrogen metabolism in the fetoplacental unit.

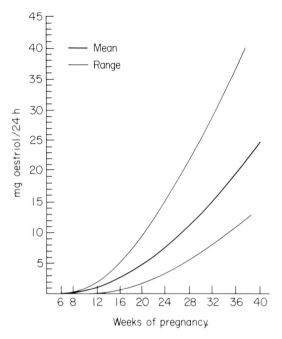

Fig. 11.4. Urinary oestriol excretion during normal pregnancy. (Reproduced from Coyle & Brown (1963), by courtesy of the Editor of *Journal of Obstetrics and Gynaecology of the British Commonwealth*.)

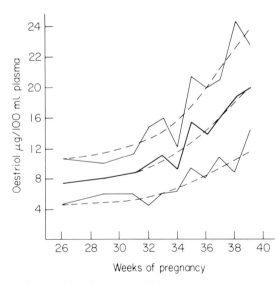

Fig. 11.5. Maternal venous oestriol after 26th week of pregnancy. The observed mean and range of one standard deviation is shown between the solid lines. The smoothed mean and range is indicated in the shaded area. (From Shearman *et al.* (1972) by courtesy of the Editor, *Journal of Obstetrics and Gynaecology of the British Commonwealth*.)

It is known that the placenta lacks α-16-hydroxylase, so is incapable itself of synthesizing oestriol. The particular role of the fetus in the synthesis of precursors of oestriol, suggested by the observations of Cassmer (1959), and extended by those of Frandsen and Stakemann (1963), has been amply confirmed. In essence, DHAS secreted by the fetal zone of the adrenal cortex is 16-hydroxylated in the fetal liver (16-OH-DHAS) and transported via the umbilical arteries to the placenta, where it is desulphated and aromatized to produce free oestriol.

The urinary excretion pattern of oestrogens in pregnancy is well documented, following the first accurate observations by Brown in 1959. Because of its widespread clinical use, urinary oestriol excretion has received particular attention, and there is a large amount of information dealing with levels in normal and abnormal pregnancy. The results obtained by Coyle and Brown (1963) are shown in Fig. 11.4.

Currently there is a great deal of interest in plasma levels of oestriol, because of the speed both of collection and following radioimmunoassay. In a qualitative sense the levels of oestriol in plasma are similar to those seen in urine (Fig. 11.5).

ENDOCRINOLOGY OF THE FETUS

As mentioned previously, it now seems apparent that even the pre-implantation blastocyst may have endocrinological actions. *In vitro* culture of fertilized ova provides no supportive evidence for production of hCG but there is clear evidence that the coronal cells of the pre-implantation blastocyst continue to produce substantial amounts of progesterone and oestradiol (Shutt & Lopata 1980). An observation of profound biological and perhaps ultimately therapeutic importance was the detection of 'early pregnancy factor' by Morton and her colleagues (1977). This factor can be detected within hours if fertilization in all species studies, including the human, and may well be important in the adaptation of the maternal environment for blastocyst implantation.

Fetal endocrinology as it relates to sexual differentiation has been discussed in detail in Chapter 3 and will not be repeated here.

Obviously a great deal more remains to be learnt about the endocrinology of the fetus both in early and mid-pregnancy. The endocrine autonomy of the fetus as it may affect the onset of labour has, however, received a great deal of attention.

It has taken more than 2000 years to confirm the

Hippocratic concept that the fetus controls the onset of labour, at least under normal circumstances. While most of the objective scientific data has come from animal studies, there is increasing evidence in the human that, in principle, the fetus does exercise control although the methods of control may differ from that so well documented in animals.

The original clinical observations relating to the effect of fetal abnormalities in cattle and sheep on prolongation of pregnancy have been discussed briefly by Liggins et al. (1973). These indicated that adrenal hypoplasia, or fetal hypopituitarism were associated with prolonged pregnancy in these two animal species. Earlier, in 1933, Malpas had indicated that in human pregnancy associated with fetal anencephaly, pregnancy was usually prolonged as long as as polyhydramnios was absent. It is rarely that an isolated case report throws light on a problem, but one such case reported by Williams and Cummins (1953) certainly indicated that the fetus must have some role in the control of labour. A twin pregnancy occurred in a patient with complete duplication of the uterus and cervix. In the 32nd week labour occurred spontaneously and one fetus was delivered followed almost immediately by a placenta. The second cervis was completely closed and remained so until the onset of spontaneous labour again 56 days later. These clinical observations suggest very strongly that in the human as well as in the experimental animal, the fetus does have some autonomy in dictating the onset of normal labour. The second of these indicates that the changes are localized within the uterus; studies of maternal peripheral blood, not surprisingly, are a very pale reflection of the central turmoil.

The role of the fetus in the onset of labour and the consequent changes in the periparturient endocrine millieu of the mother have been very well documented in the sheep by Liggins in New Zealand and in the goat by the Prospect group in Australia (Currie et al. 1973; Liggins 1974; Liggins et al. 1973). The importance of confirming these observations in the two species is that while the sheep is dependent on hormonal function from the placenta for continuation of pregnancy, the goat is dependent on persistence of the corpus luteum. In summary, in each of these species several days before the onset of labour and presumably as a result of increased fetal hypothalamic and pituitary activity the secretion rate of fetal cortisol increases rapidly. These high concentrations of cortisol in fetal blood act on the placenta or corpus luteum to reduce the secretion of progesterone and increase the secretion of oestrogens. Associated with a rising concentration of oestradiol there is a sharp increase in concentration of the prostaglandin $F_{2\alpha}$ arising from the 'maternal placenta'. The myometrium responds to the prostaglandin $F_{2\alpha}$, then as labour progresses with distension of the cervix by decent of the fetus, reflex release of oxytocin further increases the production of prostaglandin $F_{2\alpha}$. These changes are shown schematically in Fig. 11.6.

For obvious reasons the same chronic data cannot be obtained from the human fetus. However, there is suggestive evidence that although the time-scale may be different, the controlling factors in the human may be similar.

It has been shown in the human fetus that umbilical arterial corticosteroid levels and arterial cortisol levels are very substantially increased in those infants delivered vaginally after spontaneous labour when compared with infants of comparable gestational age delivered by elective Caesarean section (Shearman et al. 1974; Smith et al. 1975). Murphy (1973) has shown that this difference is not due to stress. She documented the fact that arterial cortisol levels in the human fetus after induced labour were substantially lower than the levels found in fetuses after spontaneous labour and delivery. Murphy (1983), in a comprehensive review, has pointed out the methodological pitfalls in measuring corticosteroids under these circumstances. The steep rise in fetal serum cortisol just before 40 weeks is confirmed as is the substantial difference in umbilical arterial levels in infants born after spontaneous vaginal delivery compared with those delivered by Caesarian section. Levels in fetuses delivered after induced labour are intermediate between these two.

Turnbull et al. (1974) have unconfirmed evidence of a fall in progesterone in maternal venous blood before the onset of labour and there is confirmed evidence of an increase in umbilical venous levels of oestrogens in those babies born after spontaneous labour compared with babies born by Caesarian section (Patten et al. 1973; Shutt et al. 1974). Levels of prostaglandin $F_{2\alpha}$ in liquor and its 15 keto-dihydro metabolite in venous blood increase rapidly with the onset of clinical labour.

It should be stressed that while the evidence for fetal control of the onset of labour in the sheep and goat is now overwhelming, evidence in the human at this stage remains largely inferential. While most of the objective scientific data have come from animal studies, there is increasing but still tantalizingly opaque evidence in the human that the fetus may

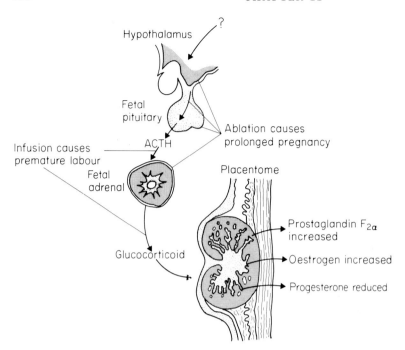

Fig. 11.6. Initiation of parturition.

play an important role in the control of the onset of labour but in a way that differs from that so well documented in animals. It does seem likely that in the human, local production of prostaglandins from the fetal membranes may be under different control from that seen in the experimental animal and this is discussed in more detail by Shearman (1979).

MATERNAL AND FETAL PITUITARY FUNCTION

There is now substantial documentation of maternal pituitary function as it relates to prolactin secretion. Prolactin levels in maternal serum increase throughout pregnancy while even higher levels (two- to ten-fold) are found in amniotic fluid (Schenker et al. 1975). Rigg et al. (1977) suggest that this maternal change is a functional reflection of hyperplasia and hypertrophy of the pituitary lactotrophes in response to 'supramaximal' oestrogen stimulation. This hypertrophy provides the basis for the well-documented enlargement of the normal pituitary in human pregnancy.

Like oestradiol, prolactin appears to regulate its own receptors (Posner et al. 1975) and increases specifically synthesis of α-lactalbumin. Oestrogens act synergistically with prolactin and other hormones,

probably progesterone and hPL, to provide prolactational changes during pregnancy, but lactation itself is not initiated until after parturition where high levels of prolactin persist in nursing mothers in a low oestrogen environment, rather like the multiple eponymic syndromes of inappropriate hyperprolactinaemia.

Oestrogens, therefore, have a dual and paradoxical effect on prolactin. They increase prolactin secretion. However, when given postpartum, although they will suppress lactation, there is no suppression of prolactin levels. That is, oestrogens antagonize the lactogenic activity of PRL on the breast (McNeilly 1975). If the mother does not breast feed, prolactin levels return to normal within two weeks. In those who breast feed on a timed basis, like many women in developed countries, prolactin levels decline much more slowly, although there are still surges of secretion during suckling.

In the fetus, prolactin levels increase throughout pregnancy until birth when they are extremely high, falling to pre-pubertal levels by the sixth week of life (Aubert et al. 1975). It is probable that most of the very high levels of prolactin seen in liquor come from the maternal rather than the fetal circulation and that once having entered the amniotic fluid, prolactin disperses very slowly. Recalling the role of prolactin as an osmoregulator in fish, it is not surprising that the first evidence is emerging for the role of prolactin in regulating amniotic fluid volume and osmolality which, in turn, has a marked effect on fetal water and electrolyte balance (Josimovich & Archer 1977). More speculatively, it might be noted that just as inappropriate hyperprolactinaemia in non-pregnant women increases DHAS levels (Carter et al. 1977), it is possible that this hormone may have some effect on the fetal adrenal in pregnancy.

It now seems likely that the site of production of the prolactin seen in such high quantities in amniotic fluid is not, at least to a major degree, the fetal pituitary but the endometrium of early human pregnancy and the deciduum of more advanced pregnancy. It also seems likely that while the control of prolactin secretion in endometrium/decidua is unknown, it is unlikely to be mediated by dopamine (Golander et al. 1979, Maslar et al. 1980).

Maternal FSH and particularly LH are known to be suppressed during pregnancy (Gaspard et al, 1976). In the early pueperium, administration of luteinizing-hormone releasing factor (LRF) is characterized by a normal or even a supra-normal FSH response, and reduced or absent LH response (Chamley et al. 1978), a pattern that becomes normal by about day 35 postpartum.

Turning to the neuro-hypophysis, there does not appear to be any specific effect of pregnancy on vasopressin. Oxytocin on the other hand is important but probably not of crucial importance. Its best-documented action, physiologically, is on milk ejection during suckling. Pharmacologically in the induction of labour there is no doubt of the role of oxytocin; its physiological role is less clear in the periparturient period (Chard 1977). Normally, oxytocin, both of maternal and fetal origin, may be the second violin to the leader of prostaglandins.

Fetal pituitary

Fetal FSH and LH cannot be detected before week 12 of gestation and there is a good correlation between pituitary, serum and amniotic fluid levels after this time (Clements et al. 1976). These in vivo data are supported by results from organ culture (Goodyear et al. 1977).

More or less at the same time, the fetal pituitary starts to produce TSH (Gitlin & Biasucci 1969), that is after the fetal thyroid starts to concentrate iodine. Before this time hCG may be the effective thyrotrophin. As discussed earlier, fetal ACTH and CLIP prob-

ably control the fetal zone of the adrenal cortex after the first trimester, but fetal hCG may play a role early in pregnancy.

Maternal adrenal cortex

ALDOSTERONE

There is a large mass of well-documented data relating to aldosterone secretion and excretion in pregnancy. The factors responsible for, and the significance of, the observed changes remain elusive.

Much of the earlier uncertainty about changes in aldosterone levels can be attributed to methodological confusion, as is so often the case. The initial observation by Venning and Dyrenfurth (1956) of an increase in pH_1 (extractable aldosterone) has been amply confirmed. Despite a marked increase in aldosterone secretion rate, there is no significant change in the protein binding of plasma aldosterone (Schteingart 1967). Neither the fetus nor placenta contribute significantly to the increased secretion rate.

CORTISOL

Changes in cortisol secretion, transport and metabolism during pregnancy are well documented and have been briefly reviewed by Schteingart (1967). The secretion rate is doubled in late pregnancy and there is an increase in plasma cortisol. The plasma half-life of free cortisol is significantly prolonged in pregnancy. It is now accepted that the most sensitive index of tissue exposure to biologically active cortisol throughout the day is measurement of urinary free cortisol. This is also increased during pregnancy.

Maternal pituitary hormones

Earlier confusion about changes in hGH (Greenwood et al., 1964) has been clarified by assays that will distinguish hGH from hPL. There is no significant increase in maternal hGH during pregnancy, but the levels in fetal blood are very high (Grumbach et al. 1968).

There is still confusion about levels of corticotrophin during pregnancy, the consensus being that there is an increase. Although it can be extracted from placental tissue, there is no evidence that the placenta produces ACTH (Diczfalusy & Troen 1961).

Odell et al. (1967) have assayed thyroid-stimulating hormone by an immunological method during pregnancy, and found it to be within normal limits.

There is a significant increase in melanocyte-stimulating hormone (MSH) in pregnancy (Hytten & Leitch 1964).

Insulin

Plasma levels of insulin, as measuured by radioimmunoassay, are increased in pregnancy (Antoniades 1968, Kyle 1968). It is known that the experimental administration of hPL to non-pregnant subjects will increase plasma insulin levels and the insulin response to hyperglycaemia (Grumbach et al. 1968). This is discussed fully by Judzewitsch (1979).

REFERENCES

ANTONIADES H.N. (1968) In Gynecologic Endocrinology (Gold J.J. ed.), p. 607. Hoeber, New York.

ASHITAKA Y. & KOIDE S.S. (1974) Fertil. and Steril., **25**, 177.

AUBERT M.L., GRUMBACH M.M. & KAPLAN S.L. (1975) J. Clin. Invest., **56**, 155.

BARLOW J.J. & LOGAN C.M. (1966) Steroids, **7**, 309.

BOLTE E. (1967) Clin. Obstet. Gynec., **10**, 60.

BRAUNSTEIN G.D., RASOR J., ADLER D., DANCER H. & WADE M.E. (1976) Amer J. Obstet. Gynec., **126**, 678.

BRINNIN J.M. (1960) In The Third Rose. Gertrude Stein and her World, p. ix. Weidenfeld & Nicolson, London.

BROVETTO-CRUZ J., MIGUEL-WENSKO C., SARDI-VALVEREE Y., UCAR D., GUISANTES J.A., GALIMIDI S. & CASTELLANO M.A. (1976) Europ. J. Obstet. Gynec. Reprod. Biol., **6**, 109.

BROWN J.B. (1959) Lancet i, 704.

CARTER J.N., TYSON J.E., WARNE G.L., McNEILLY A.S., FAIMAN C. & FREISEN H.G. (1977) J. clin. Endocr, **45**, 973.

CASSMER O. (1959) Acta endocr. (Kbh.), (Supplement), 45.

CATT K.J., TSURUHARA T. & DUFAU M.L. (1972) Biochem. et Biophys. Acta, **279**, 194.

CHAMLEY W.A., ERHARDT A., DE KRETSER D.M. & WOOD K. (1978) Personal communication.

CHARD T. (1977) Neurohypophyseal hormones. In Endocrinology of Pregnancy (Fuchs F. & Klopper A. eds), p. 71. Harper & Row, Maryland.

CHEN H.C., HODGEN C.D., MATSUURA A., LIN L.J., GROSS E., REICHERT L.E., BIRKEN S., CAUFIELD R.E., & ROSS G.T. (1976) Proc. Nat. Acad. Sci., **73**, 2885.

CLEMENTS J.A., REYES F.I., WINTER J.S.D. & FAIMAN C. (1976) J. clin. Endocr., **42**, 9.

COYLE M.G. & BROWN J.B. (1963) J. Obstet Gynaec. Brit. Cwlth., **70**, 225.

CSAPO A.I., SOUVAGE J.P. & WEIST W.G. (1970) Amer. J. Obstet. Gynec., **108**, 950.

CURRIE W.B., WONGG M.S.F., COX R.I. & THORBURN G.D. (1973) In Endocrine Factors in Labour (Klopper A. & Gardiner A. eds) p. 95. Cambridge Univ. Press.

DAWOOD M.Y. & KELMKAMP F. (1977) Obstet. and Gynec., **50**, 450.

DICZFALUSY E., CASSMER O., ALONSO C. & DE MIQUEL M. (1961) Recent Prog. Hormone Res., **17**, 147.

DICAFALUSY E. & TROEN P. (1961) Vitam. and Horm., **19**, 230.

EHRHARDT K. (1936) Muenchen. Med. Wochenschr., **83**, 1163.

ETON B. & SHORT R.V. (1960) J. Obstet. Gynaec. Brit. Cwlth., **67**, 785.

EVANS M.I., DOUGAN M-B., MOAWAD A.H., EVANS W.J., BRYANT-GREENWOOD G.D. & GREENWOOD F.C. (1983) Amer. J. Obstet. Gynec. **147**, 410.

FOTHERBY K. (1964) Vitam. and Horm., **22**, 153.

FRANSDEN V.A. (1963) The Excretion of Oestriol in Normal Human Pregnancy. Munksgaard, Copenhagen.

FRANSDEN V.A. & STAKEMANN G. (1963) Acta Endocr. (Kbh.), **43**, 184.

GASPARD U., FIRQUET J., VAN DALEM J.L., PIRRENS G. & HENNEN G. (1976) Rev. franç. Gynéc., **71**, 167.

GITLIN D. & BIASUCCI A. (1969) J. Clin. Endocr., **29**, 926.

GOLANDER A., HURLEY T., BARRETT J. & HANDWERGER S. (1979) J. Endocr., **82**, 263.

GOODYEAR C.A., HALL C.S.-G., GUDYA H., ROBERT F. & GIROUD C.J. (1977) J. clin. Endocr., **45**, 73.

GORDON Y.B., GRUDZINSKAS J.G., JEFFREY D. & CHARD T. (1977) Lancet i, 331.

GRAY E.S. & ABRAMOVICH D.R. (1980) Amer. J. Obstet. Gynec., **137**, 49.

GREENWOOD F.C., HUNTER W.M. & KLOPPER A. (1964) Brit med. J., i, 22.

GRUDZINKAS J.G., LENTON E.A. & OBIEKWE B.C. (1979) In Placental Proteins (Klopper A. & Chard T. eds), p. 119. Springer-Verlag, Berlin.

GRUDZINSKAS J.G., CHARD T. & TEISNER B. (1985) in Clinical Reproductive Endocrinology (Shearman R.P. ed). p, 224. Churchill Livingstone, London.

GRUMBACH M.M. & KAPLAN S.L. (1964) Trans. N.Y. Acad. Sci., **27**, 167.

GRUMBACH M.M., KAPLAN S.L., SCIARRA J.J. & BURR I.M. (1968) Ann. N.Y. Acad. Sci., **148**, 501.

HUDSON P., HALEY J., JOHN M., CRONK M., CRAWFORD R., HARALAMBIDIS J., TREGEAR G., SHINE J. & NIALL H. (1983) Nature, **301**, 628.

HYTTEN F.E. & LEITCH I. (1964) The Physiology of Human Pregnancy, p. 138. Blackwell Scientific Publications, Oxford.

ISMAEL A.A.A. & HARKNESS R.A. (1966) Biochem. J., **98**, 15.

JAFFE R.B. (1967) Clin. Obstet. Gynec., **10**, 7.

JOSIMOVICH J.B. (1977) In Endocrinology of Pregnancy (Klopper A. & Fuchs F. eds), 2e., p. 191. Harper & Row, New York.

JOSIMOVICH J.B. & ARCHER D.F. (1977) Amer. J. Obstet. Gynec., **129**, 777.

JUDZEWITSCH R. (1979) Thyroid and Adrenal Function. In Human Reproductive Physiology (Shearman R.P. ed.) 2e., p. 267. Blackwell Scientific Publications, Oxford.

KENIMER J.C., HERSHMAN J.M. & HIGGINS H.P. (1975) J. clin. Endocr. Metab., **40**, 482.

KLOPPER A. & BILLEWICZ W. (1963) J. Obstet. Gynaec. Brit. Cwlth., **70**, 1024.

KYLE G.C. (1968) In *Gynecologic Endocrinology* (Gold J.J. ed.), p. 607. Hoeber, New York.

LIGGINS G.C. (1974) In *Size at Birth*. CIBA Foundation Symposium No. 27, p. 165.

LIGGINS G.C., FAIRCLOUGH R.J., GRIEVES S.A., KENDALL J.Z. & KNOX B.S. (1973) *Recent Progr. Hormone Res.*, **29**, 111.

MACLENNAN A.H. (1983) *Clin Reproduct. Fertil.*, **2**, 77.

MACLENNAN A.H., GREEN R.C., BRYANT-GREENWOOD G.D., GREENWOOD F.C. & SEAMARK R.F. (1980) *Lancet*, **i**, 220.

MCGREGOR W.G., KUHN R.W., JAFFE R.B. (1983) *Science*, **220**, 306.

MCNEILLY A.S. (1975) *Postgrad. med. J.*, **51**, 231.

MALPAS P. (1933) *J. Obstet. Gynaec. Brit. Cwlth.*, **40**, 1046.

MASLAR I.A., KAPLAN B.M., LUCIANO A.A. & RIDDICK D.H. (1980) *J. clin. Endocr.* **51**, 78.

MISHELL D.R., NAKAMURA R.M., BARBERIA J.M. & THORNEY-CROFT I.H. (1974) *Amer. J. Obstet. Gynec.*, **118**, 990.

MORGAN F.J., VIRILEN S. & CANFIELD R.C. (1973) *Mol. Cell. Biochem.*, **2**, 97.

MORGAN H., ROLFE B., CLUNIE G.J.A., ANDERSON M.J. & MORRISON J. (1977) *Lancet*, **i**, 394.

MURPHY B.E.P. (1973) *Amer. Obstet. Gynec.*, **115**, 521.

MURPHY B.E.P. (1983) *Endocrine Reviews*, **4**, 150.

ODELL W.D., WILBER J.F. & UTINGER R.D. (1967) *Recent Progr. Hormone Res.*, **23**, 47.

PATTEN P.T., ANDERSON A.B.M. & TURNBULL A.C. (1973) *J. Obstet. Gynaec. Brit. Cwlth.*, **80**, 952.

POSNER B.L., KELLY P.A. & FRIESEN H.G. (1975) *Science*, **188**, 57.

QUAGLIARELLO J., SZLACHTER N., STEINETZ B.G., GOLDSMITH L.T., & WEISS M.D. (1979) *Amer. J. Obstet. Gynec.*, **135**, 43.

QUAGLIARELLO J., GOLDSMITH L., STEINETZ B., LUSTIG D.S. & WEISS G. (1980) *J. clin. Endocr.*, **51**, 74.

RIGG L.A., LEIN A. & YEN S.C.C. (1977) *Amer. J. Obstet. Gynec.*, **129**, 454.

SCHENKER J.G., BEN-DAVID M. & POLISHUK W.Z. (1975) *Amer. J. Obstet. Gynec.*, **123**, 834.

SCHNEIDER A.B., KOWALSKI K. & SHERWOOD L.M. (1975) *Endocrinology*, **97**, 1364.

SCHTEINGART D.E. (1967) *Clin. Obstet. Gynec.*, **10**, 88.

SERÓN--FERRÉ M., LAWRENCE C.C. & JAFFE R.B. (1978) *J. clin. Endocr.*, **46**, 834.

SHEARMAN R.P. (1959) *J. Obstet. Gynaec. Brit. Cwlth.*, **66**, 1.

SHEARMAN R.P. (1979) *Human Reproductive Physiology* 2e., p. 115. Blackwell Scientific Publications, Oxford.

SHEARMAN R.P., SHUTT D.A. & SMITH I.D. (1974) In *Size at Birth*, CIBA Foundation Symposium, **27**, 27.

SHUTT D.A. LOPATA A. (1981) *Fertil. and Steril.*, (in press).

SHUTT D.A., SMITH I.D. & SHEARMAN R.P. (1974) *J. Obstet. Gynaec. Brit. Cwlth.*, **81**, 968.

SIITERI P.K. & MACDONALD P.C. (1966) *J. clin. Endocr.*, **26**, 751.

SMITH I.D., SHUTT D.A. & SHEARMAN R.P. (1975) *J. Steroid Biochem.*, **6**, 657.

SOLOMON S. BIRD C.E., LING W., IWAMIYA M. & YOUNG P.C.M. (1967) *Recent Prog. Hormone Res.*, **23**, 297.

SPELLACY W.N., CONLY P.W., CLEVELAND W.W. & BUHI W.C. (1975) *Amer. J. Obstet. Gynec.*, **122**, 278.

TURNBULL A.C., PATTEN P.T., FLINT A.P., KEIRSE M.J.N.C., JEREMY J.Y. & ANDERSON A.B.M. (1974) *Lancet*, **i**, 101.

VENNING E.H. & DYRENFURTH I. (1956) *J. clin. Endocr.*, **16**, 426.

WILLIAMS H.B. & CUMMINS G.E. (1953) *J. Obstet. Gynaec. Brit. Cwlth.*, **60**, 319.

YANNONE M.E., MCCURDY J.R. & GOLDFEIN A. (1968) *Amer. J. Obstet. Gynec.*, **101**, 1058.

YKI-JÄRVINEH H., WAHLSTRÖM T. & SEPPÄLÄ M. (1983) *J. clin. Invest & Metab.*, **57**, 451.

YLIKORKALA O. (1973) *Acta Obstet. Gynec. Scand. suppl.*, **26**, 1.

YOSHIMOTO Y., WOLFSEN A.R., HIROSE F. & ODELL W.D. (1979) *Amer. J. Obstet. Gynec.*, **134**, 729.

CHAPTER 12
NORMAL PREGNANCY:
PHYSIOLOGY AND ANTENATAL CARE

D. A. DAVEY

The fertilized ovum releases messenger substances, in particular the hormone HCG, which ensure the continuation of the corpus luteum and the initiation of the changes by which the mother is prepared and adapted for pregnancy. The corpus luteum, and later the placenta, secretes a variety of hormones which produce profound changes in the genital tract and in the physiological functions of the mother. These changes represent a positive preparation and adaptation of the mother to accommodate and support the fetus as it grows and develops throughout pregnancy. At the same time the mother is prepared for the birth of the fetus at term and for the initiation of lactation immediately after delivery.

THE CHANGES IN THE MOTHER IN NORMAL PREGNANCY

The changes in the mother in pregnancy fulfil three important teleological principles.

1   *The changes in pregnancy are a temporary adaptation and produce no permanent deleterious effects in the mother.* Given a healthy mother and adequate nutrition the changes of pregnancy are not a strain on a woman's well-being. Many women feel better and happier in pregnancy in spite of the marked anatomical and physiological changes. The great majority of the structural and functional changes revert to normal once pregnancy and the puerperium are complete. Pregnancy is thus essentially a physiological and not a pathological process.

2   *The changes in the mother are a positive adaptation and prepare her to meet any possible demands of the fetus.*

(a)   The structural and physiological changes in the mother commonly occur very early in pregnancy and precede any possible need of the fetus. Renal blood flow, for example, has been shown to be increased by as much as 50% as early as the 9th week of pregnancy (Sims & Krantz 1958).

(b)   The changes in the mother are in apparent excess of the needs of the fetus. The cardiac output increases by between 27% and 64% in pregnancy (Kerr 1968), far more than is necessary to provide for the increased blood flow to the uterus, breasts, and other organs (Hytten & Leitch 1971a).

(c)   The mother accumulates reserves and anticipates the future needs of the fetus. These reserves may be accumulated early in pregnancy to anticipate a later phase of rapid growth of the fetus or to provide a reserve to meet the energy and nutritional demands of lactation. The deposition of fat, which is characteristic of the first half of pregnancy, is thought to represent a reserve store in case of nutritional deprivation either in the third trimester or during lactation. (Hytten & Leitch 1971b).

3   *The maternal internal environment is altered to create conditions favourable to the fetus.* Maternal hyperventilation, which is a normal feature of pregnancy, lowers the PCO_2 in the maternal arterial blood. The lowered partial pressure of CO_2 in the blood on the maternal side of the placenta then facilitates the transfer of CO_2 from the fetus to the mother (Prystowsky *et al.* 1961). Hytten and Leitch (1971c) have suggested that instead of preserving the 'milieu interieur' which is the most common endeavour of the body in all other situations, the physiological adaptations in the mother create a constantly changing environment appropriate to the successive changes of pregnancy and to create the conditions most favourable for the growth and development of the fetus.

The changes in the mother in pregnancy can be divided into:

(a) the changes in the genital tract to accommodate the growing fetus and to prepare for labour and delivery;

(b) the general structural changes in the mother;

(c) the physiological changes in the mother.

THE CHANGES IN THE GENITAL TRACT

Ovary

The position of the ovary changes markedly during pregnancy from being a pelvic to an abdominal structure. The ovary also becomes hyperaemic and the ovarian blood vessels enlarge to an enormous size.

CORPUS LUTEUM

The ovarian changes associated with pregnancy properly begin with the alteration of the Graafian follicle to form a corpus luteum. The corpus luteum begins to regress about the 8th day of its existence. By the 12th day, however, the secretion of chorionic gonadotrophin into the blood stream by the syncytiotrophoblast of the developing ovum is sufficient to halt this regression. Instead of shrinking, as it normally does at the end of the menstrual cycle, the corpus luteum grows and develops and becomes the 'corpus luteum of pregnancy'. At approximately the 8th week, corresponding with the rapidly increasing secretion of chorionic gonadotrophin by the placenta, the corpus luteum undergoes rapid enlargement and approximately doubles its size. After a further two weeks, however, once the peak of chorionic gonadotrophin is passed, the corpus luteum regresses relatively quickly. At the time of its greatest development the corpus luteum occupies at least a third of the entire ovary but at term it is only half this size (Nelson & Greene 1953). The corpus luteum during the first half of pregnancy is composed almost entirely of granulosa lutein cells. The theca lutein cells reach their maximum development early on in pregnancy around the 8th to the 10th week and disappear completely in the second half of pregnancy. The granulosa lutein cells contain lipoid vacuoles, colloid droplets and secretory granules. The secretory granules are present in nearly one-third of the cells up to the 24th week but disappear almost completely by term (Gillman & Stein 1941).

STROMA AND FOLLICLES

Ovulation ceases during pregnancy, but many follicles become temporarily active. Though the ova themselves in these follicles undergo cytolysis, the theca lutein cells of the follicles proliferate in pregnancy. These theca lutein cells (which are smaller, stain more deeply and have larger nuclei than the granulosa lutein cells) multiply to form a thick tunica around each atretic follicle. These masses of cells sometimes appear to lose their connection with the follicle and have then been termed 'the interstitial glands of pregnancy'. Later, however, these thecal cells undergo fatty and hyaline degeneration and form irregular hyaline bodies indistinguishable from corpora albicantia.

DECIDUAL REACTION OF CAPSULE

The surface of the ovary in pregnancy frequently undergoes a decidua-like reaction very similar to that seen in the endometrial stroma. The fibroblasts or mesenchymal cells underlying the germinal epithelium develop into ectopic decidual cells. This decidual reaction appears as velvety, reddish, convoluted ridges which bleed easily on touch and resemble freshly torn adhesions (Israel et al. 1954). Similar decidual reactions may also be seen on the posterior surface of the uterus, the uterosacral ligaments, the round and broad ligaments and even on extra-pelvic abdominal organs (Nelson & Greene 1953).

OVARIAN FUNCTION IN PREGNANCY

In early pregnancy, up to 10 weeks, the corpus luteum is an active and vital organ producing oestrogen and progesterone which assists in ensuring the continuation of pregnancy and producing many of the secondary changes in pregnancy. Removal of the corpus luteum in early pregnancy in the human, however, produces abortion in only 10% to 20% of pregnancies (Csapo et al. 1974). The human placenta normally secretes enough progesterone for the maintenance of pregnancy soon after implantation. In the human the persistence of the corpus luteum probably represents an additional safety mechanism to protect the pregnancy in the crucial period at the onset of steroid secretion by the placenta, and in cases of inadequate placentation or placental insufficiency.

Fallopian tube

During pregnancy the Fallopian tubes are pulled upwards out of the pelvis by the growth of the uterus. The tubes thus become stretched, and come to lie almost vertically alongside the uterus, and are at the same time displaced laterally by the enlarging body of the uterus. There is, moreover, a disproportionate growth of the fundus of the uterus so that in the later months of pregnancy the insertions of the Fallopian tubes and round ligaments are approximately halfway up the uterus. The Fallopian tubes become hyperaemic and congested but, surprisingly, there is little or no hypertrophy of the muscle of the tube. The epithelium of the endosalpinx is flattened and on microscopic examination the surface of the epithelium is irregular due to the bulging up of the cytoplasmic processes on the non-ciliated cells (Snyder 1924).

Uterus

In addition to the remarkable alteration in size, shape and position of the uterus in pregnancy, which is related to the increasing size of its contents, there are also changes in its blood supply, muscular arrangement and physiological behaviour. The two parts of the uterus, namely the corpus and the cervix, moreover, react very differently to pregnancy, fulfil different functions, and must be considered separately. The corpus or body of the uterus is thus composed essentially of muscle and undergoes growth, and is subject to distension. The cervix in contrast is composed essentially of connective tissue and, although it softens, it maintains its continuity as a relatively firm, closed, fibrous ring until the patient goes into labour. In labour the corpus contracts rhythmically whereas the cervix dilates to allow the passage and expulsion of the fetus and products of conception.

The corpus of the uterus

SIZE, SHAPE, POSITION AND CONSISTENCY OF THE UTERUS

Changes in size of the uterus. As pregnancy advances the uterus expands rapidly to accommodate the growing products of conception. From an organ measuring approximately $7.5 \times 5 \times 2.5$ cm and a capacity of 4 ml it expands to an organ which at term measures $28 \times 24 \times 21$ cm and a capacity of 4,000 ml or thereabouts. The wall of the uterus, which is about 8 mm thick before pregnancy, grows to about 25 mm in thickness by the 12th week. After this time, however, when the decidua capsularis fuses with the decidua vera, the wall of the uterus becomes progressively thinner as the amniotic cavity increases in size (Gillespie 1950). By the end of pregnancy the uterine wall is only 5 to 10 mm in thickness though it is strong enough to develop intrauterine pressures of 60 mmHg or so in normal labour and up to 300 mmHg in abnormal labour and the puerperium (Henricks *et al.* 1962).

Shape and position of the uterus. As the uterus increases in size it also changes in shape. For the first few weeks of pregnancy it retains its original 'pear' shape but the body of the uterus rapidly becomes progressively more spheroid as the gestation sac enlarges, until the 12th week, when the sac completely fills the uterine cavity. Thereafter the uterus increases more rapidly in length as the fetus elongates and its shape becomes increasingly more sac-like until term (Gillespie 1950; Fig. 12.1).

The position of the uterus also alters as the uterus becomes larger. Initially it is usually anteverted and anteflexed. From the 12th week onwards it is too large to remain wholly within the pelvis and the fundus of the uterus rises up into the abdomen. As it enlarges it progressively displaces the intestines to the sides of the abdomen and comes into contact with the anterior abdominal wall, exerting increasing pressure on the anterior abdominal wall and all the abdominal contents. At the same time, the round ligaments become stretched and the broad ligaments 'open out'.

The mobility of the uterus depends upon the laxity of the abdominal wall, which is generally tense in nulliparas and increases in laxity in successive pregnancies in multiparas. When a woman in late pregnancy stands upright the uterus falls forwards, particularly in multiparas. In this position the long axis of the uterus is in the same axis as the upper strait of the pelvis. The fundus of the uterus rests on the anterior abdominal wall, which, if it is very stretched and the rectus abdominis muscles are widely separated, may allow the fundus to bulge through, resulting in a pendulous abdomen or herniation of the gravid uterus (Fig. 12.2).

When a woman lies supine the uterus falls backwards and rests upon the vertebral column and may compress the inferior vena cava, causing a reduction in venous return, cardiac output and blood pressure (Kerr 1968).

As the uterus grows up into the abdominal cavity it also rotates in its long axis, usually to the right. This is attributed to the presence of the spinal column and sigmoid colon and rectum. If this dextrorotation of the uterus is not recognized at Caesarean section it may lead to misplaced incision of the uterus, possibly involving major uterine blood vessels.

Consistency of the uterus. Pregnancy causes a progressive softening of the uterus starting with the isthmus or lower part of the body. This softening of the isthmus, which commences while the cervix and fundus of the uterus are still firm, is most noticeable at the 10th week of pregnancy and is the basis of Hegar's

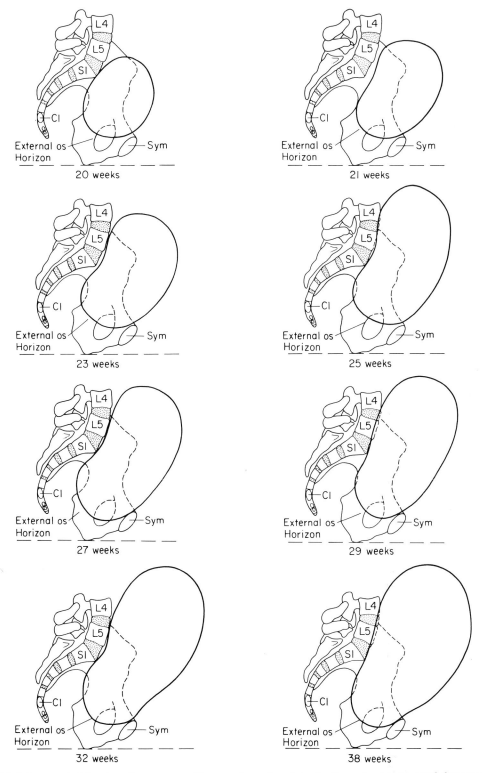

Fig. 12.1 Enlargement of the uterus in pregnancy. Diagrams drawn from lateral radiographs showing rapid elongation of uterus from twentieth to thirty-second week and increase in anteposterior diameter thereafter (Gillespie 1950).

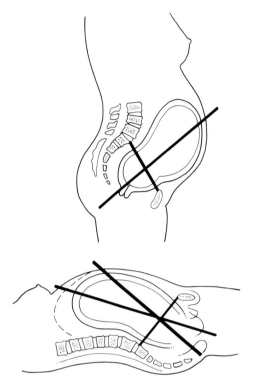

Fig. 12.2. Relation of long axis of uterus to axis of inlet in primigravidas. (a) Standing. (b) Lying flat.

sign. After the 10th weeek the cervix and fundus of the uterus become progressively softer and Hegar's sign can no longer be elicited after the 12th week. The softening of the fundus is more marked over the site of implantation of the placenta and may be associated with asymmetrical growth of the uterus. After the 24th week the uterine wall is so soft that parts of the fetus may be palpated with ease.

MUSCLE GROWTH, CHANGES IN CONTRACTILITY AND NERVE SUPPLY IN PREGNANCY

Muscle growth and arrangement of fibres. In addition to alteration in size and shape, the mass of the uterus is greatly increased in pregnancy. The weight increases from 30 g to 60 g before pregnancy to 750 g to 1000 g at term (Gillespie 1950). The increase in mass is due to the growth of the endometrium, hypertrophy and hyperplasia of the uterine muscle and connective tissue and increase in size and number of blood vessels and other tissues. Most of this growth is due to proliferation of the myometrium. In the first trimester there is actual hyperplasia of the muscle

cells and mitotic figures are common. Most of the increase is, however, due to hypertrophy of the muscle which occurs in the second, and to a lesser extent, the third trimester. The individual muscle cells increase in length from 50 μm to 200–600 μm and grow in volume to 17–40 times their non-pregnant size (Stieve 1932; Fig. 12.3).

The stimulus for this growth is chiefly oestrogen. Later in pregnancy the distension of the uterus and stretching of the muscle play an important role (Wood 1964). Distension, is, however, by no means an essential stimulus as evidenced by the considerable enlargement of the uterus which occurs in extrauterine pregnancy. It has been suggested that hyperplasia of the myometrial cells is initially due to oestrogen but that the increasing levels of progesterone later inhibit the hyperplasia and enhance the hypertrophy of the uterine muscle.

The arrangement of the muscle fibres in the uterus, both in the non-pregnant and pregnant uterus, has been studied for over 100 years or more (Helie 1864). The two chief systems of muscular fasciculi in the non-pregnant uterus result from the fusion of the two Müllerian ducts. The uterus consists of an interlacing complex of muscle fibres in which the fibres in general run spirally and have a bilateral symmetrical arrangement. The fibres tend to cross each other at right angles in the fundus but obtusely in the lower segment. In pregnancy the fibres of the upper segment preserve their original arrangement, in contrast to the fibres of the lower segment which are drawn up so that the spirals adopt a more vertical course, like that of a spiral staircase (Goerttler 1930; Fig. 12.4) thus favouring dilatation in late pregnancy and labour.

In addition to the changes in muscle fibres, there is hyperplasia and hypertrophy of the connective tissue, particularly between the muscle bundles of the uterus. There is also hypertrophy of the elastic fibres, particularly around the arteries. This increase in elastic and fibrous tissue strengthens the uterine wall, especially in the latter part of pregnancy when the muscle elements have ceased to develop.

Changes in contractility of the uterus in pregnancy. The intermittent contractions of the uterus which occur during the menstrual cycle and are noted especially at ovulation and during menstruation continue throughout pregnancy. The contractions are of two basic types, depending upon whether oestrogen or progesterone has a predominating effect on the uterus (Carey 1963).

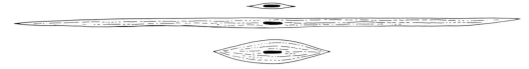

Fig. 12.3. Muscle fibres from normal non-pregnant, pregnant and pueperal uterus (Stieve 1926).

(i) Oestrogen effect—A waves

During the follicular phase of the menstrual cycle, when the myometrium is under the influence of oestrogen, the spontaneous activity of the uterus takes the form of contractions of low amplitude (0.2 mmHg intrauterine pressure) and high frequency (120 per hour) and short duration (30 seconds) which are known as A waves. At mid-cycle, corresponding with the peak of oestrogen secretion at ovulation, the frequency of the A waves increases to 240 per hour. If ovulation fails to occur and a corpus luteum is not found this pattern of spontaneous uterine activity continues throughout the cycle (Garrett 1959).

(ii) Progestogen effect—B waves

If ovulation occurs the character of the uterine contractions changes. The contractions increase in amplitude (up to 10 times), become less frequent (30 per hour) and of longer duration (2 min), and are known as B waves (Fig. 12.5).

This change in behaviour and contractility of the myometrium is believed to be due to the increased secretion of progesterone which exerts a predominating effect on the uterus in the second half of the normal ovulatory menstrual cycle. Although the secretion of progesterone drops, however, before the onset of menstruation the B wave activity continues

and is in fact maximal during menstruation and does not disappear completely until the 10th day of the next menstrual cycle.

During pregnancy from the 12th to the 14th week onwards the uterus may be felt to contract either on bimanual examination or later through the abdominal wall. The previously relaxed uterus becomes hard for a few minutes and the intrauterine pressure rises to 8 cm of water or more. These contractions, which have been known for over 100 years, are known as Braxton Hicks contractions and are characteristically sporadic, arrhythmic and infrequent until the last month or so of pregnancy when their frequency increases. Braxton Hicks contractions differ from the contractions of true labour only in that they are not regular and rhythmic, are not accompanied by dilation of the cervix, and are not painful.

The period of increasing uterine activity which occurs after the 30th week has been designated 'prelabour' by Caldeyro-Barcia and Poseiro (1959) and is accompanied by an increasing sensitivity to oxytocin (Csapo & Sauvage 1968).

The increase in size and contractility of the muscle fibres as pregnancy progresses is due to the action of oestrogen and to stretching (Csapo et al. 1965). There is an increase in actomyosin, ATP and enzyme concentrations in the muscle cells with a change in the ionic gradients and resting potential across the cell membrane. Oestrogen lowers the resting potential

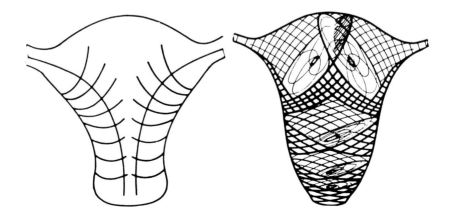

Fig. 12.4 Architecture of uterus showing arrangement of two chief systems of muscular fasciculi which result from the fusion of the Müllerian ducts. (Goerttler 1930).

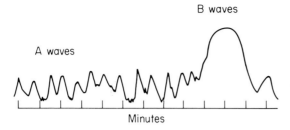

Fig. 12.5 Uterine contractions recorded by external tocography showing A and B waves (Carey 1936).

and makes the muscle more excitable but progesterone tends to raise the membrane potential. The A waves are due to the uncoordinated myogenic activity of the individual uterine muscle fibres and are probably the effect of the increased oestrogen secretion in pregnancy. The B waves, which are present only in late pregnancy, labour and the puerperium, are probably a result of the action of progesterone on the oestrogen-primed uterus and represent more coordinated activity. The smooth muscle of the uterus is not an anatomical syncytium as in the heart, but forms a functional syncytium by the electrical coupling of the branching bundles of cells at gap junctions. The formation of gap junctions is believed to be stimulated by a rise in oestrogen or a fall in progesterone levels, or both. At the present time it is uncertain how far oestrogen and progesterone have a direct action on myometrial contractility and how far the efforts are mediated or influenced by other substances such as prostaglandin and oxytocin. Much work in the last decade suggests that prostaglandins and oxytocin are intimately involved in uterine contractility and the initiation of labour (Pauerstein & Seitchik 1979, Liggins 1979, Novy & Liggins 1980). Contractions are produced by the release of prostaglandin $F_{2\alpha}$ which is synthesized in the endometrium. The control of contractions is furthermore believed to reside in the rate of prostaglandin synthesis and, in particular, in the rate-limiting enzyme phospholipase A_2 which controls the formation of prostaglandin from arachidonic acid. Oestrogens have been shown to labilize and progesterones to stabilize the intracellular lyosomes which produce phospholipase A_2. Increase in the oestrogen/progesterone ratio or withdrawal of progesterone may in this way stimulate or enhance prostaglandin synthesis and uterine contractions. Oestrogens have also been shown to stimulate and progestogens to inhibit the formation of oxytocin receptors in the endometrium. It has further been shown that oxytocin stimulates the release of

$PGF_{2\alpha}$ and that this releasing effect is maximal when oestrogen concentrations are high and progesterone concentrations are low. Oestrogen and progesterone may thus increase the uterine sensitivity to oxytocin and enhance prostaglandin release as well as prostaglandin synthesis. One of the main difficulties, however, in explaining changes in the patterns of contractions of the uterus in man, in contrast to the changes in other species such as sheep and rabbits, has been the failure to demonstrate changes either in progesterone and oestrogen secretion or in circulating oxytocin at the onset of labour. Schwarz et al. (1977), however, have shown that fetal membranes produce a progesterone-binding-protein which appears only after the 37th week of pregnancy and which could produce a progesterone withdrawal at the cellular level. Taken together, these observations suggest that the synthesis and release of $PGF_{2\alpha}$ is stimulated by an increase in the oestrogen/progestogen ratio and that this may be responsible for the increase in uterine contractility in late pregnancy and possibly for the onset of labour, though direct proof of these changes in the human is still awaited.

The nerve supply to the uterus in pregnancy. With the observation that paraplegic patients go into labour and that the uterus contracts normally, albeit painlessly, it has been assumed that the nervous system has little functional significance in pregnancy and labour. There is, however, a profuse nerve supply to the uterus from both the autonomic and central nervous systems which undergoes marked hypertrophy in pregnancy, as exemplified by the increase in size of Frankenhauser's ganglion from 2×2.5 cm to 3.5×6 cm. The sensory fibres to the uterus arise from the spinal cord through the sacral nerves and are distributed via Frankenhauser's ganglion to the cervix, where various Pacinnian-type structures have been found. The only pain to arise from the body of the uterus is thought to be ischaemic in origin and to be conducted via the sympathetic nervous system. Evidence is accumulating that motor fibres from the autonomic system may have some functional significance in the human uterus (Wood 1969). Noradrenergic nerves supplying smooth muscle fibres in the myometrium have thus been demonstrated and field stimulation and other characteristics suggest that they are of sympathetic origin (Nakanishi et al. 1969). Stimulation of the hypogastric nerve causes an increase in contractility in the luteal phase of the menstrual cycle and in early pregnancy (Alvarez et al. 1965).

In the non-pregnant uterus, noradrenergic nerves are distributed mainly to the cervix and lower part of the uterine body. Mann (1963) has shown that the isthmus of the uterus narrows during the luteal phase and opens during menstruation. The presence of the noradrenergic nerve fibres suggests that this narrowing may be due to local muscle activity resulting from nervous stimulation. Wood (1969) has suggested that this narrowing of the isthmus in the late menstrual cycle may be important in nidation and that, by closing off the lower half of the uterus, it may help to ensure that implantation of the fertilized ovum occurs in the fundus of the uterus. Implantation in the isthmus would result in abortion or placenta praevia.

In pregnancy, the distribution of the noradrenergic nerves alters and there is a relative denervation of the isthmus. The noradrenergic nerves supplying the smooth muscle become sparser so that the stimulating effect of neural noradrenaline is reduced (Nakanishi *et al.* 1969). This decrease in neural noradrenaline, coupled with the increase in circulating adrenaline, results in an inhibition of uterine contractility (Wansborough *et al.* 1967). These findings suggest that the autonomic nervous system may play a part in ensuring that implantation occurs in the fundus of the uterus and in ensuring a quiescent uterus in pregnancy.

BLOOD VESSELS, BLOOD FLOW AND OXYGEN CONSUMPTION OF THE UTERUS IN PREGNANCY

Changes in uterine blood vessels in pregnancy. The increase in the vascular system of the uterus is such that at term the placenta, uterus and associated blood vessels contain one-sixth or more of the total blood volume of the mother. In pregnancy the spiral arterioles undergo important functional and structural changes which are vital in the formation of the placenta and in ensuring an adequate chorio decidual blood flow throughout pregnancy. In the first few weeks the spiral arterioles grow towards the uterine lumen and become increasingly coiled. By mid-pregnancy this growth has stopped and with the increase in the size of the uterus the coils later become progressively 'paid out'. At the same time the number of arterioles communicating with the intervillous space decreases so that in late pregnancy the arterioles that remain are straighter and have only an occasional right-angled bend (Ramsay 1949).

The structural changes in the spiral arterioles may be divided into three phases: pre-invasive, intraluminal and wall replacement. In the pre-invasive phase, the cells lining the arterioles pile up into several layers sometimes almost occluding the lumen. The non-villous trophoblast invades the decidual segments of the spiral arterioles, and by the 12th week of gestation has colonized the whole of the basal decidual system. In the intraluminal phase, between 16 and 20 weeks, a second wave of trophoblast penetrates the spiral arterioles extending beyond the deciduomyometrial junction into the myometrial segments and replacing the endothelium. In the third phase, the trophoblast disappears from the vascular lumen and the muscular elastic elements of the arteriolar walls are replaced by fibrinoid, fibrous and amorphous tissue in which modified myometrial cells, degenerate muscle cells and trophoblastic cells are embedded. These vascular changes result in the conversion of approximately 100–150 spiral arteries into distended, tortuous and funnel-shaped utero-placental arteries that communicate through multiple openings into the intervillous space (Fig. 12.6).

The morphological changes are accompanied by a marked fall in peripheral vascular resistance in the placental bed and, by virtue of the destruction of the smooth muscle, render the spiral arterioles insensitive to circulating maternal vaso-active agents. These degenerative changes which are a normal part of placentation have been termed the 'physiological response of the spiral arteries to pregnancy' (Brosens *et al.* 1967).

The uterine veins which empty into plexuses at the side of the uterus in the medial part of the broad ligaments also undergo marked changes. Unlike the veins of the arms and legs the uterine and pelvic veins do not have a surrounding supportive fascial sheath. They can therefore dilate more easily and in pregnancy form the paminiform plexuses of the broad ligament. It is thought that these plexuses perform an important function acting as a reservoir when blood is forced out of the placenta, as for example during a uterine contraction. It has been estimated that the capacity of the uterine veins and the venous plexuses increase by more than sixty-fold by the 36th week of pregnancy compared with their non-pregnant state.

Uterine blood flow and oxygen consumption in pregnancy. A variety of methods has been used to measure the uterine blood flow but, owing to the technical difficulties of the various methods and the complexity of the uterine vascular system with uterine and ovarian arteries and veins on both sides of the pelvis, and

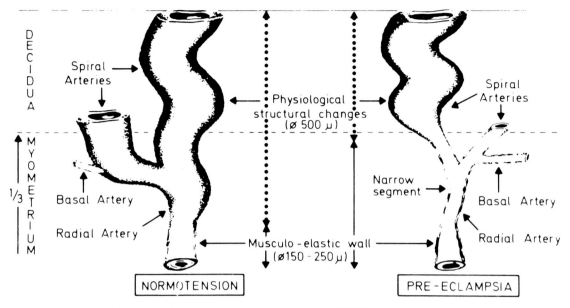

Fig. 12.6 Physiological changes in spiral arteries in pregnancy (Brosens *et al.* 1967).

numerous anastomoses, all the results so far obtained can only be regarded as a very general indication of changes of uterine blood flow. With present techniques it is also not possible to determine how much of the total uterine blood flow passes through the placental circulation and how much through the myometrium. It was estimated by Assali *et al.* (1960) that the total uterine blood flow increases from approximately 50 ml/min at 10 weeks to 185 ml/min at 28 weeks and reaches a maximum of 500–700 ml/min at term. When expressed in terms of unit weight the uterine blood flow at term is of the order of 100–150 ml/min/mg tissue, uterus, placenta and fetus (Dawes 1968). It is assumed that the major increment in blood flow throughout gestation is through the intervillous space of the placenta, though there is no information regarding the distribution of blood between the myometrium and the placenta at the various stages of pregnancy.

The effect of uterine contractions on uterine blood flow is of major importance for the fetus and there is good evidence that uterine contractions sufficient to cause a rise in uterine pressure of 20–30 mmHg cause a decrease of 10–50% in total uterine blood flow (Ahlquist 1950). The fetus nevertheless rarely seems to be compromised unless the uterus undergoes tetanic contraction when the blood flow falls over 50% (Assali *et al.* 1958).

Estimates of oxygen consumption are perhaps even less reliable than those of blood flow but from the available literature Hytten & Leitch (1971d) have estimated that the average total oxygen consumption at term is as follows:

Fetus	12.4 ml/min
Placenta	3.7 ml/min
Uterus	3.6 ml/min
Total	19.7 ml/min

If it is assumed that maternal blood O_2 content is reduced on average 5 ml/100 ml blood on passage through the uterus then the total uterine blood flow necessary to supply 19.7 ml/min is approximately 400 ml/min which is well within the observed total uterine blood flow at term.

Isthmus

The isthmus is strictly part of the body of the uterus and is defined as that portion of the uterus which joins the dense connective tissue of the cervix to the muscle fibres of the corpus. The anatomical boundaries of this zone are not well defined but its upper limit is usually considered as the constriction of the uterine cavity which marks the lower boundary of the corpus (the anatomical internal os) and its lower limit as the

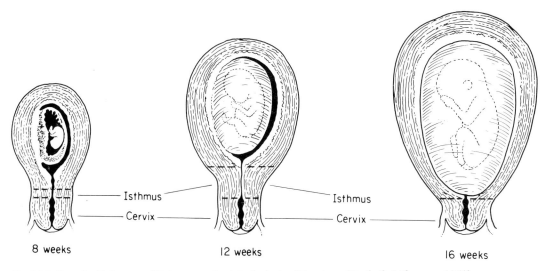

Isthmus
Cervix

Isthmus
Cervix

8 weeks   12 weeks   16 weeks

Fig. 12.7 Growth of isthmus and its incorporation into the body of the uterus (Danforth & Chapman 1950).

junction of the flattened and attentuated endometrium of the isthmus and the mucus-secreting columnar epithelium of the cervix (the histological internal os). Because the mucus-secreting epithelium
of the endocervix intermingles with the non-mucus-
secreting glands of the isthmus, often over a relatively
wide area, the lower boundary of the isthmus in particular is often ill defined. The isthmus of the uterus
nevertheless undergoes important structural and
functional changes in pregnancy. During the first
trimester it hypertrophies and elongates to three
times its original length. At the same time it becomes
soft and extremely compressible. This softening is so
great that on bimanual examination at the 10th to
12th week it feels as though the body of the uterus
and the cervix are separate entities (Hegar's sign of
pregnancy). As the gestation grows after the 12th
week the isthmus progressively opens out from above
downwards and becomes shorter. This opening out
continues until it is checked by the dense connnective
tissue ring of the cervix. At this stage the entire
isthmical canal has become incorporated in the
general uterine cavity and the isthmus becomes incorporated into and forms part of the lower segment
of the uterus. Reynolds & Danforth (1966) have defined the lower uterine segment as simply that part
of the body of the uterus which undergoes circumferential dilatation, whether this be in pregnancy or in
labour (Fig. 12.7).

Functionally, the region of the isthmus may be of
considerable importance as the muscle fibres are
arranged circularly or in a close spiral. Asplund

(1952) and Youssef (1958) have presented evidence
that this region functions as a true sphincter, contracting during the second half of the menstrual cycle
and early pregnancy under the influence of progesterone, and opening out during the first half of the
menstrual cycle under the influence of oestrogen.
This sphincteric action may be of importance in helping to retain the ovum and growing fetus within the
uterus and ensuring its implantation in the fundus.

Cervix

The cervix performs a vital function in pregnancy
and labour both in retaining the conceptus during
pregnancy, and in later dilating and allowing the
passage of the fully grown fetus through the birth
canal without structural damage to the mother.
Clinically, the cervix becomes progressively softer and
blue in colour in early pregnancy and this constitutes
one of the characteristic signs of pregnancy from the
8th week onwards. The blood and lymph vessels increase in number and size and the connective tissue
increases and alters in character. Later the glands
undergo marked proliferation so that at the end of
pregnancy the mucosa is approximately one-half of
the entire mass of the cervix.

CHANGES IN STROMA OF CERVIX

Apart from increase in vascularity and oedema, the
connective tissue of the cervix undergoes marked
changes in pregnancy and before and during labour.

On microscopy there is marked loosening and dispersion of the microfibrils and increase in the intervening clear spaces.

These spaces were originally interpreted as oedema but were later shown to be filled with ground substance composed of mucopolysaccharides or glycoaminoglycans (GAGs). Apart from dispersion the absolute amount of collagen in the cervix is decreased from 82% in the non-pregnant state to 52% at full dilatation and it is replaced by GAGs (Danforth et al. 1974). There is also a decrease in hydroxyproline content before and during labour which coincides with the period of cervical ripening (Harkness & Harkness 1959). These structural changes result in a marked change in the compliance and mechanical properties of the cervix which have been reviewed by Naftolin & Stubblefield (1980). The factors responsible for these changes probably include oestrogens and PGF$_2$ and their significance in the initiation of labour have been reviewed by Liggins (1979).

CHANGES IN EPITHELIUM AND CERVICAL GLANDS

The epithelium of the cervix and cervical canal, both squamous and columnar, is in a state of hyperactivity, probably as a result of the hormonal stimulation of pregnancy. There is hyperactivity of the squamous epithelium of the *portio vaginalis*, which may show deviations from the normal, including: basal cell hyperactivity, with irregularities in size, shape, staining and number of mitoses in the basal cells; mid-zone hyperplasia, with a high proportion of large hyperchromatic 'active' nuclei; epithelial buds extending into the underlying stroma with submucosal infiltration of lymphocytes and plasma cellls; occasional atypical mitotic figures, particularly near the squamo-columnar junction.

If present in marked degree these normal pregnancy changes may resemble carcinoma *in situ* but it is not thought that pregnancy *per se* is a cause of carcinoma *in situ* (Fluhmann 1961). Similar hyperactivity occurs in the columnar epithelium. The columnar cells are tall with nuclei elevated above the base and as a result of marked proliferation tend to become heaped up and form small projections. Squamous metaplasia and reserve cell hyperplasia, so-called 'squamo-columnar prosoplasia' where the cells enclose clear vacuoles and produce mucus are common, particularly at the squamo-columnar junction or transitory zone and more especially in cervical ectopy, where they represent an attempt of the squamous epithelium to cover the exposed columnar mucosa. The growth of the columnar epithelium is so extensive in pregnancy that the endocervical mucosa doubles in thickness from an average of 2.3 mm to 4.6 mm as measured in fixed histological specimens.

This superabundant growth of endocervical tissue may protrude from the endocervical canal producing a physiological eversion of the cervix. At the same time, under the influence of the oestrogen stimulation of pregnancy, there is extensive growth of the endocervical columnar epithelium at the squamo-columnar junction at the expense of the squamous epithelium so that the squamo-columnar junction or transitional zone moves peripherally. This peripheral displacement of the squamo-columnar junction exposes the columnar epithelium to view producing a so-called 'cervical ectopy or erosion' or 'erythroplasia' with its characteristic fiery red 'velvety' appearance around the external os. Erythroplasia of the cervix, which is present in more than 50% of women at term and over 80% in the puerperium is so common that it should be regarded as a normal phenomenon in pregnancy. It is probable that the majority of cervical ectopies arise physiologically from the increased secretion of oestrogen either in the newborn, during puberty or in pregnancy (Hellman et al. 1950).

CERVICAL SECRETIONS

In pregnancy the cervical mucus becomes thick, viscous and opaque and fills the honeycomb of the endocervix to form the so-called 'mucus plug of pregnancy'. At the same time there is a considerable increase in the mucous discharge from the cervix which may be so profuse as to constitute a considerable nuisance to the patient. Cervical mucus in pregnancy characteristically has an abundance of leucocytes, cervical epithelial and vaginal cells. It is thought that the cervical secretion and the mucus plug act as an important antibacterial and mechanical barrier to the uterine cavity.

'Ferning', which normally occurs on drying of cervical mucus in patients in whom the effect of oestrogen as compared with progesterone predominates, is characteristically absent in pregnancy; in fact, if ferning is present in the first 14 weeks of pregnancy it is thought to be pathological and indicative of progesterone deficiency as about 50% of patients abort (Ullery & Shabanah 1957). Ferning in early pregnancy is also associated with placental insufficiency in late pregnancy (MacDonald 1972).

Vagina, vulva and pelvic floor

The vagina, vulva and pelvic floor, like all other pelvic organs, undergo a profound increase in vascularity. Within a short time after the onset of pregnancy the veins become enlarged and engorged and the blood they contain is relatively deoxygenated. By the 8th to the 10th week the vagina appears cyanotic and takes on a characteristic violet, purple or deep port-wine colour. The vulva becomes similarly engorged and oedematous and the dilated vessels may become so large, particularly in mulliparae, as to constitute vulval varices. These varices usually disappear completely when pregnancy is over, sometimes even before the patient leaves the delivery room. The whole pelvic floor, including the perineum and the perineal and levator ani muscles, undergo the typical pregnancy changes, with hypertrophy of the muscles and loosening of the connective tissue. The pelvic floor thus becomes more distensible and adapted to meet the needs of pregnancy and labour.

The vagina increases in capacity and length by tissue hypertrophy and hyperplasia. The muscular fibres hypertrophy, the elastic fibres increase, and the connective tissues undergo a gradual loosening similar to that which occurs in the cervix. Because of the loosening and hypertrophy, the vagina and all its supporting structures become progressively more relaxed and distensible so that at term the vagina can readily accommodate the passage of the fetal head and trunk without rupturing. The upper part of the vagina, in particular, enlarges and is drawn up as the uterus ascends out of the pelvis as pregnancy advances. When the fetal head enters the pelvis, however, in the last month of pregnancy or in labour, the vagina may be pushed down and is sometimes thrown into horizontal circular folds. This may cause the lower part of the anterior vaginal wall to protrude to some extent through the vulval opening.

The epithelium of the vagina undergoes marked hyperplasia, the vaginal rugae deepen and the papillae enlarge, so that the surface of the epithelium becomes rough and irregular and presents a 'fine hob-nailed appearance'. The most important change in the epithelium, however, occurs in the cells of the middle layer. These cells multiply, enlarge and become filled with vacuoles which contain glycogen. With the increased activity of the epithelium these cells quickly reach the surface and are desquamated. The cells disintegrate, releasing the glycogen, which

is converted by Döderlein's bacilli (*Lactobacillus acidophilus*) into lactic acid. This results in an increasingly profuse, thick, white, highly acid discharge. Its pH varies from 3.5 to 6 and while Döderlein's bacilli thrive in this acid environment it probably plays an important role in keeping the vagina relatively free from pathogenic bacteria. The acid pH, on the other hand, does favour the growth of yeasts and for this reason *Candida albicans* infection of the vagina is common in pregnancy.

The vagina shows a gradient in the number of bacteria, decreasing from the vulva inwards, the upper part of the vagina being relatively free from bacteria. This is in spite of the heavy contamination with bacteria around the rectum and the introduction of bacteria during coitus and by the fingers. The cervical mucous plug shows a similar gradient, the lower part near the external os containing a few bacteria and numbers of leucocytes, the middle part a few leucocytes, whereas the upper part contains no leucocytes and is sterile. Thus the pregnant uterus, in the absence of interference, is kept completely free of infection.

Considerable attention has been paid to the cells desquamated from the vagina, which have been extensively studied, using the staining method of Papanicolaou (1925). In early pregnancy there are increased numbers of leucocytes and basophilic cells, the latter having curled-up edges and tending to be clumped together. As pregnancy advances, the basophilic navicular cells derived from the intermediate layer and full of glycogen are found in increasing abundance in small dense clusters (Wachtel 1964). These cells predominate over the superficial squamous and basal cells and with leucocytes and Döderlein's bacilli constitute the typical smear in pregnancy. The early pregnancy changes are the same as those which occur in the second half of the normal menstrual cycle and are due to the effect of progesterone. The absence of these typical changes suggests a deficiency in progesterone secretion. Vaginal cytology has been used as a means of detecting progesterone deficiency particularly in the cases of threatened or habitual abortion (de Neef 1967a). Vaginal cytology has similarly been used to determine the effect of, and to control treatment with, progesterone (de Neef 1967b). It has also been used as an indication of possible endocrine deficiencies at the end of pregnancy and as a guide to fetal maturity and to the prospects of labour (de Neef 1967c).

Ligaments, parametrium and peritoneum

LIGAMENTS

Round ligaments are continuous with the uterine muscle and hypertrophy with it, and in late pregnancy may be 1–2 cm in thickness. Because of the growth of the uterus their attachment becomes relatively much nearer to the midline and the direction of the ligaments becomes vertical. The round ligaments may become painful and tender during the middle trimester of pregnancy. Not only may the pain itself cause considerable distress but it may raise problems in clinical differential diagnosis.

Uterosacral ligaments are also continuous with the uterine musculature and hypertrophy in pregnancy. It has been suggested that they contract with the uterus during labour and help to keep the uterus in its proper axis.

Broad ligaments are similarly strengthened by the hypertrophy of smooth muscle cells, which thereby help to increase their usefulness as supports. The two peritoneal layers of the ligament become separated by the growth of the uterus and contain the dilated venous sinuses, arteries and other structures supplying the uterus.

PARAMETRIUM

The most striking change in the parametrium is the peculiar activity of the mesenchymal cells, which are particularly numerous around the blood vessels in earlier pregnancy. Later they change into plasmacytes and monocytes, acquire phagocytic properties and come to lie between the connective tissue fibres. They become more numerous towards term and are probably part of the mechanisms which protect the maternal organism against infection.

PERITONEUM

The peritoneum grows with the uterus and undergoes true hyperplasia. Over the developing lower uterine segment the peritoneum becomes loose and immediately after delivery is thrown into folds corresponding with the muscle fibres though the folds disappear in the first few days of the puerperium. Decidual reactions, which commonly occur in the ovary in pregnancy, also occur in the pelvic peritoneum and appear as raised, velvety, red areas particularly on the posterior surface of the uterus, the uterosacral ligaments and Pouch of Douglas.

THE GENERAL STRUCTURAL CHANGES IN THE MOTHER

The structural changes in the mother vary considerably from patient to patient, and in a few cases they may be excessive, giving rise to a variety of symptoms and to various pathological entities.

Pelvis and skeletal system

BONY PELVIS

Apart from a considerable increase in vascularity there are no marked changes in the pelvic bones in pregnancy. Occasionally there is an irregular deposit of bone under the periosteum, the puerperal osteophytes of Rokitansky.

PELVIC LIGAMENTS

In contrast to the pelvic bones, there are marked changes in the pelvic ligaments in pregnancy. The pelvic bones are held together anteriorly by the symphysis pubis and the superior and inferior pubic ligaments, posteriorly by the sacro-iliac joints which join the sacrum to the innominate bones on either side and inferiorly by the sacrococcygeal joint where the coccyx is joined to the sacrum. These joints consist chiefly of fibrocartilage with small synovial articular cavities. In pregnancy there is a marked softening and loosening of the fibrocartilage and there is an increase in the synovia and synovial fluid, resulting in a considerable increase in mobility in the sacrococcygeal, pubic and sacro-iliac joints, particularly in multiparas. This is readily demonstrable in the case of the pubic symphysis on vaginal examination (Budin 1897) and by X-rays (Borrell & Fernstrom 1957). The symphysis pubis increases in width during pregnancy and labour, increasing the dimensions of the pelvis, but returns to normal soon after delivery. There is also separation and movements of the sacro-iliac joints, with downward displacement of the sacrum on standing and upward displacement in the lithotomy position.

The relaxation of these ligaments in pregnancy not infrequently gives rise to pain and tenderness over the symphysis pubis and the sacro-iliac joints. In some cases the relaxation may be so great that the patient experiences incapacity, pain at the joints and finds it difficult, if not impossible, to walk, when the condition may be regarded as pathological and is known as 'pelvic arthropathy of pregnancy'.

The relaxation of the ligaments and separation of the pelvic joints may play an important part in pregnancy and labour in increasing the available pelvic diameters but the extent to which separation normally occurs and its importance in labour has never been properly assessed.

SKELETAL SYSTEM

As the pregnant uterus grows in the abdomen it protrudes anteriorly. This increasing protruberance, particularly on standing, causes a progressive shift in the woman's centre of gravity anteriorly. To prevent herself falling forwards the pregnant woman throws her shoulders back and straightens her back and neck and leans backwards slightly to bring the centre of gravity vertically over the pelvis. The cervical and thoracic spine is thus progressively straightened though there is, of necessity, a compensatory increase in the lumbar lordosis and rotation of the pelvis on the femurs (Fig. 12.8).

The relaxation of the pelvic joints also causes a degree of pelvic instability so that the woman in late pregnancy adopts a characteristic waddling gait or strut. Because of these changes in skeletal dynamics the pregnant woman has to make a greater effort to maintain an erect carriage. The unaccustomed posture may also cause backache by placing unusual strains on particular muscles or ligaments. These changes in skeletal dynamics and consequent strains are much greater in women with a pendulous abdomen or twins.

Skin, face and abdominal wall

The changes in the abdominal wall are in many ways the same as occur in the skin generally but the progressive distension of the abdomen gives rise to certain features which merit separate discussion.

SKIN

There is in general an increased hyperaemia and blood flow through the skin in all parts of the body. The sweat and sebaceous glands increase in activity. In some women there is an increased growth of hair and a fine lanugo appears on the face and chest, which disappears 2 or 3 months post-partum. The

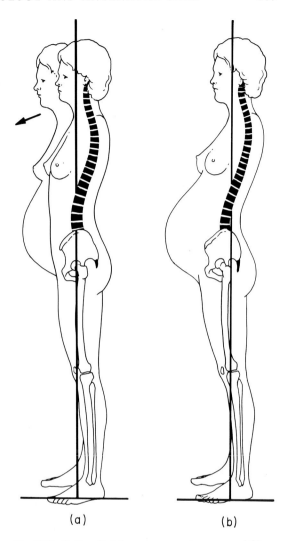

Fig. 12.8. Statics of (a) the non-pregnant woman and (b) the pregnant woman (Greenhill 1975).

subcutaneous fat becomes thicker and in late pregnancy facial features become fuller and softer, partly due to increased deposition of fat, and partly to oedema. There is often an increased pigmentation, particularly in specific areas such as the nipples, the vulva, the umbilicus and in the abdominal skin where the midline pigmentation extends from the xyphoid cartilage to the symphysis pubis, forming the linea nigra. Recent scars on the abdomen, interestingly, tend to become heavily pigmented but old scars do not.

The face is subject to a somewhat different form of pigmentation in which irregular brownish areas of varying size appear on the cheeks, the nose, the forehead and occasionally the neck, known as chloasma or 'the mask of pregnancy'. This fortunately disappears or at least regresses considerably after pregnancy. Very little is known about the nature of these pigmentary changes, which are said to be due to deposition of melanin. Melanocyte-stimulating hormone has been shown to be elevated from the 8th week of pregnancy until term. Oestrogen and progesterone, moreover, are reported to exert a melanocyte-stimulating effect (Diczfalusy & Troen 1961).

Vascular spider naevi or angiomata develop in about 60% of white and 11% of Negro women during pregnancy (Bean *et al.* 1949). They are associated with palmar erythema and are believed to be due to the effect of the high levels of circulating blood oestrogen in pregnancy. They are identical to the spider naevi and palmar erythema seen in patients with liver disease but are thought to be of no clinical significance in pregnancy. They disappear shortly after delivery.

ABDOMINAL WALL

After the 20th week, when the uterus has risen out of the pelvis, the abdominal girth increases. The abdominal wall becomes stretched and thinner. The previously depressed umbilicus usually becomes flush with the skin around the 24th week and protrudes outwards towards the end of pregnancy. Any tendency to hernia may be aggravated but usually the gravid uterus displaces the intestines and the omentum to one side which are thereby kept away from the hernial openings.

Rapid and excessive stretching of the skin is accompanied by breaking of its underlying connective tissue which gives rise to characteristic, irregular, wavy pink to purplish depressions termed striae gravidarum. These occur most frequently in the skin of the lower abdomen, over the buttocks, and along the upper parts of the thighs. They also occur on the breasts when they are arranged radially round the nipples. Blondes are said to be more affected than brunettes, primigravidas more than multigravidas, fat women more than thin women. Following delivery the striae become silvery white in appearance and resemble old scar tissue. In multiparas, both the

silvery white markings of a previous pregnancy and fresh pink to purple striae of the present pregnancy may be seen.

Identical striae may be seen in non-pregnant women with Cushing's syndrome and women who have rapidly accumulated subcutaneous fat. Striae of pregnancy are thus probably due to the increased secretion of adrenocortical hormones in pregnancy which cause marked changes in the collagen and in the ground substance of connective tissue which allow the subcutaneous fibrous tissue to rupture wherever the skin is under tension or overstretched.

Breasts

Tingling, tenseness and occasionally real pain in the breasts may be one of the earliest symptoms of pregnancy. These sensations are caused by increased vascularity and gland proliferation and are the same as those often noted in the week before menstruation. After the second month the breasts increase in size, partly from hypertrophy and hyperplasia of the glands and partly from increase in fat between the lobules and in the skin. As they increase in size delicate veins become visible just beneath the skin and as they get larger appear as bluish streaks. At the same time the nipples become larger, more pigmented and erectile and after the first few months a thick yellowish fluid, colostrum, may be expressed. The primary areola also becomes more deeply pigmented and broader and the base of the areola becomes puffed up and raised above the surface of the rest of the gland. Scattered through the areola are a number of small rounded elevations which are the mouths of hypertrophied sebaceous glands and are known as Montgomery's follicles. Later in pregnancy, around the primary areola, a secondary less pigmented areola develops. It has been described as a 'dusky paper sprinkled with drops of water'. The clear spots without pigment occur around the openings of the sweat and sebaceous glands. The depth of pigmentation varies with the patient's complexion. In blondes the areolae and nipples become pinkish, while in brunettes they become dark brown and occasionally almost black.

The breast is made up of fifteen to twenty distinct lobules embedded in a cushion of fat. Each lobule consists of a mass of branched glands or acini leading into tubules and eventually into one duct which opens on the nipple. There are thus fifteen to twenty ducts opening on the nipple, each of which is dilated in the nipple to produce a sinus lactiferous. The nipple is a muscular organ surrounded by unstriped muscular fibres which unite with those of the nipple itself to produce an erectile organ.

During the first few months of pregnancy the most prominent change is the proliferation of the glandular tissue. This is followed by a marked proliferation of the ducts. About halfway through the pregnancy the secretion of colostrum begins and continues slowly to term. Colostrum can normally be expressed but the amount present is usually not sufficient to cause spontaneous leakage from the nipple. In the last month or so of pregnancy however spontaneous leakage may occur but this has no prognostic significance with regard to lactation. As the patient reaches term breast growth and the volume of colostrum are at a maximum and the ducts hypertrophy to the point where they are ready to conduct large supplies of milk. The breasts are thus anatomically and physiologically prepared to take on the task of lactation and of supplying the infant with milk and essential nourishment once it is delivered.

PHYSIOLOGICAL CHANGES IN THE MOTHER

Widespread changes occur in the physiological functions of the mother during pregnancy. For the most part these changes are discussed in the appropriate chapters dealing with medical disorders complicating pregnancy. Here they will be summarized briefly to illustrate the main physiological changes during pregnancy and the principles underlying those changes. For comprehensive and critical discussion on specific physiological changes in pregnancy refer to Philipp *et al.* (1977), Shearman (1979), Hytten & Chamberlain (1980) and de Swiet (1984).

The blood and its constituents

BLOOD VOLUME

During pregnancy there is an increase in the total blood volume, the plasma volume and the red cell mass. Increase in total blood volume is of the order of 1250 ml in primigravida and 1500 ml in multigravida; this peak is reached about 34 weeks of pregnancy, after which there is a gradual decrease until term. Plasma volume increase (45%) is chiefly responsible for the general increase in total blood volume, the red cell mass increasing by some 18% only. The increase of red cell mass is of the order of 400 ml when iron supplements are given during pregnancy, and 250 ml when not given. The increase in plasma volume is more variable and is related to parity, fetal birth weight and number and clinical outcome. 'Poor reproducers' tend to have a smaller increase in blood volume in pregnancy (Gibson 1973). These changes are further discussed in Chapter 18 (p. 254). They are summarized in Table 12.1.

CELLULAR CONSTITUENTS

There is a marked increase in leucocyte count from around 7000/mm³ in the non-pregnant state to 10,500/mm³ in late pregnancy, due to increase in neutrophil cells; lymphocytes and other cells are unchanged. Platelets increase continuously in pregnancy and the puerperium from 187,000/mm³ in the non-pregnant to 316,000/mm³ at term and 600,000/mm³ in the puerperium. Haemodilution in pregnancy reduces blood viscosity (relative to water) from 4.61 in non-pregnant women to 3.84 in mid and late pregnancy. The erythrocyte sedimentation rate (ESR: Westergren) rises from 9.6 mm/hr to 56 mm/hr (range 30–100 mm/hr) due to increased plasma fibrinogen and globulin.

Table 12.1. Principal blood changes in pregnancy.

	Non-pregnant	34 Weeks	Increment
Total blood volume (ml)	4000	5500	+1500
Plasma volume (ml)	2500	3750	+1250
Red cell volume (ml)	1500	1750	+250
Haematocrit (whole body) %	35	30	−5
Haematocrit (venous) %	40	34	−6
Total haemoglobin (g)	510	600	+90
Total iron (mg)	1700	2000	+300

PLASMA PROTEINS

Important changes occur in plasma proteins. In general there is a fall in plasma protein concentration from the non-pregnancy value to around 6g/dl less due to haemodilution. There is a decrease in total plasma protein concentration and an alteration in the albumin/globulin ratio from 1.5 to 1 or even less, due to a fall in the albumin fraction. The globulin fraction in contrast shows a marked increase primarily due to the increase in β-globulin which are the main carrier proteins in the plasma and which rise both relatively and in absolute concentration from about 1–1.3 g/dl in late pregnancy. Fibrinogen concentration increases progressively through pregnancy and at term is about 50% greater than pre-pregnancy levels, and a part of the increase in blood coagulability.

PLASMA, LIPIDS, LIPOPROTEINS AND CHOLESTEROL

There is a marked rise in all lipids in pregnancy, with an increased ratio of β to α lipoprotein from 2:1 in the non-pregnant woman to 5:1 in late pregnancy. The total lipids increase from around 600 mg/dl in the non-pregnant woman to around 900 mg/dl in late pregnancy. This increase is predominantly in cholesterol and triglycerides; plasma phospholipid concentration increases to a smaller extent. The cholesterol figures change from around 180 mg/dl in the non-pregnant state to some 270 mg/dl near to term. These changes are all coincidental with the deposition of fat which mainly occurs in the first 20 weeks of pregnancy.

PLASMA ELECTROLYTES AND ACID-BASE BALANCE

There is a fall in total electrolytes of the order of 10 mEq/l due to haemodilution. Hyperventilation during pregnancy produces a fall in arterial blood PCO_2 from 38 to 32 mmHg. There is a partially compensated respiratory alkalosis with a fall in plasma bicarbonate. Changes in pH are of the order of 7.4 in the non-pregnant to 7.44 in the pregnant patient. Standard bicarbonate falls from some 24 mEq/l in the non-pregnant patient to 21 mEq/l in the pregnant patient. The arterial PO_2 rises from 95 mmHg in the non-pregnant to 105 mmHg during pregnancy. These changes facilitate transfer of carbon dioxide from the fetus to the mother and oxygen from the mother to the fetus.

Changes in the cardiovascular system

CLINICAL CHANGES

Pregnancy is a hyperkinetic state, similar to hyperthyroidism. This is evidenced by increased oxygen consumption, increased cardiac output and decreased peripheral resistance. Clinical changes which may be noted are: the pulse becomes bounding and partially collapsing; the apex beat is displaced upwards and outwards and the heart is dextrorotated; electrocardiography shows prominent S-wave in lead 1 and a conspicuous Q and inverted P in lead 3; the heart is slightly enlarged in diastole; a third heart sound may be heard; haemic murmurs are common; there is a slight rise in venous pressure.

CARDIAC OUTPUT

Consideration of cardiac output changes is undertaken in Chapter 17 (p. 242). These changes are summarized in Table 12.2.

Table 12.2. Summary of cardiac changes of pregnancy.

	Non-pregnant	12 weeks	36 weeks
Cardiac output (l/min)	4.5	6.0	5.5
Stroke volume (ml)	65	75	65
Pulse rate	70	80	85

There is a considerable disagreement about the timing of peak cardiac output in mid or late pregnancy. Many workers maintain that the fall in late pregnancy is due to the supine hypotensive syndrome. All are agreed that an increase occurs early in pregnancy and is more than sufficient to carry the increased oxygen consumption. Further cardiac output changes occur in labour. In the first stage of labour cardiac output increases by some 30% to 8 l/min; and in the second stage it rises by some 50% to 9 l/min.

ARTERIAL AND VENOUS BLOOD PRESSURE

The blood pressure normally falls in pregnancy by, on average, 5 mmHg systolic and 15 mmHg diastolic in normal pregnancy before the 28th week, rising to prepregnancy levels at term (Fig. 12.9; MacGillivray et al. 1969). Insufficient attention has been paid to this normal fall in blood pressure in early and mid-pregnancy, and the fact that different standards of normality need to be applied at different stages in pregnancy (Friedman 1976). The blood pressure

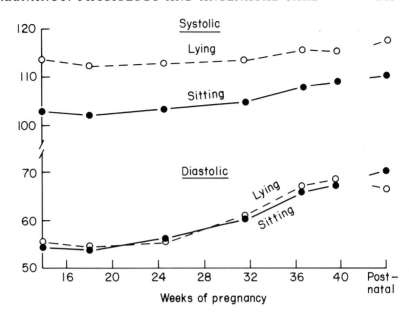

Fig. 12.9 Blood pressure trends (sitting and lying) during pregnancy (MacGillivray *et al.* 1969).

lowering effect of pregnancy means that patients who are hypertensive before pregnancy may appear normotensive when first seen in early or midpregnancy according to present-day conventional criteria. New proposed limits based on the data of MacGillivray *et al.* (1969) are set out in Table 12.3.

For practical purposes, the upper limits of lying diastolic pressure (Phase IV Korotkoff) for the different stages of pregnancy are up to 28 weeks 75 mmHg; 29–34 weeks 80 mmHg; 35 weeks to term 90 mmHg. If a standard upper limit of 90 mmHg is adopted throughout pregnancy this implies a limit 3 standard deviations above the mean in early and midpregnancy and 2 standard deviations above the mean in late pregnancy.

Venous pressure is slightly raised above the normal, except in the lower limbs where the change is greater, the pressure in the femoral veins being markedly raised up to 24 cm of water. Pulmonary artery pressures are within normal limits but show a slight rise on exercise. Peripheral vascular resistance is markedly reduced, this fall being maximal between the 25th and 28th weeks, due to dilatation of the arteries of the uterus, kidney and skin.

Changes in the respiratory system

CLINICAL CHANGES

Mechanical changes which occur in the respiratory system are some lifting of the chest cage with upward flaring of the ribs. There is elevation and increased excursion of the diaphragm, except in late pregnancy; at that time there is reduced diaphragmatic excursion, and respiratory exchange is maintained by increased thoracic movement, which may cause dyspnoea.

Table 12.3. Blood pressure in normal pregnancy. (Calculated from MacGillivray *et al.* 1969.)

	Blood pressure (mmHg)		Gestational age (weeks)		
			$\leqslant 28$	29–34	$\geqslant 35$
Systolic	Sitting	Mean	102	104	109
		+2 S.D.	122	124	131
	Lying	Mean	113	113	115
		+2 S.D.	134	134	138
Diastolic (Korotkoff Point IV)	Sitting	Mean	55	60	67
		+2 S.D.	72	80	88
	Lying	Mean	55	62	69
		+2 S.D.	75	80	92

FUNCTIONAL CHANGES

Physiological considerations include an unchanged vital capacity at 3200 ml. Tidal air is increased by some 200 ml and residual volume reduced by the same amount. Increased volume of air, together with a much smaller residual volume of air in the lungs, gives a marked improvement in gaseous exchange.

Fluid balance and weight gain

In pregnancy great changes occur in fluid balance. Hytten & Leitch (1971f) measured the total water increment of pregnancy at 7.5 l around term; of this volume it was estimated that some 5.9 l l could be accounted for in the fetus, placenta, liquor amnii, enlarged uterus, breasts, plama, and the red cells, leaving 1.6 l as increase in tissue fluid. In women with generalized oedema there was an additional increase of 3.3 l.

This tissue fluid increase is closely related to the blood volume changes discussed above. The blood volume of an average-sized non-pregnant woman is approximately 4 l, of which 2.6 l are plasma. In pregnancy the plasma volume increases beyond this figure by some 1.3 l around 34 weeks, the increase at term being lower, of the order of 1 l. Rhodes (1970) pointed out that the volume of interstitial fluid must increase if the plasma volume increases, since both are part of the extracellular fluid. Escape of the fluid from the capillaries is assisted by a reduction in the oncotic pressure which accompanies the fall in plasma protein concentration during pregnancy, and, in the lower part of the body at least, from the effect of raised venous pressure.

Weight gain is a crude but useful index of the changes in the mother and fetus during pregnancy. In general the weight gain in the first half of pregnancy is due to deposition of body fat as an energy reserve, whereas the weight changes in the second half of pregnancy are due to the increase in mass of the fetus and amniotic fluid and of the uterus and breasts and of the blood and extracellular fluid volumes. The average weight gain in a healthy patient on an adequate diet is summarized in Table 12.4.

Any weight gain in pregnancy in excess of 8 kg may be retained after the immediate puerperium and represents an accumulation of body fat which constitutes an energy reserve to meet the needs of lactation. The distribution of the weight gain at term is shown in Table 12.5.

Table 12.4. Average weight gain in healthy pregnant women on adequate diet.

Weeks	Weight (kg)		
1–12	1.0		
13–16	1.0	4.0	
17–20	2.0		
21–24	2.0		12.0
25–28	2.0		
29–32	1.5	8.0	
33–36	1.5		
37–40	1.0		

Average net loss at delivery: 8.0 kg
Average net gain: 4.0 kg

Table 12.5. Distribution of weight gain at 40 weeks (kg).

Fetal (approx. 5 kg)	Fetus	3.3
	Placenta	0.7
	Liquor	0.8
	Total	4.8
Mother (approx. 7 kg)	Uterus	0.9
	Breasts	0.4
	Blood	1.2
	ECF	1.2
	Fat	4.0
	Total	7.7
Total weight gain at 40 weeks = 12.5 kg		

Renal changes

Marked changes occur in the renal tracts in pregnancy: these are considered in detail in Chapter 19 (p. 277). Dilatation and kinking of the ureters may become pronounced, leading to stasis of urine and perhaps to urinary infection. In the kidney itself there is an increase in the renal blood and plasma flow during the first and second trimesters but a gradual fall in the total blood flow throughout the third trimester. The total renal blood flow (RBF) increases from about 900 ml/min before pregnancy to 1200 ml/min in the second trimester, falling to 1100 ml after 34 weeks. The glomerular filtration rate (GFR) increases in a similar manner reaching a figure some 50–60% higher than that of the non-pregnant state; the fall in GFR in late pregnancy is however less pronounced than the fall in RBF. The mean filtration fraction thus falls from a non-pregnant value 0.21 to 0.18 at 16 weeks, remains at this level till 28 weeks, but rises to 0.20 at term (Table 12.6).

Gastro-intestinal tract

Salivation is increased in many patients and occasionally the increase can be so great that considerable

Table 12.6. Renal function in normal pregnancy. (Data derived from Sims & Krantz 1958.)

	Approx. gestational age (weeks)			Post-partum 6 weeks	Percentage change in pregnancy
	16	26	36		
Glomerular filtration rate (inulin clearance) (ml/min)	148	147	144	92	+60%
Effective renal plasma flow (PAH clearance) (ml/min) allowing for posture	798	807	692	434	+85%
Filtration faction	0.185	0.182	0.20	0.21	?Slight decrease in early pregnancy

discomfort and annoyance is caused and the condition is then designated ptyalism of pregnancy. Reduction in the gastric acidity is also a common if not normal physiological occurrence during pregnancy, and may on occasions be pronounced. Motility of the stomach is also reduced and during labour this reduction of gastric emptying time may be very marked constituting a major hazard in general anaesthesia. There is a general diminution of bowel peristalsis, and constipation may be troublesome in some patients. These changes are in all probability due to the smooth muscle hypotonia associated with progesterone dominance in pregnancy. Towards the end of pregnancy however a mechanical factor due to pressures of the enlarging uterus on the abdominal contents may be important. Relaxation of the cardiac sphincter and pressure on the stomach may lead to regurgitation of acid stomach contents into the oesophagus and to 'heartburn' which is often a distressing symptom in pregnancy. In a few cases the enlarging uterus during late pregnancy appears to produce temporary hiatus hernia. Liver function is not significantly altered during pregnancy in normal circumstances and the blood flow through the liver appears largely unchanged (Tindall & Beazley 1965).

Metabolism in pregnancy

Metabolic rate and thyroid metabolism

The total metabolism is increased due to the demands of the fetus, the demands of the extra work of the heart and lungs, and build up of materials: this amount equals some 350 kcal/day in midpregnancy and 250 kcal/day in late pregnancy, which may in part be met by economy of activity. The increase in metabolism is probably due to anterior pituitary stimulation of the thyroid. The thyroid gland hypertrophies in the majority of patients. Changes in thyroid function noted are a rise in total T_4 due to an increase in TBG from a non-pregnant range of 4.8–11.0 g/dl to a pregnant range of 7.5–19.5 g/dl. The total T_3 also rises from a range of 90–180 g/dl to a pregnant range of 160–300 g/dl. The absolute levels of free T_3 and free T_4 do not change, and are the same as for non-pregnant euthyroid women. The thyroid hormone uptake declines as TBG increases, and the free thyroxine index remains in the normal non-pregnant range.

Metabolic balance

For the mother, pregnancy is anabolic, since she requires and retains extra material. Protein metabolism is notable for a markedly increased positive nitrogen balance throughout pregnancy. This nitrogen gain is greatly in excess of the needs of the fetus. During the puerperium there is a negative nitrogen balance, return to the normal state, however, taking some 2–3 months before it is complete. During her pregnancy the well-nourished mother deposits and stores fats, calcium and iron but probably not any other nutrients. Blood levels of nutrients and other substances are not increased, with the exception of those bound to the carrier β-globulins in the plasma, which rise during pregnancy. Some nutrients are lost in the urine, namely glucose and amino acids (particularly histidine and isoleucine), probably due to the increased glomerular filtration rate and to the excess filtration of those nutrients beyond the reabsorptive capacity of the renal tubules.

Carbohydrate metabolism

Carbohydrate metabolism is described in detail in Chapter 20 (p. 286). Briefly, there is little alteration to the glucose tolerance test or the fasting-blood sugar. Glycosuria, however, is common mainly due to the lowering of the renal threshold for glucose to well below the normal figure of 10 mmol/l. In pregnancy more glucose is utilized by the placenta, a good deal is converted into depot fat and less glycogen is probably deposited in liver and muscles.

Fat metabolism and energy reserve

As noted, approximately 4 kg of additional fat are deposited, mostly in the abdominal wall, back and thighs, during pregnancy; this deposition occurs in well-nourished women, but not when there is calorie deprivation. This stored fat provides energy which may be used in late pregnancy, labour and the puerperium, and is probably important in evolutionary terms to meet times of famine and inadequate nutritional intake.

Calcium metabolism

There is little change in calcium levels in the blood during pregnancy, despite the increased needs of the fetus. It is probable that a healthy well-nourished mother can adequately supply her fetus with the necessary quantity of calcium required, which in late pregnancy amounts to some 250 mg daily. Thirty to forty grams of calcium are deposited in the fetus during pregnancy, and this makes little alteration to the mother's calcium stores unless she is already suffering from a malabsorption syndrome.

Iron metabolism

The only common dietary deficiency is of iron and this is by far the most frequent cause of anaemia in pregnancy. Folate deficiency may also occur separately or concurrently and produce megaloblastic anaemia or a mixed type of anaemia. The incidence of iron and folate deficiency varies greatly between different geographical regions, and between and within different communities depending upon their nutritional status. Such deficiencies are much more common in multiple pregnancy, in women having repeated pregnancies or who have excessive menstrual blood loss or where haemoglobin synthesis is increased as in haemolytic type anaemias. Iron metabolism is discussed further in Chapter 18 (p. 255).

THE MANAGEMENT OF PREGNANCY

Antenatal care bestows great advantages on the fetus and the mother.

THE FETUS

The perinatal loss associated with a lack of antenatal care is some five times greater than when adequate antenatal care is provided and when antenatal clinics are attended regularly from the beginning of pregnancy. The unbooked patient is always a major hazard and a cause of high perinatal mortality. There are several reasons for this difference: diseases with an adverse effect on fetal outcome, e.g. anaemia, syphilis and rhesus disease, are detected by routine screening; mechanical problems such as malpresentations or disproportion are detected; disorders such as pre-eclampsia can be detected at an early stage; the presence of poor fetal growth and placental insufficiency recognized and appropriate management instituted. It is probable that perinatal mortality can be reduced even further by applying modern physiological understanding to the remaining major fetal risks, e.g. by the detection of inappropriately increased uterine activity and decreased fetal movements and well-being. There is however little that can be done at present to prevent fetal congenital abnormalities. Abruptio placentae, and to a lesser extent hypertension, remain continuing unsolved problems and continuing hazards to the fetus.

THE MOTHER

Antenatal clinics also constitute screening clinics because they are often the only time a young healthy woman will visit a doctor. It may be the first time a woman has been physically examined in her life. Breast palpation and cervical smears should be routine. Radiological examination of the chest has much to commend wherever there is a high incidence of tuberculosis. Incidental diseases such as diabetes, hypertension and renal disorders should be detected at a very early stage, and necessary treatment given. General advice and education should be given wherever possible to both mother and father on what to expect and do in pregnancy and labour and in the care of the infant. Pregnancy counselling should be undertaken in all women who have had a family history of any fetal abnormality, and amniocentesis for chromosomal analysis considered in all women of 35 years or older. The question of family planning and sterilization should be discussed during pregnancy and a plan made for future contraception.

Careful antenatal supervision is or should be an essential part of the management in all pregnancies. Some flexibility however is desirable depending upon the individual being cared for and the medical and nursing personnel and facilities available. For many years it has been the practice for a patient receiving antenatal care to be seen monthly until the 28th week, every 2 weeks until the 36th week, and weekly from then until she is delivered. For a healthy patient who develops no abnormality these intervals represent an ideal, but where resources are stretched they may be extended. In other circumstances, such as suspected fetal growth retardation, raised blood pressure or, failure to gain weight or any other abnormality, more frequent visits may be essential to detect a pathological deterioration in the fetal or maternal condition and to ensure timely intervention.

The first visit

At the first visit it is important to confirm the diagnosis of pregnancy and duration of gestation, make a careful review of all matters pertaining to the pregnancy and to discuss the prospects and plans for the pregnancy with the patient. Sometimes this review is best deferred to the second visit when the results of the routine and any special investigations are available.

DIAGNOSIS OF PREGNANCY

The history of amenorrhoea is important not only in the diagnosis of pregnancy itself, but in the establishment of the duration of pregnancy at any particular time. It is necessary to determine when the patient's last menstrual period was, if it was normal, and if it was preceded by other regular periods. The following points should always be elucidated:

1   the date of the last menstrual period;
2   whether it was normal in amount and duration;
3   whether it came at the correct time;
4   the cycle length;
5   whether oral contraception had been taken recently;
6   when the first symptoms of pregnancy occurred and how these compared to their time of appearance in previous pregnancies;
7   date of quickening.

The short last menstrual period, which is often disregarded in calculating gestational age of the fetus is often a more accurate index than the last normal menstrual period. With this exception, the calculated last menstrual period is probably the most accurate measure of gestational age available clinically, especially when it is in accord with clinical palpation in the first trimester.

The diagnosis of pregnancy will rest upon the finding of an enlarged soft uterus. The uterine fundus can seldom be palpated per abdomen for some 12 weeks in a patient's first pregnancy, and in most instances it will be advisable to examine the patient vaginally at her first visit. Other advantages of pelvic examination at the first visit include the recognition of other associated disorders such as fibroids, ovarian cysts and cervical polyps. A cervical smear should be taken if one has not been done recently. In cases of previous reproductive failure, the cervix should be assessed for incompetence and the cervical mucus for ferning. If the patient is nervous, it may be wiser to defer pelvic examination to the second visit in order to gain her confidence. Assessment of pelvic size should be carried out only in late pregnancy.

PREGNANCY TESTS

If there is doubt about the diagnosis of pregnancy, a pregnancy test may be performed. Immunological pregnancy tests for the detection of HCG in urine, such as the haemaglutination inhibition test, have now replaced biological ones. Immunological tests are simpler and cheaper, and in general show a higher degree of sensitivity. Most manufacturers set the sensitivity in such a manner that a reliable positive result is obtained 11 days after the missed period. Plasma β-HCG may be measured by radioimmunoassay and provide a means of detecting pregnancy very early even before the first missed period.

ULTRASOUND

Ultrasonic examination provides an alternative method of diagnosing very early pregnancy. The presence of a gestation sac may be recognizable some 6 weeks after the last menstrual period, and embryonic echoes within the sac shortly after that. The fetal head becomes recognizable at about 13 weeks. With ultrasonic apparatus now available, it is possible to identify the beating fetal heart at a very early stage and, in addition, measurement of the crown–rump length and, to a lesser extent, the sac size, enables an accurate estimate of gestational age to be made at a very early gestational age.

A good case can be made out for routine ultrasonic scanning at booking in all pregnancies, particularly in patients where the date of the last menstrual period is unknown or in doubt, or where there is some discrepancy between the size of the uterus or fetus and the gestational age. The advantages of routine ultrasonic scanning in early pregnancy are:

1   *The measurement of the size of the gestational sac, the crown–rump length, or the biparietal diameter, as appropriate, provides the most precise available guide to gestational age.* The earlier in pregnancy the measurement is performed, the more precise the estimate. This information is then available as a guide throughout the remainder of the pregnancy. In centres where ultrasound facilities are available, it is found that ultrasonic examination is requested in a third to a half of patients in pregnancy anyway.

2   *The measurement of crown–rump length or biparietal diameter provides a valuable base-line measurement for the estimation of fetal growth.* Without a base-line measurement, measurements of fetal diameter later in pregnancy are much less valuable. With a single measurement of biparietal diameter later in pregnancy, it may not be possible to distinguish between a preterm or growth-retarded fetus.

3   *The diagnosis of unsuspected abnormalities of pregnancy including:*
   (a) incomplete abortion, blighted ovum, hydatidiform mole or intrauterine death,
   (b) fetal abnormality e.g. anencephaly,
   (c) multiple pregnancy,
   (d) hydramnios,
   (e) placenta praevia,
   (f) pelvic tumours.

In many instances, where a previous pregnancy may have been abnormal, an ultrasonic examination with demonstration of the fetal heart movements and visualization of a normal fetus may provide valuable reassurance to the doctor and the patient. Routine ultrasonic screening in early pregnancy may seem a counsel of perfection, but it is nevertheless an ideal for which to strive and should be regarded as a standard procedure in virtually all pregnancies.

DIET IN PREGNANCY

During pregnancy there is a need for extra energy to supply the needs of the growing fetus and to keep pace with the increased metabolic rate and growth of tissues of the mother. The World Health Organization report entitled 'Nutrition in Pregnancy and Lactation' (1965) deals with these matters fully. The pregnant woman theoretically requires a diet of some 2500 calories daily and, in general, does not need to eat more when she is pregnant. The decreased activity of pregnancy partly compensates for the increased

needs of the fetus. The WHO group recommend, however, that some 5–6 g extra protein per day should be taken during the second and third trimester though this has been questioned. An adequate calcium intake as provided by 250–500 ml milk per day providing a total intake of 1000–1200 μg daily seems desirable. Iron supplements are required to the order of some 100 mg of elemental iron daily. Vitamin intake is adequate in most countries though folic acid deficiency may occur even in reasonably well fed communities. Supplements of folic acid (300 μg/day) may conveniently be given with iron in communities where these nutrients are deficient. In practical terms, a patient should be told that she does not require to eat more during pregnancy, but to eat wisely. A normal mixed diet, relatively high in protein (100 g) and relatively low in fat (100 g) and carbohydrate (300 g), with if necessary milk supplements, should be her aim. Supplementary iron and folic acid should be given where indicated but this does not reduce the need for routine haemoglobin checks.

GENERAL ADVICE

Many general matters may come up for discussion during pregnancy. It may be necessary to give advice about vomiting, heartburn, constipation, etc., and these are dealt with in appropriate chapters elsewhere in this book. Most women will be better for taking more rest during pregnancy, especially those who work outwith their own home. In many circumstances this may be a counsel of perfection, as in many societies women are obliged to work until term and they go into labour. Smoking has clearly been shown to be associated with limitation in fetal growth and increased perinatal mortality (Russell *et al.* 1968) and the most important advice that can be given to any patient is to stop smoking for her baby's sake if not for her own. Intercourse can safely be continued until the last few weeks of pregnancy in normal circumstances, but is probably best eschewed in cases of recurrent abortion or preterm labour.

Visits in the first two trimesters

The second trimester is usually a quiet time where attention is focused upon:
1   routine observations for the gestational age and occurrence of multiple pregnancy;
2   uterine irritability, amniotic fluid volume, and

occurrence of intrauterine growth retardation (IUGR);

3   early detection of anaemia and hypertension.

Visits in the last trimester

During the last trimester attention is focused upon:
1   fetal age, growth and maturity;
2   fetal well-being;
3   maternal complications of pregnancy and maternal well-being;
4   mechanics of pregnancy;
5   preparation for labour and induced labour;
6   education for pregnancy, labour, breast feeding, infant care and counselling in family planning.

FETAL AGE, GROWTH AND MATURITY

At each visit the precise gestational age should be calculated. If the date of the last menstrual period is certain, if there are reliable observations in early pregnancy, if ultrasonography has been performed before the 28th week and if all the observations are in agreement, the calculation may be a matter of routine. If not, the clinician must weigh the evidence and make the best estimate, as it is against gestational age that most other observations are assessed.

The size and growth of the fetus must be estimated at each visit to detect any retardation of growth, any excessive growth and any other abnormality such as hydramnios. If intrauterine growth retardation is suspected then special tests such as ultrasonic measurement of fetal biparietal diameter, head/trunk circumferences and areas, and possibly placental function tests should be performed. If there is excessive fetal growth or enlargement of the uterus, appropriate investigations such as an X-ray, or preferably ultrasound, for twins or fetal abnormality, or glucose tolerance tests should be carried out.

If termination of pregnancy by induction of labour or elective Caesarean section becomes indicated for any reason, it is important to assess the physiological development or maturity, as well as the age and size of the fetus. If dates are certain and pregnancy is well advanced (37 weeks or more), physiological maturity may be assumed. If less than 37 weeks, and in cases of doubt, amniocentesis should be performed and the amniotic fluid surfactant estimated by 'bubble stability' or 'foam' test, or estimation of the lecithin/sphingomyelin ratio, total phospholipids or phosphatidyl glycerol (Depp 1980). Amniocentesis is of particular value when induction of labour or elective Caesarean

section is contemplated and the dates are in doubt or the fetus appears small or premature. Growth retarded fetuses, furthermore, may well have an accelerated pulmonary maturity (Cunningham *et al.* 1977). In cases of oligohydramnios and in all cases of difficulty, amniocentesis should be performed under ultrasonic screening. The value and place of amniocentesis has been questioned but it is a simple, safe investigation providing direct evidence of fetal pulmonary maturity, which may be of considerable value in coming to a final decision when delivery is contemplated because of some fetal or maternal risk, and the fetus appears preterm or gestational age is uncertain.

FETAL WELL-BEING

The assessment of fetal well-being (*see also* Chapter 31, p. 447) is important and has become one of the major objectives of modern obstetric practice. In the past, insufficient attention was paid to the condition of the fetus at birth, and undue emphasis placed on the relatively crude indices of stillbirth, neonatal death and perinatal mortality. In present day obstetrics the delivery of an asphyxiated or depressed infant or an infant with impaired potential for growth and development constitutes an abnormality or deviation from the ideal or optimum. This necessitates ideal or optimum care in pregnancy and labour. Antenatally, the assessment of fetal well-being has been greatly advanced by measurements of fetal movements, by the study of fetal heart rate changes, antenatal cardiotocography or so-called 'non-stress' tests, and by ultrasonic measurements of the fetus, amniotic fluid volume and fetal breathing, and by all these measures together: the so-called biophysical profile (Manning *et al.* 1980). The indications, interpretations and details of these techniques are beyond the scope of this chapter, but it must be stressed that the practising obstetrician or midwife is not absolved from making a clinical assessment of fetal growth and well-being at each and every antenatal visit. The first step is always the clinical recognition of women in whom the fetal growth and well-being may be impaired and the selection of patients for further investigation. This clinical recognition may be assisted by identification of risk factors and simple clinical observation of weight gain, fetal movements and uterine activity.

Risk factors

Risk factors, such as advanced maternal age (35 years and over), smoking and hypertension, do provide some indication of patients in whom the fetal condition may be prejudiced. In general, however, risk factors have a low sensitivity, specificity and predictive value (Gordon *et al.* 1978). Attempts have been made to improve predictive value by adding risk factors together and calculating a risk score (Hobel *et al.* 1973, Sokal *et al.* 1977). Lists of risk factors are generally so long and risk scores are of such low predictive value that, apart from raising the 'index of suspicion', they do not contribute to the clinical management of the individual patient.

Fetal movements
Decrease in fetal movements, particularly when volunteered by the patient, has long been recognized as a sign of impending fetal death, particularly in case of rhesus-isoimmunization and diabetes. The regular recording by the patient of fetal movements has nevertheless been a significant advance in the assessment of fetal well-being and obstetric practice. The mother counts fetal movements for 30 min twice daily and the results are expressed as a number of movements for 12 hr or the time taken to feel the first ten movements of the day (Sadovsky & Polishuk 1977, Pearson & Weaver 1976). When fetal movements are not felt in the first half hour, the observation period is extended to 1 hr. When there are fewer than four fetal movements/12 hr, the situation is described as alarm. The above authors found that a significant decrease in fetal movements always preceded fetal heart rate changes by 1–4 days. When using fetal movements as a measure of fetal condition it is important to remember than any sedation given to the mother may decrease fetal activity. Movements are also decreased in quiet sleep of the fetus. Periods of quiet sleep increase with increasing maturity so that fetal movements may appear to decrease towards term, which can cause considerable anxiety. Most episodes of decreased movements prove to be false alarms, but, when fewer than 3 movements are felt per 30 min on average, then any such patient must be investigated by direct observation, real time ultrasonic scanning and/or antenatal cardiotocography. If no such facilities are available and the decreased movements are confirmed on further observation, it may be necessary to act and terminate the pregnancy. Fetal movements, however, should not be used as the sole parameter by which to assess fetal condition. A sudden marked increase in fetal movements, though much less common, is also an abnormal sign and has been observed in cord occlusion and in narcotic withdrawal in the addicted mother.

Both decrease and increase in fetal movements hence constitute a valuable warning sign and any change in movements, either spontaneously volunteered or systematically recorded by the patient, requires urgent further investigation.

Uterine activity
The marked increase of uterine contractions in late pregnancy, either volunteered by the patient or noted on clinical examination, may provide an additional guide to the condition of the fetus and of the fetoplacental unit. Uterine contractions have been less well studied in relation to fetal condition in pregnancy but increased uterine activity may indicate incipient preterm labour. In some patients this increased uterine activity and incipient labour may be secondary to fetoplacental inadequacy and, in all such cases, it is important to exclude growth retardation of the fetus and to look for evidence of impaired placental function. In other patients there may be an increased uterine activity in the presence of a normally growing fetus, suggesting 'idiopathic' preterm labour. In all patients with uterine activity which is excessive for the stage of pregnancy, a vaginal examination should be performed and the dilatation and effacement of the cervix assessed. If there is obvious increasing effacement or dilatation and the fetus is immature and in satisfactory condition, prophylactic treatment with beta-adrenergic stimulants or prostaglandin synthetase inhibitors may be indicated.

Weight gain
Lack of weight gain or excessive weight gain may provide further indications of impaired placental function and possible fetal compromise. Failure to gain weight in pregnancy at a rate of approximately 272 g or less per week from the 20th to the 36th week is associated with a trebling of perinatal mortality, primarily due to prematurity. Excessive gain in weight of 635 g or more per week from the 20th to the 36th week is associated with a trebling or perinatal mortality due to pre-eclampsia (Thomson & Billewicz 1957, Hytten & Leitch 1971f). In general failure to gain weight is much more important than excessive weight gain and is an indication of placental insufficiency provided it is interpreted intelligently. It is thus essential to question the patient on dietary habits and intake, vomiting and diarrhoea and any intercurrent illness. Any unexplained failure to gain weight then merits critical clinical examination and further investigation.

Clinical examination

Impairment of fetal growth and well-being may also be suspected on abdominal palpation. A small-for-dates fetus, a disproportionately hard or large head and a small trunk, decreased amniotic fluid or an irritable uterus are signs of possible fetal growth retardation and fetal compromise. Serial measurements of fundal height and abdominal girth, preferably by the same observer, may provide a more precise guide for the clinician conscientious enough to make these observations.

MATERNAL COMPLICATIONS OF PREGNANCY AND MATERNAL WELL-BEING

A large part of obstetrics is preventive medicine and one of the main objectives of antenatal care is the achievement of optimal health for the mother as well as for the baby. During the course of antenatal care every effort should therefore be made to detect any previously unrecognized medical disease, to correct minor ailments, and to ensure the well-being of the mother. These efforts, as well as the detection of the maternal complications of pregnancy, such as hypertension and proteinuria, constitute a considerable part of antenatal care. Small rises in blood pressure in the middle trimester may help to predict the occurrence of hypertension later in pregnancy (Page 1976, Gallery *et al.* 1977), and early antihypertensive therapy may be important in preventing later rises in blood pressure and proteinuria (Rubin 1983). The recognition and treatment of anaemia is important but requires careful interpretation of haemoglobin and haematocrit measurements. A low haemoglobin concentration may indicate anaemia but may also indicate haemodilution. A high haemoglobin value may indicate haemoconcentration and a failure in expansion of plasma volume which may be an unfavourable sign. Routine iron and possibly folate therapy, though controversial, is probably justified in most communities. The addition of fluoride 1 mg daily is even more controversial, but is the most effective way of preventing dental caries in future generations.

In late pregnancy, around the 36th week, the whole condition of the mother should be reviewed and repeat screening, for example, for abnormal red cell antibodies, performed. Repeat glucose tolerance tests in potential diabetics and repeat examination for urinary infection in patients who have had a previous urinary tract infection should be performed where indicated.

Perhaps the most important contribution in ensuring maternal health and well-being is the recognition of the woman who is thin or undernourished, as evidenced by a failure to gain weight, or who is burdened by her pregnancy and is physically stressed, as indicated by tachycardia and excessive dyspnoea or tiredness. Such women are usually found in countries or communities where nutrition or socio-economic circumstances are suboptimal and where women may be obliged to work long hours domestically, or in fields or factories. The provision of opportunity for rest and regular meals may in these circumstances make a real contribution to both maternal and fetal well-being (Raiha *et al.* 1957).

THE MECHANICS OF PREGNANCY AND DELIVERY

The mechanics of pregnancy and the timely recognition of mechanical problems such as multiple pregnancy, occipito-posterior position, breech and shoulder presentations and high head at term and cephalopelvic disproportion are an essential part of routine care. An increasing problem in modern obstetrics is that of previous Caesarean section. It must be emphasized that a decision on the management of a patient with a previous Caesarean section needs to be made antenatally, preferably as early in pregnancy as possible. The decision also needs to be discussed with the patient who frequently requires explanation and reassurance.

PREPARATION FOR LABOUR AND INDUCTION OF LABOUR

Preparation for labour from the doctor's point of view involves detecting any potential abnormality, such as cephalopelvic disproportion or abnormal presentation, ensuring that the mother and fetus are in optimal condition, and that all the arrangements for delivery are satisfactory. It also involves consideration of possible induction of labour if any abnormality is present (Davey 1980) and this subject is dealt with in another section. The advent of intravaginal prostaglandins for cervical ripening and induction of labour has, in many ways, changed the whole approach to induction of labour. Thus, if labour does not ensue following intravaginal prostaglandins, there is no commitment to proceed to delivery or to Caesarean section as is the case with surgical induction. If, on the other hand, a decision has been made to rupture the membranes artificially, this implies a definite decision to terminate the pregnancy and to Caesarean section if the induction should fail or labour be abnormally prolonged.

From the patient's point of view, preparation for labour involves knowing when labour starts, what to expect during labour and, perhaps most of all, what will be available for the relief of pain and discomfort. These questions are probably best answered at antenatal classes which should be an essential part of antenatal care. A specific question which currently arises, and on which patients require information and reassurance of the doctor, is that of epidural anaesthesia. Some patients request 'epidurals'; others wish to know whether it is available if requested. All patients appreciate being told what to do and what care will be provided when they go into labour.

ANTENATAL EDUCATION: PREGNANCY, LABOUR, BREAST FEEDING, INFANT CARE AND FAMILY PLANNING

Antenatal education for pregnancy, labour, breast feeding and infant care is an established part of the management of normal pregnancy. Newer aspects of antenatal education which may require special emphasis are: counselling following a previous perinatal loss or previous abnormal infant; breast feeding and bonding; family planning. Most patients who have had a previous stillbirth, neonatal death or abnormal infant are anxious unless they have had a subsequent normal infant. Women who have had an abnormal infant should be referred for genetic counselling, ultrasonic screening, preferably before the 12th week, and for amniocentesis. Those who have had a previous stillbirth or neonatal death may also require investigation to exclude a recurrent cause. Discussion of the plan of management of the pregnancy, a confident attitude and personal attention, should enable the patient to go through pregnancy happily and with a successful outcome.

The recognition of the psychological and physiological importance of breast feeding and of bonding between the mother and infant has received much attention in recent years. The obstetrician can assist by encouraging all women to breast feed, by attention to the breasts and nipples in pregnancy, and by ensuring that each pregnancy is a happy and rewarding experience. The aim is to ensure that each child is wanted, loved, will become part of a family and will be cared for until adulthood.

A further important aspect of antenatal education

which should be discussed individually with every patient and her partner, is family planning and contraception. Pregnancy is usually the ideal time to discuss such matters. If it is the first pregnancy, particularly an unplanned one, the whole subject of family planning and family size may need to be specifically raised. An increasing number of couples who have completed their families opt for, and request, tubal ligation, which is often most conveniently performed postpartum, but needs to be planned antenatally. Each pregnancy, normal or abnormal, and each child needs to be regarded as a part of the total reproductive life of each couple and it is the obstetrician's and midwife's responsibility to provide appropriate advice regarding each woman's whole reproductive career.

PROVISION OF ANTEPARTUM AND INTRAPARTUM CARE IN DEVELOPING COUNTRIES AND COMMUNITIES

Antepartum and intrapartum care are often described in terms of the ideal and the optimum. In fact, in many if not most, countries and communities, obstetric care and facilities and resources are far from optimal. In many instances pregnancy and delivery are conducted in the village, farm or kraal by the elder women without the assistance of midwives or doctors. In others a single midwife, who may be more or less untrained, partly trained or fully trained may serve a whole village or community. Such midwives may be stationed in areas remote from hospitals often with poor communications and limited backup in cases of emergency or major complications of pregnancy.

It must further be recognized that in many parts of the world there will in all probability not only never be enough doctors, but that there may never be enough trained midwives to conduct all the deliveries. In devising schemes of antepartum and intrapartum care in such regions, it is therefore necessary to incorporate the traditional birth attendants (TBAs). It must also be recognized that in many parts of the world there may never be enough hospitals or even enough midwife obstetric units at least for the foreseeable future. In these regions home confinement may of necessity be the norm and not a luxury.

These limitations in resources and personnel, however serious, do not negate the provision of antenatal and intrapartum care and do not prevent the implementation of schemes whereby maternal and perinatal mortality may be substantially reduced or prevented. The principles underlying such schemes include: the optimal utilization of available resources including personnel and facilities; recruitment, education and training of staff; creation of one authority to be responsible for antepartum, intrapartum and perinatal care of all the patients in a given geographical area or region. The key step is the creation of specified regions or areas of authority under the direction of one appropriately trained person or persons who must be clearly responsible and at the same time have the necessary authority over all the resources in the region. The designation of regions of obstetric responsibility and the 'regionalization' of maternity and neonatal care is not new. The importance of regionalization where facilities, personnel and resources are scarce, and where the socio-economic circumstances are poor, however, has not been sufficiently recognized.

In the USA in 1971 in response to the relatively high maternal, perinatal and infant mortality rates, as compared with many other countries, the American Medical Association, the American College of Obstetricians and Gynaecologists, the American Academy of Pediatrics and the American Academy of Family Physicians formed a Committee of Perinatal Health. The situation in the USA and many other parts of the world differ enormously, but the main recommendation of the Committee was the introduction of a regional system of maternal and perinatal care with a differentiation of facilities which were designated Level I, Level II and Level III. The final conclusion of the report 'Towards Improving the Outcome of Pregnancy' (1976), however was that:

'A major function in a regional system for the delivery of prenatal and perinatal health service is that of preparing and continuing education ... The critical factor in providing service of high quality is not electronic equipment, spacious facilities or helicopter transport. The critical factor is personnel, trained and experienced in the best professional techniques of maternity and newborn care and working in a coordinated regional plan for providing this care.'

Since the publication of this report several schemes of regional care have been introduced in the USA, and although the schemes vary they have in general been uniformly successful. The principles upon which these schemes are based are as follows.

Regionalization of maternity and neonatal care

It should be emphasized that it is not possible or desirable to separate obstetric care, the care of the newborn and family planning, and that any scheme of regionalization must incorporate all three aspects of reproductive care. Regionalization of maternity and neonatal care may be considered under facilities, personnel and organization.

OBSTETRIC AND NEONATAL FACILITIES

Any region would normally include three or possibly four levels of facilities and obstetric care, which are:
1 *Central Referral Hospital* (*Level III*) with facilities for: Caesarean section; blood bank; full laboratory facilities; investigation and treatment of complicated or high risk pregnancies; care of small, preterm and high risk neonates; specialist personnel. Normally one central referral hospital should serve in a region with at least 10–12000 deliveries per year.
2 *Community Hospital* (*Level II*) with facilities for: Caesarean section and tubal ligation; limited supplies of blood and resuscitation facilities; access to laboratory facilities; routine care and observation of mother; routine care and observation of neonate; trained but not necessarily specialist personnel.
3 *Midwife Obstetric Unit* (*Level I*). This provides facilities for: normal deliveries (24 hr stay); emergency resuscitation (not necessarily blood); essential nursing care; midwife personnel only.
4 *Peripheral Antenatal, Child Welfare, Family Planning Clinic*. This provides facilities for: antenatal care and basic medicines; child welfare clinic; family planning clinic.

In general, clinic facilities must be provided within 10 km of a patient's home where women are without transport and are obliged to walk. Depending upon the economic and physical circumstances at least 3 out of 4 types of facilities listed above would be required within each region depending upon size of population, distances and terrain. It should be noted that Levels I, II and III as set out above do not correspond with the levels as designated by the Committee of Perinatal Health.

PERSONNEL

Three levels of personnel may be distinguished, though duties and responsibilities will depend upon the need in any given situation, and the level of training provided.

Medical personnel

Medical personnel would be stationed at community (Level II) and tertiary (Level III) referral hospitals. At the community hospital, the doctor might well have other duties (surgical and medical) and would not necessarily function as a specialist but would perform operative procedures such as Caesarean sections. In certain circumstances these duties might be undertaken by medical assistants who have been trained in operative procedures. At the referral (Level III) hospital, doctors should function as specialists and work full time as obstetricians or paediatricians respectively. Ideally such individuals should have completed recognized specialist training and also have had some training in organization of schemes of obstetrical and neonatal care. These individuals would in general be the Director of the Region, or have some administrative responsibilities in addition to their clinical duties and would participate as lecturers and teachers in various training programmes throughout the region. They should also draw up schemes of management applicable throughout the region depending upon the facilities, personnel and resources available.

Midwives and trained nurses

Midwives and trained nurses would normally be the backbone of schemes of regional care and such midwives would assume primary responsibility for obstetric and neonatal care. They would not necessarily have immediate medical cover and may be in charge of units, such as antenatal clinics and of midwife obstetric units designed for the conduct of normal deliveries. They may also function in patients' homes, though this usually constitutes a relatively wasteful use of trained personnel. Midwives would normally have completed a basic nursing training and, either as part of this training or subsequently, complete one year's midwifery and pass appropriate examinations. In addition some midwives may have taken advanced training to equip them for senior positions in charge of clinics or midwife obstetric units. Such midwives may be trained to perform various procedures depending upon the needs of the particular situation. These procedures may include repair of episiotomy, forceps and vertex delivery and even Caesarean section if the circumstances demand and the health regulations permit. It is important however that the limits of responsibility in given circumstances should be clearly designated beforehand and appropriate training provided so that no individual undertakes procedures and responsibilities beyond his or her skill and competence.

Nursing assistants and Traditional Birth Attendants

Nursing assistants and TBAs can play a vital and important role in provision of obstetrical and neonatal service. In general nursing assistants can be trained to perform routine medical and nursing care, which they usually perform conscientiously and well. Clerks, domestics and drivers similarly play a vital role and may assume varying degrees of responsibility depending upon circumstances.

TBAs may similarly perform a useful and important function, particularly where there is a high proportion of home deliveries. The confidence and trust of such attendants may be gained and appropriate training in the form of 1 or 2 week courses provided in the local language so that the attendants may recognize abnormalities early and may arrange transfer to more expert care where necessary.

Organization of regional obstetrics and neonatal care

The success of regionalization largely depends upon effective organization; knowledge of the needs and facilities within a region; some regular measures of the service provided and of the outcome of pregnancy such as maternal mortality, perinatal and neonatal mortality in the various hospitals, delivery units, clinics and associated home deliveries, and in the region as a whole. The main points in effective organization are as follows:

INITIAL SURVEY OF RESOURCES, DEFINITION OF MOST ACUTE NEEDS AND FORMULATION OF SCHEME OF MANAGEMENT FOR THE REGION

The first step in implementation of regionalization must be an overall critical survey of the facilities and personnel available and needs of the situation. The needs of the situation will include:

1 *Total numbers of deliveries*, and incidences of medical disease and complicated deliveries, prematurity and intrauterine growth retardation, maternal and perinatal deaths;

2 *Hospital, midwife obstetric unit and clinic facilities* including number of beds, equipment, blood bank and laboratory facilities;

3 *Personnel*—specialist, medical, medical assistant or midwife, nursery assistants and TBAs;

4 *Communications* available, such as telephone, facilities for transmission of records, reports and specimens;

5   *Transport*—roads and distances between facilities and centres of population. Referral and transport of patients is an essential and integral part of any scheme of regionalization and the distances between centres and time taken to reach a specialist hospital from a community hospital and a community hospital from a peripheral clinic or midwife obstetric unit will largely determine the level of care to be provided in any facility;

6   *General, financial, socio-economic situation*, availability of drugs, consumables, etc.

Definition of needs

This and the submission of precise requests to funding authorities, on a realistic cost-effective basis, is an important part of initial survey. It may be necessary to recognize that it will be possible to provide a service only within a given region, and that those from outside the region may have to be excluded. It may also be necessary to recognize that it is not possible initially to meet all the needs within a given region. It is important to ensure that personnel and facilities are not over-extended leading to a breakdown in service and morale and therefore temporary limitation of service may sometimes be essential.

Formulation of scheme of management

This would include:

1   *Booking criteria* for various facilities with the aim of ensuring where possible that the high risk patients are delivered in hospital, and low risk ones delivered in midwife obstetric units or their own homes.

2   *Referral criteria* in the event of any complication or high risk situation developing in pregnancy and labour from clinic to midwife obstetric unit, midwife obstetric unit to community hospital and community hospital to referral centre. It is also important that criteria for referral to normal or low risk centres be implemented otherwise hospital and central facilities tend to be overloaded with normal patients, or with patients referred for some reason who prove to have no abnormality or do not require further investigation.

3   *Standard schemes of management* including for example pain relief in labour, prevention of postpartum haemorrhage management of hypertension, eclampsia and infant resuscitation and family planning.

Implementation of regionalization

The successful implementation and running of regional schemes of perinatal care depends upon many factors but some of the most important are:

1   *Communication*: good and easy communication by telephone (or radio) is essential, so that those working peripherally may get prompt medical or specialist advice and help; arrange patient transfer; or obtain supplies of medicines or materials including blood.

2   *Transport*: adequate transport where a mother, or sometimes neonate, develops a complication and needs transfer to a higher level facility is also vital for regionalization. Transport may include a car, 'combi' or coach to a clinic; ambulance transport to hospital and in some areas, for example the central USA, transport may include helicopters, fixed wing aircraft and even a combination. The training of drivers who can often perform vital functions should not be neglected.

In some areas an *'obstetric flying squad'* whereby an ambulance with a doctor, trained midwife, Group O Rhesus negative blood and appropriate drugs are sent to a peripheral unit to provide emergency care, and resuscitation is often the best and most effective way of providing necessary medical care. In general it is better to treat an emergency on the spot, e.g. eclamptic fit, or arrest of haemorrhage, and if shocked to resuscitate the patient before transfer, particularly if this involves a long or uncomfortable journey. In the Peninsula Maternity and Neonatal Service Region in Cape Town, a flying squad based on the Groote Schuur Hospital serves 3 midwife obstetric units, where approximately 8000 patients a year are delivered, ensures that expert medical care is available to every patient where needed in not more than 20 or 30 minutes.

3   *Good relations, exchange of staff and regular visits by senior personnel.* Good relations and trust between all levels of staff and avoidance of criteria is essential so that whatever is the best treatment for the patient is provided. Without trust and good relations there may be a temptation to 'hold on to' patients in peripheral facilities; similarly those working centrally may fail to appreciate the urgency and difficulties of those working peripherally, particularly in isolated circumstances or where the person is relatively inexperienced. Exchange of staff, if only for a few weeks, often greatly facilitates understanding and appreciation of respective difficulties and needs. Similarly, regular visits by medical or more senior experienced personnel to conduct clinics or meetings to resolve difficulties and problems on the spot are essential to ensure that a region functions as one organization and that morale is maintained.

Education, training and audit

Regionalization of perinatal care is a continuing process to meet changing needs, often with changing resources, within a region. Ideas on the best method of management of various obstetric conditions may also change. Education, training and regular 'audit' of delivery statistics, perinatal and neonatal mortality and discussion of individual cases and problems are essential. In schemes of regionalization the most important task of specialist, medical and senior midwifery staff is often the education and training of junior and untrained personnel. Apart from initial training courses, regular lectures, discussions, meetings are essential throughout the region. This will necessitate regular visits by senior personnel to peripheral units or of peripheral personnel to the main centres or both. Emphasis often has to be placed on neglected areas such as infant resuscitation, breast feeding and family planning. If midwives or medical assistants are to undertake procedures such as performance and repair of episiotomy, forceps or vertex deliveries and even Caesarean section or tubal ligation operations they must be properly trained with a full understanding of indications, complications and precautions to be followed.

Regular audit is essential in the form of: weekly or monthly perinatal mortality meetings where all stillbirths, neonatal deaths and interesting or complicated cases at each institution are discussed; regular analysis of statistics on both a monthly or yearly basis which need not be elaborate but should be promptly and readily available; yearly review of the functioning and reformulation of policies and referral criteria and patient records. In the organization the region, it is important to recognize that approximately 25% of all initially 'low risk' patients, based on epidemiological criteria, will be referred to a higher level because of some complication in pregnancy or labour. Adequate feedback of the outcome in such patients and a prompt reply by letter or telephone for patients referred for opinion is important in ensuring not only good relations, but that the region functions as an integral whole and not as isolated units.

In this discussion of regionalization of maternity and neonatal care, details of management and of particular problems have been deliberately omitted because needs and circumstances vary so greatly in different parts of the world. For more information on particular problems 'Obstetrics and Gynaecology in the Tropics and Developing Countries' by J.B. Lawson & D.B. Stewart (1967) and 'Obstetric Problems in the Developing World' edited by R.H. Philpott (1982) are strongly recommended. Apart from more strictly medical subjects, Lawson and Stewart describe the process of acceptance of antenatal care in rural and under-developed areas where deliveries were previously conducted according to traditional tribal practice and custom. Philpott enunciated some principles regarding the organization of obstetric services in the developing countries including:

1 *Community Mobilization around Obstetric Issues* —'whenever possible the members of the community should be helped to assist themselves and the paternalistic hand-down that oppresses should be avoided'; 'encouragement of childbirth within a stable family unit. This will include education on family life with the community'; 'creation of an awareness of problems of teenage pregnancies, unplanned pregnancies and venereal disease'.

2 *Education*—'educate your patients, other health workers and community leaders on basic health problems that lead to ill health'.

3 *Establish, develop and maintain a high quality clinical service*—'transitional solutions are only justifiable as long as we intend them to evolve into the type of practice we expect for ourselves'.

LEADERSHIP

In summary, not only is the obstetrician responsible for the care of the individual patient, but in developing countries at least he or she must function as the leader of the team providing maternity care for the whole area or region. The obstetrician, the paediatrician and the local medical practitioner have the responsibility for initiating, guiding and leading the efforts to provide the best possible maternity service, including neonatal care and family planning, in all the communities and regions which they serve.

REFERENCES

AHLQUIST R.P. (1950) *J. Amer. pharm. Ass. (sci Ed.)*, **39**, 370.
ALVAREZ H., BLANCO Y.S., PANIZZA V.G., ROSADA H. & LUCAS O. (1965) *Amer. J. Obstet. Gynec.*, **93**, 131.
ASSALI N.S., DASGUPTA K., KOLIN A. & HOLMS L. (1958) *Amer. J. Physiol.*, **195**, 614.
ASSALI N.S., RAUMARO L. & PELTONEN T. (1960) *Amer. J. Obstet. Gynec.*, **79**, 86.
ASPLUND J. (1952) *Acta radiol.* (Supplement) **91**, 3.

BEAN W.B., COGSWELL R.C., DEXTER M. & EMBICK J.E. (1949) *Surg. Gynec. Obstet.*, **88**, 739.

BORRELL U. & FERNSTROM I. (1957) *Acta Obstet. gynec. Scand.*, **36**, 42.

BROSENS I., ROBERTSON W.B. & DIXON H.G. (1967) *J. Path.*, **93**, 569.

BROSENS I.A. (1977) In *Clinics in Obstetrics and Gynaecology* **4**, 573.

BUDIN J. (1897) *Obstetrique*, **2**, 499.

BUTLER N.R. & ALBERMAN E.D. (1969) In *Perinatal Problems*, p. 36. E. & S. Livingstone, Edinburgh and London.

CALDEYRO-BARCIO R.R. & POSEIRO J.J. (1959) *Ann. N.Y. Acad. Sci.*, **75**.

CAREY H.M. (1963) In *Modern Trends in Reproductive Physiology*, le. (Carey H.M. ed.), Butterworths, London.

COMMITTEE ON PERINATAL HEALTH (1976) *Toward Improving the Outcome of Pregnancy*. The National Foundation—March of Dimes, New York.

CSAPO A.I., ERDOS T. & DE MATTOS C.R. (1965) *Nature (Lond.)*, **207**, 1378.

CSAPO A.I., PULKKINEN M.O. & KAIHOLA H.L. (1974) *Amer. J. Obstet. Gynec.*, **118**, 985.

CSAPO A.I. & SAUVAGE J. (1968) *Acta obstet. gynec. Scand.*, **47**, 181.

CUNNINGHAM M.D., GREENE J.W. & DUNRING J.L. (1977) *Gynecol. Invest.*, **8**, 76.

DANFORTH D.N. & CHAPMAN J.C.F. (1950) *Amer. J. Obstet. Gynec.*, **59**, 979.

DANFORTH D.N., VEIS A., BREEM M., WEINSTEIN H.G., BUCKINGHAM J.C. & MANALO P. (1974) *Amer. J. Obstet. Gynec.*, **120**, 641.

DAVEY D.A. (1980) In Clinics in Obstetrics and Gynaecology (in press).

DAWES G. (1968) *Fetal and Neonatal Physiology*, p. 62. International Year Book Publishers Inc., Chicago.

DE NEEF J.C. (1967a) In *Clinical Endocrine Cytology*, p. 216. Hoeber, New York.

DE NEEF J.C. (1967b) In *Clinical Endocrine Cytology*, p. 235. Hoeber, New York.

DE NEEF J.C. (1967c) In *Clinical Endocrine Cytology*, p. 246. Hoeber, New York.

DE SWIET M. (1984) ed. *Medical Disorders in Obstetric Practice*, Blackwell, Oxford.

DEPP R. (1980) *Sem. Perinatal.*, **4**, 229.

DICZFALUSY E. & TROEN P. (1961) *Vitam. and Horm.* **19**, 229.

FLUHMANN C.F. (1961) *Obstet. Gynec., N.Y.*, **17**, 206.

FRIEDMAN E.A. (1976) *Blood Pressure, Edema and Proteinuria in Pregnancy*. Elsevier, Amsterdam.

GALLERY E.D.M., ROSS M., HUNYOR S.N. & GYORY A.Z. (1977) *Lancet*, **i**, 1273.

GARRETT W.J. (1959) *J. Obstet. Gynaec. Brit. Cwlth.*, **66**, 602.

GIBSON H.M. (1973) *Br. J. Obstet. Gynaecol.*, **80**, 1067.

GILLESPIE E.C. (1950) *Amer. J. Obstet. Gynec.*, **59**, 949.

GILLMAN J. & STEIN H.B. (1941) *Surg. Gynec. Obstet.*, **72**, 149.

GOERTTLER K. (1930) *Gegenbaurs morph. Jb.*, **65**, 45.

GORDON Y.B., LEWIS J.D., PENDLEBURY D.J., LEIGHTON M. & GOLD J. (1978) *Lancet*, **i**, 1001.

HARKNESS M.L.R. & HARKNESS R.D. (1959) *J. Physiol.*, **148**, 52.

HELIE M. (1864) *Recherches sur la disposition des fibres musculaires de l'uterus developpee par la grossesse*. Mellinet, Paris.

HELLMAN L.M., ROSENTHAL A.H., KISTNER R.W. & GORDON R. (1950) *Amer. J. Obst. Gynec.*, **67**, 899.

HENDRICKS C.H.J., ESKES T.K.A.B. & SAAMELI K. (1962) *Amer. J. Obstet. Gynec.*, **83**, 890.

HOBEL C.J., HYVARINEN M.A., OKADA P.M. & OH. W. (1973) *Amer. J. Obstet. Gynec.*, **117**, 1.

HYTTEN F.E. & CHAMBERLAIN G.V.P. (1980) *Clinical Physiology in Obstetrics*, Blackwell Scientific Publications, Oxford.

HYTTEN F.E. & LEITCH I. (1971a) *The Physiology of Human Pregnancy*, 2e., p. 106. Blackwell Scientific Publications, Oxford.

HYTTEN F.E. & LEITCH I. (1971b) *The Physiology of Human Pregnancy*, 2e., p. 365. Blackwell Scientific Publications, Oxford.

HYTTEN F.E. & LEITCH I. (1971c) *The Physiology of Human Pregnancy*, 2e., p. 176. Blackwell Scientific Publications, Oxford.

HYTTEN F.E. & LEITCH I. (1971d) *The Physiology of Human Pregnancy*, 2e., p. 124. Blackwell Scientific Publications, Oxford.

HYTTEN F.E. & LEITCH I. (1971e) *The Physiology of Human Pregnancy*, 2e., p. 1. Blackwell Scientific Publications, Oxford.

HYTTEN F.E. & LEITCH I. (1971f) *The Physiology of Human Pregnancy*, 2e., p. 345. Blackwell Scientific Publications, Oxford.

ISRAEL S.L., RUBENSTONE A. & MERANZE D.R. (1954) *Obstet. and Gynec.*, **3**, 399.

KERR M.G. (1968) *Brit med. Bull.*, **24**, 19.

LAWSON J.B. & STEWART D.B. *Obstetrics and Gynaecology in the Tropics and Developing Countries* (1967). Edward Arnold, London.

LIGGINS G.C. (1979) *Brit. med. Bull.*, **35**, 145.

MacDONALD R.R. (1972) *J. Obstet. Gynaec. Brit. Cwlth.*, **79**, 1087.

MacGILLIVRAY I., ROSE G.A. & ROWE B. (1969) *Clin. Sci.*, **37**, 395.

MANN E.C. (1963) *Progress in Gynecology*, vol. 4, p. 123. Grune & Stratton, New York.

MANNING F.A., PLATT I.D. & SIPOS L. (1980) *Amer. J. Obstet. Gynec.*, **136**, 787.

NAFTOLIN F. & STUBBLEFIELD P.G. (1980) *Dilatation of the Uterine Cervix: Connective Tissue Biology and Clinical Management*. Raven Press, New York.

NAKANISHI H., BURNSTOCK G., McLEAN J. & WOOD C. (1969) *J. reprod. Med.*, **2**, 20.

NELSON W.W. & GREENE R.R. (1953) *Int. Abstr. Surg.*, **97**, 1.

NOVY M.J. & LIGGINS C.J. (1980) *Sem. Perinatol.*, **4**, 45.

PAGE E.W. (1976) *Amer. J. Obstet. Gynec.*, **125**, 740.

PAPANICOLAU G.N. (1925) *Proc. Soc. exp. Biol. Med.*, **22**, 436.

PAUERSTEIN C.J. & SEITCHIK J. (1979) *Human Reproductive Physiology*, p. 191. Blackwell, Oxford.

PEARSON J. & WEAVER J. (1976) *Brit. med. J.*, **i**, 1305.

PHILIPP E.E., BARNES J. & NEWTON M. (1977) *Scientific Foundations of Obstetrics and Gynaecology*, Heinemann, London.

PHILPOTT R.H. (1982) *Clin. Obstet. Gynaecol.*, **9**, ix.

PRYSTOWSKY H., HELLEGERS A. & BRUNS P. (1961) *Amer. J. Obstet. Gynec.*, **81**, 372.

RAIHA C.E., JOHANSSON C.E., LIND J. & VARA P. (1957) *Ann. Paediat. Fenn.*, **3**, 65.

RAMSAY E.M. (1949) *Contr. Embryol.*, **33**, 113.

REYNOLDS S.R.M. & DANFORTH D.N. (1966) In *Textbook of Obstetrics and Gynaecology* (Danforth D.E. ed.), p. 491. Hoeber, New York and London.

RHODES P. (1970) In *Scientific Foundations of Obstetrics and Gynaecology*, p. 440 (Philipp, Barnes and Newton Eds.). Heinemann, London.

STEEDMAN D., REID J.C. (1983) *Lancet*, **i**, 431.

RUSSELL C.S., TAYLOR R. & LAW C.E. (1968) *Brit. J. prev. soc. Med.*, **22**, 119.

SADOVSKY E. & POLISHUK W. (1977) *Obstet Gynec., N.Y.*, **50**, 49.

SCHWARZ B.E., MILEWICH L., GANT N.F., PORTER J.C., JOHNSTON J.M. & MCDONALD P.C. (1977) *Ann. New York Acad. Sci.*, **286**, 304.

SHEARMAN R.P. (1979) *Human Reproductive Physiology*, 2e. Blackwell Scientific Publications, Oxford.

SIMS E.A.H. & KRANTZ K.E. (1958) *J. Clin. Invest.*, **37**, 1764.

SINCLAIR J.D. (1963) *Modern Trends in Human Reproductive Physiology*, 1e., p. 181. Butterworths, London.

SNYDER, F.F. (1924) *Bull. Johns Hopkins Hosp.*, **35**, 14.

SOKAL R.J., ROSEN M.G., STOJKOV J. & CHIK L. (1977) *Amer. J. Obstet. Gynec.*, **128**, 652.

STIEVE H. (1932) *Zbl. Gynäk.*, **56**, 1442.

TINDALL V.R. & BEAZLEY J.M. (1965) *J. Obstet. Gynaec. Brit. Cwlth.*, **72**, 717.

THOMSON A.M. & BILLEWICZ W.Z. (1957) *Brit. med. J.*, **i**, 243.

ULLERY J.C. & SHABANAH E.H. (1957) *Obstet. Gynec. N.Y.*, **10**, 233.

WACHTEL E.G. (1964) *Exfoliative Cytology in Gynaecological Practice*, p. 77. Butterworths, London.

WANSBOROUGH H., NAKANISHI H. & WOOD C. (1967) *Obstet. Gynec. N.Y.*, **30**, 779.

WOOD C. (1964) *J. Obstet. Gynaec. Brit. Cwlth.*, **71**, 615.

WOOD C. (1969) In *Modern Trends in Obstetrics*, 4e. (Kellar R.J. ed.). Butterworths, London.

WORLD HEALTH ORGANIZATION. (1965) *Tech. Rep. Ser.*, 302.

YOUSSEF A.F. (1958) *Amer. J. Obstet. Gynec.*, 75, 1305.

CHAPTER 13
PREPREGNANCY CARE

G. V. P. CHAMBERLAIN

Prepregnancy care is the preparation of both parents for childbearing. Such management includes both physical and psychological preparation but it is mostly in the former area that prepregnancy care has been directed. The concept is a diffuse one which has been growing over the last decade. It seems to arise from a logical extension of antenatal care, an aspect of twentieth century medicine which has undoubtedly brought many benefits to women and their children. Most obstetricians consider that the prevention and early diagnosis of conditions at a presymptomatic stage has allowed more thorough and better treatment. A good example of this is the reduction in severity of pre-eclampsia because of a more thorough pickup by blood pressure estimations made at routine clinics.

THE ORIGINS OF PREPREGNANCY CARE

Antenatal care has always stressed the importance of early attendance. Several population based studies have shown the perinatal mortality rate and other indices of feto-maternal welfare to be reduced among those who attend for their first booking visit in the earlier weeks of pregnancy (before the thirteenth week). Some of this may be due to the social and biological characteristics of women who go for earlier care. They probably come from a different social, economic and educational group from those who delay antenatal care. The professionals have always stressed that early visits are important and have advanced justification for this by pointing out that such a visit allows early records of blood pressure and weight, in case these should alter abnormally in later pregnancy. Another reason advanced for care in early pregnancy is the prevention of teratogenetic activities which may lead to congenital abnormalities, such as exposure to pelvic X-rays or the taking of certain drugs in early pregnancy.

If one examines large cohorts about the frequency at which a woman appears for early organized antenatal care, in most of the United Kingdom only 15% are booked before nine weeks of pregnancy. By this time, most fissure differentiation has taken place in the fetus and organs have formed, hence contrateratogenetic advice is too late. It might be that such advice would be better given before pregnancy. Baseline measurements of the various aspects of the body (such as weight and blood pressure) could be obtained before pregnancy and these might be more valid for comparisons made later on. In addition, a woman who has a medical condition could be seen and could discuss the effects of that condition on pregnancy or pregnancy on the progress of the disease process. Part of this advice would obviously be directed to the therapy the woman is currently receiving for the disease process; this in itself may be hazardous to pregnancy, for example, a woman on long term anticoagulation with a plastic heart valve replacement needs pregnancy advice as does the diabetic mother to be. In addition, more general problems of life style and diet can be discussed.

The problems associated with the risk of recurrence of known familial abnormalities come into prepregnancy care and currently the best advice is given by a clinical geneticist. The probabilities of recurrent genetic disease need full discussion before pregnancy; with the emergence of clinical genetics as a speciality in its own right, it is correct that anyone running a prepregnancy service should invite the aid of those skilled in this subject.

The proper assessment of possible reproductive problems allows parents a wider range of options before pregnancy than does a similar discussion taking place in early pregnancy. Once pregnancy has started, there are only two options available to the couple, to let the pregnancy continue or to terminate it. If a consultation could take place before pregnancy has started, the couple may elect to remain childless (supplementing this by adoption where it is available) thus completely avoiding any risk. It may be that the couple would consider artificial insemination with donor semen or, probably in the near future, donor ova, thus avoiding the genetic risk that is carried on one or other side of the family. For a small number of metabolic conditions, special diets can be taken and this area of prepregnancy advice may expand in the next decade. Also in the future lies the whole area of gene probing and maybe gene manipulation.

ORGANIZING PREPREGNANCY CARE

These concepts have gelled into the setting up of pre-pregnancy care clinics which may act at several levels. They can provide general advice about life style and nutrition, concentrating on special problems such as alcohol taking and so may help those who have specific medical problems. At the other end of the range, they may offer specific actuarial odds about known genetic problems. Those who organize such care must be careful not to overstate what can be done in the prepregnancy clinic for much that is offered currently is without scientific basis; practice has gone ahead of knowledge in many cases.

Probably much of prepregnancy care lies in the field of education and could best be dealt with at an earlier age than those seeking pregnancy. In the schools, properly programmed teaching about education for living could include the importance of pre-paration for childbirth. While doctors themselves would not do this teaching, they can be helpful in leading and catalysing the starting of such instruction in the educational field. Prepregnancy health education would include dietary matters, cigarette smoking, alcohol, contraception and pregnancy spacing and the effect of infections such as German measles on pregnancy. All this is well within the gambit of teachers.

Such a programme could be supplemented by pre-pregnancy advisory clinics held in the community by all grades of personnel; couples could go there when they were thinking of planning a pregnancy. At these clinics, simple screening tests such as checking the titre of rubella antibodies could be performed, offering immunization to those who are still sero-negative. Anaemia and specific haematological problems such as sickling could be detected and non-specific advice about diet and occupational environment could be given. Such clinics are run by doctors in general practice, the family planning field or occupational health. There are already highly successful such advisory clinics run by nursing sisters who have taken

the trouble to acquire the knowledge in the prepreg-nancy area.

The third level of prepregnancy care would be at a specialist clinic run by obstetricians to deal with specific problems that arise. It must be stressed that this is for the minority of women and their partners to attend and should not be confused with the more general health education, best dealt by teaching at the earlier age, or with the self-referral prepregnancy advisory clinics.

RUNNING A PREPREGNANCY CLINIC

The author has run a prepregnancy clinic since 1978 and the next section is based upon his experience at such a clinic at Queen Charlotte's Hospital and latterly at St. George's Hospital, both in London. Both hospitals have a large population of mixed socio-economic background and are referral centres for tertiary health care for those with problems in obstetrics. In eight years, a wide variety of experience has been gained. This clinic started with the aim of advising those with specific medical problems but its activity has widened enormously.

The clinic on each site has been held in conjunction with clinical geneticists to whom relevant problems were referred either directly by the general practitioner or by the clinic staff themselves. In consequence, purely genetically based problems are not considered at these clinics and do not appear in the information presented in this chapter. This is not to undermine their importance but to stress that they need specialist care by clinical geneticists and at both the clinics referred to, the obstetrician was fortunate to have this service readily available.

Anyone running such a specialist prepregnancy clinic must be prepared to have statistical information which is up to date and refers to the population with which he is dealing. He will be required to give the odds about the risks of future problems; it is no good relying upon publications that have come from other countries referring to entirely different populations treated perhaps a decade ago. For example, much of our knowledge about fibroids and their behaviour in pregnancy is derived from populations that have a high Negro component. If the woman attending the prepregnancy clinic is a Caucasian, data generated from the other population might not apply and so incorrect probabilities might be offered. Sometimes such data are hard to find but can usually be derived and over the course of years the obstetrician will be able to build up his own data bank of these conditions in his own population.

We have always considered it important that couples attend this clinic rather than women alone. Often the male partner has problems he will raise which are not mentioned in the referring letter; he can assist his wife in the interpretation of any information that is given particularly in the discussions at home which usually follow such a consultation.

Good and precise communication must occur between the various doctors looking after the couple. The general practitioner should be informed of the visit, even though her referral came from a different source. He should also be told of any lines of management suggested in a subsequent pregnancy or of the actuarial risks given of recurrence of problems so that he may offer a consistent opinion to the couple. Should the woman be under the care of a consultant physician, he too should be informed fully of the discussions that have taken place in order that he can substantiate them when the woman returns to him for further care.

Running a prepregnancy clinic is a time-consuming business and the obstetrician would do well to allocate 20–30 minutes per couple seen. For convenience, the author runs his clinic weekly seeing two or three couples in the last hour or so of a pre-existing clinic However, if the load were allowed to increase greatly this would not be practical and arrangements will obviously depend upon the facilities available. No extra equipment is required more than is used in any gynaecological or antenatal clinic. The load on nursing and reception staff is minimal. The obstetrician who runs such a clinic will soon find he will have referrals to the clinic which are probably not relevant to his specialist prepregnancy area. These should be tactfully directed towards the more general area of prepregnancy education done by family practitioners or to a pregnancy advisory clinic. He should also be careful not to build up a cohort of higher risk patients to the detriment of his colleagues in a given geographical area.

The problems that present

Tables 13.1 and 13.2 indicate the type of problems that were seen in one year at the established prepregnancy clinic run by the author. In each case, a value judgement was made of the principal reason that the couple came up. Often this was not the reason written in the referral letter but for statistical simplicity each couple appears only once on these

Table 13.1. Maternal factors in 58 women attending the prepregnancy clinic at Queen Charlotte's Hospital.

Previous Problems in Pregnancy	
Pre-eclampsia	5
Antepartum haemorrhage	4
Previous Problems in Labour	
Previous operative delivery	8
Analgesia	7
Maternal trauma at delivery	3
Current Medical Problems	
Prolapse	3
Fibroids	5
Epilepsy	4
Double uterus	4
Diabetes	3
Heart disease	2
Achondroplasia	1
Future Management of Pregnancy	
Child of predetermined sex	2
Self control of labour	7
Total	58

Table 13.2. Fetal and neonatal factors in 69 women attending the prepregnancy clinic at Queen Charlotte's Hospital.

Deaths of Fetus or Newborn	
Abnormalities	
CNS	4
CVS	1
Normal singleton pregnancies	
Late abortions	12
Preterm labour	18
Normal multiple pregnancies	
Preterm labour	5
Neonatal Problems of Survivors	
Abnormalities	
CNS	3
Limb defects	2
Congenital metabolic diseases	2
Heart disease	1
Neonatal convulsions	1
Drug addiction	1
Other Problems of the Conceptus	
Recurrent early abortion	12
Fear of Down's syndrome	6
Previous hydatidiform mole	1
Total	69

tables; often discussion took place on several matters which were not considered the principal reason for the interview.

Primary maternal factors included many women who were unhappy about what happened in previous pregnancies. Detailed information about medical aspects of the pregnancy are needed to give opinions on this and it often involves writing to other hospitals and so giving re-visit appointments. Much of this could have been better done perhaps at the hospital postnatal visit, six weeks after the last delivery. All the relevant records would have been immediately available and the obstetrician probably remembered the events. However, with the demise of the hospital postnatal clinic system, this meant that women have lost the opportunity to talk to their own obstetricians about what had happened during pregnancy and childbirth while events are fresh in both their minds.

It is of interest that only a sixth of the women attending had previous medical conditions, the purpose of starting the clinic. These were the range of expected diseases more commonly found in the reproductive age group.

In Table 13.2, among the problems that arose in a previous fetus or baby, the recurrence of abnormalities is a major worry and this needs careful consideration for prognosis about future children. One should always remember that incidence of recurrence in another pregnancy depends upon not one but both parents' previous health and this should be considered in giving actuarial odds. In some conditions, there are not enough data available to discuss this field. For example, the recurrence rate of a congenital heart lesion to a family where a previous child has been born with this can be given in general. With wider and better surgical treatment of heart lesions, we are now seeing pregnancies where one or even both parents themselves have had congenital heart lesions which have been treated. This poses a new set of odds and we need to accumulate data in this group of potential parents. If the professional cannot get the exact odds, he should not guess in an optimistic way implying a more hopeful prognosis than is known.

When dealing with couples who have had a previous abnormal child, many would seek treatments to avoid the problems happening again. Since we do not know the cause of most congenital abnormalities, this is difficult, but recent publicity about some areas has led doctors into problems. A good example is the work done on the recurrence of central nervous system abnormalities after a supplementary intake of vitamins in the prepregnancy period. Several studies have shown a reduction in the expected rate of CNS abnormalities when vitamins were taken but none of these surveys is statistically perfect. In consequence, we think there may be some value in this therapy but it has not been proved. The Medical Research Council is now running a randomized control trial on the subject and an answer should be available in the next five years. Until then, doctors should consider carefully whether it is ethical to give women vitamins or folate when it has not been shown that these are going to be of any benefit. Past problems associated with the giving of large quantities of therapeutics should always be remembered when wondering if this is the right management to offer unknown but apparently harmless supplements like vitamins. Even such simple biochemicals as oxygen can be harmful in excess (retrolental fibroplasia) and there are many cited examples of vitamin excess leading to physical harm. This is an example of the problem raised earlier where prepregnancy advice might outrun scientifically acceptable background knowledge.

Another major reason for referral in the Queen Charlotte's Prepregnancy Clinic was previous pregnancies ending either in late abortion or an early preterm labour. These two conditions have similar aetiology and are only separated in time by the artificially made borderline of viability at the 28th completed week of gestation. Women are greatly worried by the thought of this happening again. There has been much discussion in the public press about the value of betamimetics and cervical encirclage so that couples attending the clinic know a certain amount of possibly biased information about these conditions. The obstetrician must be prepared to discuss these subjects fully with intelligent couples who wish for answers. Again, the state of precise knowledge about treatments such as these is exemplified by the large number of obstetricians who have willingly joined a randomized control trial on the value of cervical encirclage sponsored by the Medical Research Council and the Royal College of Obstetricians and Gynaecologists. Randomized trials have never been popular amongst clinicians and the fact that this study is proceeding so successfully indicates the state of doubt in the mind of clinical obstetricians.

The obstetrician running such a clinic is usually presented with a group of problems that the couple wish to discuss. He must take these *seriatim* and deal with them one by one, allowing time for the inevitable supplementary areas that will be brought up by the couple after the subject in the referral letter has been discussed.

The background factors affecting prepregnancy health

All the conditions mentioned above have their aetiology in a group of background factors. Rarely is one feature only responsible for the condition and the obstetrician will try to sort out the various aspects of the aetiology that are relevant. Such factors can probably best be divided into facets of aetiology which are inbuilt and cannot be changed, and those which are capable of being altered.

Among influences that one cannot change are the background biological and social background of the couple who present. For example the woman is of a certain age and parity when she sees the obstetrician and these cannot be altered. Her socio-economic background was settled many years ago and is coded at her marriage by her partner's occupation. Her race and other genetically inherited propensities were laid down at the time of her conception. The obstetrician cannot alter any of these constraints and therefore must work inside them to discuss the odds they incur, for example the chances of Down's syndrome occurring in a mother in later reproductive life.

There are however many influences that can be changed. Whilst these merge into the field of health education, we would draw attention to some of them.

Attitudes of the couple towards antenatal care and intrapartum actions can be influenced by discussion. The use of *contraception* can be altered in the prepregnancy time so that the influence for example of oral contraceptives might not be prevailing when pregnancy starts. The spacing of families according to the needs of the couple and other existing children can also be advised upon.

The *nutrition* of the woman probably bears a strong relation to what happens in a subsequent pregnancy. For a detailed discussion, the reader is referred to Rush (1986). Obvious deficiencies of some specific trace elements, vitamins or even major food groups such as protein should be corrected, if they can be detected. Intake of *alcohol* should be considered for this is a tissue poison and no assurance can be made of a safe lower level which alcohol would not have an effect on pregnancy. However, this negative advice must be tempered with practicalities (Newman 1986).

Cigarette smoking has a known and measurable effect on the fetus and probably has some effect in the prepregnancy area but this is less well measured (Sexton 1986). Like alcohol, there is no safe lower limit to cigarette indulgence and so some obstetricians would advise that no cigarette smoking should take place in the prepregnancy time. Such advice may cause more stress and potential harm than a modest intake of cigarettes and one should also remember that the effects of dragooning somebody into a line of management is different from that when it is taken voluntarily.

The effects of *work* in early pregnancy should be considered. These may be specific due to industrial hazards at the place of work (Chamberlain 1984) or less specifically due to fatigue and boredom (Mamelle & Laumon 1984). The effect of travelling to and from work is often a major feature and all these factors should be discussed to see if they are capable of modification.

A major area of influence on forthcoming pregnancies is that of *pre-existing disease* in the man or woman and the *drugs* taken for that disease. Generally the pregnancy age group is usually a healthy one and so few are chronically sick, but there are still women and their partners who have asthma, bowel inflammatory disease and urinary problems. This subject is fully discussed by de Swiet (1986). The full assessment of the effects of such diseases on metabolism and subsequent pregnancy may well lead to the obstetrician consulting with other physicians in order to give a full answer and plan a course of management in a subsequent pregnancy. This is good prepregnancy care and is helpful to both the professionals and the couple.

The effect of *infections* in early pregnancy must be dealt with in the prepregnancy clinic. The principal known one is rubella and women should be screened to check the titre of antibodies indicating previous infection. Those who are sero-negative should be offered inoculation with prevention of pregnancy for three months after such treatment.

Perhaps the most difficult area of all in the prepregnancy area is that of *stress*. This is difficult to measure and almost impossible to quantify. However, it affects every other body system and physiological function so would be strange if it did not have some influence on the early conceptus. The influence may be small and insignificant, in which case it need not concern the obstetrician, but this cannot be told, certainly in prospect. Possibly the attendance of a couple at a prepregnancy clinic to discuss matters that make them anxious is in itself a form of stress therapy. The overt airing of the problems with the professional and the private discussion with the partner which takes place subsequently may be therapeutic in their own right. This effect is being measured at one prepregnancy clinic at the moment; no results are yet available.

CONCLUSIONS

The field of prepregnancy counselling starts with good health education. As such it lies with the educators who are best trained at putting over information. Teachers are skilled in this and to them the obstetrician should turn, encouraging them to include the subject in the school curriculum. At the next layer of prepregnancy care, specific questions may have to be answered; these are often best dealt with by professionals who know the couple and meet them in other circumstances such as the general practitioner's surgery, the family planning clinic or the industrial health centre. Open access prepregnancy advisory clinics run by health professions supplement and strengthen such non-specific advice. A third and smallest group of couples are those who have specific problems and wish to consult with professionals who have taken a special interest in this field. For them, the prepregnancy clinic run in the hospital obstetrical department can be a useful and helpful aid. It should run alongside the clinical genetics department. Advice given and taken in this field could produce rewards equal to those resulting from antenatal care. It is a subject that will probably expand in the next twenty years and groups of obstetricians will become more skilled in prepregnancy care.

REFERENCES

CHAMBERLAIN G. (1984) *Pregnant Women at Work*. Macmillan Press Ltd., London.
DE SWIET M. (1986) In *Prepregnancy Care* (eds. Chamberlain G. & Lumley J.). John Wiley & Son, Chichester. In press.
MAMELLE N. & LAUMON B. (1984) In *Pregnant Women at Work* (ed. Chamberlain G.). Macmillan Press Ltd., London.
NEWMAN N. (1986) In *Prepregnancy Care* (eds. Chamberlain G. & Lumley J.). John Wiley & Son, Chichester. In press.
RUSH R. (1986) In *Prepregnancy Care* (eds. Chamberlain G. & Lumley J.). John Wiley & Son, Chichester. In press.
SEXTON M. (1986) In *Prepregnancy Care* (eds. Chamberlain G. & Lumley J.). John Wiley & Son, Chichester. In press.

CHAPTER 14
ABORTION AND ECTOPIC PREGNANCY

P. W. HOWIE

More pregnancies are lost in the early weeks than at any other stage of gestation. Three of the main categories of early pregnancy loss are spontaneous abortion, induced abortion and ectopic pregnancy and these will be discussed in this chapter. The other main cause of early pregnancy failure is hydatidiform mole which is described in Chapter 37. Although early pregnancy loss is often considered to be less important than loss of the baby in later pregnancy, this attitude is inappropriate. The loss of a wanted pregnancy is always distressing to the mother irrespective of its timing and this is particularly true in recurrent abortion. Furthermore, abortion and ectopic pregnancy can have serious maternal consequences, with appreciable risks of maternal mortality and long-term morbidity. It is likely that, as many of the problems of late pregnancy diminish in frequency, more attention will be paid to the problems of early pregnancy in the coming decades.

SPONTANEOUS ABORTION

Abortion is defined in Britith Law as termination of pregnancy before 28 weeks gestation with no evidence of life. An inherent deficiency in this definition is that many babies delivered before 28 weeks prove to be viable. In 1977, the World Health Organization (WHO) defined abortion as '... the expulsion or extraction from its mother of a fetus or an embryo weighing 500 grams or less ...' Such a definition, which uses an upper limit of fetal weight, overcomes the difficulty of defining an abortion when the gestational age is in doubt and 500 grams would usually correspond to a gestational age of 20 to 22 weeks. On the other hand, a definition of abortion based on fetal weight alone takes no account of the possibility of severe intrauterine growth failure when a very small baby may have reached a gestational age of 28 weeks or more. Many abortions in the late second trimester of pregnancy share a common aetiology

with perinatal deaths early in the third trimester and it would make sense to consider them together. It would be a useful development if a worldwide definition of abortion could be agreed so that statistical comparisons could be made between populations.

EPIDEMIOLOGY

Incidence

The incidence of spontaneous abortion is generally considered to be about 15% of all pregnancies (Roth 1963, Harlap *et al.* 1980) although some studies have estimated the incidence to be between 20 and 25% (French & Bierman 1962, Shapiro *et al.* 1963). There are several reasons why it is impossible to define exactly the incidence of spontaneous abortion. In the first place, it is quite possible for women to abort without knowing that they have been pregnant. Using the β sub-unit of human chorionic gonadotrophin (BHCG) as a marker of pregnancy, a number of studies have reported 'occult' pregnancies in which the woman is aware of no more than a slightly delayed or heavy 'menstruation' (Miller *et al.* 1980, Whittaker *et al.* 1983). The frequency of 'occult' pregnancies has varied widely in the reported studies, some of which were carried out in apparently infertile women (Chartier *et al.* 1979). It is also probable that many fertilized ova perish before implantation and are never recognized. In the second place, some women who present with vaginal bleeding are sure that they are having a miscarriage but show no confirmatory evidence of pregnancy. Some of these apparent abortions, which often occur in women who are anxious to conceive, are explained by delayed menstruation. Finally, a number of abortions which are reported to be of spontaneous origin, may have occurred as a result of deliberate interference. In many of these cases, it may be impossible to establish whether the abortion was spontaneous or not.

Factors influencing spontaneous abortion rate

Not all women have the same propensity to abort and about 25 per cent of all women will have one or more abortions (Warburton & Fraser 1964). Some studies have reported that the incidence of spontaneous abortion increases with maternal gravidity and age (Naylor & Warburton 1979) but others do not agree (for a summary of data see Huisjes 1984). The relationships between abortion, gravidity and maternal age are complex because women who are prone to abortion will have more pregnancies and reproduce for longer in order to attain their desired family size. Having allowed for this effect of reproductive compensation, it is likely that gravidity has relatively little effect on the incidence of abortion. On the other hand, maternal age over 35 years appears to be associated with an increased risk of abortion but there is no evidence that maternal age is an important risk factor in women under 35 years (Resseguie 1974). A history of having an abortion in a previous pregnancy is associated with an increased risk of abortion in subsequent pregnancies and this is discussed in more detail in the section on Recurrent Abortion later in the chapter. Spontaneous abortion is more common in multiple pregnancy (Livingston & Poland 1980) and after an earlier menarche but is not influenced by the fetal sex (Huisjes 1984) or the season of the year (Warren *et al.* 1980).

Aetiology of abortion

Spontaneous abortion has been attributed to a large number of aetiological factors although the supporting evidence for some of the alleged causes has been tenuous. Misunderstandings about the aetiology of abortion have, in some circumstances, led to inappropriate therapy with serious adverse consequences. The best-known example was the unwarranted use of diethylstilboestrol to treat mothers with recurrent abortion. Although there is an understandable desire to offer treatment to women with recurrent abortion, it is essential that any therapeutic intervention in early pregnancy should be based on a clear knowledge of the aetiological factors. Only in this way will unnecessary exposure to potentially adverse agents be reduced to a minimum. The main causes of spontaneous abortion are summarized in Table 14.1 and are discussed in this section of the chapter; any reader who wishes more detailed information is referred to the extensive review of spontaneous abortion by Huisjes (1984).

Table 14.1. Possible causes of spontaneous abortion

Abnormal conceptus	(i)	Chromosomal
	(ii)	Structural
	(iii)	Genetic
Immunological		
Uterine abnormality	(i)	Congenital
	(ii)	Fibroids and retroversion
Cervical incompetence		
Endocrine	(i)	Progesterone
	(ii)	Others
Maternal disease		
Infection	(i)	Maternal
Toxins and trauma		
Others		

ABNORMAL CONCEPTUSES

It has long been known that there is abnormal fetal development in a high proportion of those pregnancies which abort (Mall 1917); the abnormal development may manifest itself as a 'blighted ovum', which describes an empty sac in which the embryo has not developed beyond a small clump of cells. In some cases, there may be a clearly recognizable fetal abnormality, while, in others, the sac may have ruptured and the fetus is never identified. The abnormal development of the embryo or fetus may be due to a structural abnormality or to a chromosomal abnormality; it is also possible that genetic defects, leading to the absence of a specific enzyme, could cause abortion although this possibility has been little investigated. In practice, it is often difficult to identify the underlying factor in individual cases because maturation of the tissues after fetal death interferes with chromosomal analysis or adequate structural examination.

It is now generally accepted that chromosomal abnormalities account for a large proportion of all aborted conceptuses. Those studies which have reported on successful cultures have found abnormal karyotypes in about 50% of cases with a range extending from 30% (Creasy *et al.* 1976) to 61% (Boué *et al.* 1975). Differences between studies may be explained by different gestational ages because abnormal karyotypes become less common the later the pregnancy aborts. It must be remembered, however, that the 50% of abnormal karyotypes is established only for those pregnancies in which successful cell culture was possible. It may be that those aborting pregnancies in which cell culture was not possible represent a separate population with a completely different incidence of abnormal karyotypes.

Table 14.2. Distribution of types of chromosomal errors in spontaneous abortions from eight publications. From Huisjes 1984 (with permission from the author and Churchill Livingstone, Edinburgh).

	Number	%
Autosomal trisomies	1209	51.3
45,X	453	19.2
Triploidy	381	16.2
Tetraploidy	135	5.7
Structural re-arrangements	97	4.1
Others	83	4.1
	2538	100

The most commonly encountered type of chromosomal abnormality is an autosomal trisomy (Table 14.2) which accounts for more than half of the abnormal karyotypes. When a trisomy is present, it most commonly affects chromosome 16 (32%) and then chromosomes 22 (10%), 21 (8%) and 15 (7%) in that order (Huisjes 1984); other chromosomes are affected with decreasing frequency and it is presumed that the rarely detected trisomies lead to early embryonic death and unrecognized abortion. Most autosomal trisomies occur as a result of non-disjunction during the first meiotic division of the oocyte and are commoner with increasing maternal age. By contrast, maternal age is not associated with the other types of chromosomally abnormal abortions.

Monosomy X accounts for about one-fifth of abnormal karyotypes but monosomy Y is never seen because at least one X chromosome seems to be required for cell survival. Other sex chromosome abnormalities such as XXY, XXX and XYY are rarely seen in abortions and usually progress to term. Triploidy (16.2%) and tetraploidy (5.75%) are seen with reasonable frequency but those cases of triploidy in which there is a double paternal component will lead to a partial hydatidiform mole (*see* Chapter 37). The most important of the structural re-arrangements are the translocations which may be passed on by one of the parents who may be a balanced carrier; balanced translocation should be looked for in all couples who present with a history of recurrent abortion. The remaining group of abnormal karyotypes are various forms of mosaicism, double trisomies and other rare abnormalities.

It is not known why some chromosomal abnormalities, such as trisomy 21 (Down's syndrome) and monosomy X (Turner's syndrome) lead to abortion in some cases and proceed to term in others. It may be that those cases which abort have some other abnormality, in addition to the chromosomal defect, which precipitates the abortion. There is no doubt, however, that chromosomal defects play an important part in the aetiology of abortion.

STRUCTURAL ABNORMALITIES

Not all of the embryonic or fetal malformations associated with spontaneous abortion are due to chromosomal abnormalities, although the nature of these malformations have not been well documented. Neural tube defects are, however, encountered with increased frequency in spontaneous abortions. For example, in Northern Ireland, the rate was 36 per thousand (MacHenry *et al.* 1979) and, although Northern Ireland has a high incidence of neural tube defects, this incidence among spontaneous abortions was many times greater than that encountered at birth. Structural abnormalities among spontaneously aborted embryos or fetuses may be commoner than is generally realized but degeneration from maceration makes it extremely difficult to define the numbers with accuracy.

IMMUNOLOGICAL CAUSES

The immunological mechanisms which lead to the mother accepting the fetus for the duration of a normal pregnancy are not fully understood. It has been suggested that a failure of a normal immune response in the mother could be an important factor in the aetiology of abortion. This has led to an interesting new concept of stimulating immune responses in women with recurrent abortion and this subject is discussed in detail in Chapter 21 (p. 299).

UTERINE ABNORMALITIES

Uterine abnormalities result from a failure of normal fusion of the Müllerian ducts and the traditional view has held that such abnormalities predispose to abortion. Although there is reasonably strong supporting evidence, the association is by no means clear cut. A wide variety of fusion defects can occur as illustrated in Fig. 1.11 (p. 8). There has never been a detailed study of the incidence of fusion abnormalities but a general estimate is that they affect 1% of the female population (Huisjes 1984). It is impossible to calculate exactly the incidence of abortion in women with fusion abnormalities because the diagnosis will never be made in many women who have successful pregnancies. Those who have studied the problem estimate the incidence of abortion at about 30% which is double that of the normal population (Hay 1958, Heinonen *et al.* 1982). In addition, the prevalence of uterine abnormalities is about 15% amongst women presenting with recurrent abortions which is higher than that of the general population (Theo *et al.* 1979). On the other hand, many women with uterine abnormalities have unblemished reproductive careers and the risks of abortion vary according to the differing uterine shapes. Furthermore, a conservative approach may result in a successful pregnancy even after previous abortions. Paradoxically, the more severe the uterine abnormality, the less may be the risk of abortion. For example, in uterus bicornis bicollis, the outcome may be successful while a subseptate uterus may be a cause of recurrent abortion. It may be that the abnormal shape of the uterine cavity in subseptate uterus is unable to accommodate itself to the growing pregnancy. Exposure to diethyl-stilboestrol (DES) *in utero* has been shown to cause uterine abnormalities in addition to the vaginal changes which have been clearly described (Kaufman *et al.* 1977). In over 60% of women who were exposed to DES *in utero*, there were uterine defects on hysterography together with cervical abnormalities and these are associated with a doubling of the abortion rate (Mangan *et al.* 1982).

The diagnosis of uterine abnormality may be suggested by a history of abortion or transverse lie in pregnancy, or by the clinical finding of a double cervix or vaginal abnormality. The definitive diagnosis, in most cases, is made on hysterosalpingography and this should be carried out in all cases of recurrent abortion. There may be associated renal tract abnormalities and intravenous pyelography is indicated when a uterine abnormality has been detected.

Various surgical techniques for the correction of uterine abnormalities have been described. Probably the most frequently used is Strassmann's metroplasty in which a uterine septum is removed and the uterus is reconstructed. Good results have generally been claimed for reconstructive surgery, but controlled trials have not been done and it is impossible to know whether an equally favourable outcome might have resulted from conservative management (Huisjes 1984). Two aspects of metroplasty are causes of anxiety; the first is that most series have reported an incidence of subsequent infertility of about 30 per cent and the second is the potential risk of uterine rupture in any subsequent pregnancy. It is important, therefore, to perform metroplasty only in those women with a repeated history of abortion which

could not be explained on other grounds. Some women with uterine abnormalities have associated cervical incompetence and it may be worth trying cervical cerclage before proceeding to metroplasty. Nevertheless, metroplasty probably has a place in the management of uterine abnormality, although there must be careful assessment before any individual is selected for surgery.

OTHER UTERINE ABNORMALITIES

Retroversion has been implicated as a cause of abortion but the supporting evidence is very poor apart from the rare case when the retroverted gravid uterus is trapped in the pelvis. It is doubtful if ventrisuspension of the uterus is helpful in the management of recurrent abortion, although the operation has been carried out in the past for this indication. Similarly, fibroids are commonly blamed as a cause of abortion but good confirmatory evidence is lacking. It is generally presumed that submucous fibroids, by distorting the uterine cavity are the most likely fibroids to cause abortion. Fibroids, however, occur more commonly in older women and increasing maternal age is itself a contributory factor to the risk of abortion. Although myomectomy is sometimes carried out as a treatment for recurrent abortion, its efficacy has not been established.

CERVICAL INCOMPETENCE

Most obstetricians would accept that cervical incompetence can be a cause of abortion, particularly in the second trimester of pregnancy. In normal pregnancy, the cervix remains closed and retains the products of conception within the uterus. During the third trimester, the cervix softens in preparation for labour when dilatation occurs in response to uterine contractions. When cervical incompetence is present, the cervix opens prematurely with minimal or absent uterine activity and the pregnancy is expelled. Unfortunately, it has proved impossible to define cervical incompetence on objective grounds and the diagnosis has been based mainly on the clinical history. McDonald (1980) considers that the incidence varies between 1% and 2% of normal pregnancies but the condition is almost certainly over-diagnosed.

Trauma to the cervix is an important aetiological factor but gynaecologists are now well aware of the need to avoid unnecessary damage to the cervix. In the past, cervical dilatation was used to treat primary dysmenorrhoea but this procedure has now been abandoned. Cone biopsy of the cervix can undermine cervical competence and it is highly desirable that colposcopically directed local treatment of cervical lesions should replace cone biopsy whenever possible. For example, Jones et al. (1979) reported an 18% incidence of preterm delivery after cone biopsy compared with 5% among controls. If a biopsy of the cervix is required this should be as small as necessary to meet the therapeutic requirements (Leiman et al. 1980). Cervical amputation during uterine vaginal repair can also cause incompetence and this operation should be used only as a last resort in young women who have not completed their families.

In modern practice, the greatest potential surgical cause of cervical incompetence may be cervical dilatation during termination of pregnancy. In the early 1970s there were a number of reports that the incidence of mid-trimester abortion was increased among women who had undergone previous first trimester abortion (e.g. Wright et al. 1972). More recent studies, however, have failed to confirm this (Daling & Emanuel 1975, Kline et al. 1980a) including a large collaborative study by a WHO task force (1979) on the sequelae of abortion. One reason for this change may be that gynaecologists now refrain from forcible over-dilatation of the cervix, because cervical ruptures of more than 5 mm in depth were observed in 22% of uteri dilated to 12 mm Hégar (Hulka & Higgins 1961). Another factor is that the more recent studies have corrected for confounding variables such as maternal age, obstetric history and social class which were related to both spontaneous and induced abortion (Huisjes 1984). Nevertheless, it is clear that induced abortion poses a potential threat to the cervix, especially if repeated abortions are performed, and care must be taken to dilate the cervix as little as possible.

Cervical incompetence can occur even in the absence of trauma to the cervix and has been reported after exposure to diethylstilboestrol and in women with uterine abnormalities. In these cases, there may be impairment of the normal functioning of the muscular fibres round the internal os.

Management of cervical incompetence
When cervical incompetence is suspected on the basis of the clinical history and findings, cervical cerclage can be considered in subsequent pregnancies. A number of procedures have been recommended, such as Shirodkar's suture in which a strip of fascia lata was tied submucosally around the isthmus of the cervix after the vaginal mucosa and bladder had been

reflected. The disadvantage of Shirodkar's suture was that it could not be readily removed and it is now more common to tie a purse string suture round the cervix using non-absorbable material as originally described by McDonald (1957). Prior to the insertion of the suture, it is advisable to confirm fetal viability by ultrasound and to insert the suture at 14 weeks, by which time any first trimester fetal wastage could have already occurred. The McDonald suture is simpler to insert than Shirodkar's suture and can be removed at 38 weeks or at the onset of labour (whichever is the sooner) to allow a normal vaginal delivery. Cervical cerclage is not without its problems, however, and there are risks of rupturing the membranes at the time of insertion or of introducing infection which can ascend into the uterus and stimulate uterine activity (Rush et al. 1984). Furthermore, there is a risk of further cervical damage from tears, if the suture is not removed before uterine activity becomes well established during labour.

The results of cervical cerclage are difficult to assess because the diagnosis of cervical incompetence cannot be made with certainty in every case. In a literature review, Cousins (1980) reported an 82% success rate after Shirodkar's operation and 73% after McDonald's cerclage. Without a control group, however, it is impossible to know to what extent the results reflected the effect of the operation or the natural history of the treated pregnancies. It is likely that the more demanding the criteria for the diagnosis of cervical incompetence, the more valuable will be the operation of cervical cerclage. A recent survey indicated that the use of cervical cerclage varied widely among obstetricians so that there is no consensus view of its place in management. Because of the uncertain value of this procedure, the Medical Research Council is currently carrying out a multicentre randomized trial of cervical cerclage and the results are awaited with interest.

ENDOCRINE CAUSES

The corpus luteum is essential for the survival of the pregnancy during the first 8 weeks of gestation. If the corpus luteum is removed surgically before that time, abortion will occur within 4 to 7 days, an effect which can be prevented by the administration of parenteral progesterone (Csapo et al. 1973). If the corpus luteum is removed at 9–10 weeks, abortion will sometimes but not invariably occur. In addition, it has been shown that progesterone levels are lower in women with threatened abortion who proceed to inevitable abortion as compared to the progesterone levels in those whose pregnancies continue. From this evidence, the concept of hormone deficiency evolved as a possible cause of abortion and led to the widespread use of progestogens as a preventive measure.

The evidence in favour of progesterone deficiency as a cause of abortion, however, is unsatisfactory. It cannot be assumed that the effects of lute-ectomy are reproduced by any syndrome occurring naturally and the low levels of progesterone prior to spontaneous abortion are more likely to be a sign of a failing pregnancy rather than a cause of it. Nevertheless, progestogens have been used in the past, especially among women with recurrent abortion, and good results were claimed on the basis that pregnanediol levels rose in those women with continuing pregnancies. A number of controlled clinical trials, however, have failed to show any benefit of progestogen treatment as compared with the effect of a placebo (Shearman & Garret 1963, Goldzieher 1964, Klopper & Macnaughton 1965). From studies of 17α hydroxy-progesterone, which is produced by the corpus luteum and not by the placenta, it has been shown that the natural life span of the corpus luteum is the first 10 weeks after ovulation (Yoshimi et al. 1969). Before that time, the developing placenta is already producing increasing amounts of progesterone so that the possibility of progesterone deficiency can occur only at the time when the source of progesterone support for the pregnancy is changing from the corpus luteum to the placenta. Many of the regimes for progestogen therapy continued treatment well into the second trimester which cannot be justified even on a theoretical basis. Furthermore, it cannot be assumed that progestogens are without potentially harmful side-effects. Experience with diethylstilboestrol has shown that the fetus can be affected by hormones which are administered in early pregnancy and that the adverse effects may not become obvious for some years after birth. There is evidence that at least some progestogens can virilize a female fetus if given in large doses in early pregnancy (Wilkins 1960).

The story of hormone therapy in early pregnancy illustrates the need for careful evaluation of any new treatment regime. The controlled clinical trials of progestogens have played a critical role in changing attitudes to this form of treatment, and it is very doubtful if there is any place for progestogens in the prevention of abortion except after surgical removal of the corpus luteum. It is possible, however, that corpus luteum deficiency could be a cause of early pregnancy failure but this subject has been one of controversy. If corpus luteum deficiency is important, its effect would operate very early in pregnancy, usually before the prospective mother was aware of conception. The evidence to support the concept of corpus luteum deficiency is circumstantial (Jones 1976) and is, as yet, insufficient to establish it as a cause of abortion.

MATERNAL DISEASE

There have been sporadic reports that various maternal diseases such as diabetes mellitus, thyroid disease, von Willebrand's disease and systemic lupus erythematosus are associated with an increased risk of abortion. The evidence in support of these associations is flimsy and these diseases should be considered as possible, but unproven, causes of abortion.

Wilson's disease is an autosomal recessive disorder involving a disturbance of copper metabolism and accumulation of copper in liver tissue. The disease is associated with a high incidence of abortion (Walshe 1977, Klee 1979) and can be treated with penicillamine. Although Wilson's disease is rare, it can be diagnosed by a high serum caeruloplasmin level and this can be measured as part of the investigation of unexplained recurrent abortion.

INFECTION

Acute maternal infection, such as pyelitis or appendicitis, which leads to a general toxic illness with high temperature can stimulate uterine activity and loss of the pregnancy. Early diagnosis and appropriate treatment will successfully control most acute infections and forestall the occurrence of abortion.

A large number of bacterial and viral agents have been implicated as possible causes of abortion. Syphilis is one maternal infection which can spread across the placenta to cause intrauterine death and abortion although this is now a rare cause of abortion in the United Kingdom. In the majority of cases, it is very difficult to establish a direct cause and effect relationship for any particular organism. If an organism is cultured from the products of conception, it is usually impossible to establish if the colonization took place before or after the time of fetal death. Similarly, raised antibody titres merely give evidence of recent or past infection and do not establish that the organism was the causative factor. The infections which have been implicated as possible causes of abortion include listeriosis, brucellosis, toxoplasmosis and my-coplasmosis. In general, it is possible for bacteria to penetrate into the uterine cavity and cause abortion but few directly affect the fetus. It is more likely that any infection is transplacental, leading to chorioamnionitis, release of prostaglandins and preterm uterine activity. In this way, infection may prove to be a very important cause of mid-trimester abortion and preterm delivery, but further work is required to establish the significance of organisms which are isolated from preterm deliveries. In tropical countries, malaria is widely held to be an important cause of abortion in areas where the infection is endemic (Covell 1950).

Because viruses are smaller than bacteria, they can more readily cross the placenta and directly colonize the fetus. It is well known that rubella infection can cause fetal abnormality but it is difficult to determine how frequently rubella causes abortion. Cytomegalovirus, measles, herpes, influenza and other viruses can probably all cause abortion but the frequency of such occurrences is likely to be low.

TOXIC FACTORS

There is evidence that hospital staff who work in operating theatres have an increased risk of spontaneous abortion (Vessey & Nunn, 1980). It is often assumed that anaesthetic gases are responsible for this effect although conclusive proof of this is lacking (Spence 1981). Nevertheless, it is strongly advised that the air in operating theatres should be filtered to keep the concentration of gases as low as possible.

The possible harmful effects of anaesthetic gases raises the possibility that other toxic factors might cause abortion and environmental pollution is a subject of increasing public concern. There are, however, major methodological difficulties in studying the potential toxic effects of various substances upon the developing fetus. The major problem is a statistical one because large numbers would be required to establish an association between a toxic substance and abortion and many variables would confound the problem. It would be difficult to avoid bias because mothers who had experienced abortion would be more likely to recall exposure to potential toxic agents than controls who had successful pregnancies. In general, there is no clear evidence that toxic agents are a major cause of abortion in humans; on the other hand, complacency is inappropriate because the potential risk of damage to the developing fetus is ever present.

It is possible that smoking, alcohol and drug abuse can adversely affect fetal development. Women who smoke have a greater risk of abortion than non-smokers (Himmelberger et al. 1978) but it is not certain that the effect is directly due to smoking itself or to other associated factors. Similarly, there is evidence that an alcohol intake of more than two drinks per week may be related to abortion (Kline et al. 1980b). An Editorial (1980) in The Lancet recommended that, in the prevention of abortion, daily drinking of alcohol should be avoided.

TRAUMA

In general, the fetus is very well protected inside the uterus and is unlikely to be affected by trauma unless there is a direct penetrating injury. Amniocentesis appears to carry a small risk of abortion and this is generally thought to be of the order of 1% (Medical Research Council Report 1978). This means that amniocentesis is a procedure which should be carried out only when indicated by some 'risk' factor requiring precise diagnosis.

Abdominal surgery during early pregnancy may precipitate abortion and it is usual practice to delay ovarian cystectomy until 14–16 weeks if a cyst is diagnosed in the first trimester. Similarly, elective surgery should be postponed unless there is some urgency to perform the operation.

Clinical features

The traditional classification of abortion is into the categories of threatened abortion, inevitable abortion, incomplete or complete abortion and missed abortion. Septic abortion is sometimes regarded as a category of abortion but is really a complication, usually of incomplete abortion. Threatened abortion refers to bleeding from the gravid uterus before 28 weeks' gestation when there is a viable fetus and no evidence of cervical dilatation. Abortion is usually held to have become inevitable if the cervix has already begun to dilate. Incomplete and complete abortion refer, respectively, to partial and complete expulsion of the products of conception.

Threatened, inevitable and incomplete abortions are, by far, the commonest types of abortion and the usual clinical problem is to determine which is present in a woman who develops bleeding in early pregnancy. Missed abortion is relatively uncommon and will be discussed later in the chapter.

HISTORY TAKING

When a woman presents with a history of bleeding in early pregnancy, a careful enquiry should be made about the extent of the bleeding and the presence of any abdominal pain. If the bleeding is slight and there is no abdominal pain, the history is suggestive of threatened abortion; when the bleeding is heavy with passage of clots and is accompanied by cramping lower abdominal pain, the most probable diagnosis is inevitable abortion; if products of conception have been passed, the diagnosis of abortion is established. It is important to consider other possible causes of vaginal bleeding in early pregnancy in the differential diagnosis. The symptoms and signs of ectopic pregnancy are very variable, as will be discussed later in the chapter, but vaginal bleeding with or without abdominal pain may be the presenting feature; the vaginal bleeding associated with ectopic pregnancy is often very dark and is sometimes described as being 'like prune juice'.

Hydatidiform mole is another cause of vaginal bleeding in early pregnancy, and the clinical features are described in detail in Chapter 37. If the vaginal bleeding has been associated with vaginal discharge or with pruritus vulvae, a vaginitis may be responsible for the bleeding. More rarely, a cervical polyp or cervical carcinoma may explain the bleeding and in these cases the bleeding may have been provoked by intercourse. Occasionally, haematuria or rectal bleeding can be mistaken by the patient for vaginal bleeding and enquiry should be made for any associated urinary or bowel complaints. As part of the history, it is worth asking if the symptoms of pregnancy are still present, because if they have regressed, this suggests that the pregnancy may be non-viable.

CLINICAL EXAMINATION

A general clinical assessment should be made, particularly to ensure that there are no signs of shock. On abdominal examination, the size of the uterus should be assessed to see if it corresponds with the gestational age. If the uterus is smaller than expected, the pregnancy may be non-viable or the gestational age may be mistaken. If the uterus is larger than expected, a twin pregnancy, fibroids or a hydatidiform mole are some of the diagnoses to be considered; it is also necessary to ensure that a distended bladder is not the explanation of an apparently enlarged uterus. If there is tenderness on abdominal palpation, particularly in either of the iliac fossae, then ectopic pregnancy should be suspected.

Pelvic examination

A pelvic examination should be carried out in all cases as part of the full assessment, although it is important that this should be done as gently as possible. If the bleeding has been slight, a speculum should be passed to see if there is a vaginal infection or a cervical lesion which could explain the bleeding. If the bleeding is heavy, speculum examination is unlikely to be helpful as blood will obscure the view. On digital examination, the dilatation of the cervix should be assessed and, if the cervix has begun to open, the diagnosis of inevitable abortion can be made. If products of conception are present, it is worth removing as much tissue as possible as this can help to relieve discomfort. If the cervix is closed, the probable diagnosis is threatened abortion and the size and consistency of the uterus should be estimated. If there is tenderness in either vaginal fornix, this should arouse suspicions of ectopic pregnancy and may indicate the need for laparoscopy.

In a proportion of cases, the diagnosis will be established on clinical assessment alone but, in others, more detailed investigations will be required to determine the viability of the fetus. It is upon the assessment of fetal viability that the future management will depend.

ULTRASOUND

The development of ultrasound has been a major advance in the management of bleeding in early pregnancy. In many cases, the scan will demonstrate a normal intrauterine pregnancy and the fetal heart beat will be recognized. In such circumstances, the best management is to reassure the patient about the viability of her pregnancy and to advise a few days of rest until the bleeding has settled completely. If the bleeding is slight and if there is adequate home support, the rest may be taken at home. If the bleeding has been moderate or if the mother would be exposed to heavy domestic duties, it is wiser to advise rest in hospital. In addition to a viable fetus, a second empty sac is sometimes visualized within the uterine cavity. This is presumed to represent a twin pregnancy in which one of the pregnancies has developed normally and the other is a blighted ovum. There is a danger that bleeding from the non-continuing pregnancy may be prolonged and, by stimulating uterine activity, cause abortion of the viable fetus. In such a case, the correct management is expectant in the hope that the bleeding will settle and that the viable pregnancy will continue.

In a number of cases the ultrasonic picture will demonstrate an empty sac which is smaller than expected for the period of amenorrhoea with no fetal heart beat. This will usually mean that the pregnancy is not viable, although it can be confused with a very early pregnancy which has not reached a stage of development in which the fetal heart is visible. If there is any doubt about the diagnosis, it is wise to wait for a few days and repeat the scan to see if the sac is growing. A pregnancy test can be carried out but is not always helpful. A positive test does not guarantee that the pregnancy is viable although a negative test would support a diagnosis of non-viability unless the gestation was less than 6 weeks. Once it is clear that the pregnancy is not continuing it is best to evacuate the uterus. If the uterus is less than 12 weeks size, the evacuation can be carried out by dilatation and curettage but a large uterus may be more safely evacuated after the cervix has been dilated by prostaglandins as described later in the chapter.

Management of Incomplete Abortion

When the cervix is open or when products of conception have been passed, the diagnosis of incomplete abortion is established. It is important to assess blood loss and the general condition of the patient, because hypovolaemia should be treated by blood transfusion before general anaesthesia is induced. If vaginal bleeding is persisting, 0.5 mg of ergometrine should be given intravenously or intramuscularly to reduce the loss. In some cases, bleeding can be further reduced by digitally removing products of conception which are in the cervical canal and by gently rubbing the uterine fundus. Once the patient's general condition is satisfactory, her uterus should be evacuated, usually under general anaesthesia. The pregnancy uterus is soft and care must be taken not to perforate the uterine fundus. As much of the retained tissue as possible should be removed digitally and the evacuation completed by a gentle curettage. Intravenous ergometrine 0.5 mg will encourage a uterine contraction and this can be reinforced by massaging the uterus bimanually. Once the uterine evacuation is complete, the mother should return to the ward and be observed for 24 hours to ensure that bleeding has stopped.

SEPTIC ABORTIONS

Following incomplete abortion, there is always a risk of an ascending infection into the uterus which can subsequently spread throughout the pelvis. It is important that infection should be diagnosed and treated as quickly as possible. The earliest signs of infection are a maternal pyrexia, abdominal pains, persistent vaginal bleeding and offensive vaginal discharge. If any of these features are present, blood cultures and cervical swabs should be taken. If the evidence of infection is good, antibiotics are started right away and subsequently changed on the basis of the bacteriological report. The common aerobic organisms are *Escherichia coli*, *staphylococcus epidermidis* and the streptococci, whereas clostridia and bacteroidaceae are potential causes of anaerobic infection. A common initial antibiotic combination is a cephalosporin with metronidazole which will be active against both aerobic and anaerobic organisms, although other combinations may be equally effective. Postabortal infection may be due to retained products of conception and re-evacuation of the uterus should be considered to exclude a septic focus.

It is now relatively rare to see the full-blown clinical picture of septic abortion although it used to be well recognized as a potential consequence of criminal abortion. Such women are extremely ill with a high swinging temperature and acute abdominal pain. There is an offensive vaginal discharge, the vagina feels 'hot' and cervical excitation elicits exquisite tenderness. There is a danger that such women will develop bacteraemic shock and renal failure. The clinical features and the management are similar to those of puerperal sepsis which are described in detail in Chapters 32 and 41.

MISSED ABORTION

Missed abortion describes a pregnancy in which the fetus has died but the uterus has made no attempt to expel the products of conception. The diagnosis of missed abortion can be suspected if the mother notices the disappearance of the symptoms of pregnancy. Any nausea or urinary frequency may subside and the breast changes may revert to normal. The uterine size will be smaller than expected for the period of amenorrhoea and ultrasonic examination will fail to demonstrate any evidence of fetal life. If the diagnosis of missed abortion is established, it is best to evacuate the uterus without delay. The presence of a non-continuing pregnancy is upsetting to the mother and there is a small risk of a coagulation defect if the missed abortion continues for several weeks. Before proceeding to evacuate the uterus, the fibrinogen level should be checked; if this is low, and especially if there is any evidence of bruising, intravenous heparin should be given to correct the clotting defect (*see* Chapter 36).

If the uterine size is less than 12 weeks, cervical dilatation and suction curettage can be used to evacuate the uterus but if the uterus is larger than this, it is better to dilate the cervix medically before evacuating the uterus. In the past, oxytocin proved to be ineffective in most cases of missed abortion and prostaglandins are the agents of choice. In the management of missed abortion, prostaglandins, usually in the form of either PGE_2 or $PGF_2\alpha$ have been given intramuscularly (Wallenberg *et al.* 1980), extra-amniotically (Embrey *et al.* 1974) or as a viscous gel to the cervix (Ekman *et al.* 1980). A suitable regime for the management of missed abortion is by extra-amniotic prostaglandins as described in the section on induced abortion (p. 178).

Recurrent abortion

One of the most distressing problems in obstetrics is recurrent abortion, particularly in those who have no successful pregnancies. There is no precise definition of recurrent abortion, but most authorities would accept three consecutive abortions as evidence of recurrent abortion. On a theoretical basis, Malpas (1938) calculated that, after three consecutive abortions, the risk of abortion in the next pregnancy was 73%, but the practical experience in published series has indicated that the prognosis is much better than that. Warburton and Fraser (1964) reported that the chance of a further abortion in the next pregnancy after one abortion was 23.7%, which increased to 26.2% after two abortions and to 32.2% after three. Although Poland *et al.* (1977) found a rather higher figure of a 47% risk of abortion after three abortions, it was still well below the theoretical estimate of Malpas. It is not correct to assume that every woman has the same chance of a successful pregnancy after three consecutive abortions, and some individuals will have a much higher risk of abortion than others. It is necessary, therefore, to assess each woman carefully, to determine if there are any therapeutic measures which would improve their chances of successful pregnancy.

INVESTIGATION AFTER RECURRENT ABORTION

The investigations of a woman with recurrent abortion are mainly directed towards those conditions which are potentially amenable to treatment. In the first place, a careful obstetric history should be taken to see if the pattern and timing of the abortions are suggestive of any recurring factor. A history of recurrent mid-trimester abortion after previous surgery on the cervix would suggest the diagnosis of incompetence and cervical cerclage might be helpful in subsequent pregnancies. A uterine abnormality should be looked for by carrying out a hysterosalpingogram and a pelvic examination should be carried out to exclude any obvious gynaecological pathology. Blood should be sent from both parents for chromosome analysis to identify the small number of cases in which a balanced translocation is responsible for recurrent abortion. Blood can also be taken to check for systemic lupus erythematosus or Wilson's disease and a coagulation screen may be indicated if there is a history suggestive of a bleeding disorder; these conditions, however, will rarely be responsible for recurrent abortion.

The exciting new potential area of research is the question of an immunological basis for some cases of recurrent abortion. Although the place of immune factors is not yet fully understood, this aspect may become one which will deserve detailed examination in the future; the problems are discussed more fully in Chapter 21.

General advice can be given to the mother to avoid excessive smoking or alcohol intake and, if there is any suggestion of drug abuse, this will require special management in its own right. If the woman works in an operating theatre or in any situation where she might be exposed to toxins, a change of environment may be suggested.

In addition to investigations, the woman with recurrent abortion wishes to know the chances of a further unsuccessful pregnancy. She may be very despondent about her chances but the prognosis may be better than she realizes. If the previous abortion was known to be due to a chromosomal abnormality, her chances of success in her next pregnancy are better than if a normal karyotype was found (Lauritsen 1976).

Probably the most helpful advice to give a woman who has had recurrent abortions is to report for early assessment in the next pregnancy. Ultrasound can then be used to determine whether a viable pregnancy is or is not established and this will influence further management. There is a great need to offer sympathetic support to both partners because recurrent abortion is an agonizing problem which can place great stress upon a relationship.

INDUCED ABORTION

There is no aspect of obstetrics and gynaecology which has aroused more controversy than termination of pregnancy. This is not surprising because induced abortion cannot be considered in medical terms alone; it arouses strong personal emotions and involves religious and ethical considerations. From the time of Hippocrates, the consensus of medical opinion was opposed to induced abortion but the twentieth century has seen a change in this traditional stance. In the United Kingdom, prior to the 1967 Abortion Act, the law stated that induced abortion was allowed only to protect the life or health of the mother but case law had established that 'health' could be interpreted to include the mental health of the mother. Because the definition of mental health was open to wide differences of opinion, abortions were increasingly carried out on women in deprived circumstances to preserve their mental and physical health. This liberalization of attitude led to a polarization of views for and against abortion, both within and without the medical profession, a situation which exists to the present day.

LEGAL CONSIDERATIONS

In the United Kingdom, the law concerning abortion is governed by the 1967 Abortion Act, which states that abortion is allowed provided that two registered medical practitioners *acting in good faith* agree that one of certain conditions has been fulfilled. The various clauses are as follows. The practitioners have to agree that:

1   the continuance of the pregnancy would involve risk to the life of the pregnant woman greater than if the pregnancy were terminated; or
2   the continuance of the pregnancy would involve risk of injury to the physical or mental health of the pregnant woman greater than if the pregnancy were terminated; or
3   the continuance of the pregnancy would involve risk of injury to the physical or mental health of the existing child(ren) of the family of the pregnant woman greater than if the pregnancy were terminated; or
4   there is a substantial risk that if the child were born it would suffer from such physical or mental abnormalities as to be seriously handicapped.

In circumstances where an emergency procedure is required, only one registered practitioner is required to give his consent to the operation in order to save the life of the pregnant woman or to prevent grave permanent injury to the physical or mental health of the pregnant woman.

Prior to the abortion, the two registered medical practitioners, who take the view that at least one of the criteria for abortion has been met, must certify to this effect on Certificate A. The practitioner who performs the procedure, which must be done in a National Health Service Hospital or other approved place, is required to notify details of the operation, its indications and its complications within 7 days to the Department of Health on the appropriate notification form.

INCIDENCE OF INDUCED ABORTION

Following the introduction of the 1967 Abortion Act, there was a progressive rise in the number of induced abortions for several years until a plateau was reached in the mid-1970s (Fig. 14.1). Since then, however, there has been a much slower increase in the number of abortions. It is, however, notable that the proportion of abortions now being carried out on young, unmarried girls is much greater than before. By far the greatest number of abortions are carried out under the clause which is open to the widest range of possible interpretations, namely the one which permits abortion on the grounds of preserving the mental or physical health of the mother.

The risks to the mother are reduced if the abortion is induced early in the pregnancy, and most terminations are carried out during the first trimester. In some cases, delay is unavoidable and termination is performed in the second trimester but only a very small number (between 1 and 2%) are done after 20 weeks.

INDICATIONS FOR INDUCED ABORTION

Medical indications

The number of abortions which are required to protect the physical health or life of the mother are very few. Termination may be indicated, however, in malignant disease, as for example in carcinoma of the cervix or carcinoma of the breast when the tumour may develop rapidly during pregnancy. Severe cardiac disease may be an indication for pregnancy termination, but this problem is now seen less frequently following the fall in the incidence of rheumatic heart disease. Occasional cases of renal, pulmonary or gastrointestinal disease may necessitate

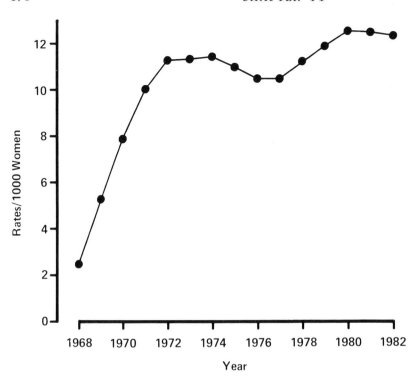

Fig. 14.1. Legal abortions to resident/non-resident women in England and Wales, 1968–82. (Rates/1000 women.)

termination of pregnancy, but the numbers will be very small.

Fetal abnormality
Recent development in the antenatal diagnosis of fetal abnormalities (see also Chapter 22) has widened the indications for induced abortion on the grounds of a serious risk of grave handicap to the baby. Evidence for the possibility of fetal abnormality can come from a variety of different sources (for further details see Chapter 22).

Blood tests. In the past, a serologically confirmed diagnosis of rubella in early pregnancy was the commonest reason for induced abortion on the grounds of fetal abnormality. It is to be hoped that the programmes to immunize schoolgirls who are not immune to rubella will reduce this indication for induced abortion. In addition, women who are found to be not immune during pregnancy, should be offered immunization after delivery.

Screening for neural tube defects. Neural tube defects are the largest group of fetal abnormalities in the

United Kingdom. Many units have instituted a programme of screening with serum alphafetoprotein, particularly in those areas of the country where the incidence is high. Screening should be carried out only with the mother's consent as mothers who have conscientious objection to termination may not wish to participate. The test should be taken at 16–18 weeks and, if a raised level is obtained, further investigation is undertaken to determine if a neural tube defect is present. The first steps are to repeat the serum alphafetoprotein and to carry out a detailed ultrasonic scan of the fetus, paying particular attention to the neural tube. If a neural tube defect is identified, the couple should be informed of the findings and the question of termination discussed. If there is doubt about the findings on the scan amniocentesis can be performed for liquor alphafetoprotein estimation. Some authorities would perform amniocentesis on all women who had two raised levels of serum alphafetoprotein and who did not reveal an explanation for the raised levels on the ultrasonic scan. The raised alphafetoprotein levels may be due to mistaken gestational age, twins or recent threatened abortion.

Amniocentesis. The commonest indication for genetic amniocentesis is maternal age but a past history or a family history of congenital abnormality may indicate the need for investigation. The risk of a live-born chromosomally abnormal child rises with maternal age from a low of 1/1923 at the age of 20, through 1/365 at the age of 35 to a high of 1/25 at the age of 46 years (Hook & Chambers 1977). The commonest abnormality progressing to live birth is Down's syndrome but other chromosomal abnormalities will be detected on chromosomal examination of amniotic fluid cells. Although different age limits have been recommended, it is a common policy to offer amniocentesis to mothers aged 35 years or more. The major disadvantage of amniocentesis is that it establishes the diagnosis of fetal abnormality only in the second trimester so that termination of pregnancy is carried out a relatively late stage. This makes the abortion itself more difficult and more unpleasant for the mother.

Other methods of investigation. In order to overcome the problems of late diagnosis, attempts are being made to obtain trophoblastic tissue at 8–9 weeks gestation. The tissue is obtained through an aspiration cannula which is passed through the cervix under ultrasound control. Although the method shows great promise it is still at the stage of development and certainly carries some risk of inducing abortion. It may prove to be the method of choice to establish the diagnosis in serious fetal conditions such as potential cases of thalassaemia major. Fetoscopy may also be used to investigate the fetus, and fetal blood can be obtained by this method. Further developments are expected in the field of antenatal diagnosis in the next few years.

Welfare of the existing children in the family
At the time of the 1967 Abortion Act, this was a particularly controversial indication for induced abortion. The intention was to help multiparous women in deprived circumstances where they found it difficult to cope with their existing families. Improvements in the family planning services and the increased use of sterilization have reduced completed family size dramatically so that this clause in the Abortion Act is now invoked much less frequently as an indication for abortion.

Mental health of the mother
The great majority of terminations are carried out under the clause which states that the procedure is justified to protect the mental health of the mother. Only a minority of these women have severe mental illness in the sense that they are likely to require treatment by a psychiatrist and criticism has been made of the extensive use of the mental health clause as a ground for termination. On the other hand, there is no doubt that unwanted pregnancy can be a cause of acute emotional distress and, in the days before the 1967 Abortion Act, this was reflected in the large numbers of women who sought the services of an illegal abortionist. One of the benefits of the freer availability of legal abortion is that the horrendous complications of illegal abortion have all but disappeared.

The issue of what constitutes a serious risk to the mental health of the mother is certain to remain a matter of controversy for many years to come.

COUNSELLING

Counselling is an important part of the management of any woman who seeks an induced abortion, whatever may be the reason. The objectives of counselling can be summarized as being: to determine the reason for the abortion request; to discuss the implications; to offer emotional support; to discuss future family planning.

Reason for abortion request
The doctor must determine the reason for an abortion request because without this information, he is unable to certify, in good faith, that the grounds for termination meet the criteria laid down in the 1967 Abortion Act. The subsequent counselling will be greatly influenced by the underlying reason for the request. If the termination is being considered because of maternal illness or suspected fetal abnormality, the medical issues should be explained carefully to the woman and her partner before the final decision is made. If the request is being considered under the clause which considers the welfare of the existing children, it may be appropriate to explore whether the mother can be given practical help and to ensure that she is receiving all the financial benefits to which she is entitled.

The majority of those who seek pregnancy termination do so because their pregnancy is unwanted. Some of the women are already clear in their decision to seek an abortion by the time they consult a doctor but others may be ambivalent. In some cases, outside pressure is being applied, possibly by the father of the pregnancy or by her parents, to make a young girl seek an abortion she does not want. In such cases, all the options should be explained and she should be helped to make the best decision in the circumstances. It is an important part of counselling to ensure that abortions are not carried out on women who do not really want them.

Discussion of the implications

Unwanted pregnancy has long-term implications for the mother whether she has an abortion, places her baby for adoption or keeps the baby herself. If the decision is to carry out a termination, the procedure should be explained so that she will know what to expect. This is particularly important if a mid-trimester abortion is being carried out when the patient will be conscious until the abortion takes place. If the alternatives of adoption or fostering are being considered, or if the patient is planning to keep the child as a single parent, the implications of these options should be discussed with her by a medical social worker. Counselling patients who are seeking an abortion can be very time consuming and the services of a medical social worker with experience in this area can be of enormous value.

Emotional support

Many of the women who seek an induced abortion are young and unmarried. Frequently, they have not discussed their problem with anyone or only with a friend who is equally young and immature. Once again, an experienced medical social worker, or some other non-medical professional, can have a valuable role by giving young girls an opportunity to discuss their feelings. In some cases, there is great anger and resentment because the young girl has been abandoned by her boyfriend when the pregnancy occurred. Although discussion may not alter the final decision to abort the pregnancy, it may help the young patient to come to terms with her feelings. In other cases, a young patient may be afraid of a termination but be seeking the operation because she is even more afraid of telling her parents. Once again, the counsellor may be able to help with this problem.

Following termination of an unwanted pregnancy, many women report a sense of relief that their immediate problem has been solved. Others report feelings of guilt or depression and, if a relationship has already been developed with a sympathetic counsellor, this can be of help.

It is important, also, to remember that women having an abortion because of a fetal abnormality may have a grief reaction, because they have lost a wanted pregnancy. Sometimes, women find it difficult to discuss their feelings with their partners because they, too, are involved. In such cases, sympathetic counselling by a third party may be of considerable value.

Family planning

Many unwanted pregnancies occur because no contraception was used or because contraception was used wrongly. An important part of counselling is to ensure that contraceptive advice is given which is appropriate to the needs of the individual patient.

METHODS OF INDUCED ABORTION

A large variety of methods have been advocated for the induction of abortion and they can be summarized as follows: curettage of the uterus; medical termination; abdominal surgical operation.

Uterine curettage

Suction curettage is the most commonly used method to induce abortion and is particularly appropriate for first trimester pregnancy termination. The operation is carried out either under general anaesthesia or using a paracervical block with the patient in the lithotomy position. The vulva and vagina should be cleaned with an antiseptic solution and an aseptic technique is used. The cervix should be dilated as little as is necessary to perform the procedure and not beyond a size 10 Hegar dilator. An oxytocic drug, such as ergometrine 0.5 mg intravenously, may be given and the suction curette introduced through the cervix. The curette is moved up and down and rotated slowly until it is felt that the uterine contents have been completely evacuated. If there is any doubt about the completeness of the evacuation, the uterine cavity can be explored with either sponge-holding forceps or a blunt curette. Care must be taken to avoid perforation of the uterine fundus. If the uterus is very small, the uterus can be evacuated by conventional curettage without the use of the suction curette.

Although most gynaecologists would limit the use of vaginal termination to first trimester pregnancy, some have employed vaginal termination in the management of second trimester pregnancies. Because of the larger size of the fetus, the bony parts of the fetus may have to be crushed before removal and there is no doubt that many would feel that the procedure had crossed the limit of what they considered to be aesthetically acceptable.

The complications of suction curettage are perforation of the uterus, haemorrhage and infection. If it is suspected that the uterus has been perforated by the suction curette, it is necessary to assess the extent of the damage. It is wise to carry out laparoscopy to inspect the fundus. If the defect is small and there is no active bleeding, no action is necessary. If the termination has not been completed, the operation can proceed under laparoscopic visualization. If the defect is large, if there is active bleeding or if there is any suspicion of injury to bowel, laparotomy must be carried out to repair the damage.

If vaginal bleeding is heavy after suction curettage, ergometrine should be given to promote uterine contraction. If this is unsuccessful, there may be retained products of conception and re-evacuation of the uterus is required. If the uterus is found to be empty and the bleeding persists, the possibility of uterine rupture should be considered and laparoscopy or laparotomy will be necessary. Infection is a potential consequence of suction termination, particularly if evacuation was incomplete. Any suggestion of infection should be investigated and treated, as required, with antibiotics. Pelvic infection carries a potential risk of tubal blockage and subsequent infertility but, in practice, the incidence of such a drastic outcome is probably very low (WHO Task Force, 1979).

Medical termination of pregnancy
In the second trimester, it is usual to employ an oxytocic drug to induce uterine contractions and thereby expel the fetus through a dilated cervix. At the same time, especially in termination after 16 weeks, a toxic solution may be introduced into the amniotic cavity to induce fetal death. Local prostaglandins have been used to soften the cervix prior to suction curettage in first trimester pregnancies but this method has not yet attracted widespread use.

The most commonly used oxytocic to induce abortion is one of the prostaglandins, usually either prostaglandin E_2 or $F_2\alpha$, although other agents which are usually one of the other prostaglandin derivatives, are also effective. The prostaglandins can be administered intra-amniotically, extra-amniotically, directly to the cervix or into the posterior vaginal fornix. The extra-amniotic route is more favoured up to 14 weeks because it may be difficult to gain access to the amniotic cavity at this stage. One recommended regime is to insert a Foley catheter through the cervix and the tip of the catheter is retained in the extra-amniotic space once the balloon of the catheter has been inflated. Prostaglandin E_2 is infused by a continuous slow-infusion pump adjusting the dose according to the uterine response. In the majority of cases, abortion will occur within about 12–18 hours and the patient taken to theatre for uterine evacuation to ensure that the cavity is empty.

Once the pregnancy has reached 15 weeks or more, it is usually possible to carry out intra-amniotic prostaglandin termination. At the same time, it is usual to instil a toxic agent such as Ureaphil® into the amniotic cavity to induce fetal death. After removing about 60 ml of amniotic fluid, an equivalent volume of Ureaphil is injected into the amniotic cavity followed by 10 units of prostaglandin E_2 in 1 ml. This is usually a highly effective regime and abortion usually follows within a few hours. Many variations on the above methods have been described but the success rates seem broadly comparable.

In the past, intra-amniotic glucose and hypertonic saline were frequently employed but have lost favour because of the risks of infection, hypernatraemia and disseminated intravascular coagulation. Medical termination of pregnancy also carries the risks of uterine rupture, haemorrhage and infection as described in the section on suction curettage. If prostaglandins are inadvertently infused into a blood vessel, there may be an acute hypotensive reaction. Fortunately, prostaglandins are rapidly removed from the circulation and the effect will be shortlived. Until she recovers, the patient should be put in the left lateral position and the end of the bed raised until the blood pressure recovers.

Abdominal surgical termination
Hysterotomy was once a common method of termination in mid-trimester pregnancies when tubal ligation was being performed at the same time. Hysterotomy was not recommended in women who had not completed their families because of the risk of subsequent uterine rupture. The complications associated with hysterotomy were greater than with other methods of termination and the operation is now performed much less commonly. In rare cases, when there is some associated pathology such as carcinoma of the cervix, termination may be accompanied by hysterectomy.

MATERNAL MORTALITY FROM ABORTION

Abortion was, until recent years, one of the most important causes of maternal mortality. Many of the deaths were associated with illegal abortion but these have now fallen to very low levels (Fig. 14.2) as

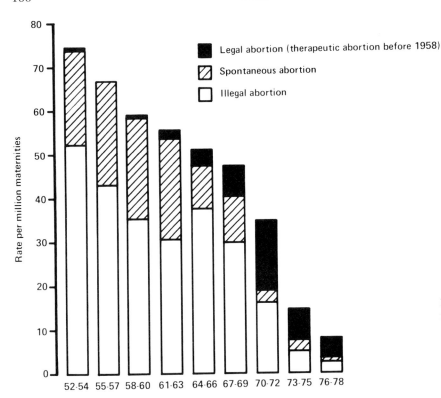

Fig. 14.2. Death rate per million maternities from abortion 1952–1978. (From *Report on Confidential Enquiries into Maternal Deaths in England and Wales, 1976–1978.*)

shown by the results from the Confidential Enquiry into Maternal Deaths in England and Wales 1976–1978. Following the 1967 Abortion Act, there was an acceleration in the decline in maternal deaths despite an increased number of deaths following legal abortion. In the triennium 1976–1978, the number of deaths from abortion had fallen to a total of 14, which was a rate of 7.4 per million maternities.

ECTOPIC PREGNANCY

Ectopic pregnancy is a major problem in gynaecology because it is often difficult to diagnose and is associated with increased risks of mortality and impaired fertility. Although the number of women who have died from ectopic pregnancy has dropped by half since 1964, the death rate has remained steady since 1972; 21 women died from ectopic pregnancy in the years between 1976 and 1978 and thus constituted 10% of all maternal deaths in England and Wales (Confidential Enquiry into Maternal Deaths 1976–1978), see Table 14.3 In some of the deaths, there were avoidable factors due to failure to investigate fully or to errors in the treatment of the bleeding so that careful clinical management is of paramount importance. Although the incidence in the United Kingdom is generally considered to be of the order of 1 per 300 mature intrauterine pregnancies the incidence of ectopic pregnancy has almost doubled in the

Table 14.3. The number of women who died from ectopic pregnancy 1952–78 (From the *Report on Confidential Enquiries into Maternal Deaths in England and Wales 1976–1978*)

Triennia	1952–1954	1955–1957	1958–1960	1961–1963	1964–1966	1967–1969	1970–1972	1973–1975	1976–1978
Maternal deaths from ectopic pregnancy	59	42	28	42	42	32	34	21	21
Registrar General's figures	78	62	42	50	49	39	36	22	21

Western World since the mid-1960s (Kadar 1983); in other communities, ectopic pregnancy is much commoner as, for example, in the West Indies where the incidence is 1 in 28 (Douglas 1963). An ectopic pregnancy is not merely an isolated episode in a woman's life. She has only a 1 in 3 chance of subsequently having a live child but a 5 to 10% chance of having another ectopic pregnancy (Grant 1972, Kitchin et al. 1979).

The site is the Fallopian tube in over 95% of cases. It may, however, be in the uterus (intramural, angular, cervical or in a rudimentary horn), the ovary, the broad ligament or elsewhere in the peritoneal cavity. These latter sites are usually secondary attachments, after extrusion from the tube. Unless stated, subsequent comments can be taken to refer to tubal pregnancy.

AETIOLOGY

It is self-evident that the condition is due to implantation of the fertilized ovum in an abnormal site. It is a matter for debate whether this is due to the tube offering a particular enticement to the ovum to implant or whether the ovum's passage has been delayed till it is at the stage for implantation and it merely 'chooses' the nearest site. The weight of evidence favours the second mechanism being the common one. The precise way in which it is brought about varies in different races and communities at different times.

Pelvic inflammatory disease
Pelvic inflammatory disease (PID) is widely regarded as the most important aetiological factor (Kleiner & Roberts 1967). In the United Kingdom the rates ·of gonorrhoea and acute salpingitis have risen sharply in the past two decades (Adler 1980), and these conditions may have contributed to the increased number of ectopic pregnancies. Tuberculous salpingitis used to be a common predisposing factor but its dwindling incidence now makes it relatively unimportant in the United Kingdom. Tissue damage from pelvic inflammation, whatever its nature, can remove the ciliated epithelium within the tube, which is so important in ovum transport. The peristaltic tubal action is also impaired and it is not difficult to appreciate how the normal progress of the fertilized ovum may be impeded.

Although there is gross or histological evidence of past pelvic infection in 30–50% of cases of ectopic pregnancy (Hallatt 1968; Westrom et al. 1981), the relationship between PID and ectopic pregnancy is not absolute. Although the overall incidence of PID has risen in recent years, the rates of increase of PID do not correlate well with the increase of ectopic pregnancy within different regions, age groups or time periods (Beral 1975). On the other hand, a cohort study in Lund, Sweden, found a much higher incidence of ectopic pregnancy in women who had laparoscopically proven PID compared with controls (Westrom et al. 1981). The data suggest that, although pelvic inflammation is an important contributor to ectopic pregnancy, other aetiological factors also operate to confound the picture.

Intrauterine contraceptive devices
If a woman with an intrauterine contraceptive device (IUCD) conceives a pregnancy, she has a high chance of an ectopic gestation. Under these circumstances, the ratio of ectopic to intrauterine pregnancies is increased by about seven times compared with conceptions in the absence of a device (Vessey et al. 1974). There is, however, controversy about the effect of IUCDs on the absolute number of ectopic pregnancies.

Methods of contraception, such as the pill and the barrier methods, which prevent fertilization will simultaneously reduce the number of intrauterine and ectopic pregnancies. On the other hand, IUCDs which may act by preventing intrauterine implantation of the fertilized ovum, might be expected to have no effect on the number of tubal pregnancies; indeed, if the IUCD interferes with tubal motility, a real increase in the number of ectopic pregnancies is theoretically possible. Lehfeldt et al. (1970) studied the number of inadvertent pregnancies in 30 000 women using an IUCD during approximately 45 000 women-years. During that time period, they calculated that 895 tubal pregnancies would have occurred without contraception, which compared favourably with the observed number of 40 tubal pregnancies in IUCD users. They concluded that IUCDs reduced the number of intrauterine pregnancies by 99.5% and the number of ectopic pregnancies by 95%.

The theoretical calculations of Lehfeldt et al. (1970) are, however, open to criticism on the grounds that IUCD users are usually women of proven normal fertility and, therefore, likely to have a lower incidence of pelvic inflammation. Thus, it is inappropriate to compare the ectopic pregnancy rates in IUCD users with the total population. After considering all the confounding variables, a Steering Committee of a WHO Task Force concluded, in 1978, that there was a real increase in the risk of ectopic pregnancy among IUCD users (Aznar et al. 1978). Since then there have been further studies, including a multi-centre case control study in the United States (Ory 1981), which have failed to confirm an increased risk of ectopic pregnancy in IUCD users. It is true that women who use oral contraceptives have a reduced risk of ectopic pregnancy as compared with IUCD users, but this is a protective effect of the pill rather than an increased risk from the IUCD. The general opinion is that the increased incidence of ectopic pregnancy in the Western World cannot be accounted for on the basis of IUCD usage (Sivin 1979, Westrom et al. 1981, Ory 1981).

Progestogen contraception
Some reports have suggested that oral progestogen-only contraception may carry an increased risk of ectopic pregnancy (Bonnar 1974, Liukko et al. 1977) although the evidence is certainly not conclusive. On the other hand, there is stronger evidence that when progestogens are added to intrauterine contraceptive devices, there is a real increase in ectopic pregnancy rates; the ectopic pregnancy rates are higher in women with these devices as compared with the rates in women who are wearing inert devices or using no contraception (Snowden 1977, Diaz et al. 1980). The mechanism of the increased risk is not known although the progestogens may have an inhibitory effect on tubal mobility which encourages a delay in transport and tubal implantation of the fertilized ovum.

Other factors
Other mechanisms which may contribute to tubal pregnancy are previous tubal ligation, and Wolf and Thomson (1980) reported that 7.4% of ectopic pregnancies were in women who had been sterilized. Reversal of tubal ligation is also associated with ectopic pregnancy as the fertilized ovum may be arrested at the site of re-anastomosis. Another theory is that of transperitoneal migration of the ovum (Berlind 1960). Schiffer (1963) found that in 21 out of 91 salpingo-oophorectomies for ectopic pregnancy, there was no corpus luteum in the ovary from the side of the ectopic pregnancy. The assumption is that the ovum came from the opposite ovary but the theory is difficult to substantiate.

CLINICAL FEATURES

Ectopic pregnancy can progress in a number of different ways. The tube may rupture or tubal abortion may occur with the gestational sac being extruded through the abdominal ostium into the peritoneal cavity. Less commonly, a tubal mole may form when there is separation of the dead conceptus from the tubal wall by layers of blood clot. The rarest outcome of all is secondary abdominal pregnancy, when partial tubal rupture occurs with the conceptus surviving and the trophoblast gaining an attachment to some other structure, such as the broad ligament or omentum.

Presentation and diagnosis
The problem of ectopic pregnancy is essentially a diagnostic one. The first feature is usually pain and this is present in 95% of cases; there is some delay in the onset of an expected period in 75% of patients followed by abnormal vaginal bleeding. Syncope may also occur. The pattern may vary greatly and the categories considered in detail below represent the commoner types.

The presentation of ectopic gestation may be acute, silent or subacute. The acute presentation is easily recognizable. It is associated with tubal rupture and massive intraperitoneal haemorrhage leading to acute abdominal pain and cardiovascular collapse. There may or may not have been some premonitory menstrual disturbance with syncope and local pain as described below under 'subacute'. Shoulder-tip or interscapular pain may be present. On examination, hypotension and tachycardia are the rule, although bradycardia is occasionally found. Generalized abdominal rigidity and rebound tenderness are present. Vaginal examination at this stage is scarcely necessary and may be unrewarding. There will usually be generalized pelvic tenderness, but the side in which the gestation has been situated may be more tender. This acute presentation without warning is particularly liable to occur if the gestation is at the utero–tubal junction.

'Silent ectopics' occasionally are detected when the patient attends the antenatal clinic for booking. Localized tenderness is elicited in one fornix, possibly with a swelling, and although there have been no symptoms other than those of pregnancy, this finding is enough to raise a high level of suspicion and may have lain dormant for a long time without detection.

It is in the subacute group that the great diagnostic problems arise. There will usually have been some vaginal bleeding, but this is generally a late and secondary feature; there is no constant pattern to the loss. Syncopal attacks may occur. The precise mechanism of these in the prehaemorrhagic state is not clear. Some degree of pain is usually the first symptom, but its degree and nature can be very variable. If free blood is in the peritoneum, referred shoulder pain may be experienced. Less well documented but frequently helpful is referred discomfort from blood in the pouch of Douglas. This may cause pain on defaecation or perineal discomfort—manifest as inability to sit square on a hard seat.

Lower abdominal tenderness and guarding may be present. On bimanual examination localized tenderness is the most significant feature. This may be in the lateral or posterior fornix. A mass may or may not be palpable. At an initial out-patient examination the patient's general apprehension and tension may interfere with localization of tenderness.

It is important to bear in mind that ectopic gestation can be simultaneously bilateral or may coincide with an intrauterine gestation.

THE SUSPECTED ECTOPIC PREGNANCY

The great clinical problem is what to do when the suspicion of ectopic pregnancy has been raised by some feature of history or examination yet the diagnosis cannot be made with confidence. The doctor cannot relax until he has clarified the situation with reasonable certainty one way or another.

The introduction of laparoscopy has greatly simplified the task of establishing the diagnosis in suspected ectopic pregnancy. The procedure is much less traumatic to the patient than laparotomy and allows the diagnosis to be made with accuracy. There is evidence that laparoscopy has improved the management of ectopic pregnancy; for example, Samuelson and Sjovall (1972) reported that, when laparoscopy was introduced on a regular basis, the proportion of ectopic pregnancies in which the diagnosis was delayed beyond a week fell from 32% to 5%. In experienced hands, the risks of laparoscopy are small but it is understandable that efforts have been made to develop non-invasive tests which could make the diagnosis with certainty.

Ultrasound is commonly used in the assessment of patients who have early pregnancy bleeding. The demonstration of a viable intrauterine pregnancy makes ectopic pregnancy very unlikely, although it is important to distinguish a pseudogestational sac which can occur in tubal pregnancy from a genuine intrauterine pregnancy. Pedersen (1980) found that adnexal or cul-de-sac masses were detectable by ultrasound in over 90% of cases of ectopic pregnancy, suggesting that negative findings made ectopic pregnancy unlikely. In very early pregnancy, an ectopic gestation may not be detected by ultrasound during the initial stages, so that a negative scan does not rule out the diagnosis with certainty (Kadar et al. 1983).

Standard urinary pregnancy tests for HCG are of relatively little value because they are frequently negative when an ectopic pregnancy is present and may be positive when there is not. There is some help when the pregnancy test is positive, because, in the presence of suspicious clinical signs, this is an additional factor indicating the need for further investigation by laparoscopy. There is more hope that the β sub-unit of HCG may be a more reliable indicator of ectopic pregnancy because some workers have shown that, using this test, there are very few false negative results (see Kadar 1983). Kadar et al. (1981) suggest, that if the serum HCG is above 6500 miu/ml and there is no intrauterine pregnancy on scan, this is indicative of ectopic pregnancy. Clearly this approach looks promising but will have to be more widely evaluated before it is generally accepted. One problem may be the provision of a rapid HCG assay service on a 7-day basis which would be required by the practising clinician.

Other aids to diagnosis have been used in the past, but, as laparoscopy has been more and more widely introduced, these are likely to disappear. The most frequently employed is needling of the Pouch of Douglas and the presence of non-clottable blood is very suggestive of ectopic pregnancy. The false positive rate of culdocentesis is, however, as high as 26% (Halpin 1970) and the test will not indicate ectopic pregnancy prior to the stage of intraperitoneal bleeding. Examination under anaesthesia is of no value because the ectopic pregnancy may not be palpable and there is a danger of rupturing the tube and causing severe haemorrhage. Although it is obviously necessary to avoid excessive use of laparoscopy, it is likely to remain the most valuable diagnostic aid for the gynaecologist who is presented with clinical problem of the 'suspected ectopic'.

TREATMENT

As soon as the diagnosis is made immediate operative treatment is essential. Difficulties arise in relation to the patients presenting with acute collapse due to massive intraperitoneal bleeding. These patients are often so ill that the anaesthetist is unhappy about administering an anaesthetic, yet no matter how rapidly blood is transfused it does not exceed the rate of intraperitoneal loss. In this situation conservatism holds no hope and the gynaecologist must persuade his anaesthetist colleague that the only prospect for the patient's survival lies in getting her to theatre as quickly as possible, opening the abdomen and arresting the source of the bleeding.

The appropriate action is to set up an intravenous infusion capable of taking a rapid flow of blood and blood, not saline or a blood substitute, should be given as quickly as possible. If the arm veins are collapsed, as may be the case, a major vein elsewhere must be used without hesitation. In the most critical cases little or no anaesthetic may be necessary.

With maximum speed the surgeon should make a vertical, mid-line subumbilical incision. Then, in the words of Lawson Tait of Birmingham, who performed the first successful operation for ectopic gestation in the 1880s, 'make at once for the source of the haemorrhage, the broad ligament, tie it at its base and then remove the ovum and debris at leisure'. Blood should be given as rapidly as possible and the patient's condition should improve immediately. Where adequate supplies of donor blood are not available, autotransfusion of blood collected from the peritoneal cavity may be lifesaving (Douglas 1963).

Type of operative procedure
Following the problem of immediate arrest of haemorrhage and resuscitation is the matter of precisely what should be done surgically. There is, however, divergence of opinion in this regard. In the early days of ectopic surgery, removal of tube and ovary was standard. Then with the Bonney era of ovarian conservation it came to be accepted that, if possible, it was right to conserve the ovary and merely perform salpingectomy. Some have pressed this further and advocated that as far as possible the tube affected should be conserved.

Jeffcoate (1955), however, pronounced a fundamentally different approach. He suggested that if the opposite appendage was normal the ovary related to the affected tube should be removed. Jeffcoate's reasoning was that:
1   ova released from the contralateral ovary will only rarely undergo transperitoneal migration and reach the opposite tube;
2   approximately half the ova are released from each ovary, and in a woman with a single tube the

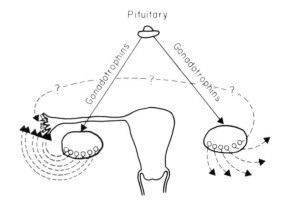
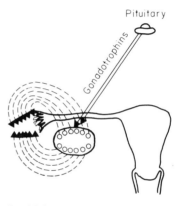

Fig. 14.3. Diagrammatic representation of the theoretical benefits of salpingo-ophorectomy as compared with salpingectomy. With salpingectomy approximately 50% of subsequent ovulations will take place from the tubeless ovary so that fertilization will occur only if transperitoneal migration takes place. If that ovary is removed, all subsequent ovulations occur from the ovary with an associated tube. (From Jeffcoate 1967.)

chances of conception would be as much as doubled if it could be arranged that each ovulation occurred from the ipselateral ovary;
3   removing the ovary with the Fallopian tube secures this effect, as the monthly pituitary stimulus for ovulation will subsequently always affect the remaining ovary which has a tube in direct relationship (Fig. 14.3).

Although the hypothetical arguments appear good, it has not been established that salpingo-oophorectomy improves the results of salpingectomy alone. Douglas *et al.* (1969) reported that, although salpingo-oophorectomy increased the conception rate, the number of subsequent live births was the same with the two procedures. In general terms, it is a bad principle to remove ovarian tissue unless it confers a clear benefit to the patient and salpingectomy is preferred by many gynaecologists to the more destructive operation of salpingo-oophorectomy. The most important factor in determining the subsequent chance of a normal intrauterine pregnancy is the health of the contralateral tube. This should be inspected before salpingectomy is carried out because, if it is grossly diseased, the question of conservative surgery to preserve the affected tube must be considered. The ectopic pregnancy may be removed after linear salpingostomy and the opening reconstituted (De Cherney & Kase 1979). There is no doubt that conservative surgery carries a high risk of recurrent ectopic pregnancy but it may give the woman her only chance of a successful pregnancy. In many cases, tubal patency is preserved and successful pregnancies have been reported (Jarvinen *et al.* 1972, De Cherney & Kase 1979). When the gestation is cornual or angular, hysterectomy will frequently be necessary or, at the least, cornual resection.

Abdominal pregnancy

A difficult obstetric problem, one to which there is no completely effective answer, is the extrauterine pregnancy which presents at an advanced stage. Though very rare in Europe, Dixon and Stewart (1960) reported ten cases occurring in relation to less than ten thousand deliveries in the West Indies. Even in modern times mortality rates range from 2 to 10% (Drury 1960, Hreshchyshyn *et al.* 1961). The condition is usually suspected by persistent abnormal fetal lie and easy palpation of fetal parts. The uterus may be felt separate from the fetus and may be enlarged by the hormonal influence to several times its normal size. There may be a history of pain early in pregnancy, representing the time of transfer of the attachment from tube to peritoneum. Abdominal discomfort may persist and slight bleeding may occur.

Radiological examination may reveal shadows of maternal intestinal gas superimposed on the fetus (Figs. 14.4[a] and 14.4[b]). A Syntocinon infusion may be employed to stimulate uterine contraction.

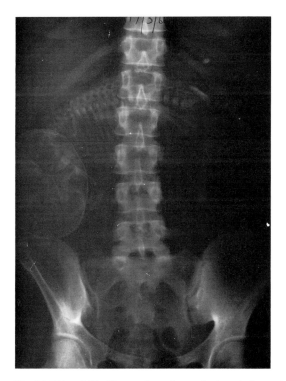 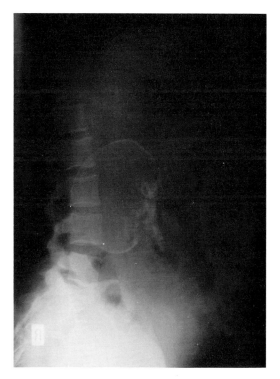

Fig. 14.4(a) and (b). X-rays of an advanced extra-uterine gestation. Note the absence of uterine contour, distorted fetal position, maternal bowel gas shadows over the fetus and, in the lateral projection, fetal skull superimposed upon the maternal spine (Photographs by courtesy of Mr G.A. Craig and Dr P.P. Franklyn.)

This will, of course, only be helpful in that if the uterus is felt to contract around the fetus, ectopic pregnancy can be excluded. Thermography, arteriography and hysterography may all give help, but the latter can be justified only when the diagnosis is virtually certain. Ultrasound can demonstrate the fetus outside the uterus.

As soon as the diagnosis is made operation is usually advisable. Very rarely it may be justified to continue the pregnancy for a short time to enable the fetus to have a more reasonable chance of survival.

The great problem at operation is whether or not to remove the placenta. Interference with it may lead to uncontrollable haemorrhage. If it is left *in situ*, the morbidity from abscess formation is high but it is usually the procedure of choice. It must be a matter for the judgement of the individual operator whether or not removal can safely be undertaken in any given case depending upon the accessibility for ligation of the maternal vessels supplying the area. Methotrexate has been used in an attempt to inactivate the trophoblast rapidly when the placenta has been left in position (Hreschchyshyn *et al.* 1965, Lathrop & Bowles 1968) and it has been suggested it be used before operation if the baby is known to be dead.

The baby delivered from an extrauterine sac often shows pressure malformation related to the lack of protection provided by the uterus; oligohydramnios seems to be the rule in these cases.

REFERENCES

Adler M.W. (1980). *Amer. J. Obstet. Gynec.*, **138**, 901.
Aznar R., Berry C.L., Cooke I.D., Cuadros A., Gray R., McNicol G.P., Newton J.R., Pizarro E., Rowe P.J., Shaw S.T., Wagatewa T., Webb F. & Wilson E. (1978). *Brit. Med. J.*, **1**, 786.
Beral V. (1975). *Brit. J. Obstet. Gynaecol.*, **82**, 775.
Berlind M. (1960). *Obstet. Gynecol.*, **16**, 51.
Bonar J. (1974). *Brit. Med. J.*, **i**, 287.
Boué J., Boué A. & Lazar P. (1975). *Teratology*, **12**, 11.
Chartier M., Roger M., Barrat J. & Michelon B. (1979) *Fertil. Steril.*, **31**, 134.
Cousins L. (1980) *Clin. Obstet. Gynecol.*, **23**, 467.
Covell G. (1950) *Trop. Dis. Bull.*, **47**, 1147.
Creasy M.R., Crolla J.A. & Alberman E.D. (1976) *Hum. Genet.*, **31**, 177.
Csapo A.I., Pulkkinen M.O. & Wiest W.G. (1973) *Amer. J. Obstet. Gynec.*, **115**, 759.
Daling J.R. & Emanuel I. (1975) *Lancet* ii, 170.
De Cherney A.H. & Kase N. (1979) *Obstet. Gynecol.*, **54**, 451.

Diaz S., Croxatto H.B., Pavez M., Quintepos E., Carrillo D., Simonetti L., Croxatto H.-D. & Rosati S. (1980) *Contraception*, **22**, 259.
Dixon H.G. & Stewart D.B. (1960). *Brit. Med. J.*, **ii**, 1103.
Douglas C.P. (1963). *Brit. Med. J.*, **ii**, 838.
Douglas E.S., Shingleton H.M. & Corst T. (1969) *S. Med. J.*, **62**, 954.
Drury K.A.D. (1960) *J. Obstet. Gynaec. Brit. Cwlth.*, **67**, 455.
Editorial (1980) *Lancet*, **ii**, 188.
Ekman G., Forman A., Ulmsten V. & Wingerup L. (1980). *Zbl. Gynakol.*, **102**, 219.
Embrey, M.P., Calder A.A. & Hillier K. (1974) *J. Obstet. Gynaec. Brit. Cwlth.*, **81**, 47.
French, F.E. & Bierman J.M. (1962) *Public Health Rep.*, **77**, 835.
Goldzieher J.W. (1964) *J. Amer. Med. Assoc.*, **188**, 651.
Grant A. (1962). *Clin. Obstet. Gynecol.*, **5**, 861.
Hallatt J.G. (1976) *Amer. J. Obstet. Gynec.*, **125**, 725.
Halpin J. (1970) *Amer. J. Obstet. Gynec.*, **106**, 227.
Harlap S., Shiono P.H. & Ramcharan S. (1980) In *Embryonic and Fetal Death* (Porter I.H., Hook, E.B., eds.). p145, Academic Press, New York.
Hay D. (1958) *J. Obstet. Gynaecol. Brit. Emp.*, **65**, 557.
Heinonen P.K., Saarikoski S. & Pystynen P. (1982) *Acta Obstet. Gynecol. Scand.*, **61**, 157.
Himmelberger D.U., Brown B.W. & Cohen E.N. (1978) *Amer. J. Epidemiol.*, **108**, 470.
Huisjes, H.J. (1984) In *Spontaneous Abortion* (series ed. T. Lind) *Current Review in Obstetrics and Gynaecology*, Churchill Livingstone, Edinburgh.
Hulka J.F. & Higgins G. (1961) *Amer. J. Obstet. Gynec.*, **82**, 913.
Hook E.B. & Chambers G.M. (1977) *Birth Defects*, **13** (13A), 124.
Hreshchyshyn M.M., Bogen B. & Loughran C.H. (1961) *Amer. J. Obstet. Gynec.*, **81**, 302.
Hreshchyshyn M.M. Naples J.D. & Randall C.L. (1965). *Amer J. Obstet. Gynec.*, **93**, 286.
Jarvinen P.A., Nummi S. & Pietila K. (1972) *Acta Obstet. Gynecol. Scand.*, **51**, 169.
Jeffcoate T.N.A. (1955). *J. Obstet. Gynaecol. Brit. Cwlth.*, **62**, 214.
Jones G.S. (1976) *Fertil. Steril.*, **27**, 351.
Jones J.M., Sweetnam P. & Hibbard B. (1979) *Brit. J. Obstet. Gynaecol.*, **86**, 913.
Kadar N., Devore G. & Romero R. (1981) *Obstet. Gynecol.*, **58**, 156.
Kadar N. (1983) In *Progress in Obstetrics and Gynaecology*, Vol 3 (Studd J. ed.) P 305, Churchill Livingstone, Edinburgh.
Kaufman R.H., Binder G.L., Gray P.M. & Adam E. (1977) *Amer. J. Obstet. Gynec.*, **128**, 51.
Kitchin J.D., Wein R.M., Nunley W.C., Thiagarajah S. & Thornton W.N. (1979). *Amer. J. Obstet. Gynec.*, **134**, 870.
Klee J.G. (1979) *Lancet* ii, 423.
Kleiner G.J. & Roberts T.W. (1967). *Amer. J. Obstet. Gynec.*, **99**, 21.

KLINE J., STEIN Z., SUSSER M. & WARBURTON D. (1980a). *Amer. J. Epidemiol.*, **107**, 290.

KLINE J., SHROUT P., STEIN Z., SUSSER M. & WARBURTON D. (1980b) *Lancet* ii, 1976.

KLOPPER A. & MACNAUGHTON M.C. (1965). *J. Obstet. Gynaec. Brit. Cwlth.*, **72**, 1022.

LATHROP J.C. & BOWLES G.E. (1968) *Obstet. Gynecol.*, **32**, 81.

LAURITSEN J.G. (1976) *Acta Obstet. Gynecol. Scand. (Supp.)*, **52**, 1.

LEHFELDT H., TIETZE C. & GORSTEIN F. (1970) *Amer. J. Obstet. Gynec.*, **108**, 1005.

LEIMAN G., HARRISON N.A. & RUBIN A. (1980) *Amer. J. Obstet. Gynec.*, **136**, 14.

LIUKKO P., ERKKOLA R. & LAASKO L. (1977) *Contraception*, **16**, 575.

LIVINGSTON J.E. & POLAND B.J. (1980) *Teratology*, **21**, 139.

MACHENRY J.C.R.M., NEVIN N.C. & MERRETT J.D. (1979). *Brit. med. J.*, **i**, 1395.

MALL E.P. (1917) *Amer. J. Anat.*, **22**, 27.

MALPAS P. (1938) *J. Obstet. Gynaecol. Brit. Emp.*, **45**, 932.

MANGAN C.E., BOROW L., BURTNETT-RUBIN M.M., EGAN V., GINNTOLT R.L. & MIKUTA J.J. (1982) *Obstet. Gynecol.*, **59**, 315.

MCDONALD I.A. (1957) *J. Obstet. Gynaecol. Brit. Emp.*, **63**, 346.

MCDONALD I.A. (1980) *Clin. Obstet. Gynecol.*, **7**, 461.

MEDICAL RESEARCH COUNCIL (1978). *Suppl. 2, Brit. J. Obstet. Gynaecol.*, **85**,

MILLER J.F., WILLIAMSON E., GLUE J., GORDON Y.G., GRUDZINSKAS J.G. & SYKES A. (1980) *Lancet*, **ii**, 554.

NAYLOR A.F. & WARBURTON D. (1979) *Fertil. Steril.*, **31**, 282.

ORY H.W. (1981) *Obstet. Gynecol.*, **57**, 137.

PEDERSEN J.F. (1980) *Brit. J. Radiol.*, **53**, 625.

POLAND B.J., MILLER J.R., JONES D.C. & TRIMBLE B.K. (1977) *Amer. J. Obstet. Gynec.*, **127**, 685.

REPORT ON CONFIDENTIAL ENQUIRIES INTO MATERNAL DEATHS IN ENGLAND AND WALES 1976–1978 (1982) HMSO, London.

RESSEGUIE L.J. (1974). *Hum. Biol.*, **46**, 633.

ROTH D.B. (1963) *Int. J. Fertil.*, **8**, 434.

RUSH R.W., ISAACS S., MCPHERSON K., JONES L., CHALMERS I. & GRANT A. (1984) *Brit. J. Obstet. Gynaecol.*, **91**, 724.

SAMUELSON S. & SJOVALL A. (1972) *Acta Obstet. Gynecol. Scand.*, **51**, 31.

SCHIFFER M.A. (1963) *Amer. J. Obstet. Gynec.*, **86**, 264.

SHAPIRO S., LEVINE H.S. & ABRAMOWICZ M. (1963) *Advances in Planned Parenthood*, **6**, 45.

SHEARMAN R.P. & GARRETT W.J. (1963) *Brit. med. J.*, **i**, 292.

SIVIN I. (1979) *Contraception* **19**, 151.

SNOWDEN R. (1977) *Brit. med. J.*, **2**, 1600.

SPENCE A.A. (1981) *Int. Anesthesiol. Clin.*, **19**, 165.

THO P.T., BYRD J.R. & MCDONOUGH P.G. (1979) *Fertil. Steril.*, **32**, 389.

VESSEY M.P., JOHNSON B., DOLL R. & PETO R. (1974). *Lancet*, **i**, 495.

VESSEY M.P. & NUNN J.F. (1980). *Brit. med. J.*, **281**, 696.

WALLENBURG H.C.S., KEIRSE M.J.N.C., FREIE H.M.P. & BLACQUIERE J.P. (1980) *Brit. J. Obstet. Gynaecol.*, **87**, 203.

WALSHE J.M. (1977) *Q. J. Med.*, **46**, 73.

WARBURTON D. & FRASER F.C. (1964) *Hum. Genet.*, **16**, 1.

WARREN C.W., GOLD J., TYLER C.W., SMITH J.C., PARIS A.L. (1980) *Amer. J. Public Health*, **70**, 1297.

WESTROM L., BENGTSSON L.P.H. & MARDH P.A. (1981). *Brit. med. J.*, **1**, 15.

WHITTAKER P.G., TAYLOR A. & LIND T. (1983) *Lancet*, **i**, 1126.

WHO TASK FORCE ON SEQUELAE OF ABORTION (1979) *Lancet*, **i**, 142.

WILKINS L. (1960) *J. Amer. Med. Assoc.*, **172**, 1028.

WOLF G.C. & THOMPSON N.J. (1980) *Obstet. Gynecol.*, **55**, 17.

WRIGHT C.S.W., CAMPBELL S. & BEAZLEY J. (1972) *Lancet*, **i**, 1278.

YOSHIMI T., STROTT C.A., MARSHALL J.R. & LIPSETT M.B. (1969) *J. Clin. Endocrinol. Metab.*, **29**, 225.

CHAPTER 15
ANTEPARTUM HAEMORRHAGE

J. S. SCOTT

Antepartum haemorrhage (APH) is still one of the gravest obstetric emergencies, though thanks to improved obstetric care the maternal mortality due to haemorrhage has dropped from 220 in the 3-year period 1952–4 to 26 in 1976–78. Eight of these were due to antepartum haemorrhage, 3.5% of the total deaths (*Report on Confidential Enquiries into Maternal Deaths in England and Wales*, 1982). To maintain and improve upon this advance it is essential to be continually alert to the possibility of severe APH and familiar with the appropriate action to deal with the problems that arise. Unlike postartum haemorrhage, which is always preceded by the adequate warning mechanism of labour, APH often occurs without warning. With dramatic suddenness a pregnant patient can become exsanguinated to the point of death. The perinatal mortality is also considerable, and if bleeding occurred at any time in pregnancy, regardless of its cause, the perinatal mortality was found to be elevated more than threefold—60.1 per thousand compared with 16.8 per thousand in non-bleeders (*British Births 1970* Vol. 2 1978). With placental abruption it was as high as 143.6 per thousand.

DEFINITION AND CLASSIFICATION

APH is here defined as haemorrhage from the genital tract after the twenty-eighth week of pregnancy but before delivery of the baby. The 28-week limit is arbitrary, related to the British legal definition of viability of the child. Precisely the same pathological types of haemorrhage can occur before 28 weeks. Severe bleeding is relatively rare then, but when it does occur the treatment is often less intensive as it is regarded lightly as a mere threatened abortion and immediate delivery for the sake of the fetus is not contemplated (Baker & Dewhurst 1963, Kinch *et al.* 1969).

Cases are sometimes divided according to the an-atomic origin of the blood into 'true' APH when from the placental site and 'false' when from lower in the genital tract. This is a distinction which is not of practical importance initially, for it must be assumed that every vaginal blood loss before delivery is coming from the placenta and appropriate action taken. If it eventually becomes clear that the condition is not one of the classical types of placental bleeding, then consideration of other possible pathology, particularly cervical, becomes appropriate.

Edward Rigby (1775) distinguished between *inevitable* APH occurring in association with a low-lying placenta and chance or *accidental* occurrence of haemorrhage from a normally situated placenta. This was a great advance in obstetric thinking. Unfortunately, 'inevitable' haemorrhage came to be spoken of as *placenta praevia*, while 'accidental' retained its name. The term 'accidental' when not opposed to 'inevitable' suggests a relationship to trauma, which is practically never present, and this has led to confusion of thought.

The current tendency is to use the clearly descriptive term *placental abruption* introduced by Couvelaire to describe the serious form of haemorrhage which may occur from the decidual attachment of a normally implanted placenta. This type of haemorrhage is self-extending, the accumulated blood clot causing more separation, and thus more haemorrhage, until the edge of the placenta is reached. After this, blood can escape via the potential space between decidua and chorionic membrane to the cervix. Haemorrhage may also occur from the edge of a normally situated placenta—'*marginal haemorrhage*' (Fig. 15.1). This was formerly referred to as 'revealed accidental haemorrhage'. It does not have the same inherent tendency to automatic self-extension as does placental abruption, as it occurs from the edge of the chorionic plate. This occurs particularly frequently in association with an extrachorial (or circumvallate) type of placenta (Scott 1960).

Placenta praevia is frequently subdivided into four

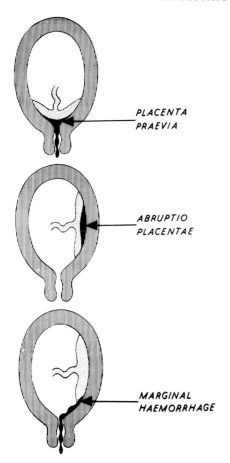

PLACENTA
PRAEVIA

ABRUPTIO
PLACENTAE

MARGINAL
HAEMORRHAGE

Fig. 15.1. A diagrammatic representation of the three anatomical types of APH. (With acknowledgement to the Editor of the *British Medical Journal*.)

grades: I, *lateral*—when the placenta extends on to the lower segment; II, *marginal*—when it extends to the edge of the internal cervical os; III, *complete (acentric)*—when it covers the internal os but is not centrally placed; and IV, *complete (centric)*—covering the internal os and centrally placed. A rare type of haemorrhage is that from a ruptured fetal vessel— *vasa praevia bleeding*. If suspected, the diagnosis can be confirmed by testing the blood for fetal haemo-globin by the Kleihauer or alkali denaturation tech-nique.

A *practical* classification of antepartum haemor-rhage *as it presents to the clinician* (Scott 1964) can be rather different, cases falling into one of three categories:

1 placental abruption;
2 placenta praevia;
3 'indeterminate APH'.

'Indeterminate' signifies a collective clinical cate-gory. It covers marginal haemorrhage, which has no positive features, and also other cases which cannot with confidence be diagnosed as placental abruption or placenta praevia. In some of these the nature and origin of the bleeding later becomes clear. It may be proved by clinical or investigative means that there is a placenta praevia, or on inspection of the placenta after delivery that there has been localized abruption. The other possibilities are that it has been a marginal haemorrhage or a 'false APH'. In this last category come bleeds from local cervical and vaginal lesions and cases in which excessive 'show' has been inter-preted as APH.

Uteri showing separation (with clot formation) of a placenta praevia and of a normally sited placenta (abruption) are shown in Fig. 15.2 (a) and (b).

Incidence

The frequency of APH varies with the age, parity and social status of the population, but a total incidence of about 3% is not unusual (5.8% of pregnancies over 28 weeks, *British Births 1970* Vol. 2 1978). Cases are approximately equally divided between the three clinical categories; abruption, placenta praevia and indeterminate.

Clinical picture

The presentation in most cases merely accords with the definition—bleeding from the genital tract after 28 weeks. Lack of pain is typical of placenta praevia and if painless haemorrhage is associated with the physical signs of placenta praevia, such as a present-ing part which is difficult to palpate or is displaced, the diagnosis is fairly certain.

Placental abruption, however, may not be asso-ciated with revealed bleeding at the outset. The patient, usually of high parity, develops pain over the uterus and this steadily increases in severity. There is usually no periodicity as with the pain of labour. Faintness and collapse may occur. There are usually signs of shock; the uterus is extremely hard and ten-der; it does not relax; fetal parts are difficult to palpate and the fetal heart may be inaudible. Unless the at-tendant is alert to the possibility the diagnosis may be missed until revealed bleeding eventually occurs. By this time the patient's general condition may have deteriorated seriously.

The differentiation of the two major types of APH is not nearly as simple in clinical practice as under-

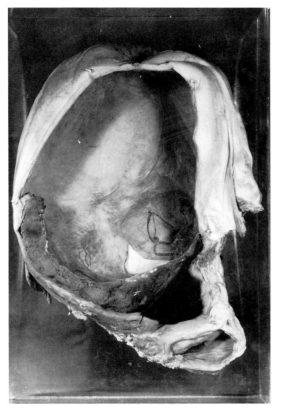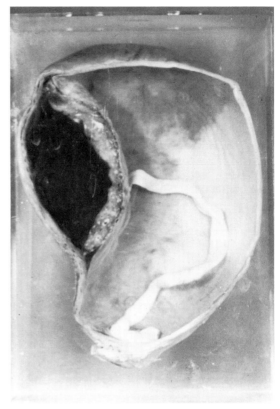

Fig. 15.2   (a) Uterus with placenta praevia (grade III) covering the external os and showing evidence of minor placental separation with clot at this site. (b) Separation of normally implanted placenta (abruptio placentae). A mass of clot has led to total separation of the placenta from the uterine wall. (By courtesy of Professor Ian MacGillivray.)

graduate texts would make it appear. Often presentation is atypical and painless losses can ultimately be shown to be due to placental abruption and painful ones to placenta praevia.

Antenatal care in relation to APH

The scope for specific prevention of antepartum haemorrhage is limited, but antenatal care has much to offer towards reducing the risks should such a complication occur. Blood group determination is a routine procedure of obvious relevance. Other important measures include: in societies where hospital delivery is not routine, booking for hospital confinement patients judged to be particularly liable to antepartum haemorrhage; prevention of anaemia; suspecting the diagnosis of placenta praevia before serious antepartum haemorrhage has occurred; early detection of pre-eclampsia and treating hypertension aggressively at an early stage; avoidance of trauma.

Booking for hospital confinement

If a woman booked for hospital confinement suffers an antepartum haemorrhage, either she will be admitted directly to the hospital or her doctor, if summoned, will be in a position to make appropriate arrangements immediately with the hospital at which she is booked. If hospital booking is not arranged, the delay in admission is likely to be longer, and even slight delays may prove fatal. Where hospital confinements are on a selective basis, women who qualify for hospital booking in this connection include those who have had previous antepartum haemorrhages (most studies show a tendency to recurrence), those of parity higher than four, and those over 35 years of age. In the high-parity group the risk of antepartum haemorrhage is very great—over 10% in O'Sullivan's (1963) series. A high proportion of deaths due to placental abruption and placenta praevia occur in women who are having their fourth or subsequent confinement (14% in *British Births 1970* Vol. 2 1978).

Prevention of anaemia

It is self-evident that the greater the degree of anaemia the lower is the ability to withstand haemorrhage. There is a strong suspicion that in the past many maternal fatalities from antepartum haemorrhage occurred in women who had been allowed to become needlessly anaemic in pregnancy. The exact policy of management of pregnancy anaemia is of less importance than the efforts which should be made to detect it at its earliest stage. Without entering into the arguments as to whether iron therapy should be given routinely in pregnancy or should always be combined with folic acid, it is relevant to bear in mind the suggested relationship between folic acid deficiency and placental abruption (*see* p. 192).

Early suspicion of placenta praevia

It is now accepted that the frequency with which the presence of placenta praevia is suspected before haemorrhage has occurred is an index of the quality of antenatal care. In modern practice when ultrasound is employed routinely this may give the first clue. It is, however, important to appreciate that scans done at a relatively early stage of pregnancy primarily to check maturity may give a false prediction of low placentation; in such circumstances the scan should be repeated later in pregnancy for confirmation. The availability of ultrasound for easy placental localization has had a major impact on obstetric practice and traditional approaches to management of APH have not yet been completely adapted to match the new technology.

In later pregnancy the physical findings which should arouse suspicion are: an abnormal or unstable fetal lie in late pregnancy—a persistent transverse lie is of the greatest significance; a presenting part which has an abnormal relationship to the pelvis—for example, held high above the brim (by a central placenta praevia), deviated from the midline (by a lateral placenta praevia), pushed forward over the symphysis (by a posterior placenta praevia), or rendered difficult to define on palpation through the anterior abdominal wall (by an anterior placenta praevia). These physical signs become more significant the longer they persist, and if they have been elicited independently at two or more separate antenatal examinations in the last 6–8 weeks of pregnancy then it is usually appropriate to take steps to exclude placenta praevia by some form of placentography. If this

is unavailable, hospital admission is indicated. If the physical signs are very definite, it may be advisable to treat the case as one of placenta praevia on this basis alone and regard placentography as superfluous.

With placenta praevia major bleeding is frequently preceded by small 'warning haemorrhages'. These haemorrhages may occur before 28 weeks and therefore be classified as threatened miscarriages. Particularly if they are repeated, they should be viewed with great suspicion and appropriate steps taken to exclude placenta praevia.

Vaginal examination is extremely hazardous in cases of possible placenta praevia, as it may provoke separation of the placenta with massive haemorrhage. Surprisingly, it is often not realized that a rectal examination is even more dangerous. Vaginally, even with only the thin glove covering the examiner's finger, there is the possibility that the placenta may not be felt before it is seriously disturbed. On rectal examination the gloved finger is covered by rectal wall, vaginal wall and intervening fascia. This makes it virtually certain that the placenta will not be detected before it is separated and serious bleeding provoked. Speculum examination is also capable of provoking bleeding from a placenta praevia and should normally be delayed until placenta praevia has been excluded by ultrasonography.

Early detection of pre-eclampsia

Early detection of pre-eclampsia is a *sine qua non* of good antenatal care. Traditional obstetric teaching is that there is an aetiological relationship between abruptio placentae and hypertensive states and it is implied that pre-eclampsia predisposes to abruption. If this is true, early detection of pre-eclampsia followed by appropriate management of the hypertensive process might be expected to result in a reduction in the incidence of abruption. It is remarkable, however, how infrequently abruption is seen in patients in whom a prior diagnosis of pre-eclampsia has been made and the existence of a significant aetiological relationshhip has been seriously questioned (Hibbard 1962, Hibbard & Jeffcoate 1966).

Avoidance of trauma

External version is a form of trauma in the antenatal period which is occasionally associated with antepartum haemorrhage. Opinion varies widely as to its place in modern obstetrics, but most obstetricians agree that, if done, it should only be attempted gently on unanaesthetized patients. If the manipulations prove difficult or cause pain, the attempt should be abandoned immediately. Naeye (1981) has drawn attention to the frequent association of APH with intercourse.

Folic acid deficiency

It has been suggested (Hibbard 1964, Hibbard & Hibbard 1963, Hibbard & Jeffcoate 1966, Streiff & Little 1967) that folic acid deficiency is closely related to occurrence of abruptio placentae. On this basis it would seem logical to expect that administration of folic acid supplements from an early stage in pregnancy might reduce the incidence. This does not appear to be the case (Willoughby 1967). It may be that the tendency to abruption is due to some metabolite, deficiency of which occurs *pari passu* with that of folic acid. Alternatively, it may be that folic acid exerts its fundamental ill-effect at such an early stage that commencing supplements at the time pregnancy is normally diagnosed is too late to be effective. The evidence, however, is conflicting and some workers (e.g. Pritchard *et al.* 1969) have failed to confirm a relationship between abruption and folate deficiency.

Decidual necrosis and smoking

Decidual necrosis has been described as being responsible for initiation of placental abruption. This is greater in heavy smokers (Naeye *et al.* 1977) so health education on this matter during the antenatal period may be beneficial.

Avoidance of sudden uterine decompression

A rare cause of placental abruption is the sudden release of liquor amnii in cases of severe polyhydramnios. The abrupt reduction in the area of the uterine wall to which the placenta is attached may result in placental separation in a manner similar to that which occurs in the third stage of normal labour after the baby has been expelled. Abdominal amniocentesis with a fine bore needle and slow release of the liquor in appropriate cases may help to prevent this.

Emergency management

On first seeing a case of antepartum haemorrhage it may be possible to conclude at once that the cause is placental abruption or placenta praevia but frequently the nature will be in doubt. Deliberation on causation is not a useful exercise. Whatever the mechanism the most important thing from the patient's point of view is to ensure that at the earliest possible moment she is brought within the availabil-

ity of a blood transfusion service, an operating theatre, and all the other resources of a fully equipped maternity hospital. In most cases the correct procedure is to arrange immediate transfer to hospital by ambulance. It must be appreciated that the only type of hospital appropriate to receive such cases is a *major* maternity hospital with full facilities, including resident staff.

In some cases where the initial blood loss has been heavy and has produced maternal shock the question may arise as to whether the Obstetric Flying Squad (OFS) should attend. It is hard to give categorical advice about this, for, unlike the situation with postpartum haemorrhage, the amount of benefit which the patient may obtain from OFS service is strictly limited. For example, with the torrential haemorrhage which sometimes occurs with placenta praevia, Caesarean section at the earliest opportunity is lifesaving; attempts at blood replacement prior to this may be futile and the delay can jeopardize life. In placental abruption, blood transfusion is unlikely to make a great contribution to improving the patient's condition unless combined with amniotomy and other measures designed to bring about speedy termination of abruption process, which can be performed satisfactorily only in hospital.

For these reasons it is often preferable to get the patient into hospital immediately rather than delay until she has been attended by the OFS. At Leeds Maternity Hospital, out of 186 consecutive attendances by the OFS only 4 were for antepartum haemorrhage. During the same period 137 antepartum haemorrhage cases were admitted directly to the hospital—without a fatality.

Management after admission

No matter what type of haemorrhage, blood replacement by transfusion is always indicated if there has been more than a slight loss or if there is any degree of shock. Blood should immediately be obtained for cross-matching and confirmation of grouping. Whether to delay administration of blood until a full cross-match has been completed, to give uncrossmatched group O Rhesus-negative blood or blood of the patient's group, is a matter for decision by the individual clinician in charge of a particular case. In cases of any severity it will often not be justifiable to await completion of the full cross-match. The *Report on Confidential Enquiries into Maternal Deaths in England and Wales 1976–78* (1982) commented that a common avoidable factor in relation to obstetric haemorrhage was lack of energy and determination in its diagnosis and management. Other measures depend upon the type of haemorrhage. In the cases where there is urgency about action the diagnosis of the type of APH is, fortunately, almost always obvious.

PLACENTAL ABRUPTION

In the case with frank clinical abruption the appropriate treatment in hospital is (1) liberal blood transfusion; (2) vaginal amniotomy; (3) oxytocin infusion; (4) sedation and analgesia.

The first and second measures are the most important. Amniotomy encourages the onset of labour and reduces the uterine tension which may contribute to two of the complications of abruption most liable to cause maternal death. These are *renal cortical necrosis*, and *coagulation disorder*. Blood transfusion is also instrumental in preventing ischaemic renal damage by maintaining the blood pressure and circulating red cell mass, and, of course, it ensures that the patient is in a better position to withstand any postpartum haemorrhage. In recent years blood has been given on a much more liberal scale in cases of abruption, and it is probable that this has contributed to the greatly improved maternal mortality figures. Only 6 maternal deaths occurred from this cause in England and Wales during 1976–8 compared with 78 in the 1952–4 period.

The mere fact that abruption can be confidently diagnosed clinically means that there has been considerable concealed blood loss and justifies the transfusion of a minimum of 1 litre (2 units) of blood regardless of the patient's general condition. The blood pressure is a notoriously unreliable guide to the extent of blood loss in these cases, as a severe degree of vasospasm or capillary bed blockage is a common response to the abruption, leading to elevated readings. The best answer to the problem of securing adequate blood replacement rests in the use of central venous pressure (CVP) monitoring as a guide (Muldoon 1969, O'Driscoll & McCarthy 1966). The average CVP in the third trimester is around 10 cm of water. This may be taken as an appropriate figure up to which patients should be transfused. Using this as a guide Muldoon (1969) found that 80% more blood was transfused, that the postnatal haemoglobin concentration was higher and that the incidence of postpartum oliguria was less. It is also possible that this policy may result in a lower incidence of coagulation disorder, for there is evidence that fibrinogen conversion is more likely to occur in the presence of hypovolaemic shock (Hardaway 1966).

With renal failure in mind, all patients with placental abruption should have careful records kept of fluid balance. Abruption is an important haemorrhagic cause of obstetric renal failure (Barry *et al.* 1964, Smith *et al.* 1968) and all the evidence suggests that hypovolaemia is the major aetiological factor. The treatment of established renal failure is a separate problem which has to be tackled after the haemorrhage has been arrested, and other than avoiding fluid overloading is not a concern during the period of active bleeding.

Coagulation disorder should always be in the clinician's mind when managing a case of abruption. The nature of the coagulation disturbance is discussed in Chapter 36. The precise mechanisms may seem of purely academic interest but rational clinical management should be related to the mechanism. Ideally the clinician would like to know which changes in the coagulation situation are harmful and which represent a beneficial function of the defence system. Unfortunately, this is not possible at present. The clinician is also faced with the problem that the coagulation disorder is developing so swiftly that results obtained from even the most rapidly efficient laboratories may bear no relationship to the situation existing when they become available.

Fibrinogen replacement was at one time recommended whenever coagulation failure became manifest, then fibrinolysis inhibitors were advised. A more mature view is that it may be wise to avoid specific coagulation therapy unless in exceptional circumstances (Bonnar *et al.* 1969, Scott 1968).

It is not sufficient justification for using a particular therapeutic factor that it should be capable of changing a disorder of the coagulation state found with abruptio placentae; *it must be reasonably certain that the change is likely to be beneficial.* This is not the case with regard to the therapies referred to. If fibrinogen is given during the thromboplastic or consumptive phase, it will undergo conversion to fibrin, with possible capillary blockage. Giving it at this stage may be compared with 'attempting to rebuild a house on fire rather than summon the fire-brigade' (Scott 1968). Conversely, giving fibrinolytic inhibitors may interfere with the mechanism by which nature is preventing intravascular occlusion (Bonnar *et al.* 1969).

In the light of the knowledge of coagulation mechanisms, heparin may be the most logical preparation to give if there is evidence of a disseminated intravascular coagulation. To administer an anticoagulant on theoretical grounds to a patient with a major APH does, however, call for a degree of courage which not all clinicians possess. F. S. Johnson (1975, personal communication) faced with a situation in Dar es Salaam where blood was not available for transfusion in adequate quantities, treated a matter of 60 severe placental abruptions with heparin and achieved improved results.

A wise approach in relation to the coagulation disorder of abruption is to concentrate on the haemorrhage *per se*. If the uterus is encouraged to empty itself rapidly, and if the blood replacement is adequate, then coagulation disorder is much less likely to occur (Basu 1969, Bonnar *et al.* 1969). The mere fact that the blood is in an incoagulable state should not be taken as an indication for therapy. One situation in which it does become of specific relevance is when Caesarean section is contemplated (see below), as surgical haemostasis is much more dependent upon the coagulation mechanism than is haemostasis in the placenta bed.

The place of Caesarean section in the management of placental abruption is difficult to define. The baby is nearly always dead in the severe case and for the mother vaginal delivery is usually safer than Caesarean section. If the child is still alive, Caesarean section may be justified in the hope that it will survive. As Lunan (1973) emphasized, the baby may be alive but the fetal heart inaudible with the monaural stethoscope due to the uterine spasm. Because of this the fetal heart, if not heard by conventional auscultation, should be sought by ultrasonic or electronic means. Unfortunately, many such babies if born alive by Caesarean section for abruptio placentae die in the early neonatal period.

There has been much debate over the years as to the place for Caesarean section to salvage the child. Hibbard & Jeffcoate (1966) calculated that in their series three baby lives *might* have been saved if 60 mothers had been exposed to the risks of Caesarean section, which may be considerable in these circumstances. Blair (1973), however, reported a Caesarean section rate twice as high as Hibbard and Jeffcoate's and concluded that it was justified in the light of the improved infant survival obtained in selected cases after the 34th week. Since then, however, improved paediatric care has made it more reasonable to perform section for the baby's sake at progressively earlier maturity. If Caesarean section is contemplated, it will usually be advisable to proceed only if the clotting is effective or can be made so.

In general, the best therapy—as well as the best prophylaxis in relation to coagulation failure—is liberal blood transfusion. If it can be obtained, fresh blood would be ideal (Bonnar *et al.* 1969), though the problems of achieving this, even with an efficient transfusion service, are considerable and blood transfusion should certainly not be delayed to await the availability of *fresh* supplies. Fresh-frozen plasma may be given to provide a range of coagulation factors and certainly should be given if more than 6 unts of blood are necessary. Transfusion of platelet concentrate may be considered if there is severe thrombocytopenia.

Usually, with the measures outlined, vaginal delivery is rapidly achieved. The most dangerous stage of labour for any patient is the third and this is particularly true if there has been significant antepartum bleeding of any type; the management described later must be rigorously applied. Frequently, the placenta has been completely separated by the abruption, and fetus and placenta are delivered synchronously. After vaginal delivery the arrest of bleeding from the placental site is mainly dependent on myometrial retraction and liberal doses of oxytocics should always be given.

PLACENTA PRAEVIA

If the case is obviously one of placenta praevia, the management depends upon the duration of the pregnancy and the extent of the haemorrhage. If the pregnancy is not far advanced in the third trimester, the usual aim is to allow it to continue until the baby has grown to a size that will give a reasonable chance of survival *ex utero*. This policy, introduced by Macafee (1945, see also Macafee 1960), has done more than anything else to reduce the fetal mortality in placenta praevia, which was mainly due to prematurity. The Macafee regime requires, for safety, strict adherence to several vital principles. From the time of the initial diagnosis of placenta praevia until delivery the patient *must* remain in a fully equipped and staffed maternity unit. This means one in which *blood is immediately available* for transfusion, in which full facilities for Caesarean section exist and in which there is, continuously throughout the 24 hours, a member of staff available to perform the operation should it prove necessary. All steps must be taken to correct any anaemia that may be present, in view of the likelihood of further haemorrhage.

This all sounds simple, but in practice it can tax to the limits the combined resources of obstetrician, midwives, family doctor and social service staff. The lives of such patients can be saved by the whole-hearted co-operation of all concerned towards keeping them contented to stay in hospital during the period of what seems to them unreasonable detention while feeling perfectly well.

Cotton et al. (1980) described an 'aggressive' form of the Macafee regime with antenatal transfusion and use of drugs to inhibit premature labour; they reported a halving of perinatal mortality with this, mainly affecting neonatal deaths. Silver et al. (1984) reported 95 cases managed in relatively recent times with increasing availability of modern technology and organization, particularly ultrasound scanning and a tertiary referral centre for intensive perinatal care. They believe from their experience that the rigid Macafee inpatient regime can be modified with safety to allow outpatient care in 'properly selected and counselled patients'.

Once the pregnancy has advanced to 37–38 weeks, or if the first haemorrhage occurs then, it has been regarded as best to deliver the baby. In minor degrees of placenta praevia, vaginal amniotomy may be sufficient to allow the head to control any bleeding in labour by pressing on the placental edge. Caesarean section is the method of delivery of choice whenever there is more than a very minor degree of placenta praevia and the baby is alive. If there is doubt about maturity, it has been thought helpful to assess the prospects for pulmonary function if the child is delivered by performing liquor phospholipid studies. However, the developments in neonatal paediatric techniques have rendered phospholipid assay almost redundant in some regions (James et al. 1983). The stage of pregnancy up to which conservative management should be persisted with is also a matter on which views are changing.

Once a decision is made to deliver the child, opinion differs as to whether vaginal examination under anaesthesia should be performed followed by Caesarean section if a major degree of placenta praevia is encountered, or a decision made on the available evidence without vaginal examination to perform elective Caesarean section. Macafee et al. (1962) attribute the improved perinatal mortality in their hospital, at least in part, to a greater use of Caesarean section, and Crenshaw et al. (1973) report similar experience, their perinatal mortality having almost halved with a doubling of the Caesarean section rate.

The Caesarean section done for placenta praevia is much more hazardous than that done for most other indications. It always tends to be haemorrhagic and

a number of different dilemmas may present which demand fine and sometimes bold judgement for their solution. It follows that the experience of the operator is of great importance. If severe haemorrhage is taking place, it may be wise to open the abdomen with a vertical midline incision rather than the normally preferable Pfannenstiel. Seconds may be vital. The next decision is whether to perform the conventional lower segment operation or elect for the classical uterine incision. The inexperienced operator may be daunted by the massive vessels sometimes evident over a lower segment on which the placenta is implanted. The experienced operator, however, will rarely regard the classical incision with its consequent disadvantages as justified. If it is felt that the time-factor should influence the decision in this regard, the patient's condition must indeed be parlous.

The next problem, if the lower segment approach is adopted, is how to deal with the placenta if it is encountered deep to the incision. If the placenta is incised with a view to delivering the baby through it, loss of fetal blood may occur and, of course, even a small quantity of this may prove fatal to the baby. On the other hand, if attempts are made to deliver the baby round the placental edge difficulties may arise which can lead to fetal death from asphyxia. As long as both hazards are borne in mind it is unlikely that either will give rise to serious trouble.

After delivery of the baby, removal of the placenta from the lower segment may prove difficult. As a consequence of the relative lack of decidua, marked adherence tends to occur and it may have to be detached piecemeal. Bleeding at this juncture may be profuse. The policy is to proceed as expeditiously as possible with placental removal and closing of the uterine incision. Often a remarkable degree of haemostasis is secured with one continuous, atraumatic suture. If control of bleeding proves difficult despite precise suturing, pressure with warm packs, oxytocics, etc., then a time will come when hysterectomy has to be contemplated. This is a decision concerning which no precise rules can be formulated. The experienced operator will know when further attempts are likely to hazard the mother's life and he will opt for the drastic action of hysterectomy before she is in extremis.

In association with the policies outlined, the perinatal mortality from placenta praevia fell in most countries. However, Hibberd (1969), dealing with a relatively poor population in Los Angeles, reported no improvement in the perinatal mortality with the use of expectant management—24.9% compared with 24.7%. Gordon's (1969) figure of 5% perinatal mortality (corrected for fetal abnormality) gives a better idea of what this approach has to offer.

INDETERMINATE APH

In cases in which the nature of the haemorrhage is not clear in the initial stages, the blood loss is not usually of an extent to cause serious concern. In all cases the usual assessment is made of the general condition and blood is taken for grouping, cross-matching and haemoglobin determination. Further action depends on the maturity of the pregnancy. If this is such that there is confidence that the baby will survive if delivered, induction of premature labour by vaginal amniotomy is usually regarded as wise. The chances are that the placenta has been to some extent damaged by the haemorrhage and its functional reserve reduced; there is also the possibility that further, more serious, haemorrhage will occur. If there is the slightest suspicion that bleeding may be due to placenta praevia, the amniotomy should be done in theatre under anaesthesia. A blood transfusion should be running and full preparations made for immediate Caesarean section should this be necessary.

In other cases, in which the maturity is less, conservative management is indicated. The patient is kept strictly at rest in bed in the hope that bleeding will cease, which it usually does. Any anaemia is corrected and after the patient has been free from bleeding for four or five days an attempt is made to determine its source. The possibility of a degree of placenta praevia is always the first thing to be excluded, and this can sometimes be done with moderate certainty by abdominal palpation. Usually, placentography is necessary to confirm the placental position and ultrasound may also detect retroplacental blood clot.

If placenta praevia is diagnosed or the suspicion of it cannot be excluded, then management is that outlined under placenta praevia. If, on the other hand, the placenta can be demonstrated convincingly on the upper segment of the uterus, it *may* be considered safe to allow the patient home. Before doing so a speculum may be gently passed to exclude a cervical cause for the bleeding. Be it noted that speculum examination is *not* recommended initially. Exposure of the pregnant cervix is difficult and could easily result in further bleeding if the placenta should be low-lying; also a cervical polyp or vascular erosion may be observed and haemorrhage attributed to this,

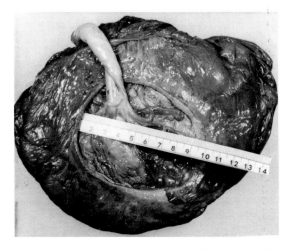

Fig. 15.3. A circumvallate (or extrachorial) placenta with which APH is particularly common. The fold at the edge of the chorionic plate, indicated by the ruler, is the site at which bleeding tends to occur.

though the real source of the trouble has been a placenta praevia.

If this policy of expectant management is implemented it must be remembered that the baby is still particularly at risk. Regular tests of placental function may be helpful and it will usually be appropriate to deliver the child when reasonable maturity is reached.

The commonest source of bleeding in the cases in this category proves to be the edge of a normally implanted placenta. In the older literature this was frequently referred to as 'haemorrhage from the marginal sinus', an apparently suitable description but for the single drawback that the weight of anatomical opinion is against the existence of such a structure. This type of haemorrhage is particularly common if the placenta is circumvallate or 'extra-chorial' (Fig. 15.3) (Scott 1960). In these placentae there is a fibrous ring round the edge of the chorionic plate which retracts, often causing repeated haemorrhages. This history of repeated haemorrhages is, in fact, highly suggestive of placenta praevia but the physical signs are absent. As Naftolin *et al.* (1973) point out, there may also be drainage of fluid per vaginam which is often described as hydrorrhoea gravidarum. This is probably serum extruded from the annular clot. Though the condition may be suspected antepartum, the diagnosis cannot be made with certainty until the placenta has been delivered and inspected. Fortunately, haemorrhages from this condition carry little risk to mother or baby. Placenta membranacea may also present in a similar way but the pregnancy is more likely to terminate in second trimester abortion (Pryse-Davies *et al.* 1973).

Testing blood for fetal origin is an important procedure for if the blood is coming from the baby, immediate delivery followed by immediate transfusion may save its life.

MANAGEMENT OF THE THIRD STAGE

'It's the APH that weakens and the PPH that kills' is a true aphorism. Not only is the woman who has suffered an APH likely to be relatively anaemic when she reaches the third stage of labour, there are also several factors which make it more likely that she will have a postpartum haemorrhage. If she has suffered a placental abruption, the whole uterus, owing to intramuscular haemorrhages or a circulating inhibitor of myometrial contraction (Basu 1969), may not contract and retract efficiently to control the blood loss. In addition, should this happen, or should there be any laceration, bleeding may be aggravated by failure of blood coagulation. If the APH was due to placenta praevia, the postpartum bleeding may be excessive owing to the fact that the lower segment to which the placenta has been attached contracts and retracts less efficiently than does the upper segment.

The third stage management is, therefore, critical in the case of the patient who has suffered an APH. By administration of an oxytocic drug such as 0.5 mg ergometrine maleate intramuscularly with the birth of the trunk, supplemented by oxytocin 5 units if necessary, every effort is made to obtain maximal uterine contraction. If need be, these drugs may be repeated several times or given intravenously. At the same time an intravenous infusion should be running through a capacious cannula and cross-matched blood available so that, if postpartum haemorrhage occurs, blood administration can be commenced immediately and given rapidly.

With regard to cases showing coagulation disorder, the arguments for withholding specific replacement coagulation therapy cease to be as strong after delivery, as the consumptive phase of the disorder is presumably over. In the relatively small proportion of cases with coagulation failure which develop postpartum haemorrhage (25%, Basu 1969) fibrinolytic inhibitors and/or fibrinogen may be given.

If despite these measures haemorrhage occurs and continues, bimanual compression of the uterus may be attempted after excluding traumatic causes for the bleeding. The most important factor in the control of postpartum blood loss is uterine retraction; redoubling of the efforts to secure this usually pays the best dividends. Very large doses of oxytocic drugs intravenously may be effective when the traditional doses have failed, and occasionally a hot intrauterine douche has a miraculous effect. Very rarely, hysterectomy may have to be resorted to as the only means of controlling the haemorrhage, but in the presence of coagulation failure this is fraught with danger.

Placental localization

Many techniques have been tried to assist the clinician in localizing the placenta when placenta praevia has been suspected. Radiological methods include those involving positioning of the mother and/or baby to demonstrate gaps between bony promontories *possibly* due to the presence of placenta; low penetration films to detect the placental shadow and aortographic techniques. This last gives excellent definition of the placenta but is associated with risk of discomfort and complications from the aortography,

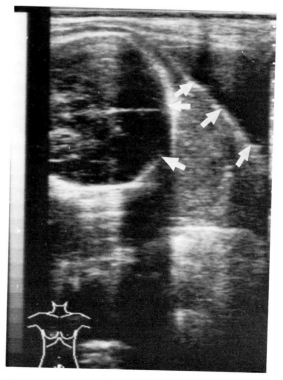

Fig. 15.4. Ultrasound scan showing major degree of placenta praevia. Arrows indicate head and bladder with placenta between.

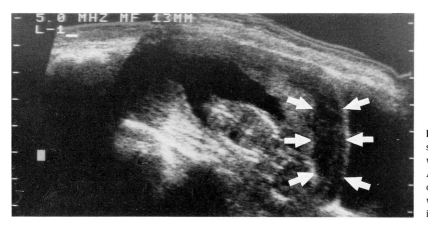

Fig. 15.5. Ultrasound scan showing retroplacental clot with a low lying placenta. Arrows indicate collection of blood. The placenta, which has a fundal implantation, is on the left.

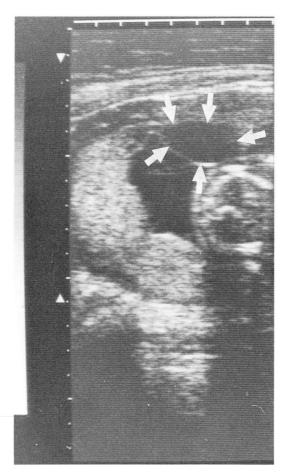

Fig. 15.6. Haemorrhage from edge of placenta which has formed a collection of blood outside the chorionic membrane demonstrated by ultrasonic scan. Arrows mark edge of collection.

quite apart from the radiation problem. The other radiological techniques were less efficient and probably did not justify the radiation exposure.

Isotope techniques were employed using albumin labelled with radiocative iodine (I^{132}) or technetium (99^mTc). The radiation involved with these techniques is minimal by comparison with radiological methods but special counting equipment is necessary.

In recent years ultrasound has become established as the method of choice in most centres. It has the great advantage of convenience and apparent lack of any fetal or maternal hazard. The convenience and efficiency has been greatly enhanced by the development of real-time scanners. As mentioned earlier, when early pregnancy scanning is performed it is likely that there will be over-diagnosis of placenta praevia.

An important part of the technique is to carry out the ultrasonic scan with the patient's bladder full, so that the relationship between the lowest point of the placenta and the cervix can readily be appreciated (Fig. 15.4).

Ultrasound may also have a role in relation to APH not due to placenta praevia. Retroplacental blood clots may be shown in abruptions and rarely intra-amniotic bleeds can be demonstrated (Jaffe *et al.* 1981. McGahan *et al.* 1982, Hill *et al.* 1984). Figures 15.5 and 15.6 show examples of, respectively, a retroplacental clot with a low-lying placenta, and formation of a subchorionic haematoma from separation of the edge of a normally sited placenta.

REFERENCES

BAKER J. L. & DEWHURST C. J. (1963) *J. Obstet. Gynaec. Brit. Cwlth.* **70**, 1063–7.

BARRY A. P., CARMODY M., WOODCOCK J. A., O'DWYER W. F., WALSH A. & DOYLE G. (1964) *J. Obstet. Gynaec. Brit. Cwlth.* **71**, 899–907.

BASU H. K. (1969) *J. Obstet. Gynaec. Brit. Cwlth.* **76**, 481–96.

BLAIR R. G. (1973) *J. Obstet. Gynaec. Brit. Cwlth.* **80**, 242–5.

BONNAR J., McNICOL G. P. & DOUGLAS A. S. (1969) *J. Obstet. Gynaec. Brit. Cwlth.* **76**, 799–805.

British Births (1970), Vol. 2, 1978. Wm. Heinemann, London.

COTTON D. B., READ J. A., PAUL R. H. & QUILLIGAN E. J. (1980) *Amer. J. Obstet. Gynec.* **137**, 687–95.

CRENSHAW C., JONES D. E. D. & PARKER R. T. (1973) *Obstet. Gynec. Surv.* **28**, 461–70.

GORDON H. (1969) In Kellar R. J. (ed) *Modern Trends in Obstetrics 4*, pp. 257–72. Butterworths, London.

HARDAWAY R. M. (1966) *Syndromes of Disseminated Intravascular Coagulation.* Chas. C. Thomas, Springfield, Illinois.

HIBBARD B. M. (1962) *J. Obstet. Gynaec. Brit. Cwlth.* **69**, 282–7.

HIBBERD B. M. (1964) *J. Obstet. Gynaec. Brit. Cwlth.* **71**, 529–42.

HIBBARD B. M. & HIBBARD E. D. (1963) *Brit. med. J.* **2**, 1430–6.

HIBBARD B. M. & JEFFCOATE T. N. A. (1966) *Obstet. and Gynec.* **27**, 155–67.

HIBBERD L. T. (1969) *Amer. J Obstet. Gynec.* **104**, 172–84.

HILL L. M., BRECKLE R. & GEHRKING W. (1984) *Amer. J. Obstet. Gynec.* **148**, 1144–5.

JAFFE M. H., SCHOEN W. C., SILVER T. M., BOWERMAN R. A. & STUCK K. J. (1981) *Amer. J. Roentgenol.* **137**, 1049–54.

JAMES D. K., TINDALL V. R. & RICHARDSON T. (1983) *Brit. J. Obstet. Gynaec.* **90**, 995–1000.

KINCH R. A. H., ROSENTHALL L. & COLLINS J. A. (1969) In Reid D. E. & Barton T. C. (eds) *Controversy in Obstetrics and Gynecology*, p. 567. W. B. Saunders Co., Philadelphia.

LUNAN C. B. (1973) *J. Obstet. Gynaec. Brit. Cwlth.* **80**, 120–4.

MACAFEE C. H. G. (1945) *J. Obstet. Gynaec. Brit. Emp.* **52**, 313–24.

MACAFEE C. H. G. (1960) *Lancet* i, 449–52.

MACAFEE C. H. G., MILLAR W. G. & HARLEY G. (1962) *J. Obstet. Gynaec. Brit. Cwlth.* **69**, 203–12.

McGAHAN J. P., PHILLIPS H. E., REID M. H. & OI R. H. (1982) *Radiology* **142**, 481–5.

MULDOON M. J. (1969) *J. Obstet. Gynaec. Brit. Cwlth.* **76**, 225–8.

NAEYE R. L. (1981) *J. Obstet. Gynaec. Brit. Cwlth.* **88**, 765–70.

NAEYE R. L., HARKNESS W. L. & UTTS JESSICA (1977) *Amer. J. Obstet. Gynec.* **128**, 740–6.

NAFTOLIN F., KHUDR G., BENIRSCHKE K. & HUTCHINSON D. L. (1973). *Amer. J. Obstet. Gynec.* **116**, 347–50.

O'DRISCOLL K. & McCARTHY J. R. (1966) *J. Obstet. Gynaec. Brit. Cwlth.* **73**, 923–9.

O'SULLIVAN J. F. (1963) *J. Obstet. Gynaec. Brit. Cwlth.* **70**, 158–64.

PRITCHARD J. A., WHALLEY P. J. & SCOTT D. E. (1969) *Amer. J. Obstet. Gynec.* **104**, 388–96.

PRYSE-DAVIES J., DEWHURST C. J. & CAMPBELL S. (1973) *J. Obstet. Gynaec. Brit. Cwlth.* **80**, 1106–1110.

Report on Confidential Enquiries into Maternal Deaths in England and Wales 1976–78 (1982) HMSO, London.

RIGBY E. (1775) *An Essay on the Uterine Haemorrhage.* Johnson, London.

SCOTT J. S. (1960) *J. Obstet. Gynaec. Brit. Emp.* **67**, 904–18.

SCOTT J. S. (1964) *Brit. med. J.* **1**, 1163–5 and 1231–4.

SCOTT J. S. (1968) *Brit. med. Bull.* **24**, 32–8.

SILVER R., DEPP R., SABBAGHA R. E., DOOLEY S. L., SOCOL M. L. & TAMURA R. K. (1984) *Amer. J. Obstet. Gynec.*, **150**, 15–22.

SMITH K., BROWNE J. C. M., SHACKMAN R. & WRONG O. M. (1968). *Brit. med. Bull.* **24**, 49–58.

STREIFF R. R. & LITTLE A. B. (1967) *New Engl. J. Med.* **276**, 776–9.

WILLOUGHBY M. L. N. (1967) *Brit. J. Haemat.* **13**, 503–9.

CHAPTER 16
HYPERTENSIVE DISORDERS OF PREGNANCY

D. A. DAVEY

Hypertension is one of the commonest complications of pregnancy and is one of the commonest causes of fetal and maternal mortality and morbidity. In 5–15% of cases it is associated with proteinuria and the fetal and maternal risks are then significantly increased. Proteinuria without hypertension is less common and is often due to chronic renal disease. In the past oedema was believed to be aetiologically and pathologically associated with hypertension and proteinuria, constituting a characteristic triad of signs. Oedema however occurs in about 80% of all pregnant women, is frequently found in normal pregnancy (Robertson 1971), and even when associated with hypertension and proteinuria it is of no diagnostic or prognostic significance (Friedman & Neff 1977a). The concept of one disease characterized by a triad of hypertension, proteinuria and oedema, with one aetiology and one pathophysiology is misleading and should be abandoned. Instead, hypertension is best regarded as the chief clinical manifestation or end result of a number of different diseases or disorders which may be either incidental or peculiar to pregnancy. Proteinuria is also best regarded as another clinical manifestation of these disorders. In summary all the evidence suggests that hypertension and/or proteinuria in pregnancy is not one single disease or disorder, as is often assumed or implied, but is due to a number of diseases or disorders which have different aetiologies, different pathophysiologies and different prognoses. They may be described collectively as the hypertensive and proteinuric disorders of pregnancy, or for short the hypertensive disorders of pregnancy, 'proteinuric' being implied. These disorders may be a direct complication or consequence of pregnancy, an exacerbation of underlying latent maternal hypertension or renal disease, or a continuation of overt chronic hypertensive or renal disease which pre-existed the pregnancy.

Definitions

It is essential to have agreed standardized methods of measurement if the incidence of hypertensive and proteinuric disorders and the results of treatment are to be assessed and compared. It is also essential that the definitions should be based on clinical observations and measurements which can be easily and reliably made, and that the criteria of normality and abnormality should be simple and unequivocal.

HYPERTENSION

Arterial blood pressure (BP) is nearly always measured in clinical practice by sphygmomanometry and the technique and conditions of measurement must be standardized if consistent results are to be obtained (O'Brien & O'Malley 1979). In non-pregnant patients the point of disappearance of Korotkoff sounds (Point V) corresponds most closely to the true diastolic blood pressure (DBP) as measured by intra-arterial catheter. In pregnancy however, the ausculated Korotkoff sounds may persist to zero due to the marked peripheral vasodilatation, and the point of muffling (Point IV) provides a better measure of the true DBP and should always be used during pregnancy and labour. Exercise, posture and stress tend to affect the systolic more than the DBP and the resting DBP provides the most reproducible and best guide to prognosis. In pregnancy BP is most commonly measured with the patient lying on a couch in an antenatal clinic or on a bed, and it is recommended that it should always be measured with the patient lying down and resting comfortably on her right side at 30° to the horizontal with the sphygmomanometer cuff at the level of the heart. The practice of measuring BP on the uppermost arm with the patient lying on either side is to be condemned as this leads to falsely low readings due to the difference (as much as 15 or 20 mmHg) in hydrostatic pressure between the level of the sphygmomanometer cuff and

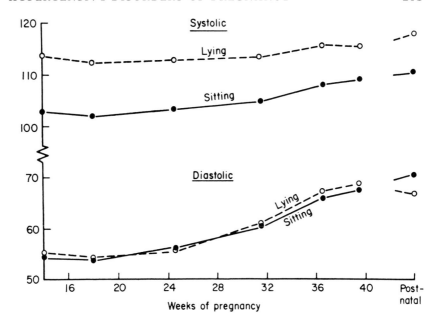

Fig. 16.1. Blood pressure trends (sitting and lying) during pregnancy. From MacGillivray I., Rose G. A. & Rowe B. (1969) *Clin. Sci.*, 37, 395–407.

the level of the heart. For the diagnosis of hypertension it is accepted practice to require two consecutive abnormally high measurements made at least 4–6 hours apart. The BP normally falls at the beginning of pregnancy and reaches its lowest level in the second trimester, when the DBP is on average 15 mmHg lower and the systolic BP 5 mmHg lower in the lying position than prepregnancy levels (Fig. 16.1; MacGillivray *et al.* 1969, Friedman & Neff 1977b). This fall in BP in the first two trimesters occurs in both normotensive and chronic hypertensive women so that chronically hypertensive women may appear normotensive at the beginning of pregnancy. It is perhaps not sufficiently appreciated that the BP normally rises in the third trimester and reaches prepregnancy levels by term. This rise to prepregnancy levels is associated with other cardiovascular changes such as a decrease in plasma volume and a reduction in renal blood flow (Davison *et al.* 1980) and is a part of the normal physiological changes in pregnancy.

MacGillivray (1961) has shown that, in terms of prognosis and management, the absolute level of BP attained is more important than the rise during pregnancy and the former should be used in the definition of hypertension. Any definition of hypertension is inevitably arbitrary, but taking a DBP (Point IV Korotkoff) of 90 mmHg or more throughout pregnancy, as originally proposed by Nelson (1955), has several advantages. It is simple and precise, and it overcomes the difficulties of using criteria based on combinations

of systolic and diastolic BP, or on derived values such as the mean arterial BP which are complicated, unlikely to be used in practice and no better than the DBP as a predictor of fetal outcome (Friedman & Neff 1977c). In the first 2 trimesters of pregnancy a DBP of 90 mmHg corresponds with about 3 SD or more above mean and after 34 weeks corresponds with about 2 SD above mean (MacGillivray *et al.* 1969, Table 16.1) which are readily understood and agreed statistical criteria. A DBP of 90 mmHg corresponds with the intersection of of the curves relating BP to perinatal mortality (Fig. 16.2) and above 85 mmHg there is a significant and progressive increase in perinatal mortality with increase in BP (Friedman & Neff

Table 16.1 Blood pressure in normal pregnancy. Mean and upper limits. (MacGillivray, Rose & Rowe, 1969.) Reprinted by permission of the Biochemical Society, London.

Period of pregnancy	Diastolic BP (Lying) mmHg			Systolic BP (Lying) mmHg		
	Mean	+2 SD	+3 SD	Mean	+2 SD	+3 SD
16 wk	55.1	73.5	82.7	113.6	135.4	146.3
16–20 wk	54.2	74.6	84.8	112.2	133.0	143.4
21–28 wk	55.7	74.9	84.5	112.9	134.5	145.3
29–34 wk	61.6	79.8	88.9	113.4	134.8	145.5
35–38 wk	67.2	88.0	98.4	115.7	138.9	150.5
39–40 wk	68.7	93.3	105.6	115.1	140.5	153.2
40+ wk	71.1	94.9	106.8	115.7	136.5	146.9
7 days postpartum	70.4	98.2	112.1	119.0	144.8	157.7
6 wk postpartum	66.5	88.5	99.5	117.8	141.8	153.8

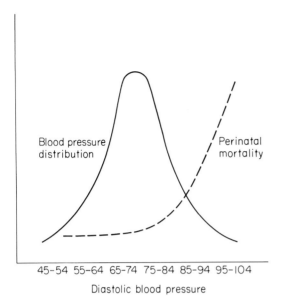

Fig. 16.2. Relationship between diastolic blood pressure and perinatal mortality. From Friedman E. A. ed. (1976) *Blood Pressure, Edema and Proteinuria in Pregnancy*, p. 279. Elsevier Science Publishing Co., Amsterdam.

1977d). In cases of severe hypertension it is frequently necessary to institute antihypertensive treatment promptly on the basis of a single blood pressure measurement and it is therefore recommended that the diagnosis of hypertension in pregnancy should be based either on two measurements of DBP of 90 mmHg or more made on 2 or more consecutive occasions 4 or more hours apart, or on one measurement of DBP of 110 mmHg or more.

PROTEINURIA

The definition of proteinuria depends upon the methods used to detect and measure it, the nature of the proteins present, and the conditions and period over which the urine is collected. A small amount of protein is normally in the urine and the average 24 hour urinary excretion in healthy non-pregnant subjects is total protein 18 mg, albumin 10 mg and beta 2-microglobulin 1–2 mg (Petersen *et al.* 1969). In pregnancy this amount may be increased up to 300 mg total protein per 24 hr. The Committee on Terminology of the American Obstetricians and Gynecologists (Hughes 1972) recommended that a total protein concentration of 300 or more mg per litre should be regarded as abnormal. In clinical practice proteinuria is most commonly detected by the use of

a dip-stick test such as Albustix or Multistix (Ames) or less commonly by the use of sulphosalicylic acid. Opinion differs as to the value and reliability of these tests. Dip-sticks may give up to 25% false positive results with a trace reaction and 6% false positives with one plus colour reaction in random urine specimens from patients with normal daily protein excretion. False positive results may also result from contamination by vaginal discharge and from urinary tract infections. Because of these difficulties, many reports on the incidence and severity of proteinuria in pregnancy must be regarded with reservation and as probable overestimates (Rennie *et al.* 1967, Shaw *et al.* 1983). The definitive test for proteinuria is quantitative measurement (using an established reliable method) of the total 24-hour excretion of protein (de Wardener 1973). This should therefore be performed on all inpatients in whom proteinuria is detected in a random urine specimen, although accurate collection of 24-hour urines presents considerable problems, particularly in outpatients. As an alternative the measurement of the urinary protein/creatinine index has been proposed (Shaw *et al.* 1983). On random specimens, this provides a useful semi-quantitative estimate of 24-hour excretion and avoids the errors of dip-stick methods. To overcome the difficulties and errors discussed above the following procedure is recommended: ensure patient has not drunk a large quantity of fluid before submitting a sample of urine; test for the presence of protein by dip-stick, and if a trace or more is detected obtain a midstream clean catch sample; test the midstream clean catch specimen with dip-stick: if this shows 2 plus or more regard it as significant proteinuria, but if there is 1 plus or a trace collect a random specimen for estimation of protein, a random specimen for estimation of protein/creatinine index or a 24-hour urinary collection for total 24-hour urinary protein. A negative dip-stick indicates that the original test was false positive.

OEDEMA, WEIGHT GAIN AND OLIGURIA

Oedema, including generalized oedema, is a normal occurrence in pregnancy, and in the absence of hypertension is associated with an above average fetal outcome (Thomson *et al.* 1967). Oedema with hypertension and/or proteinuria is not associated with increased perinatal or maternal mortality (Friedman & Neff 1977a). In normal pregnancy, increasing oedema, particularly when associated with excessive weight gain (about 0.75 kg per week, or more), may nevertheless be an early warning sign of the possible later development of hypertension and proteinuria. In hypertensive pregnancies rapidly developing generalized oedema should be regarded as a sign of imminent eclampsia, particularly when associated with epigastric pain, eye symptoms, headache, hyperreflexia or oliguria.

Classification and nomenclature

More than 100 names have been used in the English and German literature to describe the different hypertensive diseases of pregnancy and there have been almost as many classifications (Rippman 1969). Until the aetiology and pathology of hypertensive and proteinuric disorders is better understood, no classification will be entirely satisfactory.

In the meantime a practical classification, based solely on clinical criteria, is proposed (Table 16.2). It follows those of the American Committee on Maternal Welfare, as modified by the Committee on Terminology (Chesley 1978a) and Gant and Worley (1980a), but with some important differences in nomenclature. The term 'gestational' is used throughout this classification and is preferred to the term 'pregnancy induced'. The latter term implies that pregnancy may have caused the condition, whereas the occurrence of hypertension and proteinuria during pregnancy may, in some circumstances, be purely coincidental.

Gestational hypertension is diagnosed in all normotensive women who develop hypertension without proteinuria. Gestational hypertension probably includes at least three different underlying disease processes. In younger primigravid patients without a family history of hypertension it probably represents an early stage of the development of pre-eclampsia (which is diagnosed when proteinuria develops) and which might be designated pre-eclamptic hypertension. In older multigravid women with a family history of hypertension gestational hypertension is probably due to an underlying inherited tendency to hypertension which becomes overt during pregnancy and is perhaps best known as 'latent essential hypertension'. With multiple pregnancy, diabetes, rhesus isoimmunization or other forms of 'hyperplacentosis' (Jeffcoate 1966) the rise in BP probably represents an excessively good response to pregnancy and may simply be an extreme manifestation of the rise in BP which normally occurs after 34 weeks; this might be described as 'supranormal hypertension' or 'physio-logical hypertension'. Physiological hypertension may also include a raised blood pressure due to stress, exercise, pain and anxiety. Unfortunately at the present time these different underlying aetologies and pathologies cannot be clearly distinguished clinically or by current diagnostic tests.

Gestational proteinuria is diagnosed in the relatively small number of patients who develop proteinuria without hypertension in pregnancy. This group probably comprises a number of conditions including proteinuria due to false positive tests or to vaginal contamination or the presence of cells and debris from a urinary tract infection, acute or chronic renal disease or other medical conditions developing or recognized for the first time in pregnancy, or else excessive glomerular leakage of protein in otherwise normal pregnancy possibly associated with posture as in orthostatic proteinuria.

Pre-eclampsia is diagnosed in women who develop hypertension with proteinuria in pregnancy. Sheehan and Lynch (1973a) defined 'true pre-eclampsia' on the basis of characteristic changes in the renal glomeruli and found that it is almost invariably associated with albuminuria and that 'patients who do not have albuminaria do not have glomerular lesions'. Pre-eclampsia is primarily a disease of primigravidas, but much less frequently it occurs in subsequent pregnancies. It rarely occurs for the first time in second or subsequent pregnancies. It is not associated with an increased incidence of hypertension in later life except in women with pre-existing chronic essential hypertension or with a latent tendency to essential hypertension (Chesley 1978b). Because true pre-eclampsia occurs primarily in primigravidas, some abnormal immunological reaction to a first pregnancy is thought to play a key part in its aetiology (Scott & Beer 1976, Petrucco 1981).

Chronic essential hypertension. Chesley (1980) has made a strong case for the entity of latent essential hypertension in pregnancy as an initial stage in the development of chronic essential hypertension. Latent essential hypertension is characterized by the development of hypertension (but not proteinuria) in women who are normotensive at the beginning of pregnancy but who often have a strong family history of hypertension. In most cases the BP reverts to normal in the puerperium, but the hypertension recurs in subsequent pregnancies and the condition is analogous to gestational diabetes. Latent essential

Table 16.2   Clinical classification of hypertensive and proteinuric disorders of pregnancy.

Classification	Notes

1 Gestational hypertension and/or proteinuria
Hyertension and/or proteinuria developing during pregnancy in a previously normotensive nonproteinuric woman subdivided into:
 	
(a) *Gestational hypertension* (without proteinuria)
    developing during pregnancy
    developing for first time in labour
    developing for first time in puerperium
 	
(b) *Gestational proteinuria* (without hypertension)
    developing during pregnancy
    developing for first time in labour
    developing for first time in puerperium
 	
(c) *Gestational proteinuric hypertension* (Pre-eclampsia)
    developing during pregnancy
    developing for first time in labour
    developing for first time in puerperium
	(a) may be Latent essential hypertension
	    Physiological (including 'supranormal hypertension')
	    'Pre-eclamptic hypertension' (preceding pre-eclampsia)
	(b) may be Physiological (orthostatic)
	    Pyuria (pyelitis, etc.)
	    'Pre-eclamptic proteinuria' (preceding pre-eclampsia)
	    Exacerbation undiagnosed chronic renal disease
	    Acute renal disease (rare)
	    Other pathological causes (rare)
	(c) may be Pre-eclampsia, presumed diagnosis in all cases unless positive diagnosis of acute or chronic renal disease
	    Exacerbation of previously undiagnosed chronic renal disease
	    Acute nephritis (rare)

2 Chronic hypertension and chronic renal disese
Hypertension and/or proteinuria occurring during pregnancy in a woman with proven chronic hypertension or renal disease, present before, diagnosed during, or persisting after pregnancy, subdivided into:
 	
(a) *Chronic hypertension* (without proteinuria)
 	
(b) *Chronic renal disease* (proteinuria with or without hypertension)
 	
(c) *Superimposed pre-eclampsia*
    proteinuria developing for the first time during pregnancy in a woman with known chronic hypertension
	(a) may be Essential hypertension
	    Renal hypertension
	    Other known causes (coarctation of the aorta, phaechromocytoma, etc.)
	(b) may be Chronic glomerulo-nephritis
	    Systemic lupus erythromatosis
	    Other renal disease
	(c) *women found to have hypertension and/or proteinuria* at the first visit before the 20th week of pregnancy (in the absence of trophoblastic disease) are presumed to have either chronic hypertension (if they have hypertension only) or chronic renal disease (if they have proteinuria with or without hypertension) but classification may be revised if condition disappears after delivery.

3 Unclassified hypertension and proteinuria Hypertension and/or proteinuria found either at first examination at or after 20th week (140 days) pregnancy in a woman without proven chronic hypertension or chronic renal disease or where insufficient information is available to permit classification, subdivided into: (a) *Unclassified hypertension* (b) *Unclassified proteinuria* (c) *Unclassified proteinuric hypertension* (pre-eclampsia)	*Women with unclassified hypertension and/or proteinuria may be reclassified after delivery* if the hypertension and/or proteinuria disappears after delivery into 1(a) Gestational hypertension, 1(b) Gestational proteinuria or 1(c) Gestational proteinuric hypertension; or, if the hypertension and/or proteinuria persists after delivery or other tests confirm the diagnosis, into 2(a) Chronic hypertension, 2(b) Chronic renal disease or 2(c) Superimposed pre-eclampsia.

Eclampsia is regarded as one of the complications of the hypertensive and proteinuric disorders of pregnancy and is not included in the classification.

hypertension occurs in both primigravidas and multigravidas but is more common in the latter and it increases in frequency with increasing age, being commonest in women over the age of 30 (Nelson 1955). It is postulated to be due to an inherited latent tendency to hypertension which becomes overt in pregnancy (Chesley 1980). In later life there is, as would be expected, a much higher incidence of essential hypertension. In contrast, women who remain normotensive in pregnancy have a much lower later incidence of essential hypertension (Adams & MacGillivray 1961; Fig. 16.3). Latent essential hypertension and chronic essential hypertension are in all probability two phases of the same disorder. The precise nature of the inherited latent tendency is not known, but there is increasing evidence that patients

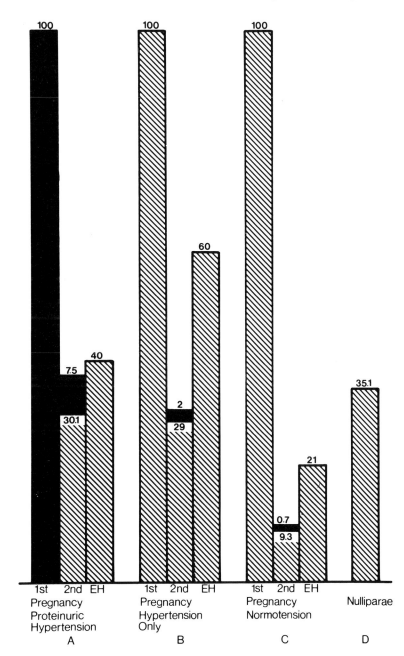

Fig. 16.3. Incidence of gestational hypertension (hatched columns) and proteinuric hypertension (solid columns) in 2nd pregnancy and of later essential hypertension in multiparae who in first pregnancy (A) developed gestational proteinuric hypertension, (B) developed gestational hypertension only, or (C) remained normotensive, together with incidence of essential hypertension in (D) nulliparae of the same age group. (Derived from Adams and MacGillivray, 1961, with permission from the *Lancet*.)

with essential hypertension have an inherited defect in the cellular transport of sodium and potassium which is related to increased contractility of vascular smooth muscle (Blaustein 1977, Kaplan 1982).

Chronic renal disease. Pregnancy may occur in women with known chronic renal disease, or this may be diagnosed for the first time in pregnancy. McCartney (1964) examined renal biopsies from 214 patients presenting with acute hypertension in pregnancy and reported that 25.8% primiparas, and 43.4% multiparas had chronic renal disease (Table 16.3). The incidence of chronic renal disease in pregnancy may therefore be much greater than is currently recognized. Clinically, renal disease may be suspected in normotensive women with proteinuria at booking or when the amount of proteinuria is out of proportion to the BP level. The aetiology, pathology and pathophysiology of the hypertension and proteinuria in chronic renal disease is probably quite different from that of other forms of pregnancy hypertension.

Table 16.3 Renal biopsies in acute hypertension in pregnancy, adapted from McCartney (1964), with permission from the American Heart Association, Inc.

Renal history	No of cases	Normal	TL	TL and CRD	CRD
Primipara	62	3 (4.8%)	43 (69.4%)	1 (1.6%)	15 (24.2%)
Multipara	152	81 (53.3%)	5 (3.3%)	16 (10.5%)	50 (32.9%)

TL = toxaemic lesion
CRD = chronic renal disease

Superimposed pre-eclampsia is diagnosed when proteinuria develops in a patient with chronic hypertension. There is some dispute as to whether the development of proteinuria represents a worsening or extension of the essential hypertension or whether it indicates the occurrence of separate pre-eclamptic disease. Altchek (1964) has produced good evidence, based on renal biopsy, that the occurrence of proteinuria in women with essential hypertension really indicates the development of a separate superimposed disorder. In either case the development of proteinuria in any women with hypertension is of major clinical and prognostic significance and merits recognition and classification as a separate clinical, if not pathological, entity of 'superimposed pre-eclampsia'.

Unclassified hypertension. Many patients book late in pregnancy and it may be impossible to determine whether hypertension and/or proteinuria was present before or developed during the pregnancy. It is generally agreed however that patients with hypertension and/or proteinuria booking before the 20th week (in the absence of trophoblastic disease) should be regarded as having chronic hypertension (if they have hypertension only) or renal disease (if they have hypertension and proteinuria, or proteinuria alone). Women who book after the 20th week and who are found to have hypertension and/or proteinuria at the first visit are diagnosed as unclassified hypertension and/or proteinuria because it is not possible to make a diagnosis or to classify them. In many instances it may be possible to reclassify such patients after delivery according to whether the hypertension and/or proteinuria disappears, or whether it persists after delivery.

CLINICAL PRESENTATION

Mild forms of hypertensive and proteinuric disorders of pregnancy are generally symptomless. In cases of severe disease women may complain of headaches, visual disturbances, epigastric pain and vomiting which are then usually indicative of imminent eclampsia. Because of the absence of symptoms, except in severe disease, the detection and recognition of the hypertensive and proteinuric disorders in pregnancy depends upon regular measurement of BP and regular urine testing for protein at each antenatal visit. Oedema and excessive weight gain are sometimes early warning signs that gestational hypertension or pre-eclampsia may occur later, and rapidly developing generalized oedema may indicate imminent eclampsia.

Diagnostic and prognostic tests
A considerable number of tests have been introduced to predict the future occurrence of hypertension or pre-eclampsia, to differentiate specific forms of hypertensive disease or to detect a specific metabolic or vascular abnormality which might provide a guide to diagnosis, prognosis or management. Most tests relate to one pathophysiological feature of the various hypertensive disorders and are of little clinical value.

Fluid retention
Many women with hypertension and/or proteinuria in pregnancy have a decreased ability to excrete a

water load and so have a tendency to retain water, particularly as extracellular fluid. This may be demonstrated by: excessive gain in weight (0.75 kg or more/week); inability to excrete water load following infusion of 5% glucose; delayed ability to excrete a water load, or abnormal urinary concentration/dilution tests. Abnormal results are not infrequent in normal pregnancy, and these tests are not sufficiently specific to predict the future occurrence of hypertension or to assist in diagnosis.

Vascular reactivity

There is much evidence that the cardiovascular system is abnormally reactive in hypertension in pregnancy, and that the increased reactivity may precede overt hypertension. Some of the tests devised to assess vascular reactivity are:

Cold pressor test is based on changes in BP which occur when one hand is placed in ice water for 1–2 minutes.

Roll over test. Gant et al. (1974) found that when patients destined to develop hypertension were turned from their sides onto their backs there was a marked rise in BP, but others have found a considerable number of false positive results (from 16%–46%). Campbell (1978) showed that the findings could be explained by the changes in sphygmomanometer height of the cuff above the level of the heart.

Response to infusion of vasoactive drugs. The test infusion causes a much higher rise in BP in hypertensive compared with normotensive pregnant women. Vasoactive substances used include vasopressin, adrenaline, noradrenaline and, more recently, angiotensin II, Gant et al. (1973) reported that primigravidas who subsequently developed hypertension showed an increase in sensitivity to angiotensin II several weeks before the development of hypertension. Further investigations have shown about 10% false negative and 10% false positive results. The tests require skilled supervision, are probably not entirely without risk and it is doubtful if they will become established as screening or prognostic procedures.

Blood biochemistry

Uric acid, the end product of purine metabolism, is a relatively insoluble substance excreted with difficulty by the kidneys, and a rise in plasma uric acid may indicate renal involvement or impairment when other metabolic end products such as plasma creatinine and urea remain within the normal range. Uric acid is primarily secreted by the distal tubules and the secretion rate is dependent upon the renal blood flow. Redman et al. (1976a) suggested that serum uric acid is a useful indicator of the risk of perinatal mortality in women with hypertension in pregnancy. They also suggested that raised serum uric acid is a specific feature of pre-eclampsia, but it may also be present in chronic essential hypertension (Messeli et al. 1980).

Deaminases. Maternal serum deoxycytidylate deaminase and serum cytidine deaminase have been proposed as routine antenatal tests to differentiate between pre-eclampsia and essential hypertension (Williams & Jones 1982). It would appear that increased levels of serum cytidine deaminase are a reflection of changes in maternal renal function rather than a specific diagnostic test for pre-eclampsia (Jones et al. 1982).

Placental protein and steroid hormones, and also of the specific placental proteins such as PAPP-A, may provide a measure of placental function or mass. In many cases of hypertension in pregnancy placental function is apparently normal so these tests are not diagnostic, but they may be of value as indicators of impaired placental function and of fetal risk.

Maternal complications

ECLAMPSIA AND IMMINENT ECLAMPSIA

Eclamptic convulsions are a major complication of pregnancy with a perinatal mortality of up to 30–40% and a maternal mortality of 3–4%. The convulsions are usually described as occurring in 4 stages:

Stage 1: Premonitory (30 seconds) with twitching of face, rolling of eyes and sometimes scratching of nose;

Stage 2: Tonic (30–60 seconds) with hypertonus of whole body with clenched jaw, clenched hands, protruding eyes, facial congestion and cyanosis;

Stage 3: Clonic: (1–10 minutes) with spasmodic contraction and relaxation of skeletal muscles, periods of apnoea and cyanosis, biting of the tongue, frothing at the mouth, often accompanied by involuntary passage of urine and faeces, and with a risk of inhalation of blood, mucus and vomit and of fracture of the long bones or other injury;

Stage 4: Coma: (minutes–hours) with stertorous breathing and sometimes cyanosis and pyrexia. Patients in coma after a fit may present a diagnostic problem because of possible associated cerebral haemorrhage and confusion with other conditions such as epilepsy and subarachnoid haemorrhage. In most cases the eclamptic fit is preceded by certain premonitory symptoms and signs. If diagnosed at this stage or if the risk of an eclamptic fit in any patient is considered to be high, the condition is called *imminent eclampsia*. The symptoms and signs of imminent eclampsia include 'aura' with increasing apprehension, anxiety and nervousness; severe increasing headache, usually frontal; visual disturbances (flashes of light, diplopia, dimness of vision, blindness); epigastric pain and vomiting (probably due to subcapsular haemorrhages or necrosis of the liver); rapid rise in BP; marked increase in proteinuria; rapidly increasing generalized oedema; oliguria; hyper-reflexia or clonus.

It is often claimed that eclampsia is a preventable condition but many patients have few or no premonitory signs or symptoms. Eclampsia without proteinuria is rare although the development of proteinuria and onset of eclampsia may be extremely rapid and measured in hours rather than days. Thus, although MacGillivray (1982) found that 27% of 66 cases of eclampsia had hypertension but no proteinuria a few days previously, Chesley (1978c) found only 2.5% of cases without proteinuria in urine examined immediately before convulsions and in 50% there was 4+ proteinuria.

CARDIAC FAILURE AND PULMONARY OEDEMA

Pulmonary oedema may be due to cardiac failure secondary to hypertension, adult respiratory distress syndrome following prolonged hypoxia, or fluid overload. Fluid overload or water intoxication can easily occur in hypertension in pregnancy, particularly if hyperosmotic infusion fluids are used, and problems in diagnosis may arise because the symptoms of water intoxication are similar to those of imminent eclampsia. Cramps or muscle weakness may provide a clue to the diagnosis, and an abnormally low serum sodium is diagnostic of water intoxication. Cardiac failure with pulmonary oedema may occur in hypertensive patients with normal hearts, and it is important to remember that pregnant women, particularly if pre-eclamptic, develop pulmonary oedema more easily than non-pregnant or normal pregnant women due to their reduced plasma proteins and plasma oncotic pressure.

CEREBROVASCULAR AND OTHER HAEMORRHAGES

Severe hypertension may cause fibrinoid change and necrosis of the walls of small arteries and arterioles which may then rupture, resulting in cerebral haemorrhage and haemorrhages in various other organs of the body. The necrosis and rupture appears to be a direct effect of vasospasm and of high BP on the vessel walls. The precise level of BP required to produce fibrinoid necrosis and rupture is uncertain but rat experiments suggest that there is a significant risk when the intra-arterial pressure rises above a level corresponding to a DBP of 130–140 mmHg (Goldby & Beilin 1972, Redman 1977).

Cerebrovascular haemorrhage may occur in eclamptic patients and is recognized by the development of localizing neurological signs. Cerebrovascular accidents may also occur in severe hypertension without eclampsia, particularly if there has been a precipitous fall in blood pressure due to antihypertensive therapy. Cerebral thrombosis or embolus complicating hypertension in pregnancy may be confused with eclampsia.

Hepatic haemorrhages and other lesions may be recognized by the occurrence of epigastric pain which is an important symptom in hypertensive disorders of pregnancy. They are characteristically periportal or subcapsular, although diffuse haemorrhages may occur. When hepatic pain is associated with abnormal liver function tests (e.g. elevated liver enzymes) a low platelet count (probably due to DIC) and haemolysis the condition is known as 'HELLP' syndrome (Weinstein 1982). The importance of this syndrome is not so much that it is a separate syndrome but that epigastric pain, elevated liver enzymes and low platelet count may occur with relatively mild or moderate degrees of hypertension. It then indicates severe disease and may be an indication for immediate delivery (MacKenna *et al.* 1983).

Other organs. Haemorrhage may occur, less commonly, in the adrenal gland, heart, intestine, kidney, spleen, stomach and retina. Blindness occurs in 1–3% of cases of eclampsia, due to partial or complete detachment of the retina, retinal arterial or venous thrombosis, retinal oedema or optic neuritis. Fortunately most retinal lesions resolve (though this may take from 2 days up to 2 months) and permanent blindness is a rare sequel of eclampsia or hypertension in pregnancy.

RENAL FAILURE

Acute renal failure complicating hypertension in pregnancy may be due to a variety of lesions, from simple ischaemia and oedema to tubular necrosis and patchy or complete cortical necrosis. There is cortical necrosis in about 25% of cases of renal failure. Although it is often fatal, recovery of renal function has been reported with oliguria lasting up to 60 days and continuing improvement up to 3 years (Walls et al. 1978). The commonest sign of renal failure is oliguria accompanied by rising serum creatinine, urea and uric acid. Oliguria is diagnosed when the urine production is less than 30 ml/hour (or 720 ml/24 hours).

DISSEMINATED INTRAVASCULAR COAGULATION (DIC)

In normal pregnancy there is both increased coagulation and increased fibrinolysis, and these processes are in balance. There is controversy as to whether intravascular coagulation occurs in all or only in some hypertensive pregnancies and, if it occurs, whether it is truly disseminated or is localized to particular organs such as the placenta and kidneys. It would appear that DIC is a common but not an essential feature of hypertension in pregnancy and that it may vary from a chronic low grade process resulting primarily in fibrin deposition (mainly in the placenta) to an acute overwhelming event resulting in complete incoagulability of the blood as in placental abruption. A decreased platelet count has been reported to be an essential feature of pre-eclampsia and to precede the onset of hypertension (Redman et al. 1978a). Pritchard et al. (1976) reported platelet counts of less than 150,000/mm³ in 26% and of less than 100,000/mm³ in 16% of eclamptic women. Other workers (Galton et al. 1971) have found no significant change in the average platelet count in pre-eclampsia, although individual cases with severe disease did have relatively low counts. Low or falling platelet counts should always be taken as an indication of severe disease and it is important that a clotting time and platelet count be performed in all cases of severe hypertension before epidural anaesthesia or any surgical procedure is performed.

MICRO-ANGIOPATHIC HAEMOLYTIC ANAEMIA

Haemoglobinaemia and haemoglobinuria have been reported in association with pre-eclampsia and eclampsia since the 19th century and the condition is now designated micro-angiopathic haemolytic anaemia (Brain et al. 1962). In a few cases of severe pre-eclampsia or eclampsia there is an acute or subacute haemolysis with the appearance of fragmented red blood cells and reticulocytes in the peripheral blood smear (Pritchard et al. 1954), associated with thrombocytopenia and renal vascular lesions, usually fibrinoid necrosis (Brain et al. 1967).

Feto-placental complications

Hypertension in pregnancy is associated with constriction of the uterine blood vessels, pathological changes in the spiral arterioles, and fibrin deposition, infarcts and other pathological changes in the placenta, resulting in retarded fetal growth, fetal hypoxia and intrauterine death.

PLACENTAL ABRUPTION

Placental abruption is regarded as a complication of hypertension in pregnancy, though only about 5% of cases are preceded by known hypertensive disease, 4% of cases occurring in primigravidas and 1% in multiparas (MacGillivray 1961). Hypertension and proteinuria however are very commonly found after placental abruption though in MacGillivray's series 38% of primigravidas and 49% of multigravidas remained normotensive. It is not certain if the hypertension and proteinuria cause placental abruption, or if the abruption and associated DIC with deposition of fibrin in the kidneys cause the hypertension or proteinuria.

INTRAUTERINE GROWTH RETARDATION (IUGR)

The occurrence of IUGR in hypertensive disorders in pregnancy is influenced by many factors such as the level of BP, the occurrence of proteinuria, smoking and nutrition. In a study in Aberdeen (MacGillivray 1977) in women with hypertension alone the mean birthweight for gestational age was the same as in normotensive women, but in women with hypertension and proteinuria the mean birthweight was reduced at all gestational ages. Long et al. (1980) found that the prevalence of small-for-dates infants (< 10th percentile) was increased in early onset pre-eclampsia (18.2%) but decreased in late onset pre-eclampsia (5.6%) compared with the rate of 8.6% in the total hospital population. Perinatal mortality was similarly increased in early onset disease (287 per

1000) births as compared with late onset disease (19 per 1000). These authors also found that patients with early onset of hypertension had significantly increased prevalences of subnormal oestriol excretion (79.5%) and hypoglycaemia (33.3%) before the onset of the pre-eclampsia. They concluded that placental insufficiency may precede the development of IUGR and pre-eclampsia and that pre-eclampsia may be secondary to placental insufficiency. The occurrence of IUGR in proteinuric pre-eclampsia indicates a significant increased risk to the fetus with increased perinatal mortality in small-for-dates infants. Thus, in Aberdeen the perinatal mortality rate in infants whose birthweight was less than the 10th centile was 17.2% compared with a rate of 4.7% in infants of greater birthweight (MacGillivray 1983a). The timely detection of IUGR and placental insufficiency is an important part of the management of hypertension in pregnancy.

FETAL ASPHYXIA AND INTRAUTERINE DEATH

One of the main complications of hypertension in pregnancy is fetal hypoxia and hypoxic intrauterine death. The occurrence of placental hypoxia as an important part of the pathophysiology of hypertension was confirmed by McLennan *et al.* (1972) who showed that ultrastructural changes in the placentas of pre-eclamptic women closely resembled those in explanted placental tissue in organ cultures subjected to hypoxia. These changes paralleled the severity of the pre-eclampsia and included thickening of the basal lamina, increased numbers of microvilli, increased subtrophoblastic space, reduction in endoplasmic reticulum, decrease in number and size of mitochondria, clumping of nuclear chromatin, thinning and degeneration of the syncytium and increased syncytial knots.

Incidence and epidemiology

The lack of an agreed classification, definitions and nomenclature, and the fact that many estimates of incidence are based on hospital admissions rather than on total populations, makes it difficult, if not impossible, to establish the true incidence. The incidence of hypertension and proteinuria in the British Perinatal Mortality Survey (Butler and Alberman 1969), in which hypertension was diagnosed on the basis of one observation of a DBP of 90 mmHg or more, is shown in Table 16.4. The overall incidence of 35.4% for all hypertensive disorders seems high,

Table 16.4 Incidence of hypertension and proteinuria in pregnancy. British Perinatal Mortality Survey from Butler and Alberman (1969).

Maternal age and parity	None %	Mild %	Moderate %	Severe %	Remainder %	All %
Primiparas (6,280 births)						
Less than 25	60.4	18.4	4.4	8.5	8.3	39.6
25 to 34	55.3	21.4	5.2	10.2	7.9	44.7
35 or more	39.0	30.9	6.8	15.3	8.0	61.0
Total	57.5	20.1	4.8	9.4	8.1	42.4
Multiparas (10,201 births)						
Less than 25	74.6	12.4	2.0	3.5	7.5	25.4
25 to 34	69.4	15.9	3.7	3.7	7.3	30.6
35 or more	60.4	19.4	4.7	6.5	9.0	39.6
Total	68.9	15.8	3.5	4.3	7.6	31.2
Total all parities	64.7	17.4	4.0	6.1	7.8	35.2
Mortality Rate	76.5	87.1	127.8	228.0	210.0	140.0

None = Normotensive Nonproteinuric
Mild = Max DBP 90–100 without proteinuria
Moderate = Max DBP 100–109 without proteinuria
Severe = Max DBP 90 or more with proteinuria or Max DBP 110 or more without proteinuria
Remainder = Proteinuria with DBP less than 90 and unclassifie
All = All hypertensive and proteinuric groups combined
Mortality Rate =

$$\frac{\text{SB and NND rate in hypertensive groups} \times 100}{\text{SB and NND rate whole population}}$$

but a similar incidence (33.8%) was found in 15,251 mothers delivered in the Cape Peninsula Maternity and Neonatal Service Region in South Africa in 1972 in whom a DBP of 90 mmHg or more on two or more occasions was used (Knutzen and Davey 1977). Both surveys included women found to be hypertensive antenatally and women who developed hypertension for the first time in labour. In the South African series the incidence of hypertension was 15.7% antenatally, and 18.1% in labour. Hypertension in labour may be a physiological or pathological occurrence and it is essential to separate patients found to be hypertensive antenatally from those found to be hypertensive for the first time in labour. A further major difficulty is that any assessment of incidence of hypertension and proteinuria will depend to a considerable extent on the number of times the BP is measured and urine is tested (MacGillivray 1983b). It is therefore difficult to make assessments or comparisons of incidence unless hypertension and proteinuria are very strictly defined and the compostition of the populations studied is known.

Wide variations in the incidence of hypertension, proteinuria and eclampsia, and in associated maternal and perinatal mortality, have been reported from different institutions in different countries, but these may result from differences in classification and definition and in methods of BP measurement. Davies (1971), who carried out an excellent survey of the literature on the incidence of eclampsia (consisting of over 170 reports from 50 countries), concluded that 'the figures and rates quoted cannot be used for international comparisons even of the grossest sort'. The most significant adequately documented change is the fall in incidence of eclampsia which is occurring in most countries. In England and Wales the deaths from eclampsia and pre-eclampsia fell from a total of 200 or 97.4 per million maternities in the years 1952–54 to 39 or 20.3 per million maternities in 1973–75. This fall is probably due to improvement in antenatal and intrapartum care and provides some measure of the overall standard of maternity services in different regions and different countries.

PREDISPOSING FACTORS

A large number of factors have been regarded as predisposing towards the occurrence of hypertension and proteinuria in pregnancy.

Age and parity

Age has an important influence on the incidence of hypertensive and proteinuric disorders and on the perinatal mortality. Young primigravidas, and both primigravidas and multigravidas over the age of 30 years have increased incidences of hypertension and hypertension with proteinuria and increased perinatal mortality. The increase in incidence of hypertension with increasing age probably reflects the increasing incidence of essential or latent essential hypertension.

Parity similarly has an important influence on the incidence of hypertension and proteinuria and on associated perinatal mortality. An analysis of 62,239 singleton deliveries in the Cape Peninsula Maternity and Neonatal Service Region in 1979–1981 is shown in Table 16.5.

Primigravidas have approximately double the incidence of hypertension and of hypertension with proteinuria, as do women in second or subsequent pregnancies. The incidence of hypertension only, however, apparently increases with increasing parity,

Table 16.5 Incidence of hypertension and proteinuria and associated perinatal mortality in 62,239 singleton births in Cape Peninsula Maternity and Neonatal Service region 1979–1981.

Type of disorder	Para 1		Para 2, 3, 4		Para 5 and over	
	Inc %	PNM/1,000	Inc %	PNM/1,000	Inc %	PNM/1,000
Hypertension only	8.3	23.7	4.7	39.1	7.4	43.2
Proteinuria only	1.0	25.0	0.9	35.1	0.9	—
Hypertension & proteinuria	4.2	55.4	1.8	79.0	2.4	72.6
All hypertension	13.7	34.8	7.4	48.8	10.7	47.3
All normotension	86.3	26.4	92.6	24.8	98.3	32.8

Inc = Incidence in %
PNM = Stillbirths plus 1st week deaths/1,000 total births
— = No perinatal deaths and number too small to calculate rate.

though analysis by age and parity shows this to be due to the concomitant increase in age, particularly over the age of 30 years, rather than the increase in parity (Fig. 16.4).

Social status

Lower socio-economic groups are reported to have a higher incidence of pre-eclampsia and eclampsia, but Duffus and MacGillivray (1968) found that differences between social class are small if allowance is made for age and parity distributions, levels of antenatal and obstetric care and smoking habits.

Race

In order to determine whether there are true differences with race, as distinct from geography and climate, it is necessary to ensure not only that the incidence of hypertensive disorders in different races in the same region are compared, but that the same standards of antenatal care and recording are applied to all races and that due allowance is made for any differences in age and parity distribution in the racial groups. In a study in Jerusalem where allowance was made for these factors and where all pregnant women received the same standard of care, Dawes et al. (1970) found that the incidence of pre-eclampsia was significantly higher in Muslim Arabs and Jews born in Iran than in Jews born in North Africa or Israel. These differences are possibly related to differences in the incidence of inherited tendencies to essential hypertension. The effect of inherited and

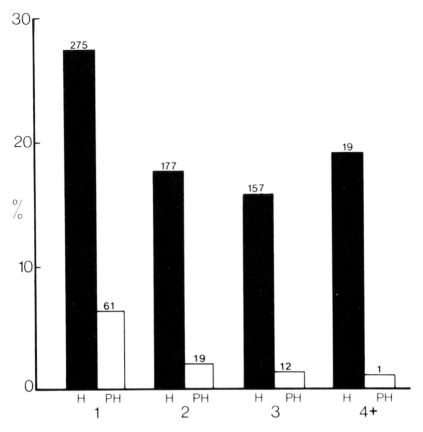

Fig. 16.4. Incidence of pregnancy-induced hypertension (hypertension only) (H) and pre-eclampsia (hypertension with proteinuria) (PH) by Pregnancy Number. From Campbell, MacGillivray and Carr-Hill (1985).

genetic racial differences are however probably small compared with differences in antenatal care and other factors in the different racial groups.

Genetic predisposition

Several hypotheses have been advanced proposing a genetic inheritance of severe pre-eclampsia including a simple recessive trait involving fetal and maternal genotypes, multifactorial inheritance, incomplete penetrance of the gene and 'variable susceptibility to fetal challenge'. This last hypothesis is consistent with the protective effect of parity and abortion, the occurrence of pre-eclampsia in parous women with new husbands, and the possible protective effect of blood transfusions prior to pregnancy. Familial and genetic factors seem to have a strong influence on the occurrence of hypertension and proteinuria in pregnancy.

Twin pregnancy

Twinning is associated with a greater incidence of proteinuric pre-eclampsia, 25.3% compared with 3.4% in singletons, and of hypertension alone which

is increased from 18% in singletons to 25% in twin pregnancies (MacGillivray 1958). The increased incidence of hypertension is postulated to be due to hyperplacentosis, increased placental hormone secretion and increased blood volume, increased cardiac output and other haemodynamic changes.

Hydatidiform mole

The occurrence and early onset of pre-eclampsia and eclampsia with hydatidiform mole is well known, but it is less well known that with small, slow growing moles there is no increased incidence of pre-eclampsia, whereas with large, rapidly growing moles the incidence of pre-eclampsia is about 70% (Page 1939). This suggests that excessive trophoblast activity and possibly excessive secretion of placental hormones may play a major role in the aetiology of pre-eclampsia. There was some doubt whether the hypertension and proteinuria associated with hydatidiform mole represented 'true pre-eclampsia' but Sanchez-Torres and Santamaria (1965) have demonstrated typical changes of pre-eclampsia on renal biopsy.

Hydrops fetalis, polyhydramnios and fetal malformations
The relationship between hypertensive disorders of pregnancy and hydrops fetalis, polyhydramnios and fetal malformations has been a matter of controversy. Scott (1958) found that 50% of pregnancies with hydrops fetalis had pre-eclampsia compared with 4.6% in haemolytic disease without fetal hydrops, so that the occurrence of pre-eclampsia may be due to the hyperplacentosis associated with hydrops fetalis. In polyhydramnios the incidence of mild and proteinuric pre-eclampsia is increased when the fetus is normal, but not when there is an associated fetal malformation (MacGillivray 1959).

Diet, vitamins and trace elements
Many aspects of dietary intake, including carbohydrate, protein and salt, have been implicated in the aetiology and pathogenesis of hypertensive disorders of pregnancy. Many workers have claimed that restriction of dietary carbohydrate, protein and/or salt prevents pre-eclampsia and eclampsia. Dietary supplementation of various nutrients, trace elements and vitamins has also been widely advocated to prevent and treat the various hypertensive disorders of pregnancy. The World Health Organization Expert Committee on Pregnancy and Lactation (1965), however, concluded that there was no scientific basis for believing that either deficiency or excess of any nutrient predisposed to, or prevented, pre-eclampsia and eclampsia.

Climate and seasons
The incidence of eclampsia, pre-eclampsia and hypertension has been reported by many authors to have a marked seasonal difference but there is no agreement on the seasonal change responsible. Changes in ambient temperature, humidity and barometric pressure have all been suggested, and there is some evidence that arterial BP is higher in cold weather possibly due to increased peripheral vasoconstriction.

Obesity
The incidence of essential hypertension and of hypertensive and proteinuric hypertension in pregnancy is significantly increased in obese women (Treharne *et al.* 1979). The influence of obesity on BP in non-pregnant subjects is well known, particularly in relation to essential hypertension, but the increase in proteinuric hypertension is surprising.

Smoking
The incidence of proteinuric hypertension in cigarette smokers is about half that in non-smokers. The difference is not related to body weight or weight gain in pregnancy (Duffus and MacGillivray 1968) but may be related to plasma volume which undergoes less expansion in smokers (Pirani & MacGillivray 1978). More important, although the incidence of pre-eclampsia is reduced, the perinatal mortality rate is approximately trebled in women with proteinuric pre-eclampsia who smoke (from 8.5% in non-smokers to 21.7% in smokers; Duffus and MacGillivray 1968). Smoking is thus a major risk factor and its importance is often underestimated in assessing the risks of hypertension and proteinuria in pregnancy.

In summary, the major identifiable predisposing and risk factors in hypertensive disorders of pregancy are age, parity, obesity, smoking and family history.

PATHOLOGY AND MORBID ANATOMICAL CHANGES

There are, in all probability, several different disease processes with different pathologies and aetiologies underlying the different hypertensive disorders of pregnancy. Moreover, not all organs and not all patients will show all the pathological features of the disorders. The pathological changes depend on the nature and extent of the underlying disorders. Much of the knowledge of the structural pathological lesions in the hypertensive and proteinuric disorders has been derived from postmortem examination of women who died of pre-eclampsia and eclampsia. Sheehan and Lynch (1973b) performed autopsies on 677 women who died in pregnancy, including 170 performed within 2–3 hours of the patient's death, most of the deaths being due to eclampsia or pre-eclampsia. They found that most of the pathological changes in women dying of eclampsia consisted of haemorrhages and oedema, although they believed that much of the oedema and accumulation of fluid was due to postmortem changes. The only organs where pathological examination has been possible in the course of the disease are the kidney and placenta, and light and electron microscopy of renal biopsy specimens have made a substantial contribution to knowledge. Pathological examination of the placenta and placental bed biopsy have yielded important information about changes in the placenta and in the underlying decidua and myometrium, but the findings tend to represent 'end stages' of the disease process and do not reflect physiological changes such as vasospasm.

Postmortem examination of stillbirths and of infants who died after delivery from hypertensive and/

or proteinuric mothers, have shown no specific pathological changes apart from those due to hypoxia and growth retardation which would be expected in infants delivered of normotensive mothers under the same circumstances. There is no increased incidence of congenital abnormalities.

PLACENTAL PATHOLOGY

Placental changes associated with hypertension and proteinuria in pregnancy include the following:

Hyperplacentosis. The presence of trophoblast is essential for the development of hypertension and proteinuria in pregnancy, and the more trophoblast that is present the greater the likelihood of hypertension and proteinuria. Hyperplacentosis is found in association with diabetes, erythroblastosis, hydatidiform mole, multiple pregnancy, thalassaemia and triploidy, and the incidence of pre-eclampsia has been reported to be increased in all these conditions.

Infarcts. True placental infarcts which are due to localized areas of ischaemic villous necrosis must be distinguished from massive intervillous fibrin deposition (Fox 1978). Placental infarcts are common in hypertensive disorders of pregnancy and the incidence is directly related to the severity of the hypertension (Table 16.6). They were once thought to have an aetiological role in pre-eclampsia, but are not an invariable feature and are probably a consequence rather than a cause of the disorder.

Table 16.6 Incidence of placental infarcts in normotensive and hypertensive pregnancies. Fox H. (1978) *Pathology of the placenta.* W.B. Saunders London, Philadelphia and Toronto, with permission.

	Generalized	Extensive
Mild pre-eclampsia	34%	2%
Mild chronic hypertension	27%	20%
Severe pre-eclampsia	60%	30%
Severe chronic hypertension	70%	66%
Normal pregnancy	25%	0%
(Extensive infarction more than 5% of villous tissue)		

Massive perivillous fibrin deposition, sub-chorionic fibrin deposition and intervillous thrombin. Fibrin may be deposited around the villi, particularly in the peripheral areas of the placenta, and the lesions macroscopically may be mistaken for infarcts. Fibrin deposits are found in 22% of placentas from full term uncomplicated pregnancies but are uncommon in

premature deliveries (6%). Their incidence is not increased in hypertensive disorders.

Histological changes in the placenta. Many histological changes have been described in placentas from hypertensive women, including syncytical degeneration, syncytical hyperplasia, syncytical knots, cytotrophoblastic hyperplasia, thickening of the basement membranes, villous hypervascularity and obliterative end-arteritis, but there is no single lesion or group of lesions characteristic of hypertension in pregnancy. These changes are probably secondary to the hypertension, and in most instances are a response to reduced blood flow and uteroplacental ischaemia, though some immunological reaction cannot be excluded particularly in association with obliterative end-arteritis.

UTERO-PLACENTAL VASCULAR PATHOLOGY

Changes in the uteroplacental vessels, particularly in the spiral arteries, may hold the key to much of the pathophysiology of hypertension in pregnancy. Reduction in calibre of the spiral arteries, due to pathological changes or spasm, must result in reduction of choriodecidual blood flow which probably causes most of the fetal morbidity and mortality. Three main vascular changes are described.

Failure of normal 'physiological' structural changes in pre-eclampsia. In early normal pregnancy cytotrophoblastic cells proliferate and invade the intradecidual portion of the spiral arteries. They spread up the lumen, invade the vessel walls, replace the maternal endothelium and destroy the elastic and muscular tissue which is replaced by fibrinoid material. This process opens up the spiral arteries, increasing the blood flow, and at the same time making them unresponsive to normal vasoconstrictor stimuli. Between 12 and 16 weeks there is a further wave of cytotrophoblastic invasion into the stroma of the myometrium and within the intramyometrial segments of the spiral arteries, extending into the distal portion of the radial arteries. This is accompanied by replacement of maternal endothelium, destruction of the muscular and elastic tissue of the media and replacement by fibrinoid material of the intramyometrial portion of the spiral arteries which further opens up the arteries to produce a further increase in choriodecidual blood flow. Both the primary and secondary waves of cytotrophoblastic invasion occur only in the vessels of the placental bed and are regarded as part of the essential physiological changes in normal pregnancy.

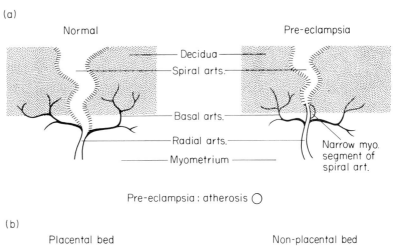

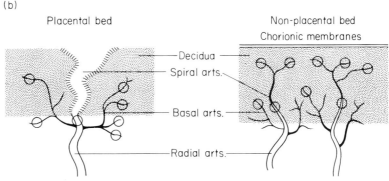

Fig. 16.5. Spiral arterioles in normal and 'pre-eclamptic' pregnancies showing (a) *extent of physiological changes* which in pre-eclampsia do not extend beyond decidua-myometrial junction leaving a constricting segment of the placental bed spiral arteries between spiral arteries and the parent radial arteries. (b) *Topography of acute atherosis,* atherotic lesions being confined to vessels unaffected by physiological changes. From Lindheimer M. D. et al. (1976) *Hypertension in Pregnancy,* p. 115. John Wiley and Sons, New York. With permission from the Publishers and Professor W. B. Robertson.

On the basis of placental bed biopsies Dixon and Robertson (1961), Brosens *et al.* (1972) and Robertson (1976) reported that in pre-eclampsia there is a failure in the second wave of trophoblastic invasion so that the musculo-elastic media of the spiral arteries in the myometrium is retained, the vessels fail to dilate and remain responsive to vasoconstrictor stimuli resulting in a decreased choriodecidual blood flow. They regard the failure of the cytotrophoblast to invade the spiral arteries and the absence of the normal vascular changes as unique and essential features of pre-eclampsia (Fig. 16.5; Robertson *et al.* 1976), but Sheppard and Bonnar (1976, 1981) reported the absence of physiological changes in normotensive pregnancies with IUGR, and they also described cases of hypertension in pregnancy in which the normal physiological changes were present. They concluded that the physiological changes of pregnancy were not restricted to decidual segments of the vessels in all pregnancies complicated by hypertension, and that there was no clearcut relationship between vascular changes in these vessels, IUGR and hypertension.

Acute atherosis. In some spiral arteries there is an accumulation of lipid in the muscle cells of the media and interna, which may be followed by necrosis releasing the lipid which is then taken up by macrophages to produce lesions which appear like atheroma, hence the name 'acute atherosis' (Zeek & Assali 1950, de Wolf *et al.* 1975). These changes may be associated with thrombosis and organization of the thrombi, resulting in vascular occlusion, and possibly placental infarction.

Acute atherosis can occur only in the musculoelastic tissues of the media of vessels which have not undergone the normal physiological changes of pregnancy. It is not found in uncomplicated essential hypertension, but similar lesions have been found in association with placental abruption (Hertig 1945).

Hyperplasia and arteriosclerosis of the basal arteries. In established essential hypertension the changes in the placental vessels are quite different from those in pre-eclampsia, the main change being a hyperplasia of the interna and media of the basal arteries of the uterus. These arteries may also show classical arteriosclerotic changes, as in the vessels of other organs in essential hypertension. These striking changes are restricted to the basal arteries where they develop fully in much shorter time, and at much lower levels of BP, than in any blood vessels elsewhere in the body. The extent and severity of the lesions in the basal arteries parallel the severity of the hypertension, and the proliferation of the fibrous and muscular tissue of the media may even lead to virtual occlusion of the vessels in severe hypertension. When pre-eclampsia is superimposed upon chronic hypertension the lesions of each disease are found in conjunction, often with exaggeration of the 'pre-eclamptic' changes, particularly acute atherosis of the arcuate and spiral arteries. This may lead to complete destruction of the spiral arteries, thrombosis and necrosis of the decidua, and decidual haemorrhage.

MATERNAL PATHOLOGY

Most of the pathological changes, being based upon postmortem findings, should be regarded as end stages or complications of the hypertensive disorders of pregnancy. In mild hypertension there may be very few, if any, pathological lesions, and in general the extent and severity of the pathological changes is related to the severity of the hypertension and/or proteinuria and the occurrence of eclampsia.

Kidney

The main renal changes in pre-eclampsia occur in the glomeruli, and Sheehan and Lynch (1973c) described ten characteristic changes which include, in order of frequency: enlargement of the glomeruli; thickening of the tuft epithelium; vacuoles in tuft epithelium; moderate or gross ballooning of loops;

swelling of endothelial/mesangial cells; fat in glomerular cells; 'pouting' of glomeruli; hyaline and fat deposition in glomeruli; foam cells in glomeruli; thrombi and deposition of fibrin in the glomerular capillaries.

Electron microscopy studies have revealed a particular form of swelling and vacuolization of the intracapillary cells of the glomeruli, together with mesangial cell proliferation, which was at one time thought to be specific to pre-eclampsia and was named glomerular capillary endotheliosis (Spargo *et al.* 1959). Robson (1976), however, whilst agreeing that there are characteristic glomerular lesions in pre-eclampsia as originally claimed by Pollak and Nettles (1960), has stressed that the lesions of pre-eclampsia are characteristic only in the sense that the glomerular changes follow a particular pattern and not because of any single unique or specific pathological feature (Fig. 16.6).

McCartney (1964) examined renal biopsies from 214 unselected cases of acute hypertension in pregnancy (Table 16.3). In 62 primiparas he found that 71% had a typical 'toxaemic' lesion, alone or combined with chronic renal disease, 24.2% had lesions suggestive of chronic renal disease and 4% had no abnormality. In contrast, of the 132 multiparas, only 13.8% had a toxaemic lesion, with or without chronic renal disease, 32.9% had chronic renal disease and 53.3% had normal biopsies suggestive of essential hypertension. The high incidence of chronic renal disease in this series has been questioned, but these findings do lend support to the concept of at least two, if not three, types of hypertension in preg-

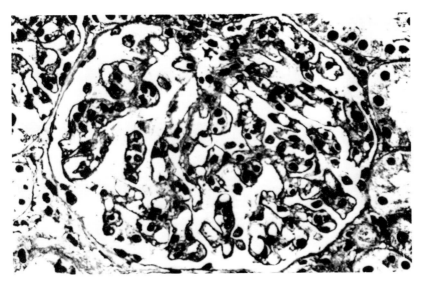

Fig. 16.6. Renal glomerulus in pre-eclampsia. The glomerulus is swollen, hypercellular and bloodless, with longitudinal expansion of the mesangium and thickened capillary cells. Mesangial/ endothelial foam cells are present at 1700, 2000 and 2200 hours. From Seymour *et al.* (1976) in Lindheimer M.D. *et al. Hypertension in Pregnancy*, 139–153. John Wiley and Sons, New York.

nancy. As already described, pre-eclampsia occurs mainly in primigravidas and is associated with proteinuria and typical renal lesions, essential hypertension occurs mainly in multigravidas without proteinuria and with normal renal biopsies, and hypertension associated with chronic renal disease occurs in primigravidas and multigravidas with the characteristic changes of chronic renal disease. Particular emphasis has been placed on the glomerular lesions in hypertensive disease in pregnancy, but it is important to note that degenerative lesions in the loop of Henle also occur, and Altchek *et al.* (1968) have claimed that the severity of these lesions is paralleled by the degree of hyperuricaemia.

Liver

Liver changes are found in 60–70% of women dying of eclampsia and pre-eclampsia, and lesions have been found on needle biopsies of the liver. The lesions are probably not specific to pre-eclampsia or eclampsia but are manifestations of vasoconstriction and disseminated intravascular coagulation. Two lesions are described: localized periportal haemorrhages which later become replaced by fibrin, and ischaemic lesions which vary from small areas of necrosis to large infarcts and are due to occlusive vasospasm of the branches of the hepatic artery (Sheehan & Lynch 1973d).

Heart and lungs

In women dying of eclampsia there are frequently subendocardial haemorrhages and scattered alveolar haemorrhages in the lungs. The lesions are not specific, but resemble the periportal haemorrhages in the liver and are due to vasoconstriction and DIC.

Adrenal gland

Adrenal haemorrhage is a rare but important complication of pre-eclampsia and eclampsia. It is recognized by the sudden onset of shock, collapse, and abdominal or lumbar pain.

Pituitary gland

Anterior pituitary necrosis may occur with severe hypertension in pregnancy, placental abruption and postpartum haemorrhage. MacGillivray (1950) described 10 cases of combined renal and pituitary necrosis associated with pre-eclampsia. Though rare, the danger of sudden falls in blood pressure, haemorrhage and shock in association with severe hypertension cannot be overemphasized.

Brain

Cerebrovascular haemorrhage is the commonest cause of death in eclampsia and pre-eclampsia. Sheehan and Lynch (1973e) found cerebral haemorrhages and softenings in 60% of eclamptic patients who died within 2 days of the onset of convulsions, but in only 20% of those who survived longer. The cerebral haemorrhage results from fibrinoid change and necrosis of the small arteries and arterioles, and is probably secondary to vasospasm which is directly related to the BP level. Thrombosis of cerebral arteries and veins may also occur, and may involve main cerebral vessels such as the vein of Galen, parietal veins and the superior sagittal sinus. Sheehan and Lynch (1973f) maintained that there is no cerebral oedema in cases of eclampsia, but recent observations using CAT scan confirm older observations of marked cerebral oedema at least in eclamptic patients presenting in coma (Richards 1985).

Pathophysiology and functional changes

As previously noted, there are several different disorders causing hypertension in pregnancy, each showing different underlying pathophysiological changes.

CARDIOVASCULAR CHANGES

Arterial BP

The arterial BP is determined primarily by the cardiac output and peripheral vascular resistance.

Cardiac output is dependent upon the heart rate and the stroke volume. Peripheral resistance is dependent upon many factors including the amount of vasoconstriction and elasticity in the peripheral arterioles and resistance vessels, the degree of filling of the vascular system determined by the blood volume and the amount of constriction and elasticity of the venous capacitance vessels, and the blood viscosity. An understanding of these changes in normal and hypertensive pregnancies is important, not only in aetiology and pathophysiology but in ensuring correct management of each hypertensive patient particularly when potent antihypertensive agents are used.

Changes in normal pregnancy. The fall in BP in normal pregnancy is due to peripheral vasodilatation as the result of decreased smooth muscle tone in arterioles possibly due to increase in circulating progesterone, and/or decreased circulating vasoconstrictor substances such as Angiotensin II and adrenaline and noradrenaline or decreased responsiveness to these substances, possibly due to increased production of vasodilator prostanoids PGE_2 or PGI_2 (Gant & Worley 1980b), and/or decreased vasomotor sympathetic nervous system activity (Assali *et al.* 1952).

In the third trimester the normal physiological rise in BP to prepregnancy levels implies a partial reversal of these changes and has some important clinical implications. These are: a rise in BP in the third trimester is a normal phenomenon, and not necessarily an indication of pre-eclampsia or other hypertensive disorders; in patients with chronic essential hypertension the BP may fall to apparently normal levels in early pregnancy but may rise to prepregnancy hypertensive levels in the third trimester; some patients (e.g. those with twins or hyperplacentosis) may have an excessive physiological rise in BP in the third trimester resulting in hypertension as defined by a DBP of 90 mmHg or more, and this 'supranormal hypertension' is associated with a marked weight gain, large increase in blood volume, large baby and a low or reduced perinatal mortality.

Changes in hypertensive disorders. In about a third of women with hypertension in pregnancy there is a reversal of the normal diurnal rhythm, and patients with severe pre-eclampsia may have a rise in BP at night (Redman *et al.* 1976b). There is also a change in the diurnal rhythm from a 24 to a 20-hour cycle with reduction in the normal fall in BP during sleep (Ruff *et al.* 1982). These changes may be due to changes in central BP regulating mechanisms or in the baroreceptor reflexes (Seligman 1971).

Changes in labour and the puerperium. Rises in BP in labour and in the puerperium are difficult to interpret. The BP may normally rise in labour because of the exertion, excitement and stress of labour, and it may be that the cardiovascular system in women with hypertensive disorders is abnormally sensitive to such external stimuli. After delivery there may be a sudden rise in BP because of the constriction of the uterine arteries and expulsion of blood into the general circulation. Administration of drugs such as ergometrine may also cause vasospasm and a rise in blood pressure.

Because of the stresses that occur in labour and the cardiovascular changes that occur at delivery, an increase in BP may not have the same clinical and pathological significance in labour and the puerperium as it has antenatally. It is necessary to subdivide all patients with hypertension into three groups: (a) those who develop hypertension antenatally (b) those who develop hypertension for the first time in labour

and (c) those who develop hypertension for the first time in the puerperium.

Cardiac output
These are major differences in the findings of different investigators with regard to the changes in cardiac output in hypertension in pregnancy. Werkö (1950) found no difference in cardiac output in pre-eclampsia and normal women at the same stage of pregnancy, the average cardiac output being 7 litres. Hamilton (1951) found that in cases of severe pre-eclampsia and of pre-eclampsia superimposed on essential hypertension the cardiac output was increased, that in cases of essential hypertension it was unchanged, and that in 6 cases of chronic nephritis it was reduced. Lim and Walters (1979), in 23 normotensive and 25 mildly hypertensive pregnant women, found that heart rate, cardiac output, stroke volume, left ventricular work index and total peripheral vascular resistance were all significantly higher in the hypertensive women. They postulated that the hypertension was due to 'hyperactivity of the sympathetic adrenergic component of the autonomic nervous system'. Benedetti *et al.* (1980), in a study of 7 severe pre-eclamptic patients in labour (using thermodilution tip pulmonary artery catheters), found that cardiac output and cardiac index, heart rate, stroke volume and total peripheral resistance were all increased compared with normotensive women in early labour. More recently, Groenendijk *et al.* (1984) using the same technique have reported a decreased cardiac output, a low pulmonary capillary wedge pressure and a high peripheral resistance in 10 patients with hypertension and proteinuria investigated antenatally. These findings suggest that there may well be differences in cardiac output with different types of hypertension, and also that cardiac output may vary at different stages of the disease and under different circumstances.

Peripheral vascular resistance, uterine vascular resistance and distribution of blood flow
The total peripheral resistance (TPR) is determined by the total of the resistance to blood flow of all the organs and tissues of the body. It is essentially a derived measurement calculated as follows:

$$\text{Total peripheral resistance} = \frac{\text{mean arterial pressure}}{\text{cardiac output}}$$

Resistance to flow is primarily arteriolar and is dependent on the cross-sectional area and length of the vessels and the viscosity of the blood. The cross-sectional area is in turn dependent on the intrinsic vascular smooth muscle tone, the vasomotor nervous system activity and the amount of vasoconstrictor or vasodilator substances released locally or circulating in the blood. In normal pregnancy the total peripheral resistance falls in the first two trimesters and progressively increases towards prepregnant values at term (Bader et al. 1955, Rovinsky & Jaffin 1965). In hypertension in pregnancy TPR is generally assumed to be increased. More important than TPR, however, is the balance of vascular resistance between different organs of the body, particularly between the uterus and the rest of the body.

This may be illustrated by the following equation:

$$\text{Uterine blood flow} = \frac{\text{uterine perfusing pressure}}{\text{uterine vascular resistance}}$$

Assuming that the uterine perfusing pressure is the same as the arterial BP, which is the product of cardiac output and TPR, the equation can be restated thus:

$$\text{Uterine blood flow} = \frac{\text{cardiac output} \times \text{TPR}}{\text{uterine vascular resistance}}$$

This means that the uterine blood flow is determined not so much by the BP per se as by the ratio of the uterine vascular resistance to the total peripheral resistance. If the main aim of treatment of hypertension in pregnancy is to increase uterine blood flow then it is essential not so much to lower BP as to produce uterine vasodilatation and reduce uterine vascular resistance. To this end it is essential that there should be a preferential vasodilatation of the uterine vessels.

Blood volume, haematocrit and blood viscosity
There is on average a reduction in *plasma volume* in the hypertensive compared with normal pregnancies of the order of 500 ml. MacGillivray (1983c), and more recently Sibai et al. (1983) have shown that this reduction is confined to the women with small-for-dates infants, and the difference in the mean values between hypertensive and normotensive pregnancies is mainly due to the greater number of such infants in the hypertensive groups. Plasma volume is also related to fetal outcome (Arias 1975, Gibson 1973) and is decreased in women who smoke (Pirani & MacGillivray 1978). These findings are important in the pathophysiology, investigation and treatment of hypertensive disorders of pregnancy. Only a minority of women with hypertension in pregnancy have reduced plasma and blood volumes, and reduction in

blood volume is not an essential feature of the condition. Estimation of plasma and blood volume in hypertensive women may provide a guide to fetal growth and fetal outcome, and measures to increase plasma volume may improve fetal growth and outcome.

In normal pregnancy the venous *haematocrit* falls from about 0.40–0.47 to a minimum of 0.31–0.34, but rises again in the third trimester (Thorburn et al. 1982). The haematocrit in severe pre-eclampsia is increased and may provide a useful index of severity and progress, as was shown 50 years ago by Dieckman (1936).

Blood viscosity is determined by the haemotocrit and by plasma macromolecules, particularly fibrinogen. In normal pregnancy low shear blood viscosity is increased towards term due to the increased haematocrit, but high shear blood viscosity is decreased due to increased erythrocyte deformability. In moderate pre-eclampsia blood viscosity is decreased due to decreased haematocrit. In severe pre-eclampsia and fetal growth retardation, however, high shear viscosity is increased due to a significant decrease in red cell deformability and this may contribute to reduced blood flow and placental insufficiency (Thorburn et al. 1982).

Organ blood flow
Most of the effects of hypertension in pregnancy are mediated by changes in blood flow in the various organs and tissues of the body.

Cerebral blood flow. McCall (1953) reported that there is no change in cerebral blood flow in normal pregnancy, but that in pre-eclampsia the blood flow and oxygen consumption may be reduced by 20%. Decreased blood flow associated with spasm of the cerebral blood vessels is probably an important factor in the aetiology of eclamptic fits and cerebral haemorrhage.

Hepatic blood flow and hepatic function. There are no detectable changes in hepatic blood flow in hypertensive compared with normotensive pregnancies, though hepatic function may be significantly impaired in both. In severe pre-eclampsia there may be a marked alteration in liver function (Ylostalo 1970) and any impairment of liver function (e.g. increased liver enzymes) indicates severe disease irrespective of the level of blood pressure.

Renal blood flow and renal function. In hypertension in pregnancy changes in renal blood flow and renal function are often marked and occur early in pregnancy. In mild essential hypertension renal plasma flow is normal or even increased, but in more severe essential hypertension it may be reduced though the filtration fraction increases so that the glomerular filtration rate (GFR) is usually unchanged. In pre-eclampsia or gestational hypertension the effective renal plasma flow (ERPF) is reduced by an average of 20% (from 750 ml/min to 600 ml/min) and the GFR is reduced by an average of 30% from 170–120 ml/min so that there is a decrease in filtration fraction, but there is great variation from individual to individual. Thus in many patients, particularly those with mild essential hypertension or pre-eclampsia, renal blood flow or function may be completely normal, whereas with severe hypertension renal they may be markedly impaired. In very severe cases this may result in oliguria, uraemia and, in a few cases, tubular or cortical necrosis.

There are other important changes in renal function in normotensive and hypertensive pregnancy, particularly in the secretion of renin, angiotensin and aldosterone which may be important in the aetiology of at least some forms of hypertension in pregnancy. Relatively large amounts of renin are also formed in the placenta (Skinner *et al.* 1968), though it is not certain whether it is an active or inactive form (Skinner *et al.* 1975). The function of the placental renin is not known, but it may serve to raise BP and so ensure adequate placental perfusion. In normal pregnancy plasma renin, angiotensinogen, angiotensin II and aldosterone are all markedly raised above non-pregnant levels and these changes may be compensatory for the increased circulating levels of progesterone (which is natriuretic and lowers BP). In normal pregnancy the opposing effects of progesterone and renin, angiotensin and aldosterone are thought to be more or less in balance, but in pre-eclampsia they may be out of balance. Reports on changes in renin concentration and activity, and in angiotensin and aldosterone levels are conflicting. Most workers (Weir *et al.* 1973, Symonds & Anderson 1974) have found them reduced, but Symonds *et al.* (1975) reported a significant positive relationship between maternal DBP and angiotensin II levels. The renin, angiotensin and aldosterone system is undoubtedly important in the aetiology of chronic hypertension but its role in the hypertensive disorders of pregnancy remains obscure.

Skin and limb blood flow is markedly increased in normal pregnancy, but limb blood flow is greatly affected by posture. Leg blood flow is increased in the lateral position and decreased in the supine position. In pre-eclampsia widely different results have been obtained by different workers. Ginsburg and Duncan (1967) found no significant changes in skin and limb blood flow in pre-eclampsia but noted that there was a marked reactive hyperaemia, suggesting that an increase in the intrinsic tone of the blood vessels which may partly explain the hypertension.

Uterine and choriodecidual blood flow. The changes in uterine and choriodecidual blood flow are the most important of all the pathophysiological changes in hypertension in pregnancy and are probably the main determinants of fetal outcome. Unfortunately there are no entirely satisfactory methods of measuring either uterine or choriodecidual blood flow in human pregnancy, but there is general agreement in the findings of the various methods that have been employed. These methods have included: clearance of nitrous oxide (Assali *et al.* 1954) clearance of 4-amino antipyrine (Huckabee 1962), clearance of radioactive sodium injected into the choriodecidual space (Dixon *et al.* 1963) and myometrium (Moore & Myerscough 1957), clearance of radioactive xenon (Xe^{133}) (Lysgaard *et al.* 1973) and indium 113M (Lunell *et al.* 1982a), metabolic clearance rate of dihydroisoandrosterone sulfate (Gant *et al.* 1977), and measurement of flow velocity waveforms in arcuate artery by pulsed doppler ultrasound (Cohen-Overbeek *et al.* 1984).

All these methods indicate that 3 or 4 weeks before gestational hypertension is recognized, utero-placental perfusion is decreased by 50–65% (Gant and Worley 1980c). These effects are in urgent need of further investigation to determine the extent of the reduction in different patients and to elucidate the effects on blood flow of such factors as posture, exercise, bed rest and antihypertensive treatment. Preliminary investigations using xenon clearance indicate that antihypertensive agents, including hydralazine (Lunell *et al.* 1983) and labetalol (Lunell *et al.* 1982b), do not produce a significant change in uterine blood flow. This suggests a high degree of autoregulation of the uterine and choriodecidual blood flow at least in man (Venuto *et al.* 1976) which maintains a relatively constant blood flow in spite of changes in BP.

BLOOD COMPOSITION

In normal pregnancy there is a generalized haemodilution and a fall in concentrations of most blood constituents. In the hypertensive disorders there is no consistent alteration in blood composition, though important changes may occur in individual patients depending upon the nature and severity of the disorder.

Plasma proteins

Plasma albumin is decreased in pregnancy and is reduced further in pre-eclampsia (Chesley 1978d). McCartney *et al.* (1971) fractionated the serum proteins of women on whom they had performed renal biopsy and found a decreased albumin but an increase in serum alphaglobulins in pre-eclampsia, and an increase in gammaglobulin and haptoglobin in nephrosclerosis and essential hypertension. Studd (1971) confirmed a fall in plasma albumin and immunoglobulin (IgG) and an elevation of alpha-2 macroglobulin and beta lipoproteins in severe pre-eclampsia, and suggested that these changes resulted from the prolonged loss of protein in the urine. The exact nature of the proteinuria in pre-eclampsia varies according to the severity of the disease, but in general shows low to intermediate selectivity, with a loss of intermediate weight proteins such as albumin, transferrin and gammaglobulin but a retention of larger weight proteins such as alpha-2 macroglobulin (McEwan 1969, Simanowitz *et al.* 1973).

Plasma colloid osmotic or oncotic pressure. An important consequence of the fall in plasma proteins, particularly plasma albumin, in normal pregnancy is the fall in plasma colloid osmotic or oncotic pressure which is decreased 20% or more. There may be an even greater fall in plasma albumin and plasma oncotic pressure in pre-eclampsia, and this may be a significant factor in the pathophysiological changes in hypertensive disorders of pregnancy including generalized oedema, a greater tendency to develop pulmonary oedema, and the development of cerebral oedema in eclampsia.

Cellular constituents

Erythrocytes. The only change in the erythrocytes is in severe pre-eclampsia in which decreased deformability may reduce tissue perfusion (Thorburn *et al.* 1982).

Leucocytes. In normal pregnancy the leucocyte count is increased from an average of 7100/mm³ in non-pregnant women to 10,500/mm³ in late pregnancy, mainly due to an increase in neutrophil polymorphonuclear cells and a small increase in lymphocytes. An increased eosinophil count has been reported in severe pre-eclampsia (Riddell *et al.* 1983) suggesting a possible allergic or hypersensitive immunological reaction.

Platelets. There is a small fall in platelet count in normal pregnancy, probably due to haemodilution, and several workers have reported a further significant decrease in pre-eclampsia and eclampsia. In women with chronic hypertension Redman *et al.* (1978a) found that the fall in platelet count occurred before the appearance of pre-eclampsia (as defined by an increase in serum urate). Although a fall in platelet count occurs fairly frequently in pre-eclampsia it is by no means an essential feature of the disorder. An abnormally low platelet count does however provide an important and useful indication of the occurrence of DIC.

Blood coagulation

The changes in blood coagulation in normal pregnancy and in hypertensive disorders of pregnancy have been reviewed by Chesley (1978e), Bonnar (1978) and more recently MacGillivray (1983d) who has postulated a series of cascades. Though typical DIC with a failure in blood clotting may occur in pre-eclampsia, particularly in association with placental abruption the DIC usually associated with pre-eclampsia and hypertension in pregnancy is essentially a chronic process with both increased fibrin deposition and increased fibrinolysis. In this chronic DIC the peripheral blood shows raised levels of cryofibrinogen, increased fibrin degradation products which may be increased three times over those found in normal pregnancy (McKillop *et al.* 1976), raised factor VIII, and reduced platelet count.

Because fibrin deposition in the placenta and kidneys is so common MacGillivray (1983e) feels that some disturbance of the coagulation/fibrinolytic system is an essential feature of pre-eclampsia. Chesley (1978f), on the other hand, noted that in patients with eclampsia and pre-eclampsia, even of severe degree, there may be no detectable signs of increased coagulation or fibrinolysis. Though common, DIC is probably a complication rather than an aetiological factor in hypertensive disorders of pregnancy.

BODY COMPOSITION AND WEIGHT GAIN IN PREGNANCY

Weight gain and water retention.

Weight gain provides an overall masure of fetal and placental growth and of changes in body composition, and it has been extensively studied in normotensive and hypertensive pregnancies. Thomson and Billewicz (1957) showed that women with high weight gain are more likely to develop pre-eclampsia though those with low weight gain had a higher perinatal mortality. MacGillivray (1961) found that 50% of women who develop hypertension and proteinuria had low weight gain. He measured the total

Table 16.7 Extracellular water (bromide Br space) and intracellular water (deuterium D₂0 space less bromide Br space) and ratio of extracellular to intracellular water (ration of Br space to D₂0–Br space) in normal pregnancy and in pre-eclampsia with and without oedema (Calculated from MacGillivray I. (1983) *Pre-eclampsia.* p. 114, Table 4.11. W. B. Saunders, London.)

Body water L litres	Normal pregnancy	Pre-eclampsia with oedema	Pre-eclampsia without oedema
Total Body Water (TBW) Deuterium (D₂0) Space L	37.2	44.8	42.2
Extracellular water bromide (Br) space L % of TBW	21.6 (58.1%)	23.5 (52.4%)	19.9 (47.2%)
Intracellular water (D₂0–Br space) L % of TBW	15.6 (41.9%)	21.3 (47.5%)	22.3 (52.8%)
Ratio intracellular/ extracellular water	0.72/1	0.91/1	1.12/1

body water in patients with hypertension and proteinuria and divided the cases into those with and without oedema (MacGillivray 1967); he also studied the distribution of body water between extracellular and intracellular space, using radioactive bromine to measure the extracellular water and deuterium to measure total body water (Table 16.7). Pre-eclamptic women showed a marked increase in intracellular water though only the oedematous patients showed an increase in extracellular water. At the same time MacGillivray measured the total body exchangeable sodium and showed that the changes in body water were paralleled by changes in body sodium and that patients with oedema retained both more extracellular sodium and more extracellular water. A more important finding, however, was that women with proteinuric pre-eclampsia also had greater intracellular sodium as well as greater intracellular water, suggesting that in severe proteinuric pre-eclampsia there is an increased leakage of both sodium and water into the cells.

Sodium and potassium retention, and sodium and potassium cellular transport

For many years excessive retention of sodium and water was thought to be a major aetiological factor in the causation of 'toxaemia', and generations of women have been treated with salt restricted diet, diuretics and other measures. The total body sodium

and potassium have been measured using radioactive sodium and potassium, and there is now general agreement that in normal pregnancy sodium is retained in proportion to the increase in extracellular water. In hypertensive disorders of pregnancy the total amount of sodium retained is similarly directly proportional to the amount of water retention so that there is no excessive retention of sodium as such. In proteinuric hypertension (pre-eclampsia), however, the amount of intracellular sodium and intracellular water appears to be increased and there is a shift of sodium and water into the cells. The intracellular sodium content of erythrocytes and leucocytes was found to be increased by Forrester and Alleyne (1981) and McMurray and Morgan (1984) respectively, but to be unchanged by Campbell and MacGillivray (1980). More recently Weissberg *et al.* (1983) have studied the sodium efflux in erythrocytes and have concluded that there is a marked increase in the ouabain sensitive sodium potassium countertransport system (or sodium/potassium pump) and a marked increase in the leakage of sodium into the cells in hypertensive women in pregnancy. Symonds (1980) suggested that the retention of sodium in the vascular smooth muscle cells in pre-eclampsia is responsible for the increased vascular tone and for altered sensitivity to infused angiotensin II, and hence for the raised BP.

Hormones and fluid retention in pre-eclampsia

Attempts have been made to relate the changes in sodium, potassium and water in normal and hypertensive pregnancies to changes in the plasma concentrations of various hormones. The findings have been unrewarding but Campbell and MacGillivray (1982) did find several interesting relationships as follows: plasma aldosterone is lower in pre-eclamptic than in normal pregnancies; plasma volume correlates with plasma aldosterone in normotensive primigravidas but not in women with proteinuric pre-eclampsia; plasma oestradiol correlates closely with prolactin in normotensive primigravidas but not in women with pre-eclampsia; women with proteinuric pre-eclampsia have lower aldosterone and higher prolactin than normotensive pregnancies. It is probable that several underlying mechanisms are involved, and there may be different underlying abnormalities in the different types of hypertension.

PLACENTAL FUNCTION AND ENDOCRINE CHANGES

The placenta must be intimately involved in the aetiology and pathophysiology of the hypertensive disorders of pregnancy. When pregnancy is terminated and the placenta removed, most hypertensive and proteinuric disorders resolve in a few hours or days, though some changes may persist for weeks and occasionally months.

Oestrogens and progestogens

These hormones are produced in large amounts in pregnancy but no consistent changes have been demonstrated in their urinary or plasma levels in the hypertensive disorders of pregnancy. Because pre-eclampsia is more commonly associated with hyper-placentosis (e.g. hydatidiform mole, twins), the hypertension and proteinuria may be due to excessive secretion of placental hormones. Gant et al. (1972) showed that women who subsequently develop pre-eclampsia had a much greater metabolic clearance of dihydroisoandrosterone sulphate (DS) than women who remained normotensive throughout the second half of pregnancy. When the pre-eclamptic women developed hypertension, however, there was a marked fall in DS clearance and in plasma oestrogen levels. Many investigators have found that the urinary excretion of oestriol, and the levels of oestriol in the plasma, are reduced in established pre-eclampsia. It could be that in the initial phases (at least in some patients who develop gestational hypertension) there is an excessive production of oestrogens which somehow triggers a secondary mechanism that causes the development of hypertension (even despite placental insufficeincy and a fall in oestrogen production).

Placental proteins

Over 30 unique placental proteins have now been identified, including the placental protein hormones human chorionic gonadotrophin (HCG), human placental lactogen (HPL), Schwangerschafts protein (SPI), pregnancy associated plasma proteins A and B (PAPP-A and PAPP-B) and placental protein S (PPS). Their functions, apart from that of HPL which is closely related to pituitary growth hormone, are largely unknown but they may play a significant role in the hypertensive disorders.

HCG. From the days of Smith and Smith (1948) it has been known that the development of pre-eclampsia is associated with a secondary rise in urinary and plasma HCG levels late in pregnancy, often together with a fall in the urinary excretion of oestrogens and pregnanediol. The rise in HCG secretion is probably secondary and compensatory for the fall in placental secretion of oestrogens and progestogens, and may help to reactivate corpus luteum function. Luteal reactivation, with increased oestrogen and progestogen production, may be an important compensatory mechanism and a first indication of placental insufficiency. Now that rapid sensitive radioimmunoassays of Beta-HCG are available, changes in HCG levels merit further investigation; they may provide an indication of impaired placental function before steroid hormone levels fall and before the fetal condition is prejudiced.

HPL inhibits the action of insulin, mobilizes free fatty acids from fat depots and is probably the main hormone ensuring an adequate supply of glucose to the fetus. Women with low serum HPL have a higher perinatal mortality (Letchworth & Chard 1972). Low levels also occur in pre-eclampsia (Spellacy et al. 1970) but probably reflect impaired placental function and consequent IUGR rather than the pre-eclamptic condition itself.

PAPP-A, PAPP-B and PPS are found only in the serum of pregnant women, and have largely unknown functions. PAPP-A is a glycoprotein with a high carbohydrate content. Its plasma concentrations rise rapidly in pregnancy till term, are highest in primigravidas and fall with increasing parity (Bischoff et al. 1980); they are raised in hypertension in pregnancy, being highest in proteinuric hypertension, and are normal or reduced in cases of IUGR (Toop & Klopper 1981). PAPP-A is an inhibitor of fibrinolysis and also of complement fixation, and may play a role both in coagulation and in immunological changes in hypertensive disorders (Bischoff 1981). The plasma levels of PAPP-B also increase progressively in pregnancy but are reduced in pre-eclampsia. Its actions are said to resemble HPL. PPS is another specific glycoprotein distinct from PAPP-A. Its plasma levels, like PAPP-A, are increased in pregnancy and increased further in pre-eclampsia. There is a close resemblance between PPS and antithrombin III, and PPS may be regarded as the placental equivalent of the latter. It could well be involved in the coagulation and immunological changes in pregnancy and pre-eclampsia.

Placental enzymes

A number of placental enzymes have been extensively studied, mainly in an endeavour to find a useful measure of placental function.

Alkaline phosphatase is a mixture of more than 20 iso-enzymes, at least one of which comes from the placenta and which is distinguished by its resistance to heat. This heat stable alkaline phosphatase (HSAP) is increased in pre-eclampsia but this is thought to be due not so much to changes in placental function but to hypoxia which causes its release from placental tissue (Curzen & Varma 1971).

Amine oxidases include monoamine oxidase (MAO) which inactivates vasoconstrictor amines such as adrenaline, noradrenaline and dopamine, diamine oxidase (histaminase) which inactivates histamine, and desoxycytidylate and cytidine deaminases which are important in the regulation of pyrimidine metabolism. *MAO* probably has only a local effect on the uteroplacental circulation and is not a factor in the pathogenesis of hypertension.

Measurements of *diamine oxidase* do not appear to be helpful in diagnosis or management (Ward *et al.* 1972) since, despite the work of Kapeller-Adler (1950), histamine does not appear to play a major role in hypertension in pregnancy.

Cystine aminopeptidase (*CAP*) is markedly increased in pregnancy but is reduced in some cases of pre-eclampsia. Watson *et al.* (1973) and Curzen and Varma (1973) found CAP to be one of the least sensitive tests with a high false negative rate.

Transaminases are produced by many different organs including the liver, kidney and placenta, and the significance of increased *SGOT* and *SGPT* in the pathophysiology of the hypertensive disorders of pregnancy is a matter of conjecture (Chesley 1978g). An increase in serum transaminase does indicate damage to tissues, to the liver in particular, and should alert the physician to possible hepatic damage and disorders (Dass & Bhagwanani 1964).

Corticosteroids

Desoxycorticosterone (DOC) and cortisol are substantially increased in normal pregnancy, but Weir *et al.* (1973) found that levels of DOC in pre-eclampsia were normal or reduced, and Kopelman and Levitz (1970) found that plasma cortisol levels and cortisol binding were the same in normal and in pre-eclamptic pregnancy.

Catecholamines

The increase in cardiac output, stroke volume, heart rate, peripheral resistance and BP in pre-eclampsia closely resemble a hyperadrenergic state, and Lim and Walters (1979) suggested that the hypertension could be due to an increase in sympathetic nervous system activity. However, it was not until the advent of sensitive radioenzymatic methods that measurement of plasma adrenaline and noradrenaline became feasible. It seems that in general there is no increase in basal circulating levels of adrenaline or other catecholamines in hypertension in pregnancy. It is therefore unlikely that increased sympathetic nervous system activity is a primary cause of this hypertension. On the other hand, the rise in plasma adrenaline following stimulation, e.g. cold pressor test, isometric hand grip (Nisell *et al.* 1985) or standing up (Marceau *et al.* 1984), does appear to be much greater in hypertensive than in normotensive women so changes in sympathetic nervous system activity or in the metabolism of catecholamines could be responsible for the rise in BP in labour and in other circumstances of stress or excitement.

PROSTANOIDS, KININS AND OTHER VASOACTIVE SUBSTANCES

At least four prostanoids are vasoactive and play an important role in the local regulation of blood flow and coagulation in various organs. They are the arachidonic acid derivatives prostaglandin E_2 (PGE_2) which is a vasodilator, prostaglandin F_2 alpha (PGF_2 alpha) which is a vasoconstrictor, the cyclo-oxygenase derivative prostacyclin (PGI_2) which is a vasodilator and inhibits platelet aggregation, and thromboxane (TXA_2) which is a vasoconstrictor and increases platelet aggregation. These substances are released locally and have a very short biological half life, with the exception of PGI_2 which is formed in the lungs and released into the general circulation. Prostanoids are formed in large amounts in the endometrium, myometrium and fetal membranes and probably have a significant role in regulating uterine blood flow. Information about levels of prostanoids in the peripheral blood is conflicting, but a diminished concentration of vasodilator in PGE_2 in the placenta has been reported (Robinson *et al.* 1979, Walsh *et al.* 1985). Others have reported an increase in vasoconstrictor PGF_2 alpha (Demers & Gabbe 1976), but Hillier and Smith (1981) were unable to confirm these findings and they doubted if PGE_2 and PGF_2 alpha are responsible for the haemodynamic changes in pregnancy and pre-eclampsia.

TXA_2 is released from the platelets and PGI_2 is the principal prostanoid synthesized in blood vessel walls. There is normally a dynamic balance in all blood vessels between TXA_2, which controls the tendency of platelets to aggregate and causes vasoconstriction, and PGI$_2$, which is antiaggregatory and vasodilatory and which is released in large amounts if blood vessels are injured or stretched.

There is considerable evidence that PGI$_2$ concentrations are decreased in hypertension in pregnancy at least locally in the placenta, fetal membranes and umbilical cord, and Lewis (1983) has suggested that deficiency in PGI$_2$ and vasodilator prostaglandins may play an important aetiological role in hypertension in pregnancy.

Bradykinin is the most potent naturally occurring vasodepressor agent. An impairment or deficiency of the kinin system e.g. deficiency in vasodilator prostanoids PGE$_2$ and PGI$_2$, could contribute to the pathogenesis of hypertension in pregnancy (Elebute & Mills 1976).

IMMUNOLOGICAL CHANGES

Circumstantial observations suggest that immunological changes play a primary role in the aetiology and pathology of pre-eclampsia. The observations considered by Beer (1978) and Thurnau (1985) respectively 'to be consistent and not consistent with an immunological basis for pre-eclampsia' are summarized in Table 16.8. Immunological changes in pre-

Table 16.8 Observations consistent and not consistent with an immunologic explanation of pre-eclampsia. From Thurnau G. (1985) in Scott J. R., Rote N. S. eds. *Immunology in Obstetrics and Gynecology*, p. 107–140. Appleton Century Crofts, New York.

Observations consistent with an immunologic explanation
Disorder primarily of primigravidas
Increased incidence in pregnancies of new paternity
Increased incidence in pregnancies with a large placental
  mass
Adaptive protection afforded by previous pregnancy of same
  paternity
Pathologic vascular changes in arterioles of the placental
  bed
Decreased incidence in consanguineous marriages
Cure following delivery of the placenta
Thrombocytopenia
Increased incidence in immunosuppressed patients
Renal pathology and pathophysiology
Disseminated intravascular coagulopathy

Observations not consistent with an immunologic explanation
Hypertension
Association with nutritional deficiencies
Oedema
Convulsion
Uniquely a disorder of humans

eclampsia include lower numbers of both B and T lymphocytes and impaired T lymphocytes in the mother, lower numbers of B lymphocytes in the father, low response in mixed lymphocyte culture between mother and father, and increased numbers of B lymphocytes in the offspring (Birkeland & Kristoferson 1979). These observations are thought to indicate maternal hyporesponsiveness and fetal hyperresponsiveness. It is postulated that in normal pregnancy maternal exposure to paternal allellic antigens in the fetus normally induces 'blocking antibodies' which block reactivity to paternal antigens. In pre-eclampsia, it is suggested that when HLA or other antigens of the father and mother are similar there may be an inadequate antigenic stimulus and inadequate production of blocking antibodies. In hyperplacentosis it is suggested that an excessively large antigenic load overwhelms the maternal immune system leaving antibodies to paternal antigens circulating freely. In both instances unblocked antibodies to paternal antigens circulate in the mother; they may attack the placenta, particularly the trophoblastic cells in the decidua and myometrium, and they may also attack the kidney, cross reacting with antigens in the renal glomeruli to produce the 'typical' glomerular changes of pre-eclampsia. Redman *et al.* (1978b) found a higher incidence of homozygosity of the LH–AB locus and a lack of HLA incompatibility between severe pre-eclamptic women and their husbands, and concluded that a maternal recessive imperfect immunoresponse may contribute to the development of pre-eclampsia. MacGillivray (1983e) concluded that 'pre-eclampsia can be considered to be a familial condition in which a faulty immune response may be triggered off by a particular male partner or be predisposed to by allergies or deficiencies, possibly of particular items of diet such as trace elements'.

Aetiology

The aetiology of the hypertensive and proteinuric disorders of pregnancy is unknown. Many theories, hypotheses and suggestions explain some features of the disorder, but the essential nature of the condition remains an enigma. Perhaps the biggest obstacle to understanding has been the tendency to regard hypertension in pregnancy as one disease with one aetiology and one pathology, whereas in reality it may be several entities with different aetiologies and different pathologies. There is also a tendency to expect all the abnormal features to be present in all

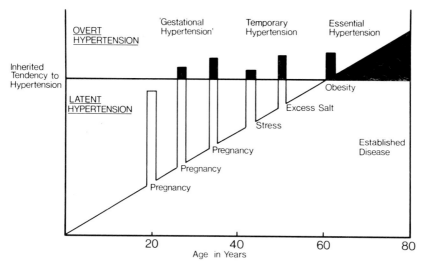

Fig. 16.7. The relationship between the effect of pregnancy in producing gestational hypertension and of other exacerbating factors in women with inherited latent tendency to essential hypertension.

cases. It is possible, as previously noted, to envisage at least three different forms of gestational hypertension characterized as follows:

LATENT ESSENTIAL HYPERTENSION

This is an inherited tendency to hypertension (possibly an abnormality in cellular sodium transport) which occurs in primigravidas and multigravidas and recurs with successive pregnancies. Its incidence increases with increased maternal age, and there may be a strong family history of hypertension. Hypertension may become overt at any stage of pregnancy, but with a tendency to above average mid-trimester blood pressure. There is an average weight gain in pregnancy, and the placenta and fetus are average in

size. Perinatal mortality is not increased. Essential hypertension often develops in later life.

The possible sequences of events by which women with an inherited latent tendency develop latent or 'temporary' hypertension in pregnancy and, subsequently, established essential hypertension are shown in Figs. 16.7 and 16.8. The effect of greater or lesser tendencies to essential hypertension and the age of development of established essential hypertension are illustrated in Fig. 16.8.

PRE-ECLAMPSIA

This may be of immunological origin with failure of second wave of trophoblastic invasion of spiral arterioles. Pre-eclampsia occurs mainly in primigravidas,

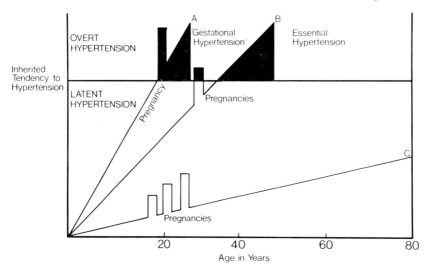

Fig. 16.8. Age of development of gestational hypertension and of essential hypertension in women with greater (A), medium (B) or lesser (C) latent tendencies to essential hypertension.

recurs in subsequent pregnancies infrequently, it has an incidence that does not increase with age, and there is usually no significant family history of the disorder. The hypertension may be of early onset (28 weeks onwards), there is below average weight gain in pregnancy, and small-for-dates placenta and fetus with more than average perinatal mortality. There is no increased tendency to hypertension in later life.

PHYSIOLOGICAL OR 'SUPRANORMAL' HYPERTENSION

This represents an excessively good response to pregnancy with excessive production of placental hormones associated with a large placenta, hyperplacentosis or excessive trophoblastic activity. It occurs in primigravidas and multigravidas, but particularly with twins, diabetic pregnancies and rhesus isoimmunization. Its incidence is not affected by age but may increase with increasing parity, and there is usually no family history. The late onset of hypertension is after 34 weeks except with hydatidiform mole, there is excessive weight gain with large-for-dates placenta and fetus and below average perinatal mortality. There is no increased tendency to hypertension in later life.

The situation may be complicated by the fact that the different forms of pregnancy induced hypertension may occur together and may not necessarily be pure forms. Differentiation between these disorders may also be made difficult because all types of hypertension may develop superimposed 'pre-eclampsia'. Renal biopsy studies (Altchek 1964, Nochy et al. 1980) have nevertheless shown that typical 'pre-eclamptic' lesions may develop in women with essential hypertension or with primary renal lesions and the pre-eclamptic lesions can be easily separated. The recognition of the different forms of gestational hypertension, gestational proteinuria and gestational proteinuric hypertension (i.e. pre-eclampsia) may nevertheless be important not only in terms of underlying aetiology and pathogenesis but also in prognosis and management.

MANAGEMENT

In the present state of knowledge the management of all the hypertensive and proteinuric disorders of pregnancy is essentially the same. The only exceptions are rare conditions such as coarctation of the aorta, phaeochromocytoma and systemic lupus erythema-

tosis which may require specific treatment. In all other cases management is essentially dependent upon the risk to the mother, the risk to the fetus, the duration of the pregnancy and associated factors such as age, parity and previous obstetric history. The aims are: (a) to protect the mother from the effects of excessively high BP and to prevent progression of the disease and the occurrence of eclamptic fits or other maternal complications; (b) to eliminate or minimize the risks to the fetus including placental abruption, IUGR and intrauterine death; (c) to deliver the fetus by the safest and most expeditious means as soon as it is mature or (even if immature) when it is judged that the risk to the fetus and/or mother if pregnancy is continued will outweigh the risks of delivery and prematurity; risk assessment being determined by the availability of expert neonatal care.

It is useful to classify hypertension and/or proteinuria in pregnancy as mild or severe according to the risks to the mother and fetus, and to the need for antihypertensive and anticonvulsant treatment. Mild hypertension in general implies minimal or no added risk to mother or fetus and no immediate indication for antihypertensive or other treatment. Severe hyper-

Table 16.9 Definition of severe hypertension, imminent eclampsia and eclampsia.

Severe hypertension (requiring anti-hypertensive therapy)
Diastolic blood pressure (DBP) 120 mmHg or more once (confirmed by competent observer after 5 min rest)
DBP 110 mmHg or more on 2 consecutive occasions 4 hr or more apart

---

Imminent eclampsia (requiring anticonvulsant therapy)
DBP of 90 mmHg or more plus a combination (usually 2 or more) of

Symptoms	severe persisting headache
	visual disturbances (flashes of light, impaired vision, diplopia)
	upper abdominal pain, nausea or vomiting
Proteinuria	increasing proteinuria (usually 3 g or more/24 hr)
Oedema	rapidly increasing generalized oedema
Oliguria	less than 30 ml/hr or 720 ml/24 hr
Hyperflexia	if unequivocal or with clonus

Change in level of consciousness or mental state unrelated to medication, either drowsiness, irritability or anxiety

---

Eclampsia (requiring anticonvulsant and ? antihypertensive therapy)
Eclampsia is diagnosed in any patient who has a fit irrespective of level of blood pressure or other findings (unless known epileptic)

---

tension implies significant risk to fetus and/or mother, and is an indication for antihypertensive or other treatment or possible termination of the pregnancy. A suggested definition of severe hypertension based on clinical criteria is shown in Table 16.9.

Prevention of hypertension and pre-eclampsia

In the past great emphasis was placed on methods to prevent pre-eclampsia, including control of weight gain, salt restriction and the use of diuretics. The evidence has been analysed by MacGillivray (1983f) and may be summarized as follows:

Control of weight gain and salt restrictions. There is no evidence that either restriction or supplementation of an ordinary diet will prevent the onset of pre-eclampsia. Nor is a low or high salt diet likely to have any influence on the development of pre-eclampsia, and pregnant women should be allowed to take salt according to taste.

Prophylactic use of diuretics. Although diuretics are effective in reducing water retention in pregnancy, they do not prevent the onset of pre-eclampsia. Furthermore there is a positive danger in giving thiazide diuretics because of their side effects on the mother and fetus.

Antenatal management

Initial assessment
All patients found to have hypertension and/or proteinuria in pregnancy should be admitted to hospital or an obstetric day unit for full initial assessment, and a plan of management should be formulated according to the severity of disease and the duration of pregnancy.

MONITORING OF FETAL AND MATERNAL CONDITION

Monitoring the condition of the fetus and mother is an essential part of the management of hypertension and/or proteinuric disorders of pregnancy. The determination of the optimum time for delivery when the risks of intrauterine death (or of some major maternal complication) outweigh the risks of prematurity is often the most important and crucial decision in the whole management.

Mild hypertension without IUGR or impaired fetal well-being
Outpatient surveillance is based on weekly antenatal visits with assessment of symptoms (e.g. headache,

epigastric pain, vaginal bleeding), fetal movements, BP, urine to detect proteinuria, fundal height, fetal size, volume of amniotic fluid. Ultrasonic measurement of fetus (e.g. biparietal diameter, head and abdominal circumference) and of amniotic fluid volume at 28 and 34 weeks, and at any time that IUGR is suspected clinically, is advisable.

Severe hypertension
Inpatient management is required, and the following observations should be made: BP every 6 hours; daily urine test for proteinuria (if present a 24 hour collection is obtained for total protein measurement; fetal movements ('kick chart'); clinical examination including fundal height measurements; serum creatine and urate weekly (or bi-weekly); weekly platelet counts; cardiotocography and placental function tests (e.g. HPL); and fortnightly ultrasonic mensuration.

Imminent eclampsia
The patient should be managed in the labour ward or other convenient intensive care area and the following observations should be made and carefully recorded: (a) half-hourly BP, pulse and respiration rates; (b) hourly fluid intake/infusion, urinary output and protein content via indwelling catheter, and central venous pressure in all cases with haemorrhage, oliguria or cardiac failure; (c) *4-hourly* general assessment including level of consciousness, symptoms, reflexes, and clinical examination of lung bases; (d) *12-hourly* full blood count including platelets, blood coagulation indices, blood urea, urate, creatine and electrolytes; (e) the dosage of all drugs administered, alterations in drip rates and results of all other observations should be recorded immediately, preferably on a flow chart.

Amniocentesis and fetal lung maturity
In selected cases amniocentesis and the estimation of the lecithin/sphingmyelin (L/S) ratio or phosphatidyl glycerol content on amniotic fluid may produce vital evidence of fetal lung maturity. In severe hypertension a mature L/S ratio or phosphatidyl glycerol before the 34th week of pregnancy may confirm pulmonary maturity. If tests are 'negative', dexamethasone, 12.5 mg 12-hourly for 48 hours, may be administered to induce pulmonary maturity and prevent respiratory distress syndrome and hyaline membrane disease. Amniocentesis should be performed only when termination of pregnancy is contemplated and where the findings will positively assist in this decision.

Amniocentesis is not usually indicated if a gestational age of more than 36 weeks is certain on the basis of the last menstrual period and ultrasonic examination, in which case fetal pulmonary maturity can be assumed.

Termination of pregnancy

In hypertensive and proteinuric disorders, when the risk of intrauterine death and placental abruption exceeds the risk of prematurity and of delivery, pregnancy should be terminated forthwith. In most cases labour should be induced by 'cervical ripening' with PGE_2 vaginal pessaries, followed 12–18 hours later by amniotomy and oxytocin infusion. When there is some additional obstetric indication such as cephalopelvic disproportion, elective Caesarean section should be performed. Elective section may also be considered in all patients less than 34 weeks on the grounds of a possible increased incidence of intraventricular haemorrhage in premature infants delivered vaginally, of difficulty in inducing labour and of an increased incidence of 'fetal distress' due to underlying placental insufficiency. Hypertensive patients should always be managed as 'high risk' in labour and given nothing by mouth so that an emergency Caesarean section can be carried out any time it is indicated.

MANAGEMENT IN LABOUR

All hypertensive patients require careful monitoring during labour, delivery and the first 24 hours of the puerperium, and all labours should be managed as 'trial labour' with facilities for immediate delivery (including Caesarean section for fetal distress or for uncontrollable hypertension).

Oral antihypertensive therapy should be discontinued at the onset of labour and intravenous antihypertensive (and/or anticonvulsion) therapy should be commenced if the hypertension becomes severe or eclampsia becomes imminent, and it should be continued for 24 hours after delivery.

Women with severe hypertension should be monitored for complications of DIC, heart failure or oliguria. Epidural anaesthesia, if indicated, should be commenced early in labour (provided DIC is excluded).

DELIVERY

An easy vaginal delivery with the assistance of forceps if necessary is the preferred method. If Caesarean section is indicated it should be performed under epidural anaesthesia if convenient, and provided there is no DIC and no immediate risk of eclampsia. If section is performed under general anaesthesia a sudden rise of blood pressure at induction of anaesthesia should be avoided. For the third stage of labour, instead of ergometrine, 5 units of oxytocin by intravenous injection or preferably an infusion of oxytocin, 40mm/l dextrose at 60 drops per minute should be given. Hypertension should be controlled with hydralazine 6.25 or 12.5 mg intramuscularly (4-hourly or as necessary). All observations must be continued for at least 24 hours.

Antihypertensive therapy

A wide variety of antihypertensive agents have been used in the antenatal management of hypertension in pregnancy (Table 16.10), but few have been

Table 16.10 Antihypertensive drugs used in the treatment of hypertension in pregnancy.

Drugs acting on vascular smooth muscle
Diazoxide
Hydralazine
Nitroprusside
Veratrum alkaloids
Ca channel blockers—Nifedipine

Adrenergic receptor blocking agents
Alpha receptor antagonists

Presynaptic and postsynaptic	Postsynaptic
phenoxybenzamine	prazosin
phetolamine	

Beta receptor antagonists

Acebutolol	Atenolol	Metroprolol
Oxprenolol	Propanolol	Stalol

Combined alpha and beta receptor antagonists
Labetalol

Drugs acting on sympathetic nerve endings
Inhibitors of noradrenaline release
Bethanidine   Debrisoqune   Guanethidine

Depletors of noradrenaline stores
Rauwolfia Serpentina

'False' Transmitters
Methyl dopa

Drugs acting on autonomic ganglia
Clonidine
Methyl dopa
Some beta adrenergic receptor antagonists e.g. Propanolol

Table 16.11 Some anti-hypertensive drugs used in controlled clinical trials in treatment of hypertension in pregnancy with main conclusions.

Anti-hypertensive drugs	Investigators		Main conclusions
a methyl dopa v placebo	Leather et al. 1968	1	Reduction in BP
	Redman et al. 1976c	2	Fewer fetal losses—mid-trimester abortions
		3	No effect fetal growth
Oxprenolol v methyl dopa	Gallery et al. 1979	1	Both control hypertension
		2	Increased fetal and placental weight
		3	Larger plasma volume
	Fidler et al. 1983	1	Equipotent lowering BP
		2	No difference in fetal of placental weight
		3	No diff. fetal outcome
Labetalol v methyl dopa	Lamming et al. 1980	1	Better control of BP
		2	Less proteinuria
		3	Improved renal function
	Redman 1981	1	Equivalent antihypertensive effect
		2	Side effects both drugs
		3	Lower umb. venous pO_2
Atenolol v placebo	Rubin et al. 1983	1	Reduce BP
		2	Prevented proteinuria
		3	Fewer admissions

subject to controlled clinical trials. Claims that have been made for some of the agents are listed in Table 16.11. Most agents lower the BP and help prevent maternal complications at least temporarily, but it remains to be shown that any of those investigated so far increase uterine or choriodecidual blood flow and significantly improve fetal growth or well-being.

Antihypertensive therapy is therefore primarily for the sake of the mother. It may prevent the peaks of BP which arise from stress and excitement, and so reduce the need for hospital admissions, and it is possible that lowering the BP in women with chronic hypertension may reduce the incidence of a super-imposed pre-eclampsia. Some investigators have further claimed that certain antihypertensive agents may improve renal function and reduce proteinuria, but it has also been suggested that they may mislead the obstetrician by masking the progress of the disease. With regard to the fetus it is possible that some antihypertensive agents may in fact do harm by reducing cardiac output and producing peripheral vasodilatation without uterine vasodilatation and so decreasing uterine blood flow. An agent which will lower BP on a long term basis and at the same time improve uteroplacental blood flow is needed. The cardiovascular changes in normal and hypertensive pregnancies, and treatment by currently available ideal antihypertensives, are illustrated in Fig. 16.9.

The use of anti-hypertensive agents in mild hypertension in pregnancy (DBP < 110 mmHG) is an open question. The obstetrician may choose either not to give an antihypertensive in the belief that it may not produce any benefit and may cause fetal and maternal side effects and possibly may also mask the progress of disease. On the other hand, he may give one or more antihypertensive agent in the belief that lowering the BP is of benefit to the mother or that there are significant benefits to the fetus which outweigh any side effects or other disadvantages.

In severe hypertension (DBP 110 mmHG or more), all obstetricians would agree that antihypertensive therapy should be commenced immediately for the benefit of the mother, even though there may be little immediate benefit to the fetus. For a detailed account of the investigation and management of severe hypertension, pre-eclampsia and eclampsia see Davey et al. (1984).

Oral therapy

Commonly used agents include the following:

Methyl Dopa (Aldomet, MSD) is primarily a central alpha-receptor stimulant which causes peripheral vasodilatation by reducing sympathetic nervous system outflow. It is safe in pregnancy but does have side effects including depression, nightmares, postural hypotension and, less commonly, cholestatic jaundice, haemolytic anaemia and a positive Coombs test. Because of the widespread experience of its use it probably remains the antihypertensive treatment of

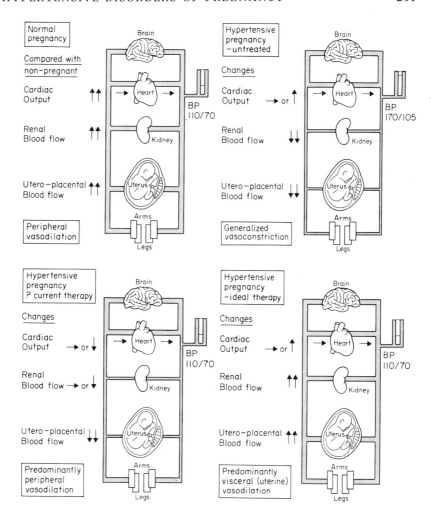

Fig. 16.9. Cardiovascular changes in normal and hypertensive pregnancy and probable effect of current and ideal antihypertensive therapy on uterine, renal and peripheral vascular resistance and blood flow.

choice, though it will probably be superseded when agents of direct benefit to the fetus become available.

Monohydralazine (Apresoline, Ciba). Dihydralazine (Nepresol) is a popular drug for parenteral use, but it has also been used orally in the form of monohydralazine (Apresoline) as supplementary therapy when other agents have failed to control the blood pressure. When given alone oral monohydralazine is a relatively weak antihypertensive agent, but it is more potent when combined with other agents such as beta-adrenergic blocking agents which also prevent its side effects (e.g. headaches, nausea and palpitations). It has the advantage of increasing cardiac output and renal blood flow as well as having a direct dilating effect on vascular smooth muscle. Its main disadvantages are the relatively high incidence of side effects and its reported tachyphylaxsis with continued use.

Beta-adrenergic blocking agents, including Atenolol (Tenormin, ICI), Labetalol (Trandate, Glaxo-Allenbury's), Oxprenolol (Trasicor, Ciba), are currently undergoing a vogue in the treatment of hypertension in pregnancy as in the treatment of essential hypertension outside pregnancy. Their mechanism of action is not fully known, but involves a central adrenergic effect, blockage of renin secretion and also reduction in cardiac output which may be an undesirable method of lowering the blood pressure as it may reduce uterine blood flow. In hypertensive pregnant rats administration of beta-blockers does produce a marked reduction in uterine blood flow (Lundgren *et al.* 1983). The exact mode of action may depend upon the particular adrenergic blocking agent used, and Labetalol has been claimed to have a particular advantage by virtue of its simultaneous alpha-adrenergic as well as beta-adrenergic blocking effect which may help to produce peripheral vasodilatation. Oxprenolol has similarly been claimed to be superior to other beta-blockers because of its intrinsic sympathomimetic activity and its effects in increasing blood volume. The rational use of beta-adrenergic blockers will depend upon a better knowledge of modes of action on the maternal circulation and particularly on uterine and chorio-decidual blood flow. Their effect on the fetal circulation is also an open question. Unlike earlier reports on propanolol, the newer beta-adrenergic blockers on the whole do not appear to cause any fetal impairment although there are reports that they inhibit the ability of the newborn infant to respond to hypoxia at delivery (Woods & Malan 1983; Woods & Morrill 1982).

In spite of good results currently reported from the use of these agents in the treatment of hypertension in pregnancy, reservations must still be expressed about their use, particularly with regard to their effects on uterine blood flow and on the fetus.

Prazosin (*Minipress, Pfizer*) is a postsynaptic alpha-adreno receptor blocking agent which produces vaso-dilation without reflex tachycardia. It also selectively inhibits visceral vasomotor activity (Moulds & Javerning, 1977) increasing visceral blood flow and possibly renal and uterine blood flow. In theory, by virtue of these actions, it is the ideal antihypertensive drug for use in pregnancy. In practice, although it effectively lowers the BP (Lubbe & Hodge 1981), it does not appear to have any special advantage of other antihypertensive agents, and there may be a tendency to tachyphylaxis with continued use. Its use in pregnancy has not yet been approved by its manufacturers, and further experience of this drug is required.

Clonidine (*Catapres, Boehringer Ingelheim*) has its main antihypertensive action via the central nervous system, and it may have a similar action to alpha-methyl dopa. It has been used in pregnancy and appears to be an effective antihypertensive, but does not seem to have any advantage over alpha-methyl dopa. It does have significant side effects, e.g. dry mouth, dizziness and sedation. Sudden cessation of therapy is reported to cause 'rebound hypertension' and, as treatment may have to be stopped in labour and quite a few patients default or discontinue treatment, its use in pregnancy seems limited.

Nifedipine (*Adalat, Bayer-Miles*) is a calcium antagonist and though very effective as an antihypertensive, its use in pregnancy and in labour is generally regarded as contraindicated because of possible inhibition of uterine contractions. Nifedipine has never-

theless been used in cases of severe hypertension in pregnancy with good results (Walters & Redman 1984). Because it is a potent agent which acts quickly and has an action different from other antihypertensive agents, it may have a place in treating patients who do not respond to other therapy or in whom a rapid response to oral therapy is required. It may have a particular place in treating severe hypertension in the puerperium when continued oral therapy may be needed.

Parenteral therapy
Parenteral therapy has an important place in the treatment of severe hypertension, particularly in labour, in the puerperium and for a 'hypertensive crisis' (diastolic BP 120 mmHG or more) as most oral therapy takes some hours (and in the case of alpha-methyl dopa some days) to become fully effective. It is advisable to commence treatment either with intramuscular monohydralazine or, if labour and delivery are contemplated, by continuous intravenous infusion of monohydralazine but intravenous bolus doses should not be given. As close control of the blood pressure is required in labour a continuous intravenous infusion until delivery is recommended; if necessary this may be continued during the first day of the puerperium. However, for patients developing hypertension for the first time in the puerperium, it is recommended that intermittent intramuscular injections should be used as the hypertension usually resolves within 24–48 hours and often only one injection is required.

The choice of parenteral antihypertensives in pregnancy is limited, and only three agents are in current use (see below). The aim is to produce a slow progressive fall in BP to safe but not necessarily normal levels, avoiding sudden falls in BP and episodes of hypotension which may do serious harm to the mother (e.g. cerebral thrombosis or haemorrhage) and to the fetus (e.g. acute distress or intrauterine death). Intravenous bolus doses should be avoided, and all antihypertensive agents should be given either by intramuscular injection or slow controlled infusion.

The recommended dosage regimes of the various drugs are as follows:

Dihydralazine (*Nepresol, Ciba*) may be given as *intramuscular* injections of 6.25 or 12.5 mg. Because of variability in response it is recommended that 6.25 mg should be given initially and repeated after 30 minutes. If diastolic BP is 110 mmHG or more intramuscular injections of 6.25 or 12.5 mg can then be repeated 4-hourly as necessary. For *intravenous infusion* 25 mg dihydralazine in 200 ml normal saline is started at a drip rate of 2.5 mg/hour and doubled every 30 min until diastolic BP is less than 110 mg, or up to a maximum dose rate of 20 mg/hour or until unacceptable side effects (e.g. headache, palpitations) develop. If diastolic BP falls below 90 mmHG the drip rate is halved and if necessary halved aagain every 30 min so as to maintain diastolic BP between 90 and 110 mmHG.

Labetalol (*Trandate, Glaxo-Allenburys*) can be given intravenously according to the method of Cummings *et al.* (1979). 200 mg labetalol in 200 ml saline is infused starting at 20 mg/hour and the drip rate and dose doubled every 30 min until diastolic BP falls below 110 mmHg or a maximum dose of 160 mg/hr (40 drops/min) is reached. If diastolic BP falls below 90 mmHg the drip rate is halved every 30 min with the aim of maintaining diastolic BP between 90 and 110 mmHg. Labetalol has been claimed to be superior to hydralazine when given intravenously in that it produces a smooth progressive fall in blood pressure without episodes of hypotension or side effects such as headaches and palpitations (Garden *et al.* 1982). Therapy with it can, if necessary, be continued orally. It is a useful alternative to hydralazine, or may be given as well if hydralazine alone fails to control the BP.

Diazoxide (*Hyperstat, Schering*) has been used as an intravenous injection, but the usual recommended dose of 150 mg may cause a precipitous fall in BP. It has been shown to reduce uterine blood flow in sheep (Brinkman & Assali 1976). Recently described regimes using repeated doses of 15–30 mg every minute are said not to cause hypotensive episodes (Maclean *et al.* 1981, Sankar & Moodley 1984). Diazoxide has however also produced reflex tachycardia, salt and water retention and hyperuricaemia. It is only rarely that the blood pressure cannot be lowered with hydralazine and/or labetalol, and the use of diazoxide should probably be restricted to these resistant cases.

Anticonvulsant therapy

Antihypertensive agents probably do not prevent eclamptic convulsions, and if a fit has occurred or eclampsia seems imminent anticonvulsant therapy should be commenced immediately. A variety of anticonvulsant regimes have been used, but the only agents in current use are clonazepam or diazepam, chlormethiazole edisylate and magnesium sulphate.

Diazepam and chlormethiazole are usually used in the United Kingdom but magnesium sulphate is used almost universally in the USA. The ideal treatment is disputed but the most important factors are the skill and experience of the obstetrician and the standard of care given to the patient.

Emergency measures
In all cases of eclampsia emergency treatment must be instituted immediately. The patient is placed flat on her side to avoid injury, and tight clothing is loosened. A free airway is ensured, the jaws are opened with a gag or spoon, the tongue pulled forward, an airway if available inserted and any secretions or vomit aspirated. Oxygen is given if patient is cyanosed, and external cardiac massage is started if there is cardiac arrest. Clonazepam 1 mg or diazepam 10 mg is given over 2 minutes as an intravenous bolus, and repeated after 10 min if fits are not controlled.

Magnesium sulphate, in a controlled intravenous infusion as described by Zuspan (1966), is preferred to intramuscular injections which are painful and do not permit the same control of dosage. The recommended regime begins with a loading dose of 4 g slowly over 20 minutes and a continuous infusion is started, giving 1.0 g/hour to a patient of less than 55 kg body weight and 1.5 g/hour if heavier. This infusion is continued for 24 hours after delivery or after the last fit. The patient is examined carefully every 4 hours for limb reflexes, respiration rate (at least 16/min) and urinary output (at least 30 ml/hour), and serum magnesium is measured if possible. If reflexes are absent, respirations are depressed or urinary output is inadequate, the infusion is discontinued, but is recommended if these signs are reversed in 4 hours' time.

If respirations are markedly depressed or cardiac arrest occurs 10–20 ml of 10% calcium gluconate is given intravenously over 10 minutes. If the diastolic BP remains 110 mmHg or more 30 minutes after starting magnesium sulphate, a dihydralazine or labetalol infusion is started. Before anaesthesia or delivery the anaesthetist and paediatrician must be fully informed because magnesium sulphate may enhance the action of curare-like and other drugs.

The advantage of magnesium sulphate is that the patient is fully conscious, the infant is not depressed and its effectiveness has been established in large series (Pritchard *et al.* 1984). Its disadvantages are the relatively close therapeutic and toxic plasma magnesium levels, the need for close supervision and the fact that magnesium sulphate may only block neuro-muscular transmission by presynaptic inhibition and may not affect cortical activity.

Clonazepam (Rivotril) or Diazepam (Valium) is given as an intravenous bolus over 2–5 minutes (1.0 mg of clonazepam, or 10 mg diazepam), followed by a continuous infusion of clonazepam 2.5 mg or diaze-pam 25 mg in 500 ml of 5% dextrose into a large vein at a rate not exceeding 0.25 clonazepam or 2.5 diazepam mg/minute, until patient is drowsy, usually a total dose of 10–30 mg diazepam (Hibbard & Rosen 1977). Infusion is then continued at a rate of 0.25–1 mg clonazepam/hour or 2.5–10 mg diaze-pam/hour to maintain drowsiness for 24 hours after the last fit or delivery. Clonazepam and diazepam are said to be very effective in stopping, but less effective in preventing, fits. They produce sedation of mother and fetus with the risk of neonatal hypothermia, hy-potonus and apnoea so that the baby may have to be artificially respired and tube fed for several days because it is unable to metabolize or excrete diazepam rapidly. It is a good drug for initial treatment of eclampsia but its effect on the neonate makes it re-latively unsuitable for long term use.

Chlormethiazole Edisylate (Heminevrin) has been shown to be an effective anticonvulsant in the treat-ment of eclampsia (Duffus *et al.* 1969) and in the treatment of status epilepticus resistant to diazepam (Harvey *et al.* 1975). It is given as an intravenous infusion of 0.8% chlormethiazole in 500 ml of 5% dextrose at a dose rate of 2–4 g/hour for first 5–10 minutes and then 0.5–1 g/hour thereafter at a rate sufficient to produce superficial (i.e. easily arousable) sleep. Although chlormethiazole is primarily a seda-tive it has a short half life (45 minutes) so that the level of sedation may be controlled precisely, and it does not produce sedation of mother and neonate when therapy is discontinued. It probably deserves to be more widely used but the complex method of mix-ing the solution is a disadvantage.

Management of complications of hypertension

Prompt detection and treatment of the major compli-cations is an important part of management of severe hypertension and eclampsia.

Pulmonary oedema and heart failure
Because pulmonary oedema may occur at relatively low levels of venous pressure due to the reduced on-cotic pressure, in all cases of severe hypertension the lung bases should be auscultated every 4 hours,

and if there is any suggestion of pulmonary oedema a central venous pressure line should be set up. Frusemide 40–80 mg should be administered intra-venously and consideration should be given to digitalization. If antihypertensive therapy is required Prazosin, which reduces excessive afterload, may be of value particularly in postpartum patients.

Renal failure
Before diagnosing renal failure it is important to en-sure that there has been adequate fluid intake and that the central venous pressure (CVP) is in the range 5–10 cm water. In all women with oligurua it is therefore important to set up a CVP line immediately: if CVP is more than 10 cm frusemide 40 mg should be given intravenously; if CVP is 5–10 cm the patient should be given 200 ml of 5% dextrose as a clear fluid challenge if she is not oedematous, or if she is oedematous 2 units of human stabilized serum (or equivalent solution) instead; if CVP is less than 5 cm 2 units human stabilized serum should be given.

The resulting diuresis, if it occurs, is reassuring and there is some evidence that maintenance of urine flow may be beneficial and may shorten the period of renal failure (Cantavorich *et al.* 1971). The preven-tion of renal failure depends upon ensuring adequate blood volume and cardiac output, so rapid restoration of blood volume is vital if antepartum or postpartum haemorrhage occurs. In hypertensive patients with oliguria requiring antihypertensive therapy, hydral-azine (which increases renal blood flow) may be of particular value, and the aim should be to maintain safe but not hypotensive levels of BP. Continued close monitoring of CVP (or of pulmonary wedge pressure) is also important to ensure continued adequate fluid replacement and to avoid fluid overload and pulmon-ary oedema. Once renal failure is diagnosed, plasma creatinine, urea and urate should be measured every 12 hours, and fluid and protein intake should be restricted. In general, haemodialysis should be started early, preferably in a renal unit, and the advice and help of a renal physician should be obtained as soon as renal failure is diagnosed.

Hepatic failure
Because of the seriousness of hepatic failure labour should be expedited and delivery effected as soon as possible.

Disseminated intravascular coagulation (DIC)
Because DIC is a common feature of severe hyper-tension, some obstetricians have attempted heparin

therapy over long periods up to 47 days (Fairley *et al.* 1976). Howie *et al.* (1975) however concluded that heparin was not an effective treatment and did not prevent the intravascular fibrin deposition or alter the course of the disease. Gill and Bonnar (1980), contrary to earlier reports, also came to the conclusion that pre-eclampsia could not be improved by heparin therapy and it would not be justified to give it as a prophylactic for pre-eclampsia.

CHRONIC MEDICAL DISORDERS PRESENTING WITH HYPERTENSION

For details of the aetiology, pathology and management of chronic renal disease and other chronic medical disorders presenting with hypertension readers are referred to larger texts on these diseases such as those by Burrow and Ferris (1982), and de Swiet (1984). Some key points in diagnosis, management and prognosis are summarized as follows:

CHRONIC RENAL DISEASE

The common forms of chronic renal disease and some of the important effects of pregnancy on the disease and of the disease on the fetus are summarized in Table 16.12 from Davison (1984) and have been reviewed by Hou (1985). The effect of pregnancy on a mother with chronic nephritis is very variable. Increased proteinuria is common and about half of these patients show a marked increase, with over 3 g/24 hours in 30% of pregnancies. Hypertension, usually mild, occurs in about 25% and is more common with diffuse glomerulonephritis and arteriolar nephrosclerosis. In spite of increased proteinuria the majority view is that, with the exception of the increased risk of pyelonephritis, pregnancy has no permanent adverse effect on the established renal disease, provided renal function is not severely compromised and hypertension is absent. Prognosis for the fetus depends upon the level of blood pressure and presence or absence of renal failure. Management, including antihypertensive therapy when indicated, is the same as for other hypertensive disorders of pregnancy. Delivery before 38 weeks may be necessary if renal function deteriorates markedly, if uncontrollable hypertension or eclampsia occurs or if there are signs of impending fetal death. The fetal prognosis is on the whole good and successful pregnancies have been reported in patients on hemodialysis and also following renal transplantation.

Table 16.12 Effects of pregnancy on pre-existing renal disease. (From Davison J. (1984) In *Medical Disorders in Obstetric Practice*, M. de Swiet ed. p. 211. Blackwell Scientific Publications Ltd, Oxford.)

Chronic glomerulonephritis and non-infectious tubulointerstitial disease	Usually no adverse effect in the absence of hypertension. Some believe that glomerulonephritis is adversely affected by coagulation changes in pregnancy. Urinary tract infections may occur more frequently.
Lupus nephropathy	Controversial: the prognosis is most favourable if the disease is in remission 6 months prior to conception. Steroid dosage should be increased in the puerperium.
Diabetic nephropathy	Probably no adverse effect on the renal lesion, although the frequency of leg oedema, pre-eclampsia and infection is higher.
Chronic pyelonephritis (infectious tubulo-interstitial disease)	Bacteriuria during pregnancy leads to more frequent exacerbation.
Polycystic disease	Functional impairment and hypertension are usually minimal in childbearing years. Probably no adverse effect.
Urolithiasis	Infections may be more frequent, otherwise ureteral dilatation and stasis do not seem to affect natural history.
After nephrectomy: solitary and pelvic kidneys	Pregnancy is usually well tolerated. Dystocia has been rarely attributed to pelvic kidneys: it can be associated with other malformations of urogenital tract.
Nephrotic syndrome	Tolerated well, infants may have low birthweight. Diuretics should not be used.

COARCTATION OF THE AORTA

Previously this condition was associated with a high enough maternal mortality for termination of pregnancy to be recommended. Maternal death is primarily due to dissection or rupture of the aorta due to cystic medial necrosis, and the risk of rupture may be increased by the haemodynamic changes of pregnancy. Recent experience is more favourable and the advisability of pregnancy depends on relative factors such as associated cardiac malformation. Pregnancy may generally be undertaken after a previous successful resection. Surgical resection during pregnancy is not usually advisable, although in a report of 10 patients requiring this 9 had uncomplicated deliveries with living infants (Hillestad 1972).

CONN'S SYNDROME

Conn's syndrome is usually diagnosed before or after pregnancy on the basis of hypertension with hypokalaemia. Diagnosis in pregnancy is difficult because of the raised plasma concentration and increased urinary excretion of aldosterone. Remission of the disorder may occur in pregnancy (possibly due to the effect of progesterone) and successful pregnancies with and without medical treatment have been reported.

CUSHING'S SYNDROME

Women with Cushing's syndrome often have amenorrhoea and are infertile. Diagnosis during pregnancy is difficult because many features of the disease resemble a normal pregnancy and plasma cortisol and urinary corticosteroids are raised in normal pregnancy. There is an increased fetal loss. Treatment is with dexamethasone. Full investigation and surgical exploration if necessary are recommended because of the relatively high incidence of primary adrenal tumours. Successful pregnancies have been reported after adrenalectomy.

NEUROFIBROMATOSIS

Hypertension is common in neurofibromatosis in pregnancy and may occur early in pregnancy, although the exact cause of the hypertension is not known. Pregnancy may cause deterioration of the disease and exacerbation of hypertension, and women with neurofibromatosis need close antenatal care (Edwards *et al.* 1983).

PHAEOCHROMOCYTOMA

Phaechromocytoma is a rare but dangerous complication of pregnancy and may closely resemble severe pre-eclampsia in presentation. Screening of all patients with severe hypertension in pregnancy for phaechromocytoma by urinary meta-adrenaline and noradrenaline excretion is recommended. Maternal mortality is as high as 50% and surgical removal of the tumour is recommended as soon as the diagnosis

is made. Adrenergic blockade is essential both to stabilize the patient before operation, during surgery and in the postoperative period. The fetal mortality rate is about 50% irrespective of when the disorder is diagnosed and treated.

FETAL AND MATERNAL OUTCOME

MATERNAL MORTALITY AND MORBIDITY

Maternal mortality from hypertension and eclampsia has shown a marked drop in most countries during recent years, and in England and Wales maternal deaths from pre-eclampsia fell from 43.8/million maternities in 1952–54 to 9.4/million maternities in 1972–75. (Reports on Confidential Enquiries into Maternal Deaths in England and Wales, 1957, 1977, 1981.) It is important to note that 'toxaemia of pregnancy' was the commonest cause of maternal death in England and Wales in 1976–78 and that avoidable factors were present in 89% of deaths from pre-eclampsia and in 62% from eclampsia. Deaths from eclampsia or pre-eclampsia are due to complications such as placental abruption, cerebral haemorrhage or renal failure. Pritchard *et al.* (1984) reported only one maternal death in 245 women with eclampsia treated in Dallas over 30 years by a standard protocol using a combination of intravenous and intramuscular magnesium and hydralazine. Maternal mortality should therefore be rare in women with eclampsia who are admitted to hospital, who are not in coma, and who are given prompt intensive skilled treatment.

PERINATAL MORTALITY

In *eclampsia* the perinatal death rate depends upon where the patient is delivered, the care given and whether the eclampsia occurred antenatally or in labour. In Cardiff Wightman *et al.* (1978) in a series of 43 women with eclampsia found a perinatal mortality of 213/1000. Templeton and Campbell (1979) in Aberdeen found a perinatal mortality from antepartum and intrapartum eclampsia of 136/1000. Most of the deaths were associated with IUGR and preterm delivery, and the perinatal mortality depended mainly on how quickly the infant was transferred to hospital and given intensive neonatal care. In 84 cases delivered between 1975 and 1983, reported by Pritchard *et al.* (1984), there were 5 intrauterine deaths before admission and 8 stillbirths or neonatal deaths in infants who were alive on admission, giving a perinatal mortality of 154 per 1000 births (101 per 1,000 in the infants alive on admission). Two of the infants weighed less than 750 g and two had congenital heart disease, so that the number of perinatal deaths due to hypertension and pre-eclampsia was in the order of 50 per 1000 births. Though eclampsia causes a significant perinatal mortality it must be remembered that fetal survival is still of the order of 90–95%.

Hypertension without eclampsia. In the British Births Survey of 1970 (Chamberlain *et al.* 1978) there was very little difference in perinatal mortality between women who were normotensive (19.2 per 1000) and those diagnosed as mild pre-eclampsia (19.5 per 1000), and patients with moderate pre-eclampsia (diastolic BP of 100–109 mmHg but no proteinuria) had a similar perinatal mortality (18.1 per 1000). Women with severe pre-eclampsia with proteinuria, however, had an almost doubled perinatal mortality (33.7 per 1000). In a large multicentre collaborative study in the USA (Friedman & Neff 1977d) the stillbirth rate rose with either a diastolic BP of at least 85 mmHg with proteinuria or at least 95 mmHg without proteinuria. In primigravidas in Aberdeen MacGillivray (1983g) found that women who had a rise in BP only at the end of pregnancy had a lower perinatal mortality rate than women who remained normotensive, but that the development of proteinuria was associated with a doubling or trebling of the rate. The overall perinatal mortality in any group of hypertensive or proteinuric women in pregnancy will of necessity depend upon the age and parity distributions and the different types and severity of hypertension and proteinuric disorders in the women studied. Failure to define the populations and groups studied has led to many discrepancies in findings and to many of the misunderstandings with regard to the significance of hypertensive disorders of pregnancy.

SOCIO-ECONOMIC IMPLICATIONS AND THE FUTURE

A great deal of time and effort goes into the diagnosis and management of the hypertensive disorders of pregnancy. Until effective means of prevention or cure are discovered it is perhaps necessary to look for more cost effective methods of management. Developments such as home monitoring of blood pressure, self-testing of urine for protein and fetal movement counting may reduce the need for inpatient hospital care. The use of obstetric day units, whereby the effect of a period of 1 or 2 hrs bed rest on the blood pressure can be assessed and all necessary investigations performed (e.g. cardiotocography, ultrasound and biochemical tests) may not only reduce the need for inpatient care but may be more acceptable to most patients. The need for bed rest and prolonged admission to hospital, except in cases of severe hypertension or hypertension with IUGR has probably been over emphasized in the past. It may even be that in some patients hypertension developing in late pregnancy is physiological. The future unquestionably lies in better knowledge of the aetiology and pathophysiology of hypertension and proteinuria in pregnancy, both in general and in the individual patient. This will lead to better and more effective methods of management, if not of prevention and cure. It is salutary to reflect that the maternal and perinatal deaths due to hypertension and/or proteinuria in most series have occurred in patients treated with all the modern techniques of monitoring and neonatal care and in spite of antihypertensive therapy, bed rest and all other currently recommended therapeutic regimes.

REFERENCES

ADAMS E. M. & MACGILLIVRAY I. (1961) *Lancet*, ii, 1373.

ALTCHEK A. (1964) *Circulation*, **29** and **30** (Suppl II): 43.

ALTCHEK A., ALBRIGHT N. L. & SOMMERS S. C. (1968) *Obstet. & Gynec.*, **31**, 595.

ARIAS F. (1975) *Amer. J. Obstet Gynec.*, **123**, 610.

ASSALI N. S., VERGON J. M., TATA U. & GERBER S. T. (1952) *Amer. J. Obstet. Gynec.*, **63**, 978.

ASSALI N. S., DOUGLASS R. A., BAIRD W. W. & NICHOLSON D. B. (1954) *Clin. Res. Proc.*, **102**.

BADER R. A., BADER M. E., ROSE D. J. & BRAUNWALD E. (1955) *J. clin. Invest.*, **34**, 1524.

BEER A. E. (1978) *Sem. Perinatol.*, **2**, 39.

BENNEDETTI T. J., COTTON D. B., READ J. C. & MILLER F. C. (1980) *Amer. J. Obstet. Gynec.*, **136**, 465.

BIRKELAND S. A. & KRISTOFERSON K. (1979) *Lancet*, ii, 720.

BISCHOFF P. (1981) *Placenta*, **2**, 29.

BISCHOFF P., HUGHES G. & KLOPPER A. (1980) *Amer. J. Obstet. Gynec.*, **138**, 494.

BLAUSTEIN M. P. (1977) *Amer. J. Physiol.*, **232**, 165.

BONNAR J. (1978) *Obstet. Gynecol. Ann.*, **7**, 195.

BRAIN M. C., DACIE J. V. & HOURIHANE D. O. (1962) *Brit. J. Haematol.*, **8**, 358.

BRAIN M. C., KUAH K. B. & DIXON H. G. (1967) *J. Obstet. Gynaec. Brit. Cwlth.*, **74**, 2.

BRINKMAN C. R. & ASSALI N. S. (1976) *Perspect. Nephrol. Hypertens.*, **5**, 363.

BROSENS I., ROBERTSON W. B. & DIXON H. G. (1972) In *Obstetrics and Gynecology Annual* (Wynn R. M. ed), p. 177. Appleton Century Crofts, New York.

BURROW G. N. & FERRIS T. F. (1982) *Medical Complications during Pregnancy*. W. B. Saunders, Philadelphia.

BUTLER N. R. & ALBERMAN E. D. (1969) In *Perinatal Problems*. p. 36. E. & S. Livingstone, Edinburgh & London.

CAMPBELL D. M. (1978) *Eur. J. Obstet. Gynaecol. reprod. Biol.*, **8**, 263.

CAMPBELL D. M. & MACGILLIVRAY I. (1980) *Clin. Exp. Hypertens.*, **2**, 897.

CAMPBELL D. M. & MACGILLIVRAY I. (1982) In *Pregnancy Hypertension* (Sammour M., Symonds E. M. Zuspan F. P. & El Tomi N. eds), p. 95. Ain Shams University Press, Cairo.

CAMPBELL D. M., MACGILLIVRAY I. & CARR-HILL R. (1985) *Brit. J. Obstet. Gynaecol.*, **92**, 131.

CANTAROVICH F., FERNANDEZ J. C., LOCETELLI A., PEREZ L. J. & CRISHOF J. (1971) *Postgrad. Med. J.*, **47** (Suppl 13): 13.

CHAMBERLAIN G., PHILIPP E., HOWLETT B. & MASTERS U. (1978) *British Births* 1970. Heinemann, London.

CHESLEY L. C. (1978a) *Hypertensive Disorders in Pregnancy*, p. 9. Appleton Century Crofts, New York.

CHESLEY L. C. (1978b) *Hypertensive Disorders in Pregnancy*, p. 40. Appleton Century Crofts, New York.

CHESLEY L. C. (1978c) *Hypertensive Disorders in Pregnancy*, p. 157, Appleton Century Crofts, New York.

CHESLEY L. C. (1978d) *Hypertensive Disorders in Pregnancy*, p. 270. Appleton Century Crofts, New York.

CHESLEY L. C. (1978e) *Hypertensive Disorders in Pregnancy*, p. 88. Appleton Century Crofts, New York.

CHESLEY L. C. (1978f) *Hypertensive Disorders in Pregnancy*, p. 104. Appleton Century Crofts, New York.

CHESLEY L. C. (1978g) *Hypertensive Disorders in Pregnancy*, p. 268. Appleton Century Crofts, New York.

CHESLEY L. C. (1980) *Clin. Exp. Hypertens.*, **2**, 777.

COHEN-OVERBEEK T., HERNANDEZ C., MEISNER I., PEARCE M. & CAMPBELL S. (1984) *Clin. Exp. Hypertens.*, **B3**, 142.

CUMMINGS A. M. M., BROWN J. J., FRASER R., LEVER A. F., MORTON J. J., RICHARDS D. A. & ROBERTSON J. I. S. (1979) *Brit. J. clin. Pharmacol.*, **8**, 359.

CURZEN P. & VARMA R. (1971) *J. Obstet. Gynaec. Brit. Cwlth.*, **78**, 686.

CURZEN P. & VARMA R. (1973) *Amer. J. Obstet. Gynecol.*, **115**, 929.

DASS A. & BHAGWANANI S. (1964) *J. Obstet. Gynaec. Brit. Cwlth.*, **71**, 727.

DAVEY D. A., DOMMISSE J., OPIE L. H. (1984) In *The Critically Ill Obstetric Patient* (Baldwin R. W. M. & Hanson G. C. eds), p. 246. Farrand Press, London, J. B. Lippincott, Philadelphia.

DAVIES A. M. (1971) *Geographical Epidemiology of the Toxemias of Pregnancy*. Thomas C. C. Illinois.

DAVISON J. (1984) In *Medical Disorders in Obstetric Practice* (de Swiet M. ed) p. 192. Blackwell Scientific Publications, Oxford.

DAVISON J. M., DUNLOP W., EZIMOKHAI M. (1980) *Brit. J. Obstet. Gynaecol.*, **87**, 106.

DAWES G. S., FOX H. E., LEDUC B. M., LIGGINS G. C. & RICHARDS R. T. (1970) *J. Physiol.*, **210**, 479.

DEMERS L. M. & GABBE S. G. (1976) *Amer. J. Obstet. Gynec.*, **126**, 137.

DE SWIET M. (1984) (ed) *Medical Disorders in Obstetric Practice*. Blackwell Scientific Publications, Oxford.

DE WARDENER H. E. (1973) In *The Kidney* 4th ed., p. 42. Churchill Livingstone, London.

DE WOLF F., ROBERTSON W. B. & BROSENS I. (1975) *Amer. J. Obstet. Gynec.*, **123**, 164.

DIECKMANN W. J. (1936) *Amer. J. Obstet. Gynec.*, **32**, 927.

DIXON H. G., BROWNE C. J. M. & DAVEY D. A. (1963) *Lancet*, **ii**, 369.

DIXON H. G. & ROBERTSON W. B. (1961) *Pathol. Microbiol.*, **24**, 622.

DUFFUS G. M. & MACGILLIVRAY I. (1968) *Lancet*, **i**, 994.

DUFFUS G. M., TUNSTALL N. E., CONDIE R. G. & MACGILLIVRAY I. (1969) *J. Obstet. Gynaec. Brit. Cwlth.*, **76**, 645.

EDWARDS J. N. T., FOOKS M. & DAVEY D. A. (1983) *Brit. J. Obstet. Gynaec.*, **90**, 528.

ELEBUTE O. A. & MILLS I. H. (1976) In *Hypertension in Pregnancy* (Lindheimer M. D., Katz A. I. & Zuspan F. P. eds), p. 329. John Wiley and Sons, New York.

FAIRLEY K. F., ADDEY F. G., ROSS I. C. & KINCAID-SMITH P. (1976) In *Hypertension in Pregnancy* (Lindheimer M. D., Katz A. I. & Zuspan F. P. eds), p. 103. John Wiley and Sons, New York.

FIDLER J., SMITH V., FAYEOS P. & DE SWIET M. (1983) *Brit. med. J.*, **286**, 1927.

FORRESTER T. E. & ALLEYNE G. A. O. (1980) *Clin Sci.*, **59**, 1995.

FORRESTER T. E. & ALLEYNE G. A. O. (1981) *Brit. med. J.*, **283**, 5.

FOX H. (1978) *Pathology of the Placenta*. p. 120. W. B. Saunders, London, Philadelphia, Toronto.

FRIEDMAN E. A. (1976) *Progress in Clinical and Biological Research*. p. 279. Alan R. Liss, New York.

FRIEDMAN E. A. & NEFF R. K. (1977a) *Pregnancy Hypertension: A Systematic Evaluation of Clinical Diagnostic Criteria*. p. 238. PSG Publishing Company Inc, Littleton, Mass.

FRIEDMAN E. A. & NEFF R. K. (1977b) *Pregnancy Hypertension: A Systematic Evaluation of Clinical Diagnostic Criteria*. p. 46. PSG Publishing Company Inc. Littleton, Mass.

FRIEDMAN E. A. & NEFF R. K. (1977c) *Pregnancy Hypertension: A Systematic Evaluation of Clinical Diagnostic Criteria*. p. 128. PSG Publishing Company Inc. Littleton, Mass.

FRIEDMAN E. A. & NEFF R. K. (1977d) *Pregnancy Hypertension: A Systematic Evaluation of Clinical Diagnostic Criteria*. p. 239. PSG Publishing Company Inc. Littleton, Mass.

GALLERY E. D. M., SAUNDERS D. M., HUNYOR S. N. & GYORY A. Z. (1979) *Brit. med. J.*, **i**, 1591.

GALTON M., MERRITT K. & BELLER F. K. (1971) *J. reprod. Med.*, **6**, 78.

GANT N. F., CHAND S., WORLEY R. J., WHALLEY P., CROSBY U. D. & MACDONALD P. C. (1974) *Amer. J. Obstet. Gynec.*, **120**, 1.

GANT N. F., DALEY G. L., CHAND S., WHALLEY P. J. & MACDONALD P. C. (1973) *J. clin. Invest.*, **52**, 2682.

GANT N.F., MADDEN J.D., SIITERI P.K. & MACDONALD P.C. (1972) In *Proceedings of the Fourth International Congress of Endocrinology*, p. 1026. Excerpta Medica, Amsterdam.

GANT N.F., PORTER J.C. & MACDONALD P.C. (1977) In *Clinics in Obstetrics and Gynecology* (Symonds E.M. ed), p. 632. W.B. Saunders, London, Philadelphia.

GANT N.F. & WORLEY R.J. (1980a) *Hypertension in Pregnancy*, p. 1. Appleton Century Crofts, New York.

GANT N.F. & WORLEY R.J. (1980b) *Hypertension in Pregnancy*, p. 34. Appleton Century Crofts, New York.

GANT N.F. & WORLEY R.J. (1980c) *Hypertension in Pregnancy*, p. 101, Appleton Century Crofts, New York.

GARDEN A., DAVEY D.A. & DOMMISSE J. (1982) *Clin. Exp. Hypertens.*, **B1**, 371.

GILL B.P. & BONNAR J. (1980) In *Pregnancy Hypertension* (Bonnar J., MacGillivray I. & Symonds E.M. eds), p. 577. MTP Press, Lancaster.

GIBSON H.M. (1973) *Brit. J. Obstet Gynaecol.*, **80**, 1067.

GINSBURG J. & DUNCAN S.L.B. (1967) *Cardiovasc. Res.*, **1**, 356.

GOLDBY F.S. & BEILIN L.J. (1972) *Cardiovasc. Res.*, **6**, 384.

GROENENDIJK R., TRIMBOS J.B.M.J. & WALLENBURG H.C.S. (1984) *Amer. J. Obstet. Gynec.*, **150**, 232.

HAMILTON H.F.H. (1951) *J. Obstet. Gynaecol. Brit. Emp.*, **58**, 977.

HARVEY P.K.P., HIGENBOTTAM T.W. & LOH L. (1975) *Brit. med. J.*, **2**, 603.

HERTIG A.T. (1945) *Clinics*, **4**, 602.

HIBBARD B.M. & ROSEN M. (1977) *Brit. J. Anaesth.*, **49**, 3.

HILLESTAD L. (1972) *Acta. Obstet. Gynecol. Scand.*, **51**, 95.

HILLIER K. & SMITH M.D. (1981) *Obstet. Gynecol.*, **88**, 274.

HOU S. (1985) *N. Engl. J. Med.*, **312**, 836.

HOWIE P.M., PRENTICE C.R.M. & FORBES C.E. (1975) *Brit. J. Obstet. Gynaecol.*, **82**, 711.

HUCKABEE W. (1962) *Amer. J. Obstet. Gynecol.*, **84**, 1623.

HUGHES E.C. (1972) *Obstetric Gynecologic Terminology*, p. 422. Philadelphia: Davis.

JEFFCOATE T.N.A. (1966) *Proc. roy. Soc. Med.*, **59**, 397.

JONES D.D., DAHIJRI S., ROBERTS E.L. & WILLIAMS G.F. (1982) *Brit. J. Obstet. Gynaecol.*, **89**, 314.

KAPELLER-ADLER R. (1950) In *Toxaemia of Pregnancy, Human and Veterinary* (Hammond J., Browne F.J. & Wolstenhome G.E.W. eds), p. 261. London, J. & A. Churchill.

KAPLAN N.M. (1982) *Clinical Hypertension*, p. 56. Williams & Wilkins, Baltimore.

KNUTZEN V.K. & DAVEY D.A. (1977) *S. Afr. med. J.*, **51**, 675.

KOPELMAN J.J. & LEVITZ M. (1970) *Amer. J. Obstet. Gynec.*, **108**, 925.

LAMMING G.D., PIPKIN F.B. & SYMONDS E.M. (1980) *Clin. Exp. Hypertens.*, **B2**, 865.

LEATHER H.M., HUMPHREYS D.M., BAKER P. & CHADD M.A. (1968) *Lancet*, **ii**, 488.

LETCHWORTH A.T. & CHARD T. (1972) *Lancet*, **i**, 704.

LEWIS P.J. (1983) In *Prostacyclin in Pregnancy* (Lewis P.J., Moncada S. & O'Grady J. eds.), p. 215. Raven Press, New York.

LIM Y.L. & WALTERS W.A.W. (1979) *Brit. J. Obstet. Gynaecol.*, **86**, 198.

LONG P.A., ABELL D.A. & BEISCHER N.A. (1980) *Brit. J. Obstet. Gynaecol.*, **87**, 13.

LUBBE W.F. & HODGE J.V. (1981) *N.Z. Med. J.*, **94**, 169.

LUNDGREN Y., LJUNGBLAD U. & KARLSSON K. (1983) *Clin. Exp. Hypertens.*, **B2**, 1.

LUNELL N.O., NYLUND L.E., LEWANDER R. & SARBY B. (1982a) *Clin. Exp. Hypertens.*, **B1**, 105.

LUNELL N.O., HJEMDHAL P., FREDHOM B.B., LEWANDER R., NISELL H., NYLUND L., PERSSON B., SANBY B., WAGER J. & THORNSTROM S. (1982b) *Excerpta Medica Congress Series*, **591**, Amsterdam.

LUNELL N.O., LEWANDER R., NYLUND L., SARBY B., & THORNSTROM S. (1983) *Gynecol. Obstet. Invest.*, **16**, 274.

LYSGAARD H., CLAVERO J.A., NEGUEREELA J., ORITZ L., DE LOS HEROS J.A. & MODREGO S.P. (1973) *Amer. J. Obstet. Gynec.*, **116**, 340.

MACGILLIVRAY I. (1950) *J. Obstet. Gynaecol. Brit. Emp.*, **57**, 924.

MACGILLIVRAY I. (1958) *J. Obstet. Gynaecol. Brit. Emp.*, **65**, 536.

MACGILLIVRAY I. (1959) *Lancet*, **i**, 51.

MACGILLIVRAY I. (1961) *J. Obstet. Gynaecol. Brit. Cwlth.*, **68**, 557.

MACGILLIVRAY I. (1967) *Scott. med. J.*, **12**, 237.

MACGILLIVRAY I. (1977) *Isr. J. med. Sci.*, **12**, 500.

MACGILLIVRAY I. (1982) In *Pregnancy Hypertension* (Sammour M.B., Symonds E.M., Zuspan F.P. & El-Tomi N. eds), p. 1. Ain Shams University Press, Cairo.

MACGILLIVRAY I. (1983a) *Pre-eclampsia.* p. 182. W.B. Saunders, London.

MACGILLIVRAY I. (1983b) *Pre-eclampsia.* p. 198. W.B. Saunders, London.

MACGILLIVRAY I. (1983c) *Pre-eclampsia.* p. 64. W.B. Saunders, London.

MACGILLIVRAY I. (1983d) *Pre-eclampsia.* p. 322. W.B. Saunders, London.

MACGILLIVRAY I. (1983e) *Pre-eclampsia.* p. 324. W.B. Saunders, London.

MACGILLIVRAY I. (1983f) *Pre-eclampsia.* p. 227. W.B. Saunders, London.

MACGILLIVRAY I. (1983g) *Pre-eclampsia.* p. 181. W.B. Saunders, London.

MACGILLIVRAY I., ROSE G.A. & ROSE D. (1969) *Clin. Sci.*, 37, 395.

MACKENNA J., DOVER N.L. & BRAME R.G. (1983) *Obstet. Gynecol.*, **62**, 751.

MACLEAN A.B., DOIG J.R., CHATFIELD W.R. & AICKIN D.R. (1981) *Aust. N.Z. J. Obstet. Gynaecol.*, **21**, 7.

MARCEAU S., MOUTQUIN J.M. & DE CHAMPLAIN J. (1984) *Clin. Exp. Hypertens.*, **B3**, 222.

MCCALL M.L. (1953) *Amer. J. Obstet. Gynec.*, **60**, 1015.

MCCARTNEY C.P. (1964) *Circ. Res.*, **29** (Suppl II): 37.

McCartney C. P., Schumacher G. F. B. & Spargo B. H. (1971) *Amer. J. Obstet. Gynec.*, **111**, 580.

McEwan H. P. (1969) *J. Obstet. Gynaec. Brit. Cwlth.*, **76**, 809.

McKillop C., Howie P. W., Forbes C. D. & Prentice C. R. M. (1976) *Lancet*, **i**, 56.

McLennan A. H., Sharp F. & Shaw-Dunn J. (1972) *J. Obstet. Gynaecol. Brit. Cwlth.*, **79**, 113.

McMurray J. A. & Morgan D. B. (1984) *Clin. Exp. Hypertens.*, **B3**, 23.

Messerli F. H., Frohlich E. D., Dreslinski G. R., Suarez D. H. & Aristimuno G. G. (1980) *Ann. Intern. Med.*, **93**, 817.

Moore P. T. & Myerscough P. R. (1957) *J. Obstet. Gynaecol. Brit. Emp.*, **64**, 207.

Moulds R. F. W. & Javernig R. A. (1977) *Lancet*, **i**, 200.

Nelson T. R. (1955) *J. Obstet. Gynaec. Brit. Cwlth.*, **62**, 48.

Nisell H., Hjemdahl P., Linde B. & Lunell N. O. (1985) Personal Communication.

Nochy D., Birembout P., Hinglais N., Freund M., Idatte J. M., Jacquot C., Chartier M. & Bariety J. (1980) *Clin. Nephrol.*, **13**, 155.

O'Brien E. T. & O'Malley K. (1979) *Brit. med. J.* **i**, 775.

Page E. W. (1939) *Amer. J. Obstet. Gynec.*, **37**, 291.

Peterson P. A., Evrin P. & Berggard I. (1969) *J. clin. Invest.*, **48**, 1189.

Petrucco O. M. (1981) In *Progress in Obstetrics and Gynaecology* (Studd J. ed.) Vol. I. p. 51. Churchill Livingstone, Edinburgh & London.

Pirani B. B. K. & MacGillivray I. (1978) *Obstet. and Gynec.*, **52**, 257.

Pollak V. E. & Nettles J. B. (1960) *Medicine*, **39**, 469.

Pritchard J. A., Cunningham F. G. & Mason R. A. (1976) *Amer. J. Obstet. Gynec.*, **124**, 855.

Pritchard J. A., Cunningham F. G. & Pritchard S. A. (1984) *Amer. J. Obstet. Gynec.*, **148**, 951.

Pritchard J. A., Ratnoff O. D. & Weisman R. (1954) *Obstet. and Gynec.*, **4**, 159.

Redman C. W. G. (1977) In *Clinics in Obstetrics and Gynaecology* (Symonds E. M. ed) Vol. 4, p. 685. W. B. Saunders Co. Ltd., London.

Redman C. W. G. (1981) In *The Investigations of Labetalol in the Management of Hypertension in Pregnancy* (Riley A., Symonds E. M. eds.) p. 101. Excerpta Medica, International Congress Series, Amsterdam.

Redman C. W. G., Beilin L. J., Bonnar J. & Wilkinson R. H. (1976a) *Lancet*, **i**, 1370.

Redman C. W. G., Beilin L. J. & Bonnar J. (1976b) In *Hypertension in Pregnancy* (Lindheimer M. D., Katz A. I. & Zuspan F. P. eds), p. 139. John Wiley, New York.

Redman C. W. G., Beilin L. J., Bonnar J. & Ounsted M. K. (1976c) *Lancet*, **ii**, 753.

Redman C. W. G., Bonnar J. & Beilin L. J. (1978a) *Brit. med. J.*, **i**, 467.

Redman C. W. G., Bodmer J., Bodmer W. F., Beilin L. J. & Bonnar J. (1978b) *Lancet*, **ii**, 397.

Rennie I. D. B., Keen H., Cohwig J., Field M. & Quartey E. (1967) *Lancet*, **ii**, 489.

Richards A. (1985) Personal Communication.

Riddell W., Campbell D. M. & MacGillivray I. (1983) In *Pre-eclampsia* (MacGillivray I. ed.) p. 84. W. B. Saunders, London.

Rippmann E. T. (1969) Gynaecologia., **137**, 478.

Robertson E. G. (1971) *J. Obstet. Gynaec. Brit. Cwlth.*, **78**, 520.

Robertson W. B. (1976) *J. clin. Pathol.*, **10**, 9.

Robertson W. B., Brosens I. & Dixon G. (1976) In *Hypertension in Pregnancy* (Lindheimer M. D., Katz I. A. & Zuspan F. P. eds), p. 115. John Wiley and Sons, New York.

Robinson J. S., Redman C. W. G., Glover I. & Mitchell M. D. (1979) *Prostaglandins Med.*, **3**, 223.

Robson J. S. (1976) In *Hypertension in Pregnancy* (Lindheimer M. D., Katz A. I. & Zuspan F. P. eds), p. 61. John Wiley & Sons, New York.

Rovinsky J. J. & Jaffin H. (1965) *Amer. J. Obstet. Gynec.*, **93**, 1.

Rubin P. C., Butters L., Clark D. M., Reynolds B., Sumner D. J., Steedman D., Low R. A. & Reid J. L. (1983) *Lancet*, **i**, 431.

Ruff S. C., Mitchell R. H. & Murnaghan G. A. (1982) In *Pregnancy Hypertension* (Sammour M. B., Symonds E. M., Zuspan F. P. & El-Tomi N. eds), p. 126. Ain Sham University Press, Cairo.

Sanchez-Torres F. & Santamaria A. (1965) Review of Obstetrics and Gynecologie, Venezuela, p. 25, 657. Quoted by Chesley L. C. (1978) in *Hypertensive Disorders of Pregnancy*, Appleton Century Crofts, New York.

Sankar D. & Moodley J. (1984) *S. Afr. med. J.*, **65**, 279.

Scott J. S. (1958) *J. Obstet. Gynaecol. Brit. Emp.*, **65**, 689.

Scott J. R. & Beer A. A. (1976) *Amer. J. Obstet. Gynec.*, **125**, 418.

Seligman S. A. (1971) *J. Obstet. Gynaec. Brit. Cwlth.*, **78**, 413.

Seymour A. E., Petrucco O. M., Clarkson A. R., Haynes W. D. G., Lawrence J. R., Jackson B., Thompson A. J. & Thomson N. M. (1976) In *Hypertension in Pregnancy* (Lindheimer M. D., Katz A. I. & Zuspan F. P. eds)., p. 139. John Wiley and Sons, New York.

Shaw A. B., Risdon P. & Lewis-Jackson J. D. (1983) *Brit. Med. J.*, **287**, 929.

Sheehan H. L. & Lynch J. B. (1973a) *Pathology of Toxaemia of Pregnancy.* p. 211. Churchill Livingstone, Edinburgh, London.

Sheehan H. L. & Lynch J. B. (1973b) *Patholgoy of Toxaemia of Pregnancy.* p. 2. Churchill Livingstone, Edinburgh, London.

Sheehan H. L. & Lynch J. B. (1973c) *Pathology of Toxaemia of Pregnancy.* p. 53. Churchill Livingstone, Edinburgh, London.

Sheehan H. L. & Lynch J. B. (1973d) *Pathology of Toxaemia of Pregnancy.* p. 398. Churchill Livingstone, Edinburgh, London.

Sheehan H. L. & Lynch J. B. (1973e) *Pathology of Toxaemia*

of Pregnancy. p. 524. Churchill Livingstone, Edinburgh, London.

SHEEHAN H. L. & LYNCH J. B. (1973f) *Pathology of Toxaemia of Pregnancy.* p. 525. Churchill Livingstone, Edinburgh, London.

SHEPPARD B. L. & BONNAR J. (1976) *Brit. J. Obstet. Gynaecol.,* **83**, 948.

SHEPPARD B. L. & BONNAR J. (1981) *Brit. J. Obstet. Gynaecol.,* **88**, 695.

SIBAI B. M., ANDERSON G. D., SPINNATO J. A. & SHAVER D. C. (1983) *Amer. J. Obstet. Gynec.,* **147**, 16.

SIMANOWITZ M. D., MACGREGOR W. G. & HOBBS J. R. (1973) *J. Obstet. Gynaec. Brit. Cwlth.,* **80**, 103.

SKINNER S. L., CRAN E. J., GIBSON R. & SYMONDS E. M. (1975) *Amer. J. Obstet. Gynec.,* **121**, 626.

SKINNER S. L., LUMBERS E. R. & SYMONDS E. M. (1968) *Amer. J. Obstet. Gynec.,* **101**, 429.

SMITH G. VAN S. & SMITH O. W. (1948) *Physiol. Rev.,* **28**, 1.

SPARGO B., MCCARTNEY C. P. & WINEMILLER R. (1959) *Arch Path.,* **68**, 593.

SPILLACY W. M. N., TEOH E. S. & BUHI W. C. (1970) *Obstet. Gynecol.,* **35**, 685.

STUDD J. W. W. (1971) *J. Obstet. Gynaec. Brit. Cwlth.,* **78**, 786.

SYMONDS E. M. (1980) *J. roy. Soc. Med.,* **73**, 871.

SYMONDS E. M. & ANDERSON G. J. (1974) *J. Obstet. Gynaecol. Brit. Cwlth.,* **81**, 676.

SYMONDS E. M., BROUGHTON-PIPKIN F. & CRAVEN D. J. (1975) *Brit. J. Obstet. Gynaecol.,* **82**, 643.

TEMPLETON A. A. & CAMPBELL D. M. (1979) *Health Bull.* (Edinb), **55**.

THOMSON A. M. & BILLEWICZ W. Z. (1957) *Brit. med. J.,* **243**, 247.

THOMSON A. M., HYTTEN F. E. & BILLEWICZ W. Z. (1967) *J. Obstet. Gynaec. Brit. Cwlth.,* **74**, 1.

THORBURN J., DRUMMOND M. M., WIGHAM K. A., LOWE C. D. O., FORBES C. D., PRENTICE C. R. M. & WHITFIELD C. R. (1982) *Brit. J. Obstet. Gynaecol.,* **89**, 117.

THURNAU G. R. (1985) In *Immunology and Obstetrics and Gynaecology* (Scott J. R. & Rote N. S. eds), p. 107. Appleton Century Crofts, New York.

TOOP K. & KLOPPER A. (1981) *Placenta,* **3** (Suppl): 167.

TREHARNE I. A. L., SUTHERLAND H. W., STOWERS J. M. & SAMPHIER M. (1979) In *Carbohydrate Metabolism in Pregnancy and the Newborn* (Sutherland H. W. & Stowers J. M. eds), p. 479. Springer, Berlin.

VENUTO R. C., COX J. W., STEIN J. H. & FERRIS T. F. (1976) *J. clin. Invest.,* **57**, 938.

WALLS J., SCHORR W. J. & KERR D. N. S. (1978) *Brit. med. J.,* **4**, 220.

WALSH S. W., BEHR M. J., ALLEN N. H. (1985) *Amer. J. Obstet. Gynec.,* **151**, 110.

WALTERS B. N. J. & REDMAN C. W. G. (1984) *Brit. J. Obstet. Gynaecol.,* **91**, 330.

WARD H., WHYLEY G. A. & MILLAR M. D. (1972) *J. Obstet. Gynaecol. Brit. Cwlth.,* **79**, 216.

WATSON D. E., SIDDIGUI S. A., STAFFORD J. E. H., GIBBARD S. & HEWITT V. (1973) *J. clin. Path.,* **26**, 294.

WEINSTEIN L. (1982) *Amer. J. Obstet. Gynec.,* **142**, 159.

WEIR R. J., BROWN J. J., FRASER R., KRAZEWSKI A., LEVER A. F., MCILWAINE G. M., HORTON J. J., ROBERTSON J. J. S., & TREE M. (1973) *Lancet,* **i**, 291.

WEISSBURG P. L., WEAVER J., WOODS K. L., WEST M. J. & BEEVERS D. G. (1983) *Brit. med. J.,* **287**, 709.

WERKÖ L. (1950) In *Toxaemias of Pregnancy Human and Veterinary* (Hammond J., Browne F. J. & Wolstenholm G. E. W. (eds), p. 155. Blakiston, Philadelphia.

WIGHTMAN H., HIBBARD B. M. & ROSEN M. (1978) *Brit. med. J.,* **2**, 235.

WILLIAMS G. F. & JONES D. D. (1982) *Brit. J. Obstet. Gynaecol.,* **89**, 309.

WOODS D. L. & MALAN A. F. (1983) *Brit. J. Obstet. Gynaecol.,* **90**, 876.

WOODS D. L. & MORRELL D. F. (1982) *Brit. med. J.,* **285**, 691.

WORLD HEALTH ORGANIZATION EXPERT COMMITTEE ON PREGNANCY AND LACTATION. (1965) Technical Report Series, 302. WHO. Geneva.

YLOSTALO P. (1970) *Acta. Obstet. Gynecol. Scand.,* **49** (Suppl 4): 1.

ZEEK P. M. & ASSALI N. S. (1950) *Amer. J. Clin. Path.,* **20**, 1099.

ZUSPAN F. P. (1966) *Clin. Obstet. Gynecol.,* **9**, 954.

CHAPTER 17
HEART DISEASE IN PREGNANCY

C. R. WHITFIELD

To understand the effects of heart disease on the pregnant patient it is necessary to know the anatomy and physiology of the circulatory system in a normal person, and the changes which occur in a healthy pregnant woman. The compensatory changes in the circulatory system which accompany pregnancy become clinically apparent only when they fail or have an adverse effect on the health of the patient. An understanding of these changes is therefore required if the patient with heart disease is to be managed effectively during her pregnancy and afterwards.

Because of modern techniques of investigation and treatment, a greater proportion of patients with heart disease are now known to have congenital anomalies than previously and many of these women can become pregnant. Diseases affecting the heart, such as acute rheumatic endocarditis, are much less frequently found although still of importance and significance.

HAEMODYNAMIC CHANGES IN PREGNANCY

With the improvement in methods of studying serially the circulatory changes in pregnant women, more information has been accumulated during the last ten years. This solves reasonably satisfactorily many of the puzzles that have been posed by previous studies and explains certain clinical observations. The main haemodynamic changes are increased blood volume and cardiac output with decreased peripheral resistance, and they are probably mediated by oestrogens and prostaglandins including prostacyclin (de Swiet 1984). The presence of an abdominal swelling of increasing size, with elevation and 'splinting' of the diaphragm and compression of the inferior vena cava when the patient is supine, also results in circulatory and respiratory changes during pregnancy.

It is well known that there is an increase in blood volume during pregnancy. It falls to below the non-pregnant level at about eight weeks' gestation due to a reduction in the red cell mass, but thereafter there is a steady increase until between the 28th and 35th week, when it is about 35% greater than the non-pregnant volume. Both the plasma volume and red cell mass are raised, the plasma volume being increased by about 40% and the increase in the red cell mass is only about 18%. The changes in total blood volume, plasma volume and red cell mass were well reviewed by Lange and Dynesius (1973); depending partly on the subject's body size, the peak total blood volume increase reaches about 1500 ml in single pregnancies, and about 2000 ml in twin pregnancies (Pritchard 1965). The total blood volume by term has shown a fall of 15–20% because of a reduction in the plasma volume. The actual circulating volume is reduced and measurement of this by a dye dilution technique in the supine position indicates a greater decrease than actually occurs, because of impairment of the venous return. The marked increase in circulating blood volume as pregnancy progresses is adequately compensated for by the healthy patient, but this may not be the case if there is impairment of cardiac function.

CARDIAC OUTPUT

Walters et al. (1966) demonstrated that there was a marked rise in cardiac output by the twelfth week of pregnancy and this work has been confirmed by other workers including Lees et al. (1967) and Metcalf et al. (1971). As there is a marked increase in oestrogen production during the early weeks of pregnancy, this might provide an explanation for the early changes observed (Ueland & Parer 1966). The increase in cardiac output, which is achieved mainly by increased stroke volume rather than heart rate, reaches its maximum of 30–40% above normal by mid-term.

Scott and Kerr (1963) showed that compression of the inferior vena cava by the gravid uterus in late pregnancy when the patient is supine may cause

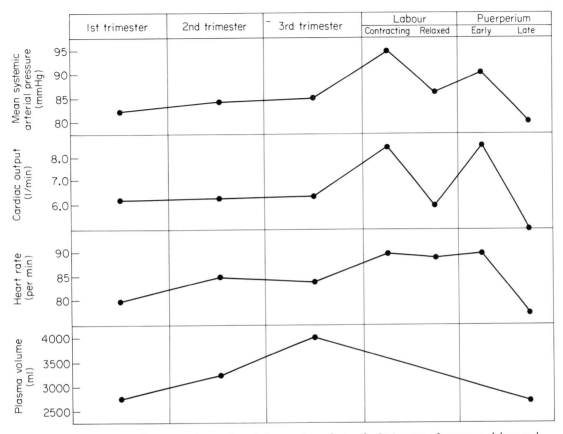

Fig. 17.1. Blood pressure, cardiac output, heart rate and plasma volume during the 3 trimesters of pregnancy, labour and the puerperium. (By courtesy of Dr M. M. Lees.)

complete occlusion, with a collateral circulation by means of the paravertebral veins being opened up. If these collateral vessels do not respond immediately the venous return to the heart is reduced and the patient develops 'the supine hypotension syndrome'. This is of importance clinically in estimating the blood pressure, and with regard to the position of the patient during labour and delivery and during Caesarean section under general or regional anaesthesia. The patient herself experiences discomfort in this position and will turn on her side or sit up if allowed to do so. The observation has helped to explain changes in haemodynamics during the last weeks of pregnancy, and now that it is appreciated false observations can be guarded against.

The observations of Lees *et al.* (1967) using an indicator-dilution method serially throughout pregnancy (Fig. 17.1) have been confirmed by Ueland and Hansen (1969) although the latter authors have found that the cardiac output at term falls slightly even when estimated in the lateral position.

During labour the cardiac output rises due to an increase in the stroke volume, the rise increasing as the intensity of the uterine contractions increases. Between contractions when the uterus is relaxed there is a fall in cardiac output to late pregnancy levels (Fig. 17.1). A further rise in the cardiac output occurs after delivery, the stroke volume being increased along with a bradycardia. The relief of supine caval occlusion and the return of blood to the general circulation as a result of contraction and retraction of the uterine muscle following expulsion of the fetus and placenta will tend to augment the cardiac output, while blood loss on delivery will tend to reduce it. These responses have been demonstrated in patients who experience pain during labour (Ueland *et al.* 1970). Lees *et al.* (1970) showed that there is a cumulative rise in cardiac output, heart rate and blood pressure throughout labour during sympathetic blockade by means of epidural anaesthesia. The changes are more dramatic following elective Caesarean section (Lees *et al.* 1968) and the administration of oxytocic substances, particularly ergometrine which has a vasoconstrictive action as well as a direct action on the myometrium, may aggravate the haemodynamic changes.

OTHER CHANGES

The heart rate shows little change during pregnancy (Fig. 17.1), an increase to no more than 10 beats per minute by term being usual. The arterial blood pressure also shows little change throughout pregnancy in the normal patient (Fig. 17.1).

Oxygen consumption is increased during pregnancy but respiratory excursion is impaired in the later weeks by the enlarged uterus. The respiratory rate increases and dyspnoea even on mild exertion is a normal feature in late pregnancy. The rise in cardiac output in early pregnancy is proportionately greater than the increase in oxygen consumption (Ueland *et al.* 1973).

In the puerperium there is a gradual return to the prepregnancy state. The arterial blood pressure and cardiac output will be elevated after delivery because of the increase in circulating volume and the raised heart rate, particularly after the administration of ergometrine. When the plasma volume falls with the post-delivery diuresis, the cardiac output, blood pressure and heart rate also fall to prepregnancy levels.

THE RESPONSE OF THE HEALTHY PREGNANT WOMAN

The changes described are usually tolerated readily by the healthy patient. They tend to be progressive and gradual, with the exception of the early rise in cardiac output but even this probably occurs over a period of time. A patient will avoid lying on her back during the latter part of pregnancy, and counteracts orthopnoea by sleeping with her head, shoulders and chest raised on pillows. She tends to restrict her activities to within her limitations, stopping on stairs and when walking if she becomes breathless.

Heart murmurs are frequently detected during pregnancy as a result of the haemodynamic changes occurring, and a third heart sound may be heard. Cardiac enlargement may be seen on radiographs and alterations of the electrocardiograph pattern are noticeable because of elevation of the diaphragm.

HEART DISEASE AND PREGNANCY

Rheumatic fever has been, at least until very recently, by far the most common aetiological factor in pregnant women with heart disease. However, the incidence of rheumatic heart disease has fallen because of the use of antibiotics in the treatment of streptococcal infection, and perhaps because the virulence of strains of streptococci associated with rheumatic fever has declined. The number of women with congenital heart lesions reaching childbearing age has increased due to improvement in the management of children with these anomalies, particularly when amenable to surgery. With more rational advice being given as to the advisability or otherwise of pregnancy when cardiac disease is known to exist and the greater use of contraception and sterilization, the number of patients who present serious problems during pregnancy has been reduced. The ratio of pregnant patients with rheumatic to congenital heart lesions was for long about 10:1, but in the United Kingdom had fallen to 3:1 or even 2:1 a decade ago (Marquis 1969), and many obstetric units now deal with as many women with congenital as with rheumatic lesions; a reversed ratio of 1 rheumatic to 2 congenital lesions was recently reported from Queen Charlotte's Hospital (de Swiet & Fidler 1981).

Examination of the patient in early pregnancy may uncover unsuspected heart disease, sometimes without any suggestive history. A primigravida may well be having her first medical examination, with auscultation of the heart sounds, since her schooldays, although it is nevertheless now much less common to find lesions of serious import which had not been detected on routine examination at school or by the family doctor. There are also fewer instances in which a woman has been labelled as having serious heart disease when no lesion exists. If a suspicious murmur is noted or the history is suggestive when the patient is seen for the first time in her pregnancy, she should be seen by a cardiologist, possibly at a combined cardiac-obstetric clinic. Close cooperation between the two disciplines has considerably reduced the morbidity and mortality from heart disease in pregnancy. It is no longer likely to be 'cost-effective' for even a large obstetric hospital to reserve a weekly outpatient session exclusively for women with cardiac problems, but it remains vital that such patients should be under close joint supervision by cardiologists with special interests and expertise in these problems during pregnancy. An effective compromise is for such cardiologists always to be present at a specific routine weekly clinic, to which all the hospital's obstetricians transfer all patients with confirmed cardiac disorders for antenatal care, and to which all women with suspected lesions or with equivocal heart sounds are referred for expert diagnosis. The same cardiologists must, of course, provide readily available care for admitted patients including during labour. Alternatively a physician specializing in maternal medicine may include cardiac disease among the medical disorders for which he takes responsibility during pregnancy.

MATERNAL MORTALITY ASSOCIATED WITH HEART DISEASE

The number of maternal deaths associated with cardiac disease has declined steadily, due mainly to a fall in the number dying from acquired forms of cardiac disease, but the maternal mortality rate for cardiac disease in association with pregnancy remains about 0.5%. The triennial Reports on Confidential Enquiries into Maternal Deaths in England and Wales (1972, 1975, 1979, 1982) illustrate very well both the steady absolute decline in mortality attributable to heart disease, and the persistence of the problem as a relatively important contributor to the very much smaller number of maternal deaths that now occur from all causes, including a significant proportion of those judged to be avoidable. During the 6 years 1973–78 cardiac disease caused 6% of the deaths reviewed. The Confidential Enquiries show that acquired forms of cardiac disease appear to be more lethal in association with pregnancy in women aged 25 years or more and in their third or later pregnancies. Congenital malformations, however, occur in younger women and in those of lower parity.

Rheumatic heart disease with lesions of the mitral valve either alone or with lesions of other valves is still the most common acquired cause. It is probable that pregnancy does not alter long-term prognosis in rheumatic heart disease provided the mother survives the pregnancy itself (de Swiet 1984). Thus, Chesley (1980) found in 38 mothers undergoing 51 pregnancies after the occurrence of severe rheumatic heart disease a mean survival time of 14 years, compared with 12 years in 96 women with comparable disease but who did not become pregnant.

The last four Reports showed that in the 12 years covered (1967–1978) coronary thrombosis was found at autopsy in 21 patients. Four patients during this period died soon after mitral valvotomy, and an-

other died under anaesthesia prior to this operation, but recently valvotomy has been performed very much less often during pregnancy and no death associated with the operation was noted in the last of these reports. Most deaths associated with acquired cardiac disease occur between 36 and 39 weeks.

Congenital malformations of the circulatory system have become of more significance with the reduction in acquired heart disease. Of the 31 deaths included in the same Reports, 9 were in patients with Eisenmenger's complex and 5 in patients with a patent ductus arteriosus. Eleven of the deaths followed abdominal surgery, 9 after Caesarean section, 1 following hysterotomy and sterilization and 1 after tubal ligation. Twenty-six of these 31 deaths (84%) were following delivery. It is interesting to note that the anaesthetic administered was not thought to have played a part in any of the deaths.

CIRCULATORY CHANGES IN HEART DISEASE OR ABNORMALITY

When stenosis of the mitral valve is present, the increase in work done by the left atrium is directly proportional to the degree of stenosis. As the cardiac output depends on the stroke volume and the heart rate, a reduction in the volume of blood entering the left ventricle has to be compensated for by tachycardia if a fall in cardiac output is to be prevented. The heart rate can be raised to a limited extent only. As the arterial blood pressure depends on the cardiac output and peripheral resistance, a fall in cardiac output will result in hypotension unless there is a compensatory vasoconstrictive rise in peripheral resistance.

The workload of the left atrium is increased considerably in the presence of mitral stenosis and complications will arise if it is unable to carry out this increased workload. The right ventricular output may be increased in an attempt to compensate for left atrial insufficiency with resultant pulmonary arterial or venous hypertension and pulmonary oedema. Subsequent failure of the right ventricle will result in congestive cardiac failure.

If there is a degree of mitral incompetence present this will result in an increase in the volume of blood in the left atrium after contraction of the left ventricle with further aggravation of the condition of the pulmonary circulation.

Stenosis of the aortic valve increases the work required of the left ventricle which hypertrophies, and there is a further increase in peripheral resistance with hypertension. Incompetence of the aortic valve will further increase the work required of the left ventricle and will aggravate left ventricular failure.

If there is a congenital abnormality of the cardio-vascular system, the effects may vary between nil or minimal and very severe. If there is a reversal of blood flow or if the oxygenation of the blood is inadequate, the patient will experience varying degrees of hypoxia and in such patients any available surgical treatment is likely to be justified. This is usually performed in childhood, but very occasionally may be necessary during pregnancy.

In *pulmonary stenosis* there is right ventricular myocardial hypertrophy with a consequent increase in right atrial pressure and eventual failure of the right side of the heart. The stenosis may involve the cusps of the pulmonary valve or occur at the conus of the right ventricle. Cyanosis is not present, but cardiac failure is likely to develop if the degree of stenosis is marked.

A *patent ductus arteriosus* results in a permanent reversed shunt, with an increase in the work of the left ventricle and pulmonary hypertension, because of the volume of blood being conveyed from the aorta to the pulmonary artery. The increased return of blood from the lungs to the left atrium and left ventricle results in left ventricular hypertrophy and eventual failure.

Coarctation of the aorta is found in the region where the ductus arteriosus joins the aorta. The disability resulting from coarctation will depend on the degree of narrowing and its length. Left ventricular hypertrophy results with hypertension in the upper parts of the body. A collateral circulation develops, but usually surgery will have been carried out prior to pregnancy if indicated by the degree of narrowing.

An *atrial septal defect* may give rise to a shunt from the left side to the right side of the heart with gradual enlargement of the right side and pulmonary artery. If the pressure is increased on the right side of the heart the shunt may be reversed, with blood bypassing the lungs and the development of cyanosis. In the left to right shunt there will be an increase in the volume of blood flowing through the right atrium, the right ventricle and the pulmonary circulation, with dilatation and later hypertrophy. The left chambers remain normal in size because the increased volume of blood returning to the left atrium once again enters the right side of the heart.

In *Lutembacher's syndrome*, mitral stenosis is associated with an atrial septal defect increasing the work done by the left atrium.

A *ventricular septal defect* means that there is a shunt from the left to the right side and may lead to pulmonary hypertension, dilatation of the right ventricle, and later to dilatation of the left atrium and left ventricle. If congestive cardiac failure develops there may be a reversal of the shunt with blood flowing from the right side to the left ventricle.

In *Eisenmenger's complex* there is an interventricular septal defect with right ventricular hypertrophy and dextrorotation of the aorta overlying the septal defect. Cyanosis is a late feature when blood passes from the right side of the heart to left ventricle. When the *tetralogy of Fallot* is present, pulmonary artery stenosis is added to the features found in Eisenmenger's complex. In this condition there may be shunting from left to right, but usually the shunt is from right to left with the development of polycythaemia and cyanosis.

EFFECTS OF PREGNANCY ON PATIENTS WITH HEART DISEASE OR ABNORMALITY

In pregnancy the increase in blood volume and therefore in cardiac output will aggravate any condition in which there is damage to the valves of the heart or an anomaly in the direction of blood flow. The degree of severity will depend on the extent of the lesion and the capacity of the heart to compensate for the congenital or acquired disability. Any additional stress or strain will tend to precipitate failure of heart action.

A woman with heart disease is less able to respond to exercise when pregnant, the degree of handicap becoming greater the more strenuous the exercise.

EFFECTS OF HEART DISEASE ON PREGNANCY

Deaths associated with heart disease have been reported in the successive Reports on Confidential Enquiries into Maternal Deaths in women who did not seek medical aid in early pregnancy or refused to accept medical advice from their family doctors, obstetricians or cardiologists. Every effort must therefore be made to diagnose early and accurately any organic cardiac lesion that may be present and to enlist the aid of a cardiologist at the earliest possible moment. There is also evidence that the infants of women with heart disease have a tendency to be born prematurely or may be 'light for dates' (Ueland et al. 1972).

Ueland et al. (1972) studied a number of pregnant patients with heart conditions and concluded that all varieties of valvular disease reduced the haemodynamic responses to pregnancy and to exertion during pregnancy. In *mitral stenosis* the increase in cardiac output was less that in normal pregnant women and the stroke volume did not increase as much as in normal patients. There was little change in the heart rate. In the presence of *aortic incompetence* the cardiac output rose normally and the heart rate was within the normal range or slightly increased. A low cardiac output was found in a patient with aortic incompetence and mitral incompetence. In patients with *aortic stenosis* and *pulmonary stenosis* the rise in cardiac output was lower than the average range in normal pregnancy, the stroke volume and heart rate increases being less also.

Antenatal management

In early pregnancy, a history of previous heart disease or of conditions which may result in heart disease, as well as a physical examination including auscultation of the heart, should alert the obstetrician to the possibility of a heart lesion being present. Prompt referral of the patient for assessment, investigation and treatment by a cardiologist or general physician, but always in preference a cardiologist with a special commitment to obstetric patients, is imperative. Various investigative measures are available but are usually best reserved for the non-pregnant state. Occasionally accurate diagnosis is required for a major decision in management to be made and cineradiography and cardiac catheterization may be essential.

The severity of heart disease is usually graded according to the classification of the New York Heart Association (1965). The grading depends on the cardiac response to physical activity, but need not bear any relationship to the extent of the heart lesions present.

Grade I Patients with cardiac disease but no limitation of physical activity.

Grade II Patients with heart disease and slight to moderate limitation of physical activity. Ordinary physical activity causes discomfort.

Grade III Patients with heart disease with marked limitation of activity. Minimal exertion gives rise to discomfort.

Grade IV Patients with heart disease who are unable to carry out any physical activity without discomfort, and have orthopnoea.

This classification is not wholly reliable since symptoms should not be used as the only guide to management (Turner & Marquis 1965). Women who

have severe cardiac lesions may be in Grades I or II in early pregnancy but may deteriorate rapidly to Grade IV. Turner (1968) considered that classification on the basis of symptoms was potentially dangerous because the false sense of security engendered by a favourable grading in early pregnancy may yet be followed by maternal death later in pregnancy. Nevertheless, when used with sensible caution, the New York classification still provides a very practical way to grade symptoms, and to draw attention to any subjective deterioration as pregnancy proceeds or that may have occurred during the interval from one pregnancy to the next.

The aims of antenatal care will be to detect obstetric complications and minimize these where possible, and also to advise the patient when and how to avoid aggravating her cardiac condition. Additional stress and strain must be avoided as these might precipitate cardiac failure. Physical activity should be restricted to well within the patient's capacity and reserves. No unnecessary activity such as 'spring cleaning', gardening, etc., should be undertaken, particularly in late pregnancy if there is any significant degree of functional impairment. Abdominal compression should be avoided, as should the supine position, as these may result in pressure on the inferior vena cava and restriction of respiratory excursion. Anaemia should be prevented by the regular and routine ingestion of iron tablets with folic acid, or treated vigorously if it does occur. The oxygen-carrying capacity of the blood should be optimal. Elastic stockings or tights are of use in preventing pooling of blood in the veins of the lower limbs. Sodium restriction and the use of diuretics may be advised. Respiratory infections should be promptly treated with antibiotics, and the administration of oxygen if there is any respiratory embarrassment. Competent dental care (comprising a full inspection, advice on oral hygiene, and any necessary dental treatment) is mandatory; tooth extractions should be 'covered' by an appropriate antibiotic.

TERMINATION OF PREGNANCY

If pregnancy is diagnosed in a patient who has circulatory decompensation, the question of termination may arise. Fortunately, with advances in treatment the necessity for this has become very uncommon. Most cardiac patients know the risks associated with pregnancy and, if appropriate, take steps to avoid becoming pregnant. Alternatively, some become pregnant and are fully aware of the potential hazards:

in these circumstances it is unlikely that termination would be acceptable to the patient.

The presence of heart disease may be a contributory factor when a patient requesting termination is being assessed. Her age and parity as well as her domestic and socio-economic position will also be considered in the assessment. The fear held by some patients that they will be persuaded or even pressed to agree to termination should be allayed as quickly as possible as the risk of termination particularly after 14 weeks is probably about equal to that of a well managed pregnancy. The patient is likely in these circumstances to cooperate fully with the obstetrician and cardiologist.

Sterilization

A patient with a heart lesion should be sterilized on request when she and her partner have decided that their family is complete. The possible problems of contraception, including excessive blood loss and coagulation defects, are relevant when a prolonged period of contraception is likely to be required; and the anxiety associated with the possibility of having an unplanned pregnancy is considerable in such patients.

Pregnancy and premarital sterilization may be reasonably suggested to patients with cyanotic congenital heart lesions as pregnancy is likely to place an intolerable burden on the circulatory system in these patients. This would not apply, of course, if surgical correction of the condition resulted in a marked improvement, but the obstetrician and cardiologist have to make a realistic decision when advice is sought in such circumstances.

MEDICAL TREATMENT

Apart from the general measures suggested, specific treatment may be required if there are complications relating to the patient's cardiac state. Disorders of rhythm may necessitate the use of digoxin, infection is vigorously treated with antibiotics, and evidence of pulmonary congestion or cardiac failure requires immediate admission and prompt treatment.

Pulmonary oedema may develop because of impedance to the outflow of blood from the left atrium or an increase in the inflow of blood to the pulmonary vascular bed. The rate at which it develops is alarming and it may manifest itself by an attack of breathlessness associated with perhaps straining at stool. Crepitations at the lung bases are a serious finding in the presence of left atrial insufficiency. The venous return to the heart is effectively reduced by the application of inflatable cuffs to the upper and lower limbs. The cuffs are inflated so that the veins are occluded and are released for 5 minutes every 15 minutes in rotation. This procedure has largely replaced venesection with the loss of red blood cells which may contribute to the patient's problems. It is now very rare for venesection to be required to relieve the pulmonary oedema. Sitting up helps the patient to breathe more easily but in advanced pregnancy brings only limited relief. Morphine or its derivatives in moderate dosage are excellent at relieving anxiety and reducing the increased respiratory rate. Digoxin is beneficial if there is a marked tachycardia or fibrillation, but some cardiologists find it of limited value in the absence of irregularities of rhythm. A quick acting diuretic, such as frusemide in a dosage of 50–100 mg intramuscularly, may help to remove excessive tissue fluid when the cuffs have been removed. Oxygen therapy will be beneficial in patients with poor oxygen transfer or frank cyanosis.

Hospital admission for assessment and treatment is imperative if there has been any deterioration in the patient's condition or any acute complication has arisen. It is also beneficial to admit the patient, for rest and assessment, for a few days before term. The dangers of venous thrombosis and pulmonary embolism must be guarded against and anticoagulant therapy may be required. Admission to hospital should not usually mean complete immobilization unless the patient's condition is very serious. Physiotherapy and ambulation with assistance should help to prevent the development of thrombosis.

SURGICAL TREATMENT

Corrective surgery is best performed in cardiac patients before the patient becomes pregnant. With a greater appreciation of the benefits of cardiovascular surgery and improvement in the techniques used, fewer women who could benefit from surgery are reaching the childbearing age without having had it performed. Some show great improvement while in others the improvement is transitory or not apparent. There may still be murmurs and anomalies after surgery, and new problems may be created by the surgical procedure should the patient become pregnant.

Surgery during pregnancy may be indicated for mitral stenosis, but is not usually recommended for the correction of congenital anomalies unless the complications are very serious and delivery of the patient is not possible. Szekely and Snaith (1977) reported that mitral valvotomy had been performed during pregnancy or early in the puerperium in 29 women in Newcastle, representing 5.5% of their mothers with pure mitral stenosis, and there was a single eventual maternal death among them. They drew attention to uncontrollable haemoptysis as an important occasional indication for the operation during pregnancy. Hasche and Dippmann (1973) reviewed their experience of 541 mitral commissurotomies in which 3 were performed as emergencies in pregnancy. The indications were that the cardiac insufficiency was resistant to treatment and that the patients had severe pulmonary congestion with recurrent lung oedema. Open heart surgery may be preferred in such life-threatening circumstances, but with the great reduction in rheumatic carditis very few operations, open or closed, are required now.

Occasionally a patent ductus arteriosus is ligated during pregnancy because of a severe degree of 'left to right' shunt. The closure of atrial or ventricular septal defects should not be undertaken during pregnancy because of the haemodynamic changes likely to be precipitated by the use of the bypass, although there have been successful operations reported. These were reviewed by Meffert and Stansel (1968).

MANAGEMENT OF PREGNANCY FOLLOWING CARDIAC SURGERY

The management of such a patient is generally the same as of any cardiac patient, in that her functional status and the nature of her lesion must be evaluated and the degree of decompensation and disability assessed. With the development of techniques for replacing heart valves, however, the problem of continuous anticoagulant therapy assumes greater importance. Long acting anticoagulants such as Warfarin are usually given until the last month of pregnancy when Heparin, which does not cross the placenta to reach the fetus, should be substituted. Despite the special risks of embolism and bacterial endocarditis, in addition to that of heart failure, the general experience is that women with prosthetic heart valves tolerate very well the haemodynamic challenge posed by pregnancy and labour (Tejani 1973, Szekely & Snaith 1974, Chew & Ratnam 1975). On the other hand, a high perinatal loss (Oakley & Doherty 1976) in patients with prosthetic valves and on oral anticoagulant therapy has been reported, and in the fetus the occasional occurrence of optic atrophy (Holzgreve et al. 1976) and chon-

drodysplasia punctata (Abbott et al. 1977) have been attributed to Warfarin.

Management of labour

The management of labour in a patient with heart disease is essentially the same as its management in healthy women, provided an active policy is practised. From the physiological point of view, the shorter the labour lasts the better as this will minimize the effect of hypoxia on the fetus. Supportive treatment is necessary throughout, particular care being taken to avoid excessive effort on the part of the patient.

She should be propped up into the most comfortable position she can find so that her breathing is made easier. Oxygen must be available and should be administered intermittently or continuously if there is any dyspnoea or any evidence of cyanosis. Pain should also be relieved effectively. Morphine and its derivatives have been traditionally advocated for 'cardiac patients' even when their use has been discouraged for others. The possibility of respiratory depression and fetal damage must be weighed against the benefits from relief of anxiety and discomfort. Continuous epidural anaesthesia has been used to good effect in patients with moderate and severe heart disease, and will usually be the method of choice. Its use prevents a cumulative increase in the cardiac output throughout labour and allows prompt intervention either by Caesarean section in the first stage of labour or by obstetric forceps in the second stage should delay or distress occur (Lees et al. 1970).

There is no evidence that patients with cardiac disease have 'easy' labours, but this impression may have resulted from the increased attention and sedation which these patients received, along with a more active approach to their management. Now that labour is not usually permitted to last longer than 12–18 hours and frequently lasts a good deal less, the management of the healthy patient more closely resembles that of the management previously given to those with cardiac lesions. There is no advantage in inducing labour because of the presence of heart disease. There are rare occasions, however, when a patient who has responded well to treatment and is near term might have her labour induced before a further circulatory crisis develops.

Similarly cardiac disease is not a specific indication for Caesarean section, but if there are obstetrical complications operation is not contraindicated. Indeed, the obstetrician should have a 'low threshold' for the option of either elective or emergency Caesarean section in such cases. If the patient fails to make progress in labour it is preferable to deliver her by early Caesarean section rather than attempt to achieve vaginal delivery at all costs. Dehydration, metabolic acidosis and infection of the genital tract are always to be avoided and particularly in patients with heart disease. It must be remembered that a stressful first stage of labour, perhaps also with some fetal hypoxia supervening, is as bad for the pregnant woman and her fetus as the inreased cardiac output during contractions in the second stage. While the second stage should be no longer than in the healthy patient, routine prophylactic forceps delivery or vacuum extraction is quite unnecessary. In labour the functional state of the patient is again of more importance than the nature of the lesion in her cardiovascular system. Most obstetricians would be unwilling to allow the patient to bear down with breath holding for more than a few contractions if she has a cardiac lesion.

The use of ergometrine with or following delivery is contraindicated in patients with cardiac disease, especially if there is tight mitral stenosis or an arterio-venous shunt, because it may precipitate pulmonary oedema. In addition to its direct action on uterine muscle, ergometrine causes vasoconstriction with an increase in both arterial and venous pressure; an immediate rise in central venous pressure of 6 cm H_2O is sustained for an hour after intravenous injection, and there is a similar although rather less immediate effect when the injection is intramuscular (Vaughan Williams et al. 1974). It is sometimes said that the use of any oxytocic drug at delivery is contraindicated in patients with more than mild cardiac disease (Barnes 1974), but the cardiovascular effects of synthetic oxytocin are quite different from those of ergometrine. With oxtytocin there is some reduction in peripheral resistance and no increase in arterial or venous pressure, so that an intravenous bolus injection of 5 units of oxytocin and/or an oxytocin infusion may be safely used in management of the third stage of labour in patients with heart disease (Moodie & Moir 1976).

The most dangerous time for the development of congestive cardiac failure or pulmonary oedema is immediately after delivery. Careful attention must be paid to patients at risk at this time. The Reports on Confidential Enquiries into Maternal Deaths during 1973–75 and 1976–78 show that the majority of the deaths associated with cardiac disease occur after delivery.

If Caesarean section is required, epidural or possibly spinal anaesthesia is preferable, particularly if this form of blockade has been used during labour, although Ueland et al. (1970) found that balanced anaesthesia (thiopentone, nitrous oxide and relaxants) was also suitable and interfered less with the patient's haemodynamics when severe heart disease was present.

The puerperium

While the necessity for rest and recovery is fully appreciated, it is essential that this is not interpreted as complete rest. Active movement in bed with regular exercising, early rising and early ambulation are to be encouraged under the supervision of the cardiologist. If immobilization in bed is deemed necessary, the possibility of anticoagulant therapy must be considered as the greatest hazard at this time is venous thrombosis and pulmonary embolism.

The administration of antibiotics routinely during labour is not thought to be necessary by all cardiologists, but these should certainly be given in the puerperium if there is any pyrexia possibly associated with uterine or urinary infection. Upper respiratory tract infections should also be vigorously treated. The danger of *subacute bacterial endocarditis* is always present and should be guarded against. It is a particular risk if the cardiac lesion is a congenital one, or when the patient has a prosthetic valve, and in such cases routine prophylactic antibiotic therapy from the start of labour is probably always indicated. On the other hand, prophylactic antibiotics were not used in a 10-year series of 387 patients with cardiac disease at the National Maternity Hospital in Dublin without bacterial endocarditis occurring (Sugrue et al. 1981). However, it should be noted that there were 11 deaths from this cause during the 9 years relating to the last three Confidential Enquiries into Maternal Deaths.

CONTRACEPTION

Sterilization may be recommended by the cardiologist, and if acceptable to the patient, the obstetrician may agree to do this by laparoscopy about six weeks postpartum. Puerperal tubal ligation is the alternative but would be advocated only if the patient had to be sterilized before leaving hospital with her baby, or if other factors precluded the safe use of the laparoscope.

If a further pregnancy has to be postponed because

of the wishes of the couple or to allow cardiac surgery to be undertaken, effective contraception should be instituted. Oral contraception or the sheath are probably preferable to the insertion of an intrauterine device. The patient's cardiac state should be assessed about six weeks after delivery and advice on cardiac surgery, the need for medical treatment, the advisability of further pregnancies and of sterilization discussed with all concerned. Some encouragement to limit family size will often be appropriate, and it is obviously desirable that the family should be completed before there is serious further deterioration in cardiac function. At the same time, optimal spacing of births will ensure that no more than one child at a time must be nursed, lifted and carried.

Acute myocardial infarction and pregnancy

It is unusual for women to develop acute myocardial infarction during pregnancy and particularly difficult to diagnose the condition. An incidence of about one case in 10 000 pregnancies, with a maternal mortality of almost 30%, has been estimated by Ginz (1970), and the relevant literature was again reviewed by Lim and Khairuddin Yusof (1973). The symptoms of upper abdominal and chest pain and flatulence are common enough in pregnancy, but electrocardiograph changes may indicate the occurrence of an infarction. If there is cardiac failure and persistence of angina, termination of the pregnancy would seem the best method of management. If the patient makes a good recovery without decompensation, the pregnancy can continue. Vaginal delivery may be attempted in a multiparous patient in whom it is thought labour will be relatively easy and rapid. If the labour is likely to be long or if cardiac decompensation is present, delivery is best effected by Caesarean section. During this procedure, hypotension should be avoided and an experienced anaesthetist should be available.

Cardiomyopathies

Although numerous papers have been published about cardiomyopathies surprisingly little is known of the causation of the disease or of its relationship to pregnancy. Cardiomyopathies may be congestive or obstructive. A primary form is confined to the myocardium, while the secondary form is associated with systemic disease.

Congestive cardiomyopathy is closely related to parturition but it is possible that pregnancy is simply a precipitating factor in a woman with a susceptible myocardium. Malnutrition and low socio-economic status may have a role in its causation. Heart failure develops acutely, angina, transient hypertension and arrhythmias are common, and sometimes a patient presents with systemic or pulmonary embolism. Its onset is in the last trimester or in the puerperium, and the outcome may be rapid death, chronic heart disease or complete recovery. It is thought to recur and progress in subsequent pregnancies, and if cardiac failure develops in the puerperium for the first time this is the likely cause. In congestive cardiomyopathy there may be no predisposing cause other than pregnancy and the only findings are of dilatation and failure of the heart.

The more usual form of pregnancy cardiomyopathy is the hypertrophic obstructive one, and Oakley et al. (1979) reported on 23 patients who had this condition and who had 54 pregnancies without any maternal or perinatal deaths, although there were 10 spontaneous and one therapeutic abortion. Heart failure is not common and the patients tend to be healthy without many symptoms. The left ventricle empties rapidly, with late systolic obstruction to further ejection and mitral incompetence accounting for mid or late systolic murmurs. There may be angina because of the increased demands of the thick myocardium, or alternatively alterations in the electrocardiogram. Confirmatory diagnosis is by angiocardiography after the pregnancy.

In the Reports for the four triennia 1967–78, 13 patients were adjudged to have died of cardiomyopathies. Rand et al. (1975) believe that there was an immunological explanation for the condition of their patient and for the stillborn fetus as high titres of antimyocardial sarcolemma antibodies were detected in the patient. A similar case was reported by Brown et al. (1967).

Caesarean section seems to be a somewhat hazardous method of treatment in the presence of acute congestive failure, and intensive treatment with diuretics and potassium supplements seems to have been successful as regards the mother. There is an increase in the work done by the left ventricle, and exercise or expulsive efforts, hypovolaemia from acute blood loss, pain and digitalis are likely to aggravate the condition. Although elective Caesarean section was recommended previously, vaginal delivery has not presented the anticipated problems and, unless there are obstetric indications for it, Caesarean section does not appear to be the method of delivery of choice in patients with this condition. It was performed in 10 of the 43 continuing pregnancies in the series of Oakley *et al.* (1979) and there were standard obstetric indications on all but 3 occasions.

Until more is known of the aetiological factors causing this condition, and the functional classification is related to pregnancy outcome on the basis of greater experience, obstetricians should be prepared to consider the diagnosis if unexplained cardiac complications occur and should apply general principles of management with the help of the cardiologist.

Beta-blocking drugs have been recommended to reduce tachycardia and the force of left ventricular ejection, but they may cause fetal bradycardia, neonatal hypoglycaemia and possibly intrauterine growth retardation, and so should be used only to control angina or arrhythmia (Oakley *et al.* 1979).

Cardiovascular hazard of beta-adrenergic drugs

Recently, a life-threatening iatrogenic variety of obstetric cardiomyopathy with pulmonary oedema has emerged as a result of the treatment of threatened premature labour by a beta-adrenergic drug, such as salbutamol or ritodrine, to inhibit uterine activity, sometimes together with a glucocorticoid, such as betamethasone, given in the hope of accelerating fetal lung maturation. Particularly in some European countries and in North America, where such combined pharmacological therapy seems to have been used widely and often continued over long periods, examples of sudden congestive cardiac failure in this circumstance have been reported (Eskes 1978, Kubli 1977, Rogge *et al.* 1979, Jacobs *et al.* 1980); there have been several fatalities, although in some at least of these postmortem examination has revealed a previously unsuspected but pre-existent cardiac lesion. Striking features in some cases have included the following: considerable overloading with intravenous fluids, massive and rapidly accumulating generalized and pulmonary oedema, prolonged membrane rupture sometimes with probable intrauterine and/or systemic infection, exacerbation or precipitation of the condition during labour or immediately following Caesarean section. The occurrence of this complication in several twin pregnancies (Elliott *et al.* 1978, Rogge *et al.* 1979, Davies & Robertson 1980) provides further suggestive evidence that maternal hypervolaemia may be an important contributory factor. In one case at least (Davies & Robertson 1980) it seems possible, indeed probable, that intravenous ergometrine given after delivery may have been the final precipitating trigger.

Further information may shed more light on the underlying aetiological process. In the meantime, it would seem prudent to avoid, or to proceed very cautiously with, this form of combined treatment over a period of more than a few days when there has been prolonged membrane rupture, when amniotic fluid from the vagina (or perhaps obtained by amniocentesis) already shows adequate or nearly adequate amounts of fetal pulmonary surfactant, when there is any suspicion of existing organic heart disease, when antihypertensive agents are being used, or in multiple pregnancies.

REFERENCES

ABBOTT A., SIBERT J.R. & WEAVER J.B. (1977) *Brit. med. J.*, **1**, 1639.

BARNES C.G. (1974) *Medical Disorders in Obstetric Practice*, 4th ed., p. 32. Blackwell Scientific Publications, Oxford.

BROWN A.K., DOUKAS N., RIDING W.D. & WYNE JONES E. (1967) *Brit. Heart J.*, **29**, 387.

CHESLEY L.C. (1980) *Amer. J. Obstet. Gynec.*, **136**,.

CHEW P.C.T. & RATNAM S.S. (1975) *Aust. N.Z.J. Obstet. Gynaec.*, **15**, 150.

DAVIES A.E. & ROBERTSON M.J.S. (1980) *Brit. J. Obstet. Gynaec.*, **87**, 539.

DE SWIET M. (1984) In *Progress in Obstetrics and Gynaecology* (Studd J. ed.), vol. 4, p. 166. Churchill Livingstone, Edinburgh.

DE SWIET M. & FIDLER J. (1981) *J. roy. Coll. Phycns.*, **15**, 183.

ELLIOTT H.R., ABDULLA U. & HAYES P.J. (1978) *Brit. med. J.*, **2**, 799.

ESKES T.K.A.B. (1978) In *Proceedings of the Study Group on Pre-Term Labour*, p. 217. Royal College of Obstetricians & Gynaecologists, London (1977).

GINZ B. (1970) *J. Obstet. Gynaec. Brit. Cwlth.*, **77**, 610.

HASCHE E. & DIPPMANN G. (1973) *Dtsch. Gesundh-wes.*, **28**, 2130.

HOLZGREVE W., CAREY J.C. & HALL B.D. (1976) *Lancet*, **ii**, 914.

JACOBS M.M., KNIGHT A.B. & ARIAS F. (1980) *Obstet. Gynec.*, **56**, 56.

KUBLI F. (1978) In *Proceedings of the Study Group on Pre-Term Labour*, p. 218. Royal College of Obstetricians and Gynaecologists, London (1977).

LANGE R.D. & DYNESIUS R. (1973) *Clinics in Haematology*, **2**, 433.

LEES M.M., TAYLOR S.H., SCOTT D.B. & KERR M.G. (1967) *J. Obstet. Gynaec. Brit. Cwlth.*, **74**, 319.

LEES M.M., SCOTT D.B., SLAWSON K.B. & KERR M.G. (1968) *J. Obstet. Gynaec. Brit. Cwlth.*, **75**, 546.

LEES M.M., SCOTT D.B. & KERR M.G. (1970) *J. Obstet. Gynaec. Brit. Cwlth.*, **77**, 29.

LIM M.A. & KHAIRUDDIN YUSOF (1973) *Med. J. Malaysia*, **28**, 129.

MARQUIS R.M. (1969) *J. roy. Coll. Phycns. London*, **3**, 121.

MEFFERT W.G. & STANSEL H.C. (1968) *Amer. J. Obstet. Gynec.*, **102**, 1116.

METCALF J., PETERSON E.N. & NOVY M.J. (1971) In *Cardiac and Vascular Disease* (Conn H.L. & Horwitz O. eds.). Lea & Febiger, Philadelphia.

MOODIE J.E. & MOIR D.D. (1976) *Brit. J. Anaes.*, **48**, 571.

New York Heart Association Inc. (1965) *Diseases of the Heart and Blood Vessels*, 6th edn., New York.

OAKLEY C. & DOHERTY P. (1976) *Brit. Heart J.*, **38**, 876.

OAKLEY G.D.G., McGARRY K., LIMB D.G. & OAKLEY C.M. (1979) *Brit. med. J.*, **1**, 1749.

PRITCHARD J.A. (1965) *Anesthesiology*, **26**, 393.

RAND R.J., JENKINS D.M. & SCOTT D.G. (1975) *Brit. J. Obstet. Gynaec.*, **82**, 172.

REPORTS ON CONFIDENTIAL ENQUIRIES INTO MATERNAL DEATHS IN ENGLAND AND WALES, 1967–69 (1972), 1970–72 (1975), 1963–75 (1979), 1976–78 (1982). HMSO, London

ROGGE P., YOUNG S. & GOODLIN R. (1979) *Lancet*, **i**, 1026.

SCOTT D.B. & KERR M.G. (1963) *J. Obstet Gynaec. Brit. Cwlth.*, **70**, 1044.

SUGRUÉ D., BLAKE S. & MacDONALD D. (1981) *Amer. J. Obstet. Gynec.*, **139**, 1.

SZEKELY P. & SNAITH L. (1974) *Heart Disease and Pregnancy*, p. 123. Churchill Livingstone, Edinburgh & London.

SZEKELY P. & SNAITH L. (1977) *Clinics in Obstet. Gynaec.*, **4**, 276.

TEJANI N. (1973) *Obstet. Gynec. N.Y.*, **42**, 785.

TURNER R.W.D. (1968) *Brit. med. J.*, **ii**, 383.

TURNER R.W.D. & MARQUIS R.M. (1965) *Scot. med. J.*, **10**, 47.

UELAND K. & HANSEN J. (1969) *Amer. J. Obstet. Gynec.*, **103**, 1.

UELAND K. & PARER J.T. (1966) *Amer. J. Obstet. Gynec.*, **96**, 400.

UELAND K., HANSEN J., ENG M., KALAPPA R. & PARER J.T. (1970) *Amer. J. Obstet. Gynec.*, **108**, 615.

UELAND K., NOVY M.J. & METCALF J. (1972) *Amer. J. Obstet Gynec.*, **113**, 47.

UELAND K., NOVY M.J. & METCALFE J. (1973) *Amer. J. Obstet. Gynec.*, **115**, 4.

VAUGHAN WILLIAMS C., JOHNSON A. & LEDWARD R. (1974) *J. Obstet. Gynaec. Brit. Cwlth.*, **81**, 596.

WALTERS W.A.W., MacGREGOR W.G. & HILLS M. (1966) *Clin. Sci.*, **30**, 1.

CHAPTER 18
BLOOD DISORDERS IN PREGNANCY

C. R. WHITFIELD

Together with disorders of the coagulation and fibrinolytic systems which are described in Chapter 36 (p. 539), anaemia and the haemoglobinopathies and rhesus isoimmunization are the most important haematological problems to complicate pregnancy and are the main topics of this chapter; leukaemia and Hodgkin's disease are also included, and thrombocytopenic purpura is dealt with in Chapter 21 (p. 301).

Blood disorders cause considerable morbidity during and after pregnancy, and they were responsible for one in every 16 of more than 1400 maternal deaths reviewed in the last three Reports on Confidential Enquiries into Maternal Deaths in England and Wales, relating to the years 1970–78. Twenty-five of these deaths were attributed to anaemia including sickle-cell disease or its complications, coagulation disorders complicated 48 cases of fatal placental abruption or a postpartum haemorrhage, and there were also 15 deaths from leukaemia and five from thrombocytopenic purpura.

ANAEMIA IN PREGNANCY

Anaemia is the commonest medical disorder to occur in pregnant women, its incidence being particularly high in many underdeveloped tropical countries where it remains a major contributing factor to maternal morbidity and mortality and it is also associated with high perinatal mortality rates. A generation ago, an incidence of 20% was usual in most of the northern industrial towns of Britain, but even in these communities there has been such a marked improvement that rates of less than 5% are now common. The three main reasons for this improvement are better living standards and nutrition, a trend to smaller and usually better spaced families with the virtual elimination of grand multiparity, and the widespread use of oral contraception which usually reduces menstrual loss.

Besides mortality, anaemia is associated with significant morbidity during and following pregnancy. It exacerbates the effects of infection and of haemorrhage, it has been thought to play a role in venous thrombosis and pulmonary embolism, it predisposes to decompensation in mothers with cardiac or respiratory disease, and it is an important factor in delayed general physical recovery postpartum especially after Caesarean section and in women of high parity and/or low socio-economic status.

Anaemia occurs when erythropoiesis is impaired, or when the marrow is unable to make up for an abnormal loss or destruction of red blood cells by haemorrhage or haemolysis. Anaemia in pregnancy is usually due to defective erythropoiesis, most often from iron or folate deficiency, or both together, although nutritional vitamin B_{12} deficiency may be important in some tropical countries. It is not intended to discuss anaemia resulting from acute obstetric haemorrhage, but attention will be drawn to the roles of chronic haemorrhage in iron deficiency and of chronic haemolysis in folate depletion.

PHYSIOLOGICAL CHANGES

An awareness of the physiological changes in the blood that occur during pregnancy, well reviewed by Lange and Dynesius (1973), and of increased requirements for iron and folic acid is essential.

Expansion of plasma volume begins in the first trimester, and it reaches a plateau between the 28th and 35th weeks of gestation when the increment is about 1500 ml in single pregnancies and about 2000 ml in twin pregnancies (Pritchard 1965), representing an increase from the non-pregnant state of about 40% in single pregnancies (Chesley 1972) and of more than 50% in multiple pregnancies. A small decline in plasma volume may occur towards term. There is considerable individual variation in these changes, with a tendency to larger increases in plasma volume in the older multiparous women, whereas unusually small increases may occur in association with placental insufficiency, fetal growth retardation, or possibly with folate deficiency.

After an initial reduction by about 100 ml before the end of the first trimester, throughout the remainder of pregnancy there is a gradual linear increase in the total red cell mass, due to increased erythrocyte production (Taylor & Lind 1979), resulting from increased secretion of erythropoietin (Mansac & Jepson 1969) possibly brought about mainly by placental lactogen. The increase in red cell volume is augmented if supplemental iron is taken, and Hytten and Leitch (1971) estimated that by term the increase was about 250 ml without supplemental iron and as much as 450 ml with it, representing increments of 18 and 32% respectively. Using the more accurate measurements made with the Coulter counter, Taylor and Lind (1979) found rather smaller normal increases of about 180 ml (14%) without supplementary iron and 350 ml (28%) when extra iron and folic acid are taken. The bone marrow becomes hyperplastic during pregnancy, but normally the red blood cells have the same haemoglobin concentration and the same survival time as in the non-pregnant state (Pritchard & Adams 1960).

The preferential expansion of plasma volume compared with red cell volume, probably resulting from increased aldosterone secretion, causes progressive haemodilution up to about the 30th to 35th week which, allowing for individual variation, may reduce the haemoglobin concentration to 11 g/dl and the haematocrit to 37%. Lower values than these cannot be accounted for by physiological changes alone, and in practice a haemoglobin concentration of 10 g/dl and a haematocrit of 35% are generally taken as the criteria for diagnosing pregnancy anaemia.

In the first 48 hours following delivery blood volume is increased by about 400 ml, with a simultaneous reduction in haematocrit, probably because of the return of interstitial tissue fluid to the circulation, but plasma volume soon falls and haemoconcentration is demonstrable from the fourth day postpartum (Pritchard 1965). The eventual return to normal non-pregnant values is a gradual process, and pregnancy induced haematological changes are still detectable six to eight weeks postpartum (Taylor & Lind 1979).

Iron deficiency

The average British diet contains 15 mg of elemental iron daily, but less is ingested by many women, especially those of poor socio-economic status and with large families to feed. Only about one-tenth of dietary iron is usually absorbed in the upper small intestine. This balances the normal daily loss of iron from the skin and the intestine, but it may barely compensate for even normal monthly menstrual loss. In some women, particularly those with menorrhagia, the iron stores of the liver, spleen and marrow may be drawn upon. Should such a negative iron balance persist, complete exhaustion of the iron stores will be followed by inadequate haemoglobin synthesis. In iron deficiency, serum iron is decreased and extra iron binding protein is free to augment the rate of absorption. In these circumstances, as much as 20% of ingested iron may be absorbed, up to a probable daily maximum of no more than 25 mg on iron medication under ideal conditions in the non-pregnant state. When iron deficiency is corrected, absorption is reduced and only very gradual replenishment of the iron stores follows restoration of the normal haemoglobin level.

The additional demands for iron during pregnancy were well summarized by Barnes (1976). The fetus and placenta (or each fetus and placenta in a multiple pregnancy) require about 500 mg of iron, and a similar amount is needed for the red cell increment. An average postpartum blood loss and lactation for six months each account for about 180 mg. From this total of 1360 mg may be substracted about 350 mg saved as a result of amenorrhoea to give an actual extra demand for about 1000 mg. This is unlikely to be provided entirely by absorption of dietary iron, but it can be mobilized from full iron stores (750–1000 mg). The requirements of a multiple pregnancy will outstrip the supply from even initially replete iron stores. Thus, it is the state of these stores that largely determines whether or not a pregnant woman becomes anaemic. The smaller her stores the earlier the anaemia occurs and, without treatment, the more severe it becomes by term. Iron deficiency anaemia at the start of pregnancy signifies already empty iron stores. Inadequate storage may reflect dietary lack, chronic menorrhagia or intestinal bleeding, haemorrhoids or hookworm infestation, or simply an insufficient interval for replenishment between pregnancies. During pregnancy, the situation may be exacerbated by poor utilization of iron by the marrow when there is a severe or chronic infection, usually of of the urinary tract, or possibly by impaired absorption.

There are no specific clinical features of anaemia due to iron deficiency. Indeed, patients usually deny even such symptoms as fatigue, giddiness and breathlessness unless the anaemia is severe.

Severity is assessed by estimation of haemoglobin concentration and haematocrit. Careful inspection of peripheral blood films is more useful than many of the electronically computed indices reported as a routine by most laboratories. Typically, there is a microcytosis and hypochromia, but, especially when iron is being given, an overactive marrow is often releasing many immature macrocytes. This results in a characteristic dimorphic appearance of the circulating red blood cell population that is easily recognized in a blood film, whereas the calculated indices are averages of the two red cell populations. Erythropoiesis remains normoblastic, and appropriate staining of the marrow smear will confirm the absence of iron. A serum iron value of $10.6 \, \mu mol/l$ or less confirms that there is an iron deficiency, but increased iron binding capacity ($> 80 \, \mu mol/l$, representing only 6.25% saturation of the binding protein) will partly reflect the normal general increase in binding proteins during pregnancy. Storage iron can be assessed by immuno-radiometric assay of serum ferritin (Jacobs et al. 1972). In iron deficiency anaemia serum iron and serum ferritin are both reduced, but the hypochromic anaemia that occurs when erythropoiesis is impaired due to infection is characterized by raised serum ferritin despite reduced serum iron.

Thalassaemia minor (see p. 263) may also present as a very mild microcytic hyperchromic anaemia in pregnancy, and this must be borne in mind in women whose ethnic origin is in the Eastern Mediterranean or Indian subcontinent (heterozygous beta-thalassaemia) or in South-East Asia or less commonly certain African countries (haemoglobin H disease). In these disorders a disproportionately low mean corpuscular volume for the haemoglobin and haematocrit values is a useful diagnostic pointer, if the haemoglobinopathy has not already been detected by routine antenatal screening. Willoughby (1977) recommended the Kleihauer staining technique, which should be in regular use in laboratories serving obstetric units, to detect the circulating red cells with fetal haemoglobin that are present in subjects with beta-thalassaemia.

MANAGEMENT AND TREATMENT

Many investigators, including Chanarin and Rothman (1971), Lund (1951) and Magee and Milligan (1951), have described convincing evidence that routine iron supplements reduce the incidence of pregnancy anaemia and also improve haemoglobin concentration, haematocrit and red cell count, even in women taking a good diet and who are not anaemic during early pregnancy. With iron supplementation the bone marrow of many women will show significant amounts of stainable iron at the end of pregnancy (de Leeuw et al. 1966).

In communities where iron deficiency is still common all pregnant women should take supplemental iron as soon as they are free from the nausea and vomiting of early pregnancy. Although this is still the policy in most antenatal clinics in Britain, the recently decreased incidence of pregnancy anaemia has tempted some to withhold supplementary iron as a routine. Abandonment of routine supplementation may seem acceptable where there are good nutritional standards, provided the blood is examined at intervals throughout pregnancy and selective prophylaxis with iron is prescribed for such groups as grand multiparas, women with multiple pregnancies, and those with a history of anaemia or menorrhagia. It is unwise in the poorer industrial areas. In Glasgow, where iron supplementation is the rule, the virtual elimination of serious iron deficiency anaemia in pregnancy, except in occasional late-booking patients, provides a good reason to persist with this cheap and effective form of prophylaxis. Even when overt anaemia does not occur, pregnancy inevitably reduces the iron stores unless supplemental iron is taken, and preservation of storage iron by supplementation during one pregnancy usually amounts to effective prevention of anaemia during the next one.

The therapeutic optimal daily intake of elemental iron is 100 mg and this is provided, together with the optimal daily requirement of $350 \, \mu g$ of folic acid, in a single tablet of several available preparations in which the iron is present as ferrous sulphate or fumarate. Intolerance is likely with larger doses which, by stimulating peristalsis, may also impede absorption. A proportion of women claim gastrointestinal intolerance to iron, but this can generally be overcome by changing to another appropriate tablet, or by reduced dosage (e.g. half a tablet per day) during the first fortnight. For the very few patients in whom gastrointestinal symptoms persist despite these simple measures, the combined chelated iron (ferrous glycine sulphate) and folic acid tablet, containing a smaller amount of elemental iron, is often tolerated.

Treatment of established iron deficiency anaemia in pregnancy is aimed at correcting the anaemia by the last month of pregnancy if possible, and then replenishing the iron stores. Specific replacement therapy with iron by mouth is preferable, but the choice of method depends on three main factors: the severity of the anaemia; the nearness to term; and the presence of additional complications. Sometimes one or more of these factors may justify parenteral rather than oral administration of iron, or occasionally blood transfusions. Because anaemia in early pregnancy is almost invariably due to iron deficiency, oral iron may be tried. If effective, this treatment may be continued for three to six months postpartum to renew the iron stores. An important proviso is that severe anaemia, even in early pregnancy, calls for full investigation to minimize the delay in starting effective therapy when the cause is not iron deficiency alone. For treatment of an existing anaemia with oral iron, it may be advisable to double the prophylactic dosage (above), but the parenteral route is indicated if supplemental iron has already proved ineffective or has not been tolerated. It is often stated that parenteral iron does not cause a significantly more rapid rise in haemoglobin concentration than does oral iron (Pritchard 1966), but this comparison refers to oral administration under ideal circumstances, i.e. in patients who remember to take, can tolerate and do absorb the therapeutic dosage of iron given by mouth. All too frequently in practice this is not the case, and the main advantage of parenteral iron therapy is the certainty of its administration and, when given by 'total dose' intravenously, the elimination of any delay in giving sufficient iron to correct the haemoglobin deficit and to fill the iron stores. Unless megaloblastic anaemia seems likely, mild or moderately severe anaemia in late pregnancy should also be treated initially with iron, but parenteral administration may again be indicated to provide quick and certain correction of the total iron deficit.

The total dosage of parenteral iron (mg) is calculated by the formula $1.4 \times W \times D$, where W is the patient's weight in kg, and D is the percentage haemoglobin deficit (below 14.8 g/dl); this allows replacement of iron stores as well as correction of the anaemia. Its administration by intravenous total dose infusion, using iron dextran in normal saline in a concentration not exceeding 5%, is particularly useful when moderate or severe anaemia is found after the 30th week and in patients unwilling or unable to complete a course of intramuscular injections. The incidence of unpleasant minor side effects (e.g. nausea, flushing, giddiness, headache and tachycardia) is minimized by resting the patient for an hour beforehand, by infusing no more than 10 drops per minute during the first 20 minutes and thereafter not exceeding 50 drops per minute, and by premedication with an anti-histamine if there is an allergic history. With these precautions, and with the patient lying on her side, hypotensive reactions are also very rare, but the pulse and blood pressure should be recorded frequently during the first hour. Should hypotension occur, despite these precautions, the infusion should be discontinued and a course of intramuscular iron given after a small test dose the following day. Iron dextran, in the same calculated total dosage, can be used for a course of intramuscular injections. Iron sorbitol is an alternative intramuscular preparation, but the urinary excretion of one-third of it must be compensated for by increased dosage.

Following total dose iron infusion or the commencement of intramuscular iron therapy, two or three weeks may pass before a significant rise in haemoglobin concentration can be demonstrated with certainty, and such delayed confirmation of a satisfactory response may be unacceptable when severe anaemia is being treated in advanced pregnancy. The reticulocytosis occurring in response to effective iron therapy is not as dramatic as that usual when the folate-deprived marrow responds to folic acid, but a moderate reticulocytosis within 7 to 10 days confirms that a satisfactory response can be awaited. However, an unsatisfactory reticulocyte response suggests that erythropoiesis may be impaired by folate depletion or chronic infection (Chan & Whitfield 1971).

Very rarely in Britain or other developed countries outside the tropics, blood transfusion may be required to treat pregnancy anaemia when the treatment determining factors are very unfavourable, e.g. when there is severe anaemia near term or when some other complication such as placenta praevia makes urgent correction of anaemia essential. In some tropical countries gross anaemia is a common complication of pregnancy, usually resulting from a combination of adverse factors such as malnutrition, too frequent pregnancies, prolonged lactation, malaria and hookworm infestation; the haemoglobin concentration may be no more than 3 g/dl, in which case to minimize the risk of cardiac failure exchange transfusion is advisable (e.g. 1300 ml of packed cells transfused simultaneously with the withdrawal of 1500 ml by venesection, an intravenous diuretic such as frusemide being given as an additional precaution).

FOLLOW-UP

Although supplementation with iron and repeated haemoglobinometry are routine practices at most clinics, follow-up management after pregnancy is usually neglected. There is insufficient realization that the occurrence of iron deficiency anaemia in pregnancy, in the absence of obstetric haemorrhage or chronic infection, means that the iron stores are completely exhausted, that they were already depleted before the pregnancy, and that they will not be replenished until after the haemoglobin deficit is fully corrected. Since the body's iron storage capacity and the extra iron demands of a single pregnancy are about equal (1000 mg of elemental iron) it follows that complete correction of iron deficiency, including the full replenishment of stores, will provide effective prophylaxis against the recurrence of this kind of anaemia in the next pregnancy. Following pregnancy and correction of the haemoglobin deficit, serum iron and iron binding values return to normal, and the small intestine's capacity for iron absorption is again reduced to about 10% of the dietary intake. It may therefore take several years to fill up the iron stores from a good diet with oral iron supplements. The great advantage of parenteral iron therapy is that replenishment of iron stores can be assured. It is also important to control menorrhagia, and to treat chronic intestinal blood loss, haemorrhoids or hookworm infestation.

EFFECTS OF IRON DEFICIENCY IN PREGNANCY

When there is anemia compensatory changes occur in the circulation in an attempt to maintain adequate tissue oxygenation. Thus, plasma volume and cardiac output rise, peripheral resistance falls, and the velocity of blood flow increases. In severe anaemia, compensation by these means cannot be adequate and high output cardiac failure is likely when haemoglobin concentration falls to less than 5 g/100 ml. This is more likely if pre-eclampsia or hypertension is present, and the anaemic patient's ability to withstand the effects of obstetric haemorrhage is of course also reduced. Severe anaemia predisposes to infection, particularly during the puerperium, and has been thought to increase the risk of thrombo-embolism. In many Third World countries it is for these reasons that anaemia, most often due to severe iron deficiency, is responsible for perhaps one-fifth of the relatively high maternal death rate. On the other hand, the effects of maternal iron deficiency on the fetus are generally negligible, cord blood serum iron being higher and iron binding capacity lower than the corresponding maternal values (Oski & Naiman 1972) and babies and mothers with iron deficiency

anaemia have normal cord blood haemoglobin levels (Pritchard et al. 1969).

Folate deficiency and megaloblastic anaemia

In non-pregnant subjects the minimum daily requirement for folate is about 50 µg (Herbert 1962), and a dietary intake insufficient to meet this is uncommon in Britain. An average daily intake of between 53 and 296 µg was found in pregnant women in London (Chanarin et al. 1968), but only 20 years ago Willoughby and Jewell (1966) found that more than half of the antenatal patients they investigated in Glasgow had an intake of less than the critical 50 µg per day, and this probably still applies in some economically disadvantaged communities. The progressively increasing needs of pregnancy, rising to 350 to 400 µg per day (Willoughby & Jewell 1966, Cooper et al. 1970), are associated with falling blood folate levels and often also with morphological changes in the circulating red and white blood cells by the end of pregnancy or postpartum. Before the introduction of folic acid supplementation in Britain incidences of megaloblastic anaemia in pregnancy varied between 0.5 and 3.0%. These changes are accentuated in multiple pregnancy, in which incidences of megaloblastic anaemia as high as 50% have been reported (Giles 1966, Whitfield 1966). The spontaneous postpartum correction of these haematological changes provides further confirmation of the role of fetal demand.

Evidence of intestinal malabsorption, including impaired folate absorption, has been found in 58% of women in whom megaloblastic pregnancy anaemia was diagnosed for the first time, and in 77% when megaloblastic anaemia recurred in a subsequent pregnancy (Whitfield 1970a), suggesting that malabsorption may largely explain the typical recurrence of megaloblastic anaemia in successive pregnancies. Gluten sensitivity is the usual cause in non-tropical countries. In epileptics the utilization of folic acid in the marrow may be inhibited by anticonvulsant drugs, and impaired utilization in the presence of infection can cause acute folate depletion and megaloblastic arrest of erythropoiesis (Chanarin & Davey 1964). Chronic haemolysis from any cause, including sickle-cell disease or beta-thalassaemia, is also likely to lead to severe folate depletion.

CLINICAL FEATURES

Although symptoms referable to the anaemia are often denied, megaloblastic anaemia in pregnancy runs a more acute, sometimes fulminant, course than does iron deficiency anaemia. Some patients are very ill with obvious anaemia and dyspnoea. The tongue is usually sore or acutely painful, it usually shows some papillary flattening, or it may be smooth and perhaps 'mapped' with dark red patches. Aphthous ulceration of the tongue and mouth is common. The liver and spleen may be enlarged, although this may not be easy to detect in late pregnancy. Retinal and subcutaneous petechial haemorrhages may be present, indicating that platelet production is also affected. There may be protracted vomiting, and anorexia is prominent in most patients. There is usually little or no weight gain, or an actual weight loss, and perhaps a history of intermittent and persistent diarrhoea, suggesting the probability that intestinal malabsorption is present. Such symptoms may have preceded the pregnancy, and a past history of proven or suspected coeliac disease is occasionally obtained.

Other obstetric complications, including antepartum haemorrhage from placental abruption, prematurity, abortion and fetal malformation, have been attributed to folic acid depletion, but most of these associations have not been found in many large reported series. The higher than average incidence of low birthweight may simply reflect the high incidence of multiple pregnancy among these patients. Regardless of the severity of maternal folate depletion, the fetus obtains enough folic acid for its own requirements, cord blood folate levels being higher than the maternal values at the time of delivery (Pritchard *et al.* 1969).

HAEMATOLOGICAL FEATURES

In his classic experiment, Herbert (1962) showed that folic acid deprivation led after several weeks to reduced serum folate, soon followed by the first recognizable morphological change in the peripheral blood, namely hypersegmentation of the neutrophils; after 19 weeks megaloblastic anaemia appeared. This experimental information may be applied to the detection of folate depletion and megaloblastic anaemia in pregnancy. Soon after neutrophil hypersegmentation appears, the blood film usually shows anisocytosis and macrocytosis, although frequently it is dimorphic due to coexistent iron deficiency; eventually occasional megaloblasts may be recognized in the peripheral film, or more often in a Buffy coat preparation which will reveal the macrocytosis and neutrophil hypersegmentation very clearly and will often show other features of folate depletion such as giant

polymorphs and erythrocytes containing Howell–Jolly bodies. The effects of folate deficiency on granulopoiesis lead to neutropenia, and in some of the more severe cases of megaloblastic anaemia, including those with haemorrhagic manifestations, there may be thrombocytopenia.

The fall in red cell (or whole blood) folate lags behind the reduction in serum folate activity. It provides useful retrospective information about the duration of the folic acid deficiency, the folate content of a red cell reflecting the availability of folate in the marrow when it was formed.

Unless there is positive evidence in the Buffy coat, megaloblastic erythropoiesis must be diagnosed by examining bone marrow, readily and preferably obtained from the iliac crest. Disordered granulopoiesis, indicated by the presence of giant metamyelocytes, is usually also present, and there is often evidence of impaired thrombopoiesis as well. Suitable staining enables the available iron stores to be assessed.

Serum vitamin B_{12} assays are also usually carried out, presumably to exclude the most unlikely possibility that the anaemia is due to a deficiency of vitamin B_{12} rather than of folic acid. However, the reduced serum vitamin B_{12} concentrations frequently seen in megaloblastic anaemia in pregnancy are restored to normal levels on treatment with small 'therapeutic' doses of folic acid alone (Whitfield 1970a). Untreated Addisonian anaemia causes infertility, and in British patients the chance that megaloblastic anaemia in pregnancy is due to vitamin B_{12} deficiency is negligible. Therefore, the risk of adverse neurological effects from treatment with folic acid in a pregnant woman suffering from combined vitamin B_{12} and folate depletion is very small indeed (Letsky 1977a).

MANAGEMENT

In communities with good nutritional standards, and provided regular antenatal haemoglobin checks are made, a case can be made for selective rather than routine prophylaxis, folic acid supplements being prescribed when there is a particular risk that folic acid deficiency may develop, e.g. because of multiple pregnancy, haemoglobinopathy, anticonvulsant therapy, or a previous history of megaloblastic anaemia. Elsewhere, routine supplementation is advisable, and the required effective dosage of 350 μg daily may be combined with the necessary iron supplement in a single tablet taken once daily.

When megaloblastosis is diagnosed, oral folic acid should be started with 2.5 mg daily, the larger doses so often recommended being almost always unnecessary. The haematological response is confirmed by reticulocyte counting on the fifth and seventh days, although improvement in the tongue, appetite and mental attitude will usually already have indicated that treatment is proving effective. A therapeutic trial with this small dosage of folic acid usually prompts an optimal response. It is also a simple method to exclude the very remote chance that the underlying deficiency is one of vitamin B_{12} since, as pointed out by Willoughby (1977), only 'pharmacological' doses of at least 5 mg of folic acid daily will induce haematological responses in true vitamin B_{12} deficiency.

Malabsorption should be tested for, but folic acid need not be withheld until this has been done. Indeed, unsuspected steatorrhoea may be revealed only when appetite and intake improve on folic acid. Other non-radioactive tests of intestinal absorption, including a D-xylose absorption and excretion test, should be carried out.

Increased doses of folic acid may be needed for an optimal response when there is impaired absorption or utilization, and the former may necessitate intramuscular administration which should also be used to start treatment when there is vomiting. Utilization of folate is often improved by elimination of infection in the urinary tract or elsewhere. In addition to starting treatment with folic acid, a packed cell blood transfusion may be required if the haemoglobin concentration is less than 6 g/dl, or less than 8 g/dl when labour occurs. With rather higher haemoglobin values, and if delivery is not imminent, cross-matched blood should be kept readily available, but a rapid haematological response may make transfusion unnecessary. Slow transfusion and an intravenous diuretic such as frusemide are obvious precautions to avoid cardiac failure if blood is required, and in the most severe cases (haemoglobin concentration < 4 g/dl) an exchange blood transfusion (Fullerton & Turner 1962) is preferable.

Even if iron deficiency is not apparent in the peripheral blood when megaloblastosis is diagnosed, it is often revealed by the absence of stainable iron in the bone marrow, or is likely to be unmasked by the demands of the very active erythropoiesis induced by folic acid. Therefore, parenteral iron is often needed if complete haematological responses are to be achieved as quickly as posssible.

Effective folic acid therapy should be continued until a full haematological response has been obtained and delivery has occurred. When absorption is unimpaired spontaneous remission will follow delivery, but it will be accelerated by giving folic acid in the standard daily supplemental dosage of 350 μg. If clinical features and biochemical tests suggest malabsorption, radioactive folic acid and vitamin B_{12} absorption tests should be performed postpartum. In the interests of future health, it may also be wise to seek direct evidence of underlying jejunal pathology radiologically and by peroral mucosal biopsy (Whitfield 1970a). If such a lesion is found, long-term gastroenterological supervision, perhaps with the exclusion of dietary gluten, is called for.

Occasionally in strict vegetarians (in Britain these are most likely to be Indian immigrants), or just as rarely in women with severe gluten enteropathy involving the ileum (where vitamin B_{12} is absorbed), megaloblastic anaemia in pregnancy may be due to true vitamin B_{12} deficiency. This is more common in certain Third World countries, as a result of tropical sprue or a severe dietary deficiency of vitamin B_{12}. If any of these possibilities is suspected, weekly injections of vitamin B_{12} 1000 μg should be given as well as folic acid until after delivery, when detailed investigation, including radioactive absorption tests, intestinal radiography, and perhaps mucosal biopsy, can be carried out to confirm or exclude either a malabsorption syndrome involving the ileum or Addisonian anaemia.

Haemolytic anaemia due to hereditary red cell disorders

Acquired haemolytic anaemia, caused by infection or a toxic chemical, is a rare complication in pregnancy. On the other hand, congenital haemolytic anaemia due to an intrinsic abnormality of the erythrocyte is a problem of increasing incidence and importance in British obstetrics as a result of large scale immigration.

CONGENITAL SPHEROCYTOSIS

In obstetrics the main importance of congenital spherocytosis lies in its dominant inheritance, there being a half chance that the baby will be affected and may develop neonatal jaundice severe enough to require exchange transfusion. Since most patients have splenectomy in childhood, with good effect, there are usually no significant maternal effects during pregnancy, but without splenectomy the accelerated red cell turnover augments folic acid requirements and predisposes to megaloblastic anaemia. Folate supplementation is therefore required, perhaps in double the normal dosage.

ENZYME DEFECTS

The most important hereditary red cell enzyme deficiency is that of glucose-6-phosphate dehydrogenase (G-6-PD), a sex-linked recessive disorder occurring quite commonly among persons of Eastern, African or Mediterranean origin. The main obstetric problem is neonatal jaundice which may require exchange transfusion. Acute haemolytic crises may be precipitated in affected male infants by certain drugs including sulphonamides and synthetic analogues of vitamin K, given directly to the infant or reaching it in the mother's milk.

HAEMOGLOBINOPATHIES

The four polypeptide globin chains of adult haemoglobin (HbA) which provides at least 95% of haemoglobin in the normal adult, are a pair of alpha-chains and a pair of beta-chains, distinguished by different amino acid configurations. In normal fetal haemoglobin (HbF), which accounts for less than 1% of haemoglobin in the normal adult, the beta-chains are replaced by two gamma-chains. There is a normal variant of adult haemoglobin (HbA$_2$) in which delta-chains replace the beta-chains. In each haemoglobinopathy, there is an inherited specific defect in globin synthesis or structure, and both homozygous and heterozygous forms occur. In homozygotes, who inherit the same abnormal globin chain from each parent, the fragility of the red cell is increased and its life span reduced so that haemolytic anaemia occurs. Heterozygotes, who inherit the abnormal globin chain from only one parent, are not overtly anaemic but are carriers of the defect. Doubly heterozygous combinations of haemoglobinopathies occur, in which the subject has inherited one haemoglobin defect from one parent and another from the second parent.

SICKLE-CELL SYNDROMES

In these autosomally inherited disorders, affecting blacks, the abnormal haemoglobin (HbS) has an amino acid substitution in the beta-globin chain that causes it to precipitate when it is in its reduced state (although not in its oxygenated form). When this occurs the erythrocytes become rigid and distorted into a characteristic sickle shape, in which form they occlude small blood vessels. The 'sickling out' phenomenon occurs typically when oxygen tension is lowered and a vicious circle, in which hypoxia and stasis reinforce one another, is readily established. The process is augmented by thrombosis at the sites of the vascular occlusions, and other exacerbating factors are acidosis and dehydration.

Sickle-cell disease (HbSS)

The features of homozygous sickle-cell disease are a severe chronic anaemia from early infancy with less pronounced symptoms than might be expected from the very low haemoglobin concentration (usually 5–9 g/dl), and acute haemolytic crises due to intravascular sickling.

There is an increased incidence of crises during pregnancy and the puerperium. They may be precipitated by hypoxia during general anaesthesia or resulting from major haemorrhage, or during severe infections, and they may be augmented by acidosis and dehydration. As well as a dramatic fall in haemoglobin and haematocrit, the occlusion of small blood vessels by sickled erythrocytes with superimposed thrombosis causes painful infarction. This is particularly likely in the kidneys, and most patients have renal complications including haematuria and progressive renal insufficiency. There is an inability to concentrate urine which augments any dehydration, and there is an increased incidence of pyelonephritis. Infarction of any abdominal organ may suggest a surgical emergency, thrombotic bone pains are common, and pulmonary embolism may occur. The maternal mortality rate in women with this disease in England and Wales has been estimated to be about 6% (Tuck 1982). A massive sickling crisis in association with acute infection is the most frequent cause of death. Abortion and stillbirth, prematurity and intrauterine growth retardation, and intrapartum fetal distress are likely complications, and pregnancies complicated by sickle-cell disease carry a fourfold increase in perinatal mortality (Tuck & White 1981).

Sickle-cell trait (HbAS)

Heterozygous HbS carriers may pass on the carrier state to their offspring, and if married to another carrier there will be a one-in-four risk that any child will have sickle-cell disease. Carriers of the trait are not anaemic, and sickling occurs only exceptionally when, during a surgical or anaesthetic accident for example, there is very severe anoxia.

Sickle-cell haemoglobin C disease (HbSC)
This sickling disorder is doubly heterozygous, for HbS and for HbC, and it may go undiagnosed because between crises there is at most only mild anaemia. However, crises may be very severe and they become more likely during pregnancy, labour and the puerperium. Especially during general anaesthesia, an unexpected life-threatening crisis may occur before the obstetrician or the patient herself is aware that she has the disorder.

Sickle-cell beta-thalassaemia disease
This disorder is also doubly heterozygous for HbS and beta-thalassaemia. Its variable severity depends on the degree of beta-chain suppression. With complete suppression, no HbA is formed and the clinical features are those of sickle-cell disease. If suppression is incomplete, the clinical course is milder, but dangerous crises may occur during pregnancy.

Screening and diagnosis
About 10% of blacks living in the United Kingdom are carriers of HbS, and the blood of all black women attending antenatal clinics should be screened for its presence. The 'Sickledex' test is a quick and reliable method for doing so. It does not distinguish between any of the different sickling disorders, so Sickledex-positive patients and their partners should have the specific diagnosis made by haemoglobin electrophoresis. In the newborn, HbS can be demonstrated in cord blood and sickle-cell disease can be distinguished from the trait (Huntsman *et al.* 1972). The newborn inheriting a sickling disorder has no clinical manifestations, and is not anaemic because most of its haemoglobin is in the form of fetal haemoglobin which lacks the beta-chains in which the sickling defect occurs.

Management
There is no specific treatment to correct the abnormal haemoglobin or its intrinsic liability to cause sickling. By maintaining a high proportion of the circulating haemoglobin as stable HbA and also by reducing the stimulus to erythropoiesis so that production of further sickle cells is diminished, repeated blood transfusions throughout pregnancy reduce the likelihood of crises in women with sickle-cell disease. A haemoglobin concentration of 10.5–12.5 g/dl with 60% as normal HbA is an acceptable target, and an aggressive approach to achieve this from early pregnancy has been suggested in the interests of fetal well-being (Tuck 1982). Weekly small transfusions of fresh packed red cells may be required, and the exchange technique is of particular value during a crisis or if the patient presents with severe anaemia near term (Buckle *et al.* 1969).

In any of the sickling disorders, the avoidance of hypoxia, acidosis and dehydration, and also the effective antibiotic treatment of urinary, pulmonary and other infections, are important measures to reduce the risk of crises. Increased red cell turnover may lead to folate deficiency which, in turn, would augment any anaemia, so that therapeutic doses of folic acid should be prescribed. However, because of the risk of haemosiderosis, iron should be given parenterally only when a coexistent iron depletion has been demonstrated with certainty. Should general anaesthesia be needed, preoperative blood transfusion, the services of an expert anaesthetist, and postoperative vigilance to avoid anoxia, are all essential. If appropriate epidural analgesia should be used instead.

During crises alkalis, anticoagulants, plasma expanders, vasodilators, and hyperbaric oxygen have all been tried without proven advantage, and the most effective measure is the maintenance of fluid balance (Letsky 1977b). Electrolyte balance, particularly the prevention of acidosis, is also important. Blood transfusion is required (above). Pain from vascular occlusions calls for effective analgesia without respiratory depression. Heparin is indicated for bone pain or if there is evidence of pulmonary embolism (Hendrickse *et al.* 1972). In sickle-cell trait no special antenatal management is needed except that an increased incidence of pyelonephritis calls for regular examination and culture of the urine, and prompt treatment if infection does occur. If general anaesthesia is required, it must be remembered that a dangerous crisis can occur in these patients if there is very severe anoxia, so that skilled anaesthesia and close postoperative supervision are essential.

THALASSAEMIA

In the thalassaemias there is partial or complete suppression of the synthesis of either the alpha- or the beta-globin chains, resulting in reduced haemoglobin content in the red cells which have a shortened life span.

Beta-thalassaemia
In Britain this is the commonest variety, affecting mainly immigrants of Mediterranean origin, particularly Greeks and Greek-Cypriots and to a lesser extent Italians and Sicilians, and its occurrence in a

doubly heterozygous combination with HbS as sickle-cell beta-thalassaemia has been noted (above).

Most affected subjects have 'thalassaemia minor', the heterozygous form of beta-thalassaemia, in which, although the degree of suppression of beta-chain synthesis varies very considerably, the haemoglobin concentration is usually 10 g/dl or more. The red cells show hypochromia, anisocytosis and poikylocytosis. As a compensatory process, there is continued production into adult life of significant amounts of fetal haemoglobin and of a variant of adult haemoglobin (HbA_2), neither of which contains beta-chains. The disorder may not be diagnosed until the anaemia becomes overt as a result of some 'haematological stress' such as pregnancy. The increase in red cell mass that is usual during pregnancy does not occur so both haemoglobin concentration and haematocrit fall. These patients are of course genetic carriers of the defect.

Homozygous beta-thalassaemia is a crippling disorder with severe anaemia, leading to death during childhood unless regular blood transfusions are given, and these transfusions carry their own eventual lethal consequence of haemosiderosis.

Alpha-thalassaemia

In this defect, which occurs mainly among people of certain Oriental regions including South-East Asia, alpha-chain synthesis is suppressed. The homozygous form is incompatible with life because normal fetal (or adult) haemoglobin cannot be made and, although there is a small amount of HbH having only beta-chains, an invariably lethal fetal hydrops occurs. In heterozygous alpha-thalassaemia, the degree of suppression of alpha-chain synthesis is usually insufficient to cause symptoms or anaemia. However, there is an overt variant, HbH disease, in which the clinical problem is like that of the more severe examples of beta-thalassaemia minor and in which there is persistent synthesis of unstable HbH.

Detection and diagnosis

Occasionally when a hyperchromic anaemia proves refractory to iron during pregnancy, especially in a woman of Mediterranean or Oriental stock, a very low mean corpuscular volume, and perhaps the presence of erythrocytes containing fetal haemoglobin (revealed by Kleihauer staining), may suggest the likelihood of thalassaemia minor. Demonstration of the characteristic microcytosis, using an automated cell counter, is a simple screening procedure when these women first attend the antenatal clinic, or there may be a known family history of thalassaemia. When any of these circumstances suggest the possibility of thalassaemia trait, or of other or combined haemoglobinopathies, a definitive diagnosis should be made by haemoglobin electrophoresis, and the husband's blood should be tested in the same way.

Management of thalassaemia

Very occasionally there is an accompanying iron deficiency, as seen for example in South-East Asia when a woman has both alpha-thalassaemia minor and hookworm infestation. Iron therapy, particularly parenteral, should otherwise be avoided. If the serum iron concentration is not elevated, routine iron supplements should be prescribed. Treatment with folic acid is important, therapeutic doses (2.5 mg daily) rather than routine supplementation being required. Blood transfusion is sometimes necessary.

Diagnosis of haemoglobinopathy in the fetus

The specialized operative procedure and laboratory techniques, available at a limited number of centres, for the diagnosis of haemoglobinopathies in the fetus to permit selective termination of pregnancy, and prospects for their further development are outlined in Chapter 22 (p. 322).

Aplastic anaemia

Rarely, pregnancy may occur in a patient with chronic aplastic anaemia, or the disease may appear during pregnancy. Recurrences in subsequent pregnancies have been reported (Taylor et al. 1968) and there is generally pancytopenia with anaemia, agranulocytosis and thrombocytopenia. Anaemia, haemorrhage and infection are the main dangers. Only 12 mothers survived in forty cases reviewed by Fleming (1973), and five years previously Evans (1968) found that survival had been reported only after spontaneous or therapeutic abortion.

With improving methods of management, the prognosis for these patients has become rather less unfavourable, and when the diagnosis is made early during pregnancy therapeutic abortion need no longer be regarded as always necessary. Repeated transfusions of packed cells and sometimes platelet and granulocyte transfusions, strict asepsis at all times with antibiotic cover and perhaps laminar flow isolation at and after delivery, and an uncomplicated vaginal delivery if possible, are the main lines of treatment.

Leukaemia and Hodgkins' disease

Leukaemia

The leukaemias are seen infrequently in pregnancy. The review by Ask-Upmark (1961) of 57 reported cases of acute leukaemia and 61 of chronic leukaemia, confirmed that pregnancy has no effect upon the disease, but maternal death was common at or following delivery, and acute leukaemia was associated with a high fetal wastage. More recently, Willoughby (1977) has noted an improved prognosis due to newer methods of treatment such as platelet transfusions and laminar flow isolation.

The obstetrician must seek the help of a physician or haematologist with special expertise in these disorders. Antitumour drugs are teratogenic, and in chronic myeloid leukaemia (also malignant melanoma and chronic lymphocytic leukaemia) chemotherapy may be deferred until after delivery because, while eventual cure cannot be expected, some delay in starting treatment is not likely to have a serious effect on the clinical course. In acute leukaemia chemotherapy should be started at once since, without it, survival to term is most unlikely; abortion is likely to occur as a result of the chemotherapy. In acute lymphoblastic leukaemia, especially late in pregnancy, steroids may achieve a short remission, and antitumour drugs and/or radiotherapy are then given after delivery which can be effected early to minimize delay.

Hodgkins' disease

The course of Hodgkins' disease is not affected by pregnancy. When pregnancy occurs in a patient known to have the disease, radiotherapy will usually have been completed and, unless the disease is advanced, she is not usually still receiving chemotherapy. In such cases no additional complications need be anticipated, and the pregnancy and delivery are managed normally. Indeed, pregnancy need no longer be discouraged in women with local disease in remission. The treatment of advanced Hodgkins' disease in pregnancy is therapeutic abortion followed by chemotherapy.

FETO-MATERNAL BLOOD GROUP INCOMPATIBILITY

In response to the introduction of foreign protein, antibody to neutralize it is made in the immune system of the recipient, and immunization occurs in this way in pregnancy when fetal red cells bearing antigen foreign to the mother enter her circulation, or exceptionally nowadays such immunization may follow incompatible blood transfusion. The antibody will combine with any antigen-carrying red cells that are still present in, or which subsequently enter, the recipient's circulation, and will cause them to be sequestered in the reticulo-endothelial system. During pregnancy, including subsequent pregnancies, the IgG antibody fraction will cross the placenta. If the fetus is 'positive' for the antigen in question, the antibody will combine with antigens on the fetal erythrocytes which then undergo haemolysis. The results of this haemolytic reaction are erythroblastosis fetalis and haemolytic disease of the newborn.

ABO and other non-rhesus incompatibilities

In ABO incompatibility the maternal serum contains antibody to the A or B antigen present on the fetal erythrocyte. Ascari (1977) pointed out that two-thirds of all cases of erythroblastosis fetalis are due to incompatibility in this system. Anaemia in the newborn is generally very mild or absent, despite the usual early occurrence of jaundice, and in most cases this incompatibility goes unrecognized. Phototherapy is sometimes required to control hyperbilirubinaemia, especially if the baby is also premature. Only rarely does the baby require blood transfusion of any sort, but one reported intrauterine fetal death has been attributed to ABO incompatibility (Miller & Petria 1963).

The usual mildness of haemolysis due to ABO incompatibility is not simply because naturally occurring anti-A and anti-B isoagglutinins are mainly the larger IgM and thus do not cross the placenta. Immune antibodies are made in response to the entry of A or B antigen-bearing fetal red cells into the mother's circulation and, since these are mainly IgG, they cross the placenta freely. The explanation lies in other peculiarities of the ABO system that are not shared by most blood group antigens, and these were described by Ascari. One such difference from rhesus (Rh) incompatibility is that intrapartum 'boosting' of immune anti-A and anti-B antibodies does not occur. Therefore, the progression in severity of the disease in successive babies that is typical of Rh disease does not occur in ABO incompatibility. Indeed, an affected baby may be followed by an unaffected one of the same ABO blood group.

Very occasionally haemolytic disease of the newborn is the result of maternal immunization to a blood group antigen that is not part of either the ABO or Rh system. An example is the Kell antigen, immunization to which most often results from incompatible blood transfusion since Kell-typing is not usually undertaken prior to transfusion and since 10 per cent of the population, and therefore of blood donors, are Kell-positive. Haemolytic disease of the newborn due to Kell incompatibility is usually very mild and transfusion of the baby is needed only very occasionally. However, the recently reported death of the fetus rendered hydropic by anti-Kell antibodies (Whitfield 1983) and another baby dying from haemolytic disease caused by anti-Duffy (anti-Fy^a) antibodies (Hardy & Napier 1981) provide a warning that non-Rh antibodies can kill babies.

Rhesus immunization and incompatibility

In the Rh system the $Rh_o(D)$ antigen is by far the most important, and its presence or absence is used to categorize a patient as Rh-positive or Rh-negative respectively. Antibodies to other Rh antigens (rh'(C), rh''(E), hr'(c), and hr''(e)) may develop, but the most commonly formed Rh antibody is anti-Rh_o (anti-D), sometimes with one or more of the others. The ability of the other Rh antigens to produce significant immunization is said to be less than that of the D antigen, but the presence of maternal antibodies to them can cause severe erythroblastosis in the fetus and serious haemolytic disease in the newborn. As a result of anti-D immunoprophylaxis, an increasing proportion of Rh haemolytic disease is caused by antibodies other than anti-D (O'Sullivan 1982). Anti-c is the most likely to do so (Fraser & Tovey 1976, Hardy & Napier 1981) even though it is present in fewer mothers than is anti-E. With modern methods of blood matching it is rare for Rh(D)-positive blood to be given to an Rh(D)-negative female under the age of 50 years, but usually no attempt is made to match donor blood for the other Rh factors such as C or e, and immunization to these factors occasionally occurs when the recipient lacks them.

FETO-MATERNAL HAEMORRHAGE

The Kleihauer-Betke technique (Kleihauer et al. 1957), or a modification of it, can be used to demonstrate fetal erythrocytes in the mother's blood. In contrast to the 'ghosted' maternal cells from which adult haemoglobin has been eluted, the uneluted HbF maintains the colour of the fetal red cells.

While so-called 'silent' feto-maternal haemor-

rhages may occur during pregnancy in the absence of any clinically obvious complication, these transplacental bleeds are much more likely to occur in association with certain complications or procedures. Following spontaneous abortion there is a 3 or 4% risk of immunization in a Rh-negative woman unprotected by the administration of anti-D immunoglobulin (Freda et al. 1970, Queenan et al. 1971a). It is unlikely that spontaneous abortion in the early weeks of pregnancy leads to enough feto-maternal bleeding to sensitize the mother, but the risk increases through the second trimester. Significant transplacental bleeds are even more likely to occur during therapeutic termination of pregnancy which, without prophylactic anti-D immunoglobulin, has been shown to carry a 5.5% risk of immunization (Queenan et al. 1971b). Feto-maternal haemorrhage may also follow antepartum haemorrhage, particularly when due to a major placental abruption, or it may complicate pre-eclampsia, external version or amniocentesis. It is also much more likely to occur following Caesarean section or manual removal of the placenta than after normal delivery of the fetus and placenta. Knox et al. (1961) showed that many of these complications and procedures predisposed to Rh immunization, and subsequently this has been confirmed in many other reports. In fulminant pre-eclampsia, placental abruption, Caesarean section and manual removal of the placenta, and also in multiple births, not only is there a high incidence of feto-maternal bleeding, but the amount of blood transferred across the placenta is sometimes relatively very large. This may result in 'vicious sensitization' of the mother so that the next Rh-positive fetus (i.e. the first affected one) may be critically or fatally affected by haemolytic disease (Whitfield 1976). At Caesarean section not only is it common to carry out a hurried manual removal of the placenta but unless the uterus is 'packed off' carefully there may be considerable spilling of blood, including fetal blood, into the peritoneal cavity from which its absorption readily occurs.

DEVELOPMENT OF Rh ANTIBODIES

Whether or not an 'at risk' Rh-negative woman becomes Rh-immunized depends on a number of factors. Firstly, it depends on her inborn ability to respond to the Rh antigenic stimulus, about two-thirds of Rh-negative women being responsive (WHO Scientific Group Report 1971). Secondly, there is significant protection against immunization when there is also ABO incompatibility between the fetal red cells and the mother; this reduces the incidence of Rh immunization to about one-tenth of that when they are ABO-compatible. Thirdly, there is some variation in the strength of the Rh antigenic stimulus, depending on the Rh genotype of the fetal blood, e.g. R′r (CDe/cde) genotype is relatively 'strong' (Murray 1957). Fourthly, the volume of fetal blood entering the maternal circulation is very important, with 0.25 ml representing a critical sensitizing volume and with the likelihood and severity of sensitization increasing with greater volumes.

Levine (1943) first drew attention to the relative protection against immunization afforded by ABO incompatibility between mother and fetus, pointing out the ABO compatibility between the father and mother were associated with an increased risk of Rh haemolytic disease in their baby. Nevanlinna and Vainio (1962) noted that when mother and fetus have the same ABO group (or when the fetus is group O) Rh immunization is more likely to occur than when there is ABO incompatibility between them (e.g. a group A or B fetus, and a group O mother having naturally occurring anti-A and anti-B glutinins). When ABO-incompatible Rh-positive fetal red cells enter the mother's bloodstream they combine with her natural anti-A and/or anti-B antibodies, and are then soon sequestered in her liver; unless there has been a large transplacental haemorrhage, Rh antigen particles are unlikely to reach enough immunologically competent maternal cells to cause an antibody response. Occasionally there is sufficient contact between Rh antigen and immunologically reactive lymphocytes for immunization to occur despite ABO incompatibility.

However, if ABO-compatible Rh-positive fetal red cells enter the mother's blood, they persist there for their remaining normal circulating lifespan until they are removed by the mother's reticulo-endothelial tissues where they are broken up and Rh antigen is liberated. Depending on the responsiveness of the reticulo-endothelial system, the chance of immunization occurring is directly related to the number of Rh antigens liberated and therefore to the number of fetal red cells that have entered the mother's blood. Because of the time involved in this process, immunization before delivery in a first or sensitizing pregnancy is unlikely, unless feto-maternal bleeding is considerable. Thus, fewer than 1% of patients at risk develop detectable antibodies by the time of delivery of their first Rh-positive infants (see example a in Fig 18.1). Presumably the same percentage are primarily immunized during the course of any subsequent Rh-positive pregnancies. It is much more usual for fetal erythrocytes, or at least for the critical sensitizing volume, to reach the maternal circulation during labour, commonly after placental separation during the third stage. For this reason, immunization is much more likely to occur after delivery, and antibodies can be detected in up to 10% of at risk mothers six months after delivery (example b in Fig 18.1). Other patients are immunized but the amount of circulating antibody is too small for detection by the usual tests (example c in Fig 18.1). In such patients the antibody level may have been detectable at some time postpartum, but without a further antigenic

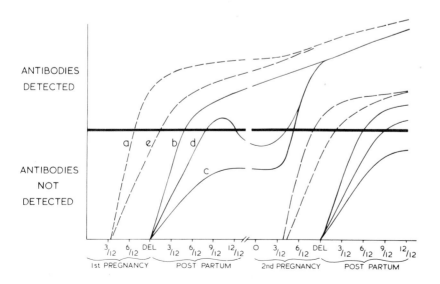

Fig. 18.1. Timing of development of Rh immunization (see text). a and e = immunization during pregnancy; b, c and d = immunization following delivery.

stimulus it then falls below the sensitivity of the laboratory tests (example d in Fig. 18.1); an important consequence is that a woman may become immunized during pregnancy, but the amount of antibody present at delivery is still too small for detection (example e in Fig. 18.1) so that prophylactic anti-D immunoglobulin is given, but will fail to protect the already immunized patient, and this is often wrongly regarded as a 'protection failure'.

If a patient has been immunized, detectably or undetectably, in one pregnancy, then antibodies are likely to be demonstrable from an early stage during the next pregnancy, especially if the fetus is Rh-positive, but even if it is Rh-negative (the so-called anamnestic response). By the end of the second pregnancy 17% of at risk mothers have detectable antibodies, mostly the result of immunization by the first pregnancy with a small proportion (perhaps 1%) becoming primarily immunized during the second one. The same possibilities arise after the delivery of any subsequent Rh-positive baby as arose after the first. Thus, some women will fail to respond to the antigenic stimulus for the same reasons as before, some will respond slowly so that immunization will not become apparent until yet another pregnancy, while yet others will be immunized strongly enough to show it if tested six months after delivery.

As with most immune responses, IgM anti-Rh antibodies develop first, but thereafter IgG antibodies are formed and will persist at a higher concentration in the mother's blood for a considerable time after the IgM can no longer be detected. A further Rh-positive pregnancy will stimulate a very rapid rise in IgM antibodies as well as the more sustained increase in IgG.

FETAL AND NEONATAL EFFECTS

Anti-Rh IgG crosses the placenta but will not affect a Rh-negative fetus. However, if the fetus is Rh-positive, the IgG molecules become attached to the antigen sites on the surfaces of its erythrocytes which will then give a positive direct antiglobulin or Coombs' reaction. Only a small proportion of these sites needs to be occupied in this way for the cell to be rapidly removed from circulation by the reticulo-endothelial system. The removal and destruction of fetal red cells, the number depending on the amount of IgG reaching the fetus and the ability of the fetal tissue to remove the 'coated' cells, results in anaemia with the release of increased amounts of unconjugated bilirubin. In response to this anaemia, a marked compensatory haemopoiesis occurs and immature erythroblasts enter the circulation.

In the very mildly affected fetus, increased haemopoiesis may maintain a satisfactory haemoglobin concentration, and the baby may be just slightly anaemic at birth or may develop anaemia during the first few weeks of life. In such cases the baby may not require blood transfusion of any sort, and hyperbilirubinaemia is usually controllable by phototherapy.

Excessive removal of circulating red cells leads to severe anaemia with hypoxia affecting all tissues. Placental hyperplasia occurs to increase the transfer of oxygen, but as the fetal anaemia tends to be progressive, the number of oxygen-carrying erythrocytes continues to be reduced. Cardiac and circulatory failure may occur, with generalized oedema, ascites and/or hydrothorax in addition to placental oedema, and in such cases there is metabolic failure with acidosis. The generalized oedema is termed hydrops fetalis, and although recovery has been reported as a result of energetic treatment when frank hydrops has been said to be present, death in utero or immediately after birth is the almost invariable result. Close scrutiny of the records of most 'hydropic survivors' shows that generalized hydropic change, including obvious scalp oedema, had not yet occurred.

Excessive red cell destruction results in the level of unconjugated bilirubin rising, but most of this can be passed into the maternal circulation by the placenta. Some of the bilirubin enters the amniotic fluid, perhaps from the fetal lung or though its skin, as well as across the surfaces of the placenta and umbilical cord. There is usually some elevation of unconjugated bilirubin in the cord blood at the time of birth in babies that are more than just mildly affected. After delivery and clamping of the umbilical cord, with continuing haemolysis, the bilirubin concentration rises and jaundice develops very rapidly in the most severely affected babies. This is due to inability of the liver, particularly that of a premature baby, to conjugate the excessive amount of bilirubin. If the level rises too high, bilirubin crosses the blood-brain barrier to stain and damage the basal nuclei of the brain, resulting in permanent neurological disorders and mental impairment which may be very severe. This is the condition of kernicterus, and it is prevented by maintaining a concentration of toxic unconjugated bilirubin below the danger level, usually taken as 310–345 μml/l, by exchange transfusion. This procedure may have to be repeated several times, especially when the baby is very premature and/or haemolysis is very severe. Once bilirubin is conjugated it is soluble and non-toxic, and the amount of bilirubin bound to protein is disregarded in deciding to carry out exchange transfusions.

PREVENTION OF Rh IMMUNIZATION

In 1960, having shown that feto-maternal ABO incompatibility brought about rapid removal of fetal erythrocytes from the maternal blood after delivery, Finn and his associates in Liverpool suggested that specific anti-Rh antibodies might be injected into the mother to neutralize Rh-positive fetal cells entering her circulation before they could induce immunization (Finn *et al.* 1961). Finn's reasoning was that the temporary passive immunity provided in this way would be more effective in preventing lasting active Rh immunization than would the natural protection afforded by ABO incompatibility. Successive experimental studies of Rh immunoprophylaxis in male volunteers soon followed in Liverpool and in New York. In both these cities during 1964 anti-D IgG was used to prevent immunization of Rh-negative women after delivery, and the efficacy of this prophylaxis was demonstrated by the first reported clinical trials (Freda *et al.* 1966, Combined Study from Centres in England and Baltimore 1966). Since then, a vast amount of reported and unreported experience confirmed that, when given intramuscularly within 72 hours of delivery, anti-D IgG will prevent development of antibodies if the patient has not already been immunized and if enough immunoglobin is given to neutralize the volume of fetal red cells reaching the mother's circulation. It is probable that, when given in this way, the anti-D binds onto antigen (D) sites on the cell membranes of the fetal erythrocytes, and that the occupation of even only 10% of these sites is sometimes sufficient to prevent active immunization (WHO Scientific Group 1971).

In the early 42-centre trial of prophylaxis in the United States, a dose of $300 \mu g$ of RhoGAM (Ortho Diagnostics) was used, and $200 \mu g$ was given in the early British prophylactic programmes (these doses being equivalent to 1500 and 1000 iu respectively). Following the reported findings of the Medical Research Council Working Party (1974) the standard British dose is 500 iu, and a smaller dose of 250 iu is used following abortion before 20 weeks gestational age. In the Medical Research Council trials the failure rate was similar in women receiving the equivalent of 1000, 500 and 250 iu doses, but higher when only 100 iu was injected.

An approximate estimate of the volume of fetal blood in the mother's circulation is provided by a Kleihauer test in which, for example, by counting the number of dark staining fetal red cells in 50 low power microscope fields, Woodrow and Finn (1966) found that five fetal cells in 50 low power fields represented a transplacental haemorrhage of 0.25 ml of fetal blood, and that following a feto-maternal haemorrhage of less than this volume it is exceptional for antibodies to be detectable six months after delivery. However, the real test of prophylaxis is the absence of Rh antibodies at the end of the next Rh-positive pregnancy, and when the sensitizing feto-maternal bleed is less than 0.25 ml a small but significant incidence of delayed immunization becomes detectable when boosted by this further Rh stimulus. Women immunized by larger volumes of fetal blood usually develop detectable antibodies by six months postpartum without further stimulus.

Since Pollack *et al.* (1971) showed that 1500 iu of RhoGAM can be relied upon to neutralize 15 ml of Rh-positive blood (corresponding to 100 iu for every 1 ml) the standard British dose of 500 iu for an estimated transplacental bleed of up to 4 ml leaves a safety margin to spare. It is injected when it becomes known that a baby of an as yet unimmunized Rh-negative women is Rh-positive; a Kleihauer count should be made, and if a large transplacental bleed is demonstrated 500 iu should be given for every calculated 4 ml, or fraction of 4 ml, of fetal blood in the mother, 4 ml being equivalent to 80 fetal red cells in 50 low power fields.

The smaller available dosage (250 iu), used when a pregancy ends before 20 weeks, will 'cover' a transplacental haemorrhage of up to 2 ml of fetal blood, it being quite exceptional for larger volumes to reach the mother's circulation in these circumstances.

Anti-D immunoglobulin should also be given to any at risk Rh-negative woman when there has been a procedure or complication likely to be associated with feto-maternal bleeding due to placental separation or trauma, giving 250 iu before 20 weeks and 500 iu after that time. Such potential immunizing events include threatened as well as spontaneous or induced abortion, antepartum haemorrhage, external version and amniocentesis. Particularly following a placental abruption, a Kleihauer count should be made because a larger transplacental haemorrhage may have occurred and would require more than the standard prophylactic dosage.

Immediately before the administration of anti-D immunoglobin in any of these circumstances, maternal blood should be sent for antibody testing so that, in the event of apparent failure of prophylaxis, it will become known if immunization had in fact occurred already.

A fail-safe system of clinical documentation is essential to eliminate failures to give anti-D immunoglobulin whenever indicated. It should draw attention to the need for and the results of the tests described, and provide a clear indication that anti-D immunoglobulin has or has not been given.

In addition to rigorous implementation of the immunoprophylaxis programme, particularly after abortion when omissions are most likely or following large transplacental haemorrhages, the obstetrician is sometimes able to reduce the chance of a transplacental haemorrhage occurring or to minimize its amount. Thus, at Caesarean section in Rh-negative patients the placenta should not be hurriedly removed manually after the baby is delivered, and care should be taken to avoid spillage of blood into the peritoneal cavity. Amniocentesis should always be performed under direct ultrasonic guidance to avoid the placenta.

Failures of protection
Information presented at the McMaster Conference on Rh Prevention (Davey & Zipursky 1979) and from Yorkshire (Tovey *et al.* 1978) showed that, while incompatible blood transfusion still caused occasional Rh immunizations and in about one-third of pregnancies complicated by Rh antibodies immunization had occurred before anti-D immunoglobulin became available, in another one-third there had been a failure to give this following previous births, 13% represented true therapeutic failures of postpartum prophylaxis given as indicated, and in 20% there had been antepartum immunization. In an analysis of stillbirths and deaths from Rh haemolytic disease in England and Wales, Clarke (1982) reported similarly on the frequencies of these causes of immunization. A more recent analysis of causes of Rh immunization relating to 210 pregnancies managed at the Queen Mother's Hospital, Glasgow, during the years 1977–83, showed that antepartum immunization during either a previous or the current pregnancy was a more frequent cause (in 38%) than was either failure of postpartum prophylaxis to protect (in 14%) or omission to give it (in 9%). Incompatible blood transfusions should no longer occur, progressively fewer women immunized before the introduction of immunoprophylaxis are now having further pregnancies, and the failure rate from standard postpartum pro-

phylaxis is very low (0.9% according to Tovey *et al.* 1978). Therefore, the main problems of prevention relate to the failure to implement postpartum prophylaxis and to antepartum immunization which occurs more frequently than is generally recognized.

Antepartum administration of anti-D immunoglobulin
To reduce the risk of antepartum immunization, Zipursky and Israels (1967) gave anti-Rh immunoglobulin to Rh-negative women without antibodies at about the 36th week of gestation. This reduced the incidence and amount of detectable fetal cells in the maternal circulation after delivery, and it caused no complications in any babies although some Rh-positive infants gave a weak positive reaction to the direct Coombs' test. Bowman and Pollock (1978) reported on more than 1000 as yet unimmunized Rh-negative mothers who gave birth to Rh-positive babies after receiving a single injection of $300\,\mu g$ of anti-D immunoglobulin (i.e. 1500 iu) at 28 weeks' gestation; none of these mothers had evidence of Rh immunization at delivery, and neither did more than 500 of them when re-tested six months later. Based on previous experience, had this large series of Rh-negative women not been given antepartum prophylaxis, 14 would have been expected to be Rh-immunized by the time of delivery and a further six of those re-tested six months after delivery would have shown antibodies then. These workers attributed a reduction in the incidence of Rh isoimmunization in Manitoba from 3.5 to only 2.0 per thousand total births to their introduction of antepartum prophylaxis. Similarly, in Yorkshire a controlled trial in Rh-negative primigravidas confirmed the efficacy of antepartum prophylaxis when standard 500 iu doses are given at 28 and 34 weeks (Tovey *et al.* 1983). In this trial two treated and 18 control patients out of groups of about 2000 developed antibodies in the studied pregnancy, and in 16 of the untreated controls the baby was affected by haemolytic disease (two requiring exchange transfusion) while 11 further immunizations became apparent when 582 of the control patients were followed through further Rh-positive pregnancies, compared with only two new immunizations in further Rh-positive pregnancies in 325 of the treated patients.

In Britain, introduction of antenatal prophylaxis would produce a significant reduction in new Rh immunizations, but the logistic and financial demands of the necessary fourfold increase in harvesting anti-D immunoglobulin would be very considerable. Further, the supply of anti-D immunoglobulin depends increasingly on post-menopausal (or sterilized) Rh-negative women and Rh-negative men volunteering for hyperimmunization and regular donations of blood; but boosting injections of Rh-positive cells may cause the development of other antibodies in these donors to put them at risk should they themselves require transfusion, and there are also the at least theoretical risks of transmitting hepatitis or other viral diseases.

Provided nearly all failures to give prophylaxis have been eliminated, the selective antenatal administration of anti-D immunoglobulin to all at risk Rh-negative women without a previous successful pregnancy, and perhaps also the use of the smaller (250 iu) available dosage, would represent an acceptable compromise. In the future, monoclonal techniques may obviate the need for donors, and might even become less expensive.

MANAGEMENT OF PREGNANCY COMPLICATED BY Rh IMMUNIZATION

An overall strategy for serological surveillance and the management of pregnancies complicated by Rh

immunization is outlined in Fig. 18.2, which also includes the standard British scheme for immunoprophylaxis.

Antibody screening

The blood of all pregnant women should, at the first possible attendance, be screened for the presence of irregular antibodies including all varieties of Rh antibodies and non-Rh antibodies such as anti-Kell. They may have been immunized already but have an undetectable antibody level at booking, although enzyme tests (e.g. using papain-treated red cells) will often detect a low level of antibody that is undetectable by the more often used indirect Coombs' test. Because initially weak sensitization by a previous pregnancy may become detectable only later during the current pregnancy, these patients should have antibody tests repeated at monthly intervals from the 20th week of pregnancy. Rather less frequent repeat testing may seem adequate for Rh-negative primigravidas, but one may not be aware of a previous pregnancy (perhaps terminated) and a standard screening system regardless of parity is more effective.

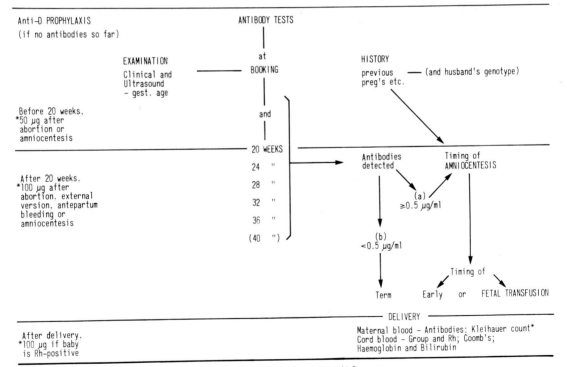

*N.B. Kleihauer count to indicate (>80 fetal red cells/50 LPF) need for extra anti-D.

Fig. 18.2. Rh disease—outline plan for the obstetric management and for prophylaxis. Reproduced from Whitfield (1982) in *Progress in Obstetrics and Gynaecology*, Volume 2, p. 48. Studd, J. W. W. (ed). Churchill Livingstone, Edinburgh.

Management following detection of Rh antibodies

Once a woman has developed antibodies, her pregnancy should be supervised from a centre providing all aspects of care for the Rh problem. When there were still relatively large numbers of cases 'Rh mortality', defined as all abortions, stillbirths, and neonatal and later deaths due or partly due to the disease or its attempted treatment, was reduced to a rate of 9% at a number of centres providing such regionalized ultraspecialist care (Liley 1963, Freda 1964, Whitfield 1970b). Now, because of prophylaxis, each region has only a small, and still decreasing, number of these patients, and it is becoming impossible to maintain the former level of experience and expertise (obstetric, laboratory, ultrasound, paediatric) at more than a very few centres, and even at these with some difficulty. The case for regionalized care is unanswerable, and the remainder of this chapter is written accordingly.

As soon as maternal antibodies are detected they should be quantitated. The partner's probable Rh genotype should be established, and the patient should be seen as soon as possible at a regional Rh clinic to plan the management of the pregnancy. Repeated titration in an albumen medium measures the amount and trend of anti-Rh IgG, but the results of titration lack good reproducibility and must be interpreted with caution. Automated measurement of antibody protein (specifically anti-Rh D) provides a much more accurate test which is now available at every regional blood transfusion centre. Thus, in the author's previous experience of repeated measurements in more than 400 Rh-immunized women, term delivery without prior amniocentesis was shown to be safe provided, on repeat testing, the level of the antibody in the maternal serum never exceeded 2.5 iu/ml. On the other hand, particularly in first affected pregnancies, levels exceeding 20.0 iu/ml are usually associated with very severe haemolytic disease, and a very sharp rise in antibody over a four-week period (e.g. from < 25 to > 50 iu) suggests that an acute fetal haemolytic crisis may require immediate intervention. This experience of the value of automated quantitative antibody tests is in close agreement with that of Fraser *et al.* (1972) and similar to the findings in a more recently reported smaller series (Bowell *et al.* 1982).

Although Rh genotyping does not give results of absolute certainty, and although the father of the fetus is not necessarily the mother's husband, knowledge that a fetus may be Rh-negative (i.e. because the husband is probably heterozygous Rh-positive) is

sometimes helpful in management, e.g. when amniotic fluid analysis suggests a less serious prognosis than does the previous history.

Obstetric management of these pregnancies is based on the optimal timing of intervention by delivery or, when the fetus is very severely affected, by intrauterine blood transfusion. From the previous history, the level of maternal antibody, and other factors including accurate confirmation of gestational age by ultrasound, the first decision is when to perform the initial amniocentesis (unless antibody levels are persistently below the critical value, see above). Previous experience of the great variety of patterns of severity of Rh disease is perhaps the most important factor in making these decisions, and this is why reference to a central Rh clinic as early as possible is vital.

Amniocentesis

Amniocenteses, which should always be performed under ultrasound direction to locate a suitable pool of fluid while avoiding the placenta, are timed in accordance with the previous Rh history, unless a sudden rise in antibody (see above) calls for an earlier than planned first tap. The following guidelines were developed for use with the Action Line method for timing intervention (Whitfield 1970b), but are applicable to most other prediction and management systems.

To give adequate warning of very severe haemolysis, the first amniocentesis is performed 10 weeks before the time of the earliest previous intrauterine death from Rh disease, of the earliest previous birth of a fatally or very severely affected baby (cord blood haemoglobin < 10.0 g/dl), or of the earliest fetal transfusion during a previous pregnancy, but not usually before 20 weeks' gestation since intrauterine transfusion by the traditional intraperitoneal technique is not a feasible procedure before 22 weeks. Without such a previous history of very severe Rh disease, the first amniocentesis is carried out between 28 and 30 weeks and is usually followed by a second test three or four weeks later; this interval usually avoids difficulties arising from spectrophotometric distortion due to previous 'bloody taps', it minimizes the effects of possible small measurement errors, and it is long enough to reveal clearly the amniotic fluid bilirubin trend that is of so much more prognostic importance than is a single estimation. Reduced intervals between amniocenteses, or additional taps, are required if the bilirubin value is already close to the critical level for the stage of gestation, if the trend between separate estimations has been rising sharply, or sometimes to confirm a favourable trend when severe Rh disease is expected from the history.

Amniotic fluid analysis

The semi-quantitated method of Liley (1961), whereby the height of the optical density deviation at the wavelength of 450 nm (ΔOD 450) is measured, is the most widely used method of estimating the amount of bilirubin in the amniotic fluid. ΔOD 450 values are plotted against the gestational age on whichever 'prediction chart' is used. A number of modifications of Liley's widely used prediction zones have been described. These include various critical levels or zones indicating the need for fetal transfusion, almost all of which coincide with the demarcation between Liley's upper and middle zones before 33 weeks. Except when intrauterine transfusion is indicated, the disadvantage of all these methods is that the prediction of severity of the haemolytic process at birth has to be converted into a decision on when to intervene. An essentially different approach was introduced by Freda (1965) whose grading of the ΔOD 450 indicates the current condition of the fetus in terms of the allowable 'safe' interval before further amniocentesis or intervention is called for. The Action Line method (Whitfield 1970b and 1976), devised to determine in advance the gestational age at which intrauterine transfusion or delivery would become safer to the fetus than continued non-intervention, was used in Belfast as the basis of the management of almost 1400 pregnancies complicated by Rh immunization during two successive three-year periods. By extrapolating to the Action Line the trend between separate measurements of ΔOD 450, this method combines Freda's concept of the need for continuing assessment (usually with much fewer amniocenteses) with the accuracy of Liley's methods, and it provides an effective and easily understood system for translating predictions of severity into optimal timing of intervention. For a detailed description of these and other systems, the interested reader is referred to the excellent reviews by Robertson (1978) and Queenan (1977). In all these methods, allowance is made for the gradual decline during the last trimester of the 'physiological' component of the amniotic fluid bilirubin. Accurate determination of gestational age, best made by ultrasound measurements in early pregnancy, is therefore essential in interpreting the level and trend of the 'pathological' bilirubin component that alone reflects the severity of the haemolytic process.

Delivery

When any Rh-immunized mother is approaching delivery, skilled paediatric help should be called to the labour ward. If severe Rh disease is expected, this should include a paediatrician experienced in dealing with the particular problems of the Rh-affected newborn. Neonatal management, including simple and exchange transfusion, the full range of intensive resuscitation and care, and the use of phototherapy, is outwith the scope of this chapter. In labour the obstetrician should ensure that the baby is born in the best possible condition apart from its haemolytic disease. Because the anaemic fetus is predisposed to intrapartum distress, and because hypoxia and acidosis impair further the baby's ability to conjugate bilirubin, there should be a 'low threshold' for delivery by Caesarean section if continuous intrapartum monitoring shows any evidence suggesting fetal distress. With this important proviso, induction of labour by standard methods will be the usual means of effecting delivery when intervention is indicated after 35 weeks, or when it is indicated between 31 and 35 weeks and adequate fetal pulmonary maturation has been confirmed by measuring the lecithin/sphingomyelin ratio, or other phospholipid index of fetal lung maturation in the amniotic fluid. Using the lecithin/sphingomyelin ratio in this way to make the decision between delivery and intrauterine transfusion, when action was needed between 31 and 35 weeks, was largely responsible for a significant reduction in neonatal deaths from the combined effects of haemolytic disease and severe respiratory distress syndrome in the second three-year Rh series in Belfast (Whitfield 1976).

Intrauterine fetal blood transfusion

Techniques used for intrauterine fetal transfusion by the intraperitoneal route have been described in detail by Friesen (1971), Bowes (1971), Queenan (1977), Whitfield *et al.* (1972) and others, and the reader requiring more information on the procedure is referred to these sources. With refinements the principle is that used by Liley (1963) who performed the first such fetal transfusion. Packed compatible Rh-negative blood is infused slowly through a catheter that has been threaded through an introducing needle inserted into the fetal abdominal cavity under radiographic guidance, or more commonly nowadays under combined X-ray and real-time ultrasound guidance, or indeed with real-time ultrasound imaging alone (Cooperberg & Carpenter 1977, Frigoletto *et al.* 1978 & 1981, Harman *et al.* 1983).

Successful ultrasound-guided transfusion directly into the dilated hepatic part of the umbilical vein of a severely affected fetus at 29 and 30 weeks was reported by Bang *et al.* (1982) in Copenhagen.

The first large review of intrauterine transfusion was the cooperative survey from 15 American centres reported by Queenan (1969). In a single-centre series in Belfast in which 364 transfusions were performed on 226 fetuses (Whitfield 1976) the eventual survival of 40% of them, including 47% of those not already grossly hydropic, was similar to the success rates being achieved at that time at other referral centres. Previous experience at the centres concerned suggests that, without intrauterine transfusion, most of these fetuses would have died. The survival of fetuses with significant ascites at the time of transfusion was almost as good as the survival of infants without demonstrable ascites or generalized hydrops, but none of the 34 fetuses with radiological evidence of generalized hydrops including gross scalp oedema survived. However, recently reported results of a 'refined management plan' in Winnipeg, based on close teamwork and intensive use of ultrasound to assess the fetal condition, to guide intrauterine transfusion and to determine the interval between these transfusions in the light of a favourable response or further deterioration in the fetus, are most encouraging (Harman *et al.* 1983); six of eight fetuses already hydropic at the first transfusion, and all of 16 non-hydropic fetuses, eventually survived, there being no neonatal deaths and no traumatic deaths following the transfusion.

Alternatives for the critically affected fetus

With improved results when intervention can be delayed beyond 30–32 weeks, the main obstetric challenge posed by Rh disease today is the fetus that is already critically affected, perhaps even developing hydrops, before this stage of gestation. Intraperitoneal transfusion *in utero* remains the mainstay of management in such cases, but in certain circumstances there are now additional and alternative methods to be considered.

Early rescue to intensive neonatal care. Reference has already been made to the improved salvage that followed the revised, more flexible, policy of delivery instead of intrauterine transfusion when intervention is indicated as early as 31 weeks and adequate surfactant has been demonstrated in the amniotic fluid; and the occasional survival of severely affected babies born even earlier, sometimes when intrauterine transfusion has apparently provoked very premature

labour before a further transfusion is due to be performed, is well recognized.

Therefore, if amniotic fluid analysis reveals that the fetus is likely to die soon, but has satisfactory or 'marginal' surfactant, perhaps as early as 28 or 29 weeks, immediate delivery by Caesarean section may be considered the safest course. Skilled ultrasound imaging is essential in making this decision, and such planned early rescue to intensive neonatal care probably offers the only hope for a fetus that is already frankly hydropic or, as shown by rapid accumulation of fluid in the body cavities, is threatening to become so.

Fetoscopic transfusion. Fetoscopy now makes possible direct intravascular transfusion of the fetus before intraperitoneal transfusion would be feasible (i.e. before 22 weeks). At King's College Hospital Rodeck *et al.* (1981) first reported the use of their expertise in fetoscopic diagnosis in this way, having injected blood into an umbilical cord vessel under fetoscopic vision on two occasions in each of two fetuses. The experience of Rodeck's team now extends to 109 such intravascular transfusions, given to 42 fetuses, followed in 11 instances by aspiration of ascitic fluid sometimes proceeding to an additional intraperitoneal transfusion (Rodeck & Nicolaides 1984). Their results when the first intravascular transfusion was not given until after 25 weeks have been disappointing, but the eventual survival of 27 out of 32 fetuses (84%) first transfused in this way before 25 weeks suggests that this may be a feasible way to treat the fetus likely to die before intraperitoneal transfusion is possible or likely to be easy. Particularly encouraging is the fact that some of the survivors had shown varying degrees of hydrops and fluid accumulations which reduced after transfusion and intravascular injection of digoxin. The phenomenon of quite large ascitic accumulations disappearing has often been observed after intraperitoneal transfusions, and regardless of the route by which the fetus is transfused the most important point is to be sure that the transfusion cannot be postponed safely to a later stage or perhaps may not be required at all. It should also be borne in mind that these excellent results, achieved by expert fetoscopists, do not quite match the remarkable recent survival rates from ultrasound-guided intraperitoneal fetal transfusion achieved by very experienced teamwork in Winnipeg (see above).

Fetal blood sampling and selective termination of pregnancy. Fetoscopic blood sampling, at about 18 weeks, makes possible Rh typing of the fetus. When there have been previous early intrauterine deaths due to Rh incompatibility and the partner is probably heterozygous Rh-positive, continuation of a proven Rh-negative pregnancy but termination of one shown to be Rh-positive may be acceptable to some couples. If ultrasound examination shows the placenta to cover the anterior uterine wall, placentocentesis might provide a more suitable way to obtain the sample of fetal blood.

Artificial insemination. If, however, the partner is probably homozygous (DD) Rh-positive, a couple with a very bad history may opt for artificial insemination with sperm from a Rh-negative donor.

Intensive plasma exchange. The attempted reduction of very high antibody levels by frequent repeated plasma exchanges during pregnancy when severe Rh disease is anticipated, was first used in Winnipeg (Bowman *et al.* 1968) and subsequent reports of its use in this way include those of Pole *et al.* (1974) and Fraser *et al.* (1976). The procedure is much more effective in maintaining an initial reduction in antibody if a continuous flow cell separator is available, but even with this equipment antibody 'escape' often occurs. Where success has been claimed, close examination of the data reported usually shows clearly that the eventual survival rates fall short of those being achieved at many referral centres not using this expensive and logistically demanding therapy. Indeed, one advocate of intensive plasma exchange in the management of Rh disease (Robinson 1984) has compared survival rates from 35 pregnancies recently treated in this way with the results achieved in more than 1000 pregnancies complicated by Rh disease 30 or more years ago (Walker & Murray 1956); the latter results were of course achieved before the introduction of predictive amniocentesis, intrauterine transfusion or anything resembling modern intensive neonatal care.

Attempted desensitization during pregnancy. Following claims that the daily oral administration of gastric acid-resistant capsules of group O Rh (D)-positive erythrocyte membranes to Rh- immunized mothers may reduce the expected severity of haemolytic disease in the fetus (Bierme *et al.* 1979), a multicentre trial of this therapy was initiated in the United States. Confirmation of any beneficial effect is awaited with interest, although 'no amelioration of the disease process could be determined' in five cases treated in this way by Gold *et al.* (1983). A potential advantage of such treatment, if proved effective, would be its application to mothers strongly immunized with Rh antibodies other than anti-D, or indeed with anti-Kell, and likely to bear severely affected babies.

Counselling and contraception
Counselling on the risks of future pregnancies and contraceptive advice must be an integral part of any Rh service, in which referring obstetricians and family doctors also have important roles to play. A sympathetic but unvarnished explanation of the prognosis for a future pregnancy is invariably welcomed by the patient and her husband even when it has to be given shortly after an unsuccessful pregnancy. An exact statistical prognosis is not possible because the pattern of Rh disease varies very greatly from patient to patient and because management, especially of the newborn, has improved so very considerably since the large series, on which predictive guidelines are based, were reported. Fifteen years ago, the following Rh mortality rates were reported from the first three-year series (666 cases) in Belfast; almost 4% when no previous baby had been affected; 6% when at least one had been affected but survived without exchange transfusion, 10% when there had been no previous Rh death, but at least one baby required exchange transfusion; and just over 50% when one or more of previous babies had died of Rh disease or its treatment. Significantly better mortality rates should now be achievable by improved obstetric and neonatal methods in the hands of experienced teams in patients referred to them early during pregnancy, perhaps ranging from 2% when no previous baby has been affected to about 35% when there has been a previous Rh death. These estimates may serve as helpful guidelines for Rh counselling today.

REFERENCES

ASCARI W. Q. (1977) In *Modern Management of the Rh Problem* (Queenan J. T, ed.), 2e, pp. 5 & 240. Harper and Row, New York.

ASK-UPMARK E. (1961) *Acta Med. Scand.*, **170**, 635.

BANG J., BOCK J. E. & TROLLE D. (1982) *Brit. med. J.*, **284**, 373.

BARNES C. G. (1976) *Medical Disorder in Obstetric Practice*, 4e, p. 189. Blackwell Scientific Publications, Oxford.

BIERME S. J., BLANC M., ABBAL M. & FOURNIE A. (1979) *Lancet*, **i**, 604.

BOWES W. A. (1971) *Clin. Obstet. Gynec.*, **14**, 561.

BOWMAN J. M. & POLLOCK J. M. (1978) *Canad. Med. Ass. J.*, **118**, 627.

BOWMAN J. M., PEDDLE L. J. & ANDERSON C. (1968) *Vox Sang.*, **15**, 272.

BOWELL P., WAINSCOAT J. S., PETO T. E. A. & GUNSON H. H. (1982) *Brit. med. J.*, **285**, 327.

BUCKLE A. E. R., PRICE T. M. L. & WHITMORE D. N. (1969) *Postgrad. med. J.*, **45**, 722.

CHAN W. H. & WHITFIELD C. R. (1971) *J. Obstet. Gynaec. Brit. Cwlth.*, **78**, 632.

CHANARIN I. & DAVEY D. A. (1964) *Brit. J. Haemat.*, **10**, 314.

CHANARIN I. & ROTHMAN D. (1971) *Brit. med. J.*, **ii**, 81.

CHANARIN I., ROTHMAN D., PERRY J. & STRATHFULL D. (1968) *Brit. med. J.*, **ii**, 394.

CHESLEY L. C. (1972) *Amer. J. Obstet. Gynec.*, **112**, 440.

CLARKE C. (1982) *Maternal and Child Health*, **7**, 4.

Combined Study from Centres in England and Baltimore (1966) *Brit. med. J.*, **ii**, 907.

COOPER B. A., CANTILIE G. S. D. & BRUNTON L. (1970) *Amer. J. clin. Nutr.*, **23**, 848.

COOPERBERG P. L. & CARPENTER C. W. (1977) *Amer. J. Obstet. Gynec.*, **128**, 239.

DAVEY M. G. & ZIPURSKY A. (1979) *Vox Sang.*, **36**, 50.

DE LEEUW N. K. M., LOWENSTEIN L. & HSIEH Y. S. (1966) *Medicine*, **45**, 291.

EVANS I. L. (1968) *Brit. med. J.*, **iii**, 166.

FINN R., CLARKE C. A., DONOHOE W. T. A., MCCONNELL R. B., SHEPPARD P. M., LEHANE D. & KULKE W. (1961) *Brit. med. J.*, **i**, 1486.

FLEMING A. W. (1973) *Clinics in Haemat.*, **2**, 477.

FRASER I. D. & TOVEY G. D. (1976) In *Clinics in Haematology, Blood Transfusion and Blood Products* (Cash J. B. ed.), Vol. 5, p. 149. W. B. Saunders, London.

FRASER I. D., TOVEY G. H., LOCKYER W. J. & SOBEY D. F. (1972) *J. Obstet. Gynaec. Brit. Cwlth.*, **79**, 1074.

FRASER I. D., BOTHAMLEY J. E., BENNETT M. O., AIRTH G. R., LEHANE D., MCCARTHY M. & ROBERTS F. M. (1976) *Lancet*, **i**, 6.

FREDA V. J. (1964) In *Proceedings of 10th Congress Internat. Soc. Blood Transfusion*, p. 919. Karger, Basel.

FREDA V. J. (1965) *Amer. J. Obstet. Gynec.*, **92**, 341.

FREDA V. J., GORMAN J. G. & POLLACK W. (1966) *Science*, **151**, 828.

FREDA V. J., GORMAN J. G., GALEN R. S. & TREACY N. (1970) *Lancet*, **ii**, 147.

FRIESEN R. F. (1971) *Clin. Obstet. Gynec.*, **14**, 572.

FRIGOLETTO F. D., BIRNHOLZ J. C., ROTHCHILD S. B., FINBERG H. J. & UMANSKY I. (1978) *Amer. J. Obstet. Gynec.*, **131**, 273.

FRIGOLETTO F. D., UMANSKY I., BIRNHOLZ J. C., ACKER D., EASTERDAY C. L., HARRIS G. B. C. & GRISCOM N. T. (1981) *Amer. J. Obstet. Gynec.*, **139**, 781.

FULLERTON W. T. & TURNER A. G. (1962) *Lancet*, **i**, 75.

GILES C. (1966) *J. clin. Path.*, **19**, 1.

GOLD W. R., QUEENAN J. T., WOODY J. & SACHER R. A. (1983) *Amer. J. Obstet. Gynec.*, **146**, 980.

HARDY J. & NAPIER J. A. F. (1981) *Brit. J. Obstet. Gynaec.*, **88**, 91.

HARMAN C. R., MANNING F. A., BOWMAN J. M. & LANGE I. R. (1983) *Amer. J. Obstet. Gynec.*, **145**, 823.

HENDRICKSE J. P. DE V., HARRISON K. A., WATSON-WILLIAMS E. J., LUZZATTO L. & AJABOR L. N. (1972) *J. Obstet. Gynaec. Brit. Cwlth.*, **79**, 410.

HERBERT V. (1962) *Arch. int. Med.*, **110**, 649.

HUNTSMAN R. G., METTERS J. S. K. & YAWSON G. I. (1972) *J. Pediat.*, **80**, 279.

HYTTEN F. E. & LEITCH I. (1971) *The Physiology of Human Pregnancy*, 2e, p. 24. Blackwell Scientific Publications, Oxford.

JACOBS A., MILLER F., WORWOOD M., BEAMISH M. R. & WARDROP C. A. (1972) *Brit. med. J.*, **iv**, 206.

KLEIHAUER E., BRAUN H. & BETKE K. (1957) *Klin. Wschr.*, **35**, 637.

KNOX G., MURRAY S. & WALKER W. (1961) *J. Obstet. Gynaec. Brit. Cwlth.*, **68**, 11.

LANGE R. D. & DYNESIUS R. (1973) *Clinics in Haemat.*, **2**, 433.

LETSKY E. (1977a) *Brit. J. hosp. Med.*, **15**, 357.

LETSKY E. (1977b) In *Contemporary Obstetrics and Gynaecology* (Chamberlain G. V. P. ed.), p. 95. Northwood Publications, London.

LEVINE P. (1943) *J. Hered.*, **34**, 71.

LILEY A. W. (1961) *Amer. J. Obstet. Gynec.*, **82**, 1359.

LILEY A. W. (1963) *Brit. med. J.*, **ii**, 1107.

LUND C. J. (1951) *Amer. J. Obstet. Gynec.*, **62**, 947.

MAGEE H. E. & MILLIGAN E. H. M. (1951) *Brit. med. J.*, **ii**, 1307.

MANSAC B. & JEPSON J. (1969) *Canad. Med. Ass. J.*, **100**, 687.

Medical Research Council Working Party (1974) *Brit. med. J.*, **ii**, 75.

MILLER D. F. & PETRIE S. J. (1963) *Obstet. Gynec.*, **22**, 773.

MURRAY S. (1957) *Brit. J. Haemat.*, **3**, 143.

NEVANLINNA H. R. & VAINIO T. (1962) *Proceedings of 8th Congress of Internat. Soc. Blood Transfusion* (Holland L. ed.), p. 231. Karger, Basel.

OSKI F. A. & NAIMAN J. L. (1972) *Haematologic Problems in the Newborn*, p. 33. W. B. Saunders, Philadelphia.

O'SULLIVAN J. F. (1982) In *Clinics in Obstetrics and Gynaecology* (Harley J. G. MacD. ed.), Vol. 9, No. 1, p. 91.

POLE J. R. G., BARR W. & WILLOUGHBY M. L. N. (1974) *Lancet*, **i**, 1051.

POLLACK W., ASCARI W. Q., KOCHESKY R. J., O'CONNOR R. R., HO T. Y. & TRIPODI D. (1971) *Transfusion*, **11**, 333.

PRITCHARD J. A. (1965) *Anesthesiology*, **26**, 393.

PRITCHARD J. A. (1966) *J. Amer. Med. Ass.*, **195**, 717.

PRITCHARD J. A. & ADAMS R. H. (1960) *Amer. J. Obstet. Gynec.*, **79**, 750.

PRITCHARD J. A., WHALLEY P. J. & SCOTT D. E. (1969) *Amer. J. Obstet. Gynec.*, **105**, 388.

QUEENAN J. T. (1969) *Amer. J. Obstet. Gynec.*, **104**, 397.

QUEENAN J. T. (1977) In *Modern Management of the Rh Problem* (Queenan J. T. ed.), 2e, p. 73. Harper and Row, New York.

QUEENAN J. T., GADOW E. C. & LOPES A. C. (1971a) *Amer. J. Obstet. Gynec.*, **110**, 128.

QUEENAN J. T., SHAH S., KUBARYCH S. F. & HOLLAND B. (1971b) *Lancet*, **i**, 815.

REPORTS ON CONFIDENTIAL ENQUIRIES INTO MATERNAL DEATHS

IN ENGLAND AND WALES, *1970–72* (1975), *1973–75* (1979) and *1976–78* (1982). HMSO, London.

ROBERTSON J. G. (1978) In *Amniotic Fluid* (Fairweather D. V. I. & Eskes T. K. A. B. ed.), 2e, p. 165. Excerpta Medica, Amsterdam.

ROBINSON E. A. E. (1984) *Plasma Therapy and Transfusion Technology*, **5**, 7.

RODECK C. H., HOLMAN C. A., KARNICKI J., KEMP J. R., WHITMORE D. N. & AUSTIN M. A. (1981) *Lancet*, **i**, 625.

RODECK C. H. & NICOLAIDES K. (1984) Personal communication.

TAYLOR D. J. & LIND T. (1979) *Brit. J. Obstet. Gynaec.*, **86**, 364.

TAYLOR J. J., STUDD J. W. W. & GREEN I. D. (1968) *J. Obstet. Gynaec. Brit. Cwlth.*, **75**, 963.

TOVEY L. A. D., MURRAY J., STEVENSON B. J. & TAVERNER J. M. (1978) *Brit. med. J.*, **ii**, 106.

TOVEY L. A. D., TOWNLEY A., STEVENSON B. J. & TAVERNER J. (1983) *Lancet*, **ii**, 244.

TUCK S. M. (1982) *Brit. J. hosp. Med.*, **28**, 125.

TUCK S. M. & WHITE J. M. (1981) In *Progress in Obstetrics and Gynaecology* (Studd J. ed.), Vol. 1, p. 70. Churchill Livingstone, London.

WALKER W. & MURRAY S. (1956) *Brit. med. J.*, **1**, 187.

WHITFIELD C. R. (1966) *J. Obstet. Gynaec. Brit. Cwlth.*, **73**, 586.

WHITFIELD C. R. (1970a) *J. Obstet. Gynaec. Brit. Cwlth.*, **77**, 577.

WHITFIELD C. R. (1970b) *Amer. J. Obstet. Gynec.*, **108**, 1239.

WHITFIELD C. R. (1976) *J. Clin. Path. 29 Suppl. (Roy. Coll. Path.)*, **10**, 54.

WHITFIELD C. R. (1983) In *Recent Advances in Perinatal Medicine* (Chiswick M. L. ed.), No. 1, p. 95. Churchill Livingstone, Edinburgh.

WHITFIELD C. R., THOMPSON W., ARMSTRONG M. J. & REID M. McC. (1972) *Brit. J. Obstet. Gynaec.*, **79**, 931.

WILLOUGHBY M. L. N. (1977) *Clinics in Obstet. Gynaec.*, **4**, 371.

WILLOUGHBY M. L. N. & JEWELL F. G. (1966) *Brit. med. J.*, **ii**, 1568.

WOODROW J. C. & FINN R. (1966) *Brit. J. Haemat.*, **12**, 297.

WHO SCIENTIFIC GROUP REPORT (1971) *WHO Technical Report Series No. 468.* Geneva.

ZIPURSKY A. & ISRAELS L. G. (1967) *Canad. Med. Ass. J.*, **97**, 1245.

CHAPTER 19
URINARY TRACT DISORDERS IN PREGNANCY

D. W. WARRELL

A knowledge of the physiological and anatomical changes which occur during pregancy allows a more rational approach to the diagnosis and treatment of urologic problems in pregnancy.

CHANGES IN THE URINARY TRACT IN PREGNANCY

There are three main areas of change: (a) kidney function, in which renal blood flow and glomerular filtration rate (GFR) increases up to 50%; (b) hormonal changes and pressure effects of the gravid uterus on the collecting system of the kidney resulting in dilatation of the ureters, kidney, pelvis and calyces; (c) changes in bladder and urethral function consequent on damage sustained at parturition.

CHANGES IN RENAL FUNCTION

Pregnancy increases the renal workload markedly and it is fortunate that the kidneys have considerable reserve. Effective renal plasma flow (ERPF) and GFR increase by up to 50% in pregnancy. Early reports on the timing of these changes produced confusing literature. However, more recent investigations (Davison & Noble 1981) have shown changes starting soon after conception which become well established by the end of the first trimester (Dunlop 1981). Towards the end of pregnancy there is a moderate fall in both ERPF and GFR. During pregnancy there is an increase in total body water of 6–8 litres, the majority of which is extracellular. There is a cumulative retention of between 600 and 900 MEq of sodium, distributed between the products of conception and the maternal extracellular fluid. The result is physiological hypervolaemia. However, the volume receptors in pregnancy adapt and regard the changed state as normal. The causes of the changes in the blood flow and GFR are uncertain. Attempts to relate to cardiac output, heart size and blood volume to renal haemodynamics are unconvincing (Gylling 1964). En-

docrine changes accompanying pregnancy such as increased secretion of aldosterone, prolactin, cortisol and placental lactogen are possible but unproven causes (Katz & Lindheimer 1977). The changes return to normal in the puerperium. The increased GFR produces an increased filtered load which may exceed the resorptive capacity of the renal tubules. The best known example is that of glycosuria of pregnancy in which the excretion of glucose may be up to ten times that of the non-pregnant woman (Davison & Hytten 1975). However, it is important to appreciate that other substances such as water-soluble vitamins and amino acids may be lost in pregnancy (Davison 1975). The increase in GFR has other important clinical implications. Since the production of creatinine and urea is not significantly altered the serum levels of these solutes decrease. Creatinine falls to reach a level of between 40 and 50 per mol/L in the third trimester. Plasma uric acid concentration falls by at least 25% in early pregnancy. Robertson and Cheyne (1972) reported average plasma levels of 3.5, 3.3 and 3.1 mmol/l in the three trimesters. Thus levels considered normal in non-pregnant women may reflect decreased renal function in pregnancy.

One other change in renal function of which the pregnant woman is aware is that of a disturbed circadian rhythm. In non-pregnancy more urine is produced by day than at night. In pregnancy when erect various mechanisms combine to increase sodium retention. With recumbency at night urine secretion is increased giving nocturnal frequency (Parboosingh & Doig 1973).

CHANGES IN THE COLLECTING SYSTEM

There is no doubt that hydronephros and hydro-ureter occur in pregnancy. These changes are evident by 10th–12th week of pregnancy and even at this early stage are more marked on the right than the left. The change progresses during the pregnancy so that at least mild hydronephros is seen in 90% of women in the right kidney and in 67% on the left side (Peake *et al.* 1983). Ureteric dilatation is much more marked above the pelvic brim than in the pelvis again particularly on the right. It is suggested that these differences may be explained by pressure from the right ovarian vein which crosses the ureter, while on the left side the ovarian vein runs parallel to it. Also the left ureter may be protected by the descending colon.

It seems likely that both hormonal and mechanical factors play a part in the aetiology of hydro-ureter. It is probable that the hormonal changes alter the compliance of the excretory ducts so as to allow mechanical factors to have an increased effect. Hydronephros and hydro-ureter can be documented by X-ray and scan techniques. Studies of ureteric function are much more difficult to make. However Mattingly and Borkowf (1978) report that pregnancy produces no change in the frequency or amplitude of ureteric contractions. Indeeed there is hypertrophy of ureteric smooth muscle and increased tone in the upper portion of the ureter. Early concepts of hypotonic ureters with inefficient contraction resulting in urinary stasis have not been substantiated. However the dilatation results in considerable enlargement of the 'dead space' in the urinary tract. This when combined with the alterations in urine secretion dependent on posture may lead to errors in tests based on timed urine collection e.g. 24 hour creatinine or oestriol excretion.

The errors may be minimized by increasing fluid intake so as to produce a high urine flow and lying the pregnancy woman on her side for an hour before and at the end of urine collection. Rarely pregnancy may reveal a previously compensated pelviureteric obstruction and precipitate an acute hydronephrosis (Mears 1978).

The dilatation of the collecting system seen in pregnancy is slow to return to normal after delivery. Intravenous pyelography should not be performed before four months postpartum for if it is carried out earlier and if dilatation of the collecting system is seen it is not possible to say whether the dilatation is pathological or a relic of the physiological changes of pregnancy. Vesicoureteric reflux may appear for the first time in pregnancy; usually in the last trimester. Heidrick et al (1967) report a prevalence of 3%–4%. The cause is uncertain as is the relevance of the reflux to acute pyelonephritis in pregnancy. Vesicoueteric integrity is restored with involution of the uterus.

CHANGES IN BLADDER AND URETHRAL FUNCTION

Frequency of micturition and incontinence of urine are well known and common problems in pregnancy. Usually frequency begins early in pregnancy (Francis 1960a) and has resolved by the time of the first postnatal visit. It seems likely that it is due, certainly in early pregnancy, to increased urine secretion rather than to a reduction in functional bladder capacity (Fancis 1960a). Assessment of bladder function by the technique of retrograde cystometry contains conflicting reports as to the changes that occur. Youssef (1956) and Marchent (1978) both report increased bladder capacities in pregnancy while Francis (1960b) reports a decrease in the third trimester.

There is an agreement that intravesical pressure measured when the bladder is full is raised in pregnancy. Pressures of 20cms H_2O, i.e. double the nonpregnant normal value, are found (Clow 1975 and Iosif *et al.* 1980). This increase in pressure is probably due to the changed position of the bladder which becomes an intra-abdominal organ as pregnancy advances and to the increase in intra-abdominal contents.

Delivery commonly blunts bladder sensation and impairs the capacity to micturate. Bennets & Judd (1941) found decreased bladder sensation and increased capacity in over 80% of patients in the early puerperium; findings substantiated by Marchant (1978) and Grove (1973). The conclusion is that delivery damages the autonomic nerve supply to the bladder. Usually the damage is short lived, and bladder sensation and contractility return to normal a few days after delivery. However, this is not always so and the author has encountered a number of women who date a permanent impairment in the capacity to void from their delivery.

Stress incontinence is a common symptom in pregnancy occurring in about 50% of primigravida and the majority of multipara (Francis 1960b). The cause of this symptom is unknown. The facts are that most women who suffer from stress incontinence date its appearance to pregnancy rather than to parturition (Francis 1960b) yet the evidence is that it is parturition rather than pregnancy that damages the urinary sphincter mechanism. Iosif *et al.* (1980) report normal urethral closure pressures in pregnancy. There is a decrease in urethral closure pressures postpartum except in women delivered by Caesarean section. Further evidence supporting the concept of delivery damaging the sphincter has been produced by

Snooks *et al.* (1984) who report an impaired conduction time in the perineal branches of pudendal nerve (i.e. the nerve supply of the striated muscle of the urethra) as a result of vaginal delivery. It may be that stress incontinence experienced in pregnancy has a different cause to stress incontinence of later life. Further studies in this field are needed.

Urinary infection

The term urinary infection conjures the image of an ill woman suffering from frequency and painful micturition, whose urine contains significant numbers of pus cells and bacteria. There is a general impression that in pregnancy infection is more common and more serious than in non-pregnancy, threatening the well-being and sometimes the life of both mother and fetus. In fact the prevalence of asymptomatic bacteriuria is very similar in pregnant and non-pregnant women, increasing with both age and parity (Kunin 1979). Infection in pregnancy presents in different forms, some of which are serious and others of small consequence. Clearly it is the duty of the obstetrician to assess the problems and risks and organize the care of the patient whose pregnancy is complicated by a urinary infection.

ASYMPTOMATIC SIGNIFICANT BACTERIA

Kass (1956) introduced the concept of asymptomatic significant bacteriuria (10^5 organisms per ml of urine) to aid in the diagnosis of urinary tract infection, stating that this number was reliable evidence of bacteria multiplying in the urine thus helping distinguish infection from contamination. In a later publication Kass (1960) suggested that up to a half of the women who were found to have asymptomatic significant bacteriuria in early pregnancy would if untreated develop pyelonephritis. He also suggested an association with prematurity as defined by a birth weight of less than 2500 g. These observations sparked off a host of reports.

The prevalence of asymptomatic significant bacteriuria varies with the population studied and the method of the collection and handling of specimens. Opinions vary whether the patient should clean the vulva and then catch the first urine voided in a sterile container, or if the vulva should be uncleansed and an effort made to catch a genuine mid-stream specimen. Often the technique is unspecified. The handling of the specimens is important. Urine left at room temperature will allow multiplication of bacteria. There

is no doubt that urine should be transported to the laboratory and examined fresh. If that is not possible it should be refrigerated until examination.

Prevalence rates of up to 12% are reported (Chng & Hall 1982). The importance of the finding of a significant number of bacteria in an asymptomatic pregnant woman varies according to the site of infection. In about 25% the urine will have cleared by the time a second specimen has been examined (De Alvarez 1976) suggesting either error in handling the specimen or that the bacteriuria was a transient phenomenon and as such not important. Attempts have been made to localize infection using ureteric catheterization (Fairley *et al.* 1966), bladder wash-out techniques (Heineman & Lee 1973) and bacterial fluorescent techniques (Harris *et al.* 1976). Kidney infection is reported between 25% and 50% and bladder infection in about 40%.

Infection in the upper renal tract is often associated with a structural abnormality of the kidney and may also be associated with hypertension or anaemia. It is thus a much more serious condition than that of bacteria multiplying in the bladder, the main risk of the latter being that of ascending infection.

Since localization of infection is not a practical proposition in everyday practice, the clinician must have a scheme of management for patients with asymptomatic bacteriuria. The first question to be decided is whether bacterial examination of the urine is a worthwhile screening procedure to undertake in early pregnancy. There are three main areas of discussion. The first is whether identification and treatment of women in early pregnancy will reduce the incidence of overt infection later in pregnancy. The evidence is that bacteriuric women, if untreated, are about four times more likely to develop a symptomatic infection in pregnancy than bacteriuria-negative women. However, since at least 90% of women will be bacteriuria-negative in early pregnancy, the majority of women who develop symptomatic proven infection in pregnancy will have started pregnancy without bacteriuria. At best screening will pick up no more than a third of patients who are likely to develop an overt infection. However, it seems clear that bacteriuric women are at an increased risk of infection and that treatment reduces the chance of covert infection developing. The second point is whether identification and treatment of bacteriuric women can reduce the risk of pregnancy complications. This seems not to be so. Kincaid-Smith and Bullen (1965) reported an increased prematurity rate and fetal loss in this group. Treatment did not improve the outlook for the fetus. Thirdly, perhaps the most cogent reason for screening is the detection of kidney abnormalities, such as pyelonephritis and stone, frequently found in women with persistent bacteriuria (Gower *et al.* 1968, Whalley 1967). Many such patients are symptom free and would be detected only by a screening procedure. In these women pregnancy is the event which is most likely to bring them under medical care and allow recognition of a serious health problem. Though the high hopes with which screening was introduced have not all been realized nevertheless it is a worthwhile exercise.

Management of asymptomatic significant bacteriuria
A midstream specimen of urine should be examined fresh at the first visit. Of those negative, 98% will remain negative and about 2% will develop a symptomatic infection. If positive, a second specimen should be obtained. If still positive, it is worth prescribing antibiotics for a week. Sulphonamides, trimethoprim, ampicillin and Furadantin are the drugs of choice, as being relatively safe and non-toxic in early pregnancy. About 80% will respond to a short course of treatment, and of these about 80% will remain uninfected. In these the majority view is that treatment has prevented the discomforts of an overt infection and in a large proportion the risks of pyelonephritis. Women with persistent bacteriuria are likely to have a renal structural abnormality and to suffer increased fetal loss. There is no evidence that antibacterial treatment will improve the outlook of this group. However, it is important to identify an at risk group of women and to focus obstetric care on them. After delivery it is in their health interests to evaluate the urinary tract.

SYMPTOMATIC INFECTION

These may be of the lower or upper urinary tract. Lower urinary tract symptomatology may be due to urethral or bladder infection. The latter willl usually be found to have greater than 10^5 per ml bacteria in a fresh midstream urine. Urethral infection may be difficult to substantiate by microbiological investigation. A midstream urine may contain white cells but few bacteria and may contain neither. It is not possible to differentiate on clinical grounds alone between patients with cystitis and bacteria multiplying in the bladder and patients whose symptoms arise in the urethra and in whom evidence of infection is often lacking. It is important to make this distinction because patients with bacterial infection are at risk of ascending infection, while patients with symptoms arising from the urethra are by and large not at risk of serious bacteriurial infection.

All patients with acute lower urinary tract symptoms should have their urine cultured. All should be encouraged to drink at least 1.5 litres of water a day and potassium citrate prescribed. Ideally antibiotic therapy should be delayed for a day until the urine culture is known. If this is not practical a few days' treatment with antibiotics may be prescribed.

Acute pyelonephritis is a serious condition. Regrettably identification and treatment of patients with significant bacteriuria early in pregnancy does not greatly reduce the number of patients who will develop a covert urinary infection at some time in the pregnancy, because in the majority of cases this occurs out of the blue' in patients who have had a sterile urine early in pregnancy (Chng & Hall 1982). Two-thirds of the attacks take place before the 28th week of the pregnancy. The attack threatens the life of the patient and may be complicated by shock and respiratory insufficiency (Cunningham *et al.* 1984). A typical history is of malaise, fever and localizing symptoms of loin pain and less commonly dysuria. On examination the patient is toxic, pyrexial and often dehydrated. One kidney is usually acutely tender and may be accompanied by lumbar spasm on the affected side. The patient should be managed in hospital. Treatment should be active, with intravenous rehydration, pain relief by intramuscular injection and antibiotic therapy. Ampicillin is the drug of choice unless an organism insensitive to this drug is identified. There is a substantial risk of re-infection so patients should be treated for at least two weeks and their urine regularly cultured for the remainder of the pregnancy. An intravenous urogram should be performed after delivery for about one-third will have an abnormal urogram. The latter investigation must be delayed until all the pregnancy effects on the urinary tract have subsided.

Conclusion
The acute onset in pregnancy of symptoms suggestive of urinary infection may be due to acute renal infection with an appreciable fetal and maternal morbidity and mortality, or to a non-serious cause such as urethritis. The clinician needs to be aware of the spectrum of disease and active in diagnosis and treatment.

Urinary calculus

Calculus disease is uncommon during pregnancy, probably affecting no more than 0.2% of all pregnancies (Lattanzi & Cook 1980). Calcium stones, either oxalate or phosphate, are the most common. Uric acid stones are much less common. Stones formed of magnesium ammonium phosphate are sometimes known as 'infection stones' because they commonly form in association with organisms that split urea e.g. *proteus mirabilis*.

The common presentations are those of a persistent ache in the renal area or a colicky pain of ureteric distribution. These symptoms, particularly if accompanied by a persistent infection, are strongly suggestive of stone. In these circumstances it is worth taking a plain large film of the abdomen for modern X-ray techniques allow a reduction in radiation to the fetus to insignificant levels. If the stone is small and the urine sterile treatment should be conservative and consist of a 3 litre/day fluid intake in the expectation that the stone will pass spontaneously. Patients with non-obstructing stones accompanied by infection should receive antibiotics in an attempt to keep the urine sterile until delivery. Untreated the caculi may enlarge and cause obstruction or pyonephrosis. These complications need surgical management and are fortunately very rare. When a stone is found serum calcium levels should be measured. As serum calcium levels normally drop in pregnancy even a borderline elevation is significant. If raised, the serum parathyroid hormone level should be measured. If elevated, it is virtually diagnostic of primary hyperparathyroidism. The baby of a mother with this disorder should be monitored with care because the maternal calcium crosses the placenta to the fetus with consequent suppression of fetal parathormone levels leaving the neonate at risk of tetany.

Haematuria

Clinical haematuria is uncommon in pregnancy. However the presence of a non-haemolysed trace of blood discovered by the sensitive 'dip-stick' tests is much more common.

Visible blood in the urine may often have a source in the genital tract, so that when haematuria is suspected it is worth occluding the vaginal introitus with a swab and testing a second specimen. If there is doubt about the source a catheter specimen should be obtained and tested. If there is no doubt the patient has clinical haematuria the source must be found. The causes are infection, tumour and stone.

If the patient does not have an infection and an X-ray of the abdomen is negative cystoscopy should be performed under anaesthesia. The bladder is distorted by the pregnancy but it is usually possible to make an adequate examination. Often no cause is found and the worry is that the bleeding is coming from a renal tumour.

An ultrasound scan of the kidneys should be performed, but in the absence of other indications an intravenous urogram should be delayed until the puerperium for renal tumours are extremely rare in young women. Often no cause is found and the suggestion is the bleeding has come from an area of increased vascularity in the kidney. Blood detected by dip-stick alone almost never has a serious cause. In the author's experience it is almost always an association of urethritis. Haematuria in labour is a different sort of problem, it is an extremely grave physical sign and indicates impending rupture of the lower uterine segment, particularly if the patient has previously been delivered by lower segment Caesarean section.

Chronic renal disease

As renal function declines the ability to conceive and sustain a viable pregnancy decreases. It appears that when renal function prior to conception declines to a degree where serum creatinine and urea nitrogen exceed 3 and 30 mg/100 ml respectively normal gestation is rare (Bear 1976). Thus it is of interest that pregnancy may be jeopardized by degrees of functional impairment that do not cause symptoms and do not overtly disrupt homeostatic functions in non-pregnant women. The obstetrician may be asked to advise on the risks of pregnancy in a woman with chronic renal disease and the likelihood of a successful outcome for the pregnancy. These risks are dependent on the rate of disease progress in the particular patient, the amount of renal damage and the presence or absence of hypertension. The latter seems the major risk factor, for if a pregnant mother comes to harm or the fetus dies, they do so more commonly as a complication of hypertension than of renal failure.

The features in favour of a satisfactory outcome to pregnancy are a stable and not progressive disease process, renal function only minimally or moderately compromised and normal blood pressure.

Chronic glomerular nephritis is a term encompassing many aetiologically different entities. It seems unlikely that pregnancy affects the natural history of the disease process (Katz *et al.* 1980, 1981). A review of eight published series of 424 pregnancies in 365 women with chronic glomerular nephritis reported no maternal deaths. Fetal survival was 93% in 176 normotensive gravidas. In contrast 45% of the fetuses of women whose renal disease was complicated by hypertension died (Lindheimer & Katz 1977).

The main risk to the pregnant woman with chronic renal disease is that of hypertension which is present in about 25% of pregnancies. Katz *et al.* (1980, 1981) reported that approximately 1–10% were diagnosed on clinical grounds as having developed pre-eclampsia. The GFR in women with renal disease is usually lower than that of healthy pregnancies. However pregnancy still causes an increase. Towards term the GFR tends to fall mildly but recovers after delivery. The most common event is that of increased protein excretion. Major amounts, i.e. exceeding 3g a day, complicate about a third of pregnancies and often lead to nephrotic oedema. Perinatal mortality and the incidence of small-for-dates babies are mildly increased. It is crucial for success that there is close cooperation between mother, obstetrician and renal physician, and meticulous care of the pregnancy.

THE NEPHROTIC SYNDROME

This is the triad of heavy proteinuria with secondary hypo-albuminaemia and generalized oedema. Most reports agree that the outlook for pregnancy in this condition is good provided hypertension is absent and that renal function is good. The keystones of care are frequent observation of blood pressure and renal function as judged by creatinine clearance and measurements of urea and electrolytes. The patient should spend much of the pregnancy recumbent. Complications, particularly the appearance of hypertension, demand instant recognition and meticulous control. It is important for these patients to receive a high protein diet: above 3gm per kilo body weight per day is advised. Diuretics should be avoided for nephrotic patients are oligaemic and diuretics will increase this problem.

Acute renal failure

Acute renal failure is a clinical syndrome characterized by a sudden and marked decrease in glomerular filtration, rising blood urea nitrogen and serum creatinine levels and usually by a decrease in urine output to below 400 ml/day.

Usually this entity occurs in women with pre-

viously healthy kidneys, but it may be a complication in patients with pre-existing renal disease.

There are three patterns of disease which probably are different areas in a spectrum of increasing severity of the same pathogenic mechanism of renal hypoperfusion with preferential cortical ischaemia. These are prerenal failure, acute tubular necrosis and renal cortical necrosis.

Prerenal failure is the mildest of these illnesses and is due to slight to moderate degrees of renal hypoperfusion. It is a disturbance of function with no changes in renal morphology. Rapid improvement in renal perfusion reverses the condition. If renal ischaemia is more severe or persists acute tubular necrosis occurs. Recovery can be expected after a period of renal shutdown. Persistent or severe degrees of ischaemia produce cortical necrosis from which recovery is very rare. Acute renal failure follows excessive blood loss, dehydration and vasoconstriction. The common obstetric causes are septic abortion, severe pre-eclamptic toxaemia with placental abruption, placenta praevia and postpartum haemorrhage. The end result of these conditions is hypotension, the cause of which may be simple blood loss, sepsis with endotoxic shock and coagulation disorders. Most clinical problems possess more than one factor.

In the Western world the incidence of acute renal failure as a complication of pregnancy is declining. Two decades ago the incidence was about 0.02% to 0.05% (Kerr & Elliot 1963). The current incidence is now probably less than 0.01% (Lindheimer *et al.* 1982). Therapy should be extremely active and consist of fluid replacement monitored by a central venous pressure line, antibiotics where appropriate and corticosteroids if shock is a dominant factor. Renal function is assessed by urine output and the blood chemistry. Homeostasis is maintained by renal dialysis until renal function returns. This vigorous treatment has produced a significant improvement in prognosis over the last two decades.

PREGNANCY IN PATIENTS WITH A RENAL TRANSPLANT

Life expectancy and the quality of life have improved so much for patients where renal failure is treated by transplantation that their hopes and aspirations now include pregnancy and child rearing. The world experience in this topic has been reviewed by Davison and Lindheimer (1982). In order for pregnancy to stand a good chance of success the following criteria should be fulfilled.

First of all the transplanted kidney should be stable and not likely to be rejected. It is customary to advise against pregnancy for two years after transplantation for this reason. The patient should be normotensive. Residual hypertension is the major reason why pregnancy may be unsuccessful.

There should be sufficient reserve function in the transplanted kidney to allow for the increased metabolic demands of pregnancy. If these criteria can be met then it is reasonable to allow the patient to try to conceive, and if successful for pregnancy to go ahead. The risks associated with pregnancy are hypertensive problems, renal failure (about 10% of patients show evidence of this), and infection mainly with cytomegalovirus or herpes as a consequence of immunosuppressive therapy.

In order to minimize risks the patient should be cared for jointly by the renal transplant team and a concerned obstetrician. Tests of renal function, viral antibody titres and tests of urine and saliva for evidence of virus infection need to be performed at least every 4 weeks throughout the pregnancy. If the pregnancy has been uneventful it is reasonable to aim for vaginal delivery. The site of the transplant in the false pelvis should not mechanically affect vaginal delivery. Corticosteroids need to be increased in labour.

In women fulfilling the above criteria the chances of successful pregnancy are about 90%. Having said that, many of the pregnancies are eventful with premature labour and intrauterine growth retardation as common problems. The utmost care is needed to achieve this success rate.

Immunosuppressive therapy with corticosteroids and azothiaprim does not cause a material increase in fetal abnormality. However the long term well-being of children born to immunosuppressed mothers must contain a question mark which will not be answered for several decades.

REFERENCES

BEAR R.A. (1976) *Obstet. and Gynecol.*, **48**, 13.

BENNETTS F. A. & JUDD G. E. (1941) *Amer. J. Obstet. Gynec.*, **42**, 419.

CHNG P. K. & HALL M. H. (1982) *Brit. J. Obstet. Gynaecol.*, **89**, 8.

CLOW W. M. (1975) *Urol. Int.*, **30**, 9.

CUNNINGHAM F. G., LEVANO K. J., HANKINS G. D. V., WHALLEY P. J. (1984) *Obstet. and Gynecol.*, **63**, 121.

DAVISON J. M. (1975) *Clin. Obstet. Gynaecol.*, **2**, 365.

DAVISON J. M. & HYTTEN F. E. (1975) *Brit. J. Obstet. Gynaecol.*, **82**, 374.

DAVISON J. M. & LINDHEIMER M. D. (1982) *Nieren und Hochdruckk Rank Heiten*, **11**, 258.

DAVISON J. M. & NOBLE M. C. B. (1981) *Brit. J. Obstet. Gynaecol.*, **88**, 10.

DE ALVAREZ R. (Ed.) (1976) *The Kidney in Pregnancy*. John Wiley & Sons, New York.

DUNLOP W. (1981) *Brit. J. Obstet. Gynaecol.*, **88**, 1.

FAILEY K. F., BUND A. G., ADEY F. D. (1966) *Lancet*, **i**, 939.

FRANCIS W. J. A. (1960a) *J. Obstet. Gynaecol. Brit. Emp.*, **67**, 353.

FRANCIS W. J. A., (1960b) *J. Obstet. Gynaecol. Brit. Emp.*, **67**, 899.

GOWER P. E., HASWELL B., SIDAWAY M. E. & DE WARDENER H. E. (1968) *Lancet*, **i**, 990.

GROVE L. H. (1973) *Brit. J. Anaesth.*, **45**, 1147.

GYLLING T. (1964) *Acta. Obstet. Gynaec. Scand.*, **40**, (Suppl. 5).

HARRIS R. E., THOMAS D. L., SHELOKOV A. (1976) *Amer. J. Obstet. Gynec.*, **126**, 20.

HEIDRICK W. P., MATTINGLEY R. F. & AMBERG J. R. (1967) *Obstet. and Gynecol.*, **29**, 571.

HEINEMAN H. S. & LEE J. H. (1973) *Obstet. Gynec. N.Y.*, **41**, 22.

IOSIF S., INGERMARSSON I. & ULMSTEN U. (1980) *Amer. J. Obstet. Gynec.*, **137**, 696.

KASS E. H. (1956) *Trans. Assoc. Amer. Phycns.*, **69**, 56.

KASS E. H. (1960) *Arch. intern. Med.*, **105**, 194.

KATZ A. I., DAVISON J. M., HAYSLETT J. P. SINGSON E. & LINDHEIMER M. D. (1980) *Kidney Int.*, **18**, 192.

KATZ A. I., DAVISON J. M., HAYSLETT J. P. & LINDHEIMER M. D. (1981) *Contrib. Nephrol.*, **25**, 53.

KATZ A. I. & LINDHEIMER M. D. (1977) *Ann. Rev. Physiol.*, **39**, 97.

KERR D. N. S. & ELLIOTT R. W. (1963) *Practitioner*, **190**, 459.

KINCAID-SMITH P. & BULLEN M. (1965) *Lancet*, **i**, 395.

KUNIN C. M. (1979) *Detection, Prevention & Management of Urinary Infection*, 3rd ed. Lea & Febiger, Philadelphia.

LATTANZI D. R. & COOK W. A. (1980) *Obstet. and Gynecol.*, **56**, 462.

LINDHEIMER M. D. (1982) In *Acute Renal Failure*. (BRENNER D. M., LAZARUS J. M. & MYERS B. D. Eds.) W. B. Saunders & Co., Philadelphia.

LINDHEIMER M. D. & KATZ A. I. (1977) *Kidney Function and Disease in Pregnancy*, p. 154. Lea & Febiger, Philadelphia.

MARCHANT D. J. (1978) *Clin Obstet. Gynaec.*, **21**, 3.

MATTINGLEY R. F. & BORKOWF H. I. (1978) *Clin. Obstet. Gynec.*, **21**, 863.

MEARS E. M. (1978) *Clin. Obstet. Gynec.*, **21**, 907.

PARBOOSINGH J. & DOIG A. (1973) *Amer. J. Obstet. Gynec.*, **116**, 609.

PEAKE S. L., ROXBURGH H. B. & LANGLOIS S. P. (1983) *Radiology*, 146.

ROBERTSON E. G. & CHEYNE G. A. (1972) *Brit. J. Obstet. Gynaecol.*, **79**, 769.

SNOOKS S. J., SETCHELL M., SWASH M. & HENRY M.M. (1984) *Lancet*, 546.

WHALLEY P. (1967) *Amer. J. Obstet. Gynec.*, **97**, 723.

YOUSSEF A. F. (1956) *Obstet. and Gynec.*, **8**, 181.

CHAPTER 20
DIABETES AND OTHER ENDOCRINE
DISEASES COMPLICATING PREGNANCY

J.W.K. RITCHIE

INTRODUCTION

Before the discovery of insulin in 1921 by Banting and Best the life expectancy of the diabetic was short, children living little more than a year after the onset of the disease and adults on average only six years (Best 1945). Few diabetic women conceived, and in those who did pregnancy was often disastrous, nearly 30% of mothers dying in diabetic coma as a direct result of pregnancy, while many more died within two to three years of confinement from concurrent tuberculosis (Williams 1909). The perinatal mortality rate ranged between 40 and 60%.

After the introduction of insulin the incidence of pregnancy in diabetic patients rose steadily and maternal mortality fell dramatically, although fetal loss remained high. By the 1950s the perinatal mortality rate had fallen to 25% and a decade later had fallen further, ranging from 10 to 15% (Peel 1962, Harley & Montgomery 1965). This reflected increasing teamwork in the care of the pregnant diabetic and her newborn which continues to be the cornerstone of management, and is responsible for rates reported in most recent series of less than 5%.

CLASSIFICATION AND DIAGNOSTIC CRITERIA

Much confusion and little agreement exists about the classification and diagnostic criteria for carbohydrate intolerance in pregnancy (Beard & Hoet 1982). This is mainly because the range of abnormality is wide and the effect on pregnancy is variable. Also there is still debate about which pregnant women should have a formal test of carbohydrate tolerance. Fortunately there have been recent attempts to break traditional ground and to gain a measure of consensus (World Health Organization 1980). Accordingly these recommendations will be adopted here.

Insulin-dependent diabetes (IDD)

Most often the diagnosis of IDD will have been made before pregnancy, the patient presenting with the classical picture of weight loss, thirst, polyuria with glycosuria, hyperglycaemia and a tendency to keto-acidosis. Insulin therapy will already have been commenced. The more severe kind of carbohydrate intolerance occurs chiefly in younger patients who will have little or no circulating insulin. These have been called type I or insulin-dependent diabetics (World Health Organization 1980). The older obese diabetic (type II, non-insulin-dependent diabetes) has a less severe variety of intolerance; fasting insulin levels may be normal but there is increased insulin resistance. The pancreas is easily exhausted and the response to a glucose load is impaired. In Western society the type I diabetic is commonly encountered below the age of 40, but in other cultures, e.g. in some parts of the Middle East and the USA, type II diabetes may be commonly found in younger people. Although outside pregnancy normoglycaemia may be maintained by other means, during pregnancy the latter type may require treatment with insulin.

Some women may develop symptoms or signs of diabetes for the first time during pregnancy and require treatment, usually in the form of insulin, to achieve normoglycaemia. The criteria by which diabetes may be diagnosed are based on the fasting plasma glucose concentration and the 2-hour level after a glucose tolerance test (GTT). The values are shown in Table 20.1.

The standard test now recommended is 75 g of glucose in 250–350 ml water taken orally over 5–15 minutes after an overnight fast (World Health Organization 1980). It should be pointed out that slightly different criteria are in use in the USA based on data for a 100 g GTT from O'Sullivan and Mahan (1964).

Table 20.1. WHO criteria for diagnosis of diabetes and impaired glucose tolerance using a 75 g oral GTT (WHO 1980).

	Venous plasma glucose level (mmol/l)	
	Fasting	2 h post glucose
Diabetes	≥ 8.0	≥ 11.0
Impaired glucose tolerance	< 8.0	≤ 8.0 to < 11.0
Normal	< 6.0	< 8.0

Gestational diabetes

Gestational diabetes may be defined as that meeting the WHO criteria for diabetes during pregnancy but with glucose tolerance reverting to normal after the puerperium. It follows that all women developing diabetic symptoms during pregnancy or who have an abnormal GTT should be followed up after the puerperium and have their current carbohydrate metabolism checked. The WHO criteria suggest that, in the absence of symptoms, at least one additional abnormal plasma glucose value during the GTT is required to confirm the diagnosis of gestational diabetes, e.g. 1-hour post-glucose of 11.0 mmol/l or more.

Impaired glucose tolerance (IGT)

Some women may develop a mild glucose intolerance during pregnancy without symptoms. The criteria for making this diagnosis are given in Table 20.1 Rarely, the mild intolerance persists and requires long-term treatment.

Gestational impaired glucose tolerance

Commonly the mild intolerance returns to normal after the puerperium (when it should be checked again by GTT) in which case the condition may be called gestational IGT.

In an attempt to relate the severity of carbohydrate abnormality to fetal outcome and to simplify the reporting of results White (1965) suggested a classification grouped according to the age at onset and duration of the disease together with the presence of diabetic complications. This was a useful exercise at the time, but there are considerable drawbacks to its use today. This is partly due to disagreement about the definition of 'class A' and who should be included in it. Also, there has been a tendency to report 'class A' results together with those from insulin-dependent

diabetics, which confuses interpretation. Most importantly, it is now recognized that the effect of maternal age and of the duration of maternal diabetes are better considered separately. The fetal outcome is not closely related to the 'severity' or class of the disease in the great majority of diabetic mothers (UK Diabetic Pregnancy Study, Lowy & Beard, unpublished data). For these reasons many specialists in pregnancy complicated by diabetes would prefer a simple classification such as that given in Table 20.2 which takes into account only the WHO classification and the duration of insulin treatment.

Table 20.2. Classification of carbohydrate intolerance in pregnancy.

1	Impaired glucose tolerance
2	Insulin-dependent diabetes (IDD) of duration less than 10 years
3	IDD for 10 to 19 years
4	IDD for 20 years or more

INDICATIONS FOR GTT

Most would now accept that all women should have a preliminary test of glucose tolerance by estimating the random venous plasma glucose at booking, which may be repeated at 28 weeks' gestation. If the plasma glucose concentration is 7.2 mmol/l or greater there is an indication to carry out a GTT. This cut-off point has been determined after careful study of the normal distribution of random plasma glucose concentrations in a large series of consecutive mothers at first visit to the antenatal clinic and represents three standard deviations above the mean (Hadden 1980).

Other indications for GTT have been put forward in the past and those mothers included have been termed 'potential diabetics'. This is now recognized as rather strong terminology since it would appear that there is no greater incidence of diabetes eventually developing within this group than one would expect in the general population, at least in the first 10 years of follow-up (Hadden 1980). Nevertheless, from an obstetrical point of view the indications traditionally used to perform a GTT have singled out a high risk group of mothers. This is self-evident, since it includes mothers with a previous unexplained perinatal death or abnormal baby, and it is not surprising that in the past the perinatal mortality in so-called 'potential diabetics' has been reported as being twice the overall hospital rate. Because these patients deserve special attention further study of their carbohydrate metabolism is still recommended. The indications for GTT usually adopted are as follows:

1   a history of diabetes in a first degree relative;
2   glycosuria on two or more occasions (second specimen taken after fasting);
3   maternal weight greater than 90 kg;
4   a previous baby weighing 4.5 kg or more;
5   a previous unexplained intrauterine death or early neonatal death;
6   congenital abnormality in a previous pregnancy.

Within this group approximately 20–25% of mothers will have an abnormal GTT. No single indication has been found to be more or less useful than another as an index of carbohydrate intolerance although when more than one indication is present an abnormal GTT is more likely (Hadden & Harley 1967).

INCIDENCE OF ABNORMAL CARBOHYDRATE METABOLISM

The incidence of diabetes in pregnancy is approximately 1 in 1000 of the overall number of pregnancies for a given population (Hadden 1980). Less than 10% of pregnant mothers will have an indication for a GTT and of these 20–25% will be abnormal. Only a small number will be so severely abnormal as to fall within the diabetic range, the vast majority being classified as impaired glucose tolerance (IGT).

PREGNANCY AND CARBOHYDRATE METABOLISM

Pregnancy alters carbohydrate metabolism, but adaptation normally occurs without adverse effect on mother or fetus. In some the maternal response to these changes is abnormal, which without careful management would lead to increased fetal risk.

Perhaps the major change is the decreased sensitivity to insulin with increasing gestation. In early pregnancy fasting serum insulin concentration and the peak achieved after a glucose load are similar to those in the non-pregnant state. These levels are higher in late pregnancy (Lind et al. 1973), and there is a tendency to postprandial hypoglycaemia. Thus, if normal glucose homeostasis is to be achieved more insulin must be secreted. Most patients have an adequate reserve of pancreatic beta cell activity, but the few who do not develop impaired glucose toler-

ance. The cause of this alteration in sensitivity is an increase in factors antagonizing the action of insulin, such as cortisol, oestrogen, progesterone and human placental lactogen (hPL), together with the degradation of insulin by the placenta.

Human placental lactogen is a glycoprotein produced by the syncytiotrophoblast (Higashi 1961, Josimovich & MacLaren 1962), and has a structure and function similar to that of growth hormone. It affects protein, fat and carbohydrate metabolism, being growth-promoting, lactogenic and luteotrophic. It plays a major role in the diabetogenic effect of pregnancy and contributes to the difficulty in controlling blood glucose in the pregnant diabetic. Thus in the insulin-dependent diabetic the dose of exogenous insulin must be increased, sometimes two or threefold as pregnancy advances, as a result of the diminished sensitivity.

Pregnancy can reveal a tendency to carbohydrate intolerance which may be expressed in the first instance by the birth of a baby weighing more than 4.5 kg. The incidence of babies weighing 4.5 kg or more is about 1.5% of all births, whilst among the children of women who later develop diabetes the figure may be as high as 30% (Pyke 1962). There is no clearcut evidence to support the idea that the proportion of heavy babies increases as the time of diagnosis draws near, suggesting that genetic factors (such as maternal age and parity) are more important than environmental factors (such as maternal hyperglycaemia). Maternal environmental factors do influence birth weight; the babies of women whose diabetes is very carefully controlled are lighter than those of similar women who are less well controlled (Pyke 1968).

Blood glucose and insulin relationships in mother and fetus

The observation by Cardell (1953) that babies dying in association with diabetic pregnancy commonly have histological evidence of pancreatic beta cell hyperplasia suggested that maternal hyperglycaemia might be affecting carbohydrate metabolism in the fetus. Furthermore surviving babies often show an increased tendency to neonatal hypoglycaemia (Baird & Farquhar 1962, Gilmer et al. 1975) and a more rapid absorption of glucose than normal (Isles et al. 1968).

In the normal pregnant woman there is a continued demand by the fetus for glucose as an energy substrate, and it crosses the placenta by facilitated diffusion. During fasting (e.g. overnight), maternal glucose may fall significantly, but in diabetes glucose levels are usually maintained and may be high without adequate insulin therapy. The fetal blood glucose concentration closely follows that of the mother, and if hyperglycaemia occurs it stimulates hypertrophy of fetal pancreatic islet cells resulting in insulin release, particularly towards the end of pregnancy. Insulin produced by the fetus is a potent stimulus to growth, causing macrosomia and organomegaly (especially of the liver) due to glycogen synthesis and increased protein synthesis and deposition of fat. Strict control of maternal glucose concentration should prevent fetal hyperinsulinaemia and result in infants of normal weight.

The effect of pregnancy on diabetes

Control. The considerable effects of pregnancy on carbohydrate metabolism, particularly the lowered renal threshold for glucose and the diminishing sensitivity to insulin as pregnancy advances, render the control of diabetes more difficult. Poor control increases the incidence of maternal and fetal complications and is the single most important factor influencing the outcome of the pregnancy.

The potentially harmful effect on the fetus of poorly controlled maternal plasma glucose underlines the importance of teamwork between the patient and an obstetrician and a physician with a special interest in diabetes in pregnancy, working together with an experienced neonatologist. The recent UK Diabetic Pregnancy Study (Lowy & Beard, unpublished data) suggests that best results have been obtained where the numbers of patients dealt with have been sufficient to allow considerable accumulation of experience. Constant availability of the team managing the pregnancy and attention to detail are of paramount importance.

Careful plasma glucose control is mandatory because of the adverse effects of hyperglycaemia and ketosis on the fetus. This is particularly difficult and needs special attention in early pregnancy when nausea and vomiting are common or when infection of any kind occurs and also during labour. Early hospitalization is essential when control becomes a problem.

Retinopathy. It is now accepted that careful ophthalmic assessment is necessary for all diabetics likely to have retinal damage and particularly for those women entering pregnancy. Less severe background retinopathy is not uncommon and should be monitored carefully.

Whilst the incidence of pregnancy complications is related to the degree of retinal damage the perinatal outcome is still relatively good. In those with proliferative retinopathy there may be progression of the lesion during pregnancy but the current policy of careful observation and prompt treatment with laser photocoagulation seems to give satisfactory results (Price *et al.* 1984). Previously proliferative diabetic retinopathy was considered a serious hazard in pregnancy in terms of maternal sight and fetal prognosis. On this basis termination of pregnancy has been considered, but this would now seem unnecessary on ophthalmic grounds alone (Hadden 1982).

Nephropathy. Diabetic nephropathy may be difficult to diagnose in pregnancy if the patient is not seen early. The signs may be confused with the hypertension and proteinuria associated with pre-eclampsia.

It is important to assess renal function since a major reduction due to established end-stage renal disease seriously affects the fetal prognosis. A creatinine clearance of less than 20 ml/min or a blood urea persistently above 30 mmol/l indicates the approach of end-stage disease, and some would advise termination of pregnancy although others would not (Hadden 1982). Renal transplantation may be available to the young diabetic with this degree of renal disease.

Surprisingly the fetal outcome in pregnant diabetics with nephropathy allows for cautious optimism, particularly if pre-eclampsia does not supervene and plasma glucose control is good. There is no evidence that pregnancy causes a permanent deterioration in renal function.

The effect of diabetes on pregnancy

SPONTANEOUS ABORTION

The incidence of spontaneous abortion may be higher in the poorly controlled diabetic; this may be attributable to the associated increase in abnormality rate.

INFECTION

Urinary tract infection is more common in pregnant diabetics than in non-diabetics (Pedersen 1977) and asymptomatic bacteriuria should be sought at booking, 28, 32 and 36 weeks. Any sign of infection must be vigorously treated with parenteral antibiotics since pyelonephritis seriously influences pregnancy outcome (Pedersen 1977). In particular, pre-existing nepropathy should be remembered as a differential diagnosis of proteinuria in the patient seen in pregnancy for the first time.

MONILIAL VAGINITIS AND VULVITIS

The increased glucose content of the vaginal epithelium and the presence of glycosuria make infection with Monilia commonplace. Awareness of this allows early recognition and treatment with nystatin or miconazole vaginal pessaries and vulval cream.

PRE-ECLAMPSIA

Pre-eclampsia has a deleterious effect on the pregnancy and may affect blood glucose control. This complication occurs in up to 8% of cases (Oakley 1965), and the perinatal mortality can be doubled, mostly due to the need for elective preterm delivery.

The difficulty of accurate diagnosis of each of the component signs of pre-eclampsia should be remembered. Hypertension (a blood pressure of 140 mmHg and 90 mmHg diastolic on two separate occasions) is more commonly encountered, and occurs in about a quarter of diabetics in early pregnancy. Oedema may be accentuated by the presence of a large baby or polyhydramnios. Proteinuria may occur as a result of urinary tract infection or diabetic nephropathy.

POLYHYDRAMNIOS

In the past polyhydramnios was found frequently, often in association with poor control, a large baby and large placenta. There is a theoretical possibility that it is caused by fetal polyuria. The amniotic fluid in diabetes has a high glucose content, but there is no direct relationship between this and the amount of liquor present.

PERINATAL DEATH

Before the use of insulin perinatal loss was over 50%, but most recent series now report a rate under 5%. The incidence of unexplained still-birth and idiopathic respiratory distress syndrome (IRDS) has fallen, but congenital abnormality has assumed greater importance. The latter is thought to be associated with the degree of plasma glucose control in the first trimester, and when this is kept as strictly controlled as possible the incidence of abnormality is said to be lower (Miller *et al.* 1981).

Unexplained stillbirth now occurs less frequently because of better control, and is thought to be due to a fetal metabolic disturbance rather than to placental insufficiency. Intrauterine death may result from an episode of hyperglycaemia in the presence of hypoxia, the combination of which leads to severe fetal acidosis (Shelley *et al.* 1975). More recently, fetal blood hyperviscosity has been suggested as a possible cause of sudden intrauterine death (Foley *et al.* 1981).

MACROSOMIA

With more rigid plasma glucose control the birthweight of infants of diabetic mothers (IDM) has decreased. If a large baby is suspected clinically or on ultrasound examination precautions should be taken to avoid prolonged labour, shoulder dystocia and traumatic delivery.

CONGENITAL MALFORMATION

The incidence of congenital malformation in diabetes is increased to about three times the expected rate and more so in those patients with poorly controlled plasma glucose levels. The commonest abnormalities encountered are those of the cardiovascular, skeletal and central nervous systems. The caudal regression syndrome, with agenesis of the sacrum and hypoplasia of the lower limbs, occurs most often in association with diabetes.

FETAL LUNG MATURITY

There is a well established relationship between maternal diabetes and neonatal idiopathic respiratory distress syndrome (Roberts *et al.* 1976, Tsang *et al.* 1981). Various explanations for this effect have been put forward such as the comparative immaturity of the baby at birth, an enhanced effect of birth asphyxia and the higher incidence of delivery by Caesarean section. There is evidence from *in vitro* studies that insulin antagonizes the action of cortisol on lecithin synthesis by cultured fetal lung cells (Smith *et al.* 1975). It has therefore been suggested that fetal hyperinsulinaemia may delay the maturation of surfactant production systems and in particular the appearance of phosphatidyl glycerol (PG). Recently this view has been challenged and it would appear that there is no such delay in the appearance of phosphatidyl choline (PC), phosphatidyl inistol (PI) and phosphatidyl glycerol (James *et al.* 1984).

Nevertheless the amniotic fluid lecithin/sphingomyelin (L/S) ratio is less reliable in predicting fetal lung maturity in diabetic women than might be expected (Dahlenburg *et al.* 1977, Mueller-Heubach *et al.* 1978). For this reason the presence of PG in amniotic fluid has been recommended as an indicator of lung maturity (Whittle *et al.* 1983) but the presence of PC (>2 mg/l) is said to be even more helpful (James *et al.* 1984)

With the advent of ultrasonic scanning, better blood glucose control and the tendency to allow pregnancy to continue towards term the incidence of IRDS has fallen.

THE PLACENTA

The placental size is closely related to the size of the baby, which in part is related to plasma glucose control. Placental function does not seem to be compromised unless hypertension or vascular complications are present, in which case intrauterine fetal growth retardation may result.

Management of pregnancy complicated by diabetes

COMBINED CARE

The best results are obtained when antenatal care is undertaken at a combined clinic where the physician and obstetrician can see the patient together. Visits are more frequent than usual, the minimum being every two weeks up to 28 weeks and weekly thereafter. If any obstetrical or diabetic complications arise it is best to admit the patient to hospital for further assessment. If, on the other hand, the pregnancy continues without complication many would now defer admission to hospital and await spontaneous labour up to 40 weeks' gestation (Drury *et al.* 1983). It cannot be overemphasized that the management of each patient needs to be tailored to her individual needs as assessed by experienced personnel.

FOOD PLAN

During pregnancy the carbohydrate content of the patient's usual food plan is increased to between 150 and 250 g per day. No restriction is placed on fat or protein intake unless weight gain is excessive.

MEDICAL CARE

The vast majority of diabetics require insulin therapy during pregnancy and even those who can be con-

trolled by diet while not pregnant are better controlled by having this therapy started; all patients should receive two daily injections of a short-acting and a longer-acting insulin. Insulin requirements usually rise progressively, and are often increased by 50–100% by term. Oral hypoglycaemic agents are almost never used, since they can cause severe neonatal hypoglycaemia, particularly the long-acting chlorpropamide.

The aim is to keep preprandial plasma glucose concentration between 4 and 6 mmol/l. This degree of control is now achieved by self-monitoring of capillary blood glucose before each meal, using an impregnated paper strip (e.g. Dextrostix, Ames Co. or BM Strips, Boehringer Ingleheim). The accuracy of these readings is improved by the use of a simple reflectance meter which may be lent by the hospital to each patient during her pregnancy. The control obtained using this method should be checked by a laboratory plasma glucose estimation at appropriate times prior to each antenatal visit. If the equipment for home monitoring is not available, or the patient is unwilling or unable to use it, a series of four preprandial plasma glucose values once a week is used to check control. The testing of urine for glucose and ketones, together with random plasma glucose estimations does not give precise enough control for management of the pregnant diabetic.

HAEMOGLOBIN A₁ (HbA₁)

Glucose influences the slow glycosylation of haemoglobin during the life cycle of the red cell so that a high HbA_1 level reflects a high average plasma glucose concentration. In non-diabetics the level is about 5%, but may be as high as 20% in newly diagnosed diabetics.

In normal subjects the HbA_1 level averages 6% throughout pregnancy. It is raised in diabetics, and although it falls as pregnancy advances it is always higher than normal (Leslie *et al.* 1978). In diabetic pregnancy the level should be as near to 6% as possible, and values above 10% should be viewed with concern.

Obstetric management

ANTENATAL

Strict control of plasma glucose around the time of conception reduces the incidence of congenital malformation (Fuhrmann *et al.* 1983), and when continued throughout pregnancy the risk of developing other complications such as pre-eclampsia, polyhydramnios, preterm labour and fetal macrosomia is reduced.

Early booking and dating of the pregnancy is important. The latter is confirmed by two ultrasonic measurements of the biparietal diameter (BPD) between 14 and 24 weeks. One measurement is usually made around the 16th week when major congenital malformation may be diagnosed, although cardiac and skeletal abnormalities are often difficult to exclude even by expert ultrasonography. Serum alpha-fetoprotein estimation may be performed at the same time.

As pregnancy progresses antenatal care should be provided at two-weekly intervals, with a view to early detection of maternal complications and assessing fetal welfare. After 24 weeks estimates of fetal growth are performed at least monthly, the most useful methods being measurement of the BPD and the trunk. If plasma glucose control is good and fetal growth follows a normal pattern, and the amniotic fluid volume is consistent with gestational age the fetal condition should be satisfactory. When doubts about the fetal condition arise further investigation is required. Measurement of oestriol and hPL to assess placental function is unsatisfactory. Of much greater value is the fetal kick chart combined with antepartum cardiotography. The use of ultrasound to make further fetal measurements and to assess fetal movement and breathing is valuable in cases of suspected fetal compromise. These procedures are described more fully in Chapter 31 (p. 448).

In late pregnancy admission to hospital at 36 weeks has been the practice until recently, but if control is good and no complications have arisen admission to hospital may be further delayed.

DELIVERY

Timing

The timing of delivery is not as rigid as heretofore, and much depends upon the patient's cooperation regarding control of her diabetes and the absence of pregnancy complications. It is now the practice to tailor the timing of delivery to the individual, and where pregnancy is apparently normal it may be allowed to continue up to 40 weeks. This practice allows many more patients to go into spontaneous labour with an improved chance of delivering vaginally (Drury *et al.* 1983). In more complicated cases delivery is usually at 38 weeks, and occasionally elec-

tive preterm delivery becomes necessary, most often because of pre-eclampsia. It is essential that the timing of delivery is made in conjunction with the neonatologist so that the special care baby unit is prepared for the infant. When delivery has been decided upon before 37 completed weeks an amniocentesis should be performed to measure the L/S ratio and assess whether PG is present or not. Where pregnancy has progressed beyond this time the procedure is unnecessary.

Mode of delivery

Formerly many diabetic women were delivered by Caesarean section, but increasingly pregnancy is allowed to continue, which has resulted in a rise in the number delivered vaginally. In most centres the Caesarean section rate is now less than 30% in primigravidas and less than 50% overall. Caesarean section may be indicated when complications dictate urgent delivery or when a malpresentation is present. Occasionally extenuating factors such as age, previous infertility or pregnancy loss may influence the decision. Caesarean section is not indicated on account of diabetes alone.

Spontaneous labour

Spontaneous labour is managed in the usual way (Chapter 24, p. 349) and the membranes ruptured to assess the amount and colour of the liquor and to permit the application of a fetal scalp electrode. If progress is slow despite acceleration with oxytocin, Caesarean section is indicated. Fetal distress and acidosis confirmed by fetal scalp pH require prompt action. During the second stage difficult forceps delivery should be avoided and the possibility of shoulder dystocia remembered if the fetus is large.

Induction of labour

On the morning of induction half the usual insulin dose is given and an intravenous infusion of 5% dextrose is set up to run at a rate of 500 ml every 4 hours. A plasma glucose estimation is performed, and capillary blood glucose levels checked hourly thereafter by the labour ward staff, using a reflectance meter. Rapid-acting insulin may be added to the infusion (6 units per 500 ml) or given via motorized syringe at 1–2 units per hour as required.

If the cervix is favourable induction is best carried out by artificial rupture of the membranes and intravenous oxytocin. Internal fetal heart rate monitoring is mandatory. When the cervix is less favourable induction with a 3 mg prostaglandin E_2 vaginal tablet at 0700 hours is more convenient, in which case the fetal heart rate should be monitored externally. The aim is to achieve delivery within 12 hours as plasma glucose control becomes increasingly difficult thereafter. Failure to progress quickly enough is therefore a common indication for Caesarean section in labour.

Caesarean section

Insulin therapy is managed in the same way as that already described for induction of labour, and elective Caesarean section is carried out at 0900 hours; intravenous dextrose and insulin are continued until oral fluids are restarted. Epidural analgesia, which is useful in the management of spontaneous and induced labour, is particularly effective as there is less interference with peristalsis postoperatively, and oral feeding can begin almost immediately. Insulin requirements usually fall rapidly after delivery and the patient can be commenced on her prepregnancy regimen which is adjusted as necessary.

Preterm labour

Preterm labour is nearly twice as common among diabetic mothers as in the general hospital population. After 34 weeks there is little point in attempting to stop labour with beta adrenoceptor agonists. Indeed, before 34 weeks the potential hazard of such drugs in combination with corticosteroids, together with their effect on plasma glucose by causing hyperglycaemia suggests there is little place for their use in diabetic patients in preterm labour. If they must be used, an amniocentesis to check that the L/S ratio is less than 2 provides a reason to continue their use. To counteract the effect on plasma glucose it is suggested that up to 20 units per hour of insulin may be required during treatment (Barnett *et al.* 1980).

POSTPARTUM CARE

Care of the mother

Insulin requirements fall rapidly in the first few days of the puerperium and doses should be titrated against the results of frequent glucometer readings.

Food intake may need to be adjusted by the dietician. Breast feeding is more commonly practised now and an increase of 50 g in carbohydrate in the daily food plan is suggested (Whichelow & Dodderidge 1983).

Care of the baby

It is now unusual to encounter the overweight plethoric infant of the diabetic mother (IDM) with rounded face, buried eyes and abundant hair and in which all the organs except the brain are enlarged excessively. When such a baby is born maternal control must be questioned, since the most constant feature is the increased number, size and granularity of pancreatic islet cells (Cardell 1953). The plethoric appearance is due to polycythaemia, and mild degrees of this may be present in the baby who is not particularly overweight. For this reason it is unwise to strip the umbilical cord of blood into the baby at delivery, a procedure which only serves to increase the polycythaemia. The high viscosity resulting from this condition can cause vascular problems in the infant, and exchange transfusion is indicated if the haematrocrit is greater than 65%.

Respiratory system. The IDM does not withstand birth asphyxia well and this may precipitate or exacerbate the IRDS which is six times more common than usual in IDM (Roberts *et al.* 1976) because of delayed surfactant maturation, a situation compounded by the fact that immature surfactant is unstable in the presence of birth asphyxia. The incidence of IRDS appears to have decreased in keeping with better control of maternal plasma glucose and later delivery.

Transient tachypnoea of the newborn (TTN) also occurs more frequently, possibly in association with the high incidence of delivery by Caesarean section. The condition is unrelated to gestational age and, although initially presenting in a similar manner, has characteristic lung changes on X-ray and normally settles within 6–12 hours.

Hypoglycaemia. A low blood glucose concentration 60 minutes after birth is common and it usually rises gradually over the next 6 hours. Asymptomatic hypoglycaemia can occur in 14% of IDM, while a further 12% may have symptoms (Essex *et al.* 1973). Symptomatic hypoglycaemia may be expected when maternal control has been poor or when sulphonylurea drugs (which cross the placenta) have been used.

Blood glucose may be as low as 0.25 mmol/l by 2 hours after birth, rising to 1.1 mmol/l by 4 hours of age. All infants should have capillary blood glucose checked by reflectance meter at 2, 4, 6 and 12 hours of age, and if less than 2.5 mmol/l a laboratory measurement of capillary blood glucose should be done. Any infant developing symptoms or with a capillary blood glucose 1.4 mmol/l or less by 4 hours of age should have an intravenous infusion of 10% dextrose.

Feeding should begin by 2 hours of age and continue at three to four hour intervals.

Hyperbilirubinaemia. About 25% of IDM have at least one serum biluribin value over 170 mmol/l. Bruising, polycythaemia, IRDS and prematurity predispose to jaundice, whereas early feeding reduces the incidence of jaundice and the degree of hyperbilirubinaemia. Vitamin K 1 mg is given intramuscularly at birth and phenobarbitone (2.5–5 mg/kg daily in three divided doses) orally if severe bruising is present. Phototherapy is used if the bilirubin concentration is greater than 170 mmol/l and rising. Exchange transfusion is indicated if the level continues to rise.

The mean packed cell volume (PCV) is high in IDM and when severely polycythaemic the infant may appear plethoric and develop fits, heart failure and IRDS; treatment by plasma exchange is required. Capillary haematocrit (which is 15% higher than venous) should be checked at 2 hours of age.

Hypocalcaemia. This is more common in infants who are hypoglycaemic and acidotic and may cause neuromuscular excitability, apnoeic spells and fits.

General. Serum calcium, magnesium, blood glucose and PCV should be estimated in any IDM with hypotonia, irritability, cyanotic attacks or convulsions. Intracranial haemorrhage should also be excluded.

OTHER ASPECTS

Pre-pregnancy counselling
Diabetic clinics and general practitioners should be made aware of the advice to offer the young non-pregnant diabetic woman, since good diabetic control at the time of conception and in the first trimester leads to a decrease in the congenital abnormality rate (Miller *et al.* 1981). Those diabetic patients contemplating pregnancy should be instructed in the technique of home monitoring of capillary blood glucose and control should be good before trying to conceive. This may be checked by estimation of HbA_1, which should be less than 10%.

Contraception
Uncomplicated diabetes is not a contraindication to the combined contraceptive pill but it is suggested that the progesterone-only pill might be preferable (Oakley & Beard 1975). Although the pill marginally impairs carbohydrate tolerance it does not usually increase insulin requirements.

A diabetic woman has to take more care of her health than others, and a large family should be discouraged. Most are content with two or three children, with permanent contraception in the form of sterilization thereafter. The risk to offspring of becoming a diabetic in later life is abut 1 in 100, which compares to the risk of 1 in 1000 of any child developing IDD in the general population, and is not in itself a valid reason for advising family restriction.

Contraindications to pregnancy
Serious complications of diabetes such as retinitis proliferans and nephropathy are grounds for advising against becoming pregnant. They are not grounds for termination of pregnancy, except in the worst cases. Minor degrees of retinopathy are often present in patients with long-standing diabetes and do not usually have any prognostic importance for pregnancy.

Management of impaired glucose tolerance (IGT)
Plasma glucose control, as judged by serial measurement, is maintained within the normal range. This can often be achieved by adjusting the patient's diet but occasionally insulin therapy may be required. The decision to use insulin in such patients is normally based on plasma glucose results.

The same care afforded to patients with IDD should be given to patients with IGT (whether or not they are receiving insulin) even though the incidence of complications and the perinatal mortality is less. It is the practice not to allow the pregnancy to go beyond 40 weeks' gestation.

Management of 'potential diabetes'
As has been suggested earlier, patients who have been selected for a GTT because of the given criteria constitute a high risk obstetrical group. Those with an abnormal GTT are treated as already suggested. Those with a normal GTT require little interference other than attentive antenatal care, but it is usual to place those who are obese on a 1500 calorie diet. Pregnancy is not normally allowed to go beyond 40 weeks' gestation.

THYROID DISORDERS IN PREGNANCY

The control of thyroid activity

Thyroid disease in pregnancy can affect both mother and fetus. In normal pregnancy maternal thyroid function is altered, with an increase in gland size, a rise in basal metabolic rate and, under the influence of oestrogen, an increase in total serum thyroxine concentration due to the increase in thyroxine-binding globulin. The thyroid uptake and clearance of iodide is increased, matched by an increased renal iodide clearance. The placenta produces thyroid stimulating hormone (Tunbridge & Hall 1975), which may explain the increased thyroid stimulating activity of plasma in pregnant women and the increase in gland size.

The thyroid gland synthesizes and releases thyroxine (T_4) and tri-iodothyronine (T_3). Of the two substances T_3 is approximately three times more potent than T_4 and is less firmly bound to plasma proteins. It seems likely that most of the T_3 in the blood arises from the peripheral conversion of T_4 and that T_3 is the metabolically active thyrooid hormone at cellular level. The formation of these two hormones by the thyroid is normally under the control of the pituitary through thyroid stimulating hormone (TSH). This in turn is secreted under the influence of a tripeptide releasing hormone (TRH) formed in the hypothalamus and transported to the anterior pituitary via the portal vessels. The action of TRH on the pituitary and the release of TSH are inhibited by T_3 and T_4 so that a feedback controlling mechanism operates which keeps the secretion of TSH constant under normal conditions. Radioimmunoassay of plasma TSH shows raised levels in patients with primary hypothyroidism and undetectable levels in patients with hypothyroidism secondary to pituitary disease. In thyrotoxicosis, plasma TSH is almost always undetectable, confirming the importance of abnormal thyroid stimulators or autonomous hyperfunction as the main factors in this disorder. Hyperthyroid Graves' disease, an organ-specific autoimmune disease, is probably due to autoantibodies which, by binding in the region of the thyroid follicular cell thyrotrophin receptor, stimulate thyroid function (Adams 1980). These thyroid specific immunoglobulins (TSI) will cross the placenta and are the cause of transient neonatal hyperthyroidism in infants of mothers with this form of hyperthyroidism.

Thyroid function in pregnancy

Circulating thyroxine is strongly associated with plasma binding proteins and free plasma hormone makes up only a small fraction of the total circulating level. The major binding protein is thyroxine binding globulin (TBG), whose production by the liver is increased when the blood oestrogen level rises. When this happens in pregnancy (or on oestrogen therapy, e.g. the contraceptive pill) the proportion of protein-bound thyroxine rises and that of free thyroxine falls. The feedback mechanism now comes into play with an increase in TRH activity and TSH production by the anterior pituitary. This, in turn, leads to thyroid hyperplasia and a consequent return of the free thyroxine level to normal although the protein-bound thyroxine level remains above the normal level. Thus, the free thyroxine available to the tissues is unaltered by pregnancy in spite of the hyperplasia of the gland and the raised protein-bound thyroxine. Enlargement and increased vascularity of the thyroid is common in normal pregnancy. The basal metabolic rate rises after twelve weeks and increases to 20% above normal by the last trimester. This rise is attributed to oxygen consumption by the fetus rather than to an increase in maternal metabolism.

ASSESSMENT OF FUNCTION

Mild forms of hyperthyroidism in pregnancy are difficult to diagnose because pregnancy itself may lead to thyroid enlargement, tachycardia, emotional lability, warm extremities and increased pulse pressure.

A raised concentration of serum-free thyroxine is indicative of thyrotoxicosis but low levels are less reliable in the diagnosis of hypothyroidism; thus the TSH level should also be measured. In all cases the results of laboratory investigations need to be interpreted carefully in the light of the clinical findings and physical signs such as weight loss or failure to gain weight, heat intolerance, high sleeping pulse rate or exophthalmos should not be overlooked.

Table 20.3. Thyroid disase in pregnancy.

1	Simple (non-toxic) goitre
2	Hyperthyroidism
3	Hypothyroidism
4	Other thyroid enlargements

A classification of thyroid disease in pregnancy is given in Table 20.3.

A diffuse enlargement of the thyroid gland occurs normally in pregnancy. Nodular goitres usually enlarge but do not need treatment unless thyroid function is altered or obstructive symptoms appear. Haemorrhage into a cyst, hypothyroidism and malignant change may also be present and require further investigation and treatment.

Hyperthyroidism

Hyperthyroidism is nearly as common as diabetes in pregnancy, but there is no evidence that the overactivity is made worse by pregnancy. Fertility may be impaired and abortion more common when the disease is untreated. Graves' disease is the most usual form encountered, but toxic nodular goitre may occur.

Treatment of the disease in pregnancy carries extra risks, and the choice lies between antithyroid drugs, with or without thyroid hormone replacement, and subtotal thyroidectomy.

Surgery is rarely indicated when medical treatment has failed because too large doses have to be used, the patient is unwilling or unable to comply or toxic reaction to antithyroid drugs occurs. Subtotal thyroidectomy is also indicated when obstructive symptoms arise due to a large goitre. Pre-operative preparation with antithyroid drugs, iodides and propranolol is necessary, and surgery, while relatively safe in the first two trimesters, may precipitate premature labour in the last trimester and for this reason may be deferred.

Medical treatment with antithyroid drugs is the more usual course, but the place of thyroxine replacement is controversial, though both regimens appear to achieve good results. Carbimazole, which acts by blocking thyroid hormone synthesis, is the drug of choice, 30 mg daily being given initially, decreasing to 20 mg daily or less once control has been achieved. Propranolol is occasionally used for a short time to control the peripheral effects of the disease. Propylthiouracil is an alternative drug to carbimazole. Thyroxine (0.1–0.2 mg daily) may be used to keep the mother euthyroid. Both drugs can be reduced and usually stopped before delivery as hyperthyroidism usually becomes milder towards the end of pregnancy. The principle of treatment is to use the smallest dose necessary to maintain a normal maternal concentration of free thyroxine. Serial TSH measurement is also useful, a rise indicating overtreatment.

Antithyroid drugs cross the placenta and may cause abortion, hypothyroidism and goitre in the fetus. They are excreted in very small amounts in breast milk, and breastfeeding is usually contraindicated.

If the euthyroid state has been maintained throughout pregnancy the infant may be expected to be normal. Maternal pretibial myxoedema and exophthalmos are associated with the presence of thyroid stimulating immunoglobulins which can cause exophthalmos, a goitre and congenital thyrotoxicosis in the infant. All infants should be examined carefully for hyperthyroidism, which if present usually remits within four to six weeks when maternal immunoglobulins are eliminated from the neonate's circulation. When neonatal symptoms are severe propranolol is now the treatment of choice (Pemberton et al. 1974).

Medical treatment of hyperthyroidism carries some fetal risk even when the disease is well controlled. In one study of 53 pregnancies so treated four infants were lost (7.5%), three of whom had major congenital abnormalities, giving a corrected loss of 1.8%. Another three infants had goitre and neonatal Graves' disease (Montgomery & Harley 1977).

It is uncertain whether there is a real increase in congenital abnormalities, but growth and psychological development in children born to mothers treated with carbimazole is normal (McCarroll et al. 1976). A higher than expected incidence of low birth-weight infants has been reported (Niswander & Gordon 1972).

Hypothyroidism

Women with serious hypothyroidism rarely conceive, and the incidence of abortion and stillbirth is increased. Pregnancy may occur in the presence of mild thyroid insufficiency (diagnosed on TSH measurement), during which the symptoms improve. Substitution therapy with thyroxine should be given, and adjusted to achieve normal thyroid function assessed by clinical and biochemical methods. Information about the long-term outlook for children of hypothyroid mothers is imprecise, but it is suggested that a normal infant should be expected (Ect & Doss 1963, Montgomery & Harley 1977).

Other thyroid enlargements

HASHIMOTO'S DISEASE

Autoimmune thyroid disease can be differentiated from simple goitre by the finding of antibodies to thyroglobulin and thyroid microsomes in high titre in the patient's serum. Although these antibodies can cross the placenta they do not seem to affect the fetal thyroid. The importance of making the diagnosis in the pregnant woman is that the characteristic firm enlargement of the gland can be reduced without the need for surgery by the administration of adequate amounts of thyroxine.

THYROIDITIS

Subacute thyroiditis rarely complicates pregnancy but when it does hyperthyroidism or less commonly hypothyroidism can occur. Treatment involves administration of corticosteroids, but antithyroid drugs and thyroxine may be required.

ENDEMIC GOITRE

Endemic goitre and cretinism is found in areas of iodine deficiency, e.g. the Andes, the Congo, the Himalayas and New Guinea. Treatment of mothers with iodized salt or with an injection of iodized oil intramuscularly reduces the incidence of sequelae, particularly of congenital hypothyroidsm in the infant.

ADRENAL GLAND DISORDERS

The normal response of the maternal adrenal gland to pregnancy and the disorders which affect it have been reviewed by Montgomery and Harley (1977). The two major adrenal cortex steroids, cortisol and aldosterone, are produced in increased quantities from the enlarged adrenal gland during pregnancy via cholesterol, progesterone and $17\alpha OH$ progesterone.

Much of the cortisol rise is due to an increase in binding globulin under the influence of oestrogen, but free cortisol also increases. Central obesity, striae formation and glucose intolerance may in part be due to the effect of cortisol. Aldosterone concentration increases markedly after the 16th week, partly in response to a rise in plasma renin. Catecholamine production and metabolism remain unchanged in pregnancy. Disorders of the adrenal cortex in pregnancy are rare and include adrenal failure (Addison's disease) and excessive secretion (Cushing's syndrome). Disorders of the adrenal medulla include excessive catecholamine secretion from a phaechromocytoma.

Adrenocortical hyperfunction

CUSHING'S SYNDROME

Excessive adrenal activity (due to adenoma or carcinoma of the adrenal cortex, or bilateral adrenal hyperplasia with an ACTH-secreting pituitary tumour) is rarely compatible with pregnancy. Hypertension is the major hazard, and the incidence of abortion, placental insufficiency, intrauterine death and premature labour is high (Grimes et al. 1973). Successful management with metyrapone, a drug inhibiting adrenal cortisol production, has been achieved in a pregnancy associated with an active adrenal adenoma (Gormley et al. 1982).

In treated cases hydrocortisone therapy will be given in the same way as in cases of adrenal insufficiency.

CONGENITAL ADRENAL HYPERPLASIA

Children with congenital virilizing adrenal hyperplasia have been successfully treated now for some years, and an increasing number of these patients are becoming pregnant. The condition is commonly due to 21-hydroxylase deficiency (or less commonly 11-hydroxylase deficiency) and treatment with prednisone 5 mg at night and 2.5 mg in the morning suppresses the overproduction of ACTH which originally caused the inappropriate androgen excess.

In these patients treatment is continued throughout pregnancy with supplementary steroid cover being given during labour as discussed later. Mothers with congenital adrenal hypoplasia have a 1 in 4 risk of passing the condition on to the fetus, but prenatal diagnosis is available by demonstrating an excess of 17-hydroxyprogesterone in amniotic fluid at amniocentesis at 16–18 weeks' gestation.

Adrenocortical hypofunction

ADDISON'S DISEASE

Pregnancy is rare in the untreated state. If it does occur, Addison's disease carries serious maternal risk as a result of vomiting in early pregnancy, infections and the stress of labour.

Most treated cases are now due to autoimmune disease, and pregnancy does not carry a significant risk to mother or fetus. Therapy consists of a daily replacement dose of hydrocortisone 30 mg with a small maintenance dose (0.1 mg) of 9-α-flurohydrocortisone. Parenteral supplementation is required when vomiting occurs, particularly in the three special circumstances mentioned previously.

Suppression of fetal ACTH and hence adrenal insufficiency at birth has not been observed with replacement doses of cortisol (Montgomery & Harley 1977). When given in addition to normal maternal adrenal function such doses cause a decrease in fetal adrenal precursor production resulting in a fall in maternal oestriol production (Ohrlander *et al.* 1975). Delivery of the mother should be by the vaginal route unless obstetrical complications supervene, but it should be borne in mind that an increased incidence of low birthweight has been reported in infants of mothers with Addison's disease (Osler 1962).

The administration of corticosteroids in pregnancy

Patients who are receiving large doses of corticosteroids for serious medical conditions such as rheumatoid arthritis, bronchial asthma or collagen diseases can safely continue to do so when they become pregnant. With the increased output of endogenous corticosteroids as pregnancy advances the dose of administered hormone can often be decreased as the medical condition improves. It should not be drastically reduced or withdrawn, however, because the patient's adrenals may then fail to respond adequately when faced with stress, for example in labour. The slow recovery of normal adrenal function after a course of administered corticosteroids means that patients who have received such a course of treatment in the preceding twelve months should be given hydrocortisone cover in labour. If more than a year has elapsed, such treatment is unnecessary but careful watch should be kept on any patient who has had previous corticosteroid therapy in times of stress. Unexplained failure to respond to such stress calls for the immediate administration of hydrocortisone. The dose normally given is hydrocortisone 50 mg intramuscularly and 50 mg six hourly thereafter for 24 h.

A few cases of cleft palate and hare lip have been reported in infants of mothers receiving corticosteroids (Davis & Plotz 1956) and for this reason corticosteroids should be given in early pregnancy only for serious medical problems. In practice the normal daily doses of corticosteroids (50–100 mg hydrocortisone or 5–20 mg prednisolone) constitute a

very small additional risk of congenital abnormality and can safely be continued in early pregnancy if the medical condition makes it desirable.

Adrenal medulla

PHAEOCHROMOCYTOMA

This tumour of the adrenal medulla is rare, but may develop or become active in pregnancy, when it carries a high risk of fatality for both mother (48%) and fetus (58%) (Shenker & Chowers 1971). The diagnosis should always be suspected in those with sustained or intermittent hypertension. Convulsions, or symptoms due to the metabolic effects of adrenaline mimicking thyrotoxicosis, diabetes mellitus or an anxiety state may occur. A 24-hour collection of urine for catecholamine metabolites and plasma for catecholamine concentration should be carried out before commencing treatment for serious hypertension, particularly when episodic. Other symptoms include skin pallor, sweating, palpitations, epigastric pain and chest discomfort. The episodes may be triggered by exercise, loin palpation or labour. Treatment of prolonged episodes of hypertension requires initial alpha blockade with phentolamine followed by beta blockade with propranolol. Surgical removal is recommended, and can be performed safely during pregnancy.

PITUITARY DISORDERS

Functioning and non-functioning adenomas and deficiency of one or more pituitary trophic hormones may rarely be encountered during pregnancy. The prolactin-secreting adenoma, which may be large or small, is now the most common pituitary problem in pregnancy. This has arisen because adenomas producing prolactin, although causing the amenorrhoea-galactorrhoea syndrome and infertility, may be treated and normal pregnancy achieved. Microadenomas have been treated successfully with bromocriptine, and in over 1200 pregnancies there has been no increase in the rate of abortion, multiple conception or congenital abnormality when compared to the normal population (Griffith *et al.* 1978, McGregor & Ginsberg 1981).

Careful follow-up by serial serum prolactin tests and observation of the visual fields for clinical signs of pituitary fossa enlargement during pregnancy is essential. In most centres treatment with bromocriptine is continued into the later stages of pregnancy in an attempt to avoid this risk, and the dose is titrated against the prolactin concentration. Alternative methods of treatment (hypophysectomy or radiotherapy) have been used for larger tumours, but fertility is not as commonly restored. If pregnancy does occur in the presence of a prolactinoma the risk of expansion is present and great care is required throughout.

ACKNOWLEDGEMENTS

The help of Professor J.M.G. Harley and Dr D.R. Hadden in the preparation of this chapter is gratefully acknowledged.

REFERENCES

ADAMS D.D. (1958) *J. clin. Endocr. Metab.*, **18**, 699.

BAIRD J.D. & FARQUHAR J.W. (1962) *Lancet*, **i**, 71.

BARNETT A.H., STUBBS S.M. & MANDER A.M. (1980) *Diabetologia*, **18**, 365.

BEARD R.W. & HOET J.J. (1982) *Diabetologia*, **23**, 307.

BEST C.H. (1945) *Can. med. J.* **III**, 204.

CARDELL B.S. (1953) *J. Path. Bact.*, **66**, 335.

DAHLENBURG G.W., MARTIN F.I.R., JEFFREY P.E. & HORACEK I. (1977) *Brit. J. Obstet. Gynaec.* **84**, 294.

DAVIS M.E. & PLOTZ E.J. (1956) *Obstet. Gynec. Surv.*, **2**, 1.

DRURY M.I., STRONGE J.M., FOLEY M.E. & MACDONALD D.W. (1983) *Obstet. Gynec. N.Y.*, **62**, 279.

ECT C.R. & DOSS J.F. (1963) *Obstet. Gynec., N.Y.*, **22**, 615.

ESSEX N.L., PYKE D.A., WATKINS P.J., BRUDENELL J.M. & GAMSU H.R. (1973) *Brit. med. J.*, **4**, 89.

FOLEY M.E., COLLINS R. STRONGE J.M., DRURY M.I. & MACDONALD D. (1981) *J. Obstet. Gynaecol.*, **2**, 93.

FUHRMANN K., REIHER H., SEMMLER K., FISCHER F., FISCHER M. & GLÖCKNER E. (1983) *Diabetes Care*, **6**, 219.

GILMER M.D.G., BEARD R.W., BROOKE F.M. & OAKLEY N. (1975) *Brit. med. J.*, **iii**, 399.

GORMLEY M.J., HADDEN D.R., KENNEDY T.L., MONTGOMERY D.A.D., MURNAGHAN G.A. & SHERIDAN B. (1982) *Clin. Endocrin.*, **16**, 283.

GRIFFITH R.W., Turkalj I. & BRAUN P. (1978) *Brit. J. clin. Pharmac.*, **5**, 227.

GRIMES E.M., FAYEZ J.A. & MILLER G.L. (1973) *Obstet. Gynec., N.Y.*, **42**, 550.

HADDEN D.R. (1980) *Diabetes Care*, **3**, 440.

HADDEN D.R. (1982) *Clin. Obstet. Gynec.*, **9**, 29.

HADDEN D.R. & HARLEY J.M.G. (1967) *J. Obstet. Gynaec. Brit. Cwlth.*, **74**, 669.

HARLEY J.M.G. & MONTGOMERY D.A.D. (1965) *Brit. med. J.*, **i**, 14.

HIGASHI K. (1961) *Endocr. Jap.*, **7**, 288.

ISLES T.E., DICKSON M. & FARQUHAR J.W. (1968) *Paediat. Res.*, **2**, 198.

JAMES D.K., CHISWICK M.L., HARKES A., WILLIAMS M. & TINDALL V.R. (1984) *Brit. J. Obstet. Gynaec.*, **91**, 325.

JOSIMOVICH J.B. & MacLAREN J.A. (1962) *Endocrinology*, **71**, 209.

LESLIE R.G.D., JOHN P.N., PYKE D.A. & WHITE J.M. (1978) *Lancet*, **ii**, 958.

LIND T., BILLIEWICS W.Z. & BROWN G. (1973) *J. Obstet. Gynaec. Brit. Cwlth.*, **80**, 1033.

McCARROLL A.M., HUTCHINSON M., McAULEY R. & MONTGOMERY D.A.D. (1976) *Arch. Dis. Child.*, **51**, 532.

McGREGOR A.M. & GINSBERG J. (1981) *Brit. J. Hosp. Med.*, **25**, 344.

MILLER E., HARE J.W., CLOHERTY J.P., DUNN P.J., GLEASON R.E., SOELDER J.S. & KITZMILLER J.L. (1981) *N. Engl. J. Med.*, **304**, 1331.

MONTGOMERY D.A.D. & HARLEY J.M.G. (1977) *Clin. Obstet. Gynaec.*, **4**, 339.

MUELLER-HEUBACH E., CARITAS S.N., EDELSTONE D.I. & TURNER J.H. (1978) *Amer. J. Obstet. Gynec.*, **130**, 28.

NISWANDER K.R. & GORDON M. (1972) *The Women and their Pregnancies*, p. 246. W.B. Saunders, Philadelphia.

OAKLEY W.G. (1965) On the nature and treatment of Diabetes, p. 673. Excerpta Medical Foundation, Amsterdam.

OAKLEY N.W. & BEARD R.W. (1975) In *Early Diabetes in Early Life* (Proceedings 3rd International Symposium Madeira 1974) (Camerini-Davalos R.A. & Cole H.S. eds.), p. 345. Academic Press, New York.

OHRLANDER S.A.V., GENNSER G.M. & GRENNERT L. (1975) *Amer. J. Obstet. Gynec.*, **123**, 228.

OSLER M.J. (1962) *Acta Endocrin.*, **41**, 67.

O'SULLIVAN J.M. & MAHAN C.M. (1964) *Diabetes*, **13**, 278.

PEDERSEN J. (1977) *The Pregnant Diabetic and her Newborn*, 2nd ed., p. 101. Munksgaard, Copenhagen.

PEEL J. (1962) *Amer. J. Obstet. Gynec.*, **53**, 847.

PEMBERTON P.J., McCONNELL B. & SHANKS R.G. (1974) *Arch. Dis. Child.*, **49**, 813.

PRICE J.H., HADDEN, D.R., ARCHER D.B. & HARLEY J.M.G. (1984) *Brit. J. Obstet. Gynaec.*, **91**, 11.

PYKE D.A. (1962) *Disorders of Carbohydrate Metabolism*. Pitman, London.

PYKE D.A. (1968) In *Clinical Diabetes* (Oakley W.G., Pyke D.A. & Taylor K.W. eds), Ch. 9. Blackwell Scientific Publications, Oxford.

ROBERTS M.F., NEFF R.K., HUBBELL J.P., TAEUSCH H.W. & AVERY M.E. (1976) *N. Engl. J. Med.*, **294**, 357.

SHELLEY H.J., BASSETT J.M. & MILNER R.D.G. (1975) *Brit. med. Bull.*, **31**, 37.

SHENKER J.G. & CHOWERS I. (1971) *Obstet. Gynec. Surv.*, **26**, 739.

SMITH B.T., GIROUD C.J.P., ROBERT M. & AVERY M.E. (1975) *J. Pediatr.*, **87**, 953.

TSANG R.C., BALLARD J. & BRAM C. (1981) *Clin. Obstet. Gynec.*, **24**, 125.

TUNBRIDGE W.G.M. & HALL R. (1975) *Clin. Obstet. Gynec.*, **2**, 381.

WHICHELOW M.J. & DODDERIDGE M.C. (1983) *Brit. med. J.*, **287**, 649.

WHITE P. (1965) Pregnancy and Diabetes. Medical Aspects. *Medical Clinics of North America*, **49**, 1015.

WHITTLE M.M., WILSON, A.I. & WHITFIELD C.R. (1983) *Brit. J. Obstet. Gynaec.*, **90**, 134.

World Health Organisation Expert Committee on Diabetes Mellitus (1980) Technical Report Series 646. WHO, Geneva.

WILLIAMS J.W. (1909) *Amer. med. J. Science.*, **137**, 1.

CHAPTER 21
IMMUNOLOGICAL DISORDERS IN PREGNANCY

J.S. SCOTT

INTRODUCTION

In the last few decades there has been a gradual realization that in most human biology and pathology, immunological factors or systems are involved. Confusion has existed, and still does to some extent, as to what constitutes an immunological disease. It is now appreciated that in very many diseases, deviations of measurable immunological factors from normal are merely Nature's response to the disease and do not indicate it is primarily an immunological disorder.

Because of concern to overcome the barrier to organ transplant between immunologically different individuals, many scientists have concentrated their attention on pregnancy as this apparently represents a successful natural 'graft' upon the mother of the fetus and placenta which possess 50% 'foreign' antigens derived from the father: a semi-allograft. How Nature has apparently abrogated the laws of tissue immunology to allow pregnancy to be successful is still not entirely clear. At least some of the evidence suggests that the delay in getting an answer is due to the wrong question having been asked. It may be more appropriate to consider to what extent tissue immunology is essential to the occurrence of successful pregnancy.

There are a number of specific immunological disorders related to pregnancy and of these the best known is Rhesus sensitization which is dealt with in Chapter 18 on 'Blood Disorders'. This highlights the demarcation problems. Rhesus disease is a precisely defined immunological disorder but its effects are almost all mediated through the blood system.

Iso(allo)immunity refers to the development of immunological reactions to an antigen not carried by the individual concerned but by other members of the same species. Rhesus sensitization induced by pregnancy or blood transfusion is the classic example of an isoimmune disease. There is no basic disorder of the immune system itself, it is a normal response to a foreign antigen.

Autoimmunity refers to inappropriate immunological responses to antigens carried by the individual concerned; Graves' disease and myasthenia gravis are examples. Usually there is an abnormal response to a range of antigens rather than a single one as is common in isoimmunity. Autoimmunity, unlike isoimmunity, usually represents a disorder of the immune system which permits the unfavourable immunological response.

In this chapter a general review will be given of iso(allo)immunity considering the ways in which it may be detrimental or beneficial to pregnancy. Autoimmunity will be considered in relation to the way the diseases may have detrimental effects on pregnancy and also how observations in pregnancy can contribute to elucidating the mechanisms of such diseases. Finally, attention will be given to pregnancy disorders which may have an immunological basis but for which scientific proof is currently lacking.

ISO(ALLO)IMMUNITY

Rhesus sensitization remains the outstanding example of iso(allo)immunity and it serves as a model for other forms. The Rhesus negative host is challenged by the Rhesus antigen which she herself does not possess and responds by antibody formation. In reproductive terms, the challenge is usually from a fetus which carries the positive antigen determined by a paternal gene. It may also be as a consequence of transfusion. The initial response is with an IgM antibody which does not cross the placenta but later there is usually IgG production and this does cross to the fetus. The time scale is such that the sensitizing event may be so late in pregnancy that noxious IgG is not produced, or not at significant levels, until after the confinement. A subsequent fetus, if it possesses the relevant antigen, will be likely to be affected by the antibody. Furthermore it may be that a Rhesus positive fetus will itself lead to increased antibody production by causing further sensitization.

In fact the most dramatic events in the history of the subspecialty now referred to as 'reproductive immunology' have been the unfolding of the story of Rhesus sensitization, uniting under a single cause the various disparate forms of haemolytic disease of the newborn and erythroblastosis fetalis and the development of means of prevention of Rhesus sensitization by the administration of anti-D gamma globulin (*see* Tovey & Moroni 1976 for review).

The question arises in considering Rhesus disease as to why iso(allo)immune pathology appears to be confined to reactions to red blood cells and to a very small group of closely related antigens. The answer is that iso(allo)immune reactions are not nearly as restricted as is often imagined. They do occur to a much wider range of antigens carried on blood cells. Platelet iso(allo)immunity occurs which has entirely predictable effects producing a simulation of Rhesus disease but on the platelet system; sophisticated techniques are required to differentiate it from autoimmune thrombocytopenia (see later).

Iso(allo)immunity also occurs to leucocyte antigens and the sera used for detecting various HLA (human leucocyte associated) antigens are mainly derived from pregnant women sensitized to a paternally derived antigen carried by a fetus. However, only rarely do these white cell antibodies produce any demonstrable effect upon the child.

Iso(allo)immunity can also occur to humoral substances which are antigenic such as specific allotypes of antibody carried by the child and not the mother but these also are of little or no pathological significance.

AUTOIMMUNE DISEASE

Knowledge of the mechanisms of many autoimmune diseases has expanded and still is expanding as a consequence of observations made when the diseases occur in pregnancy. The recording of the improvement in pregnancy of rheumatoid arthritis, now known to be an autoimmune disease, led to the development of corticosteroid therapy 40 years ago. Pregnancy also provides an opportunity to discover if an IgG antibody is involved in the pathological process. IgA and IgM molecules do not cross the placenta whereas IgG ones do. This is not merely a question of molecular size but is related to molecular configuration with a 'key' specificity analogous to a Yale lock. Trophoblast carries receptors to which the Fc portion of the IgG molecule may attach and antibody transfer follows from this.

If a patient with an autoimmune disease mediated by an IgG antibody is pregnant, the child may show effects of the disease provided the child carries the relevant antigen. The degradation time of IgG is about 3 months so it would be expected that any effects on the baby would be likely to diminish in the early weeks of life. If the antibodies have produced irreversible tissue damage, however, the effects may rarely be permanent. Effects may sometimes not be obvious until some time after birth: if drugs given to treat the mother have also crossed the placenta exerting a protective effect initially but having a shorter half-life than the antibody; or if the mechanism requires some other exogenous influences such as ultraviolet light to produce full expression of the pathology.

Pregnancy can thus be regarded as an experimental model (Fig. 21.1). Nature programmes the experiments in a capricious way but otherwise it is an excellent system because, being human, the findings apply to humans and a single observation on it may be superior to very many on animals.

With dizygotic twins, one fetus may carry the relevant antigen and show disease effects while the other lacks it and is unaffected. If the disease involves a specific organ, surgical removal of that organ from the mother may alter the whole picture; she may still

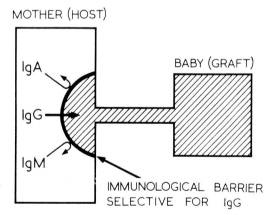

Fig. 21.1. A schematic representation of the situation which exists in pregnancy with the feto-placental system represented as a graft on the mother. The placenta is a barrier to IgA and IgM but not to IgG antibodies. IgG-mediated diseases may result in an effect of the antibody being exerted on the baby *in utero*. This will usually disappear gradually in the weeks after birth as degradation of the passively transferred IgG takes place. Immunologically, this can be regarded as 'Nature's experimental system'.

possess the noxious antibodies but show no effect as she lacks the target organ but the baby, having that organ, may show effects. Also an IgA or M 'blocking' antibody not able to cross the placenta, may prevent any maternal effects of an IgG antibody but the baby will show them. A similar paradoxical effect, simulating iso(allo)immunization, may occur if the mother for some reason is not expressing the relevant antigen yet the baby does so.

It is important to differentiate between: aetiological or initiating factors, which may be genetic or environmental; mechanisms of disturbance of tissue or of function, which appear to be immunological in all the conditions discussed; and how the disease produces its clinical effects, which may be endocrinological, cardiac, neurological etc.

Antibodies *per se* usually produce little damage but the nonvariable Fc end of the molecule may bind to non-specific Fc receptors and set up various reactions. Involvement with complement can produce effects through specific antigen-antibody-complement immune-complex formation. Ultimately there may be lysis of cell membrane and tissue damage. Prostaglandin activation may lead to inflammation and pain.

Two important points underlie the apparent contradictions and confusions:—

'Families' of antigens may be involved in single diseases but not all are pathogenic. The antibody first discovered and measured may be the close 'cousin' of the practically important one. For example, in Graves' disease there was confusion between long-acting thyroid stimulator (LATS), the first stimulator antibody detected and measured but which it eventually became clear does *not* stimulate the *human* thyroid, and long-acting thyroid stimulator-protector (LATS-P) which is very closely related and does so. Systemic lupus erythemotosus (SLE) is another disease in which irrelevant antibodies were measured initially (*see* p. 305).

Even if the correct (pathogenic) antibody is being measured, the results may not correspond with the disease activity. Antibody may be detected in the circulation only when all the antigens have been bound and in that case the disease may present before the antibody is measurable. The reverse may also happen and antibody be present in measurable amount yet the disease be inactive. This happens with hyperthyroid disease sometimes because of damage inactivating the target organ.

The diseases to be considered can be regarded broadly as mistakes or errors of the immunological system. They can be categorized as: *Tissue (or organ)-specific diseases*, and *Multisystem (or multitissue) diseases*.

Immune thrombocytopenic purpura

Immune (formerly 'idiopathic') thrombocytopenic purpura (ITP) is now recognized as an autoimmune disease. This arose from finding that babies born to mothers with the disease showed thrombocytopenia. It was found that infusing plasma from individuals with the disease into healthy persons produced thrombocytopenia and there is now good evidence that an IgG antibody against a platelet-associated antigen is present (McMillan 1983). But for the pregnancy observations the search might well have been abandoned. Van Leeuwen *et al.* (1981) using fluorescein labelled specific antiglobulins confirmed that IgG antibodies crossed the placenta to cause fetal/neonatal disease. As referred to previously, iso(allo)antibodies may also form in the maternal system reacting specifically with fetal platelets.

A normal platelet carries 6–12,000 molecules of IgG in its surface and in ITP this is increased up to twentyfold; C_3 is also concentrated on the cell surface and the combined effect produces accelerated clearance in spleen and liver. The blood film shows an increased number of large platelets and marrow specimens show an increase in megakaryocytes. Splenectomy not only removes the major site of platelet destruction but also a major source of antibody production. Steroid therapy reduces platelet clearance and antibody production but when C_3 platelet-binding is a major factor it is less effective. Another method of treatment is the intravenous administration of a high dose polyvalent, intact immunoglobulin (Imbach *et al.* 1981); how this works is unknown. Cytotoxic agents such as azathioprine may sometimes have a place.

ITP carries risk to the baby at delivery. Abortion is increased and overall perinatal mortality of the order of 16% was recorded (Scott 1966), the major factor being death due to intracranial haemorrhage. With the physical stresses and strain of delivery together with the transient hypoxia, small petechial haemorrhages which are normal for a newborn may, if there is thrombocytopenia, extend into massive bleeds. If not fatal these can produce severe cerebral damage. Scott *et al.* (1983) have shown that while maternal platelet antibody determinations can indicate whether the baby *may* have thrombocytopenia, even if the antibodies are measured by sophisticated quantitative techniques, the findings do not correlate well with the fetal platelet count. It seems that unknown antigenic characteristics of the fetus may be relevant to the degree of effect the antibodies exert.

Surprisingly, maternal haemorrhage does not often cause major problems about the time of delivery. When it occurs it is usually related to lacerations or incisions rather than arising from the placental site. Nowadays, platelet concentrate is available for transfusion if the blood loss is severe. It is prudent to contact the transfusion service when a patient with ITP is about to be delivered to ensure availability of platelets.

Management

Steroid therapy should be given regardless of the pregnancy if it is otherwise indicated (Handin 1981). It has dramatically reduced the maternal risk and it has been claimed that it will also improve the baby's platelet count. The precise place for splenectomy in pregnancy is not agreed but if clinical deterioration occurs despite medical therapy it is no longer necessary to regard pregnancy as a contraindication, thanks to the availability of platelet concentrate.

With the high perinatal mortality from intracranial haemorrhage, the question arises as to whether Caesarean section should be routine to achieve the gentlest possible delivery. Some claim that if the mothers' platelet level is reasonable ($\geq 100,000$ per cubic mm) the risk is less but others find no correlation between levels of platelets in mother and child (Scott *et al.* 1983).

Even if a woman is clinically cured of ITP by splenectomy any subsequent child is likely to be affected as the antibody will still be present, the baby's platelets alone being subject to splenic destruction, so Caesarean section has been advocated for all such women regardless of the maternal platelet count (Carloss *et al.* 1980, McMillan 1981 a & b). Scott *et al.* (1980) have used fetal blood scalp sampling in early labour to obtain a direct count of the baby's platelet level; if the count is below 50000 per cubic mm they advocate Caesarean section.

Treatment may be required for a newborn child with a very low platelet count or with evident haemorrhage. Corticosteroids may be used, 12 mg intravenous hydrocortisone 12 hourly for 2–3 days followed by oral prednisolone 1 mg per kilogram per day. The steroids act by reducing both antibody binding and the rate of splenic sequestration with destruction of platelets. Platelet transfusion may be needed, 2 platelet packs every 6–8 hours (McMillan 1981a); rarely, exchange transfusion which removes antibody may be required.

The differentiation of auto- and iso(allo)immune neonatal thrombocytopenia is not an academic issue. In the iso(allo)immune type the best treatment is to transfuse some of the mother's platelets to the baby as they are not affected by the antibody (Kelton *et al.* 1980). With the autoimmune type the antibody is often anti PL^{A1} and theoretically the best course is to transfuse PL^{A1} negative platelets but only a few laboratories can test for this antigen. If there is doubt as to whether it is an auto- or an iso(allo)antibody, measurement of platelet-associated IgG and serum platelet bindable IgG may help to give the answer (Kelton *et al.* 1980).

Autoimmune haemolytic anaemia

Autoimmune haemolytic anaemia is a typical immunological disease in that it develops mainly in young females and therefore sometimes coincides with pregnancy, but it is exceptional in that it tends to be worse during pregnancy. This behaviour has led to use of the term 'relapsing haemolytic anaemia of pregnancy' though whether this is a distinct entity is uncertain. Many cases have negative antiglobulin tests but complement-fixing antibody consumption tests indicate that despite the negative Coombs test, the haemolysis has an immune basis (Yam *et al.* 1980). Leucopenia and thrombocytopenia may occur suggesting that antigens not confined to red cells are involved. Haemoglobin may drop in pregnancy to below 5 g/dl and this can carry a hazard to the mother but sometimes haemolysis is present without the patient being anaemic. Death *in utero* may result from the hypoxia of the maternal anaemia and from IgG antibody crossing the placenta and causing haemolysis of fetal red cells. One estimate of the risk to the baby is of a 35–40% chance of stillbirth or severe neonatal anaemia (Chaplin *et al.* 1973).

MECHANISM OF EXACERBATIONS IN PREGNANCY

One suggestion as to why the anaemia worsens in pregnancy is that fetal red cells cross the placenta and stimulate the autoimmunity in some undefined way. However, measurable antibody levels and intensity of positive antiglobulin tests do not correlate directly with the degree of haemolysis in pregnancy (Chaplin *et al.* 1973). Changes in cellular immune function in pregnancy may lead to accelerated destruction of antibody-coated red cells. There may be a response to a substance specific to pregnancy such as a hormone or trophoblast microvillus antigen which is also injurious to red cells. There is a relationship between this type of anaemia and ovarian teratoma and it may be that this association with a tumour of embryonal tissue has a similar basis.

'Warm', 'cold' and 'mixed' antibodies are described. In a series of 865 patients the mixed types seemed to carry a bad prognosis (Sokol et al. 1981). 'Cold' agglutinins are usually IgM and therefore unlikely to affect the fetus. Splenectomy, sometimes the chosen therapy, is of little benefit with such an antibody as the erythrocytes are destroyed in the liver and steroids are also relatively ineffective (Dickson & Barlow 1981). However, plasmapheresis is relatively more effective as the IgM molecule tends to remain in the intravascular compartment. In 'warm' agglutinin anaemia the antibody is usually IgG and the fetus is liable to be affected because of transplacental passage of the antibody. Steroids are relatively effective and splenectomy is also beneficial, often leading to a stable state with a lower dosage of corticosteroids. They act by suppressing antibody production, by altering avidity for the antigen and by diminishing the reticulo-endothelial clearance of antibody-coated cells.

DIAGNOSIS

Diagnosis stems from the demonstration of a normochromic, normocytic anaemia with high reticulocytosis, high unconjugated bilirubin in the plasma and urobilinogen in the urine. It is then a matter of excluding haemoglobinopathies, enzyme defects, hereditary spherocytosis, paroxysmal nocturnal haemoglobinuria, folate deficiency and infections. Drug induced sensitization (methyldopa) should be differentiated. Specific evidence of an immune process should be sought by an antiglobulin (Coombs' test) or other more refined technique and by complement studies.

MANAGEMENT

Once the diagnosis is made, close monitoring of the haemoglobin and reticulocyte levels is required. Antibody level measurement may be of value and certainly identification of its type is important. Corticosteroids are indicated to try to keep the haemoglobin level above 10 g/dl. In severe cases vigorous blood transfusion and premature delivery may save the mother's life. Obtaining entirely suitable blood for transfusion is difficult and it is usually a matter of using the least incompatible available. Plasmapheresis and splenectomy may be worth considering in a difficult case.

If there is a haemolytic IgG antibody in a significant titre then spectrophotometric analysis of amniotic fluid should be performed to assess fetal haemolysis and then plans for management are made on the same basis as with Rhesus isoimmunization (Chapter 18, p 265).

Myasthenia gravis

Myasthenia gravis is not common (incidence circa 1 in 30 000), but two-thirds of cases occur in women and the peak onset is in the twenties so it is relatively frequent in pregnancy. The effects are of weakness of voluntary muscles ultimately involving those of respiration. The association of thymic abnormalities has long been known and the observation that transient myasthenia was sometimes evident in newborn children of women with the disease was correctly interpreted as indicating that an immunoglobulin was involved (Simpson 1960). This stimulated one of the most exciting sequences of expansion of knowledge in modern medicine. It was discovered that a fraction of a snake venom (alpha-bungarotoxin) bound to acetyl choline receptors. These were found in, and extracted from, the electric eel using the snake venom. Immunizing rabbits with these receptors stimulated antibody formation and a myasthenic syndrome developed. Similar antibodies were then found in most myasthenic patients. Neonatal myasthenia is associated with presence of the antibody and the level falls as the infant's condition improves (Vincent et al. 1978).

MANAGEMENT

The diagnosis of myasthenia can be confirmed with a test done with the rapid anticholinesterase drug edrophonium chloride (5–10 mg intravenously). Then long acting drugs such as pyridostigmine are used. Immunosuppressive drugs, corticosteroids, plasmapheresis and thymectomy also have a role. Myasthenic patients are sensitive to analgesics, etc. as used in labour so care is necessary with preparation for controlled ventilation if required. Uterine action in labour is normal but forceps delivery is wise to minimize voluntary muscle effort. Puerperal deterioration may occur so careful supervision is required in this period.

The transient neonatal form occurs in about 12% of cases (Namba *et al.* 1970); the essential thing is to be aware that it may happen. It usually presents as respiratory failure within a few hours of birth; the baby probably has initial protection from the maternal anticholinesterase drug which has crossed the placenta. If there is any doubt a test dose of edrophonium chloride (0.5–1 mg subcutaneously) may be given. Ventilation may be required initially but with appropriate dosage of a longer acting drug the baby should be able to breathe unaided. The dosage can be reduced as the antibody effect wears off; thereafter the baby should be normal. If affected by the transient form of the disease the babies are usually 'light for dates' as occurs with other 'transient transferred' neonatal forms of immunological disease (Scott 1976).

Thyroid disease

Thyroid disease is normally regarded as an endocrinological problem and as such is considered elsewhere (p. 293). However, it is now accepted that most forms have an immunological basis. This springs from the observation by White (1912) that the baby of a mother with Graves' disease may show a transient form. This effect on the baby was also noted after the mother had been rendered *hypo*thyroid by thyroidectomy. Early searches for the cause concentrated on thyroid stimulating hormone (TSH) but as it does not cross the placenta, it could not be responsible. Ultimately, using mice, a thyroid stimulatory substance with a longer action than TSH was noted in sera from Graves' disease patients, and christened long-acting thyroid stimulator (LATS). LATS was shown to be an IgG antibody and, being capable of placental transfer, was presumed to cause the fetal/neonatal form of the disease. It was noted, however (see Scott 1977, for review), that it was not always present when the baby was affected and it was eventually discovered that LATS was only stimulatory in the mouse system and not in the human. Then the closely related member of the thyroid stimulatory antibody (TSAb) family, LATS-P (protector), was found and its presence correlated closely with fetal/neonatal effects. LATS-P is a human thyroid stimulator which derived its contradictory name from its first detection as a substance which protected against stimulation by LATS in animals. These antibodies were shown to be specific for the TSH receptor

and Graves' disease became the first and best defined cell receptor antibody disease and also the first example of a disease in which antibodies stimulate hyperactivity.

A differential effect has been observed with Graves' disease and binovular twins, one showing severe and the other mild thyrotoxicosis. This is in keeping with the fact that only a small proportion of babies of mothers with Graves' disease show frank manifestations of the transient-transferred form of the disease.

Thyroid binding inhibiting immunoglobulins (TBIIs) exist which may block TSH stimulation of the normal thyroid (Endo *et al.* 1978) and can cause transient fetal/neonatal *hypo*thyroidism. In a screening programme for neonatal hypothyroidism, Lazarus *et al.* (1983) have described finding elevation of the neonatal TSH level due to maternal IgG antibody which bound to and inhibited human TSH. This is important to recognize in order to prevent unnecessary and inappropriate thyroxine replacement therapy. Recently it has been shown that there are antibodies which can stimulate or block thyroid growth, which may account for goitre or gland shrinkage with myxoedema (Drexhage *et al.* 1981).

It is now appreciated that Graves' disease, Hashimoto's disease and primary myxoedema represent different facets of a spectrum of immunologically-mediated disease. The story indicates that closely related antibodies may have opposite effects. The 'Yale lock' analogy is still pertinent: some molecules will enter receptors and turn the lock to produce stimulation but others will only be sufficiently similar in configuration to fit the lock but not turn it, possibly 'blocking' a more specific 'key' from entering.

Evidence is accumulating that pregnancy may affect the natural history of thyroid disease (Amino *et al.* 1978, Fein *et al.* 1980) and this may be another immunological effect. Disordered thyroid function represents a dynamic spectrum and manifestations may swing from *hyper*thyroid to *hypo*thyroid and the reverse; these reports indicate that after delivery there may be transient hypothyroidism or hyperthyroidism or one preceding the other. Estimation of antithyrotropin receptor antibodies in late pregnancy may help to predict the state of the child (McGregor *et al.* 1984).

OTHER TISSUE SPECIFIC IMMUNOLOGICAL DISEASES WHICH MAY HAVE EFFECTS IN PREGNANCY

There are a number of other tissue specific immunological diseases which may have effects on the child in pregnancy as they are mediated by an antibody, often to a specific receptor. One is *diabetes mellitus with acanthosis nigricans* in which there is antibody to insulin receptors (Hall 1981). This may have a bearing on the mystery of the rare transient form of neonatal diabetes which has been described in babies born to non-diabetic mothers (Scott 1976). A retrospective review of diabetic pregnancies occurring 30 years ago indicated that in cases in which the mother has in the interval developed an immunological disease (hyper- or hypothyroidism, pernicious anaemia, etc.) the perinatal mortality was significantly greater (Beral *et al.* 1984). Given the strong association between different immunologic diseases it is likely that in most, if not all, of these women the diabetes also has an immunological basis. This suggests that immunological as opposed to metabolic factors may be important in the perinatal mortality associated with diabetes.

Allergic rhinitis and asthma may sometimes be due to a B_2-adrenergic receptor antibody (Fraser *et al.* 1981) which could, theoretically at least, affect the baby transiently as could *parathormone receptor antibody*. *Pernicious anaemia* is very rare in pregnancy not only because of its relatively late age incidence but because it exercises a rather specific anti-fertility effect. There is some evidence (*see* Scott 1976) that IgA antibody in breast milk may produce a form of the disease in the baby if breast feeding takes place.

Systemic lupus erythematosus and related connective tissue diseases

Systemic lupus erythematosus (SLE) is the major member of a group of immunological diseases affecting connective and other tissues. The group also includes scleroderma, Sjögren's syndrome, dermatomyositis and rheumatoid arthritis (RA). The observation of the frequent improvement of RA in pregnancy resulted in the development of corticosteroid therapy with a major impact on medical practice (Hench 1938) but the related forms of connective tissue disease do not all show this tendency. Most observations relate to SLE in pregnancy but it is reasonable to regard closely related forms of connective tissue disease (CTD) as an entity for the present purpose.

There is profound immunological disturbance in SLE with many antibodies directed against a wide and changing spectrum of antigens. Immune-complex formation and deposition occurs, complement levels are reduced and cellular immunity is deranged; apparently a deficit of 'T' cell function allows the abnormal humoral activity. The female preponderance is about 9:1 and it is particularly common in the childbearing age group. Antibodies initially associated with the condition (antinuclear factor and LE factor) were observed to cross the placenta but produced no observable effect on the baby so it was assumed that antibodies were of little or no relevance (*see* Scott 1984 for review). It is now known, however, that these particular antibodies are mere epiphenomena and apparently irrelevant to the pathogenesis.

Reports indicated that the fetal wastage is very high (Mor-Yosef *et al.* 1984), 36% in 630 pregnancies (Chesley 1978) and this could not be attributed to maternal renal or cardiovascular involvement. Cases were reported of babies born to mothers with SLE showing the classical SLE 'butterfly' rash (Fig. 21.2) and sometimes other manifestations suggestive of a transient form of the disease. A few cases were also recorded of the baby having congenital heart block (CHB). Subsequently it was shown that about 1 in 3 babies with CHB are born to mothers who have, or later develop, evidence of CTD (Esscher & Scott 1979). CHB is permanent because, unlike the other transplacental immunological disease effects, the damage to the cardiac conduction system is irreversible. A baby with CHB may be born before the mother has any signs of SLE. Therefore if a healthy woman delivers a baby with CHB she should be watched for signs of SLE developing, just as the mother of an overweight baby is watched for diabetes.

Abortion is common with SLE and anti-trophoblast antibodies have been inculpated (Bresnihan *et al.* 1977) as have immune complexes in trophoblast and decidual vasculopathy. Frequently immune and coagulation systems ultimately interact in pathogenesis and some SLE antibodies have an effect on coagulation. In particular an antibody 'lupus (LE) anticoagulant' has such an effect and paradoxically acts *in vivo* by causing thrombosis which, if in the placenta, may result in fetal death. Control of the antibody level may allow successful pregnancy (Lubbe *et al.* 1983).

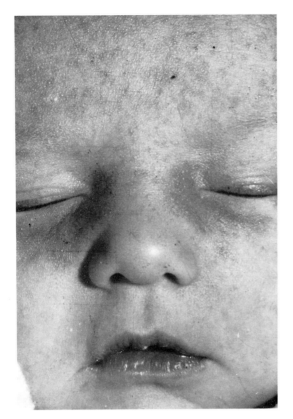

Fig. 21.2 Butterfly rash on the face of a newborn child whose mother had systemic lupus erythematosus. The rash gradually disappeared by 3 months of age. Such rashes may not be evident until a few days after birth, some exposure of the skin to ultraviolet light being relevant.

MANAGEMENT OF PREGNANCY

Prepregnancy advice

The patient should be advised about the high fetal wastage, mainly associated with abortion which, as it carries little maternal risk, is not a reason for a discouraging attitude and the same is true of the problems of drug therapy. If there is severe renal and/ or cardiovascular involvement it may be prudent to advise avoidance of pregnancy. Swings of exacerbation and remission occur and ideally a pregnancy would be timed during a remission.

Early pregnancy

Very rarely SLE may be regarded as an indication for termination though there is no reason to expect any therapeutic benefit and abortion may be followed by exacerbation. The high spontaneous abortion risk may be regarded as a reason to advise restricted activity. A fall in serum C_3 level during pregnancy is often followed by a 'flare-up'; serial measurements form a basis for predicting exacerbation and organizing attempts at their prevention by adjustment of therapy.

Late pregnancy

Corticosteroids given for the disease may be associated with poor fetal growth though this is a feature with immunological diseases even in the absence of therapy (Scott 1976). If the patient is not on steroids, any exacerbation may be an indication for starting them, using the smallest effective dosage. Steroid dosage over 55 mg cortisol (or its equivalent) per day may interfere with oestriol determination as a measure for assessing fetal well-being.

Renal and vascular effects of the disease may be mistaken for pre-eclampsia. If lupus nephritis develops, steroid therapy may diminish the maternal risk. Fetal heart rate should be counted frequently and a consistent rate of 60–70 per minute interpreted as probably due to CHB. It is not, in these circumstances, an indication for Caesarean section. During labour or operative delivery corticosteroid supplementation should be given as necessary.

Postnatal care

Steroid therapy should only be reduced slowly. CHB has to be regarded as permanent and each case assessed individually as to the necessity for a pacemaker.

New developments

New immunological prospects for determining causes for fetal loss in SLE are opening up and recent discoveries on SLE in pregnancy seem likely to have an important bearing on understanding of the pathogenesis; it now seems that some IgG antibodies, though not those usually measured, may produce serious effects.

It was suggested some years ago that anti-Ro (SS-A), an antiribonucleoprotein antibody, might be involved when lupus effects were manifest in the baby. It is now known that when the child has congenital CHB there is a very high incidence of anti-Ro antibodies in maternal serum suggesting that anti-Ro, or some closely related serological factor, is involved in the pathogenesis (Scott *et al.* 1983). Further study seems likely to define precisely the immunological factors involved in CHB and other ill-effects.

With wider application of immunological laboratory techniques, SLE has come to be diagnosed more frequently, often in women who are only mildly ill. This is reflected in a recent report (Varner *et al.* 1983) which showed only a minimal increase in pregnancy morbidity and mortality over the general figures.

SLE and RA differ in that the latter tends to improve in pregnancy. Recently it has been suggested that the alteration in disease activity is related to pregnancy associated alpha$_2$-glycoprotein (Unger *et al.* 1983).

The female-dominant sex ratio observed in the adult disease is not seen in the transient-transferred neonatal forms, indicating that the sex factor operates at the level of the initiation of the disease process and not at the level of the tissue damage. The variability in the extent to which the baby is affected, even between binovular twins, points to the likelihood that some cellular antigen such as HLA may play a part.

PREGNANCY DISORDERS WHICH MAY HAVE AN IMMUNOLOGICAL BASIS

Herpes gestationis (pemphigoid gestationis)

A rare (1 in 3–5000 pregnancies) but fascinating disease, herpes gestationis falls in the category of 'probably immunological', possibly in the iso-(allo)immune category. It presents in pregnancy usually with pruritus and papules, vesicles and bullae appear. Resolution occurs afterwards with variable rapidity. Rarely, infants born to affected mothers show this disease in a transient form and the babies are frequently small for dates (Holmes & Black 1984). Eosinophilia is a feature. Immunohistology shows IgG and IgM in the basement membrane zone.

Recurrence with subsequent pregnancies is usual but not invariable. Relapse may occur with oral contraceptive usage and with taking oestrogens only. The natural ovulation/menstruation cycle may also be associated with variation in severity. Whether it is oestrogen or progestogen which is more important has been uncertain but the current evidence points to oestrogen (Holmes *et al.* 1983). Change of partner may play a role. There is an association with HLA antigen DR3, an antigen with a high frequency in relation to a number of immunological diseases. Patients affected by herpes gestationis have a raised incidence of autoimmune diseases and autoantibodies. A circulating herpes gestationis (HG) factor which is an IgG antibody has been demonstrated in 80% cases and may have pathogenic importance.

The mainstay of treatment is the administration of corticosteroids.

Pre-eclampsia

The one major disease specific to pregnancy is pre-eclampsia. Its aetiology stands out as being completely unknown, beyond the obvious fact of its association with pregnancy. In the last decade or so many diseases which were still resting in the 'unknown aetiology' category have been demonstrated to have an immunological basis. It is therefore not surprising that such an aetiology should have been sought for pre-eclampsia, particularly as it has this specific association with Nature's great immunological enigma: pregnancy. Added to that is the puzzling fact that pre-eclampsia is much more common in first pregnancies (about tenfold, Redman 1981).

Many of the studies undertaken showed immunologic abnormalities compared with controls. However, few of these were such that one could say that they pointed to an immunological cause of the disease; many could be a consequence of it or of treatment (*see* MacGillivray 1983, for review). However, some of the studies done with the idea in mind that there might be an abnormal immunological *hyper*reactivity of the mother to the fetus showed exactly the reverse: a *hypo*responsiveness (Scott *et al.* 1978). These observations pointed to an idea hitherto unconsidered but which has since received much attention: that the immunological reaction of mother to fetus may be beneficial in terms of successful viviparity. This, however, largely remained a theoretical concept as nothing developed which pointed to a means of treatment.

An exception to this was the observation that abortion occurring prior to the first pregnancy proceeding to maturity conferred a degree of protection as also did previous blood transfusion (Feeney *et al.* 1977), rather as transfusion preceding renal transplantation improves graft survival prospects. These findings, when considered in immunological terms, suggested the possibility that prior exposure of a woman to foreign tissue antigens, particularly those derived from the father of her child, might reduce her chances of pre-eclampsia when she became pregnant. Unfortunately ethical reasons made it unreasonable to embark upon a programme of prophylactic injection of foreign tissue antigens to simulate the immunologic effects of an abortion or a blood transfusion. However, such an approach has been followed in relation to recurrent abortion, a similar mechanism having been postulated (see below).

Therefore, although pre-eclampsia still appears to be asking to be classified as an immunological disease, the verdict on the scientific evidence remains 'not proven' and for further practical information Chapter 16 should be consulted.

Retarded fetal growth

As indicated, the transient-transferred forms of auto-immune disease, (Graves' disease, myasthenia gravis, thrombocytopenic purpura and systemic lupus erythematosus) tend to be associated with the babies being 'light for dates' (Scott 1976). This points to an immune mechanism for at least a proportion of cases of retarded fetal growth.

Recurrent fetal loss possibly due to immunological factors

Excluding severe iso(allo)immunization to red cell antigens such as the Rhesus one, which is virtually always identified today, immunological hypotheses for recurrent fetal loss cover a *damaging autoimmune effect* on the conceptus and the *lack of a favourable iso(allo)immune response* to it.

Autoimmune factors, which are considered earlier, account for only a small proportion of recurrent fetal losses but the evidence on them is stronger than that on the category attributed to defective iso(allo)immune response. The background facts have been established on LE anticoagulant. It is an antibody which may be an IgG or IgM molecule. *In vitro* it is an anticoagulant interfering with phospholipid-dependent coagulation tests such as the kaolin cephalin clotting time (KCCT). This effect persists when the plasma is mixed with normal plasma but is abolished by the presence of platelets. *In vivo*, however, it acts as a *coagulant* probably also by an antiphospholipid effect interfering with the release of arachidonic acid from cell membranes producing a prostacyclin-thromboxane-alpha$_2$ imbalance (Scott 1984). This may account for the frequent association with massive placental thrombosis. Despite some imprecision of certain aspects of the evidence it does seem that if circulating LE-anticoagulant is present the prospect for a successful pregnancy is poor but if the antibody is suppressed by therapy, with or without aspirin to counter the thrombotic tendency, a live baby is much more likely.

The principal iso(allo)immune hypothesis is that some antibody which promotes tolerance of the con-

ceptus is lacking but that production of it can be stimulated by an antigen in transfused blood. The idea is alluring to the immunologist as it offers a 'raison d'être' for tissue immunogenicity other than it merely being Nature's impediment to transplantation work; the notion also matches with the unconfirmed observation made with regard to pre-eclampsia that prior blood transfusion appears to have a beneficial effect on reproductive performance (Feeney *et al.* 1977).

Factors which block immune reaction to paternally-derived or other allo-antigens *in vitro* have been detected in pregnant women and absence of these factors has been reported in association with recurrent abortion (Rocklin *et al.* 1976). However, demonstration of these factors has not been consistent and it has not been shown whether their absence from serum of aborting women is cause or consequence of the abortions (Stirrat 1983).

Evidence which relates to HLA typing is not capable of being influenced by the abortion process. Some groups have found that there is an increased degree of HLA sharing between parents in cases of recurrent abortion but this is not a universal finding (Stirrat 1983).

Against this background of incomplete, and to some extent contradictory, evidence a number of groups have embarked upon programmes aimed at stimulating immune responses in women with unexplained recurrent abortion. The methods chosen include injecting pooled donor leucocytes, or paternal lymphocytes. The regimes used have frequently been followed by successful pregnancies but the placebo effect in this situation is strong and there are potential hazards to such procedures (Lancet 1983, Bastian *et al.* 1984). Mowbray *et al.* (1985) reported a double-blind trial of treatment with husband's leucocytes in which 17 out of 22 had successful pregnancies, compared with 10 out of 27 controls. More such studies are required.

'Unexplained recurrent abortion' is a term covering an assortment of mechanisms, varying with current knowledge and the intensity of investigation but still amounting to around 50% of cases of repeated fetal loss. 'Patient perseverance' has been the gist of the advice given to these women and those who could accept the stresses involved in applying it were often rewarded with a live child. If there be a category of recurrent abortion due to lack of iso(allo)immunity, the women who eventually carry a child surely belong to it as the incidence of detectable iso(allo)immunity rises with gravidity order. Assessment of treatment results must take into account that, on the postulate advanced, those treated mothers who succeed in carrying a pregnancy would have had an increased chance of doing so *without* specific therapy as each pregnancy is itself a natural unit of 'treatment'.

A report covering 195 couples with recurrent abortion emphasizes how extraordinarily good results would have to be to carry conviction. In 37 couples with 3 consecutive, spontaneous, unexplained abortions, 32 (86%) had a successful pregnancy with 'tender loving care' alone (Stray-Pedersen & Stray-Pedersen 1984). Any study to assess whether immunotherapy is more effective faces major statistic and logistic problems.

REFERENCES

AMINO N., YABU Y., MIYAI K., FUJIE T., AZUKIZAWA M., ONISHI T. & KUMAHARA Y. (1978). *Lancet* 2, 344–6.

BASTIAN J.E., WILLIAMS R.A., ORNELAS W., TANI P. & THOMPSON L.E. (1984) *Lancet*, i, 1435–37.

BERAL V., ROMAN E. & COLWELL L. (1984) *Lancet*, i, 4–7.

BRESNIHAN B., GRIGOR R.R., OLIVER M., LEWKONIA R.M., HUGHES G.R.V., LOVINS R.E. & FAULK W.P. (1977) *Lancet*, ii, 1205–6.

CARLOSS H.W., MCMILLAN R. & CROSBY W.H. (1980) *J. Amer. med. Ass.* 244, 2756–8.

CHAPLIN H. JR, COHEN R., BLOOMBERG G., KAPLAN H.J., MOORE J.A. & DORNER I. (1973). *Brit. J. Haematol.* 24, 219–29.

CHESLEY L.C. (1978) *Hypertensive Disorders in Pregnancy.* Appleton-Century-Crofts, New York.

DICKSON C.Z. & BARLOW J.F. (1981) *South Dakota J. Med.* 34, 23–8.

DREXHAGE H.A., BOTTAZZO G.F., BITENSKY L., CHAYEN J. & DONIACH D. (1981) *Nature* 289, 594–6.

ENDO K., KASAGI K., KONISHI J., IKEKUBO K., OKUNU T., TAKEDA Y., MORI T., TORIZUKA K. (1978) *J. clin. Endocrinol. Metab.* 46, 734–9.

ESSCHER E. & SCOTT J.S. (1979) *Brit. med. J.* i, 1235–8.

FEENEY J.G., TOVEY L.A.D. & SCOTT J.S. (1977) *Lancet* i, 874–5.

FEIN H.G., GOLDMAN J.M. & WEINTRAUB B.D. (1980) *Amer. J. Obstet. Gynec.* 138, 504–510.

FRASER C.M., VENTER J.C. & KALINER M. (1981) *New Engl. J. Med.* 305, 1165–1170.

HALL R. (1981) *Hospital Update* 7, 161–172.

HANDIN R.I. (1981) *New Engl. J. Med.* 305, 951–3.

HENCH P.S. (1938) *Proc. Mayo Clinic* 13, 161.

HOLMES R.C., BLACK M.M., JURECKA W., DANN J., JAMES D.C.O., TIMLIN D. & BHOGAL B. (1983) *Brit. J. Dermatol.* 109, 131–9.

HOLMES R.C. & BLACK M.M. (1984) *Brit. J. Dermatol.* 110, 67–72.

IMBACH P., BARANDUN S., D'APUZZO V., BAUMGARTNER C., HIRT A., MORELL A., ROSSI E., SCHÖNI M., VEST M. & WAGNER H.P. (1981). *Lancet* i, 1228–31.

KELTON J.G., BLANCHETTE V.S., WILSON W.E., POWERS P.,

MOHAN PAI K.R., EFFER S.B. & BARR R.D. (1980) *New Engl. J. Med* 302, 1401–3.

LANCET, Editorial. (1983) *Lancet* ii, 1175–6.

LAZARUS J.H., JOHN R., GINSBERG J., HUGHES I.A., SHEWRING G., SMITH B.R., WOODHEAD J.S. & HALL R. (1983) *Brit. med. J.* 286, 592–4.

VAN LEEUWEN E.F., HELMERHORST F.M., ENGELFRIET C.P. & VON BORNE A.E.G.K. (1981) *Brit. med. J.* 283, 104.

LUBBE W.F., PALMER S.J., BUTLER W.S. & LIGGINS G.C. (1983) *Lancet* i, 1361–3.

MACGILLIVRAY I. (1983). *Pre-eclampsia. The Hypertensive Disease of Pregnancy.* W.B. Saunders Co. Ltd., London, Philadelphia, Toronto.

MCGREGOR A.M., HALL R. & RICHARDS C. (1984) *Brit. med. J.* 288, 1780–1.

MCMILLAN R. (1981a) *New Engl. J. Med.* 304, 1135–47.

MCMILLAN R. (1981b) *New Engl. J. Med.* 305, 831.

MCMILLAN R. (1983) *Clin. Haemat.* 12, 69–88.

MOR-YOSEF S., NAVOT D., RABINOWITZ R. & SCHENKER J.G. (1984) *Obstet. Gynecol. Survey* 39, 67–84.

MOWBRAY J.F., GIBBINGS C., LIDDELL M., REGINALD PW., UNDERWOOD J.L. & BEARD R.W. (1985) *Lancet*, i, 941–3.

NAMBA T., BROWN S.B. & GROB D. (1970) *Pediatrics* 45, 488–504.

REDMAN C.W.G. (1981) *Contr. Nephrol.* 25, 120–27.

ROCKLIN R.E., KITZMULLER J., CARPENTER B., GAROVOY M. & DAVID J.R. (1976) *New Engl. J. Med.* 295, 1209–13.

SCOTT J.R., CRUIKSHANK D.P., KOCHENOUR N.K., PITKIN R.M. & WARENSKI J.C. (1980) *Amer. J. Obstet. Gynec.* 136, 495–99.

SCOTT J.S. (1966) *Brit. med. J.* i, 1559–67.

SCOTT J.S. (1976) In *Immunology of Human Reproduction* (eds. Scott J.S. & Jones W.R.) p. 229, Academic Press, London.

SCOTT J.S. (1977) In *Progress in Allergy* (eds. P. Kallos *et al.*) 23, 321–66.

SCOTT J.S. (1984) *Amer. J. Reprod. Immunol.* 6, 19–24.

SCOTT J.S., JENKINS D.M. & NEED J.A. (1978) *Lancet* i, 704–6.

SCOTT J.S., MADDISON P.J., TAYLOR P.V., ESSCHER E., SCOTT O. & SKINNER R.P. (1983) *New Engl. J. Med.* 309, 209–12.

SIMPSON J.A. (1960) *Scot. med. J.* 5, 419–36.

SOKOL R.J., HEWITT S. & STAMPS B.K. (1981) *Brit. med. J.* 282, 2023–7.

STIRRAT G.M. (1983) *Brit. J. Obstet. Gynaecol.* 90, 881–3.

STRAY-PEDERSEN B. & STRAY-PEDERSEN S. (1984) *Amer. J. Obstet. Gynec.* 148, 140–6.

TOVEY L.A.D. & MORONI E.S. (1976) In *Immunology of Human Reproduction.* (eds Scott J.S. & Jones W.R.) Academic Press, London.

UNGER A., KAY A., GRIFFIN A.J. & PANAYI G.S. (1983) *Brit. med. J.* 286, 750–2.

VARNER M.W., MEEHAN R.T., SYROP C.H., SROTTMAN M.P. & GOPLERUD C.P. (1983) *Amer. J. Obstet. Gynec.* 145, 1025–40.

VINCENT A., NEWSOM-DAVIS J. & MARTIN V. (1978) *Lancet* i, 1254.

WHITE C. (1912) *J. Obstet. Gynaec. Brit. Emp.* 21, 231–3.

YAM P., WILKINSON L., PETZ L.D. & GARRATTY G. (1980) *Amer. J. Hematol.* 8, 23–29.

CHAPTER 22
ANTENATAL DIAGNOSIS OF FETAL ABNORMALITIES

C.R. WHITFIELD

Fetal abnormalities are sometimes recognized during the later months of pregnancy or occasionally during labour, but the usual purpose of antenatal (prenatal) diagnosis is to detect lethal or severely handicapping anomalies and disorders so that selective abortion of affected pregnancies can be offered, and to do so as early as possible to simplify and reduce the risks of therapeutic abortion for mothers choosing that option. The abnormality under consideration is, of course, more often excluded than shown to be present, and, in this way, the availability of antenatal diagnosis with selective termination enables many at risk couples to fulfil their wishes to have families of healthy children.

For each abnormality or group of related disorders a two-tier diagnostic system is the ideal requirement, consisting of a primary screening procedure to select at risk mothers (and families) and a secondary definitive method to identify the affected fetus. Ideally the primary screening procedure, which may be clinical or based on either laboratory testing or ultrasound imaging, must have acceptable sensitivity and specificity; the secondary diagnostic investigation, which may be an invasive one, should be accurate and safe. Rhesus disease has provided a good model for two-tier antenatal diagnosis of this sort, with rhesus-typing and antibody testing as the primary screen to identify all at risk pregnancies, followed by amniocentesis and amniotic fluid tests as the second step to make the definitive diagnosis that a fetus is affected and how severely. The analogy goes further in that the eventual understanding of the pathophysiology of rhesus immunization and its perinatal effects led not only to useful diagnostic methods but to usually successful treatment and ultimately to prophylaxis. We must hope that, similarly, an understanding of the disorders causing fetal abnormalities, such as cystic fibrosis, muscular dystrophies, neural tube and other malformations, will make possible not only diagnosis *in utero* but treatment or prevention instead of selective abortion.

In this chapter, after outlining a strategy for screening and describing the diagnostic methods that are already available or under development, the most important abnormalities will be considered in turn. Opportunities for intrauterine treatment and for transfer *in utero* for immediate specialized management in a neonatal referral centre will be noted, as will the diagnosis of fetal abnormalities during late pregnancy.

SCREENING FOR FETAL ABNORMALITIES

Clinical markers: history and maternal age

The initial screening stage begins at the clinical level, when the mother presents for antenatal care or even beforehand as part of preconceptional counselling by an informed family doctor or at one of the prepregnancy clinics that obstetricians are at last beginning to establish (*see* Chapter 13). The mother's age, her medical history and recent drug treatment and alcohol consumption are noted, her family history and that of her husband elicited, and the outcome of any previous pregnancies recorded.

At present, documentation of family and obstetric histories is all too often a hurried routine, in which the mother may not understand the relevance of potentially useful information and so does not volunteer it, while the 'recorder' may not have the knowledge or experience to complete an effective enquiry. A more thorough historical record, than is now to be found in most case notes, should become standard practice, beginning with an easily comprehended questionnaire for the mother to complete and which could be posted to her with her booking appointment so that she has time for careful consideration and consultation with other family members. In this way more accurate medical, obstetric and family histories are likely to be obtained, especially when established or possible reasons for unsuccessful pregnancies (including abortions) or serious disorders in offspring were explained at the time or have been properly documented. Thus, even the simple knowledge of where and when an unsuccessful pregnancy ended, or where a disabled child is under supervision, may start an enquiry that will sometimes establish that the current pregnancy is at risk of a fetal disorder amenable to prenatal diagnosis.

COUNSELLING

The information provided may call for genetic counselling and perhaps family studies, or these may have already been carried out following a previous pregnancy with fetal abnormality or as part of the investigation of familial disease in a relative or either parent. Detailed investigation and counselling of this sort is the field of the specialist in clinical genetics, but every obstetrician should have a broad practical knowledge of inheritance and recurrence rates, especially for the commoner abnormalities (*see* Chapter 2).

In single gene disorders of known inheritance (X-linked or autosomal; recessive or dominant) recurrence risks are precise and, provided an accurate diagnosis of the disorder has been made, can easily be explained to couples one or both of whom are carriers (or are affected, e.g. haemophilia). Carrier testing is available for some disorders (e.g. Duchenne muscular dystrophy, by measuring serum creatinine kinase, see below) and if this is negative anxiety about the fetus can be dispelled and there is no need to offer prenatal diagnosis.

The increasing maternal age risks for bearing a child with trisomy 21 Down's syndrome or one of the least common chromosomal aberrations (e.g. trisomy 13 or 18, XXY) are also well established (*see* p. 321), and (excluding the older mothers) the chance of recurrence of these non-inherited chromosomal aberrations when a previous baby has been affected is generally about 1.5%. For balanced or unbalanced inherited chromosomal rearrangements, expert genetic counselling and family studies are essential, as they may be in assessing the recurrence risks for disorders of multifactorial inheritance. In the latter the recurrence risk increases with the number and closeness of affected relatives, but it is usually less than 1 in 20 with one affected first degree relative (e.g. for NTD) although it becomes significantly worse when more than one such family member has been affected (e.g. when two previous babies have had NTDs).

Explanatory pamphlets about prenatal diagnosis, dealing particularly with the significance of high maternal age and with maternal serum alpha-fetoprotein (MSAFP) screening, are found useful and reassuring by most mothers, and can be provided with each historical questionnaire. At hospitals serving immigrant communities it may be useful to have translations of questionnaires and antenatal information, although there may be other educational and cultural difficulties to overcome.

Blood tests

MATERNAL SERUM ALPHAFETOPROTEIN (MSAFP)

Measurement of MSAFP is by far the most useful screening blood test. It is now offered as a routine service in many parts of Britain, especially but not only where there is an unusually high incidence of neural tube defect (NTD). Apart from anencephaly and open spina bifida, which together account for more than 90% of fetal anomalies associated with high MSAFP, other less common malformations that may have this association include Meckel's syndrome (encephalocoele, polydactyly and polycystic kidneys), abdominal wall defects (exomphalos or gastroschisis), Turner's syndrome, haemangioma of the placenta or umbilical cord, and teratoma. High MSAFP may result from threatened or missed abortion, presumably because chorionic separation has caused fetomaternal bleeding, and higher than normal values are often present in multiple pregnancies.

MSAFP rises throughout most of pregnancy (from about 12 to 32 weeks) and there is overlap between values in normal pregnancies and those associated with NTD (especially before 16 weeks). In practice therefore accurate determination of gestational age is very important, and the chosen cut-off limit, above which a value is to be regarded as abnormal and calls for further investigation, is a compromise between sensitivity and specificity. The cut-off is usually set at between 1 and 3 multiples of the median (MOM), and the optimal time for screening was shown by the UK Collaborative Study (1977) to be 16–18 completed weeks of gestation. In the West of Scotland the 97th percentile (approximately 2.5 MOM) between 16 and 20 weeks is used, and if this is again exceeded in a second blood sample obtained a week later, confirmation or exclusion of an abnormality by detailed ultrasonic inspection of the fetus and/or amniocentesis is called for. This policy has kept the need for amniocentesis to below 1% of all pregnancies screened in this way. The importance of

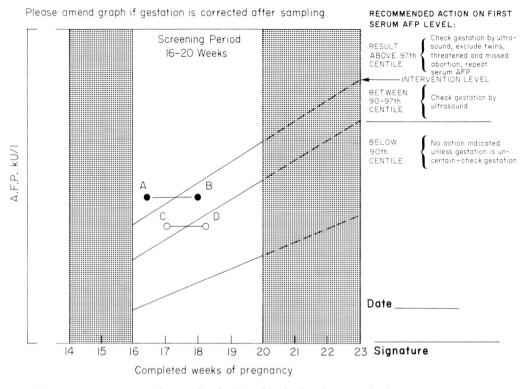

Fig. 22.1 The MSAFP screening report form used in the West of Scotland, with 2 examples showing the importance of accurate determination of gestational age. In the upper example if the true gestational age is 16 weeks and 3 days MSAFP is above the 97th centile cut-off (A), but if it is overestimated to be 18 weeks the same value would be regarded as a borderline result (B); conversely if a true gestational age of 18 weeks (B) is underestimated by the same interval (A) a borderline MSAFP value is made to appear abnormally high. The lower example shows how plotting the same MSAFP value at different gestational ages only a week apart gives either a borderline result (C) or a normal one below the secondary cut-off at the 90th centile (D).

precise determination of gestational age is illustrated in Fig. 22.1 which shows the MSAFP report form used in the West of Scotland; even a small underestimation of gestational age may 'convert' a value from just below the cut-off to just above it, and likewise a similar error of overestimating gestational age may conceal an abnormal value by moving it below the cut-off. For this reason a secondary cut-off, the 90th percentile, is used to indicate the need to confirm gestational age as precisely as possible; skilled ultrasonic measurement of the fetus for this purpose is therefore recommended whenever an intermediate MSAFP value (90th–97th percentile) is reported.

The UK Collaborative Study (1977) showed that 88% of anencephalic fetuses and 79% of those with open spinal defects could be 'detected' by MSAFP screening between 16 and 18 weeks of pregnancy. With its slightly different policy (see above) the West

of Scotland regional service, for a population of almost 3 million and some 37,000 births annually, achieved sensitivities of 97% for anencephaly and 72% for open spina bifida and, as the annual proportion of pregnancies screened reached almost 75%, the estimated proportion of 'affected births avoided' by prenatal diagnosis and selective abortion rose to 72% (Ferguson-Smith 1983).

From more than 200 MSAFP-screened twin pregnancies, Ghosh *et al.* (1982) reported 11 in which one fetus had a NTD and in which MSAFP was more than 5 MOM. This value is a practical cut-off for twin pregnancies in which the median MSAFP value approximates to the singleton cut-off of 2.5 MOM.

Other MSAFP-predicted risks
In the absence of fetal anomalies, high MSAFP values continue to have some prognostic value for the out-

come of pregnancy, there being increased rates for late abortion, perinatal mortality and low birthweight (Brock *et al.* 1977 and 1982, Wald *et al.* 1977). Although predictive sensitivity and specificity for these outcomes is disappointingly low, Hamilton *et al.* (1985) found that spontaneous labour before 34 weeks was 38 times more common when the screening MSAFP value was above the 97th percentile cut-off than when a normal value had been obtained. Likewise in twin pregnancies, Ghosh *et al.* (1982) reported an eventual fetal wastage of more than 50% when the MSAFP screening value had been above 5 MOM, while Redford and Whitfield (1985) noted that when the screening value had exceeded 4 MOM 40% of normally formed twin fetuses were stillborn or died later as a result of perinatal causes, whereas only 3% died when the screening MSAFP was less than 2 MOM.

HAEMOGLOBINOPATHY SCREENING

This should be carried out whenever an ethnically predisposed woman first attends for antenatal care or prepregnancy advice. In Britain, sickle-cell disease or trait should be sought in blacks, and beta-thalassaemia in those whose ethnic origin is in Eastern Mediterranean or Middle East. The very simple sickledex test is used for the former (p. 262), and the demonstration of microcytosis (mean corpuscular volume of 70 fl or less, compared with a normal value of about 90 fl) on routine Coulter blood counting is the first step towards identifying a mother carrying beta thalassaemia. When a mother is sickledex-positive or has been shown to have microcytosis, her husband's blood should be tested in the same way, and if the same result is obtained they should both have haemoglobin electrophoresis and haemoglobin A_2 quantitation (increased in beta-thalassaemia). This procedure has been established at all antenatal clinics in the North-East Thames region, and during three years only one child with beta-thalassaemia trait has been born to an undetected couple of carriers, although two were born to detected and counselled couples who chose not to proceed to definitive prenatal diagnosis by fetal blood sampling (Modell 1984).

OTHER BLOOD TESTS

Apart from MSAFP and haemoglobinopathy screening (and rubella and syphilis serology, *see* below) as yet no other maternal blood tests are established as useful universal routine methods to identify pregnan-

cies at risk of fetal abnormalities. In European (Ashkenazi) Jews, carrier (heterozygote) status for the rare but fatal autosomal recessive metabolic disorder known as *Tay-Sach's disease* is identified by demonstrating reduced hexosaminidase A activity in serum (or in leucocytes or platelets during pregnancy or when an equivocal serum result is obtained). This screening may be carried out when a couple are both Jewish, whether or not there is a known family history of the disease, but screening programmes among Jewish communities in several countries have failed, largely because of poor participation (Hecht & Cadien 1984). Serum creatinine kinase levels are raised in carriers of *Duchenne muscular dystrophy*, but they vary from time to time, fall during pregnancy and are higher in healthy teenage girls than in healthy women; there is also very considerable overlap between carrier and control values so that both sensitivity and specificity fall far short of the requirements for antenatal or prepregnancy carrier screening. There is urgent need for such a test, and also for one to detect carriers of cystic fibrosis. Eventually identification of the underlying gene abnormality and further developments in diagnostic DNA technology should provide these as well as carrier tests for the less common X-linked and autosomal disorders.

CONGENITAL INFECTION

This may be included in a list of fetal disorders for which blood tests are available for maternal screening, although lesions may not appear until some time after birth. Screening for syphilis is a long established antenatal practice; and there is increasing awareness of the importance of 'TORCH' infections as causes of fetal abnormalities and neurological and mental impairment as well as stunted growth, abortions and perinatal deaths.

The Venereal Disease Research Laboratory (VDRL) test is now the standard British test for routine screening for *syphilis* in the mother, and should be performed quantitatively whenever a positive result is obtained by any of the other available tests.

The main purpose of maternal *rubella* antibody screening is to select non-immune mothers for vaccination during the puerperium, although knowledge of the mother's 'rubella status' is helpful in the event of her becoming a rubella contact or developing an illness that might be rubella. Testing for *cytomegalovirus* (CMV) antibody is not a routine screening procedure but it is available, an 'ELISA' test probably being the method of choice, and might be introduced in communities with high carrier rates or in which nore than an occasional case of congenitally acquired CMV infection is known to have occurred. It is, of course, the sero-negative woman who is at risk of primary infection in pregnancy, with fetal infection in about one-third of them and defects occurring in about half of the infected babies, amounting to more than 500 per year in England and Wales (MacDonald & Tobin 1978). An ELISA test is also available to screen for mothers susceptible to *toxoplasmosis*, and, if effective treatment becomes possible, routine screening may be introduced in some countries although avoidance of cats and uncooked meat would be more logical and less costly.

In conclusion, while routine antenatal screening for syphilis and rubella is worthwhile, and in England Wales can be expected in each year to avoid more than 100 cases of congenital syphilis (by maternal and neonatal treatment) and about 100 cases of congenital rubella in subsequent pregnancies (following vaccination) universal antenatal screening for teratogenic infections is either not available or would probably not be cost-effective (Sequeira & Tobin 1984). The expected development of an effective vaccine would, of course, make the case for serological CMV screening.

Routine ultrasound scanning

The introduction of easily operated and relatively inexpensive high resolution real time ultrasound systems has made feasible routine scanning in pregnancy, and at least two-thirds of British obstetric units operate such a policy. Better general provision of equipment and increased numbers of well trained operators (obstetricians, midwives, and radiographers) would allow every antenatal clinic to have its own on-site scanner and every mother to have the benefits of routine ultrasound examination. Some clinics prefer to scan routinely at first attendance, and this has some clinical and organizational advantages; but for the specific purpose of scanning for fetal abnormalities 16–20 weeks is a better time, it is also the optimal time for MSAFP screening, and it is not unreasonably late for terminating the pregnancy if necessary. The ideal would be a booking scan to confirm viability of the early pregnancy and to establish its gestational age with precision, followed by more detailed imaging of the fetus at the same time as MSAFP screening. At present few units are able to implement this. Whatever routine policy is adopted, the clinic scanning team must have support from a

second tier ultrasound team, at the same hospital or a referral centre, expert in difficult and detailed imaging and measurement and in the definitive invasive methods for prenatal diagnosis (*see* below).

The results obtained at King's College Hospital by a first tier clinic scanning team of midwives, radiographers and technicians is a good example of what can be achieved in this way (Campbell & Smith 1984). In 11664 pregnancies scanned routinely at 16–18 weeks, 34 fetal anomalies, including all open NTDs, were suspected and then confirmed by the expert obstetric ultrasound team, at the cost of one misdiagnosis of hydrocephalus leading to the abortion of a normal fetus and of 5 undiagnosed abnormalities (microcephaly: renal agenesis; 3 cardiac).

DEFINITIVE DIAGNOSIS

The definitive diagnosis of fetal abnormalities in at risk mothers selected by screening, as described above, or occasionally when one develops a clinical feature sometimes associated with an anomaly (e.g. oligohydramnios or polyhydramnios), is by detailed ultrasonic inspection of the fetus and by invasive procedures to obtain fetal cells, fluid or tissue for laboratory analysis. The invasive techniques are themselves best guided by ultrasound which, therefore, has a central role in prenatal diagnosis from screening and 'second level' scanning with amniocentesis in most obstetric units to very expert 'third level' capabilities, including the full range of invasive sampling methods, provided by specialized teams at regional referral centres. Close liaison between such a referral team and a medical genetics centre, preferably at the same location, forms the focus of an effective regional organization, the genetics side providing its skilled counselling and family screening services and the special expertise of its laboratories, as well as access to a national and international network of such centres that ensures diagnostic support for even the rarest of detectable inborn disorders.

Fetal inspection by ultrasound

For detailed descriptions of the recognition of fetal abnormalities by expert imaging with high resolution real time ultrasound, readers are referred to Campbell and Pearce (1983) and to sections of the proceedings of a study group of the Royal College of Obstetrics and Gynaecologists relating to cranio-spinal abnormalities (Campbell *et al.* 1984), cardiac lesions

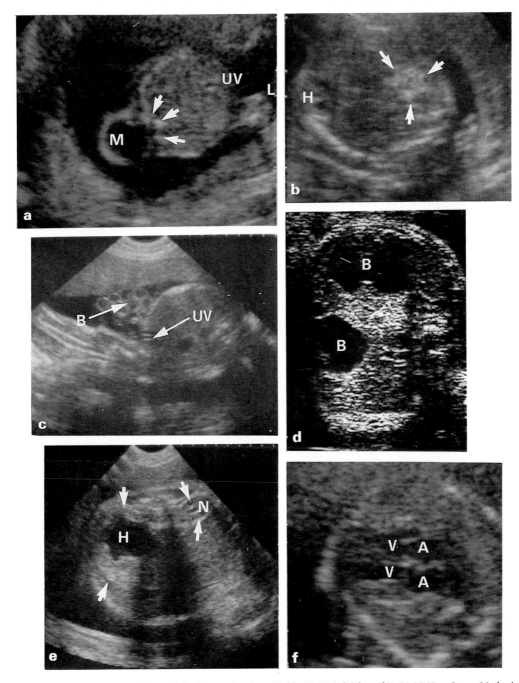

Fig. 22.2 Examples of ultrasound-detected fetal anomalies (provided by Dr M. Whittle and Dr M. McNay, Queen Mother's Hospital, Glasgow). (a) Open thoraco-lumbar spina bifida at 18 weeks. Transverse scan showing splayed out vertebral ossification centres (arrows) at the defect (M = meningocoele; UV = umbilical vein; L = limb). (b) Meconium ileus at 18 weeks. Longitudinal scan showing clumped echoes (arrows) from meconium-loaded bowel; (H = heart); cystic fibrosis confirmed following therapeutic abortion. (c) Gastroschisis at 28 weeks; bowel (B) free in amniotic cavity without an enclosing sac and separate from umbilical cord (UV = umbilical vein). (d) Intestinal atresia at 36 weeks showing 'double bubble' (BB); duodenal atresia associated with trisomy 21. (e) Unilateral hydronephrosis (H) at 34 weeks, with normal contralateral renal pelvis (N); arrows mark kidney surfaces. (f) Normal fetal heart at 21 weeks (4-chamber view; VV = ventricles, AA = atria).

(Allan 1984), skeletal dysplasias (Little 1984a) and anomalies of the gastrointestinal tract (Little 1984b) and urinary tract (Pearce & Campbell 1984). A few examples of ultrasound-detected fetal malformations are shown in Fig. 22.2.

In Britain by far the largest referral service for detailed ultrasound examination of mothers suspected or at high risk of carrying an abnormal fetus is provided by the academic obstetric department at King's College Hospital, where Campbell and Pearce (1983) described the results, summarized in Table 22.1, in 1737 such patients referred before 26 weeks during a recent 5-year period. Abnormalities were present in 262 of the fetuses (15%) and 244 of these (93%) were detected including all but 8 of 174 NTDs and other cranio-spinal anomalies, at the cost of 6 false positive diagnoses in normal fetuses. Seventeen undetected lesions included 6 open spina bifidas, 3 renal dysplasias or agenesis, and 2 abdominal wall defects.

Similarly at the Queen Mother's Hospital, Glasgow, during 1983 and 1984, 288 booked mothers and 167 referred from other hospitals had detailed ultrasound examinations because a previous baby was abnormal, MSAFP was high, or because there was some clinical pointer (e.g. high maternal age). There was an abnormality in 110 of the fetuses (24%) and it was recognized by ultrasound in 104 of them (95%) including 54 NTDs; 5 abnormal fetuses went undetected (aortic valve atresia; tracheo-oesophageal fistula; renal agenesis and spina bifida; trisomy 18; trisomy 21). Although no abnormality was diagnosed when there was none, a large mesenteric cyst in a

Abnormality	Detected	Not detected
Craniospinal (1084 referrals)		
Anencephaly	41	–
Open spina bifida	73	6
Closed spina bifida	4	–
Encephalocoele	13	1
Isolated hydrocephaly	16	–
Other	19	1
Sub-total	166	8
Gastrointestinal (172 referrals)		
Abdominal wall defects	21	2
Atresias	3	1
Other	6	–
Sub-total	30	3
Renal and urinary tract (99 referrals)		
Renal agenesis/dysplasia	4	3
Polycystic/multicystic kidney	11	–
Other renal cysts	2	–
Obstructive lesions	11	–
Cloacal extrophy	1	–
Sub-total	29	3
Cardiac anomalies (261 referrals)	8	2
Limb deformities (92 referrals)	13	–
***Fetal tumours** (19 referrals)	16	–
All referrals = 1737	262	16

Table 22.1 Details including detection, of fetal abnormalities in 1737 at risk pregnancies referred for detailed ultrasound at King's College Hospital, 1978–82 (adapted from Campbell & Pearce 1983)

* includes cystic hygroma and other neck swellings

twin was mistaken for obstructive dilatation of the urinary tract, the co-twin having a correctly diagnosed hydrocephalus.

Thus in both these centres, and elsewhere, it has been shown that expert imaging can achieve a diagnostic sensitivity of about 95% (excluding any further anomalies that may become apparent later in life) with a specificity exceeding 95.5% (1815 of 1821 normal fetuses in both series correctly diagnosed as such).

Ultrasound has roles in prenatal diagnosis other than routine scanning early in pregnancy and the search for abnormalities in high risk mothers referred for this purpose. Sometimes when performed for another indication, it will show an unexpected fetal malformation or will reveal some feature that may be associated with one (e.g. abnormal liquor volume, stunted growth or a placental abnormality). The accurate determination of gestational age is important in interpreting not only MSAFP values but also fetal measurements such as head and brain size, limb lengths and dimensions of particular organs (e.g. kidney) when a related anomaly is under consideration. Ultrasound also provides the essential guidance for the invasive diagnostic procedures described below.

Amniocentesis

The hazards of second trimester amniocentesis were the subject of a multicentre assessment by the Medical Research Council (1978), and by collaborative surveys in Canada (Simpson *et al.* 1976) and the United States (NICHD 1976). For more recent descriptions of technique, safety, indications and available amniotic fluid tests, the reader is directed to reviews by Ritchie and Thomson (1982), Turnbull and Mackenzie (1983) and McNay and Whitfield (1984).

The optimal timing of amniocentesis for prenatal diagnosis is 16 weeks' gestation, earlier than which it may be less easy to obtain liquor and cell growth in culture may be unsatisfactory. Especially when diagnosis depends on first establishing cell cultures, delay beyond this time progressively reduces the simplicity and safety and increases the emotional stress of terminating pregnancy (if required) or may even make it inappropriate.

Although amniocentesis for this purpose was established before ultrasound became generally available, it is now mandatory to perform it under direct ultrasound guidance to locate a suitably placed pocket of fluid for aspiration and to avoid the placenta while doing so. Multiple pregnancy, the placental site or early oligohydramnios may make

amniocentesis difficult, but with expert ultrasound guidance it is usually possible to obtain liquor from each of twins, to bypass the edge of an anterior placenta, or to find at least a small pocket of fluid that can be aspirated. Oligohydramnios at this stage, which is not infrequently associated with high MSAFP, is an ominous sign, but sometimes postponement of amniocentesis by a week or two may make sampling easier. The same may apply with an extensive anterior placenta, which may no longer guard the whole amniotic cavity as the pregnancy grows, or if necessary the deliberate transplacental insertion of the needle into an identified pool of liquor is usually safe and successful. In the latter circumstance, if the mother is rhesus-negative she should be protected by an injection of anti-D immunoglobulin (p. 268), and as part of 'defensive medicine' this precaution is wise even when ultrasound shows the placenta to be well clear of the needle.

Apart from rhesus-immunization, exsanguination following puncture of a placental or umbilical vessel has been a very rare cause of fetal death, and a variety of fetal traumas have been described. With adequate ultrasound all such complications are avoidable. Likewise, an expert ultrasound/amniocentesis team can reduce the risk of subsequent abortion to a rate of less than 0.5%. Increased perinatal mortality following amniocentesis mainly concerns pregnancies with raised MSAFP, which even without amniocentesis have increased wastage and low birthweight rate (Read *et al.* 1980), the latter probably also explaining an apparent increased risk of neonatal respiratory difficulties. The importance of operator experience is illustrated by the excess wastage rates (attributable to the procedure) from late abortions and perinatal deaths of only 0.3% at centres in the West of Scotland where large numbers of amniocenteses are carried out, compared with an overall rate of 0.7% in the region (Ferguson-Smith & Ferguson-Smith 1983).

Table 22.2 summarizes the indications for prenatal diagnosis by analysis of amniotic fluid and its cells and the related risk rates for the fetus to be affected; the categories of test available in the medical genetics laboratory, with examples of lethal or handicapping disorders detectable by them, are also shown.

In offering couples the option of amniocentesis followed by selective abortion of an affected fetus, or of a male fetus when the risk is a recessive X-linked disorder for which there is no specific diagnostic test, full account must be taken of their attitudes and preferences. Their decision must be guided by sensitive

Table 22.2 Indications for amniocentesis for prenatal diagnosis of fetal abnormalities, with risk rates and types of test

Indication	Risk	Amniotic fluid test	
High MSAFP	1/7 (mostly NTD)	Supernate	Alphafetoprotein Acetylcholinesterase
NTD in previous pregnancy	1/20 recurrence	,,	,,

Maternal age, e.g. at 35 years
          at 37 years
          at 40 years
	1/213
	1/125 } for trisomies
	1/63 } 21, 18, 13
		Cell culture	Karyotype

Trisomy in previous pregnancy	1/67 recurrence	,, ,,	,,
Either parent carrying balanced chromosomal structural rearrangement	varies from 1/5 (Robertsonian 21q 22q) to 1/62 (Robertsonian 13q 14q)	,, ,,	,,
Mother carrying X-linked recessive disorder (e.g. Duchenne muscular dystrophy, or haemophilia)	1/2 if male	Uncultured cells Cell culture	Sex chromatin (provisional) Karyotype
Either parent carrying detectable recessive disorder	1/4	Supernate (occasionally) Cell culture	Enzyme ,, DNA (e.g. sickle-cell disease & thalassaemia)
Sibling of either parent with detectable recessive disorder	Varies with carrier incidence in general population	,, ,,	,, ,,
	1/132 recurrence for cystic fibrosis	,, ,,	,, ,,

and informed clinical and genetic counselling. Close cooperation between the obstetric and genetic teams is, of course, as essential in relation to the newer techniques of fetoscopy and chorion villus sampling, described below, in which on-the-spot laboratory involvement is also required.

Fetoscopy

Endoscopy through the uterine wall, exposed at laparotomy prior to hysterotomy-termination, had been used to view the fetus and obtain samples of its blood and skin (Valenti 1972, Scrimgeour 1973), but it was the introduction by Hobbins *et al.* (1974) of percutaneous transabdominal fetoscopy, using fibre-optic illumination, that made possible the clinical exploitation of this new approach to intrauterine diagnosis. Further improvements of technique and equipment have been matched by the development of appropriate laboratory methods for testing the small samples of blood or tissue obtained. The most extensive experience has been at the referral centre at King's College Hospital, and this was the basis for a useful review by Rodeck and Nicolaides (1983) of fetoscopic techniques and their application in the in-

vestigation of 700 at risk pregnancies (summarized in Table 22.3).

The optimal time for inspection of the fetus for an anatomical abnormality, perhaps a facial or digital defect as a visible syndrome marker, is 15–18 weeks, but fetoscopy is less often used for this purpose than might be expected because most important malformations are detectable by ultrasound and because, especially if there is oligohydramnios, it may be difficult or impossible to view the fetal part in question. For blood sampling, which is the indication for most fetoscopies and in which the samples are obtained from either end of the umbilical cord, the optimal time is 18–20 weeks; earlier than this excessive bleeding from the punctured vessel is more likely, and later there is increasing turbidity of the liquor, although for the treatment of severe rhesus disease fetoscopically directed intravascular transfusion has been performed as late as about 30 weeks (p. 273). Apart from the detection of disorders requiring blood or tissue samples, fetoscopy has the further advantage over amniocentesis that it permits rapid lymphocyte culture for karyotyping within 2 or 3 days. Thus, when an at risk mother attends late (e.g. 20 weeks), or when very occasionally amniotic fluid cells

Diagnostic method	Examples of condition at risk
Fetal inspection (64 cases)	Facial defects ⎫ Limb ,, ⎬ e.g. as syndrome markers Digital ,, ⎭ NTD Abdominal wall defects Sex-linked
Fetal blood sampling (534 cases)	Haemoglobinopathies Coagulation disorders Metabolic disorders Chromosomal anomalies Severe combined immunodeficiency
Fetal skin biopsy (15 cases)	Epidermolysis bullosa letalis
Fetal liver biopsy (5 cases)	Rare metabolic disorders ?Phenylketonuria

Total pregnancies	618
Failed fetoscopy	3
Diagnostic error	1
Operative loss (<48 hours)	3
Termination of pregnancy	176
Intended continuing pregnancy	439
Spontaneous abortion	8 (1.8%)

Table 22.3 Possible indications for fetoscopic diagnosis of fetal abnormalities in 618 pregnancies referred to King's College Hospital (adapted from Rodeck & Nicolaides 1983)

have failed to establish satisfactory cultures, fetoscopic blood sampling may be preferred to amniocentesis to avoid further significant delay should termination become necessary.

No associated maternal mortality or significant morbidity has been reported, and Nicolaides and Rodeck (1984) reported only 4 operative fetal losses (within 48 hours) after fetoscopy in 707 pregnancies (a rate of 0.6%), and in the 512 continuing pregnancies with an unaffected fetus there were only 11 subsequent spontaneous abortions (2.1%) although delivery before 37 weeks occurred in 12% of those followed up to confinement.

Chorionic villus sampling

Chorion is a fetal tissue reflecting the chromosomal, DNA and biochemical constitution of the fetus. Its recent, now increasing, use for first trimester prenatal diagnosis has been reviewed by Rodeck and Morsman (1983). Its sampling, optimally at 8–11 weeks and ideally from the rapidly proliferating chorion fron-

dosum from which the placenta is forming, provides actively dividing mesenchyme cells for culture. DNA analysis, and also chromosomal and biochemical studies, are then possible within less than 2 weeks, and techniques have been developed for direct karyotyping and enzyme determinations without prior culture (Simoni et al. 1983) with results being reported within 2 days. Various transcervical sampling techniques have been used, including blind aspiration, intrauterine lavage, endoscopic biopsy with or without ultrasound guidance, and ultrasound-directed needle aspiration or biopsy. None of these procedures requires general anaesthesia. Increasingly the preferred technique has been aspiration through a plastic or malleable metal cannula inserted into the chorion under guidance by real time ultrasound used by the operator or by an assistant. This can produce sufficient viable material, uncontaminated by decidua, for successful culture in more than 90% of cases. The success rate is improved by immediate on-site microscopy to verify the presence of villi in the aspirated sample (Fig. 22.3).

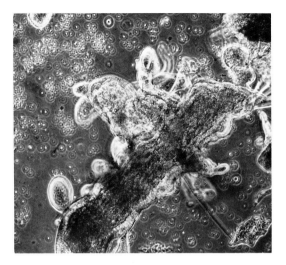

Fig. 22.3 A branching chorionic villus in an aspiration biopsy sample.

Chorion cultures are suitable for DNA analysis for the diagnosis of haemoglobinopathies and of an increasing number of serious disorders for which gene probes are becoming available or can be expected to be developed in future (Humphries & Williamson 1983). Until specific gene probes become available, fetal sexing makes possible early selective abortion of males at 50% risk of an X-linked disease (e.g. Duchenne muscular dystrophy) and when adequate samples contain sufficient mitoses for direct karyotyping this is feasible by the 10th week.

Some vaginal bleeding is not uncommon following chorion sampling, but the risks of penetrating the gestation sac or introducing infection seem to be negligible. The important hazard is spontaneous abortion, but this risk is reduced by operator experience which should always be gained in patients about to have termination of pregnancy. Information from an international registry shows that in more than 4000 pregnancies intended to continue following diagnostic sampling, of which more than 1300 have proceeded to delivery, a fetal loss rate of 4.1% had been notified (Jackson 1985). Therapeutic abortion was carried out on 9% of all the patients registered, and sampling failed in 2.2%. The effect of operator experience with high quality ultrasound guidance is underlined by sampling failures. The results at 4 centres, each of which registered more than 500 patients, show this very clearly: their combined sampling failure rate was only 1.4%, and the fetal loss rate in the intended continuing pregnancies was only 3.2%. However, an important caution is that at 6 centres, each with between 50 and 100 patients registered, 3.5% of attempts to sample failed and in the intended continuing pregnancies, only 16% of which had so far proceeded to delivery, a fetal loss rate of 7.5% had already been reported.

DIAGNOSTIC STRATEGIES FOR PARTICULAR ABNORMALITIES

In practice NTDs and Down's syndrome are the most common detectable abnormalities that may lead to handicap in surviving infants. Strategies for their diagnosis, and for the detection of other specific abnormalities or groups of disorders, and progress towards this goal in relation to several outstanding major problems, will be outlined.

Neural tube defects (NTD)

In some regions the incidence of NTD may be as high as 4 or 5 per 1000 births. Since fewer than one in 20 babies born with anencephaly, encephalocoele or spina bifida have been preceded by a previous sibling with a NTD, routine estimation of MSAFP is in most parts of Britain the mainstay of screening to identify pregnancies at unexpected risk of these defects, although routine ultrasound scanning at the same gestational age may now be just as effective. Because closed spina bifida and a few, usually small, open defects are not accompanied by raised MSAFP, and because small lesions may also go undetected at ultrasound screening, it is best to use both methods if available. Confirmation that NTD (or other relevant abnormality) is present is by detailed ultrasound examination and/or amniocentesis for the measurement of alphafetoprotein and detection of acetylcholinesterase bands in the liquor, the latter marker (a second, fast moving band) being particularly useful when the AFP value is raised but no lesion has been seen by ultrasound or when either or both of these have given uncertain results. Although amniocentesis was once the main method for definitive diagnosis, it is an invasive procedure and amniotic fluid AFP measurement gives some false negative and false positive values. In most centres it has therefore been used less and less as ultrasound equipment and scanning expertise have improved, even to the point where reliance on ultrasound alone has been suggested (Campbell & Pearce 1983). However, at least for some time, amniocentesis and ultrasound should be regarded as complementary methods which, together with MSAFP screening, can detect almost all open NTDs.

OTHER CRANIO–SPINAL DEFECTS

Hydrocephaly. The ultrasonic detection and assessment of hydrocephaly is made by displaying and measuring the lateral ventricles, including their anterior and posterior horns, and the surrounding mantle of cerebral cortex. If isolated hydrocephalus develops it is almost always detected too late for termination of pregnancy, and serial measurements should be made at regular intervals. Near term, if the cortex is thinning, it may be decided, after paediatric and surgical consultation, that the baby should be delivered so that a shunt may be inserted. Insertion of a tube to drain the ventricle into the amniotic fluid has been carried out in a few cases, but prognosis has remained poor and long-term follow-up is probably very unlikely to support a case for this intrauterine procedure.

Microcephaly. The usual warning that microcephaly may develop is provided by a previous affected baby, and this defect cannot usually be detected with certainty in time for therapeutic abortion to be an option. Serial head measurements are made and can be compared with normal dimensions and growth rates, but to distinguish this defect from severe intrauterine growth retardation the ratio between the head and abdominal circumferences should be measured (serially) and compared with normal values.

Down's syndrome and other chromosomal abnormalities

Trisomy 21, Down's syndrome, is the commonest seriously handicapping chromosomal disorder, affecting about 1 in 800 liveborns and accounting for 1 in 4 children with severe mental impairment. Its incidence is well known to rise with increasing maternal age, as do the rates for the less common trisomy 18 and trisomy 13 and for the abnormal sex chromosome syndromes XXY (Klinefelter's) and XXX. Other unbalanced chromosomal aberrations, leading to variable but sometimes severe disability or to 'natural wastage' by spontaneous abortion, are unrelated to maternal age.

As a practical guide for obstetricans, Table 22.4 summarizes maternal age specific rates for trisomy 21 alone, for trisomies 21, 18 and 13 together, and for all unbalanced aberrations, over the age range (35–40 years) in which most obstetricians will choose a threshold at which to offer amniocentesis. It is adapted from the data of a European collaborative study of more than 50 000 pregnancies coming to amniocentesis and karyotyping (Ferguson-Smith & Yates 1984). Based on this information, the detection rate for trisomy 21 rises from 0.35%, or 1 in 286, in women aged 35 years to 1.23%, or 1 in 81, at the age of 40 years, the corresponding combined rates for all 3 autosomal trisomies being 0.47% (1 in 213) and 1.6% (1 in 63) respectively, while the detection rate for all unbalanced aberrations increases from 0.9% (1 in 111) at 35 years of age to 2.14% (1 in 47) at 40 years.

Subsequent to amniocentesis, however, some 30% of trisomy 21 pregnancies will end in spontaneous abortion or stillbirth, with higher wastages in trisomies 18 and 13 (and generally lower but variable rates applying to the other abnormalities). By subtracting 30%, it is possible to calculate approximate risk rates for the livebirth of babies with these syndromes, and these are perhaps the most valid rates to use when counselling on the option for amniocentesis which carries its own attributable fetal loss rate of about 0.5 or 1.0%. Thus at 37 years,

Maternal age	Trisomy 21	Trisomies 21, 18, 13	All unbalanced
35	0.35 = 1/286	0.47 = 1/213	0.90 = 1/111
36	0.57	0.68	1.10
37	0.68 = 1/147	0.80 = 1/125	1.21 = 1/81
38	0.81	1.00	1.39
39	1.09	1.34	1.88
40	1.23 = 1/81	1.60 = 1/63	2.14 = 1/47
45	4.53 = 1/22	5.12 = 1/20	7.28 = 1/14

Table 22.4 Maternal age specific rates (%) for chromosomal abnormalities, in the usual range (35–40 years) for amniocentesis because of maternal age, adapted from European Collaborative Study (Ferguson-Smith & Yates 1984)

which is regarded by many as a reasonable threshold at which to offer amniocentesis and selective abortion, without such intervention 1 in 179 mothers (0.56%) will give birth to a live baby with Down's or one of the other trisomy syndromes, and 1 in 115 (0.87%) will go on to livebirth of an infant with some sort of unbalanced chromosomal anomaly.

As a further guide, a recurrence rate of 1.5% can be used, independently of maternal age, when there has been a previous child with Down's or other autosomal trisomy syndrome. When some other chromosomal abnormality has been found in a previous offspring, or was established as the cause of an earlier unsuccessful pregnancy, or has been identified in a close relative, expert genetic counselling is needed to determine the likelihood of recurrence and the probable severity of disability that may result.

For some time at least, amniocentesis will remain the mainstay of antenatal diagnosis of chromosomal disorders. Nevertheless, there is a case for fetoscopic blood sampling and immediate karyotyping when a mother at risk does not present until 20 weeks or so in her pregnancy, or if amniotic fluid cell culture has already failed. In older very high risk mothers (e.g. aged 40 years or more) attending very early in pregnancy, perhaps as a result of prior counselling to do so, the balance of risks may be judged to favour chorion villus sampling with direct karyotyping, followed by immediate termination of an affected pregnancy, as an alternative to having a diagnosis 2 months later from cultured cells obtained by amniocentesis. When a centre has been able to establish chorion biopsy as a standard technique with acceptably low failed sampling and attributable fetal loss rates, the age threshold may be reduced, and, depending on the eventual results of a planned multicentre controlled trial to compare it with amniocentesis, chorion sampling may become the preferred method in most patients attending before the 12th week of pregnancy.

X-linked recessive disorders

Prenatal diagnosis of these disorders depends on whether or not a specific diagnostic test is available. If it is not, as in *Duchenne Muscular Dystrophy*, fetal sexing followed by abortion of a male fetus with a 50% chance of being affected is the best that can be offered, although gene linkage studies may be approaching a successful diagnostic technique. Sex chromatin analysis on cells obtained by amniocentesis provides a rapid provisional indication of fetal

sex, but this should be confirmed by karyotyping cultured cells. At fetoscopy blood samples can be taken for rapid karyotyping, and fetal sex can be determined by direct karyotyping of chorionic villus cells.

When a specific diagnostic test is available (haematological, enzymatic or by DNA analysis) this should be carried out as soon as a male fetus has been identified. An example is the measurement of clotting factors in blood from a fetus at a risk of haemophilia or certain other bleeding disorders.

FRAGILE-X SYNDROME

This may have a frequency as high as 1 per 1000 male births. and is perhaps second only to Down's syndrome as a cause of mental retardation in males. In affected males a fragile site can be demonstrated in the X-chromosome in a proportion of cultured peripheral blood leucocytes, using special folate-deficient media, but is much less reliably detected in cultures of amniotic cells so that false negative results may be reported. It is to be hoped that chorion villus sampling will provide cultures amenable to inducing and detecting X-chromosome fragility.

Screening of mentally retarded males for fragile-X would lead to the identification of some obligatory female carriers who would be offered prenatal diagnosis.

Haemoglobinopathies

Carrier screening for thalassaemia and sickle-cell anaemia, described on p. 313, has become an important part of antenatal care in Britain as a result of immigration. Definitive diagnosis in the fetus is by fetoscopic blood sampling to measure Haemoglobin S (in sickle-cell disease) or Haemoglobin A (halved in amount in thalassaemia trait; absent or virtually so in thalassaemia major). There is some overlap in Haemoglobin A values between normal fetuses and those with beta-thalassaemia trait, but a demarcation between beta-thalassaemia major and the trait. In more than 500 diagnostic cases at University College Hospital, London, there were only 6 misdiagnoses and fetal losses attributed to the fetoscopic procedure were reduced from 10 to 3% (Modell 1984).

Methods of DNA analysis have been developed for the diagnosis of sickle-cell disease and beta-thalassaemia and can be used in samples of chorionic villi. They may well come to replace fetoscopic blood sampling for the detection of these crippling diseases in well counselled and screened at risk ethnic communities, in which most known carrier mothers may be motivated to report very early in pregnancy.

Inherited metabolic errors

Some of the earliest successful prenatal diagnoses were made in fetuses with inborn metabolic disorders, and there is now a list of at least 60 such diseases (Patrick 1983) that can be detected by demonstrating the underlying enzyme defect in cultures of amniotic fluid cells, or less often in the amniotic supernate or in uncultured cells which may give an immediate provisional diagnosis requiring confirmation in culture. Most of these disorders are rare, but may be lethal or crippling, many are untreatable and, being mostly recessively inherited, carrier parents have a 1 in 4 risk of recurrence.

Fetoscopy also has a role. Enzymatic tests can be performed on blood samples, and some of these disorders including severe haemolytic anaemias can be diagnosed only in this way. Fetoscopic skin biopsy makes possible the diagnosis of epidermolysis bullosa letalis and other grave skin disorders, and liver biopsy can be used for the detection of rare errors expressed in that tissue.

Enzymatic tests can be carried out on chorion villus samples, although it remains to be shown that these will reflect properly the biochemical constitution of the fetus and that there is no overlap between normal, heterozygous and homozygous values. It is to be expected that DNA analysis with specific gene probes and linkage techniques will also find practical application in the diagnosis of metabolic disorders in chorionic samples.

CYSTIC FIBROSIS

The development of a test to detect cystic fibrosis, a recessively inherited disease with a birth incidence in Caucasians of about 1 in 2000, is arguably the most important clinical challenge in prenatal genetic research. The underlying biochemical defect is still unknown, but low amniotic fluid values of several enzymes produced in the microvilli of epithelial membranes have been found. Brock *et al.* (1985) have used a monoclonal antibody for specific measurement of alkaline phosphatase of intestinal origin and, with a cut-off at half the median value for gestational age, they reported 91% sensitivity in the diagnosis of cystic fibrosis in live fetuses and abortuses in which the disorder was confirmed by bio-

chemical analysis of meconium in the ileum; specificity was 95%. While, therefore, there was some overlap producing false negative and false positive results, parents known (because of a previous affected child) to have a 1 in 4 chance of recurrence may well find this an acceptable test, especially when gestational age can be confirmed with precision to allow for the changing normal range of values between 16 and 20 weeks. A carrier test to identify other at risk couples is needed, and it is hoped that DNA analysis will eventually become available to make an accurate diagnosis of the disorder, including in chorion villus samples.

Ultrasound may come to have a complementary role in the intrauterine diagnosis of cystic fibrosis. A report from Paris described ultrasound findings consistent with meconium ileus just before termination of pregnancy, and this was confirmed by post-mortem examination (Muller *et al.* 1984), and in Glasgow similar localized 'clumping' of echoes in the fetal abdomen (Fig. 22.2[b]) had been seen prior to amniocentesis, and meconium ileus was confirmed by post-mortem examination after termination.

Abdominal wall defects and other gastrointestinal anomalies

Exomphalos and gastroschisis

The possibility of an abdominal wall defect is usually suggested by raised MSAFP and also, when a small defect is not then seen by ultrasound, by abnormally high alphafetoprotein in the amniotic fluid, although there will not be 2 bands of acetylcholinesterase unless there has been contamination with blood. Usually the defect can be seen and the herniated abdominal contents identified by ultrasound. A correct diagnosis in 17 of 23 abdominal wall defects at a mean gestational age of 19 weeks was reported recently (Hutson *et al.* 1985).

In exomphalos gut, sometimes liver and even heart, and the umbilical vessels, herniate through a defect in body stalk closure and within a membrane which usually remains intact. A high mortality is largely explained by the frequent presence of other major abnormalities particularly trisomies. Associated abnormalities are much less common and mortality is much lower with gastroschisis; in this condition the defect is beside the umbilical cord, and there is no covering membrane so that ultrasound shows widely separated and mobile loops of bowel in the amniotic cavity.

If exomphalos is diagnosed early in pregnancy termination may be considered, and associated chromosomal or structural anomalies must always be searched for. Otherwise, delivery must take place where neonatal intensive care and surgery are available. For gastroschisis it seems sensible to deliver by Caesarean section to protect the exteriorized bowel, but this may not be necessary; following birth progressive reduction of the herniation can be achieved, using a silastic bag to contain the bowel until the abdominal cavity is large enough to accommodate it.

Atresias

It is polyhydramnios that usually draws attention to *oesophageal atresia*, which may be associated with a tracheo-oesophageal fistula, and repeated ultrasound examinations will confirm the absence of fluid in the stomach and gut.

Duodenal and jejunal atresias, with which other anomalies frequently coexist, also cause polyhydramnios, and ultrasound reveals the now classical 'double bubble' of fluid (Fig. 22.2[d]) retained in the stomach and duodenum (or more than 2 bubbles in some jejunal atresias).

Diaphragmatic hernia and colonic obstruction

These may also be recognized by ultrasound, but prognosis may be poor because of pulmonary hypoplasia in association with the former and bowel necrosis with perforation in the latter.

For these lesions too, unless other major malformations have been found and dictate management, delivery must be planned to take place where expert neonatal care and surgery can be provided.

Renal and urinary tract anomalies

Using ultrasound the normal fetal kidney, with the echo-free renal pelvis at its centre, can be outlined by the 18th week at the latest, and intermittent filling of the bladder can be observed by 14–16 weeks. Kidney dimensions may be compared with established normal values at different gestational ages.

Renal agenesis

Attention to the possible presence of renal agenesis is usually drawn by oligohydramnios which, however, together with the usual fetal hyperflexion that results, may make the diagnosis by ultrasound difficult. The fetus is usually very small, and severe growth retardation without a recognized malformation may be reported, but absence of bladder filling should also suggest the correct diagnosis.

Cystic kidneys

Congenital polycystic kidney disease is one of the fetal anomalies associated with raised MSAFP which is the usual clue leading to its detection by ultrasound. However, sometimes the cysts are very small and may not be recognized easily. This is a bilateral, recessively inherited disease of grave prognosis, for which no obstetric intervention is indicated other than termination if the diagnosis is made early enough in pregnancy.

Multicystic kidneys, by contrast, are usually unilateral, with good prognosis although eventually nephrectomy is often necessary. The cystic spaces may be quite large, and easily recognized on ultrasound examination. *Isolated cysts*, which do not affect renal function, are occasionally detected.

Obstructive lesions

High obstruction at the pelvi-ureteral junction, due to a neuromuscular defect or an aberrant renal artery, is the most common of these lesions. It is usually a chance finding by ultrasound, is usually unilateral and/or incomplete, and causes mainly extrarenal enlargement of the renal pelvis without much thinning of the renal cortex or impairment of function. Intrauterine decompression by insertion of a vesico-amniotic shunt is not therefore required. However, if appreciable cortical thinning is occurring towards term, early delivery and neonatal surgery may be the best course.

By contrast, *low obstruction* in male fetuses, due to urethral valves or stenosis, is usually complete so that there is very severe oligohydramnios which is the usual indication for ultrasound examination; this shows the grossly dilated bladder with bilateral hydroureter and hydronephrosis, and with little kidney tissue. With posterior urethral valves obstruction may be intermittent and/or incomplete, oligohydramnios may be less marked, but there is usually obvious bladder distension; hydroureter and hydronephrosis vary in degree, as do the effects on the cortex and on kidney function. Other anomalies including trisomy-18 and 'prune belly' may be present, and another hazard is pulmonary hypoplasia. Decompression by insertion of a double pigtail ended catheter, as a vesico-amniotic shunt, has the two aims of protecting renal function and allowing lung development, but the value of this procedue remains uncertain.

Congenital cardiac lesions

Major cardiac anomalies are present in 4 of every 1000 liveborns, although they are not always detected until some time after the neonatal phase. With ultrasound a good 4-chamber view of the fetal heart can usually be obtained by 20 weeks, but cardiac scanning requires more skill and experience than does that of other fetal organs. Allan (1984) has described the correct diagnosis of 26 cardiac anomalies, missing only 4 minor lesions, in 1000 pregnancies in which the fetal heart was scanned in detail by a specialized team; the indication for the examination was either an environmental risk (e.g. family history, diabetes, exposure to a teratogen or viral infection) or because fetal ascites, arrythmia or growth retardation had been detected. It is unlikely that such results will be obtainable at more than a few centres specializing in this form of obstetric imaging. Most of the diagnoses will be made too late to permit therapeutic abortion, but will provide a useful warning to the neonatal team and should ensure delivery in a hospital with full facilities for cardiological investigation and treatment including surgery. The great majority of mothers can be reassured that their babies do not have serious cardiac defects.

Skeletal dysplasias

Some 'short limbed dwarf' deformities may be diagnosed *in utero* in time for termination of pregnancy, using ultrasound to measure the length of the fetal long bones, particularly the femur, and comparing these measurements with established normal values. Examples are osteogenesis imperfecta and homozygous achondroplasia. In heterozygous achondroplasia, obvious limb shortening is not present until about 24 weeks, and in some other deformities it occurs later still.

Inspection of the fetal hands by ultrasound may reveal 'lobster claw' deformity, polydactyly or syndactyly as external markers of rare syndromes in which other anomalies are the more important. Unilateral shortening of a limb may be a similar syndrome marker, or it may be caused by an amniotic band.

DIAGNOSIS LATE IN PREGNANCY AND FURTHER MANAGEMENT

Before the development of ultrasound, X-ray was used to demonstrate deformities of the fetal skull, spine or long bones, and some soft tissue malformations were sought by amniography and fetography after injecting radio-opaque contrast into the amniotic fluid. The latter techniques (Queenan & Gadow 1970) may still be useful when polyhydramnios is being investigated but high quality ultrasound is not available, and are therefore worth describing briefly. Water-soluble contrast disperses quickly throughout the amniotic cavity and an external abnormality such as encephalocoele, meningomyelocoele or cystic hygroma may be outlined as a filling defect, or the following day the absence of contrast from the fetal stomach and/or bowel may confirm the presence of an oesophageal or high intestinal atresia. Lipid-soluble contrast is taken up by the vernix caseosa to outline the fetal skin so that an externally protruding deformity may be more easily recognized by X-ray on the following day. Where an effective ultrasound service is available, these radiographic techniques will be needed rarely if at all. Instead, with further developments in techniques and equipment, the scope for ultrasonic diagnosis of even small defects will increase, while the coming of nuclear magnetic resonance promises much for the detailed imaging of most fetal organs.

For fetal abnormalities requiring further investigation and/or intensive care after birth, and perhaps surgical correction, reference has been made several times to the need to ensure that delivery takes place where there are all the facilities needed. Team work is essential in deciding the timing and method of delivery. Decisions should be made only after full assessment of risks, the presence of any additional abnormalities, the likely disability and prognosis with and without treatment, and of alternative methods of management including, occasionally, a very cautious consideration of intrauterine decompression by insertion of a shunt. The parents should be counselled carefully, and their own informed preferences taken into account. The conclusions of an interspecialty group in Glasgow, describing the management of 35 babies born alive with major anomalies detected during pregnancy (and also 15 terminated pregnancies, and two ending in spontaneous abortion or stillbirth) are summarized below.

To build up an experienced team, and to gather as much information as possible to guide future decisions and developments, there should be a referral system for the small number of fetuses with nonlethal or treatable malformations diagnosed during pregnancy, to a centre where all the disciplines involved are represented, work closely together and have all the diagnostic, medical and surgical facilities that may be needed (Hutson et al. 1985).

The obstetric management of hydrocephaly and

other fetal deformities causing, or likely to cause, dystocia is described in Chapter 26 (p. 382).

REFERENCES

ALLAN L.D. (1984) In *Prenatal Diagnosis: Proceedings of 11th Study Group* (Rodeck C.H. & Nicolaides K.H. eds.), p. 285. RCOG, London.

BROCK D.J.H., BARRON L., JELEN P., WATT M. & SCRIMGEOUR J.B. (1977) *Lancet*, ii, 267.

BROCK D.J.H., BARRON L., WATT M., SCRIMGEOUR J.B. & KEAY A.J. (1982) *Brit. J. Obstet. Gynaec.*, 89, 348.

BROCK D.J.H., BEDGOOD D., BARRON L. & HAYWARD C. (1985) *Lancet*, i, 1175.

CAMPBELL S. & PEARCE J.M. (1983) *Brit. med. Bull.*, 39, 322.

CAMPBELL S. & SMITH P. (1984) In *Prenatal Diagnosis: Proceedings of 11th Study Group* (Rodeck C.H. & Nicolaides K.H. eds.), p. 325. RCOG, London.

CAMPBELL S., SMITH P. & PEARCE J.M. (1984) In *Prenatal Diagnosis: Proceedings of 11th Study Group* (Rodeck C.H. & Nicolaides K.H. eds.), p. 245. RCOG, London.

FERGUSON-SMITH M.A. (1983). *Brit. med. Bull.*, 39, 365.

FERGUSON-SMITH M.A. & FERGUSON-SMITH M.E. (1983) In *Developments in Human Reproduction and their Eugenic and Ethical Implications* (Carter C.O. ed.), p. 187. Academic Press, London.

FERGUSON-SMITH M.A. & YATES J.R.W. (1984) *Prenatal Diagnosis*, 4, Spec. Iss., 5.

GHOSH A., WOO J.S.K., RAWLINSON H.M. & FERGUSON-SMITH M.A. (1982) *Brit. J. Onstet. Gynaec.*, 89, 817.

HAMILTON M.P.R., ABDALLA H.I. & WHITFIELD C.R. (1985) *Obstet and Gynec.*, 65, 465.

HECHT F. & CADIEN J.D. (1984) In *Antenatal and Neonatal Screening* (Wald N.J. ed.), p. 128. Oxford Univ. Press, Oxford.

HOBBINS J.C., MAHONEY M.J. & GOLDSTEIN L.A. (1974) *Amer. J. Obstet. Gynec.*, 118, 1069.

HUMPHRIES S.E. & WILLIAMSON R. (1983) *Brit. med. Bull.*, 39, 343.

HUTSON J.M., McNAY M.B., MACKENZIE J.R., WHITTLE M.J., YOUNG D.G. & RAINE P.A. (1985) *Lancet*, i, 621.

JACKSON L. (1985) *Chorionic Villus Sampling Newsletter*. Personal communication through Gilmore D.H.

LITTLE D. (1984a) In *Prenatal Diagnosis: Proceedings of 11th Study Group* (Rodeck C.H. & Nicolaides K.H. eds.), p. 301. RCOG, London.

LITTLE D. (1984b) In *Prenatal Diagnosis: Proceedings of 11th Study Group* (Rodeck C.H. & Nicolaides K.H. eds.), p. 307. RCOG, London.

MACDONALD H. & TOBIN J.O'H. (1978) *Developmental Med. Childh. Neurol.*, 20, 471.

McNAY M.B. & WHITFIELD C.R. (1984) *Brit. J. hosp. Med.*, 31, 406.

MEDICAL RESEARCH COUNCIL (1978) *Brit. J. Obstet. Gynae.*, 85, Suppl. 2.

MODELL B. (1984) In *Prenatal Diagnosis: Proceedings of 11th Study Group* (Rodeck C.H. & Nicolaides K.H. eds.), p. 93. RCOG, London.

MULLER F., FROT J.C., AUBRY M.C., BOUE J. & BOUE A. (1984) *Lancet*, i, 223.

NICHD National Registry for Amniocentesis Study Group (1976) *J. Amer. med. Assoc.*, 236, 1471.

NICOLAIDES K.H. & RODECK C.H. (1984) *Brit. J. hosp. Med.*, 31, 396.

PATRICK A.D. (1983) *Brit. med. Bull.*, 39, 378.

PEARCE J.M. & CAMPBELL S. (1984) In *Prenatal Diagnosis: Proceedings of 11th Study Group* (Rodeck C.H. & Nicolaides K.H. eds.), p. 313. RCOG, London.

QUEENAN J.T. & GADOW E.C. (1970) *Obstet. and Gynec.*, 35, 648.

READ A.C., DONNAI D., HARRIS R. & DONNAI P. (1980) *Brit. J. Obstet. Gynaec.*, 87, 372.

REDFORD D.H.A. & WHITFIELD C.R. (1985) *Amer. J. Obstet. Gynec.*, in press.

RITCHIE J.W.K. & THOMPSON W. (1982) In *Recent Advances in Obstetrics and Gynaecology* (Bonnar J. ed.), p. 47. Churchill Livingstone, Edinburgh.

RODECK C.H. & MORSMAN J.M. (1983) *Brit. med. Bull.*, 39, 338.

RODECK C.H. & NICOLAIDES K.H. (1983) *Brit. med. Bull.*, 39, 332.

SCRIMGEOUR J.B. (1973) In *Antenatal Diagnosis of Genetic Disease* (Emery A.E.H. ed.), p. 40. Churchill Livingstone, Edinburgh.

SEQUEIRA P.J.L. & TOBIN J.O'H. (1984) In *Antenatal and Neonatal Screening* (Wald N.J. ed.), p. 358. Oxford Univ. Press, Oxford.

SIMONI G., BRAMBATI B., DANESINO C., ROSELLA F., TERZOLI G.L., FERRARI M. & FRACCARO M. (1983) *Human Genetics*, 63, 349.

SIMPSON N.E., DALLAIRE L., MILLER J.R., SIMINOVICH L., HAMERTON J.L., MILLER J. & McKEEN C. (1976) *Canadian med. Assoc. J.*, 115, 739.

TURNBULL A.C. & MACKENZIE I.Z. (1983) *Brit. med. Bull.*, 39, 315.

UK Collaborative Study, First Report (1977) *Lancet*, i, 1323.

VALENTI C. (1972) *Amer. J. Obstet. Gynec.*, 113, 851.

WALD N., CUCKLE H., STIRRAT G.M., BENNETT, M.J. & TURNBULL A.C. (1977) *Lancet*, ii, 268.

CHAPTER 23
MISCELLANEOUS DISORDERS COMPLICATING PREGNANCY

C. R. WHITFIELD

VIRAL AND OTHER INFECTIONS

Excluding the common cold, a maternal viral illness probably occurs in about 5% of pregnancies (Sever & White 1968) but the true incidence of either overt or subclinical infection is uncertain and can be expected to vary from time to time and from place to place. The fetus is not usually affected, but, particularly in relation to certain viruses including those of the 'TORCH' group, transplacental infection may occur during maternal viraemia at any stage of pregnancy, and later the fetus may be infected from the birth canal either as an ascending infection after rupture of the membranes or by direct contact during birth. The incidence of fetal infection, and of consequent abortion, stillbirth, congenital abnormality or some other serious effect also remains uncertain. In addition, even without infection of the fetus, any acute or sustained pyrexial illness may be complicated by abortion, premature labour or occasionally by intrauterine death.

Torch infections

During recent years increasing attention has been directed to the so-called 'TORCH' syndrome of serious fetal, perinatal and residual effects of intrauterine infection by Toxoplasmosis (TO) and the viruses of Rubella (R), Cytomegalovirus (C) inclusion disease and Herpes (H) simplex.

RUBELLA

The teratogenicity of viral infection was first revealed in Australia when Gregg (1941) reported the association between maternal rubella and congenital cataract. It soon became clear that there was a similar association with other malformations including cardiac lesions, and subsequently with a whole range of deformities depending on the stage of organogenesis at the gestational age when the short period of maternal viraemia occurs (for no more than a week before symptoms, until almost as soon as the rash has developed). Following on possibly a particularly virulent epidemic of rubella in the United States during 1964, when 30 000 deformed babies were born despite very many terminations of pregnancy, mental retardation and defective hearing were found in infants without anatomical abnormalities, and the *expanded rubella syndrome* (characterized by hepatosplenomegaly, thrombocytopenic purpura and defective bone formation) was described. The symptomatic rubella attack rate is about 1 per 1000 pregnancies rising to 22 per 1000 during epidemics (Sever & White 1968), and it is almost always a primary maternal infection that damages the fetus with a 10–50% chance of severe lesions when infection occurs during the first trimester (Sever 1979). Since rubella may be symptomless, or virtually so, its true incidence during pregnancy must be even greater and the contribution by maternal rubella to congenital disease, particularly to impaired hearing (Iuorio *et al.* 1984), is almost certainly underestimated. Asymptomatic 'recurrence' of rubella occasionally occurs, being more likely following vaccine-induced immunity than after naturally occurring infection, but it very rarely causes intrauterine infection. Similarly, despite fears to the contrary, experience in both America and Europe indicates that there is no significantly increased risk of fetal defects in rubella-susceptible mothers inadvertently receiving rubella vaccine within 3 months before or after conception (Centres for Disease Control 1984, International Symposium on the Prevention of Congenital Rubella Infection 1984) so that routine termination of pregnancy in this circumstance need not be considered, although it remains sensible to regard known pregnancy as a contraindication to vaccination.

The most common clinical problem arises when a mother has been, or may have been, exposed to rubella (most often in her own children) early during pregnancy. Because the fetal risk depends on her immune status and gestational age, knowledge of these may be all that is needed to allay her fears and exclude therapeutic abortion from consideration, for example if routine screening earlier in pregnancy or a blood sample obtained within 10 days of exposure showed that she is already immune to rubella, or if the pregnancy was beyond 16 weeks (preferably confirmed by ultrasound) at the time of contact. Otherwise, decisions must be based on serial testing to reveal seroconversion or rising titres, or on the detection of 'recent antibodies' (i.e. antibody-specific IgM, significant levels of which persist for only 2–3 months after infection), in which circumstances therapeutic abortion will usually be offered and accepted.

Prevention

Congenital rubella is preventable by vaccination but, because the protection afforded may not be as lasting as that conferred by naturally acquired infection, vaccination may have to be repeated especially when, as in the United States, the aim is to achieve 'herd immunity' by vaccinating all children during the second year of life (reinforced by the denial of admission to primary school without evidence of vaccination against rubella and other infections). The more selective British policy of voluntary vaccination of schoolgirls is more likely to give lasting protection during their reproductive years, but is less effective because of disappointing uptake rates. Mothers found to be seronegative in pregnancy are offered vaccination during the puerperium.

For serological screening, the older haemagglutination inhibition (HAI) test, which gave some false positive results, has generally been replaced by the reliable single radial haemolysis (SRH) test, with which an arbitrary antibody level of 15 iu/ml is usually taken to be protective. Following vaccination antibody levels may very gradually decline to below this limit (O'Shea *et al.* 1982) so it is necessary to repeat serological screening, with postpartum revaccination if indicated, in every pregnancy. Screening, and vaccination of those found not to be immune, could usefully be extended to family planning clinics (after first excluding pregnancy), well women clinics (for those still in the reproductive years), infertility and prepregnancy clinics and, despite administrative difficulties related to short stay in hospital, also to women whose pregnancies have failed before they have booked for antenatal care (spontaneous abortions and ectopic pregnancies).

CYTOMEGALOVIRUS INFECTION

Cytomegalovirus (CMV) is an antigenically distinct member of the herpes group of viruses, usually causing a symptomless infection in adults but occasionally a non-specific febrile illness or one that resembles glandular fever. Spread may be by contact with infected urine or saliva but is usually venereal from the infected cervix in women. As with herpes simplex but unlike rubella, reactivation of latent virus occurs and this is largely responsible for high rates of infection (including maternal and perinatal infection) in some low socio-economic populations.

Intrauterine infection occurs via the placenta, but its incidence is less than that of maternal infection, particularly recurrent infection when there is considerable, but not complete, passive antibody protection from the mother. Cervical infection with CMV at some time during pregnancy has been reported in between 3 and 28% of mothers (Waterson 1979) and the infant may be infected in the birth canal during delivery, or the newborn may acquire CMV in breast milk or by exchange transfusion (King-Lewis & Gardner 1969). In one American study, the incidence of primary infection in susceptible (i.e. seronegative) pregnant women was about 1.5% and fetal infection occurred in about half of these pregnancies, compared with less than 2% of those in which there was recurrent infection (Stagno *et al.* 1982). In the same investigation and in two recent studies in London (Peckham *et al* 1983, Griffiths & Baboonian 1984) some 45% of women in early pregnancy did not have antibodies to CMV and were therefore susceptible, but with very high antibody-positive rates (90%) in Asian mothers. Varying rates of maternal and fetal infection, and perhaps also of fetal damage when intrauterine infection has occurred, probably reflect different host responses between communities, different socio-economic and hygiene standards which may influence the proportion of primary and reactivated infections, as well as different overall carriage rates and viral strains.

It is generally believed that, as in rubella, the earlier in pregnancy that fetal infection occurs the more severe are likely to be its effects, but this is not certain (Griffiths & Baboonian 1984); it may simply reflect a relatively high proportion of primary infections in early pregnancy compared with later on. Intrauterine effects include fetal death, retarded growth, purpura, hepatosplenomegaly with jaundice, and involvement of the central nervous system which may present as microcephaly (detectable *in utero* by ultrasound), choroidoretinitis, optic atrophy, deafness and other severe mental handicap; periventricular calcification may be seen in the brain by X-ray, and fetal hydrops with histological evidence of inclusion disease has been described (Morton & Mitchell 1983). Sometimes there are also severe congenital malformations including cardiac and intestinal defects. The fully developed picture of congenital CMV inclusion disease is rarely seen, and infection late in pregnancy or at delivery is often 'silent' (Monif et al. 1972), but even these infections may be the cause of deafness and mental retardation discovered later in childhood (Hanshaw et al. 1976) and infants with proven or possible CMV infection should remain under developmental follow-up for this reason. In England and Wales each year about 400 babies are born mentally retarded as a result of primary maternal infection by CMV (Waterson 1979) and the disease is numerically more important than rubella (MacDonald & Tobin 1978).

At present there is no treatment of congenital CMV infection, nor when a mother is infected is there any generally available way to confirm fetal infection or to assess its likely effects. Antenatal screening for CMV antibodies, with repeated serological testing of susceptible women, has been advocated (Lancet 1977), but until a safe and effective vaccine can be introduced for prophylaxis, along the lines of rubella immunization, a good case cannot be made for routine screening. Nor is the recommendation of termination after a recent infection valid. Thus for example, in more than 10,000 pregnancies Griffiths and Baboonian (1984) identified 30 with evidence of recent infection (i.e. seroconversion or specific IgM) at a stage when termination could be offered, and from these there were only 2 surviving infected children (both developing normally at the time of report); there were in addition 5 perinatal deaths, but 23 uninfected normally developing infants would have been sacrificed. The identification of specific IgM antibody in fetal serum (Lange et al. 1982) may in future provide an acceptable means of verifying fetal infection in these circumstances, but fetoscopic blood sampling is not yet available generally. CMV has been cultured from amniotic fluid (Davis et al. 1971) but the reliability of this as a diagnostic test is not known. Furthermore, positive results from either amniotic fluid or fetal blood would not indicate if, or how severely, an infected fetus might be damaged. It should also be borne in mind that probably as many primary maternal infections occur after, as before, the time limit for legal abortion.

The case for delivery by Caesarian section to avoid infection when CMV has been isolated from the cervix remains to be substantiated. It is also not yet established if there is a danger of transmission of CMV from an infected infant to susceptible attendants, but it might be advisable to screen medical and nursing staff and any who are shown to be seronegative should be excluded from the care of clinically affected or virus-excreting infants which should be isolated (Waterson 1979).

HERPES INFECTION

The Herpes-virus hominis (HVH) or herpes simplex virus (HSV) is very common in the female genital tract where it is usually the serotype HSV2 that is present and this infection can be recognized in cervical smears by the expert cytologist or can be identified by culture, but increasingly some genital herpes infections are by HSV1 which is the usual cause of oral infection. Antibodies to one strain do not confer immunity against the other, although they may reduce the severity of its effects. Latency in the posterior root ganglia, with reactivation and recurrent attacks of genital or extragenital herpes is the rule, but it is a primary infection transmitted via the placenta in early pregnancy that is of most danger to the fetus and newborn. Infection usually occurs by contact with active genital lesions during delivery, when perhaps as many as 40% of babies may be infected (Nahmias et al. 1971). Transplacental infection is less common, but a primary infection transmitted this way early in gestation may result in abortion, or it may cause growth retardation and involve the central nervous system causing microcephaly and choroidoretinitis.

When herpetic lesions are visible on the mother's external genital and anal region, or when HSV has been cultured from the cervix of women with a history of recurrent herpes, delivery by Caesarean section may prevent infection of the baby, but, especially if the membranes have ruptured some time beforehand, this cannot be guaranteed. Treatment with topical acyclovir reduces symptoms, promotes healing and shortens the time of virus shedding, and may therefore be of value when birth is expected soon.

Neonatal infection is rarer than might be expected from the general prevalence of herpes infection, but it may become commoner as prevalence rates increase. Besides surface lesions such as conjunctivitis, it carries a high mortality because of overwhelming systemic infection with shock, thrombocytopenia, encephalitis and residual brain damage. Administration of non-specific immunoglobulin is ineffective, but treatment with antiviral drugs may ameliorate some. of the effects of neonatal herpes; the most appropriate therapy with antivirals has still to be established. It is to be hoped that an effective non-oncogenic in-activated subunit vaccine against HSV2 will become available, and will protect against both muco-cuta-neous and latent ganglion infection (Skinner et al. 1978).

TOXOPLASMOSIS

Toxoplasmosis, a protozoal infestation, is included with the viral infections of the TORCH group because of the similarity of their perinatal effects. Maternal manifestations are also similar, sometimes being absent or so mild as to pass unnoticed, but in other cases causing a 'flu-like' illness with specific diagnosis depending on laboratory investigation.

Infection by *Toxoplasma gondii*, caused by ingestion of raw or undercooked meat containing toxoplasma cysts or food contaminated from cat faeces, is often symptomless in the mother, but congenital toxoplas-mosis can be the most severe of the TORCH syndromes. Fetal infection is via the placenta, and it occurs only during the primary parasitaemia so that there is no risk in women who are seropositive before conception, including of course those who have al-ready given birth to a child with the disease. Infection during early pregnancy is the most damaging although abortion is not common. When infection occurs during the first trimester one-fifth of the babies will show the full syndrome (Kovar & Harvey 1981) in which choroidoretinitis, hydrocephaly and patchy cerebral calcification are associated with impaired vision, convulsions and severe mental handicap, and in which there is hepatomegaly and sometimes also lymphadenopathy and pneumonitis. Infection late in pregnancy is usually subclinical at birth, but most of these children develop convulsions and other neuro-logical sequelae (Wilson et al. 1980), in a minority going on to severe psychomotor retardation, serious visual impairment and other features such as jaun-dice, blood dyscrasia and pneumonitis.

Specialized laboratories may be able to culture the parasite from the baby's blood (including cord blood) or cerebrospinal fluid, or from the placenta, and sig-nificant antibody levels (rising during, or persisting after, the first year of life) or specific IgM would also confirm the diagnosis.

Serological screening

Routine serological screening might be worthwhile where toxoplasmosis is unduly prevalent, e.g. in Paris where 75% of all patients of childbearing age have antibodies (Roux et al. 1976) or in Brussels where they are present in 53% of antenatal patients and there are two clinically manifest cases of congenital toxoplasmosis per 1000 births (Foulon et al. 1984). Repeated testing of susceptible mothers would detect seroconversion due to primary infection, or initially high antibody titres would indicate that toxoplasma infection may have occurred early in pregnancy or just before conception (Foulon et al. 1984). In Britain where meat is usually well or over-cooked, preva-lence rates are lower (although susceptibility rates are therefore high) and routine serology would not be cost-effective in a strictly fiscal sense (Beattie 1984). For example, in the West of Scotland only 25% of the population have antibodies and the sero-conversion rate in pregnancy is only 0.2% (Williams et al. 1981) compared with 0.4 and 0.67% respec-tively in the French and Belgian studies quoted above, and the incidence of congenital toxoplasmosis is only 0.06 per 1000 births (Williams & Williams 1979).

Management and prevention

When seroconversion occurs in the first 20 weeks of pregnancy it is doubtful if therapeutic abortion should be suggested. Thus, in the Brussels series, toxo-plasma was not isolated from the placenta in 7 such early seroconverters having abortions performed, while 2 out of 10 early seroconverters continuing their pregnancies and 2 of 17 women with initially high antibody titres gave birth to infected babies, with choroidoretinitis and cerebral calcification in one, convulsions in two and with only serological evidence of the disease in the fourth baby.

Antenatal drug treatment has some value in pre-venting transplacental infection when it is known (how else than by serological screening?) that a pri-mary maternal infection has occurred, especially in the most dangerous early months of pregnancy. Fou-lon et al. (1984) used spiramycin cyclically (3-week courses with 1-week intervals), while reduced neo-natal infection rates have been reported with either spiramycin (Desmonts & Couvreur 1979) or pyri-methamine plus sulphadiazine (Thalhammer 1979). However, since neonatal treatment improves the immediate prognosis in acute disease but does not reduce subsequent ill health and brain damage (Kovar & Harvey 1981), the efficacy of antenatal prophylaxis in this way must await long-term follow-up studies. The most important preventive measures remain as follows: (1) avoidance of contact spread and careful handwashing in the kitchen; (2) avoidance of cat faeces in the home, garden and elsewhere; (3) inclusion of only well-cooked meat in the diet during pregnancy or when conception is planned.

Other viral infections

VARICELLA

Varicella-zoster, a DNA virus of the herpes group, causes chicken-pox as a primary infection and zoster (shingles) as a reactivation. Most women have had chicken-pox as children but a few, especially among immigrants, may not be immune. There is a common, but unsubstantiated, view that the disease is more severe when it occurs in pregnancy, but the virus is less teratogenic than the other herpes viruses, CMV and HSV. However, a very few cases of congenital varicella syndrome have been described (Dudgeon 1976), the abnormalities being microcephaly, convulsions, impaired vision and mental retardation, and also limb deformities (hypoplasia and scars). If a pregnant woman who is not known to have had chicken-pox previously has been in contact with a case, zoster-immune globulin given within 3 days of exposure will probably protect the fetus from the maternal viraemia should she become infected (Waterson 1979).

Congenital chicken-pox later in pregnancy is also rare but may be lethal, with necrotic lesions in the lungs and brain, especially if the baby is born before there is protection from the rising maternal antibody levels, and babies born within 4 days of the mother's rash appearing should be given zoster-immune globulin.

POLIOMYELITIS AND OTHER ENTEROVIRUSES

Pregnant women may be more liable to infection with poliomyelitis, and its effects may be worse in pregnancy. Transplacental infection may occur, possibly resulting in abortion or stillbirth, but these losses may be due to the maternal febrile illness rather than to intrauterine infection. Neonatal poliomyelitis has a grave prognosis.

Other enteroviruses, including Coxsackie B, echovirus and rotavirus may cause clinical or subclinical neonatal infection, but there is no certain evidence that they have serious effects.

INFLUENZA, MUMPS AND MEASLES

These infectious diseases may be associated with an increased fetal loss as a result of the mother's febrile illness. Apart possibly from growth retardation and an as yet uncertain association between maternal mumps and endocardial fibroelastosis in the baby (Kovar & Hardy 1981) there would seem to be no teratogenic or other adverse effects attributable to transplacental infection.

HEPATITIS B VIRUS

Hepatitis B virus is a DNA virus with several marker antigens: surface (Australia) antigen (HBsAg), core antigen (HBcAg) and e-antigen (HBeAg). Acute hepatitis is rare in pregnancy, but, besides its maternal effects and increased risks of prematurity and retarded fetal growth, when it occurs in the last trimester or puerperium placental transmission of the preceding heavy viraemia will usually cause infection in the newborn, which may be symptomless, chronic with elevation of liver enzymes or acute perhaps with fatal liver failure. In these circumstances the newborn should receive specific hyperimmune globulin as prophylaxis. When a mother has acute hepatitis B in early pregnancy the risk of fetal infection is for some reason only about 10% (Schweizer et al. 1973) and this may be due to relative protection by increasing maternal antibodies against the HB antigens. There is no evidence that hepatitis B virus is teratogenic.

The chronic carrier state with HBsAg is more common in pregnancy than is acute hepatitis, but there is a low rate of fetal infection except among Chinese or when HBeAg is also present; once again it is perhaps the transplacental passage of maternal antibody that gives considerable protection. It is not yet known if administration of hyperimmune globulin to the baby of a carrier will augment this protection, but it should be given.

Hepatitis B virus is highly contagious, and either acute disease or the HBsAg carrier state at delivery presents an important hazard of infection by contact with the mother's blood, not only to the baby during birth but to the obstetric attendants who must take strict precautions to avoid this risk and, if possible, should be selected from staff known to be immune. If there is accidental contact with maternal blood the attendant should receive hyperimmune globulin.

Sexually transmitted disease in pregnancy

While *syphilis* and *gonorrhoea* have no particularly
adverse effects on the mother during pregnancy, if
untreated the former will almost invariably infect the
fetus and this may be fatal when the disease has been
acquired recently, while the latter is likely to cause
ophthalmia neonatorum. Despite suggestions that
routine antenatal serological screening for syphilis
should be abandoned as no longer cost-effective, the
continued occasional occurrence of syphilis in many
obstetric units makes this unwise, and the disease is
still a relatively common problem in some other
countries. The Venereal Diseases Reference
Laboratory (VDRL) test has displaced the Wasser-
mann and Kahn reactions for serological screening
for syphilis, with specific confirmation of positive
results by the Treponema Pallidum Haemagglutinat-
ing Antibody (TPHA) test or Fluorescent Treponema
Antibody Absorption (FAA-ABS) test. Treatment of
the mother with large doses of penicillin should begin
as soon as the diagnosis is confirmed. Treatment, or
retreatment (which is probably always advisable in
previously treated women), will usually prevent congenital syphilis with its developmental, haematological, neurological and bony manifestations, but the
baby should be examined clinically and serologically
and treated if evidence of infection is found (specific
IgM, or higher titre of IgG than in the mother). Erythromycin provides alternative treatment if there is
penicillin allergy.

   Treatment of proven gonococcal infection is also
by penicillin or, if there is bacterial resistance to penicillin, with another appropriate antibiotic.

   Treatment of these diseases should be carried out
in consultation with, or by, a clinic for sexually transmitted diseases, which will also have the necessary
organization for follow-up and for family and contact
tracing.

   'Non-specific' genital infection by *Chlamydia trachomatis* is now increasingly a recognized cause of
ophthalmia neonatorum, although the nasopharynx
is the predominant site of seeding from which there
may be further spread to internal organs, e.g. causing
chlamydial pneumonitis (Harrison *et al.* 1978). Treatment of chlamydial infection in the mother (when
cultured from the cervix) or newborn is by erythromycin (topical suspension for ophthalmia). The roles
of *Ureaplasma urealyticum* and *Mycoplasma hominis* in
maternal infection, including chorioamnionitis associated with preterm labour in the case of U. urealyticum (Shurin *et al.* 1975), and in neonatal infection,

and the possible advantages of prophylactic therapy
when they are isolated from the mother's genital
tract require further detailed study.

Acquired immune deficiency syndrome

Infection by Type III Human T-cell Lymphotrophic
Virus (HTVL-III) may be asymptomatic or cause
minor illnesses with lymphodenopathy, and a minority of infections go on to the fully developed acquired
immune deficiency syndrome (AIDS) characterized
by severe immunosuppression leading to opportunistic bacterial infections, and quite often also viral, fungal and toxoplasma infections, and sometimes rare
tumours (e.g. Kaposi's sarcoma and B-cell lymphoma). This 'new' disease appeared first in homo-
sexual men in California in 1981, and the first case
in Britain was reported in the same year. It carries a
mortality of about 50%. It is fortunate that pregnancy is uncommon in some of the high risk groups,
but in the United States AIDS has been reported in
infants whose parents had the disorder. Although
some of these mothers belonged to at risk categories
including intravenous drug abusers and sexual contacts of bisexual males, transplacental infection may
have occurred in some cases, or there may have been
infection in the birth canal or breast milk or by close
parental contact with the newborn (Cowan *et al.*
1984).

   If AIDS or a HTLV-III-related infection is suspected
in pregnancy, urgent referral to an infectious diseases
or genito-urinary medicine unit is required. A specific
diagnostic antibody test should soon become
generally available. When blood samples, for this or
other purposes, or other samples are taken, strict precautions against chance infection are required, and
must also be observed at delivery and in the neonatal
period. Safety guidelines have been issued by the
Government Health Departments (Advisory Committee on Dangerous Pathogens 1984), and the
patient and her family would require careful counselling. The case should be reported in confidence to
the Communicable Disease Surveillance Centre. It is
to be hoped that an effective vaccine against HTLV-
III will eventually be developed. In the meantime
some obstetric units will be faced with the task of
managing pregnancy and delivery in HTLV-III carriers, with or without related diseases, and also
occasionally in women with manifest AIDS.

Bacterial infections in pregnancy

Bacterial infection in the genital tract during pregnancy has particular importance in relation to spontaneous premature rupture of the membranes and chorioamniotis with its significant associated perinatal mortality. Management of neonatal infection is dealt with in Chapter 34 (p. 496) and urinary tract infection in Chapter 19 (p. 277). Bacterial infection is not teratogenic, most of the antibiotic drugs are free of adverse fetal effects, and the general principles of antibiotic therapy hold good in obstetrics. There are, however, some contraindications, including long acting sulphonamides which displace bilirubin from binding protein and may provoke significant neonatal hyperbilirubinaemia, tetracycline which discolours the infant's teeth permanently and may affect bone formation, and cotrimoxazole which is a folic acid antagonist. When it is necessary to achieve effective antibiotic levels in the fetus, ampicillin or a first generation cephalosporin may be chosen, adding gentamycin or kanamycin to cover enterobacter infection if that is considered important; clindamycin may be added if infection with anaerobes such as Bacteroides fragilis is a risk. When the risk of fetal infection is acute, treatment should begin by parenteral administration. There should be a hospital policy for all these circumstances, which is decided and updated in consultation with a specialist microbiologist to take into account changing patterns of infection and sensitivity and new antibiotics as they become available.

Pulmonary tuberculosis is now often ignored as a possible problem in pregnancy in Britain, but there is a significant small incidence among certain immigrants. Routine chest X-ray (usually by mass miniature radiography) was abandoned some time ago, but standard chest films should be obtained after the first trimester when there is a recent family history of tuberculosis or recent contact with a case, and in some recently arrived immigrants unless it is known that a recent film shows no active lesion or there is proof of successful BCG vaccination. When tuberculosis is present during pregnancy streptomycin should not be used for treatment because of the risk of nerve deafness in the baby, but with today's range of available antituberculous drugs this is not a serious disadvantage. If there is open lung disease the infant should be vaccinated with BCG and separated from the mother for 6–8 weeks.

MEDICAL AND SURGICAL DISORDERS COMPLICATING PREGNANCY

Any disease or surgical problem that occurs during the childbearing years may of course complicate pregnancy, and those most important in clinical obstetrics are dealt with in separate chapters on heart disease (p. 242), blood disorders (p. 254), thromboembolism (p. 539), endocrine disorders including diabetes (p. 284) and urinary tract disorders (p. 277), while puerperal depression is considered in Chapter 32 (p. 463) and aspects of pregnancy associated with genital tract lesions are dealt with in Chapter 23 (p. 327). For detailed description of the underlying pathophysiology, presentation and course and management of other disorders occurring in pregnancy the reader is referred to such recent volumes as *Medical Complications during Pregnancy* edited by Burrows and Ferris (1982) and *Medical Disorders in Obstetric Practice*, edited by de Swiet (1984). Also, since much of what is appropriate in the management of these disorders in the non-pregnant subject is also appropriate in the pregnant woman, and is described thoroughly in well known standard textbooks, these general aspects will not be considered here. Consultation with whichever general or specialist physician or surgeon is appropriate, leading often to joint management, should be the working rule with overall maternal and fetal responsibility remaining with the obstetrician. It is here that advantages accrue from close teamwork with other specialists who themselves have developed particular experience and interests in the management of 'their disorders' when they occur in pregnancy.

Two disorders that do merit some remarks here are jaundice appearing in pregnancy and the management of the pregnant epileptic.

Jaundice in pregnancy

Jaundice is not common in obstetric patients, occurring about once in every 2000 pregnancies, although there is much higher frequency in countries where the general incidence of hepatitis is increased.

Various causes, of which a viral hepatitis is the most common, are found to explain the symptom. Other conditions include haemolytic jaundice, recurrent cholestatic jaundice of pregnancy, jaundice occurring in association with treatment with drugs such as chlorpromazine and, now very rarely, jaundice in severe cases of excessive vomiting or eclampsia.

Viral hepatitis does not appear to occur more frequently in pregnancy than at other times, nor is it significantly different in its course or management so far as the mother is concerned. An increased mortality during pregnancy has often been described, but there is considerable geographic variation and the mother's nutrition may well play a large part in the outcome. The resistance of the pregnant woman will be similar to that of others who are not pregnant; in areas of poor nutrition, however, an increased mortality has been reported (Naidu & Viswanathan 1957).

Management of the patient is not influenced by pregnancy, and similar treatment should be given then as in the non-pregnant.

The outcome for the fetus may be a little less favourable. Prematurity and stillbirth are more common if the disease occurs later in pregnancy; if jaundice occurs earlier, however, it appears to be less harmful. Neither hepatitis B (p. 331) nor hepatitis A virus causes congenital abnormalities, and infection during pregnancy is not an indication for termination (Waterson 1979).

Jaundice due to gallstones obstructing the common bile duct is rare in pregnancy, but if it does occur from this cause and removal of a stone would otherwise be indicated, this should be carried out.

A variety of jaundice which is now more widely recognized than formerly is recurrent jaundice which may be seen towards the end of several pregnancies. The jaundice is accompanied by considerable pruritus which may be the only feature. If the condition has been present in the previous pregnancy, its recurrent nature, combined with pruritus, will be sufficient to permit the diagnosis on purely clinical grounds. The most consistent abnormalities on liver function testing are a slightly raised serum bilirubin and a significantly raised alkaline phosphatase. The jaundice is obstructive in origin, and is due to intrahepatic cholestasis. The general view is that this type of jaundice is benign for both mother and baby, but after delivery the pruritus disappears quickly and the jaundice more slowly, although patients affected with a recurrent cholestatic jaundice may experience similar effects when taking oral contraceptives (Drill 1974).

ACUTE HEPATIC FAILURE

Rarely, in late pregnancy, a patient will develop vomiting, upper abdominal pain and jaundice; these features are quickly followed by headaches, mental confusion, coma and death. The whole duration of the disease may be merely a few days. The urine is bile-stained and the stools are pale, indicating the jaundice to be obstructive in type. Obstetric acute yellow atrophy and the acute fatty liver of pregnancy are names which have been applied to this condition. Whether pregnancy can, in any way, be considered an essential feature of the disease is open to question, however. Acute liver failure of this type arises at other times following (although not by any means immediately following) drugs or various poisons; tetracyclines have been incriminated (Kunelis et al. 1965). In other cases, however, a cause may not be discovered.

The most prominent histological feature is fatty degeneration in the centre of the liver lobule; necrosis of liver cells is not a marked feature and the picture is not the same as that of acute hepatic necrosis of viral origin.

The progress of the condition is so rapid that effective treatment may be almost impossible. Early delivery is indicated at the first appearance of jaundice.

Epilepsy in pregnancy

The effect of pregnancy on epilepsy is unpredictable, fits becoming more frequent in some patients, and seemingly less frequent in others, with little obvious change in the majority.

Advice should be sought from a physician when an epileptic patient becomes pregnant, and any change in the pattern of fits may require an alteration in treatment. In general, the drugs employed to control epilepsy in the non-pregnant patient are used during pregnancy also. Phenytoin is often the mainstay of treatment, but it is an anti-folic acid agent, although normal folic acid supplementation will usually prevent megaloblastic anaemia. This antifolic acid activity may be an important factor in the doubled incidence of congenital malformations in the children of epileptics (Speidel & Meadow 1972, Lowe 1973). Alternatively the anticonvulsants used in treatment may be the most likely aetiological factor, phenytoin in particular having been incriminated. Fedrick (1973), in reporting similar findings, comments that until more is known about genetic linkage between epilepsy and other abnormalities, this problem will not be solved but present evidence does suggest that anticonvulsant drugs may have a substantial teratogenic effect.

Epileptics contemplating pregnancy should consult their physicians about its advisability or should be referred to a prepregnancy clinic, and they should then be informed about possible risks. If pregnancy is planned, phenytoin at least should be stopped if possible, particularly before 16 weeks of gestation. Anticonvulsants should not be discontinued entirely during pregnancy because the risk of uncontrolled epilepsy may be high and that of congenital abnormality is low (de Swiet 1979).

INCARCERATION OF THE RETROVERTED GRAVID UTERUS

Mention must be made of this problem, so often described in considerable detail in the textbooks of 50 or more years ago, but now an apparently disappearing problem; perhaps with the passing of gross flattening of the pelvic brim due to rickets, the enlarging uterus can always escape from incarceration in the pelvis.

Most retroverted uteri will correct themselves without any difficulty as the enlarging uterus grows upwards out of the pelvis during the fourth month. If, exceptionally, incarceration of the retroverted gravid uterus occurs, between the 12th and 16th weeks the patient may become aware of difficulty in passing urine, leading eventually to an episode of acute retention. The uterus has become large enough to fill the pelvis, and the urethra may become mechanically obstructed or may be unduly elongated upwards with the displaced cervix.

The physical signs will be the presence of a lower abdominal cystic swelling, the distended bladder, and there will be a swelling palpable vaginally in the posterior fornix, the retroverted fundus. The cervix may be so high that it is elevated beyond reach.

Management is to pass a catheter to empty the bladder, and to leave it in place with the patient nursed in a prone position. It is extremely uncommon for this simple treatment not to be successful. If the bladder is kept empty by continuous drainage, the enlarging uterus will raise itself out of the pelvis and become palpable abdominally within 24–48 h in nearly all cases. Digital pressure with the patient occupying the knee/chest position has been described, but how frequently this is really necessary is open to conjecture. It has never been necessary in the author's experience, or in that of the previous editor, to carry out measures other than the simple treatment by continuous bladder drainage as described above.

MATERNAL ALCOHOL CONSUMPTION

Since alcohol was believed to be a teratogen by the ancient Greeks and Phoenicians, and in 1834 evidence to a committee of Parliament noted that infants of alcoholic mothers appeared 'starved, shrivelled and imperfect' (Jones et al. 1973), it is strange that hard facts about serious fetal effects have only quite recently emerged. Indeed, much uncertainty still remains about a range of such effects in relation to the amount and pattern of maternal drinking and the importance of other related factors.

Fetal alcohol syndrome

What is now certain is that a proportion, perhaps 10–20% (Jones et al. 1974), of babies born to alcoholic mothers show a group of effects now recognized, and named by Jones et al. (1973), as the Fetal Alcohol Syndrome (FAS). It was suggested by Halliday et al. (1982) that the risk of FAS occurs when there is a regular daily consumption during pregnancy of 80 g of alcohol (equivalent to 10 measures of spirits, or 5 pints of beer), but a lower daily critical intake of 6 measures of vodka (about 50 g of absolute alcohol) has been reported (Beattie et al. 1983). There is considerable geographic variation in the incidence of FAS, ranging from 1 per 50 births in some American Indian reservations (Rosett et al. 1981) to only 2 cases from 25,000 births at two London hospitals (Wright et al. 1983a) and significant underdetection from lack of familiarity with the syndrome is probably still widespread. In the West of Scotland 40 infants with FAS, born during the 10 years between 1971 and 1981 but with more than half being born in the last 2 years of this period, were traced by Beattie et al. (1983) through paediatricians in and around Glasgow, reflecting both increasing awareness of the condition and the increasing northward prevalence within Britain of alcohol-related problems in general.

FAS is characterized by four categories of abnormalities (Hanson et al. 1976): (1) typical craniofacial appearances with microcephaly and midfacial dysmorphism; (2) retarded growth in utero and continuing after birth; (3) neurodevelopmental dysfunction ranging from hypotonia or hyperactivity and uncoordination to serious retardation; (4) increased frequency of major and minor congenital abnormalities including cardiac defects. Criteria for the diagnosis of FAS, requiring signs in each of the first 3 categories, have been defined (Rosett 1980). Understandably

obstetricians are even less familiar than are paediatricians with the facial characteristics, so it is likely
that there is a significant under-reporting of FAS
as a cause of stillbirths attributed to 'unexplained'
intrauterine growth retardation. In regard to this
probability, in a review of 9000 pregnancies in France,
Kaminiski *et al.* (1976) reported a higher stillbirth
rate in mothers consuming more than 30 g of alcohol
(i.e. 4 drinks or more daily), and also lower birth
and placental weights among heavy drinkers.

A synergism between heavy drinking and smoking
has been established (Wright *et al.* 1983b; Beattie *et
al.* 1983) and the Glasgow series showed a clear bias
towards the lowest socio-economic group, with more
than half the mothers being single parents, and with
high rates for other alcohol-related morbidity and
mortality (2 suicides and 1 liver failure in 39 mothers). Elsewhere, however, it has been established that
the group with the highest proportion of heavy drinkers (as opposed to alcoholics) may be the smoking
mothers of social classes I and II (Wright *et al.*
1983b).

Occasional 'binge' drinking is probably also harmful, as it has been reported to be associated with
reduced birthweights (Streissguth *et al.* 1981). More
information on the fetal effects of this pattern of
drinking by pregnant women is required.

EFFECTS OF LESS SEVERE ALCOHOL CONSUMPTION

Wright *et al.* (1983a & b), in reviewing the drinking
habits of 900 antenatal patients in London, found
that among the 20% which they classified as 'heavy
drinkers' on the basis of a weekly consumption of at
least 100 g of alcohol (roughly equivalent to 1–2
drinks each day; or more exactly to 12 drinks per
week where a drink is a half-pint of beer, a measure
of spirit or 60 ml of wine) there was more than a
doubled risk of the baby being of low birthweight for
gestational age (< 10th centile) when compared with
light drinkers (0–50 g of alcohol per week). Their
other findings, and those of their review of the literature, seem to indicate that moderate drinking in pregnancy (50–100 g of alcohol per week) does not carry
increased risks of congenital abnormality or retarded
growth in the fetus, or of spontaneous abortion.
There was also no evidence that reduction of initially
heavy drinking to more moderate consumption later
in pregnancy had any benefit. Their suggested 'safe'
level of no more than 1 or 2 drinks per day is the
same as the lowest harmful daily intake of 1.5 units

(1 unit = 1 drink as defined above) in several American and French reports reviewed by Plant (1984)
who, somewhat surprisingly, found that this amount
was exceeded by fewer than 2.0% of the women she
studied in antenatal clinics in Edinburgh. It seems
therefore that the advice of the Surgeon General in
the United States (1981) that pregnant women
should observe complete abstinence may be unnecessary and also unduly alarmist. As with smoking, it
may be more effective to encourage pregnant women
to moderate rather than eliminate alcohol consumption, and an average of 1 drink per day with no more
than 2 drinks on any one day would make a very
simple and easily understood message. Even more importantly, and whenever possible, this advice should
be given at family planning and prepregnancy clinics
and it should also become part of general health ed-
uction.

REFERENCES

ADVISORY COMMITTEE ON DANGEROUS PATHOGENS (1984). *Ac-
quired Immune Deficiency Syndrome (AIDS)—Interim Guide-
lines*, DHSS, London.
BEATTIE C.P. (1984) *Brit. J. Obstet. Gynaec.*, **91**, 417.
BEATTIE J.O., DAY R.E., COCKBURN F. & GARG R.A. (1983)
Brit. Med. J., **287**, 17.
BURROW G.N. & FERRIS T.F. (1982) *Medical Complications
during Pregnancy*. W.B. Saunders, London.
CENTERS FOR DISEASE CONTROL (1984) *Morbidity and Mortal-
ity Weekly Report*, **33**, No. 22.
COWAN M.J., HELLMANN D., CHUDWIN D., WARA D.W.,
CHANG R.S. & AMMANN A.J. (1984) *Pediatrics*, **73**, 382.
DAVIS L.E., TWEED G.V., CHIN T.D.Y. & MILLER G.L. (1971)
Amer. J. Obstet. Gynec., **109**, 1217.
DESMONTS G. & COUVREUR J. (1979) In *Perinatal Medicine* (6th
European Congress of Perinatal Medicine), p. 51 (Thalham-
mer O., Baumgarten K. & Pollak A. eds.). George Thieme,
Stuttgart.
DRILL V.A. (1974) *Amer. J. Obstet. Gynec.*, **119**, 165.
DUDGEON J.A. (1976) *Brit. Med. Bull.*, **32**, 77.
FEDRICK J. (1973) *Brit. med. J.*, **ii**, 442.
FOULON W., NAESSENS A., VOLKAERT M., LAUWARS A. & AMY
J.J. (1984) *Brit. J. Obstet. Gynaec.*, **91**, 419.
GREGG N.M. (1941) *Transactions of the Ophthalmological
Society of Australia*, **3**, 35.
GRIFFITHS P.D. & BABOONIAN C. (1984) *Brit. J. Obstet. Gy-
naec.*, **91**, 307.
HALLIDAY H.L., REID M.McC. & McCLURE G. (1982) *Brit. J.
Obstet. Gynaec.*, **89**, 892.
HANSHAW J.B., SCHEINER A.P., MOXEY A., GAEN L., ABEL V.
& SCHEINER B. (1976) *New Engl. J. Med.*, **295**, 468.
HANSON J.W., JONES K.L. & SMITH D.W. (1976) *J. Amer. Med.
Assoc.*, **235**, 1458.

Harrison H.R., English M.G., Lee C.K. & Alexander E.R. (1978) *New Engl. J. Med.*, **298**, 702.

International Symposium on the Prevention of Congenital Rubella Infection (1984) *Reviews of Infectious Disease*, **7** (suppl.).

Iuorio J.L., Hosking C.S. & Pyman C. (1984) *Brit. Med. J.*, **289**, 1566.

Jones K.L., Smith D.W., Streissguth A.P. & Marianthopoulos N.C. (1973) *Lancet*, **i**, 1267.

Jones K.L., Smith D.W. & Streissguth A.P. (1974) *Pediatric Research*, **8**, 440.

Kaminski M., Rumeau-Rouquette C. & Schwarz D. (1976) *Rev. Epidemiol. Sante Publique*, **24**, 27.

King-Lewis P.A. & Gardner S.D. (1969) *Brit. Med. J.*, **ii**, 603.

Kovar I. & Harvey D. (1981) In *Progress in Obstetrics and Gynaecology*, **vol. 1**, p. 39 (Studd J. ed.).

Kunelis C.T., Peters J.L. & Edmondson H.A. (1965) *Amer. J. Med.*, **38**, 359.

Lancet (1977) Editorial, **ii**, 541.

Lange I., Rodeck C.H., Morgan-Capner P., Simmons A. & Kangro H.O. (1982) *Brit. med. J.*, **284**, 1673.

Lowe C.R. (1973) *Lancet*, **i**, 9.

MacDonald H. & Tobin J.O'H. (1978) *Developmental Med. Childh. Neurol.*, **20**, 471.

Monif R.G., Egan E.A., Held B. & Eitzman D. (1972) *J. Pediatrics*, **80**, 17.

Morton R. & Mitchell I. (1983) *Brit. J. Obstet. Gynaec.*, **90**, 276.

Nahmias A.J., Josey W.T., Naib Z.M., Freeman M.G., Fernandez R.J. & Wheeler J.H. (1971) *Amer. J. Obstet. Gynec.*, **110**, 825.

Naidu S.S. & Viswanathan R. (1957) *Indian J. med. Res.*, **45** (suppl.) 1.

O'Shea S., Best J.M., Banatvala J.E., Marshall W.C. & Dudgeon J.A. (1982) *Brit. med. J.*, **285**, 253.

Peckham C.S., Chin K.S., Coleman J.C., Henderson K., Hurley R. & Preece P.M. (1981) *Lancet*, **i**, 1352.

Plant M.L. (1984) *Brit. J. Addiction*, **79**, 207.

Rosett H.L. (1980) *Clin. Exper. Res.*, **4**, 119.

Rosett H.L., Wiener L. & Edelin K.C. (1981) *Obstet. Gynec.*, **57**, 1.

Roux Ch., Desmonts G., Mulliez N., Gaulier M., Tufferand G., Marmor D. & Herbillon A. (1976) *J. Gynecol. Obstet. Biol. Reprod.*, **5**, 249.

Schweitzer I.L., Dunn A.E., Peters R.L. & Spears R.L. (1973) *Amer. J. Med.*, **55**, 762.

Sever J. & White L.R. (1968) *Ann. Rev. Med.*, **19**, 471.

Sever J.L. (1979) *Clinics in Perinatology*, **6**, 347.

Shurin P.A., Alpert S. & Rossner B. (1973) *New Engl. J. Med.*, **293**, 5.

Skinner G.R., Williams D.R., Buchan A., Whitney J., Harding M. & Bodfish K. (1978) *Med. Microbiol. Immunol.*, **166**, 119.

Speidel B.D. & Meadow S.R. (1972) *Lancet*, **ii**, 839.

Stagno S., Pass R.F., Dworsky M.E., Henderson R.E., Moore E.G., Walton P.D. & Alford C.A. (1982) *New Engl. J. Med.*, **306**, 945.

de Swiet M. (1979) *Prescribers Journal*, **19**, 59.

de Swiet M. (1984) *Medical Disorders in Obstetric Practice*. Blackwell Scientific Publications, Oxford.

Streissguth A.P., Martin D.C., Martin J.C. & Barr W.M. (1981) *Neurobehav. Toxicol. Teratol.*, **3**, 223.

Surgeon General's Advisory Committee on Alcohol and Pregnancy (1981) *FDA Drug Bulletin*, **11(2)**, 9.

Thalhammer O. (1979) In *Perinatal Medicine (6th European Congress of Perinatal Medicine)*, p. 44 (Thalhammer O., Baumgarten K. & Pollak A. eds.). George Thieme, Stuttgart.

Waterson A.P. (1979) *Brit. med. J.*, **ii**, 564.

Wright J.T., Barrison I., Toplis P.J. & Waterson J. (1983a) *Brit. J. Hosp. Med.*, **29**, 260.

Wright J.T., Waterson E.J., Barrison I.G., Toplis P.J., Lewis I.G., Gordon M.G., MacRae K.D., Morris N.F. & Murray-Lyon I.M. (1983b) *Lancet*, **i**, 663.

Williams K.A.B., Scott J.M., Macfarlane D.E., Williamson J.M.W., Elias-Jones T.F. & Williams H. (1981) *J. Infect.*, **3**, 219.

Williams K.A.B. & Williams H. (1979) *Brit. med. J.*, **i**, 561.

Wilson C.B., Remington J.S., Stagno S. & Reynolds D.W. (1980) *Pediatrics*, **66**, 767.

CHAPTER 24
NATURAL LABOUR AND ITS ACTIVE MANAGEMENT

J. M. BEAZLEY

Labour is the whole process whereby the products of conception are expelled from the mother. In humans the process begins naturally about term.

CHANGING ATTITUDES TO LABOUR

During the last 30 years obstetric developments in this country have significantly influenced the attitudes of all those associated with parturition. Each triennial report on Confidential Enquiries into Maternal Deaths in England and Wales has revealed a steady decline in this frightful hazard. The risk of maternal death is now so low that it has ceased to serve as a reliable index of obstetric progress. Whereas women were thankful to accept advice which helped to avoid death, their attitude, rightly, has steadily changed to one in which they not only expect to survive childbirth in good health, but also to enjoy all the emotional satisfaction of the processs. The time will come, perhaps, when a Confidential Enquiry will seek to analyse not the avoidable causes of morbidity and mortality but of more positive aspects of maternal well-being, both physical and mental (Barron 1973).

Perinatal Mortality Reviews have, in more recent years, largely taken over the role of providing the index of satisfactory care in labour. The approach remains a statistical one, and as circumstances rapidly improve the usefulness of the method becomes less. Already obstetricians look towards reports which dwell less on the advent of failure and more upon the promotion of good fetal health.

The concepts of health are important to obstetrics, and schematically, one is outlined in Fig. 24.1. Women, naturally concerned about the recent technical developments in obstetrics, and particularly in parturition, may legitimately ask, 'Is pregnancy an illness?' Some would go so far even as to object to being called a 'patient'. But labour, as an intensive-care situation, which it is, or, in the author's view, should

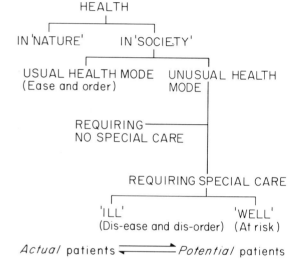

Fig. 24.1. A view to emphasize that, in society, pregnancy is an unusual mode of health in which women require special care of they are to remain 'well' and not become actual patients.

be, does not mean that it also has to be depersonalized. As the figure tries to illustrate, the woman in pregnancy, and especially the parturient woman, however well she may be in labour, is potentially at risk from unpredictable acute emergencies. These include fetal distress, prolapsed cord, occasionally shoulder dystocia, apnoea in the newborn, uterine inertia, retained placenta, or postpartum haemorrhage. Any one of them can quickly convert a 'potential patient' into a 'real patient' with a serious, even lethal, problem. This is a concept which both the patient and her attendant ought to appreciate. The accoucheur should recognise the woman's need to enjoy her labour with the minimum interference compatible with safety. The woman should understand the doctor's dilemma of balancing obstetric risks against maternal comfort and satisfaction. Regrettably, intertwined with this patient–doctor interface, there is now the

338

ever increasing medico-legal problem of responsibility. Who is responsible for the child's well-being *in utero?* The mother, the attendant, or hopefully, both? A certain mutual flexibility, based on the concepts of health and safe care, will go a long way towards retaining emotional satisfaction for women in parturition without endangering the baby or compromising the authority of the attendant.

Against the background of changing maternal and obstetric attitudes to childbirth, numerous implications arise which affect the following.

THE PLACE OF BIRTH

The unforeseeable hazards of labour assume their greatest proportions when they occur where facilities are limited or unavailable, and especially when medical aid is remote. Barry (1980) argues that the onus of proof lies with those who advocate hospital confinement for all women if at all possible. He also describes three maternal deaths at home due to postpartum haemorrhage, when there was no contraindication to home confinement! As Beazley and Lobb (1983) point out, regarding the proposal to organize randomized controlled studies to evaluate the relative risks of selected home versus hospital confinement, 'was such a trial ever organized to evaluate the parachute?' Surely the Obstetric Flying Squad attests to the seriousness of unforeseen obstetric emergencies. Yet unforeseen problems are not the same as unavoidable ones.

While being a dedicated advocate of hospital delivery, the author also believes firmly that compassionate understanding of a woman's natural antipathy to hospital confinement demands of the obstetrician time spent in explanation. Hopefully this can avoid polarizing her initial uncertainties into those extreme views which prompt her to accept an increased perinatal risk at home, rather than undergo confinement in a consultant unit with a resident doctor, or, perhaps, in a general practitioner unit suitably sited adjacent to a consultant unit and full hospital facilities.

LABOUR SUITE ATTITUDES

A 'birthing room' which combines the relaxed atmosphere of home with the safety of hospital delivery is appreciated by many mothers. To include a birthing room within the labour suite has the advantage of employing its staff and resources economically. It also ensures that adequate back-up facilities are quickly available if required. Needless to say, delivery of a woman in a birthing room in no way diminishes the need to keep the area clean, or for assistants to be meticulous about their principles of hygiene and sterility.

It is now quite common practice in many obstetric units for husbands (or sometimes another close relative) to be present at the delivery, unless it is operative. Unfortunately he still is often required to adopt a gown and mask, although the obstetric attendants move to and from the labour room and all parts of the hospital in apparel which is certainly no less 'bug-ridden' than the clothes of a well groomed and neatly dressed relative. The belief that the labour room is a sterile area is quite incorrect. Indeed, the organisms harboured there may be significantly more injurious to the patient and her husband than any commensals he introduces. In such matters flexibility with safe care is perhaps the key to progress.

CONTROLLED PARTURITION

While it is important to ensure that labour retains its emotionally satisfying character, it must not be overlooked that the present safety of parturition is the result of significant obstetric progress, in the past 50 years especially. Much of what has been achieved is embodied in the concept of Controlled Parturition, and therefore it is important this term should not be misunderstood by patients. It is not 'taking over' childbirth, nor is it 'conveyor-belt' obstetrics. Even less is it a policy of 'convenience' for either the patient or the obstetrician. It *is* a term which expresses firstly the idea that 'masterly inactivity' is no longer an acceptable method of securing feto-maternal safety, and secondly, that sensible anticipation, based on accurate diagnosis and a knowledge of modern delivery techniques, is preferable. Diagrammatically, this is expressed in Fig. 24.2, which emphasizes initially the important influence which antenatal events have upon the method of delivery. (In some labour suites this important matter is further emphasized by the use of Labour Prediction Scores.) Spontaneous labour should follow an active obstetric decision, made antenatally, that it is in the best interests of the mother and baby, and preferable to one of the forms of planned labour.

In the case of any proposed vaginal delivery, a policy of active management is now thought to be safer than a policy of 'wait and see'. And here it is worth pointing out that in contrast to earlier develop-

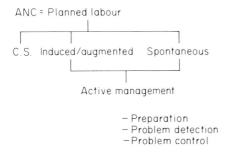

ANC = Planned labour

C.S. Induced/augmented   Spontaneous

Active management

– Preparation
– Problem detection
– Problem control

Fig. 24.2. Aspects of controlled parturition.

ments, there now seems less justification than was previously thought for classifying obstetric situations as 'high' or 'low' risk with regard to labour room management. It is not that the idea is invalid, but experience reveals that it is all too easy for patients in the low risk category to receive less than adequate attention, and patients in the high risk category to be over-treated. A sensible and flexible use of obstetric commonsense is more valuable than rigid and brittle labour room policies. It also facilitates kind and personal care to the individual, which rule books tend to omit.

Labour—an intensive care situation

In Britain the concept of labour as an intensive care situation is fundamental to the policy of active management in labour. Parturient women require the undivided attention of their attendants. (Interestingly, it was the dangers of the third stage of labour which promoted an active approach to patient management, long before active management of the first and second stages of labour was seriously considered.) The Irish School point out forcibly that no patient should compete for the attention of labour room staff who does not require their specialized skills immediately. Only patients in labour should occupy the intensive care beds of the labour room. Those women not in labour should be elsewhere.

The active management of natural labour

The active management of natural labour is a policy which contrasts sharply with the 'watchful expectancy' of former years. The concept is based not on an idea of normal labour but on the idea of minimal risk labour. Normal labour can be diagnosed with confidence only in retrospect. Active management implies sensible anticipation of the patient's progress in labour.

In this country we are fortunate in the ready availability of national and international statistics which draw attention to the real and potential hazards of obstetric management. Reports on Confidential Enquiries into Maternal Deaths in England and Wales, or the National Brithday Trust publications entitled Perinatal Mortality and Perinatal Problems, facilitate assessment of the risks involved in the many circumstances which influence pregnancy and parturition. This statistical information, when combined with the evidence of personal obstetric experience and knowledge of the obstetric environment, enables each consultant to deduce, in a meaningful way, the minimal risk situation for his patient. Naturally, the different environments in which obstetrics has to be practised alter the minimal risk situation in each area of the world. Nevertheless the overall concept of minimal risk should be invariable.

The active management of natural labour includes the following features.

PATIENT PREPARATION

The transition from antenatal care to care in labour is continuous. Each obstetrician has the duty to record in some obvious place in the antenatal notes any significant features of labour which he believes may occur. This includes the anticipation of both a minimal risk situation and any departure therefrom.

Routine practices of the past, such as an enema on admission (and even castor oil!) have, rightly, been eradicated. They achieve little except the aggravation of painful piles, and, in promoting involuntary defaecation, confuse inexperienced patients about the desire to bear down. A glycerine suppository, if spontaneous bowel action cannot be encouraged, is usually all that is required to avoid soiling at delivery.

Shaving of the patient's pubic hair is unnecessary. The procedure often traumatizes the skin, and significant irritation of the area is often experienced during regrowth. Shaving offers no advantages of sterility. All that is necessary is sufficient trimming of the vulvo-perineal area to ensure good vision for delivery and care of the perineum should an episiotomy or stitches be required afterwards.

Low amniotomy is a debatable preparatory procedure. Certainly control of the duration of labour has altered the need to preserve the forewaters. The 'fluid wedge' theory of cervical dilatation is less often invoked than the theory of mechanical advantage which is believed to be secured by the presenting part being firmly implanted within the pelvis, thereby enabling the fetal body to act as a firm central pole within the uterus from the upper end of which the fundus can gain the necessary purchase to take up the lower segment and cervix during retraction. Of course, low amniotomy as a preparatory procedure can be performed only when there is some cervical dilatation, and should be performed only when the head is within the pelvis and well applied to the cervix in order to minimize the risk of cord prolapse. The subsequent advantages to the fetus are that meconium stained liquor is quickly revealed, and, if necessary, a fetal-scalp clip is readily applied.

On admission to hospital patients in suspected labour should be treated as though, at some time during the next 12 hours, a Caesarean section will be necessary. If it is deemed necessary to supply the patient with her necessary calories and fluid by parenteral infusion, considerable care must be taken not to overload the circulation unnecessarily (Lind 1983). Apart from avoiding solid food by mouth, it is also wise to ensure that the patient has some antacid mixture by mouth. In the event of an unforeseen emergency requiring anaesthetic this helps to prevent the inhalation of acidic gastric contents and the subsequent development of Mendelson's syndrome.

As a preparatory procedure, should epidural analgesia be desired later in labour, it is often advantageous to insert the epidural catheter in early labour when the mother is still comfortable and well able to cooperate. Subsequently the analgesic agent can be easily introduced as required.

THE COMPONENTS OF NATURAL LABOUR

The powers

PRIMARY FORCES

Forces that expel the baby, its placenta and membranes, through the various maternal passages are, in the first part of labour, derived from the action of the uterus. To be effective, this primary uterine power has to function in a particular way.

The muscle fibres of the upper uterine segment must possess the facility not only to contract and relax, but also to retract, i.e. after relaxation they retain a length which is not so great as before the contraction began. The process of retraction must be progressive.

The power generated by the upper uterine segment must be associated with a degree of uterine polarity whereby the retractile effects of the uterine fundus can overcome the stretching and relaxation properties of the lower uterine segment and cervix.

Braxton–Hicks contractions, which may be observed during the latter part of pregnancy, and which precede labour, are ineffective with regard to cervical dilatation or descent of the presenting part. Moreover they do not increase their frequency or duration. In these respects they differ from the primary forces of parturition. Nevertheless the primary powers appear to develop from the pattern of uterine contractility established in the later part of pregnancy, and, whatever may be the factor which ultimately precipitates their expulsive efficiency, no significant difference has yet been discovered between the basic natures of these two types of contraction.

The primary forces of labour gradually increase their frequency, duration and power. Eventually they occur approximately one every three minutes, for approximately one to two minutes, and there is one to two minutes' effective relaxation between them. The fibres of the lower segment become elongated and thinned during the process, and gradually incorporate the supra-vaginal portions of the cervical canal. Subsequently the infra-vaginal cervix, which is at first effaced, dilates progressively. Studies performed in Liverpool suggest that the mechanism of cervical effacement necessitates a relatively rapid uptake of peripheral cervical substance, thereby preserving the integrity of the internal os until the last. Correct pressure relationships between the fetal head and the lower uterine segment are important to this mechanism (Beazley 1979).

Measurements obtained during labour indicate that uterine contractions probably begin at the cornual regions of the uterus, from where, in a circular distribution, they spread outwards and downwards as a peristaltic wave. Intrauterine pressure recordings taken during natural labour indicate that the resting tone is usually about 5 mm of mercury (0.67 kPa) and does not increase by more than about 5–10 mm of mercury (0.67–1.3 kPa) between contractions. Cervical dilatation is associated with intrauterine pressures above 20 mm of mercury (2.67 kPa), and it may be observed that patients often experience abdominal discomfort when pressures exceed 25 mm of mercury (3.33 kPa). Forceful uterine contractions may increase the intrauterine pressure to about 75 mm of mercury (10.0 kPa) above the resting tone. To exceed this is unusual.

SECONDARY FORCES

After the primary forces of labour have achieved full dilatation of the cervix and descent of the fetal presenting part to the pelvic floor, the patient in natural childbirth experiences a spontaneous and overwhelming desire to contract the voluntary muscles of her diaphragm and abdominal wall, in an effort to expel the baby from her body. These secondary powers now take on an unaccustomed and almost involuntary role which, if the patient is to bear down effectively, she must try to coordinate towards that purpose.

The passages

The passages through which a mother expels the baby from her body during natural labour, include the soft passages of the birth canal, supported by ligaments, fascia and fat, and the hard bony passage of the pelvis.

The bony passages
The pelvis resembles a basin. It is divided into a true and false portion which are separated from one another by the pelvic inlet. Only the true pelvis concerns the obstetrician. It may be divided into an upper, mid, and lower pelvic strait (Figs. 24.3, 24.4 and 24.5).

The upper strait
The circumferential boundary of the upper strait runs

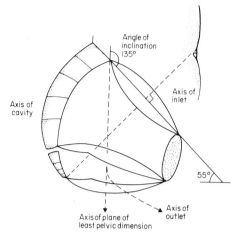

Fig. 24.4. Shows the axes of the pelvis described in the text.

from the centre of the anterior surface of the sacral promontory along the ilio-pectineal lines and around to the posterior aspect of the upper surface of the pubis. This upper strait has a real, though immeasurable, depth and may be thought of as a thin bony oval whose longest diameter runs transversely. The axis of the plane of this inlet follows a line which

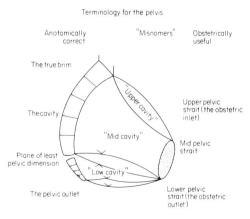

Fig. 24.3. The terminology on the left correlates satisfactorily with terms used in Anatomy text books. On the right side are terms that are used in this chapter. The central terms are not as correct as either of the other two, for, in practice, the upper pelvic strait is not a cavity at all.

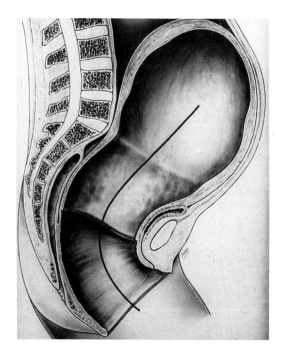

Fig. 24.5. Shows how these axes unite to form the uteropelvic axes of the birth canal.

extends from the normally situated umbilicus to the tip of the coccyx. In the anatomical position an angle of approximately 135° exists between the plane of the pelvic inlet and a vertical line drawn through the spine.

The lower strait

The lower strait is a cavity whose anterior wall is missing. The strait lies between the 'plane of least pelvic dimension' (i.e. bounded by the lower border of the symphysis pubis, the ischial spines and the tip of the sacrum), and the anatomical outlet of the pelvis (which stretches between the lower border of the symphysis pubis along the pubic rami to the ischial tuberosities and backwards along the sacrotuberous ligaments to the top of the coccyx). The normal axis of entry to the lower pelvic strait follows a line from the sacral promontory through the centre of the plane of least pelvic dimension. The axis angles downwards thereafter and curves forwards, through the centre of the lower pelvic strait towards the centre of the anatomical outlet.

Along the line of the plane of least pelvic dimension the levator ani muscles largely originate. Internal rotation of the presenting part normally occurs at this station of the pelvis. After passing through it, the presenting part is required to follow a curved axis.

The mid strait

The cavity of the pelvis lies between the pelvic brim and the plane of least pelvic dimension. The anterior surface of the sacrum comprises the posterior wall of the cavity. Anteriorly it is bounded by the posterior surface of the symphysis pubis. The posterior wall of the cavity is much longer than the anterior wall. The plane in the middle of the cavity is usually larger than any of the other pelvic planes.

The pelvic axis

From the plane of the pelvic brim to the plane of the anatomical outlet, the pelvic axis crudely resembles that of a drainpipe end or even a Wellington boot. The axes of the upper two pelvic straits are relatively linear when compared with the sharp forward angulation and the subsequent curve of the axis of the lowest pelvic strait.

Pelvic shapes and sizes

Each of the pelvic straits may be considered as a hoop, thus, at the inlet as an oval whose longest diameter lies transversely; in the middle as a circle; and at the lower end as an oval whose longest diameter runs antero-posteriorly. The normal diameters of the bony pelvis at these different planes are:

Upper strait:	anteroposterior	11.5 cm
	transverse	13.6 cm
Mid strait:	all diameters	12.0 cm
Lower strait:	anteroposterior	12.5 cm
	transverse (at level of ischial spines)	10.5 cm.

The fetal head which passes through these imaginary hoops while following the pelvic axis downwards, naturally undergoes a screw action imposed by the pelvic anatomy.

Alterations in the basic shape of the pelvic inlet (gynaecoid) may be described more scientifically as android, platypelloid or anthropoid (Fig. 24.6). For precise details of these pelvic types the reader is referred to the standard works of Caldwell *et al.* (1940). Simply, the android type means the pelvic inlet resembles a triangle. The rest of the pelvis resembles a male pelvis, which is rather like the long section of a short cone. The brim of the platypelloid pelvis is a wide but rather flat oval, whereas, in the anthropoid pelvis the oval of the pelvic brim is rather narrow side to side but has a long diameter antero-posteriorly. The anthropoid pelvis is also associated with a deep pelvic cavity because the angle of inclination between the vertical line of the spine and the plane of the pelvic brim exceeds 135°. This abnormality usually results from high assimilation, i.e. the sacral body is incorporated with the fifth lumbar vertebra.

The diameters usually observed between the different points of the bony pelvis have been given earlier. It is the shape of the pelvis, however, that determines the availability of these pelvic diameters. In addition to the shapes considered so far there is one other that deserves special mention.

At the plane of the anatomical outlet the sub-pubic arch may be unduly narrow. When a circular disc, diameter 9.3 cm, is fitted to the arch subtended by the descending rami of the pubis, as shown in Fig. 24.7 it becomes evident that the narrower the arch the less the disc is able to fit into it. The unusable space is referred to as the Waste Space of Morris, and normally it does not exceed 1 cm (Fig. 24.8). If the waste space is greater, the available diameter between the tip of the sacrum and the rami of the pubis will be significantly shorter than the absolute measurement.

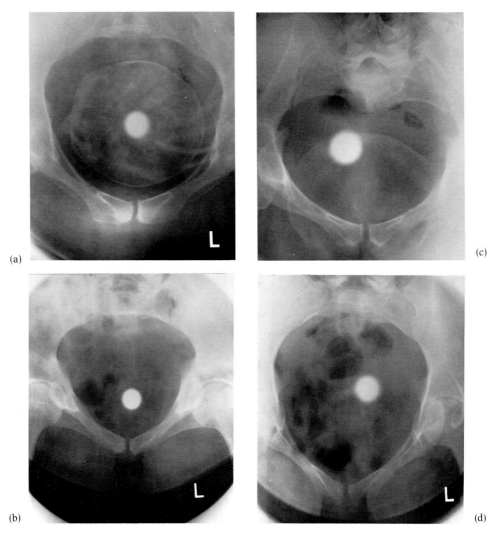

(a)

(c)

(b)

(d)

Fig. 24.6. A radiograph of the brim of (a) a gynaecoid pelvis; (b) an android pelvis; (c) a platypelloid pelvis; (d) an anthropoid pelvis.

The soft passages

During natural parturition the child must pass from the upper into the lower uterine segment and continue downwards, through the fully dilated cervix and the distensible vagina, to pass ultimately through the vulval introitus. Congenital anomalies of these structures may significantly alter the manner in which the fetus normally passes through the genital tract (cf. Chapters 1 and 27). Also the thickness of the soft passages, together with their supporting tissues undoubtedly influence the pelvic dimensions available to a child during its birth.

The passengers

The nature of the fetus as an inanimate passenger to be extruded through the birth canal will be considered here. The delivery of the placenta and membranes which are equally important passengers will be described later.

It is the size of the fetal skull that usually determines the ease with which parturition occurs. Availability of pelvic diameters is only ever of significance in as much as they relate to the dimensions of the child's head. Although many clever methods based

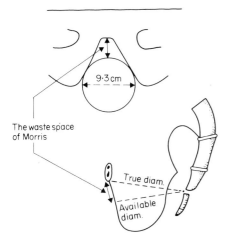

Fig. 24.7. Measuring the Waste Space of Morris (see text).

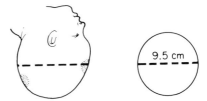

(a) Suboccipito bregmatic

Fig. 24.8. (a) A well-flexed head which presents to the brim as a circle of 9.5 cm diameter. The presenting diameter is suboccipito bregmatic.

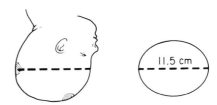

(b) Occipitofrontal

Fig. 24.8. (b) A deflexed head which presents as an oval with a longer occipitofrontal measurement of 11.5 cm.

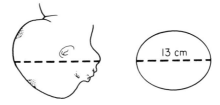

(c) Mentovertical

Fig. 24.8. (c) Greater deflexion resulting in a brow presentation; the oval is still bigger, its long diameter (mentovertical) being 13 cm.

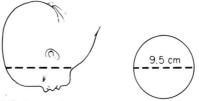

(d) Submento bregmatic

Fig. 24.8. (d) A fully extended head which again presents as a circle of diameter 9.5 cm; the presenting diameter is the submento bregmatic.

on detailed calculations of the pelvic dimensions have been used to anticipate cephalo-pelvic disproportion, it is the functional and not the absolute capacity of the pelvis which truly matters.

At the onset of labour it is usual for the fetus to lie longitudinally in a flexed attitude, with its head presenting over the pelvic brim. When well flexed, the vertex of the skull, i.e. that area which lies between the biparietal eminences, and the anterior and posterior fontanelles, normally enters the true pelvis first. Extension of the fetal head will alter the shape, and increase the diameters of that portion of the skull which enters the pelvis first (Fig. 24.8 a–d).

The extent to which the presenting fetal part has successfully negotiated the three pelvic straits is usually expressed by describing the 'station' of the presenting part, i.e. the level within the pelvis to which a known fetal landmark has descended. The ischial spines are usually taken as the maternal reference point.

The fetal head is said to be engaged when the presenting plane of the skull at the level of the biparietal diameter is at, or has passed, the plane of the pelvic brim. Passing downwards from the upper into the lower part of the pelvic cavity the biparietal plane next enters the lower pelvic strait via the plane of least pelvic dimension. Emerging from the pelvic outlet the biparietal plane next arrives at the maternal introitus. When the fetal head no longer recedes from the introitus between uterine contractions, the bipar-

ietal plane is at or has passed the anatomical outlet, and the head is said to be crowned.

Although the station of the fetal head is usually expressed as the level of the leading part of the skull in relation to the ischial spines of the maternal pelvis, the experienced obstetrician will recognize that this custom can be misleading. For example, the foremost part of the fetal skull may be distorted by caput succedaneum and/or moulding. To express the station of the fetal head meaningfully it is essential to have a visual image of both the fetal size and the pelvic capacity. A more accurate impression can then be obtained of what is happening at the level of the biparietal diameter and not just at the level of the leading part of the fetal skull.

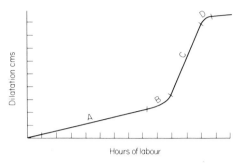

Fig. 24.9. Freidman's graph of labour (see text).

THE COURSE AND MECHANISMS OF NATURAL LABOUR (STAGES 1 AND 2)

It cannot be stated too often that the safe passage of the fetus through the pelvis is dependent less upon their absolute measurements and more upon five unknown factors of labour, viz the efficiency of the uterine contractions, the 'give' of the pelvis, the moulding potential of the fetal head, the fortitude of the mother, and the adaptability of the child's physiology.

The course of labour

Parturition is usually a continuous process, but traditionally it is divided into three stages. The first stage continues up to full cervical dilatation; the second stage terminates when the child is fully expelled; the third stage concerns the separation and expulsion of the placenta and membranes.

The time of onset of spontaneous labour is difficult to determine. Commonly, early in the first stage, the mucous plug within the cervix is extruded and appears at the vulva as a jelly-like substance streaked with red blood. Anything more should be considered an antepartum haemorrhage. Rupture of the membranes can occur at any time during the first or second stage. Usually, they rupture spontaneously in the later part of the first stage. The nature of the uterine contractions, and the discomfort caused by them, also provide unreliable guides to progress. Throughout the first stage contractions increase their frequency and duration slowly and steadily. During the second stage they become most powerful and cause most pain.

Progress during the first and second stages of labour is determined by dilatation of the cervix, and/or descent of the presenting fetal part through the maternal pelvis. In the early phase of labour the cervical state is commonly utilized as an index of progress. During the second stage of labour, when the cervix cannot be felt, descent of the presenting part becomes the most reliable index.

Friedman (1955, 1956) analysed the progress of spontaneous labour by plotting, graphically, cervical dilatation against time. He described (a) a latent phase of variable duration followed by (b) a phase of acceleration at about 2–3 cm dilatation of the cervix, (c) the phase of maximum dilatation, followed by (d) a short deceleration phase which led to full cervical dilatation (Fig. 24.9).

Friedman's work has influenced all subsequent thoughts on the natural course of spontaneous labour. Nevertheless several clinicians have since undertaken similar analyses and have been unable to confirm a deceleration phase prior to the onset of full cervical dilatation. Also, the standard deviations in Friedman's original graph are too wide for it to assist with clinical practice (see later).

Traditional teaching on the duration of the second stage of labour implies that it should continue no longer than one hour in multipara or two hours in primigravidas. A recent review of the second stage of labour by Stewart (1984) showed that the mean duration in primigravidas was 39 minutes, and in multiparas 15 minutes, which compares closely with other studies. The onset of the second stage, however, was, apparently, diagnosed by the urge to push, or else predicted from previous cervicographic progress. These methods are indirect, and, prospective studies in Liverpool, designed to determine when the cervix actually assumed full dilatation, revealed mean durations of the second stage which were unexpectedly much longer than this (102.5 ± 54.3 minutes in primigravidae, 47.0 ± 40.8 minutes in multipara). Until accurate means are available to diagnose the onset of full dilatation in a reasonable number of patients undergoing spontaneous labour, the actual duration of the normal second stage will remain in doubt. Meanwhile Stewart's report provides helpful practical information. It should be remembered, however, that, without continuous assessment of the cervical state, full dilatation is as difficult to diagnose as the onset of labour and certainly the mother's desire to 'bear down' cannot be taken as equivalent to the onset of full cervical dilatation.

CERVICAL DILATATION

The mechanism by which the cervix dilates deserves consideration. Myometrial contraction and retraction, even in the presence of polarity and fundal dominance, are unlikely to promote significant cervical dilatation unless the upper uterine pole is fixed relative to the lower one. The fetus probably acts as a central column for the uterus. Thus while the head cannot escape from the lower uterine area, myometrial retraction occurring in the upper segment pulls upwards the more elastic tissues of the lower uterine segment. Eventually, when the cervix is fully dilated, myometrial retraction continues but the stretched lower pole of the uterus now becomes fixed relative to its upper pole, so the fundus is pulled gradually downwards. Clinical evidence which supports this mechanism includes the poor dilatation which occurs with a transverse lie of the fetus, the increase in cervical dilatation which normally follows stabilization of the fetal column by amniotomy, rupture of the uterus, or the formation of Bandl's retraction ring in neglected cephalo-pelvic disproportion, and the increase in myometrial efficiency that occurs when the utero-pelvic axis facilitates optimal thrust along the fetal column.

Research in Liverpool has indicated that in the relationship between the forces generated in the uterine fundus, and the process of cervical dilatation, normal progress necessitates a head-to-cervix pressure gradient which is maximal at the level of the biparietal diameter, and minimal at the cervical rim. Reverse pressure gradients are associated with delayed labour (Beazley 1979).

The mechanisms of labour

The mechanisms of labour concern alterations in the attitude and position of the fetus, especially its presenting part, during passage through the birth canal. In a cephalic presentation, the fetal head usually enters the pelvic brim with the occiput directed laterally to the left or right (i.e. left or right occipitolateral position, 'LOL', 'ROL'*). Occasionally, the occiput lies in one of the anterior quadrants of the pelvis (LOA, ROA) or, less commonly, in one or other of the posterior quadrants (LOP, ROP).

Throughout labour, uterine activity promotes descent of the presenting fetal part. One of the first effects of descent is to cause increased flexion of the fetal head. The diameter of the head anterior to the fulcrum of the atlanto-axial joint is normally greater than the diameter posteriorly. Thus, on meeting the resistance of the pelvic tissues, the natural lever effect on the fetal head is to promote flexion (Fig. 24.10).

Consideration of the three hoops of the pelvis through which the fetus must travel will reveal that their disposition promotes a screw action as the head descends through them. Superiorly the oval lies transversely. Inferiorly the oval lies anteroposteriorly and, between the two, the pelvic cavity is basically circular. Thus flexion of the head in the occipitolateral position at the brim facilitates its passage into the circle of the pelvic cavity, wherein the fetal head may rotate to an occipitoanterior position. Rotation within the pelvis largely depends upon the gutter shape of the pelvic floor with its forward and downward slope. This shape promotes anterior rotation of the fetal part which first contacts either side of the pelvic floor. The rebound effect of the pelvic floor, which occurs during the time of uterine relaxation, also assists forward movement of the presenting part. As it recoils from the pressure enforced by the uterine contraction, the sloping and downward angle of the pelvic gutter tends to cast the presenting part forwards and to the opposite side.

After completion of internal rotation, the fetal vertex can enter the plane of least pelvic dimension along the axis of the lower pelvic strait, a movement which promotes extension of the fetal head. The presenting antero-posterior diameter of the skull increases during extension causing great distension of the maternal perineum and introitus at the moment of crowning. The fetal shoulders, which by now have entered the pelvic cavity, are undergoing similar movements to those recently undertaken by the fetal head. When the fetal skull escapes from the introitus the natural tendency is for it to restitute, so that it

---

* Sometimes the term occipitotransverse is used. In the author's view this is incorrect. Consistency demands the pelvic areas in which the occiput may lie are described as anterior, lateral or posterior. Pelvic planes may be described as horizontal or vertical and their direction as sagittal, transverse or oblique.

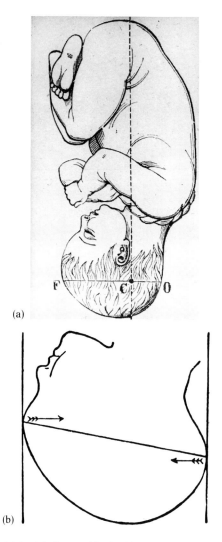

(a)

(b)

Fig. 24.10. (a) Flexion of the fetal head. The occipital 'arm' O–C is much shorter than the frontal 'arm' F–C.
(b) Flexion of the fetal head. Lateral pressure from the birth canal serves to keep the fetal head flexed.

the introitus without causing undue damage to the maternal perineum.

During passage along the birth canal the fetal head is subject to considerable pressures. An area of oedema called the caput succedaneum forms in the scalp where it protrudes through the ring of the dilating cervix. It is unusual to find a significant caput until after the membranes have ruptured.

A more important change in the fetal skull is that of moulding, i.e. movement of the skull bones in the spaces created by the fontanelles and wide suture lines. Skull bones which can slide and bend a little in this way facilitate an easier and safer delivery than skull bones which are more fixed and rigid. Usually the edges of the occipital and frontal bones pass under the edges of the parietal bones. The two parietals pass one under the other in the region of the sagittal suture. It is wonderful that, in contrast to an adult skull, a fetal skull can accommodate its shape and dimensions to the canal through which it must pass without causing damage to the delicate brain tissue it contains. Alterations of 4 mm in fetal skull

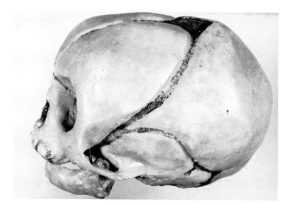

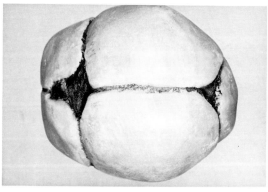

Fig. 24.11. (a) The fetal skull, lateral view.
(b) Superior view. The broad sutures and large fontanelles permit moulding during labour. For details see text.

occupies the normal right-angle relationships to the line of the shoulders. Restitution indicates, by the movement of the fetal occiput, the position of the fetal back and, therefore, the position of the anterior fetal shoulder. The shoulders descend into the lower pelvic strait and, as they occupy the antero-posterior oval of the obstetric outlet, the fetal head rotates externally. Next, the anterior shoulder escapes from under the symphysis pubis. Acute lateral flexion of the baby's body over the mother's abdomen now permits the posterior fetal shoulder to be expelled from diameter occur commonly during natural birth. Where there is significant cephalo-pelvic disproportion skull diameters may be altered by as much as 6–7 mm. This degree of moulding is incompatible with fetal safety (Fig. 24.11).

THE ONSET AND MAINTENANCE OF LABOUR

The factors which start the process spontaneously have not yet been elucidated. One surprising feature of pregnancy is that although smooth muscle usually contracts when stretched, in most women effective uterine contractions do not begin before term. Whether progesterone, secreted by the placenta or by the ovaries, inhibits uterine activity during pregnancy remains unanswered. There is some evidence that prior to the onset of labour progesterone secretion diminishes, and, at the same time, oestrogen output increases significantly. The effect of oestrogens on the myometrium is contrary to that of progesterone. It may be, therefore, that it is not the absolute concentration of either of these two hormones that really is important, but the ratio of one to the other. In some animal species, especially the sheep, a critical ratio between ·oestrogen and progesterone is associated with the relatively quick appearance of prostaglandins in the myometrium. These substances may sensitize the uterus to the effect of circulating oxytocin, or stimulate it directly.

The central role of prostaglandins in the onset of labour relates to their known action as myometrial stimulants, their ability to change cervical compliance and especially reduce its resistance, and their influence on gap junction formation in the myometrium. Husslein (1984) suggests that $PGF_{2\alpha}$ (rather than PGE_2) is the effective prostaglandin in spontaneous labour, its stable metabolite increasing during spontaneous and induced labour.

Prior to the onset of parturition there is no more than a low constant concentration of oxytocin in the blood stream, and Sellers et al. (1981) believe that the initiation of labour does not result directly from the stimulus of maternal plasma oxytocin, though it may be involved in some facilitatory mechanism.

Much work has been done to evaluate the hypothesis that the fetus in utero is chiefly responsible for triggering the onset of labour. The fetal hypothalamic/pituitary/adrenal axis in particular has been studied in detail. In sheep prolonged pregnancy results from fetal hypophysectomy while the administration of corticogrophin or corticosteroids stimulates premature delivery. Whether, in the human, corticosteroids are a trigger for the onset of labour, or simply a protective mechanism for the maturation of the fetal lung, has yet to be decided (Bzörkhem et al. 1978). It is known that there is release of fetal oxytocin during labour, but whether this release is a consequence of labour or a direct stimulant to the process is also undecided.

Clinical evidence to support the idea that the onset of labour, and its subsequent maintenance, involve separate mechanisms, is obtained from daily observation that labour induction usually requires a much higher concentration of intravenous oxytocin than the maintenance of labour.

The mechanisms of the onset of labour have not yet been fully elucidated. The enormous quantity of literature now available on the subject is beyond the scope of this chapter. The interested reader is referred to useful articles in the Lancet (1974), the book Endocrine Factors in Labour edited by Klopper and Gardener (1973), to Control of Parturition (1973), the article by Schwarz (1982) and to Chapter 11 (p. 115).

THE DIAGNOSIS OF LABOUR

As the onset of labour is usually a self-diagnosis it is not surprising that it is often incorrect. Confirmatory objective evidence of labour must, therefore, always be sought by the medical staff. On admission to the delivery suite, pelvic examination is performed. When cervical dilatation confirms the symptoms of labour, the diagnosis should be accepted. Should the cervix be closed, however, a 'show' or evidence of spontaneous rupture of the membranes provides confirmatory evidence. When none of these confirmatory signs is present, the patient should be transferred to an antenatal ward for observation. There she can rest more comfortably until parturition is established.

According to a report by Quinn et al. (1981), in 'false' or 'spurious' labour painful contractions are no longer recognized within 1 hour of admission in 85% of patients. When painful contractions do continue, but labour does not progress, patients deserve special attention, for a significant number of them will develop meconium stained liquor.

Recent interest has centred upon maternal posture during labour. According to McManus and Calder (1978) there are no differences, following labour induction, in the length of labour, mode of delivery, requirements of oxytocic and analgesic drugs, fetal and neonatal condition, between women who labour in an upright posture and those who are recumbent. By contrast, in another study of ambulation in labour, Flynn *et al.* (1978) investigating only women whose labour began spontaneously, observed that, in the ambulant group, the duration of labour was significantly shorter, the need for analgesia significantly less, and the incidence of fetal heart abnormalities significantly smaller. These investigators accepted, however, that nursing of the ambulant patient in labour is different though not necessarily more complicated than in the conventional recumbent position, and radio-telemetry is required to undertake continuous monitoring.

Ambulation is unsuitable for any mother receiving epidural analgesia. Moreover, amongst women without an epidural blockade Calvert *et al.* (1982) found only 45% who were offered the possibility of mobility elected to get out of bed, and then only for short periods.

It is now well recognized that patients confined to bed, perhaps because of epidural analgesia or fetal monitoring, should be nursed in a lateral position, or sitting up, in order to avoid the hazard of vena caval compression. Supine hypotension can compromise the baby.

Alternative birthing positions have received considerable publicity of late. Some of the upright, gravity assisted, positions are reported to have uterine and pelvic mechanical advantages (Stewart 1984) which have led to an increased use of the Birthing Chair or Borning Bed. The advantages of alternative

position may not always outweigh the disadvantages of poor visibility and access to the perineum during delivery. Also, fetal monitoring may be difficult to continue, and patients with epidurals may find birthing chairs unsuitable.

MONITORING

Reference to the impact made by Friedman's graphical presentation of the course of labour was made earlier. More suitable partographs, of varying complexity, are now available for clinical use (Studd 1975). They all present visually the rate of progress in low risk labours. By the direction taken of a patient's graph of progress modern partographs facilitate the early recognition of any departure from the low risk situation. Acceleration of labour is not a feature of the active management of normal labour. Usually it is a treatment reserved for labours which have become prolonged. Personally the author favours those charts which are simple to use. In my view the more complicated the partograph, the less frequently it is employed, and even then with no great accuracy. An example of the partograph now used commonly in this department is shown in Fig. 24.12.

Eighty per cent of labours in patients in a low risk category may be expected to follow a course whose graph lies on or to the left of the lines shown. This particular type of partograph begins at 2 cm cervical dilatation and should be utilized only when a positive

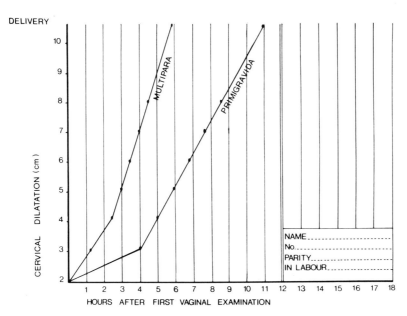

Fig. 24.12. One type of partograph (see text).

diagnosis of labour has been made. It will be noted that for primigravidas the subsequent duration of labour is approximately 11 hours. In multiparas it is only 6 hours.

The predictive value of cervimetric labour patterns (especially in primigravidas) has recently been re-emphasized by Cardozo et al. (1983).

MATERNAL COMFORT

Fear and pain are often closely associated in a patient's mind. Pain is a personal symptom. Although, on occasion, the doctor may choose to ignore his patient's complaint of pain, it is not a symptom which he can deny. Fear is dispelled, perhaps, partly by good antenatal care. During pregnancy time should have been taken to inform the patient of what is likely to happen to her in labour, to show her the labour room area and to introduce her to some of the staff who will be caring for her. During her time in labour fear can be further allayed by the ready availability of a competent personal nurse. Regrettably, in many hospitals such an arrangement does not seem to be possible. In other centres, the presence of the husband, to support his wife during labour, is favoured. The Irish school have shown convincingly that a personal nursing service can be achieved in labour rooms where there is no competition for attention from patients who are not in labour.

In the past it has always been the patient's prerogative to accept or decline an offer of analgesia during labour. Today the situation remains the same. In the author's view, however, the doctor now has a duty to recommend to his patient that labour be pain-free in order to facilitate better control of monitoring techniques. A patient undistracted by pain is able to remain much calmer throughout parturition. It is then much easier to detect problems which may arise in either the mother or her baby.

Elective epidural analgesia, though requiring specialized facilities, remains, in the author's view, one of the most valuable forms of pain relief during parturition. It is often convenient to arrange for the insertion of the epidural catheter prior to induction of labour, when this form of management is appropriate. Where epidural analgesia is used frequently it is essential that nursing and medical personnel are familiar with the care of patients receiving this form of treatment. Otherwise, maternal supine hypertension, or caval compression problems, including the discrimination between genuine and apparent fetal distress, will prove to be troublesome problems.

FETAL WELL-BEING

Modern technology should now be utilized to support sound clinical judgement. Appropriate monitoring equipment should be available for everyone. Continuous fetal heart monitoring, supported when necessary by fetal blood scalp sampling, is a far better method of monitoring fetal well-being in labour than simply recording the fetal heart rate at intervals of 15–20 minutes with a Pinard stethoscope. Details of modern techniques are described in Chapter 31 (p. 455). Here it is important only to draw attention to the debate for and against the effectiveness of continuous fetal heart rate monitoring in comparison with more traditional methods. Parer (1979), in an excellent review of the situation, concludes that, despite all the difficulties of obtaining adequate data, there is good evidence to support the view that continuous monitoring reduces intrapartum deaths by 1–2/1000 and neonatal deaths by as much as half. In my view, these benefits outweigh any difficulties inherent in monitoring techniques, which particularly include fetal scalp damage from electrodes, and subsequent infection. Furthermore, continuous fetal heart monitoring, if supported by fetal blood sampling when necessary to confirm anoxia, has been shown to reduce the incidence of Caesarean section (Edington et al. 1975, Boehm et al. 1981, Low et al. 1981).

Conclusion

Active management of labour takes advantage of the past years of clinical research, and the advent of modern technology. Machines are utilized to do their job effortlessly and continuously, thereby relieving compassionate nurses to go about work for which they were trained and which they do better than anyone else. In the future, an increased use of centralized monitoring suites may be envisaged. These will tirelessly and accurately monitor all patients in labour. With the help of appropriate data logging and computer equipment it will be possible to make meaningful use of information such as maternal temperature, pulse and respiration, the dip area under changes observed in the fetal heart tracings, the maternal blood pressure, and cervical dilatation.

Active management can convert one of the most important times in a family's life into a safer situation. Physiological facts are translated into measured parameters. These facilitate analysis and, therefore, better obstetric judgement. Active management relieves neither the doctor nor the nurse from the responsibility of making clinical and scientific judgements. Nor does it remove from the family unit the wonderment and emotion of childbirth.

THE THIRD STAGE OF LABOUR

The third stage of labour commences with the delivery of the infant and ends with the delivery of the placenta, and is thus an event related to the process of labour. From the practical point of view, however, the efficient management of the third stage begins much earlier, during the course of labour, and some of the problems of management continue after the delivery of the placenta.

The main complication of the third stage is blood loss and this may be excessive before the delivery of the placenta and for a period of time afterwards. Retention of the placenta may lead to, or even exaggerate, uterine bleeding but the continued presence of the placenta within the uterus has no known direct deleterious effect.

Physiological mechanisms involved in the delivery of the placenta

Uterine contractions have been shown to continue after the birth of the infant and, although the patient may feel little discomfort, the intrauterine pressure continues to be rhythmically raised. Possibly during, and certainly after, delivery the uterine muscle fibres contract and retract, with a resultant reduction in the size of the upper segment. This shortening reduces the area of the uterine surface to which the relatively incompressible placenta is attached. Separation of the placenta through the spongy layer of the decidua basalis occurs as a result of this retraction, and the consequent reduction in intrauterine volume tends to force the placenta into the relaxed lower segment, as well as assisting in the separation process. Retroplacental bleeding may play a part in this separation, but it seems that the lower edge of the placenta becomes detached first in most instances and so the concept of central separation and retroplacental bleeding is less likely (Macpherson & Wilson 1965).

When placental separation is complete and the placenta is forced into the lower segment and vagina it may be delivered spontaneoulsy by maternal effort, the lower edge presenting first at the vulva (the Matthews Duncan method of expulsion). If traction is exerted on the umbilical cord or the uterine fundus is forcibly compressed, the fetal surface may appear first, with the membranes covering the maternal surface (the Schultz method).

The continued retraction of the uterine muscle is of paramount importance in minimizing the blood loss during and after this stage. The blood vessels supplying the placental site are compressed by the oblique fibres of the middle layer of the myometrium. This mechanism of controlling bleeding is only effective if the uterine muscle is capable of efficient contraction and retraction, and any impairment of this will predispose to haemorrhage.

Most patients can be delivered without undue blood loss, but because the consequences of severe haemorrhage are very serious, firstly, obstetric 'flying squads' were introduced, and secondly, the prophylactic use of oxytocics was recommended. With the marked reduction in the number of women having their infants in other than specialist maternity units, the role of the 'flying squad' has changed considerably. The use of prophylactic oxytocics is now widespread and has certainly reduced the incidence of serious postpartum haemorrhage. The Report on Confidential Enquiries into Maternal Deaths in England and Wales 1967–69 (HMSO 1972) indicated that out of approximately 2.5 million births there were 16 maternal deaths directly due to postpartum haemorrhage and in nine others this was an important factor. Little or no real improvement is seen in the 1973–75 report in which were 13 deaths directly due to postpartum haemorrhage, which was also a contributory factor in another 13.

Management of third stage

ACTION OF OXYTOCIC DRUGS

The drugs used are oxytocin and ergometrine given alone or in combination. They may be given intravenously or intramuscularly, and the injection may be administered with the 'crowning' of the head, with the delivery of the head, with the delivery of the anterior shoulder, after the delivery of the infant or after the delivery of the placenta.

Oxytocin produces rhythmical contractions of the uterus augmenting retraction, and its effect is noticeable about 3 minutes after intramuscular injection (Embrey 1961). An injection of 5 units of oxytocin produced effective contractions for about 15 minutes. Ergometrine by injection results in a more prolonged contraction with retraction, and its effect is noticeable about 7 minutes after intramuscular injection. When either drug is given intravenously, the uterine contraction commences in about 30–40 seconds.

Obviously the drugs will affect only the upper segment, and the uterus below the retraction ring will not respond because of the absence of muscle fibres.

USE OF OXYTOCIC DRUGS IN MANAGEMENT

The prophylactic use of oxytocic drugs is now well established, but differences in technique and in the selection of the drug used still exist. The theoretical object of prophylactic oxytocics is to ensure efficient contractions of the uterus after the delivery of the infant, thus minimizing the amount of blood loss due to failure of occlusion of the capillaries in the placental site, and to promote rapid separation and descent of the placenta. If an oxytocic drug is given before the delivery of the placenta, the routine procedure for its subsequent delivery must be strictly adhered to, otherwise the placenta may be retained and blood loss may not be prevented.

Intravenous oxytocics are given with the delivery of the anterior shoulder, and the resulting contraction should follow very soon after the one which delivers the infant. If the placenta is partially or completely sheared off the uterine wall at the time of delivery of the infant, a further contraction should complete its separation and encourage its descent into the lower segment or vagina. It is necessary to anticipate this process by assisting the delivery of the placenta immediately after delivery of the infant, and before the uterine contraction prevents complete descent of the placenta as may sometimes happen (see below). As soon as the umbilical cord has beeen clamped and separated from the infant the placenta is delivered.

If the injection is given intramuscularly (and Syntometrine, Syntocinon 5 units and ergometrine 0.5 mg [Sandoz], is commonly used) delivery of the placenta can be achieved only by administering it at the 'crowning' of the head or after its delivery and allowing an interval of about 2 minutes before completing the delivery of the infant. If Syntometrine is given with the delivery of the anterior shoulder (in a vertex or face presentation) this is comparable to administering the injection after the infant is delivered. Time must then be allowed for the uterus to respond to the preparation and for delivery of the placenta to be accomplished. Gibbens et al. (1972) using a radioimmunoassay for oxytocin found that following an intramuscular injection of Syntometrine an effec-tive plasma level of oxytocin was achieved almost as rapidly as following an intravenous injection. In view of the haemodynamic consequences of intravenous oxytocin in certain circumstances it would seem that intramuscular Syntometrine is just as effective, almost as rapid and is to be preferred. As discussed in Chapter 17, ergometrine may be contraindicated in patients with heart disease but oxytocin may be safely given.

When oxytocin is not given until after the delivery of the placenta, it is necessary to rely on uterine contractions to separate the placenta completely from its attachment and then to expel it into the vagina. Because the uterine contractions are sometimes inefficient and ineffective, there is a greater risk of haemorrhage in these circumstances and injection before placental separation is preferred.

Delivery of the placenta
Separation of the placenta may be accompanied by a little vaginal bleeding. Descent of the placenta into the vagina is followed by a narrowing of the uterine body palpable in the abdomen, increased mobility of the uterus and lengthening of the umbilical cord. However, if oxytocic drugs are given prophylactically it is not necessary to wait for these signs before effecting delivery of the placenta. When the uterus is felt to contract, the patient can be encouraged to bear down and expel the placenta by increased intra-abdominal pressure. In many patients this is not sufficient, and pressure with the hand by attendant is required.

A more active policy is often considered advisable. When the uterus is felt to contract after the delivery of the infant, it can be pushed towards the umbilicus by a hand on the lower abdomen while the cord is held taut at the vulva as described by Andrews (1940) and Brandt (1933). Alternatively the cord may be gently and gradually pulled downwards and posteriorly with one hand while the uterus is pushed upwards (Fig. 24.13) as practised by Fliegner and Hibbard (1966). A further modification of this cord-traction technique is to initiate descent of the placenta by applying pressure to the fundus at the same time as cord traction is commenced, provided the uterus is contracting. Once the placenta is felt to be descending, the abdominal hand 'peels' the uterus off the placenta as previously described. It is essential that the uterus is contracted whenever cord traction is practised. Energetic traction of the cord, with a relaxed fundus may invert the uterus.

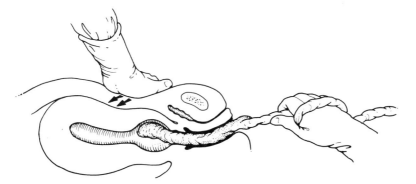

Fig. 24.13. Illustration of controlled cord traction.

CLAMPING OF THE CORD

The necessity for clamping the maternal end of the divided cord has been questioned, as has the timing of clamping and dividing the cord in order to separate the infant. Botha (1968) has reported a reduction in the incidence of retained placental and post-partum blood loss in Bantu women who squat in order to deliver their infants and later deliver the placenta without first separating the child from it. This results in an increase in the blood volume of the infant, and others have commented on the beneficial effects of this procedure. The exsanguinated placenta is thought to separate more readily and to be more easily delivered. If the infant is separated from the placenta soon after delivery, the blood in the placenta may be allowed to flow into a receptacle while a uterine contraction and the delivery of the placenta are awaited.

Yao and Lind (1969) have shown the effect of gravity on the volume of placental transfusions. When the infant was 40 cm below the introitus, the placental transfusion was complete in 30 seconds, so waiting 3 minutes before clamping the cord was not beneficial. If the infant was held above the introitus, placental transfusion was lessened or prevented. At Caesarean section, raising the infant might result in hypovolaemia and ideally the infant should be held 20 cm below the level of the placenta for 30 seconds before clamping. Yao et al. (1969) also have shown that the distribution of infant–placental blood volume at birth was 67% to 33%. At 15 seconds it was 73% to 27%, at 1 minute 80% to 20% and at 3 minutes 87% to 13%. No significant change in distribution was achieved by delaying clamping for longer than 3 minutes. Yao and her colleagues (1968) also demonstrated that postnatal transfer of placental blood was rapid and amounted to 55% of the infant's blood volume at birth. More than one-quarter of the blood was transferred with the contraction resulting in delivery while the remainder of the blood was transferred at 1 minute after a contraction if ergometrine had been given. If no oxytocin was given, the transfer took three minutes. They could not demonstrate any direct significant influence of respiration on placental transfusion, as had been suggested by Redmond et al. (1965). Philip et al. (1969) concluded that placental transfusion occurred as a result of fetal asphyxia before delivery in patients with fetal distress. Although asphyxia is frequently found before the development of the respiratory distress syndrome, the haematocrit tends to be low in the infants suggesting that an intrauterine placental transfusion has not occurred. These studies would indicate that it was theoretically beneficial to allow as much placental blood to enter the infant as possible after delivery by delaying clamping for 3 minutes and holding the infant below the introitus. In fetal asphyxia the fetus may trigger off a transfusion of blood from the placenta to the fetus, an increase in 'venous return'. The finding of intrauterine fetal respiratory gasps and asphyxia may be relevant (Boddy & Dawes 1975).

In diabetic patients it is preferable to reduce the volume of the placental transfusion as far as possible because of the risk of vascular thrombosis in the infant. Early clamping is advocated for infants suspected of having haemolytic disease of the newborn, as in affected infants late clamping results in the serum bilirubin levels being higher.

Saigal et al. (1972) found that while most of the blood had been transferred in one minute in term infants, this was not the case with premature infants. A placental transfusion in premature infants increased the severity of neonatal hyperbilirubinaemia and the incidence was directly related to the time elapsing before the cord was clamped.

EXAMINATION OF THE PLACENTA

The placenta should be examined after it has been delivered to ensure that the cotyledons are all present and that the placenta is complete. A succenturiate lobe may have been missed and retained in the uterus, and vessels ending abruptly on the fetal surface of the placenta may suggest this. Immediate exploration of the uterus is required if it is certain that placental tissue is missing, or if the nature of the delivery of the placenta makes it likely that a cotyledon is retained. The completeness of the membranes is less easy to assess and less important; a fragment may be detected on vaginal examination and removed with long artery forceps but exploration of the uterus is not required.

The vessels of the umbilical cord should be examined and any anomaly, including absence of an umbilical artery, should be reported to the paediatrician. If an artery is absent, the incidence of congenital abnormalities in the child is about 30% (Benirschke 1965), especially those involving the renal and cardiovascular systems.

Blood loss after delivery of the placenta
Estimation of the blood lost in the third stage is grossly inaccurate when this is done by inspection alone. Although it is possible to collect some of the blood lost before and during the delivery of the patient, and allowances can be made for contamination by amniotic fluid and the soiling of bed linen, bleeding from the uterus occurring during the 24 hours after delivery is not usually measured accurately unless the loss is considerable and replacement is required. An appreciable fall in the haemoglobin level may occur without any single episode of haemorrhage. Exact measurement is not necessary provided the patient's blood pressure and pulse rate are unchanged, but if there is excessive bleeding and she shows evidence of shock, the amount of blood to replace is important.

Brant (1967) described a method for calculating the loss at delivery using a 'washing machine' method for bed linen and drapes, and confirmed the impression that when the actual loss was over 300 ml the attendants underestimated the volume of the loss. A more accurate method of determining the effects of blood loss and the amount to be replaced involves the measurement of the central venous pressure (O'Driscoll & McCarthy 1966).

REFERENCES

ANDREWS C.T. (1940) *Sth. Med. Surg.*, **102**, 605.
BARRON D. (1973) *Lancet*, **ii**, 555.
BARRY C.N. (1980) *J. roy. Coll. gen. Practit.*, **30**, 102.
BEAZLEY J.M. (1975) *Amer. J. Obstet. Gynec.*, **122**, 161.
BEAZLEY J.M. (1979) *Amer. J. Obstet. Gynec.*, **133**, 723.
BEAZLEY J.M., LOBB M.O. (1983) *Aspects of Care in Labour.* (Lind T. ed), p. 13. Churchill Livingstone, Edinburgh.
BENIRSCHKE K. (1965) *Birth Defects* (original article series), p. 53. The National Foundation, March of Dimes.
BJÖRKHEM I., LANTTO O., LUNELL N.O., PSCHERA H. (1978) *Brit. J. Obstet. Gynaec.*, **85**, 446.
BODDY K. & DAWES G.S. (1975) *Brit. med. Bull.*, **31**, 3.
BOEHM F.H., DAVIDSON K.K., BARRET J.M. (1981) *Amer. J. Obstet. Gynec.*, **140**, 295.
BOTHA M.C. (1968) *S. Afr. J. Obstet. Gynaec.*, **6**, 30.
BRANDT M.L. (1933) *Amer. J. Obstet. Gynec.*, **25**, 662.
BRANT H.A. (1967) *Brit. med. J.*, **i**, 398.
CALDWELL W.E., MOLOY H.C. & D'ESOPO D.A. (1940) *Amer. J. Roentgenol.*, **40**, 558.
CALVERT J.P., NEWCOMBE R.G. & HIBBARD B.M. (1982) *Brit. J. Obstet. Gynaec.*, **89**, 285.
CARDOZO L.D., GIBB M.F., STUDD J.W.W., VASANT R.V., COOPER D.J. (1982) *Brit. J. Obstet. Gynaec.*, **89**, 33–8.
CONTROL OF PARTURITION (1973) *Journal of Reproduction and Fertility*, Supplement No. 16, Blackwell Scientific Publications, Oxford.
EDINGTON P.T., SIBANDA J., BEARD R.W. (1975) *Brit. med. J.*, **iii**, 341.
EMBREY M.P. (1961) *Brit. med. J.*, **i**, 1737.
FLIEGNER J.R. & HIBBARD B.M. (1966) *Brit. med. J.*, **ii**, 622.
FLYNN A.M., KELLY J., HOLLINS G. & LYNCH P.F. (1978) *Brit. med. J.*, **ii**, 591.
FRIEDMAN E.A. (1955) *Obstet. Gynec.*, **6**, 567.
FRIEDMAN E.A. (1956) *Obstet. Gynec.*, **8**, 691.
GARFIELD R.E., KANNAN M.S., DANIEL E.E. (1980) *Amer. J. Physiol.*, **238**, C81.
GIBBENS D., BOYD N.R.H., CROCKER S., BAUMBER S. & CHARD T. (1972) *J. Obstet. Gynaec. Brit. Cwlth.*, **79**, 644.
HMSO (1972) *Report on Confidential Enquiries into Maternal Deaths in England and Wales 1967–69*, p. 27. London.
HUSSLEIN P. (1984) *Brit. J. Obstet. Gynaec.*, **91**, 228.
KLOPPER A. & GARDENER J. (eds) (1973) *Endocrine Factors in Labour.* Cambridge University Press.
LANCET (1974) (*Leader*), **1**, 124.
LIND T. (1983) *J. roy. Soc. Med.*, **76**, 870.
LOW J.A., COX M.J., KAREHMAR E.J., McGRATH M.J., PANCHAM S.R., PIERCY W.N. (1981) *Amer. J. Obstet. Gynec.*, **139**, 229.
McMANUS T.J. & CALDER A.A. (1978) *Lancet*, **i**, 72.
MacPHERSON J. & WILSON J.K. (1956) *J. Obstet. Gynaec. Brit. Cwlth.*, **63**, 321.
O'DRISCOLL K. & McCARTHY J.R. (1966) *J. Obstet. Gynaec. Brit. Cwlth.*, **73**, 923.
O'DRISCOLL K. & STRONGE J.M. (1975) In *Clinics in Obstetrics and Gynecology* (Beazley J.M. ed.), p. 3., W.B. Saunders Co., Philadelphia.

PARER J.T. (1979) *Lancet*, **ii**, 632.

PHILIP A.G.S., YEE A.B., MOOTHEDAN ROSY, NERGESH SURTI, TSAMTSOURIS A. & INGALL D. (1969) *Brit. med. J.*, **ii**, 11.

QUINN M.A., MURPHY A.J., GALLAGHER J. (1981) *Aust. N.Z. J. Obstet. Gynaec.*, **21**, 167.

REDMOND A., ISANA S. & INGALL D. (1965) *Lancet*, **i**, 283.

SCHWARZ B.E. (1982) In *Progress in Obstetrics and Gynaecology* (Studd J. ed), p. 1, Churchill Livingstone.

SAIGAL S., O'NEILL A., SUREINDER Y., CHUA L. & USHER R. (1972) *Pediatrics*, **49**, 406.

SELLERS S.M., HODGSTON H.T., MOUNTFORD L.A., MITCHELL M.D., ANDERSON ANNE B.M., TURNBULL A.C. (1981) *Brit. J. Obstet. Gynaec.*, **88**, 725.

STEWART K.S. (1984) In *Progress in Obstetrics and Gynaecology*, vol. 4. (Studd J. Ed.) p. 197. Churchill Livingstone, Edinburgh.

STUDD J. (1975) In *Clinics in Obstetrics and Gynecology* (Beazley J.M. ed), p. 127. W.B. Saunders Co., Philadelphia.

YAO A.C., HIRVENSALO M. & LIND J. (1968) *Lancet*, **i**, 380.

YAO C. & LIND J. (1969) *Lancet*, **ii**, 505.

YAO A.C., MOINIAN M. & LIND J. (1969) *Lancet*, **ii**, 871.

CHAPTER 25
SPECIAL CIRCUMSTANCES AFFECTING LABOUR

J. M. BEAZLEY

THE INFLUENCE OF AGE

Children and young teenagers

CHILDREN

Premenarcheal pregnancy is a fascinating condition. A child aged $5\frac{1}{2}$, thought to be the youngest mother in the world, was delivered in Peru by Caesarean section. The baby weighed 2.7 kg. A German child aged $6\frac{1}{2}$ years delivered a 3 kg child normally. Twins have been delivered to a girl aged $7\frac{1}{2}$ in Brazil and a 7-year-old Mohammedan girl is described who was delivered of a child weighing 2 kg by Caesarean section. The youngest English mother is reported to have been 9 years old at the time of delivery (Dewhurst 1963, Huffman 1968). Bender (1969) describes an uneventful pregnancy in a girl aged 13 years 8 months. Labour lasted 18 hours and 50 minutes, and was terminated by a compassionate low forceps delivery under general anaesthesia followed by a necessary manual removal of the placenta. Her baby weighed 3.7 kg. Reference is made by James (1969) to a former case report in which a girl, aged little more than 11 years, ultimately had a spontaneous delivery after a normal pregnancy and labour.

Both James (1969) and Bender (1969) refer to the minimal psychological effects of pregnancy in the premenarcheal age group and comment upon medicolegal aspects of this kind of problem. They also re-emphasize the tendency for these very young mothers to be free from obstetrical problems. The Caesarean section rate seems to be particularly low.

YOUNG TEENAGERS

In England and Wales 1974–78 there were 18851 pregnancies in schoolgirls aged 15. Of these, 12873 were terminated. There has been a sevenfold true increase in the number of pregnant 15 year olds in England and Wales since 1950 (Russell 1983). Data derived by Smith (1983) from an enquiry into teen-

age mothers under 20 revealed that only 43% had used birth control at the first coitus, 35% had intended to become pregnant, only 4% had not, and the remaining 61% had mixed feelings about becoming pregnant. In the USA today one in five births is to women aged 18 or younger, and in the 15–17 age group the pregnancy rate is almost four times more for black than for white girls.

It is important to distinguish between older teenagers (age 17–19), whose reproductive capacity is good, and those aged 16 and less, in whom obstetric complications are significantly greater. Lewis (1967) has reported the results of study of 103 primigravid patients plus one multigravid patient who were under the age of 16 at the time of conception. They were all delivered in one obstetric unit between 1 January 1963 and 20 September 1966. An increased incidence of pre-eclampsia was observed in this group although the perinatal mortality rate was only 1%. Easy spontaneous vaginal delivery was the rule. The incidence of forceps deliveries was 10% and Caesarean section rate 4%. Although the greatest obstetric hazard was pre-eclampsia, grave sociological problems complicated the pregnancy in many of these young mothers. Utian (1967) also emphasized pregnancy toxaemia as a complication of young motherhood. In a consecutive series of 100 white primigravid patients aged 13–16 years he observed an increased incidence of prematurity.

Emotional and psychological sequelae were obviously harrowing features of pregnancy in four girls aged 13–15 described by Russell (1969). Whereas, from the obstetric viewpoint, the complications in such patients are minimal, Russell re-emphasizes that occasionally there may be an element of disproportion found, in which instance, especially if the girl is very young or of small stature, Caesarean section should not be avoided.

Three leaders (*Brit. med. J.* 1971, 1980a, *Lancet* 1983) have taken a less sanguine view than former writers on the hazards of teenage pregnancy. It is clear however that pregnancy in young patients is associated with definite risks of hypertension and tox-aemia. There is also a lower incidence of engagement of the fetal head before labour and a higher incidence of operative delivery. Infants are more likely to be premature and carry a high perinatal mortality espe-cially in the under 15 age group. Congenital malfor-mations are a larger cause of infant death than pre-viously has been recognized. The risk of maternal self-harm, including suicide, is greater than may have been imagined from previous reports, and should the pregnancy be allowed to continue, poor social relationships at home can lead to baby batter-ing and severe disturbances of maternal behaviour.

In a recent clinical study of pregnancy in 263 young teenagers in Liverpool, Elliott and Beazley (1980) found that, although prematurity continued to remain a problem, many of the other hazards of pregnancy were no greater in the general population. It was emphasized that this observation probably re-flects better antenatal care, which this group of patients now receives.

The older mother

Age can be expected to be associated with increased risks for the pregnant woman. With advancing age progressive diseases get worse, e.g. mitral stenosis, diabetes, chronic bronchitis, chronic pyelonephritis, etc. The commonest maternal complication over the age of 45 is hypertension (Rahman *et al.* 1983). Other problems include the development of uterine fibroids, or degenerative changes in the joints of the lumbosacral spine and pelvis. These trends will be aggravated by a poor social environment, poor nutrition, or excessive childbearing. The incidence of some congenital abnormalities, especially Down's syndrome, increases significantly with maternal age.

One category of older mothers who are particularly at risk is the women who conceive for the first time in later life. An important distinction should be made, however, between women who marry late but be-come pregnant quickly after marriage, and women who, although married for quite a long time, fail to become pregnant despite attempting to do so for sev-eral years. In both instances the future chances of pregnancy are diminished when compared with young women. Nevertheless, in the former group a high degree of fertility has been retained, and further successful pregnancies are likely to be the rule. In the latter group fertility is low, and the chances of future pregnancies are remote.

A third group is those who simply have a pro-longed interpregnancy interval. Opaneye (1983) compared the labour and delivery of 60 women with an interpregnancy interval greater than 7 years and found no significant difference from a control group with a shorter interpregnancy interval.

An 'elderly primigravida' used to be characterized as being over the age of 40 years. By general consent the age has now been lowered to 35 years. On this basis the incidence of elderly primigravidity is now of the order of 0.64%.

The obstetric outlook for elderly primigravid patients of high fertility, and who remain compara-tively unaffected by the influence of age upon their physiology, is extremely hopeful. The imagined risks stemming from maternal anxiety, or loss of elasticity in the soft and bony passages, are more theoretical than practical. The hazards from possible abortion, prolonged pregnancy, uterine inertia and puerperal psychosis tend to be over-exaggerated. By contrast, the patient of low fertility who becomes pregnant may well suffer from complications related to the cause of her infertility. Thus, endocrine disorders tend to be more common, there is an increased risk of miscarriage, the date of gestation is often unknown, mild pelvic abnormalities may promote malposition of the fetal head or even result in cephalo-pelvic dis-proportion. Maternal mental attitudes may aggravate minor emotional problems. Fetal distress and peri-natal mortality occur more frequently. The need for operative delivery is usually increased. There is often difficulty is establishing breast feeding in the puerper-ium.

THE INFLUENCE OF PARITY

Primigravidity

Primigravidas are a group at risk. Their capacity for childbearing has never previously been put to the test. They cannot be relied upon to run 'true to form'. In 1959 the Cranbrook Committee made it clear that 70% of all confinements should take place in hospital and that all primigravidas should be included in this proportion. The perinatal surveys of 1958 (Perinatal Mortality, published 1963; and Perinatal Problems, published 1969) both reaffirmed that primigravidity was itself a risk, and that hazards were increased as social class diminished and/or patient's age increased. In 1962 the Royal College of Obstetricians and Gynaecologists recommended that no primigravida should be booked for a General Practitioner (GP) maternity unit who was over the age of 30 years, below 5 ft tall, or who had any obvious medical problem such as obesity, essential hypertension, infertility, cephalo-pelvic disproportion, or pre-existing disease. Fetal malpresentation, or the development of raised blood pressure during pregnancy, and any complications such as antepartum haemorrhage, or obstetric problems like hydramnios, multiple pregnancy and even non-engagement of the fetal head near term, were also contraindications to confinement outside a hospital. Hobbs and Acheson (1966) expressed the view that whereas the perinatal mortality rate in mothers booked for GP care was equal to that in mothers booked for consultant care, the evidence also revealed a selection of unfavourable cases among primigravidas for consultant care. This finding, together with the very high rate of emergency transfer to consultant care of women booked for GP care, suggested that primigravidas should be cared for in fully equipped obstetric units. A review by Cooper (1969) reaffirmed the findings of the earlier perinatal mortality survey, namely, that of the primigravid patients originally booked for GP care, one in four were subsequently transferred as emergencies to hospital. He also pointed out that the standard of obstetric care today cannot be satisfactorily measured by perinatal and maternal mortality rates alone. Morbidity, if it can be evaluated, is probably a better index of the standard of care. Certainly, any hospital in which regular meetings are held to study the obstetric care of babies with a low Apgar score at birth, will recognize that for every stillbirth or neonatal death which occurs, there are many near deaths occurring. This is especially true in first births.

Primigravidity is associated with an increased incidence of pre-eclamptic toxaemia, suspected cephalo-pelvic disproportion, apparent prolongation of pregnancy, prolonged labour, forceps delivery (to expedite the second stage of labour or to correct a malposition of the fetal head), and difficulty with baby management during the first week of life. For these, and other less significant reasons, most consultant obstetricians share the view that all primigravidas should be booked for hospital confinement, and delivered in a correctly equipped hospital unit.

Multiparity

In terms of the minimal risk concept, the safest babies to have are the second, third and fourth. The hazards are greater for women in their fifth pregnancy.

The term 'grande multipara' has frequently been used to identify women of high parity. It is not a particularly good term in the author's view though, by common usage, it will probably be retained.

Cluster analysis of multiparity reveals a close association between five children or more, a maternal age in excess of thirty-five, maternal obesity, a low socio-economic status of the mother, an increased incidence of minor obstetric problems, e.g. iron deficiency anaemia, bad teeth, varicose veins, haemorrhoids, lumbar lordosis, and backache with or without spondylolisthesis. Naturally, these associations are not invariable. With modern family planning and good antenatal care amongst women who choose to have larger families complications are less now than they used to be.

Significant problems which are seen quite frequently amongst high parity groups include an increased incidence of multiple pregnancy, placenta praevia, and fetal malpresentation. Unstable lie is a particularly common hazard. The risk of minor cephalo-pelvic disproportion increases with multiparity not only because of spondylolisthesis, but also because babies tend to increase in size with subsequent pregnancies. The uterus of the multiparous woman, when faced with even minor degrees of cephalo-pelvic disproportion, has the tendency to increase its action and rupture. Paradoxically, in the third stage of labour, the uterus tends to be inert and postpartum haemorrhage is common. It is hardly surprising that, amongst women of high parity there is an increased maternal and perinatal mortality.

Feeney and Green (1970) published an interesting report from Ireland on the problems of high parity. In their hospital they regard as a 'grande multipara' a woman who has already been delivered of seven or more babies at or past twenty-eight weeks' gestation. For the purposes of their paper they included deliveries by Caesarean section in the qualification of grande multiparity but excluded abortions, miscarriages, vesicular moles and ectopic pregnancies. Their national incidence of grande multiparity had varied during 40 years from 8 to 13% of all deliveries, with an average of 10%. At the Coombe Lying In Hospital, from 1929 to 1969 inclusive, the overall maternal mortality fell from 5.3 per 1000 to 0.8 per 1000. Nevertheless, the deaths amongst grande multipara, when expressed as a percentage of all deaths, was never less that 22% and sometimes as high as 40%. Emphasized amongst the features of management of patients of high multiparity are the need for improvement in the socio-economic state of the less privileged. The importance of income, housing, employment, home help, medical and nursing services, education and family planning are also stressed. The individual care of the patient necessitates that she be delivered in a maternity hospital, with mobilization, where possible, of the various voluntary services to assist with problems at home. Defaulters at the antenatal clinic should be reviewed regularly, and communications between practitioners, midwives and consultants must be impeccable to avoid the errors of split responsibility. Clinics for the special care of varicose veins are recommended, as is attention to general hygiene, especially the care of teeth, breasts, bowels, nutrition and general cleanliness. Sympathetic attention to the minor disorders of pregnancy, which may include constipation, heartburn, insomnia and depression are greatly appreciated by the patient. Rest in hospital from the 37th week of gestation may be particularly welcomed by the harassed mother. Naturally, the supervision in labour, especially monitoring of the maternal and fetal condition, must be continuous. These patients are 'at risk'. Active management is mandatory, but this rarely necessitates the use of oxytocic stimulation.

Postnatally, the opportunity to discuss family planning or even sterilization, is usually welcomed by multiparous women. When the decision has been made, sterilization should be undertaken expeditiously. Discussion with both the husband and wife during the antenatal period may facilitate either a vasectomy during the remaining months of pregnancy, or a tubal occlusion procedure in the early puerperium.

THE INFLUENCE OF MATERNAL WEIGHT

Between successive pregnancies the maternal weight lost by multiparous women diminishes progressively until, after the fourth pregnancy, the postnatal weight usually exceeds the weight at the 20th week of gestation. The biggest increment in weight occurs, usually, in the interval between the end of the first pregnancy and the 20th week of the second. This is especially noticeable in obese multiparae (Beazley & Swinhoe 1979).

UNDERWEIGHT

Pregnancy in the underweight woman i.e. who is 10% or more below the standard weight for height before pregnancy, is associated with an increased risk of complications for both the mother and baby (*Brit.*

med. J. 1980b). These include an increased incidence of prematurity, with subsequent delay in neurological development and inadequate growth. The mothers exhibit an increased incidence of anaemia, but are less prone to develop pre-eclampsia. Antenatal care of such patients should attend particularly to any smoking habits or chronic infection which may be associated with poor nutritional status.

OVERWEIGHT

Fat women are an obstetric hazard. To quibble about who is fat and who is not is unhelpful. There are multiple criteria of obesity—fashionable, social, functional, etc. For practical purposes it is useful to keep in the antenatal clinic acceptable statistical tables which indicate the weight range, within or above which a women of medium frame and given height may be considered to be obese. Such tables provide a useful criterion for comparison. The tables used in my own clinic are based on the idea that obesity is weight which, at the beginning of pregnancy, is 20% in excess of an ideal.

As pregnancy itself has been shown to be a direct cause of obesity (Sheldon 1949) it is not surprising that fat women attending the antenatal clinic are often multiparous. In the presence of obesity a clinical diagnosis of pregnancy is sometimes difficult to make. As the pregnancy proceeds it may be equally difficult to evaluate the size of the fetus, to determine the presenting fetal part, to detect the fetal heart, or recognize the presence or absence of hydramnios. In later pregnancy, wherever there is doubt about the normality or presentation of the fetus, an abdominal X-ray can be invaluable in obese women. Because latent diabetes tends to be associated with both obesity and increasing age, the fat multiparous patient should be suspected of having a baby of larger than average size.

Cephalo-pelvic relationships are difficult to estimate, with any clinical accuracy, when patients are fat. In practice, cephalo-pelvic disproportion is relatively uncommon in obese women. Nevertheless the potential risk is always present particularly as multiparity, and the increased lordosis caused by obesity, are both predeterminants of spondylolisthesis.

Maternal blood pressure is difficult to determine when the upper arm is fat. When the circumference of the upper arm is gross it is sometimes advocated that a correction be made to the systolic and diastolic values recorded (*Lancet* 1966). This is rarely necessary in obstetric practice where changes in the blood pressure are of more significance than the precise value of the systolic and diastolic measurements.

Because antenatal diagnosis is often difficult, induction of labour sometimes has to be considered in obese women on the grounds of suspected pre-eclampsia, suspected prolonged pregnancy, or suspected latent diabetes. It can be mechanically difficult to establish an intravenous infusion in a fat limb. Also, it is difficult to appreciate if the infusion needle has escaped from the vein, or if fluid is running into the maternal tissues. There are difficulties too in monitoring maternal and fetal well-being.

Fortunately, most obese patients make good progress in labour. Usually they deliver spontaneously. If Caesarean section is necessary, and there is a natural hesitancy to operate on obese patients, the hazards of both surgery and anaesthesia are increased. In the fat abdomen a transverse incision is often more useful than a longitudinal incision. The incision should not, however, be made in the abdominal skin crease above the symphysis pubis. Depending upon the site of the abdominal wound, there may be delayed healing due to haematoma formation or sweating. During the puerperium there is an increased risk of deep vein thrombosis.

Direct management of obesity during pregnancy, specific dieting, does not significantly alter the hazards of antenatal care and parturition. Moreover, in a report by Blumenthal (1976) it is suggested that dietary restriction of women with excessive weight gain during pregnancy probably impairs fetal growth and results in a persistent height and weight deficit in the child. Thus, an attempt to control or reduce the patient's weight is best made between pregnancies.

THE INFLUENCE OF THE TIME OF ONSET

The early onset of labour

'Term' is now defined as the interval from 37 to less than 42 completed weeks. The word is often confused with the calculated date of confinement. 'Preterm' is less than 37 completed weeks. The lower limit is still undecided, but in practice what matters is whether or not the child is viable. The infant weighing less than 2.5 kg should be termed 'low birth weight' rather than 'premature'. Less than 1.5 kg is 'very low birth weight', and less than 1 kg, 'extremely low birth weight'. 'Dysmaturity' signifies an infant whose weight is less than the 10th centile for its gestational age. 'Light for dates' is an alternative term.

The 50th percentile of birth weight uncorrected for sex or maternal parity is 2.3 kg at the onset of the 36th week of gestation, and 2.5 kg at the end of it. In general it is acknowledged that babies weighing less than 2.5 kg who are born preterm are 'at risk', but the hazards relate very much to where the child is born. Concepts about the risks of preterm labour, whether spontaneous or induced, are continually being modified. Today, in a good perinatal unit, the uncorrected survival figures are expected to be 100% at 2001 gm or above, and about 90–100% between 1501–2000 gm, 75–85% between 1101 and 1500 gm, and 50–70% between 751–1000 gm. Fetal handicap is therefore a more important index now of improved care.

The very important improvements in paediatric expertise have significantly altered obstetric views about when preterm labour should be stopped. Any child suffering from growth retardation who is 34 weeks old or more or weighs more than 2 kg is now more likely to benefit from expert care in a special care baby unit than from continued existence *in utero*. *In utero* transfer is better than transfer after delivery.

There are other groups of patients for whom pharmacological treatment of spontaneous preterm labour is best avoided. Zlatnik (1927) lists amongst the reasons for not postponing delivery the following conditions: an estimated fetal weight greater than 2.5 kg, rupture of the membranes, multiple gestation, third trimester bleeding, intrauterine growth retardation, Rhesus isoimmunization.

Caution must be exercised to avoid maternal pulmonary hypertension, which can occur quite acutely when corticosteroids are combined with beta-sympathomimetics in treatment of preterm labour. The symptoms of pulmonary oedema may not become clinically manifest until 12 hours after treatment ceases.

In most units today steroids are advocated only if they can be given more than 24 hours before delivery, if the gestation interval is less than 34 weeks, and if the membranes are intact. After consultation with the paediatrician, it may be wise in some patients to delay labour for 24 hours in order to employ corticosteroids, but this is unusual. More commonly, they are given prior to the induction of premature labour.

When unavoidable premature labour is anticipated, features of management include the sparing use of analgesic drugs. Morphine is now considered to be inappropriate therapy. Premature labour often proceeds much more quickly than expected and maternal morphine administration within 6–7 hours of birth may well depress fetal respiration severely. Moderate doses of pethidine are preferable. When the facilities are available, epidural analgesia may be desirable. The delivery itself requires careful consideration. For the preterm child delivered vaginally the author favours the use of an episiotomy and obstetric forceps to avoid sudden changes in the skull shape and to control the rate of delivery of the fetal head. He accepts there is little hard data to support this view. Nevertheless, it seems sensible to him to use forceps to *reduce* the speed of delivery of a small fetal head when there is otherwise a danger of an uncontrolled expulsion. Traction is rarely required.

Some very low birth weight infants are perhaps better delivered by Caesarean section, but it is by no means certain this improves their chances and it certainly compromises the uterus, the lower segment of which is often barely formed at the time of surgery (Beazley & Lobb 1983).

It is well established that the effect of adrenaline upon myometrial activity is to promote relaxation. During the last ten years a number of other pharmacological agents have been investigated which also produce a sympathomimetic action upon the contracting uterus. These preparations are chiefly stimulators of beta receptors in the uterus, e.g. isoxsuprine hydrochloride, orciprenaline, ritodrine hydrochloride and salbutamol. There is little evidence to support that they significantly reduce perinatal mortality. Nor do they significantly reduce the incidence of preterm birth, though they may well delay it for 72 hours or more.

Fuchs (1967) described the use of ethyl alcohol in the treatment of premature labour. Ethyl alcohol is believed to act centrally by inhibiting the release of oxytocin from the pituitary. The alcohol (9.5% alcohol in 5% dextrose) is infused intravenously in sufficient quantity to increase the blood alcohol concentration to 80 mg per 100 ml. (A simple and useful measure of this critical level can first be achieved with the help of the normal 'breathalyser' used by the police!) Blood concentrations of alcohol in excess of 100 mg per 100 ml promote significant inebriation.

Isoxsuprine therapy begins with an initial infusion rate of 0.2 mg per minute, increasing gradually to 0.8 mg per minute. The limiting factor to treatment is chiefly in hypotension when possible treatment is continued until contractions are controlled. Thereafter it is usual practice to give intramuscular injections, or, more commonly, oral isoxsuprine, from about the 3rd day, in doses of 10 mg 4-hourly.

Treatment of premature labour with orciprenaline has been described by Baillie *et al.* (1970) and Tyack *et al.* (1971). The effective dose varies between 10 and 20 μg per minute, and the inhibition of uterine contractility is dose dependent. Treatment promotes maternal tachycardia and a slight increase in the fetal heart rate. Accordingly, only 20 minute infusion periods were used in some studies, though later reports suggested these could be extended.

Treatment with ritodrine by intravenous infusion for 24–28 hours, followed by oral administration for 5–7 days, has been described by Wesselius-de Casparis *et al.* (1971). The drug is used now quite frequently in clinical practice, though its efficacy appears to remain unverified by controlled clinical trials (Hemminki & Starfield 1978, O'Connor *et al.* 1979). Furthermore, there have been disturbing reports of pulmonary oedema in mothers following its use in conjunction with betamethasone to suppress premature labour (Elliott *et al.* 1978, Tinga & Aarnoudse 1979), and one of ritodrine-induced acidosis in pregnancy (Desir *et al.* 1978).

A report by Liggins and Vaughan (1973) on the use of salbutamol, suggests that this drug is a safe and effective means of inhibiting uterine contractions for limited periods of time. In 15% of the patients studied, salbutamol failed to delay delivery for at least 24 hours. In these women the maternal pulse rate increased to 140 beats per minute before incomplete inhibition of uterine activity occurred, and treatment was stopped.

Salbutamol, diluted in 5% dextrose solution to a concentration of 25 mg per 500 ml, was infused continously into a forearm vein. The initial dose was 1.8 μg/min. At 5-minute intervals the dose was increased by 50% until a rate of 43 μg/min was reached. If uterine activity ceased prior to this infusion rate or the maternal pulse rate increased to 140/min, further increments of salbutamol were withheld.

These authors suggest that in contrast to other uterine inhibitors salbutamol was reasonably effective in the presence of ruptured membranes and was also successful in two-thirds of patients in whom the cervix was more than 3 cm dilated. It is their impression that salbutamol is more effective and better tolerated than ethyl alcohol, and that it is probably at least five times more potent than ritodrine.

A comparison of salbutamol and ethanol in the treatment of preterm labour, by Sims *et al* (1978) revealed no statistically significant differences between their efficacy, and although salbutamol acted more rapidly, it also produced more cardiovascular side effects.

The use of prostaglandin inhibitors to suppress premature labour is not advised at present. Indomethacin, for example, has been implicated in intrauterine closure of the fetal ductus arteriosus (Goudie & Dossetor 1979, *Lancet* 1980).

The late onset of labour

When the date of confinement is calculated in the normal manner, it is found that only about 4% of patients deliver on the expected day. Park (1968), studying the time of delivery of 2100 patients whose confinement date was known with reasonable accuracy, showed that, in 68% of these women, spontaneous parturition occurred after the calculated date, and only in 32% before the calculated date. When considered in relation to the calculated date of confinement, prolonged pregnancy is a common occurrence.

Pregnancies continuing beyond the end of the 42nd week of gestation are described as 'postterm'. Prior to that time the hazards of intrauterine anoxia are minimal, and the features by which paediatricians recognize 'fetal postmaturity' are rarely seen. Thus, when the date of confinement can be calculated accurately, or may be accurately known by ultrasound, when the antenatal history is uncomplicated, when, statistically, the patient falls into a low-risk category, it is reasonable to wait until the end of the 42nd week of gestation for parturition to begin spontaneously. Labour occurring up to this time should be conducted actively in the usual manner. If pregnancy is not of the low-risk type, to induce labour about term is better than to wait until the end of the 42nd week.

Homburg *et al.* (1979) who argue against the concept of routine induction of labour at an agreed gestational age, devised a scheme for monitoring pregnancy by amioscopy or amniotomy, (to detect meconium), oxytocin challenge tests, 24 hour urinary oestriol estimations and fetal movement counts. Of 50 patients with normal tests, 49 had uneventful labours. In 47 other patients, the colour of the amniotic fluid and the result of the oxytocin challenge test proved most helpful. In England liquor estimation is uncommon now, and oestradiol estimations and fetal movement counts have proved much less reliable than originally anticipated. Greater reliance is placed on antenatal cardiotocography.

Two studies, by Noble (1981) and Gibb *et al.*

(1982), appear to present conflicting views on the management of postterm labour. In a series of 2000 patients, 350 had labour routinely induced at 41 weeks (by ultrasound) with prostaglandin E2 vaginal pessaries, followed a day later by low amniotomy in 40%. Noble reports that the incidence of Caesarean section in these 350 patients was 5.7% and none for failed induction. Perinatal death, respiratory distress syndrome, and neonatal jaundice proved to be no problem. It seems that the essence of these good results rests upon accurate ultrasound diagnosis, and the avoidance of potential problems associated with 42 weeks' gestation.

The study by Gibb *et al.* (1982) was controlled but not randomized. 'Certain postmaturity' was diagnosed in 4% of 2000 patients, and in 30 of these 81 women labour was induced. Thrice-weekly antenatal cardiotocography was performed in the other 51 until labour began spontaneously in them all by 44 weeks. There were no perinatal deaths. However after inducing labour more babies were delivered with low Apgar scores at one minute, and significantly more mothers were delivered by Caesarean section. When 'postmaturity' was 'uncertain' these differences were even more noticeable. Gibb and co-workers conclude, therefore, that there is no case for induction of labour in uncomplicated prolonged pregnancy (Cardozo *et al.* 1983).

The conservative management of prolonged pregnancy using antenatal cardiotocography is also advocated by Cairo (1984) who reports a prospective study of 80 patients with prolonged pregnancy. Tests were introduced at term plus 14 days and performed thrice weekly. Nine patients (11.2%) required Caesarean section, five for fetal distress, two for failure to progress in labour, and two for a positive stress test.

In the absence of any detectable abnormality by antenatal cardiotocography it is the practice on our own unit to initiate labour artificially at about 10 days postterm when this is reliably known. It has been our experience that this approach is not attended by problems where controlled parturition policies are sensibly employed. Also it has seemed better to act before the onset of intrauterine anoxia than to await signs of deterioration in the fetal heart tracings.

THE INFLUENCE OF THE RATE OF PROGRESS

Slow labour

No one can treat prolonged labour. Prolonged labour is not a diagnosis, it is an abnormality which may be

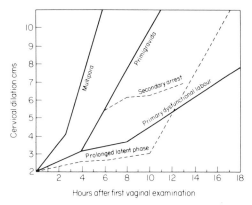

Fig. 25.1. Partographic analysis of prolonged labour (after Studd 1975).

detected during parturition, and for which a cause must be found by examining the patient clinically.

Jeffcoate (1961) described the important factors commonly associated with prolonged labour at that time. Developments which have since altered the approach to the problem include a further consideration of uterine action, the administration of oxytocics and methods of fetal and maternal monitoring.

Prolonged labour necessitates careful evaluation of at least five important features, namely, an evaluation of the powers (both voluntary and involuntary), the passages (both hard and soft), the passengers (mainly the fetus, but also the placenta, membranes and liquor amnii), and the state of the maternal and fetal conditions. In Chapter 26 problems are considered in which the passages or passenger may be chiefly responsible for prolonged labour. In this chapter emphasis is placed on inefficient uterine action.

The partographic analysis of labour now facilitates the early detection of prolonged labour. Moreover as Studd (1975) has shown, the form taken by the partograph in prolonged labour will distinguish between secondary arrest, primary dysfunctional labour, and a prolonged latent phase of labour (Fig 25.1). Inasmuch as this broad distinction may suggest to the accoucheur the most likely cause of the problem, partographs facilitate diagnosis.

In former years attempts were made to distinguish inefficient uterine action into a hypo- and hypertonic type, both of which affected the uterus generally. A variety of localized, incoordinate types of uterine action were also described which resulted in conditions such as reversed uterine polarity and constriction ring. The present trend is not to distinguish between such varieties of uterine activity, but to speak of them collectively under the general term of 'inefficient uterine action'.

Emphasis in the management of prolonged labour has changed during recent years from hastening delivery in the second stage to accelerating labour during the first stage. Naturally obstetricians are still required to be skilled in the use of forceps and the ventouse (Chapter 30). Nevertheless, whenever augmentation is feasible, the correction of delay by propulsion rather than by traction is favoured.

It is now widely accepted that in the absence of efficient uterine activity, problems like malposition disproportion cannot be truly assessed. Thus, whenever it can be shown that prolonged labour is associated with inefficient uterine action, the present trend, in primigravid patients, is to correct this inadequacy first, by the judicious use of oxytocics; details of administration are given later in this chapter (p. 367). If, by that means, the normal rate of labour cannot be restored, attention is again given to possible remaining causes. In practice, it is surprising how often correction of inefficient uterine action resolves the situation satisfactorily.

Conditions which respond particularly well to oxytocic augmentation of existing uterine contractions include, in primigravida, prolonged 'latent phase' of labour, and secondary arrest of uterine activity occasioned by fetal occipitoposterior position. In multiparous women, great care must be taken before augmenting uterine action with oxytocics. In multiparas it is much less likely that inefficient uterine action is the cause of prolonged labour. Because there is a grave risk of causing uterine rupture in multiparas by the injudicious use of oxytocics, detailed consideration of both maternal passages and the passenger are always necessary before administration.

The idea of labour progressing for longer than 12 hours is now virtually unthinkable. Prolonged labour cannot only be detected early but the methods used to correct it can be monitored partographically to ensure that they are effective (Fig. 25.2). When methods of correction fail, early recourse to Caesarean section is usually advised.

The manner in which corrective measures operate is of considerable importance. The purpose of augmentation is not solely to promote an increased rate of labour, but to do so in an acceptable manner. For example, during augmentation, intrauterine pressure should be monitored to ensure that adequate myometrial relaxation is occurring between contractions. If the resting uterine tone is increased to an undesirable level by the oxytocics, or, perhaps, they promote

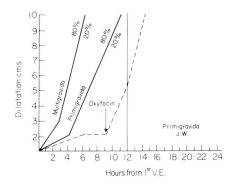

Fig. 25.2. Monitoring the effect of oxytocin administration.

contractions which are too frequent or too prolonged, the complications of management will soon outweigh the advantages of acceleration. It is also clear, from the work of Steer *et al.* (1975), that to continue to increase oxytocin stimulation of the inefficient uterus, once stable uterine activity has been achieved is both useless and dangerous.

Fetal scalp blood sampling and/or continuous fetal heart monitoring, should be undertaken regularly whenever augmentation of uterine action is used. The measurements obtained may indicate the need to reduce the rate of infusion. Alterations in the pattern of the fetal heart rate can, of course, be produced simply by pressure of the uterus upon the maternal vena cava. This is likely to happen when the patient is nursed in the supine position. Thus, when labour is prolonged, and particularly if epidural analgesia has been used as part of the management, it is important to nurse the patient in a more lateral position. A left lateral tilt of about 15 degrees is usually sufficient to prevent caval compression. If, despite these measures prolonged labour continues or fetal distress supervenes, Caesarean section is advocated, and it is important that the patient is transferred to theatre, and operated upon, with the lateral tilt maintained.

Amniotomy has traditionally been accepted as an important surgical method of hastening labour. Certainly it is a useful adjunct to oxytocic stimulation of uterine activity. Recent studies in this department have shown, however, that in normal labour, amniotomy alone improves uterine activity in only about 50% of primigravid women, whereas, in multiparous women, it results in some acceleration of labour in more than 80%. No direct correlation can be made between the use of amniotomy in normal labour and prolonged labour, but this result lends support to the idea that, in primigravida, amniotomy should always

be utilized with concomitant uterine stimulation, whereas, in multipara, if amniotomy fails to promote acceleration, oxytocics should be utilized only with great care.

Vibratory techniques to dilate the uterine cervix have been described by Tokuyama and Fujimoto (1968) and Dahlgren (1972) and Brandt and Lachelin (1974). More recent preliminary investigations, in which a vibrator with a frequency range from 73–102 Hertz, driven by a variable speed 60-watt electric motor, and utilizing a metal spatula 3 cm broad which is introduced into the cervix, has been described by Alderman (1975). He comments that the technique is simple enough to be clinically attractive and is acceptable to the patient. Its efficacy however is dependent upon the fetal head being continually applied to the cervix after vibration has increased the dilatation of the os.

Cervical vibration may confidently be expected to result in cervical dilatation to an extent that could not be achieved by any other method in the same amount of time. In a small number of suitable patients, therefore, it may form a useful alternative to Caesarean section.

Rapid labour

Labour that occurs extremely rapidly, especially if it also occurs unexpectedly, can result in a child being born prior to arrival at hospital. Sometimes precipitate labour occurs at home. If the labour is unattended, it may be associated with postpartum haemorrhage, maternal injuries such as third degree perineal tears, or even uterine inversion (cf. Chapter 29). The baby too may be damaged, either by rapid passage through the birth canal, or because it drops unattended to the floor, or sometimes into the toilet! Fortunately, such disasters are rare.

In a paper by Hughes and Hamlett (1975), rapid labour is defined as labour in which the first and second stages together last two hours or less. The onset of painful uterine contractions was taken as a cardinal feature of the establishment of labour. Among 17031 patients who were delivered at Mill Road Maternity Hospital between 1967 and 1971, rapid labour occured in 4.3%. During this interval, mainly as a result of rapid deliveries following induction of labour, the incidence of rapid labour increased from 3.8 to 6.8% per annum. A careful review of complications, including second or third degree lacerations of the perineum, postpartum haemorrhage, cervical lacerations, fetal morbidity, perinatal and neonatal mortality, revealed that there was no significant maternal or fetal risk from rapid labour, so long as it occurred in a fully equipped obstetric unit with patients under close supervision.

Rapid labour is a most unusual occurrence in a first labour. Multiparous women, whose history suggests a previous rapid labour, should be admitted to hospital towards term to await the onset of spontaneous parturition. Iatrogenic rapid labour, caused by the over-enthusiastic use of active management, must be avoided.

INDUCTION OF LABOUR

Planned delivery

'Planned delivery' signifies the induction of parturition, as an elective procedure, at a predetermined time. In contrast to some American literature, the term 'elective' is not intended here to mean 'socially indicated'.

The safety and reliability of induction of labour has greatly increased in recent years. The incidence of planned delivery also increased for a time but has now declined.

In recent years the major fetal and maternal indications for induction of labour have not altered greatly. They still include pre-eclampsia and hypertension, dysmaturity, Rhesus incompatibility, diabetes mellitus, prolonged pregnancy, gross fetal abnormality, antepartum haemorrhage, and sometimes fetal death *in utero*. In addition, however, induction of labour is often performed now for cumulative indications, any of which, if considered in isolation, would probably constitute an insufficient reason, e.g. increasing maternal age, previous infertility, poor obstetric history, etc.

The concept of minimal risk labour has also influenced the approach to labour induction. If it can be shown, for example, that it is in the patient's best interests to deliver her baby when all the facilities of an intensive care unit are available, delivery must be planned in advance, with due regard to the workload on obstetric, anaesthetic, paediatric, and labour room personnel, labour room beds and hospital services. Because planned delivery facilitates a predictable workload, it tends to improve obstetric efficiency. This, in turn, improves the quality of patient care.

Factors influencing induction of labour

The expected date of confinement may be unknown. In approximately 22% of patients attending antenatal clinics it is impossible to calculate the expected date of confinement by the traditional method. The patient may be uncertain when her last menstrual period began, or her menstrual cycle may be prolonged and irregular. Sometimes conception occurs before menstruation, or late in the puerperium, or during the months of breast feeding.

Clinical assessment of the uterine size is an unreliable method of determining fetal maturity. Ultrasound assessment is more accurate. Towards term radiological assessment of fetal maturity may be of value but is now rarely required. Cytological examination of the liquor, or biochemical assay of its constituents are now largely outmoded.

The gestational age of the fetus is of less concern to the obstetrician than the functional maturity of the baby's lungs. In normal pregnancy the concentration of lecithin (a surfactant within the alveoli of the newborn lung) increases to 8.8 ± 3.0 mg per 100 ml about term. When the ratio of lecithin to sphingomyelin (another surface active phospholipid within the fetal lung) exceeds two, respiratory distress syndrome is unlikely to occur.

A simple 'bubble test' to assess lecithin/sphingomyelin ratio depends upon the ability of lung surfactants to generate a stable foam in the presence of ethanol. When a complete ring of bubbles persists for 15 minutes around the meniscus of liquor in a test tube at a dilution of 1 in 2 the bubble test is regarded as positive (i.e. 'safe'). As this test takes 20 minutes only it has a significant practical advantage over more complicated chemical analyses.

False-negative values are rather common with the bubble test (i.e. a negative result is obtained even though the fetal lung is functionally mature). Liquor contamination, with blood or meconium, makes the test unreliable.

With the dramatic improvements which have occurred in recent years in obstetric assessment of fetal maturity and paediatric care of the immature or small baby, the use of tests to assess lung maturity have diminished.

THE STATE OF THE CERVIX

There is little doubt that a 'ripe' cervix usually indicates labour may be induced without undue difficulty. Regrettably, the converse is not true. Despite the presence of an 'unripe' cervix labour can often be induced with comparative ease by modern methods.

Beazley and Alderman (1976), using a standard induction regimen, described a graph (the 'Inductograph') which defines the rate of progress of the latent phase of labour in 80% of a group of patients selected from a 'low risk' category. Progress is measured clinically by changes in the cervix, evaluated by a modified Bishop scoring system. The graph facilitates early detection of delay in augmented labour (Beazley 1977). Even more precise control of parturition has recently been achieved by combining the inductograph with a plot of uterine activity (Gee & Beazley 1980). These graphs together make it clear that delayed progress may be associated with optimal, inefficient, or sometimes excessive uterine activity, and the patterns described facilitate early recognition and management of such clinical problems as cephalo-pelvic disproportion, undue cervical resistance, inadequate myometrial activity, and impending fetal distress.

The application of real time microcomputer monitoring to the surveillance of induced labour by uterine activity quantitation (Tromans & Beazley 1983) also makes it clear that additional problems which can be readily detected include excessive uterine sensitivity to oxytocin in early labour following the pre-induction use of prostaglandins to ripen the cervix. The increase in uterine activity which attends unexpected cephalo-pelvic disproportion, especially in the late first and the second stage of labour is also readily detected.

In recent years ripening the unfavourable cervix by the use of local prostaglandins has received a good deal of attention (Gordon & Calder 1983, Read & Mattock 1982, Quinn et al. 1981, Stewart et al. 1981). A comparative study in Liverpool of the efficacy of both PGE$_2$ (4 mg) and oestradiol (150 mg) applied locally to the cervix, reveals no significant differences with regard to the efficacy of the two substances, but prostaglandins appear to achieve their effect by stimulating significant uterine activity, whereas oestrogens appear to ripen the cervix chiefly by softening it (Tromans et al. 1981, Jagani et al. 1982, Stewart et al. 1981). The use of prostaglandins may promote fetal distress and even fetal death (Quinn & Murphy 1981) particularly in the presence of intrauterine growth retardation, and the investigators recommend fetal monitoring whenever prostaglandins are used.

Preparation for induction

Labour suites which have adopted the principles of intensive care during labour usually favour the insertion of epidural catheters in the morning, prior to amniotomy and the establishment of an intravenous infusion. Patients also welcome this order of events as it avoids the need for inserting the catheter after labour has commenced, when the patient already has discomfort, and an intravenous infusion is attached to her arm.

To facilitate engagement of the fetal head, and also to safeguard against undue soiling of the perineum during delivery, a small and gentle enema prior to the induction of labour can sometimes benefit the patient. Usually this treatment is unnecessary.

The techniques of induction

Traditionally, the surgical and medical methods of inducing labour are considered separately. In modern practice this division is somewhat artificial. There is now an abundance of literature which confirms that amniotomy or oxytocics alone can induce labour satisfactorily when conditions are optimal. Unless methods are used in combination, the duration of labour remains uncertain.

At term, when the cervix is 'ripe', 70–80% of patients will go into labour with amniotomy alone. Only about 35% of these patients will deliver in less than 12 hours. A further 30% will continue to labour for more than 24 hours even if an oxytocic is added to the regime after the first 12 hours. Oxytocin alone, if used in accordance with modern regimes can be equally effective. Thus, with doses of oxytocin ranging from 2–64 milliunits per minute, 70% of patients will deliver in less than 12 hours when all conditions are favourable.

The method of oxytocin administration may significantly influence the success of the induction regime. If it is assumed that the sensitivity of the uterine myometrium determines the success of induction procedures, it follows that the first important principle of oxytocin administration is to discover the dose which will initiate effective uterine contractions. The modern techniques by which this is achieved involve increasing the rate of oxytocin infusion incrementally at intervals of 15–20 minutes. If, therefore, for safety's sake, the infusion is commenced at 1 milliunit per minute and doubled every 20 minutes, the patient will be receiving oxytocin at the rate of 32 milliunits per minute after 2 hours. In most women labour has already commenced by the time they are receiving 16 milliunits per minute. Monitoring of uterine contractions, or frequent examination of the cervix in the early part of labour, is a helpful guide to management. Only occasionally is it necessary to exceed a dose of 16 milliunits per minute, and doses of 32 or 64 milliunits per minute should not be utilized without accurate quantitation of uterine activity.

A second method of labour induction involves oxytocin titration. With the help of an automatic infusion pump (e.g. Cardiff infusion system Mark III) a very smooth dose increase of oxytocin is achieved. The infusion concentration recommended is 10 units of oxytocin in 500 ml of 5% dextrose or 0.9% saline. The infusion range is from 1 milliunit to 32 milliunits per minute. The dose rate is doubled every 12.5 minutes and an effective dose of oxytocin is achieved quickly. The rate of infusion may be controlled by intrauterine pressure, which can be measured via an intra-amniotic catheter. When the intrauterine pressure exceeds or falls below a predetermined level the infusion stops.

A full review of the advantages and disadvantages of the modern techniques of induction of labour is provided by Clarke (1975). In Liverpool we favour the incremental method of oxytocin administration and prefer to use infusion pumps rather than automated titration methods or 'gravity feed' intravenous drips. We consider that the induction of labour frequently requires a high concentration of oxytocin, and should be differentiated from the maintenance of labour, which requires no more than 7 milliunits per minute. In practice, this means that once labour has progressed to the stage of 5 cm dilatation of the cervix, infusion rates in excess of 7 milliunits per minute should be reduced to that dose or even less (Beazley et al. 1975).

The administration of oxytocin by the intranasal and oral routes have been reported in the literature. Within the modern concept of the active management of labour these routes offer less accurate control than intravenous infusion. It would also appear that whatever advantage may be gained by the ease of administration, the lack of predictability with regard to absorption and control remains a serious disadvantage of these routes. If the cervix is unfavourable at the onset of labour, the disadvantages are especially important.

PROSTAGLANDINS

It is now well established that both PGE_2 and $PGF_2\alpha$ can induce labour by the intravenous route. Numerous reports have compared the efficacy of protaglandins with that of oxytocin. When administered in equally effective doses, and in comparable clinical situations, both drugs appear to be equally efficient

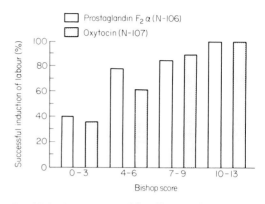

Fig. 25.3. A comparison of the efficiency of axytocin and $PGF_{2\alpha}$ in clinical situations of comparable difficulty (from Spellacy et al. (1973) Obstetrics and Gynaecology, **41**, 14).

for the induction of labour (Fig. 25.3). At present, for the routine induction of labour, there is little reason to justify a change from intravenous oxytocin, the efficacy and safety of which are well known.

In selected patients, especially multiparas in whom the conditions for induction of labour are favourable, oral prostaglandins are strongly recommended by some clinicians. As a routine method of inducing labour, oral prostaglandins are not favoured. Certainly, they can have unpleasant side-effects on the gastrointestinal tract.

Prostaglandins, particularly those of the E group, can be used in small quantities to increase the sensitivity of the myometrium to the effects of oxytocin administered either at the same time (potentiation) or afterwards (enhancement). The possibility of utilizing prostaglandins in this way, to minimize the dose of oxytocin necessary to induce labour is readily appreciated by those who employ prostaglandin pessaries to ripen the cervix. There is also the danger of initiating unduly strong contractions with oxytocin, unexpectedly, after initial treatment with prostaglandin E_2. Prostaglandins may be used to obviate the neonatal hyperbilirubinaemia which can be associated with a maternal oxytocin infusion of more than 20 units (Beazley & Alderman 1975, Friedman et al. 1978). According to Buchan (1979) it is the vasopressin-like activity of oxytocin that causes osmotic swelling of erythrocytes, leading to decreased deformability and more rapid destruction, with resultant hyperbilirubinaemia in the neonate. Neonatal hyperbilirubinaemia does not appear to be associated with the use of prostaglandin E_2 (Beazley & Weekes 1976, Chew 1977).

CHOICE OF METHOD

When the conditions for induction of labour are favourable, almost any of the accepted methods of induction will prove successful. Induction of labour is probably best undertaken, however, in controlled circumstances and after adequate preparation of the patient. Low amniotomy facilitates detection of any prolapse of the fetal cord and permits the liquor to be examined for the presence of meconium. Oxytocin infusion, following immediately upon low amniotomy, offers the best chance of success in most instances. The dose, in milliunits per minute, should be administered with regard to the uterine response. Controlling the infusion rate by means of a constant infusion pump is perhaps the most efficient technique.

Prostaglandins may be the drug of choice whenever it is necessary to minimize the risk of neonatal hyperbilirubinaemia. Otherwise, prostaglandins offer no significant advantage at present over oxytocin. Their oral use can be of value in a busy unit in selected multiparous women.

LIQUOR AND MEMBRANES

The fetus lives in a private pond of amniotic fluid, the constituents of which are regularly exchanged via the membranes and uterine wall as well as by mechanisms such as fetal swallowing, urination and respiratory movements. Some of these methods are non-selective. The fetal membranes are the major route of water transfer in both directions. Liquor volume, however, may be secondary to variations in its constituents, especially proteins. The amniotic fluid volumes in normal pregnancy exhibit a wide variation, but the mean volume increases from approximately 239 ml at 15–16 weeks to 669 ml at 25–26 weeks, and 984 ml at 33–34 weeks. It then decreases slightly to 836 ml at term and 544 ml at 41–42 weeks (Queenan et al. 1972, Nelson 1972, Smith 1971).

Polyhydramnios

Polyhydramnios is usually a clinical diagnosis although today it may more reliably be diagnosed ultrasonically. It signifies an excess of liquor which is likely to influence the usual course of pregnancy. According to Scott and Wilson (1957) the clinical diagnosis should be based on observations made by independent observers on at least two occasions. This avoids the easy error of diagnosing polyhydramnios at about 32–34 weeks' gestation when the normal liquor to baby ratio is maximal. The recovery of more than 1500 ml of liquor at amniotomy is a further index of polyhydramnios, but is seldom, if ever, used now.

Excessive fluid accumulation is associated especially with barriers to fetal ingestion (e.g. anencephaly or oesophageal atresia), presumably because this interferes with absorption mechanisms. About half the cases of polyhydramnios are associated with fetal abnormality, but in the remaining cases alternative mechanisms resulting in excessive formation or deficient disposal have been invoked. In addition to the above, other associated fetal abnormalities include iniencephaly, but not usually hydrocephaly; duodenal atresia; functional obstruction of the oesophagus associated with significant deflexion of the head (Hibbard 1962); hydrops fetalis. Acute polyhydramnios can be associated with monozygous twin pregnancies (Weir et al. 1979), and with large placental chorio-angiomas. Hibbard (1962) suggests that the mechanism may be via large arterio-venous shunts causing fetal cardiac decompensation.

It is difficult to distinguish clinically between polyhydramnios and the presence of two sacs in twin pregnancy. When maternal diabetes is associated with polyhydramnios the mechanism is obscure and does not appear to be an osmotic effect of glucose excreted by the fetus into the liquor. Nor has any significant relationship been found with the hourly urine fetal production rate (Van Otterlo et al. 1977). In many instances no satisfactory cause for polyhydramnios is discovered.

The clinical problems associated with polyhydramnios apart from fetal abnormality are maternal discomfort, difficulty in examining the baby clinically, and the serious risk of premature labour associated with early spontaneous rupture of the membranes. Sudden release of liquor, accompanied by significant reduction in uterine volume may precipitate an abruption of the placenta. Should it be deemed necessary to perform amniotomy to promote labour, an attempt should be made to release liquor slowly, via a Drew–Smythe catheter, from the hindwaters. Often this intention does not succeed. Transabdominal amniotomy in an attempt to promote maternal comfort or to avoid the onset of premature labour is rarely effective for longer than a few hours. Withdrawal should be slow and no more than 500 ml over half an hour should be removed.

Oligohydramnios

It is now well recognized that oligohydramnios is associated with dysmaturity, and especially when this is associated with the abnormalities of renal agenesis or lower urinary tract obstruction (Jeffcoate & Scott 1959, Wladimiroff & Campbell 1974, Van Otterlo et al. 1977). Urinary tract dysplasia accounts for about half the cases of serious oligohydramnios. Renal agenesis is characteristically associated with the facies described by Potter; low-set ears, epicanthic folds, flattening of the nose and micrognathus. This facial appearance is not pathognomonic of renal agenesis.

The ultrasonic assessment of early pregnancy now quickly detects oligohydramnios and can assess when it is associated with absent bladder filling, or, occasionally, an abnormally large bladder due to urethral obstruction. It is sometimes advised that chromosome analysis should be obtained in such cases, but it can be difficult to obtain liquor samples, even under ultrasound control.

Amnion nodosum is a condition associated with oligohydramnios. The amnion shows areas containing small nodules, a millimetre or two in size, and yellowish in colour. They are formed by aggregations of squames in an amorphous matrix and are often seen in cases of oligohydramnios whatever the cause. Scanning electron microscopy of the amnion revealed a predominance of two of the four patterns seen in normal amnion, and intercellular canals were sparse which could limit the fluid exchange through the amnion in this condition. These changes were not discovered in the amnion from patients with polyhydramnios (Pollard et al. 1979).

Premature rupture of the membranes

The fetal membranes rupture spontaneously before labour in 6–12% of pregnancies. At term labour usually follows or is easily stimulated with oxytocin to avoid possible infection. In about 2–3% of pregnancies the membranes rupture spontaneously before 37 weeks' gestation, and its management raises difficult questions (Drife 1982).

The aetiology of the condition is largely unknown, though it may be associated with an incompetent cervix, an unstable lie, or polyhydramnios. Amnionitis is more common when membranes rupture before the onset of labour, which suggests that local infection may play a part in the aetiology, but recent work by Zaaijman et al. (1982), suggested this is unlikely. The diagnosis can be difficult when a direct view of the cervix by sterile speculum examination reveals no liquor draining through the cervical os. Alternative methods of diagnosis include amniotic fluid arborization, but false positives are common. Staining techniques with Nile Blue Sulphate, or pH tests with Nitrazine yellow, or the measurement of substances such as Diamine oxidase, or even prolactin have all been tried but are not completely successful (Friedman & McElin 1969, Elmfors et al. 1974, Koninckx et al. 1981).

The chief obstetric problems associated with this condition are intrauterine infection, premature labour, and pulmonary hypoplasia.

Fliegner et al. (1981) emphasized the association of severe pulmonary hypoplasia with oligohydramnios in infants without renal anomalies. Prolonged rupture of the membranes was the cause in 8 of 10 patients they described, and 7 of the 8 babies died of respiratory failure within 24 hours of delivery. They recommend that ultrasonic assessment of the thoracic cage volume may help to assess the prognosis before delivery.

The duration of membrane rupture does not appear to be closely associated with whether or not intrauterine infection occurs. Some patients are infected quickly, others not at all. There is only a poor correlation between vaginal bacteriology and infection in the baby. In the absence of signs of infection, or unless labour starts more than 24 hours after membrane rupture, antibiotics are of little value. When infection does supervene, it is far more likely the baby will have a better chance with the paediatrician than continuing in utero under antibiotic cover given to the mother. Therefore should infection occur after 34 weeks' gestation, pregnancy should be terminated. Prior to that time consultation with the paediatrician should be undertaken about the best management. Caesarean section may be considered for very small babies but the value of this method has yet to be proved. However, in a small infant compromised by infection, it may be important to effect delivery quickly and as atraumatically as possible, and sometimes this indicates the need for Caesarean section. The paramount need is to *avoid* intrauterine infection if at all possible. Hence admission to hospital is important and the avoidance of all but essential diagnostic speculum examinations under sterile conditions.

Premature labour has been discussed previously. Here it is necessary only to emphasize that often in the presence of ruptured membranes there is no advantage in delaying labour, and there may even be significant disadvantage. Following membrane rupture of longer than 24 hours, there is no value in administering corticosteroids to improve fetal lung function. Also unless corticosteroids are administered at least 24 hours prior to delivery they are probably valueless.

REFERENCES

ALDERMAN B. (1975) In *Clinics in Obstetrics and Gynaecology* (Beazley J.M. ed.). W.B. Saunders and Co. Ltd., London.

BAILLIE P., MEEHAN F.P. & TYACK A.J. (1970) *Brit. med J.,* **4**, 154.

BEAZLEY J.M. (1977) *Brit. J. Hosp. Med.,* **17**.

BEAZLEY J.M. & ALDERMAN B. (1975) *Brit. J. Obstet. Gynaec.,* **82**, 265.

BEAZLEY J.M. & ALDERMAN B. (1976) *Brit. J. Obstet. Gynaec.,* **83**, 513.

BEAZLEY J.M. & LOBB M.O. (1983) *Aspects of care in labour.* (Lind T. ed.). Churchill Livingstone, London, p. 109.

BEAZLEY J.M. & SWINHOE J.R. (1979) *Acta Obstet. Gynaec. Scand.,* **58**, 45.

BEAZLEY J.M. & WEEKES A.R.L. (1976) *Brit. J. Obstet. Gynaec.,* **83**, 62.

BEAZLEY J.M., BANOVIC I, & FELD M.S. (1975) *Brit. med. J.,* **2**, 248.

BENDER S. (1969) *Brit. med. J.,* **1**, 760.

BLUMENTHAL I.L. (1976) *Brit. med. J.,* ii, 733.

BRANDT H.A. & LACHELIN G.C.L. (1974) *J. Obstet. Gynaec. Brit. Cwlth.,* **81**, 278.

Brit. med. J. (1971) Editorial, **2**, 602.

Brit. med. J. (1980a) Editorial, **1**, 1061.

Brit. med. J. (1980b) Editorial, **1**, 1153.

BUCHAN P.C. (1979) *Brit. med. J.,* **11**, 1255.

CAIRO G.M. (1984) *Brit. J. Obstet. Gynaec.,* **91**, 23.

CARDOZA L., PEARCE J.M., FYSH J. (1983) *J. Obstet. Gynaec.,* **4**, 69.

CHEW W.C. (1977) *Brit. med. J.,* ii, 679.

CLARKE J.F.B. (1975) In *Clinics in Obstetrics and Gynaecology* (Beazley J.M. ed.). W.B. Saunders and Co. Ltd., London.

COOPER J.A. (1969) *Brit. J. Clin. Pract.,* **23**, 107.

CRANBROOK, EARL OF (1959) *Report on the Maternity Services Committee.* HMSO, London.

DAHLGREN S. (1972) *Proceedings of the International Symposium on the Treatment of Fetal Risks* (Baumgarten K. & Wesselius-de Casparis A. eds. p. 118). The University, Vienna.

DESIR D., VAN GOEVORDEN A., KIRKPATRICK C. & GAUFRIEZ A. (1978) *Brit. med. J.,* ii, 1194.

DEWHURST C.J. (1963) *Gynaecological disorders of infants and children.* Cassell, London.

DRIFE J.O. (1982) *Brit. med. J.,* **285**, 583.

ELLIOTT H.R. & BEAZLEY J.M. (1980) *J. Obstet. Gynaec.,* **1**, 16.

ELLIOTT H.R., ABDULLA U. & HAYES P.J. (1978) *Brit. med. J.,* ii, 799.

ELMFORS B., TRYDING N., TUFVESSON G. (1974) *J. Obstet. Gynaec.,* **81**, 361.

FEENEY J.K. & GREENE A.T. (1970) *Brit. J. Hosp. Med.,* **4**, 351.

FLIEGNER J.R., FORTUNE D.W. & EGGERS T.R. (1981) *Aust. N.Z. J. Obstet. Gynaec.,* **21**, 77.

FRIEDMAN L., LEWIS P.J., CLIFTON P. & BULPITT C.J. (1978) *Brit. med. J.,* **i**, 1235.

FRIEDMAN M.L. & MCELIN T.W. (1969) *Amer. J. Obstet. Gynec.,* **104**, 544.

FUCHS F. (1967) *Amer. J. Obstet. Gynec.,* **99**, 627.

GEE H. & BEAZLEY J.M. (1980) *Brit. J. Obstet. Gynaec.,* **87**, 115.

GIBB D.M., CARDOZA L.D., STUDD J.W.W., COOPER D.J. (1982) *Brit. J. Obstet. Gynaec.,* **89**, 292.

GORDON A.J. & CALDER A.A. (1983) *Brit. J. hosp. Med.,* **30**, 52.

GOUDIE B.M. & DOSSETOR J.F.B. (1979) *Lancet,* ii, 1187.

HEMMINKI E. & STARFIELD B. (1978) *Brit. J. Obstet. Gynaec.,* **85**, 411.

HIBBARD B.M. (1962) *Clin. Obstet. Gynec.,* **5**, 4, Harper & Row, U.S.A. p. 1044.

HOBBS M.S.T. & ACHESON E.D. (1966) *Lancet,* **1**, 761.

HOMBURG R., LUDOMIRSKI A., INSLER V. (1979) *Brit. J. Obstet. Gynaec.,* **86**, 759.

HUFFMAN J.W. (1968) *The Gynaecology of Childhood and Adolescence.* Saunders, Philadelphia.

HUGHES T.B.J. & HAMLETT J.D. (1975) *Aust. N.Z. J. Obstet. Gynaec.,* **15**, 15.

JAGANI N., SCHULMAN H., FLEISCHER A., MITCHELL J., RANDOLPH G. (1982) *Obstet. Gynaec.,* **59**, 21.

JAMES J.R.E. (1969) *Brit. med. J.,* **i**, 51.

JEFFCOATE T.N.A. (1961) *Lancet,* ii, 61.

JEFFCOATE T.N.A. & SCOTT J.S. (1959) *Can. Med. Ass. J.,* **80**, 77.

KARIM S.M.M., RATNAM S.S., PRASAD R.N.V. & WONG Y.M. (1977) *Brit. J. Obstet. Gynaec.,* **4**, 269.

KONINCKX P.R., TRAPPENIERS H., ASSCHE F.A.V. (1981) *Brit. J. Obstet. Gynaec.,* **88**, 607.

Lancet (1966) **i**, 414.

Lancet (1973) Editorial, **i**, 924.

Lancet (1979) **i**, 364.

Lancet (1980) **ii**, 185.

LEWIS B.V. (1967) *Brit. med. J.,* **i**, 733.

LIGGINS G.C. & HOWIE R.N. (1972) *Paediatrics,* **50**, 515.

LIGGINS G.C. & VAUGHAN G.S. (1973) *J. Obstet. Gynaec. Brit. Cwlth,,* **80**, 29.

MACKENZIE I.Z. & EMBREY M.P. (1977) *Brit. med. J.,* ii, 1381.

MACKENZIE I.Z. & EMBREY M.P. (1978) *Brit. J. Obstet. Gynaec.,* **85**, 657.

MACLENNAN A.H., GREEN R.C., BRYANT-GREENWOOD G.D., GREENWOOD R.C. & SEAMARK R.F. (1980) *Lancet,* i, 200.

NELSON M.M. (1972) *J. Obstet. Gynaec. Brit. Cwlth.,* **79**, 50.

NOBLE A.D. (1981) *J. Obstet. Gynaec.,* **2**, 88.

O'CONNOR M.C., MURPHY H. & DALRYMPLE I. (1979) *Brit. J. Obstet. Gynaec.,* **86**, 706.

OPANEYE A.A. (1983) *Brit. J. Obstet. Gynaec.,* **90**, 1180.

PARK G.L. (1968) *Lancet,* ii, 1388.

PERINATAL MORTALITY (1963) *The First Report of the 1958*

British Perinatal Mortality Survey (Butler & Bonham eds.), Livingstone Ltd., London.

PERINATAL PROBLEMS (1969) *The Second Report of the British Perinatal Mortality Survey* (Butler & Alderman eds.), Livingstone Ltd., London.

POLLARD S. M., SYMONDS E. M., AYE N. N. (1979) *Brit. J. Obstet. Gynaec.,* **86,** 228.

QUEENAN J. T., THOMPSON W., WHITFIELD C. R., SHAH S. I. (1972) *Amer. J. Obstet Gynec.,* **114,** 34.

QUINN M. A. & MURPHY A. J. (1981) *Brit. J. Obstet. Gynaec.,* **88,** 650.

QUINN M. A., MURPHY A. J., KUHN R. J. P., ROBINSON H. P., BROWN J. B. (1981) *Brit. J. Obstet. Gynaec.,* **88,** 644.

RAHMAN J., RAHMAN M. S., HISHAM AL-SIBAI, M., BUTALACK F. (1983) *J. Obstet. Gynaec.,* **4,** 7.

READ M. D. & MATTOCK E. J. (1982) *J. Obstet. Gynaec.,* **3,** 71.

Recommendations on the Principles of Organisation of G.P. Maternity Units and their relation to Specialist Maternity Units. (1962) London, Royal College of Obstetricians and Gynaecologists.

RUSSELL J. K. (1983) *Brit. J. Hosp. Med.,* **i,** 159.

RUSSELL T. K. (1969) *Lancet,* **i,** 365.

SCOTT J. S. & WILSON J. K. (1957) *Lancet,* **ii,** 569.

SHELDON J. H. (1949) *Lancet,* **ii,** 869.

SHEPHERD J., SIMS C. & CRAFT I. (1976) *Lancet,* **ii,** 709.

SIMS C. D., CHAMBERLAIN G. V. P., BOYD I. E. & LEWIS P. J. (1968) *Brit. J. Obstet. Gynaec.,* **85,** 761.

SMITH C. A. (1983) *J. Obstet. Gynaec.,* **3,** 553.

SMITH D. L. (1971) *Amer. J. Obstet. Gynec.,* **110,** 166.

STEER P. J., LITTLE D. J., LEWIS N. L., KELLY M. C. M. E. & BEARD R. W. (1975) *Brit. J. Obstet. Gynaec.,* **82,** 433.

STEWART P., KENNEDY J. H., BARLOW D. H., CALDER A. A. (1981) *Brit. J. Obstet. Gynaec.,* **88,** 236.

STUDD H. (1975) In *Clinics in Obstetrics and Gynaecology* (Beazley J. M. ed.). W. B. Saunders & Co. Ltd., London.

TINGA K. J. & AARNOUDSE J. G. (1979) *Lancet,* **i,** 1026.

TOKUYAMA T. & FUJIMOTO J. (1968) *Jap. J. Obstet. Gynaec.,* **35,** 31.

TROMANS P. M. & BEAZLEY J. M. (1983) *Brit. J. Obstet. Gynaec.,* **90,** 40.

TROMANS P. M., BEAZLEY J. M. & SHENOUDA P. I. (1981) *Brit. med. J.,* **282,** 679.

TYACK A. J., BAILLIE P. & MEEHAN F. P. (1971) *Brit. med. J.,* **ii,** 741.

UTIAN W. H. (1967) *Brit. med. J.,* **i,** 734.

VALENTINE B. H. (1977) *Brit. J. Obstet. Gynaec.,* **84,** 846.

VAN OTTERLO L. C., WLADIMIROFF J. W., WALLENBURG H. C. S. (1977) *Brit. J. Obstet. Gynaec.,* **84,** 205.

WEIR P. E., RATTEN G. J., BEISCHER N. A. (1979) *Brit. J. Obstet. Gynaec.,* **86,** 849.

WESSELIUS DE CASPARIS A., THIERY M., YO LE SIAN A., BAUMGARTEN K., BROSENS I., GAMISANS O., STOLK J. G. & VIVIER W. (1971) *Brit. med. J.,* **iii,** 144.

WILSON P. D. (1978) *Brit. J. Obstet. Gynaec.,* **85,** 941.

WLADIMIROFF J. W. & CAMPBELL S. (1974) *Lancet,* **i,** 151.

ZAAIJMAN J. DU T., WILKINSON A. R., KEELING J. W., MITCHELL R. G., TURNBULL A. C. (1982) *J. Obstet. Gynaec.,* **2,** 155.

ZLATNIK F. J. (1972) *Amer. J. Obstet. Gynec.,* **113,** 704.

CHAPTER 26
DYSTOCIA CAUSED BY THE PASSAGES OR PASSENGER

J.M. BEAZLEY

Dystocia signifies difficult labour. A difficult labour is one where the hazards significantly exceed those of minimal risk labours. In this chapter problems will be discussed which arise chiefly from abnormalities in the hard and soft passages, or from difficulties caused by the fetus.

The trials of labour

The term 'trial of labour' was originally used to describe the management of patients with cephalo-pelvic disproportion at the pelvic brim. The deformity commonly resulted from rickets. In terms of its original meaning the phrase is now obsolete and present-day trials are conducted to put to the test numerous features other than pelvic capacity. In trial of breech, for example, there should be no suggestion of cephalo-pelvic disproportion. It is the efficacy with which the powers will dilate the cervix and cause descent of the breech, which remains to be tested. If the principal problem is the integrity of a uterine scar, attention should be drawn to the problem by admitting the patient for a 'trial of scar' procedure. Other problems detected antenatally can be similarly emphasized by utilizing terms such as 'trial of occipitoposterior position', 'trial of face presentation', 'trial of unstable lie', etc. Each problem has its specific requirements, and they do not relate necessarily to cephalo-pelvic disproportion.

In Britain, minor degrees of cephalo-pelvic disproportion occur either at the pelvic brim or the obstetric outlet. If just the pelvic brim is to be tested, 'trial of inlet' seems an appropriate term. If cephalo-pelvic disproportion is suspected at the outlet, the term 'trial of outlet' seems more pertinent than 'trial of forceps'. The latter may involve quite separate procedures.

Each trial should have a beginning and an end. Thus, 'trial of the inlet' for example, should finish when the plane of the biparietal diameter has passed the plane of the pelvic brim. The 'trial of the outlet' does not begin until the plane of the biparietal dia-

meter reaches the plane of least pelvic dimension. It finishes when the head is safely delivered through the anatomical outlet. The term 'trial of labour' should be reserved for patients in whom the whole process of expelling the products of conception from the mother is put to the test. Such a trial cannot end until parturition is complete.

THE HARD PASSAGES

There is no substitute for clinical examination of the patient. This aphorism includes the antenatal assessment of pelvic capacity. It has long been recommended that about 36 weeks' gestation clinical pelvimetry be performed. If, however, the fetal head is already engaged at that time there is no point, clinically, in attempting to assess, by digital examination, the diagonal pelvic conjugate. Manual examination can be restricted to an evaluation of the pelvic outlet. This, too, is of extremely limited value for until moulding of the fetal head has occurred, and the 'give' of the pelvic ligaments has been evaluated, no meaningful judgement can be made about cephalo-pelvic relationships at the lower pelvic strait. Final judgement must be reserved for labour.

Average pelvic dimensions are given in Chapter 24 (p. 343). Pelvic size, however, is not the only important feature; pelvic shape must be considered also. Neither is of great value without reference to the size of the fetal head.

Accurate measurement of pelvic size, if required, is now made by antero-posterior and lateral X-rays of the pelvic bones. Any maternal pelvis with an obstetric diameter less than 10 cm should be viewed with suspicion.

A lateral X-ray of the pelvis provides information about all the antero-posterior diameters, the angle of inclination of the brim, and the angle at which the fetal head is negotiating the pelvic inlet. The depth of the pelvis can also be assessed, as can the size of the sacro-sciatic notches. A particular feature of interest is the shape of the sacrum.

Clinical information which is obtained only from a lateral X-ray is limited (Rubin & Francis 1967). Full radiological assessment of the pelvis always necessitates an antero-posterior view in addition. The transverse pelvic diameters are much more difficult to evaluate clinically than the antero-posterior diameters, and asymmetry of the pelvis is easy to miss. Antero-posterior X-rays of the pelvis avoid these errors.

At all planes of the pelvis the fetal head is the best pelvimeter. In obstetric practice a trial of cephalopelvic disproportion is justifiable now only if pelvic contraction occurs in one plane and in one diameter of that plane.

An approach to pelvic abnormality

The pelvis is a variable skeletal entity. Most pelves have a similar shape. The factors that influence this shape, or determine pelvic size, can be considered in the following way.

CONGENITAL INFLUENCE

If the sacrum is incorporated in the fifth lumbar vertebra the sacral promonotory will be higher than usual (high assimulation pelvis). There is an apparent lengthening of the sacrum, and the pelvic brim has a steeper angle of inclination. In the patient who has only four sacral vertebrae the pelvic brim lies almost horizontally. The sacrum is short and its promontory is lower than usual (low assimilation pelvis).

Much rarer congenital conditions that effect the pelvis include the Otto pelvis (protrusio ascetabulae) in which deep acetabula protrude medially to encroach on and distort the cavity of the true pelvis. The condition is hereditary and familial (Francis 1959). Diaphyseal aclasis is also an inherited condition. It affects women only rarely. The long bones are most affected, but nodular osteomata formation may encroach on the true pelvic cavity, and there may be pelvic asymmetry with narrowing (Adey & Kneale 1966). Classical rarities include malformations of one or both sacral alae resulting in gross pelvic narrowing of the Naegele or Robert type. In ectopia vesicae the pelvis is split and held together by fibrous tissue which replaces the pubis.

ACQUIRED INFLUENCE

Alterations in pelvic shape and size may be the primary result of an acquired problem. More commonly, acquired pelvic defects are secondary, resulting from problems that primarily affect the spine or lower limbs.

The spine
Kyphosis of the thoracic spine usually promotes a compensatory lumbar lordosis. This results in contraction of the antero-posterior diameter of the pelvic outlet, and an increase in the angle of inclination of the pelvic brim. Kyphosis of the lumbar region promotes an almost horizontal pelvic inlet. Scoliosis produces an unequal pelvic shape, which particularly affects the contour of the pelvic inlet.

Kyphoscoliosis is a clinical problem. It affects not only the size and shape of the pelvis but also results in significant maternal cardiovascular complications. Because of these, and also because of the short distance between the xiphisternum and the pelvic brim, the enlarging uterus is accommodated only with difficulty. The anatomical distortion may complicate Caesarean section (Fig. 26.1).

Spondylolisthesis is the condition in which the fifth lumbar vertebra rides forwards on the upper surface of the first sacral vertebra. The result is to produce an artificial promontory which significantly reduces the antero-posterior diameter of the pelvic inlet. The condition is usually associated with multiparity. The spondylolisthesis follows continued softening of the spinal ligaments and recurrent lordosis of pregnancy (Fig. 26.2).

The lower limbs
Conditions that arise during childhood and which may, thereby, secondarily affect the development of the pelvis, include unrecognized hip dislocation, local diseases such as tuberculosis, suppurative arthritis (Perthe's disease), or limping secondary to poliomyelitis. Pelvic size may not be significantly reduced by these complications. Disuse atrophy, however, may result in an alteration of the pelvic shape.

The pelvis
Direct pelvic trauma may cause fractures that alter the shape of the pelvis, or result in the development of hard ridges along the fracture line. Pelvic neoplasms are extremely rare and so is degenerative atrophy (Foruhan & Jennings 1978).

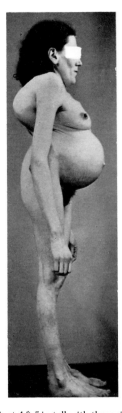

Fig. 26.1. A patient 4 ft 5 in tall with thoracic kyphoscoliosis.

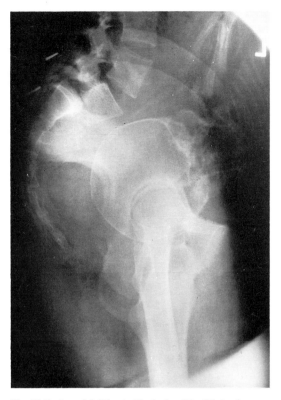

Fig. 26.2. Spondylolithesis. The body of the 5th lumbar vertebra has slipped forward for a distance equivalent to almost half its antero-posterior diameter.

Metabolic influence on the pelvis can be quite dramatic. Depending upon the age at which it operates the effects on the pelvis differ. Tall women of superior physique and good health, who normally enjoy an upper class environment, usually have a pelvis with good diameters. Women of lower socio-economic status, who are usually less than 153 cm tall, of poor physique and health, often have a pelvis of small diameters with some antero-posterior flattening.

Major metabolic variants, such as the low calcium disorders are rarely seen in England today. Rickets used seriously to affect the development of the pelvis during childhood. The sacral promontory was pushed forward, which narrowed the antero-posterior diameter of the pelvic brim so that the inlet appeared kidney shaped. The angle of inclination of the brim was diminished. The sacrum itself tended to move backwards and the pelvic cavity was usually sizeable. To negotiate the pelvic brim the fetal head would tip laterally. This asynclitism would result in one of

the parietal bones becoming the presenting part. The supra-infraparietal diameter is about 1 cm less than the biparietal diameter. Anterior asynclitism, i.e. when the anterior parietal bone first enters the pelvis, is a favourable situation. It permits the posterior parietal bone to slip into the hollow of the sacrum. If the posterior parietal enters the pelvis first, the anterior parietal bone overlaps the symphysis pubis and becomes lodged against its upper surface.

In undernourished countries osteomalacia affects adults. The pelvic deformity caused by osteomalacia differs from that of rickets. The sacral promontory is pushed forward, but in addition the sides of the pelvis are also pushed inwards. The fore pelvis becomes 'beaked' and the pelvic outlet is narrowed in its transverse diameters.

Hormonal influence

Secondary sexual characteristics are reflected in the basic differences between the male and female pelves. The pelvic brim is less triangular in the female. Also, the female pelvis is not so deep. It is lighter than the male, less funnel shaped, and the sciatic notches are much wider. The ischial spines and tuberosities are more everted in the female and the subpubic arch is wider.

In contrast to the male pelvis, which has been described as the long section of a short cone, the female pelvis has been described as the short section of a long cone.

Pelvic contraction

Pelvic contraction is best described as a reduction in one or more of the diameters, to such an extent that the normal mechanism of labour is adversely affected.

At the pelvic inlet, significant diminution of diameters is associated with an android or anthropoid pelvis, or spondylolisthesis.

The pelvic cavity is seriously compromised when the sacrum is flat. Also, its diameters may be minimal, even though the shape remains gynaecoid, if the mother is less than 5 feet tall.

The pelvic outlet is contracted in a high assimilation pelvis, e.g. in the anthropoid pelvis, or a patient with kyphoscoliosis. The available antero-posterior diameter of the outlet is reduced when the subpubic arch is narrow. Deformity of the coccyx, especially forward angulation, may constrict the antero-posterior diameter of the outlet. Prominent ischial spines diminish the transverse diameter of the plane of least pelvic dimension.

The active management of cephalo-pelvic disproportion

The first principle of management in cephalo-pelvic disproportion is to make an accurate assessment of (a) the pelvic level at which the disproportion occurs, (b) the diameter in which it occurs, and, (c) the degree of disproportion suspected. This necessitates not only careful X-ray evaluation of the available pelvic diameters at the appropriate plane, but also accurate assessment of the biparietal diameter just prior to the onset of labour. Ultrasonic measurement of the fetal head, and X-ray and clinical measurement of some of the bony landmarks of the maternal pelvis, can now be made at the same time.

Antenatal X-ray evaluation does not often alter the proposed direction of clinical management (Hanna 1965). Careful evaluation, however, converts clinical suspicion into facts which will either support a decision in favour of elective Caesarean section, or else enable a clinician meaningfully to pursue an appropriate trial of labour.

Any trial of labour should be designed to find out what a woman can accomplish rather than what she can endure. In former years the procedure was hesitant and uncertain. Labour was expected to begin spontaneously. Uterine stimulations were frowned upon because of the fear of the risk of uterine rupture. Much attention was paid to the difference between hypo- and hypertonic uterine inertia. Artificial rupture of the membranes was not favoured because of the risks of intrauterine infection. In labours prolonged beyond 24 hours the statistical risk of infection was increased. Caesarean sections were undertaken as much on the basis of time as for reasons like slow progress, fetal or maternal distress.

Today, controlled methods of oxytocin administration, partographs, the ready availability of fetal and maternal monitoring devices, and a different approach to uterine dysfunction, have radically altered the management. It is now the policy to be more active. In primigravidas some of the fundamentals that justify this change include, (a) the pelvic capacity is largely an unknown entity, (b) prolonged labour is a fairly common feature of parturition, (c) prolonged labour, if it occurs, can be related chiefly to pelvic factors rather than fetal factors, (d) uterine rupture following oxytocin stimulation is extremely rare, (e) the potential for childbearing is determined by the outcome of the first labour.

In multiparous women the patient's pelvic capacity is, largely, understood. Moreover, prolonged labour is unusual in multipara. When it does occur, there is commonly a fetal factor involved, and oxytocin, if used carelessly, can promote uterine rupture. It is the previous labours that chiefly influence the conduct of parturition, not the future capacity for childbirth.

The Irish School have been largely responsible for establishing many of these points as they have clearly demonstrated that minor cephalo-pelvic disproportion in a primigravid woman with a vertex presentation may be treated confidently by active management, whereas in multiparous women active management should be used only after the most careful and thorough individual appraisal.

Traditionally the three main components of dystocia are inefficient uterine action, minor cephalo-pelvic disproportion, and functional difficulties in the mechanism of labour associated with malposition of the fetal head. The interrelationship between these components is such that, in the presence of uterine contractions of the usual type, dystocia, arising from either cephalo-pelvic disproportion or occipito-posterior positions, is very uncommon. It may be thought, therefore, that there is no particular merit in distinguishing between occipito-posterior position and minor cephalo-pelvic disproportion. This is not a view the author shares. Cephalo-pelvic disproportion and malpositions of the fetal head are problems associated with different potential hazards. The conduct of labour is managed differently in the two instances.

The following features of the active management of minor cephalo-pelvic disproportion are now frequently utilized.

PLANNED DELIVERY

In contrast to the days when spontaneous labour was the best start to a trial of labour, it is now the practice to induce labour as a planned procedure about term. All too often previously a tired patient was admitted during the night in desultory labour to a unit, unprepared for her particular problem at that time, and unable to control the inflow of competitive patients to the labour room. Despite everybody's best efforts, hazards were imposed by overwork, shortage of night-time personnel, and delays in mobilizing laboratory or X-ray facilities.

A planned procedure ensures that labour can be undertaken during a time that will enable the patient to make maximum use of her energy, and, at the same time, conserve her resources, for the subsequent care of her baby. Not least amongst the advantages of a planned procedure is the ready availability of a full-time anaesthetic service that can assist with epidural analgesia when it is required. It is often a great advantage for the patient undergoing a trial to have an epidural catheter inserted prior to the induction of labour so that she may receive good analgesia early in the process.

Induction of labour used to be performed in the hope that a softer, and smaller fetal skull, would pass more easily through the pelvis. The difference, which occurs in the measurement of the biparietal diameter during the last 2–3 weeks of pregnancy, is too small to be of real significance with regard to disproportion.

Induction of labour

In former years it was considered unwise to rupture membranes prior to engagement of the fetal head. Also, during a trial of labour, membranes were preserved as long as possible to diminish the risk of intrauterine infection. Both these concepts have changed.

The hazard of cord prolapse is most likely to be recognized if the accoucheur is undertaking a pelvic examination at the time of amniotomy. The contractile pattern of the uterus is minimal at this time, and the dangers of cord compression are less. Should such an accident befall the patient Caesarean section can be undertaken without delay.

High amniotomy, using a Drew Smythe catheter, is used much less frequently now than in previous years. Nevertheless it remains a useful instrument, in my view, particularly for reducing the liquor volume when the fetal head is not engaged at the time of induction of labour. The risk of cord prolapse seems to be diminished, and, once the head has settled against the pelvic brim, the subsequent gush of liquor, following low amniotomy, is less. This too further diminishes the risk of cord prolapse.

After successful amniotomy uterine stimulation should be utilized to maintain good contact between the fetal head and the pelvic inlet.

Uterine stimulation

The medical induction of labour is discussed in more detail in Chapter 25. Here it is necessary only to re-emphasize that modern technology, and modern oxytocics enable the obstetrician to stimulate the myometrium with fine control, and great safety. Effective contractions can be promoted before, or after amniotomy. In cephalo-pelvic disproportion intravenous infusion of oxytocin immediately after amniotomy is most effective, and gives the best chance of success.

Oral oxytocic agents may be suitable for induction of labour in some circumstances, but never during a trial of labour.

Partography

The modern partograph and inductogram (cf. Chapters 24 and 25) provide useful measures against which the progress of induced labour can be assessed during a trial. Lack of progress, despite adequate uterine stimulation, is quickly revealed and raises for consideration the need for early Caesarean section. If a satisfactory rate of progress changes suddenly, it is essential to re-evaluate the whole obstetric situation to detect an unforeseen problem.

Some delay in the rate of progress may be expected throughout the duration of a trial. When the trial is over, however, the rate of progress should return to the usual rate indicated by the partograph.

Monitoring

The unknown factors, which justify a trial of labour,

include the physiological ability of the mother and baby to withstand the procedure safely. Monitoring of the maternal condition and fetal well-being has, therefore, always been an integral part of the trials of labour.

The timescale of modern trials, from induction of labour to delivery, is much shorter than in former years. Deterioration in maternal and fetal well-being occurs less commonly, but can arise quickly. Intermittent monitoring is, therefore, no longer satisfactory. Continuous monitoring, especially of the fetus, is now considered mandatory.

Early rupture of the membranes enables the fetal heart rate to be monitored continuously throughout labour, by fetal scalp electrode. Transcervical catheters inserted into the intra-amniotic cavity provide excellent recordings of uterine activity.

External monitors are valuable in early labour when it is impossible to apply fetal scalp electrodes or introduce transcervical intra-amniotic catheters. Unfortunately the recording obtained by external monitors often becomes increasingly difficult to interpret as labour progresses.

Data logging equipment, with computer analysis of the information obtained, provides the best record of time relationships between uterine contractions and changes in the rate of the fetal heart. Additional, and often more meaningful information, such as the dip area under the graph of the fetal heart rate, can readily be analysed by computer and correlated with such parameters as intrauterine pressure and the infusion rate of oxytocin. Until sophisticated monitoring equipment and visual display units are generally available, maximum use should be made of simpler recording devices plus fetal scalp blood sampling. Intrapartum fetal surveillance is described in detail in Chapter 31 (p. 442).

Assistance

Forceps. The modern use of oxytocics has reduced the need for forceps delivery in minor cephalo-pelvic disproportion at the brim, and for patients with occipitoposterior position. Nevertheless, recent reports on the use of Kielland's forceps continue to indicate the relative danger of this procedure when it proves necessary (Chiswick & James 1979). It should not be assumed, however, that Caesarean section is necessarily a better recourse, for to disengage from above a fetal head impacted in the pelvis carries significant fetal risks (*Brit. med. J.* 1979). According to Davidson *et al.* (1976) the more the interval from 7 to 10 cm dilatation of the cervix exceeds two hours, the greater

is the proportion of Kielland's forceps deliveries that may be classed as moderately difficult or difficult.

Early assistance during the second stage of labour is commonplace today as part of the management of trials of labour. When there is any doubt about the safety of the lower uterine segment, or simply to minimize the time during which the lower segment is subject to its greatest strain, forceps delivery is desirable.

When a patient has successfully completed a trial of labour it is unreasonable and unnecessary to subject her to the further expenditure of energy entailed in bearing down. In fact, the use of epidural analgesia for many labour trials considerably diminishes the patient's desire to expel her fetus and assistance with forceps becomes obligatory towards the end of labour.

Many of the more difficult vaginal procedures that were formerly performed in the later stages of labour to help overcome cephalo-pelvic disproportion, have now been made obsolete by the increased safety and freer use of Caesarean section. Nevertheless, the cephalo-pelvic relationships at the lower pelvic strait must sometimes be tested. Even in the absence of disproportion it is sometimes desirable to utilize more than one pair of forceps to correct the fetal position and effect delivery. Often these procedures are best undertaken in theatre under general anaesthesia.

The basis of a trial of forceps, or a trial of outlet, is not so much to pull the baby out, as to draw the fetal head safely through the pelvis. A successful outcome is most likely to be achieved if the patient is put into an exaggerated lithotomy position and a generous episiotomy made. An experienced operator, who understands the axis and shape of the pelvic outlet, should perform the task.

Caesarean section

Minor cephalo-pelvic disproportion is rarely the sole indication for elective Caesarean section in modern practice. Suspected minor cephalo-pelvic disproportion may figure frequently, however, with additional indications such as poor previous obstetric history, elderly primigravidity, relative infertility, or some unstable condition like pre-eclamptic toxaemia. Caesarean section for failed induction of labour is now a most infrequent occurrence.

The purpose of the active management of cephalo-pelvic disproportion is not simply to reduce the incidence of Caesarean section for this condition. In fact, though the proportion of elective to emergency operations has not appreciably altered, the indications for Caesarean section are now more liberal and the absolute number of operations is increasing. This trend is reflected in figures quoted recently by Sutherst and Case (1975) who show that in 1970, prior to the adoption of a policy of active management of labour, 66.7% of patients coming to an emergency Caesarean section had been in labour for more than 12 hours. By contrast, in 1973, when active management was the rule rather than the exception, only 24.7% of such patients had been in labour for 12 hours or more. They stress that the obstetrician's aim should now be to deliver every woman within 12 hours of the onset of labour and to perform Caesarean section at that time unless delivery is imminent. Their comments are not restricted to patients with cephalo-pelvic disproportion but they might apply equally well to this condition.

THE SOFT PASSAGES

Dystocia caused by problems arising in the soft passages is not common in this country. They may occur from congenital abnormalities of the genital tract or acquired anomalies.

The vulva

Previous episiotomy scars provide no problem during labour. If there is any doubt about their integrity, a repeat episiotomy should be performed.

Vulval varicosities can prove to be a nuisance (Fig. 26.3). Despite fears of extensive haemorrhage from an episiotomy or perineal laceration it is uncommon for this to occur. Pressure of the fetal head around

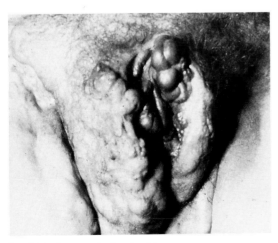

Fig. 26.3. Severe vulval varicosities.

the vulva at the time of delivery collapses the veins considerably, and the stitches of the normal repair, which can be inserted without difficulty, secure any venous oozing.

Bartholin's cyst is uncommon prior to delivery but may be treated by marsupialization if there is a fear that it will impede delivery.

Oedema of the vulva is observed from time to time during otherwise normal labour. If the oedema is gross, multiple puncture of the skin surface under analgesia and in clean conditions may be necessary. The free escape of fluid reduces the oedema considerably.

Female circumcision and imfibulation may complicate delivery. The circumcized mother is unlikely to deliver herself. Without assistance, severe perineal lacerations, fistulae, haemorrhage and infection are common sequelae. An episiotomy sufficient to divide the circumcision scar is necessary in all patients. Adhesions that extend forwards from the region of the fourchette sometimes require antenatal surgery. Antenatal treatment is not required for adhesions which begin at the front of the vulva and extend backwards (Daw 1970, Egwuatu & Agugua 1981).

Pregnancy following radical vulvectomy for carcinoma of the vulva has been reviewed by Gemmell and Haines (1960). Delivery was not invariably by Caesarean section.

The vagina

Serious prolapse of the anterior or posterior wall of the vagina may cause delay in labour, especially if the bladder or rectum is full. Scars from a previous anterior or posterior colporrhaphy may give way under the distension caused by passage of the fetal head. Such an occurrence is extremely uncommon. Unusual cases from underdeveloped countries have been described in which utero-vaginal prolapse has resulted in full dilatation of the cervix occurring outside the vulva.

In developed countries obstetricians may expect to treat patients who have had a previous vaginal repair. Cervical amputation and/or surgical treatment to correct stress incontinence of urine may have been performed at the same time. High cervical amputation is more likely to result in premature labour than cervical dystocia. Pregnancy may well cause some deterioration in a patient's urinary control. If it is considered that delivery vaginally may further aggravate the situation, elective Caesarean section about term should be considered. Caesarean section is mandatory when a previous vesico-vaginal fistula has been successfully repaired. It is often desirable also after a successful repair of a serious recto-vaginal fistula. A previous third degree tear can be managed easily by the use of a generous episiotomy.

Congenital anomalies of the vagina include complete duplication, which rarely causes a problem. A partial mid-line septum might get in the way of a descending fetal head. It will not cause obstruction but is likely to produce an unpleasant tear in the anterior or posterior vaginal wall. The vagina becomes so distensible near term that often the septum can be pushed to one side. Surgical removal of the septum as an interval procedure between pregnancies is required in some patients. Removal of the septum during pregnancy is usually unnecessary and may be a rather haemorrhagic procedure.

A transverse membrane in the upper part of the vagina, just below the normal cervix, may create some diagnostic difficulty when first seen. The condition has been incorrectly called 'cervical phimosis'. It is not a condition of the cervix. Only vaginal epithelium is involved, and after full cervical dilatation the transverse membrane can be incised, allowing passage of the fetal head. Subsequently, examination and suture of the upper vaginal epithelium should be undertaken.

Traumatic or congenital strictures involving the upper portions of the vagina or resulting perhaps from reconstruction of the vagina may seriously impede labour. Moreover, because of the close proximity of the bladder anteriorly, strictures of this kind constitute a significant maternal hazard if vaginal delivery occurs. Caesarean section is usually the treatment of choice in patients with such a problem.

The cervix

Cervical dystocia is a situation which may be said to exist when, in an otherwise normal labour, and despite adequate and effective uterine contractions, the cervix fails to dilate. The condition may result from cervical scarring following amputation, deep cervical cauterization or trachelorrhaphy. Two recent reports (*Brit. med. J.* 1980, McLaren *et al.* 1974) also indicate that following cone biopsy of the cervix, there is an increased incidence of Caesarean section, due in some instances to cervical stenosis. Cryotherapy of the cervix is reported to have no effect on the onset or progress of labour (Hemmingson 1982).

Circumstances arise, though infrequently, when

dilatation of a normal cervix appears to stop towards the end of the first stage of labour. The cervix may be incised with reasonable safety so long as the biparietal diameter has passed below the level of the vaginal vault. If, however, the biparietal diameter is above the vaginal vault at the time of cervical incision, lacerations tend to extend upwards as far as the widest part of the fetal head. This will result in severe maternal damage or haemorrhage. It is traditional to site the one inch incisions at 2 o'clock and 10 o'clock, to avoid injury to the bladder, ureters or uterine vessels. Forceps delivery must be undertaken subsequently, and very slowly. In modern practice the vacuum extractor has made nearly obsolete the need for cervical incisions.

Cervical carcinoma during pregnancy is extremely malignant and has a very poor prognosis. In this country it is no longer a cause of dystocia because treatment of the malignancy takes precedence over everything else. In the event of a late discovery, treatment will usually be by Caesarean section followed by immediate radical hysterectomy with node dissection, although radiotherapy is an alternative (*see* Chapter 50, p. 780).

The uterus

As a generalization it may be said that the more complete the uterine malformation, the less likely dystocia is to occur. Complications such as obstructed labour, caused by the non-pregnant uterus of a patient with complete duplication of the genital tract, are more imagined than real.

Partial division of the uterine cavity, or the presence of a mid-line septum, may prevent the fetus from lying longitudinally. Sometimes it prevents spontaneous antenatal version to a cephalic presentation. Habitual abortion, malpresentation and retained placenta are found more frequently in association with uterine anomalies. Dystocia, however, is uncommon if the patient proceeds to term with a cephalic presentation.

A cervical fibroid necessitates Caesarean section. Fibroids situated in the upper uterine segment may be associated with problems such as red degeneration, or retained placenta, but they are not significant causes of dystocia.

Retroversion of the uterus in early pregnancy, with subsequent sacculation is theoretically possible. Exciting descriptions of anterior wall sacculation, with the uterine cervix tucked high under the symphysis pubis and carriage of the bladder upwards into the lower abdomen, may be found in older textbooks. With modern antenatal care retroversion of the uterus in early pregnancy is no longer a problem (Weeks *et al.* 1976).

The ovary

Ovarian cysts which lie below the pelvic brim and do not rise into the abdomen with the uterus as it increases in size may constitute an obstruction to delivery. Heavy tumours on a long pedicle, such as dermoid cysts, may complicate pregnancy in this way. If, as usually happens, the cyst is detected in early pregnancy, laparotomy is undertaken between the 16th and 20th week and the tumour is removed. In the unlikely event that the cyst is not detected until labour has commenced Caesarean section is usually necessary. Prior to surgery, with the patient anaesthetized and in a Trendelenburg position, it is reasonable to attempt to ease the cyst above the pelvic brim from below. Care must be taken not to rupture the cyst. For the same reason it is always incorrect to force a fetal head downwards past a cyst which is fixed within the pelvic cavity.

Ovarian cysts which escape above the pelvic brim do not cause dystocia. They may, however, undergo torsion or be damaged during the conduct of labour. Such cysts are usually removed surgically in the early part of the puerperium.

Pelvic kidney is a condition which has no definitive signs or symptoms. The diagnosis is established only by pyelography or exploration. It is easy for a gynaecologist to mistake a pelvic kidney for the more common conditions of fibroids, dermoids or even intraligamentous cysts.

An ectopic kidney is fixed below the pelvic brim as a soft tissue mass, and will usually impede descent of the fetal head during labour at term. Should the condition be recognized before labour commences, Caesarean section is the treatment of choice. Vaginal delivery has occurred without undue difficulty, but in modern practice this should be reserved for very premature babies which can bypass the obstruction without the slightest difficulty. Vaginal interference in any other situation is frequently followed by serious consequences.

Rarer soft tissue tumours, which sometimes utilize the space within the pelvic cavity, include retroperitoneal masses such as ganglioneuromata or even chordomas (Freeth & Mair 1951).

DYSTOCIA CAUSED BY THE PASSENGERS

Hazards to the first and second stages of labour may be caused by unusual conditions of the placenta, its membranes and vessels, or the umbilical cord. Placenta praevia, or a succenturiate lobe of the placenta with vasa praevia, or a cord presentation, will create difficulties during parturition.

In this chapter consideration will be given to difficulties in labour caused by general enlargement of the fetus, and local fetus deformities.

Generalized fetal enlargement

In mothers of average size, an unusually large baby develops most often as a result of heriditary influences. Latent or overt diabetes may also result in the development of a large baby. Hydrops fetalis, caused by severe rhesus isoimmunization, is now a less common cause of fetal enlargement than in recent years. Pregnancy prolonged by 10–14 days may be associated with a large fetus, but growth has occurred throughout pregnancy and not just after term.

Antenatal detection of a relatively large child is not easy. An unconfirmed suspicion of hydramnios, or a uterus slightly larger than expected for the period of gestation, or late engagement of the fetal head in an otherwise normal woman, should raise the suspicion of a child of excessive weight. Unfortunately, there are no really helpful confirmatory tests. Antenatal X-ray near term may reveal generalized fetal enlargement, with radiological signs of advanced bone development, an unusually thick fat shadow, or even oedema of the abdominal wall or scalp.

During labour a partograph which indicates slow general progress in a mother whose pelvis and baby seem otherwise normal, should raise the suspicion of an unusually large child, and a difficult delivery.

Otherwise, Lobb and Beazley (1984) reporting on a retrospective study of the delivery of 118 consecutive infants of birth weight more than 4.5 kg, found no major obstetric or neonatal complications. The management of the large fetus should not differ from that of the fetus of average size.

SHOULDER DYSTOCIA

Problems experienced during the delivery of an unusually large baby are chiefly cephalo-pelvic disproportion and shoulder dystocia. These complications can also occur when a child of average build has to escape from the genital tract of a relatively small mother. Like uterine inertia, maternal or fetal distress, cord prolapse, and antepartum haemorrhage, shoulder dystocia still constitutes one of the unsuspected hazards of an otherwise well-conducted pregnancy and labour.

Although shoulder dystocia may be unsuspected the astute obstetrician can often foresee the problem while he is delivering the fetal head. Despite good maternal effort, and seemingly good advance of the fetal vertex, there is often some difficulty in achieving 'crowning' of the head. Perineal pressure to prevent recession of the vertex between contractions is often required. Even an episiotomy does not facilitate the extension which normally leads to delivery of the child's face. Assisting extension of the fetal head by hand proves to be more difficult than expected.

As the baby's face appears it is obvious that it has fat cheeks and a double chin. These are made even more pronounced by the manner in which the chin presses down firmly against the perineum. The fetal head does not restitute and with the ensuing contraction no obvious external rotation occurs.

Time is of the essence. The accoucheur is faced with the difficulty of discovering on which side the fetal back lies. He must exclude any unsuspected localized abnormality which may be affecting the neck, chest or abdomen. There is little enough time to make even a cursory examination. Not only is the fetal cord compressed but also the fetal chest. Neither clearing the nasal and oral massages of mucus, nor the insertion of an oral airway will enable the child to breathe. If the baby is to be saved, prompt action is required.

The most important principle of management is to create as much space as possible posteriorly. Meanwhile a runner, if one is available, should be dispatched to summon the immediate arrival of an anaesthetist.

The two methods of increasing space posteriorly are, firstly, to position the patient correctly and, secondly, to make a large episiotomy or increase the size of the existing one. Putting the patient in the lithotomy position is best. If that is not possible, she should lie on her left side, across the delivery bed.

The position of the fetal back can now be determined by vaginal examination. A firm attempt is made again to rotate the fetal head in the normal manner. Excessive rotation or traction must not be used as it is easy to fracture the cervical vertebrae, or tear the brachial plexus and leave the child with a permanent Erb's palsy. Abdominally an extra hand is useful to push the child's anterior shoulder for-

wards off the pelvic brim and down into the pelvic cavity. The aim of these manoeuvres is to adduct the shoulders so that their diameter across the pelvic brim is minimized. Pressure applied in the wrong direction will abduct the shoulders and make matters worse.

If positioning and an adequate episiotomy does not allow sufficient rotation and downward traction to be made, even with assistance from above, the accoucheur must insert a hand posteriorly into the hollow of the sacrum and move it upwards to grasp the posterior fetal arm. This should be flexed and brought down through the pelvis posteriorly. The child is then manhandled through 180 degrees, to adduct the shoulders and take the anterior arm to the back. The arm is now brought down, through the pelvis as before, by the accoucheur once again entering his hand into the uterus via the pelvic curve.

These procedures are not possible without sufficient space behind the vagina to perform the appropriate manipulations. They cause a good deal of maternal distress. Indeed without an anaesthetic they may be impossible. If access is impossible, it will be necessary to divide the child's clavicles with a large pair of scissors.

Localized fetal deformity

HYDROCEPHALY

Antenatal detection of gross hydrocephaly is not difficult clinically. There is obvious disproportion between the size of the fetal head and the fetal body. Ultrasonic examination will confirm an abnormally large biparietal diameter. The condition can be visualized on X-ray (Fig. 26.4) or ultrasound.

Hydrocephalus is often diagnosed prior to term, but even in labour the diagnosis is not difficult. A large fetal head is palpated above the pelvic brim. The head does not engage and on vaginal examination wide suture lines are palpable. An inexperienced obstetrician may at first be confused by the findings on vaginal examination, as, in gross hydrocephaly, a portion of the head often manages to squeeze down into the upper part of the pelvis giving the impression of reasonable descent. Consideration of the level of the biparietal diameter rather than the leading portion of the head will soon reveal the error.

Whenever the diagnosis of hydrocephalus is confirmed an appropriate form of management has to be considered. If the condition is detected antenatally, the author allows the patient to continue with preg-

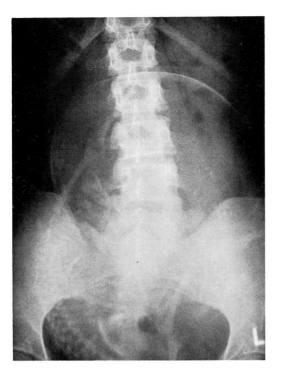

Fig. 26.4. Hydrocephaly in a breech presentation.

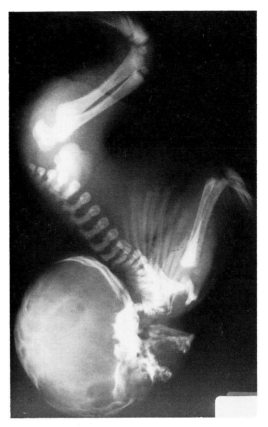

Fig. 26.5. Iniencephaly.

nancy until it seems certain that induction of labour can be achieved successfully. The patient's admission is arranged if possible without explaining to her the precise nature of the problem. By contrast, the author tries to make sure the partner fully understands the difficulty. The induction of labour is expedited and shortly after labour has been successfully established the problem is explained to the mother as kindly as possible. Reasonable sedation is then prescribed and at 3–4 cm dilatation of the cervix arrangements are made for decompression of the fetal head.

Antenatal growth of the fetal head to such a size that there is real danger of rupturing the lower uterine segment is rare. The condition may be treated, however, by inserting a needle through the maternal wall of the abdomen and tapping fluid from the fetal head via one of the wide suture lines. There is, of course, a danger of breaking the needle during this procedure.

On humanitarian grounds the author favours decompression of the fetal head in labour, as an elective procedure under a general anaesthetic. This is not necessary, however, and decompression in labour may be achieved successfully under epidural analge-

sia. From below, fluid can be withdrawn from the fetal head by an appropriate needle and syringe. This method may be preferred when the accoucheur wishes to preserve the child's heart beat. Simpson's perforator is a preferred alternative. With the help of a good light and an optimal visual field, the fetal scalp may be grasped between two pairs of straight forceps, and the fold of skin cut with scissors. Into this small 'button-hole' is passed the point of the perforator. The 'button-hole' secures its point and prevents its blades from slipping towards the bladder as they are pushed into the fetal skull. It is of little concern whether the perforation occurs through a suture line or one of the cranial bones. The hole may be kept open with a short length of rubber pressure tubing until the skull collapses. A Drew Smythe catheter can be most useful when decompressing the fetal head. The pointed tip of the catheter can be inserted easily into the scalp 'buttonhole', then pushed into the cranial cavity to allow the escape of cerebrospinal fluid. After all the fluid has been withdrawn the catheter may be used to destroy the vital centres of the medulla.

When the fetus presents by the breech decompression of the fetal head can be more difficult to achieve. Sometimes there may be an associated spina bifida, in which case it may be possible to insert a metal cannula into the open spinal canal. Otherwise it is necessary, while applying traction to the breech to keep the fetal head against the pelvic brim, to cut transversely between the cervical vertebrae and expose the dilated spinal cord. This is more difficult than it sounds. A Drew Smythe catheter can then be introduced through the space between the cervical vertebrae and guided into the cranial cavity. An alternative technique is to insert a wide bore needle through the suture lines via the maternal abdomen. The author does not favour this method, as it may compromise the maternal bladder or promote bleeding from the partially retracted uterus.

Although it is unusual to detect minor degrees of hydrocephalus before labour, Caesarean section is probably the treatment of choice in these suspicious circumstances.

INIENCEPHALY

Because of the gross extension of the head caused by this abnormality the practical problem is one of an unremediable brow presentation (Fig. 26.5). Accordingly, Caesarean section is necessary unless labour begins extremely prematurely.

ANENCEPHALY

The anencephalic fetus may develop to become a large baby. The absence of the fetal skull results in a face presentation. This is rather a poor dilator of the soft passage and prolonged labour may occur.

The main problem is that of shoulder dystocia. This can be difficult to overcome by the methods described previously. However, as there is no urgency to deliver the baby the problem can be dealt with slowly, if necessary as an elective procedure under general anaesthesia. There should be no hesitation in fracturing the fetal clavicles.

OTHER ABNORMALITIES OF THE FETUS

Congenital goitre or a lymphangioma may give rise to a face presentation. Abdominal enlargement caused by ascites, bladder distension, renal tumour, enlargement of the liver or spleen, or even a gross umbilical hernia, may cause dystocia. When there is doubt about this type of abnormality an X-ray can sometimes prove helpful for it may reveal the traditional Buddha position with flaring of the fetal ribs and arms away from the body and the legs abducted and flexed.

Cystic abnormalities can be reduced by needle aspiration but evisceration may be required for the firmer tumours.

MONSTERS

Conjoined twins, in which survival seems possible, are best delivered by Caesarean section about 38 weeks' gestation. In the unlikely event that conjoined twins have remained undiagnosed until the second stage of labour, examination under anaesthesia will prove necessary. If the second twin is contained in a sac of membranes, there is obviously no union between the babies. If, however, no sac of membranes is felt or one of the twins is lying transversely, suspicion will be aroused. When an unsuspected diagnosis of double monster has to be seriously entertained it is in the mother's best interests to abandon any attempt at vaginal delivery and undertake Caesarean section.

Teratomas of the jaw or sacrum do not usually cause a significant problem. When they are too large to be rotated into the sacrum and removed, Caesarean section is advisable to safeguard the mother from undue damage during labour.

REFERENCES

ADEY D. & KNEALE B. (1966) Aust. N.Z. J. Obstet. Gynaec., 6, 80.
Brit. med. J. (1979) i, 362.
Brit. med. J. (1980) i, 1393.
CHISWICK M.L. & JAMES D.K. (1979) Brit. med. J., i, 7.
DAVIDSON A.C., WEAVER J.B., DAVIES P. & PEARSON J.F. (1976) Brit. J. Obstet. Gynaec., 83, 279.
DAW E. (1970) Practitioner, 204, 559.
EGWUATA V.E. & AGUGUA N.E.N. (1981) Brit. J. Obstet. Gynaec., 88, 1090.
FORUHAN B. & JENNINGS P.J. (1978) Brit. J. Obstet. Gynaec., 85, 231.
FRANCIS H.H. (1959) Surg. Gynec. Obstet., 103, 295.
FREETH A. & MAIR J. (1951) Brit. med. J., i, 512.
GEMMELL A.A. & HAINES M. (1960) J. Obstet. Gynaec. Brit. Emp., 67, 199.
HANNA W.J. (1965) Amer. J. Obstet. Gynec., 91, 333.
HEMMINGSON E. (1982) Brit. J. Obstet. Gynaec., 89, 675.

Lobb M.O. & Beazley J.M. (1984) *J. Obstet. Gynaec.*, **4**, 181.

McLaren H.C., Jordan J.A., Glover M. & Attwood M.E. (1974) *J. Obstet. Gynaec. Brit. Cwlth.*, **81**, 383.

Rubin E.L. & Francis H. (1967) *Clin. Radiol.*, **18**, No. 2, 213.

Sutherst J.R. & Case B.D. (1975) In *Clinics in Obstetrics and Gynaecology* (Beazley J.M. ed) 2e, p. 241. W.B. Saunders, London.

Vaclavinkova V. (1973) *Acta Obstet. Gynec. Scand.*, **52**, 161.

Weekes A.R.L., Atlay R.D., Brown V.A., Jordan E.C., Murray S.M. (1976) *Brit. med. J.*, **i**, 622.

CHAPTER 27
MALPOSITIONS OF THE OCCIPUT AND MALPRESENTATIONS

J. W. K. RITCHIE

Introduction

Malpositions and malpresentations carry an increased risk for both mother and fetus which is greatest when the mother is unattended or is managed during labour by inexperienced personnel.

The maternal risks include prolonged labour, which may lead to infection and, if neglected, can result in obstructed labour. General anaesthesia may be required at short notice when the mother is in poor condition and difficult vaginal delivery or Caesarean section may result in trauma leading to haemorrhage. In the puerperium venous thrombosis and fatal pulmonary embolism may occur as a result of damage to the pelvic veins. In developing countries obstructed labour may cause tissue necrosis and lead to vesico-vaginal and recto-vaginal fistula.

Perinatal mortality and morbidity associated with malposition or malpresentation are high, partly because fetal malformation, intrauterine death and extreme prematurity go hand in hand. Malpresentations predispose to cord prolapse, abnormal uterine action and prolonged or obstructed labour, all potent causes of fetal hypoxia which may be fatal. In addition the fetus is at risk of infection after prolonged rupture of the membranes and also meconium aspiration. Finally, traumatic delivery, maternal hypoxia or hypotension during anaesthesia and maternal ketosis and dehydration may further endanger the fetus.

For optimal results it is necessary to follow early diagnosis by skilled assessment and planned delivery by experienced staff working in proper surroundings. It should be stressed that for these most difficult cases experienced anaesthetists must be available. If vaginal delivery is decided upon, vigilant supervision, full use of available monitoring methods and the facility to perform immediate operative delivery or Caesarean section are mandatory. Review of progress and necessary intervention by currently active and dextrous senior staff members should be the rule.

Cross-matched blood should be readily available throughout 24 hours.

Many of these points are emphasized by the Reports on Confidential Enquiries into Maternal Deaths in England and Wales (HMSO 1969, 1972, 1975, 1979). Although the number of deaths from ruptured uterus have fallen dramatically over recent years it is unfortunate that a significant proportion still result from unwise management of a malpresentation or malposition.

OCCIPITO-POSTERIOR POSITIONS AND DEEP TRANSVERSE ARREST

When the head engages the occiput is usually lateral, but will rotate anteriorly during labour in four cases out of five. Very rarely the head is born with the occiput lateral and occasionally it will rotate to an occipito-posterior position.

In about one-fifth of cases the occiput is posterior during early labour with the sagittal suture in one or other oblique diameter, usually the right. A left occipito-posterior position is rare, possibly because the colon occupies the left posterior pelvic quadrant and also because the uterus usually shows dextro-rotation. Should flexion increase during labour the occiput may become the leading part and rotate anteriorly on reaching the pelvic floor. When deflexion persists, or increases, the bregma will be the part which first reaches the pelvic floor, by which it will be rotated forwards so causing the occiput to rotate backwards.

The head can enter the brim in the direct occipito-posterior position when the fetus is small and the pelvis capacious, or when a larger fetus engages in an anthropoid pelvis which possesses a long oval inlet and generous measurements (especially of the hind pelvis). Under such favourable circumstances the head descends without rotation and can be born with ease face-to-pubis. In these patients the perinatal mortality and morbidity and the duration of labour are no greater than with occipito-anterior positions, nor does the incidence of operative delivery rise (Calkins 1953).

When there is delay in spontaneous labour an occipito-posterior position is one of the three possible causes, the others being cephalo-pelvic disproportion and inefficient uterine action. This position of the occiput is more common in primigravidas in whom inefficient uterine action should be treated with intravenous oxytocin. With this cause of delay in labour removed it becomes a relatively simple matter to decide which of the two remaining problems are accounting for failure to progress normally. Although there is bound to be some overlap it does not affect management, as O'Driscoll and Meagher (1980) have pointed out, and the differential diagnosis should be based entirely on the position of the occiput.

Aetiology

An anteriorly situated placenta or a pelvic brim which is longer antero-posteriorly than transversely is said to predispose to an occipito-posterior position. If the back of the fetus comes to lie along the front of the maternal spine, normal fetal flexion will be decreased. The resulting deflexion of the head tends to maintain the occipito-posterior position. This effect is less in a multipara whose abdominal muscles tend to be lax.

Much less emphasis has been placed on abnormal pelvic shapes in modern obstetrical practice because of their rarity, but two main types have an inlet in which the antero-posterior diameter equals or exceeds the transverse; the anthropoid and the android.

The anthropoid pelvis has a longitudinally oval

inlet, large measurements (especially the posterior sagittal diameters), wide greater sciatic notches and an adequate subpubic arch. Even if there is high assimilation a direct occipito-posterior position in the pelvis may be regarded as normal and safe delivery face-to-pubis can be expected. This will be true for any capacious pelvis with a small baby. The android pelvis, however, favours an oblique occipito-posterior position. The relatively flat sacrum, reduced posterior saggital diameters, small sacrosciatic notches and prominent ischial spines make anterior rotation less likely, and cessation of progress with the occiput posterior or transverse will occur much more frequently. The report of Holmberg et al. (1977) reviewed these features in 68 consecutive cases which were studied by X-ray pelvimetry.

It is now recognized that many such mechanical problems may be overcome by efficient uterine action (O'Driscoll & Meagher 1980).

Diagnosis

There may be visible flattening of the abdomen below the umbilicus, and in direct occipito-posterior positions a dip may be palpable. Limbs are felt anteriorly, the anterior shoulder being palpated at some distance from the mid-line. The back is often difficult to define but can usually be identified well round in the flank, where the fetal heart is best heard. Deflexion is revealed when the prominences of sinciput and occiput can both be felt at the same level above the symphysis pubis (Fig. 27.1), and the head will feel relatively large from side to side. Extreme deflexion may result in the fetal heart tones being best heard anteriorly in the midline, albeit faintly.

Vaginal examination in early labour reveals a high

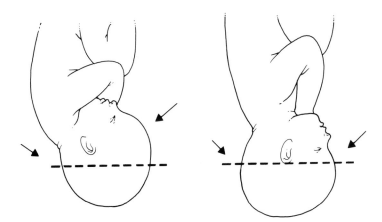

Fig. 27.1. The hands palpating a well-flexed head (left) are at different levels; those palpating a deflexed head (right) are at the same level

deflexed head, the anterior fontanelle occupying the centre of the pelvis whilst the posterior lies at a higher level and is difficult to reach. The sagittal suture may occupy an oblique diameter or may run antero-posteriorly.

Anterior rotation will be preceded by increased flexion so that the posterior fontanelle becomes progressively easier to feel lower and more centrally in the pelvis, whilst the anterior recedes. Continuing deflexion, however, is associated with posterior rotation.

In late labour, when forceps are to be applied, landmarks may be obscured by moulding and caput. The occipital bone is, however, the only one which is overriden by both its neighbours. Furthermore, if two adjacent fingers are drawn along the length of the sagittal suture, with one on either side of it, they must either cross the lambdoid suture and reach the occipital bone or alternatively traverse the coronal suture to reach the frontal bone. The frontal bone unlike the occipital bone is in halves separated by the frontal suture. The two parts of this bone can be made to move one upon the other by gentle pressure with the adjacent fingers. If still in doubt, an ear should be sought, both tragus and pinna being identified.

One has a final opportunity to correct misdiagnosis when applying forceps. With an unrecognized and uncorrected occipito-posterior position the forceps will lock with difficulty or not at all. Traction will need to be greater than anticipated, the perineum will stretch and the anus gape while the presenting part is still high, and the forceps will not sweep forwards as the head descends.

The earlier delay in labour is treated the less difficulty is encountered with moulding and caput as these are much reduced.

Features of labour

Backache and incoordinate uterine action are not infrequent, but Friedman and Kroll (1972), using the grapho-statistical method, emphasized that these abnormalities are often indicative of associated disproportion. The occipito-transverse position shows a persistent prolongation of all phases, and an occipito-posterior one is characterized by a lowered maximum slope and slower active phase. Premature rupture of membranes is common, and may lead to problems of prolapsed cord and infection. Miller (1930) emphasized that when the membranes rupture prematurely the chance of spontaneous delivery

is much reduced. Deep perineal laceration may occur unless the child is small and the patient multiparous. Early distension of perineum and dilatation of anus with the head comparatively high will suggest that face-to-pubis delivery is likely.

Treatment

Attempts at antenatal correction have been abandoned.

During labour, interference may be called for because of fetal hypoxia, cessation of progress, or incidental complications the most important of which are prolapse of the cord and cephalopelvic disproportion. Cessation of progress is usually associated with abnormal internal rotation due to poor uterine action. Slow progress in the first stage of labour due to posterior position of the occiput in primigravidas should be treated with intravenous oxytocin infusion to augment uterine contractions. If satisfactory progress is not achieved delivery by Caesarean section is indicated.

In the second stage if the occipito-posterior position exists it is mandatory to ensure that uterine contractions are efficient, and again oxytocin is used to achieve this. When strictly carried out this regimen results in surprisingly few cases in which rotation and extraction with forceps are necessary. In the presence of efficient uterine action this position of the occiput adversely affects the outcome of labour in about 1 in 250 primigravidas, encouraging some obstetricians to adopt a policy of delivery by Caesarean section when it persists for more than one hour in the second stage, unless the head is on the pelvic floor and delivery can be effected by forceps directly face-to-pubis or after easy manual rotation (O'Driscoll & Meagher 1980).

It is now recognized that transverse arrest of the occiput is not the result of obstruction in the vast majority of cases, but the result of inadequate forces of expulsion which can be overcome by augmentation with oxytocin. This procedure is safer than attempts at rotation and traction on a head still at the level of the ischial spines, and it is usually effective.

All patients require careful, frequent and expert assessment of progress by abdominal and vaginal examination. Cervical dilatation is best recorded graphically. Adequate intravenous fluid replacement, to avoid ketosis, and fetal monitoring by the best available method are essential. Epidural analgesia is especially helpful where backache is a problem or augmentation with oxytocin is being carried out. Paracervical block is no longer used because it has been reported to produce frequent (7%) fetal brady-cardia and occasional fetal death.

Assisted delivery

CAESAREAN SECTION

This may be performed for disproportion, associated conditions not due to the malpresentation, prolapsed cord or fetal distress. For the last indication it will certainly be the correct method if the cervix is less than 5 cm dilated. In developed countries the tendency is towards more Caesarean sections and fewer difficult forceps deliveries which have in the past been shown to carry a risk of cerebral damage of 7.3% (British Congress in Glasgow 1965).

Traumatic intracranial haemorrhage is a well recognized complication of forceps delivery (O'Driscoll *et al.* 1981).

VENTOUSE DELIVERY

The ventouse takes up no space necessary for rotation, can be used under pudendal block or perineal infiltration, and encourages flexion. It allows the occiput to rotate in the direction most suitable for delivery through a particular pelvis. Thus 5% of occipito-transverse and one-third of occipito-posterior positions rotate to direct occipito-posterior and are delivered as such. In his series Chalmers (1968) found that instrumental delivery was needed in 11.1% of occipito-transverse or occipito-posterior positions. The ventouse alone was successful in 85.8% of occipito-posterior and 89.6% of occipito-transverse positions. It was not employed by him if the head was high, disproportion was present, or the cervix was less than half dilated. Most obstetricians would reserve ventouse delivery for cases where the cervix is fully dilated or almost so, preferring to manage delay with oxytocics. A reduced perinatal mortality has been claimed for the ventouse, as compared to the obstetric forceps, though as with all instruments its unwise application or unskilled use can cause grave fetal damage.

FORCEPS ROTATION AND EXTRACTIONS

Kielland's forceps have been deservedly popular with those obstetricians trained to use them properly. They can be used with local anaesthesia, but epidural, spinal or general anaesthesia is preferable. Correct cephalic application is followed by disimpaction and rotation at the level of optimal diameters and extraction without reapplication. For the android pelvis, it is a disadvantage to rotate until the presenting part is very low (d'Esopo 1941). Contrary to general teaching, it is not necessary to perform episiotomy before application, or even before rotation. Indeed it is an advantage to defer episiotomy until rotation has been performed, so reducing the danger of spiral vaginal tears. It is usually helpful to re-examine the patient when rotation has been half completed as a final check that all is well.

Parry-Jones (1968) reviewed the use of Barton's forceps for the occipito-transverse position. These instruments must be used only by properly trained operators.

Other types of forceps demand more than one application in a Scanzoni manoeuvre. They include Shute's forceps, which are little used in Britain.

The perinatal mortality figures are today too crude an index of fetal outcome. In a review of the relative results of mid forceps operations and Caesarean section for malrotation at full dilatation, Hughey *et al.* (1978) found a less than ideal outcome in 30.8% of infants delivered by forceps especially when growth retardation, prematurity, extremes of maternal age, very small or very large infants and other risk factors were present. In a report from Manchester (Chiswick & James 1979), attempted Kielland's forceps delivery was associated with an increased perinatal morbidity, including a neonatal mortality of 3.49% when compared with vaginal delivery. Unfortunately this was not a valid comparison, since the results of delivery by Kielland's forceps must be compared with those of alternative methods of delivery. Certainly, Healey *et al.* (1982) were unable to show any difference in neonatal outcome when rotation with Kielland's forceps was compared with other methods of rotation and delivery.

Traub *et al.* (1984) examined the outcome in newborns following Kielland's forceps delivery and in those where Caesarean section was performed in the second stage of labour, and no significant difference could be demonstrated. They concluded that in well trained hands there is still a place for the use of this instrument in properly selected cases. However, training of younger obstetricians in their use has become increasingly difficult because of the decrease in the number of suitable cases.

This method is favoured by some who feel it is more gentle than rotation with forceps. It suffers from the disadvantages that deep general anaesthesia may be necessary. The hand itself diminishes the available space, displacement of the head can only be upwards so that it can never be drawn down to a more favourable level for rotation. Excessive displacement of the head can cause cord prolapse or may tempt the operator to perform the dangerous high forceps delivery. Despite these disadvantages it is still a very useful technique, particularly as experience with Kielland's forceps diminishes.

Manual rotation and forceps delivery of a right occipito-posterior position will be facilitated by putting the patient in the exaggerated left lateral position, if the operator is familiar with the technique.

FACE PRESENTATION

Friedman (1967) calculated an incidence of 1 in 496 from a review of literature totalling 1645 face presentations. Incidences of 1 in 596, 1 in 443, 1 in 380 and 1 in 305 have been reported by Cruickshank and White (1973), Agüero and Kizer (1972), Posner *et al.* (1963) and Mostar *et al.* (1966).

Aetiology

In early labour minor deflexion attitudes are common, especially with occipito-posterior positions and multiparity (Fig. 27.2). In such cases uterine contractions often cause increased flexion, but occasionally extension will increase so producing successively a brow presentation and finally the fully extended face. Most face presentations are thus secondary, becoming evident only in established labour.

Anencephaly, stated by earlier authors to be one of the commonest causes, has since been reported in less than 10% of cases. With wider use of alphafetoprotein estimations and ultrasound the number of pregnancies with anencephaly reaching later pregnancy has fallen. Should a face be felt during vaginal examination the possibility of anencephaly must be considered, but when discussing the management and outcome of face presentation it is usual to exclude consideration of the anencephalic fetus.

In many series no cause could be found in almost half the cases.

Prematurity is a definite association occurring in 34% of the cases of Posner *et al.* (1963). Friedman (1967) quoted a 25% incidence of prematurity in his patients with face presentation, against a generally expected incidence of 9.8%.

A large baby (3.7 kg or over) does not seem to be a constant feature.

In the past contracted pelvis was diagnosed, but this is not a common association in more recent reviews (Cruickshank & White 1973, Agüero & Kizer 1972).

Multiple pregnancy is a frequent cause (Posner *et al.* 1963). This may act by causing hyperextension, although other mechanisms may be involved.

Other possible fetal factors include the presence of several loops of cord round the neck, tumours such as goitre and an unduly large thorax. Polyhydramnios, pelvic tumours, bicornuate uterus, uterine obliquity and placenta praevia may each account for the occasional case. Primary extensor tone is well documented, but the proportion of cases thought to be caused by it varies widely.

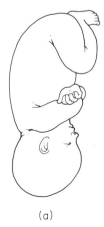 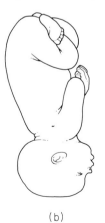 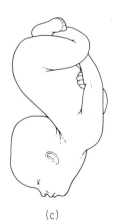

Fig. 27.2. Deflexion attitudes. In (a) the child is in the military attitude of early deflexion often associated with the occipito-posterior position; in (b) there is more deflexion amounting almost to brow presentation; in (c) extension is complete and the face presents.

(a)   (b)   (c)

The importance of multiparity in producing face presentation is difficult to assess, but Posner *et al.* (1963) found that over 70% of their patients were multiparae. Increasing numbers of face presentations have been reported as maternal age rises.

Dolicocephaly is probably a result of face delivery and not its cause. Rapid recovery of normal skull shape after birth is usual.

Positions

Posner *et al.* (1963) found that 77% of face presentations were mento-anterior. The results of X-ray examination suggest that more mento-transverse positions would be present if diagnosis were made earlier (Borrel & Fernstrom 1960).

Diagnosis

The majority of face presentations are secondary and arise in labour. Primary face presentations will oc-

casionally be diagnosed on antenatal radiographs taken because of a high head or bizarre abdominal findings (Fig. 27.3).

In half the cases the diagnosis is not made until delivery is imminent (Posner *et al.* 1963).

ABDOMINAL FINDINGS

The well rounded breech is prominent in the fundus. The fetal back can be felt easily near the breech but recedes from the examining hand and is difficult to define in the lower half of the uterus. Limbs are felt anteriorly, usually to one side of the mid-line. In vertex presentations one can distinguish a triangular pool of liquor bounded by the fetal arms, legs and body, but in face and brow presentation this triangle is absent. Between the anterior shoulder and the head prominence there is a characteristic deep depression in which no fetal part can be felt. A large amount of the head is palpable on the same side as the back, but no cephalic prominence can be felt on the same side of the pelvic inlet as the limbs. Fetal heart sounds transmitted through the thorax are heard most clearly on the same side as the limbs, which is also the side opposite the maximum cephalic prominence. Palpation of the lower pole of the fetus may be rendered difficult by overdistension, spasm or tenderness of the lower segment.

VAGINAL FINDINGS

During this examination one should avoid damaging the eyes by trauma or antiseptics. In early labour the presenting part will be high. Landmarks are the mouth, jaws, nose, malar and orbital ridges. The presence of alveolar margins distinguishes the mouth from the anus. It also helps to remember that mouth and maxillae form the corners of a triangle, whilst the anus is on a straight line between the ischial tuberosities; this is especially helpful when oedema is present. Vaginal examination must include a thorough search for cord presentation or prolapse.

Labour in face presentation

As the face is incompressible and irregular it might be expected to exert little stimulus on the lower segment and so predispose to inertia. However, Friedman (1967) suggests that abnormal uterine action usually results from associated bony dystocia and not the malpresentation itself. The poor line of thrust between body and head of the fetus usually results in

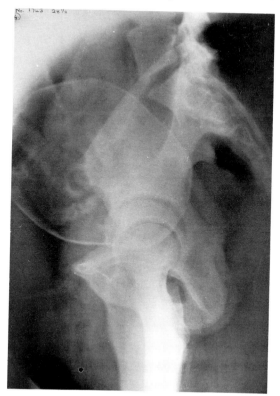

Fig. 27.3. A lateral X-ray showing a fetus presenting by the face. Note the narrower bifrontal diameter at the lowest level and the wider biparietal diameter above the pelvic brim.

prolongation of the second stage of labour. Early rupture of membranes may occur.

Descent occurs, followed by internal rotation, the chin passing anteriorly. It must be remembered that the biparietal diameter is 7 cm behind the advancing face, so that even when the face is distending the vulva, the biparietal diameter has only just entered the pelvis (see Fig. 27.3). Descent is thus always less advanced than vaginal examination would suggest, even when one allows for the gross oedema which is usually present. The value of abdominal examination in such cases cannot be overstressed. Anterior rotation having occurred, the neck comes to lie behind the symphysis and the head is born by flexion, causing considerable perineal distension in the process. The shoulders and body are then born in the usual way.

In cases of persisting mento-posterior position the neck is too short to span the 12 cm of the anterior aspect of the sacrum. Delivery is impossible unless, as can happen with a very small fetus or one which is macerated, the shoulders can enter the pelvis at the same time as the head. With satisfactory uterine action and a mento-anterior position, spontaneous or easy 'lift-out' assisted delivery ensues in 80% or more. Even with mento-posterior positions, anterior rotation will occur in the second stage in 45–65% of cases, so that persistent mento-posterior position or mento-transverse arrest are encountered in only 10% of face presentations.

Management

Fetal abnormality and contracted pelvis must first be excluded. One then considers: the patient's age and parity; the previous obstetric history; whether the uterus is scarred from previous surgery; whether complications such as pre-eclampsia or placenta praevia co-exist and, finally, whether the child is thought to be larger than 3.5 kg. It may now be evident that elective Caesarean section is wise.

In cases where elective Caesarean section is not necessary, labour is carefully supervised, progress being assessed by careful examination per abdomen as well as per vaginam; continuous fetal monitoring is valuable. With mento-anterior positions no interference is necessary whilst satisfactory progress continues and there is no fetal distress or cord prolapse. Generous episiotomy is always necessary.

Assistance is required if progress ceases, a mento-posterior position persists or if fetal distress occurs. The choice then lies between forceps rotation and extraction, or Caesarean section. Before contemplating the former one must be certain that the cervix is fully dilated and that there is no suspicion of cephalo-pelvic disproportion. The Caesarean section rate in this type of case is from 25 to 30%. A vertical lower segment incision may sometimes be useful.

In a neglected case with an impacted dead fetus, the choice between craniotomy and Caesarean section is influenced by local conditions.

Internal version and breech extraction are dangerous both to mother and child. They have no place in treating face presentation.

After birth, the oedema and bruising of the child's face can persist for some days and may make feeding difficult.

Increasing use of Caesarean section and the avoidance of complicated vaginal manoeuvres have reduced the perinatal mortality to a figure similar to that for occipito-posterior positions of the vertex. The mother is liable to all the puerperal complications which can follow prolonged labour, instrumental delivery, deep perineal laceration and bruising.

BROW PRESENTATION

This extension attitude arises between deflexed vertex and face presentations. An incidence of 1 in 1050 deliveries was quoted by Berger et al. (1967), reviewing the literature of the last 30 years. Many brow presentations early in labour are transient, proceeding to full deflexion or alternatively undergoing spontaneous flexion and correction to vertex.

Aetiology

The causes are those of face presentation and will not be repeated. Prematurity is twice as common as expected (Berger et al. 1967, Meltzer et al. 1967). Contracted pelvis is less commonly reported than before but has been found in 10.9% of cases (Meltzer et al. 1967). Even this was four times the expected incidence in their practice.

Diagnosis

Abdominal findings resemble those in face presentation. The fetal back is very difficult to feel except near the breech and the fetal heart is best heard on the same side as the limbs, whilst the maximum head prominence is on the side opposite the limbs. Unlike face presentation, however, a head prominence is

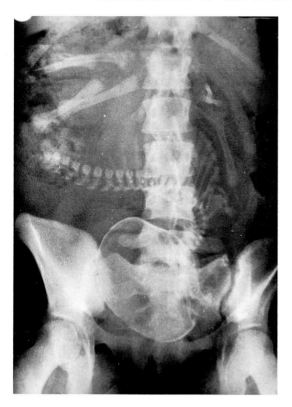

Fig. 27.4. An antero-posterior X-ray showing marked deflexion of the fetus and a brow presentation.

palpable on the same side as the limbs and the groove between anterior shoulder and head, though distinct, is less marked. The head feels large from side to side, so that hydrocephaly may be suspected. Many cases are diagnosed by X-ray for 'high head' at term or in early labour (Fig. 27.4).

On vaginal examination a hard, high, rounded part presents, the bregma occupying the centre of the dilating cervix. Frontal suture, anterior fontanelle, orbital ridges and nasion can be identified, but nose, mouth and chin cannot be felt. In labour a large caput succedaneum may make diagnosis almost impossible. The nasion is more often found anteriorly than posteriorly.

Course of labour

Prolonged and complicated labour has often been described (Madden 1956, Posner et al. 1957). More recent studies suggest that prolongation of the second stage and of the phase of deceleration in the first stage are the only consistent features and that other abnormalities in the first stage such as incoordinate action or arrest of dilatation are indicative of disproportion (Friedman 1967, Posner et al. 1963). There is a slightly increased incidence of premature rupture of membranes.

In persisting brow presentation the mento-vertical diameter has to engage, which is unlikely, but may be possible with a capacious pelvis and a small fetus, which becomes markedly moulded. Following engagement, anterior rotation will occur and the forehead, orbital ridges and nasion will appear at the vulva. The maxilla then becomes fixed against the lower part of the symphysis pubis, and by flexion of the head the brow, anterior fontanelle, vertex and occiput successively appear. Finally the face and chin slip out from behind the symphysis. Occasionally following engagement spontaneous correction to a vertex will occur in the pelvis. In patients with contracted pelvis or when a large or average size fetus is present with a normal pelvis, engagement may be impossible. The case then becomes one of obstructed labour.

Prognosis

Should the brow presentation be transient, the first stage of labour of average length and moulding not excessive the prognosis for the infant is that of the face or vertex presentation which ensues. In persistent brow presentation the outlook is best where the fetus is small and the pelvis large. With a term fetus of average size the factor of disproportion is all important and fetal mortality will rise because of gross moulding, early rupture of membranes, long labour and the need for operative delivery. These will also contribute to maternal morbidity.

Management

Fetal abnormality and pelvic contraction must first be excluded. This done, no treatment is necessary if labour progresses normally, especially if the infant is small. In all 11 such cases described by Posner et al. (1963) vaginal delivery proved possible. In assessing progress, however, it must be remembered that increasing caput succedaneum can produce a false impression of descent of the presenting part.

Pelvic contraction, associated disease or a term infant persisting as a brow presentation are best treated by Caesarean section. Should delay in labour or fetal distress become evident then again Caesarean section is the best treatment.

OTHER POSSIBLE COURSES OF ACTION

Conversion manoeuvres

Thorn's manoeuvre attempts a radical conversion to vertex presentation. It is performed under general anaesthesia and demands not only an adequate amount of liquor (i.e. membranes should be intact or only recently have ruptured), but also the cervix dilated enough to allow a hand to be introduced into the uterus. The occasions on which it can safely be attempted are, therefore, extremely rare. Conversion to a face presentation is feasible even less often. Both manoeuvres have largely been abandoned.

Forceps or ventouse extraction

By rotation with Kielland's forceps, which allows increasing flexion of the head, or through increased flexion produced by the ventouse, delivery of the deeply engaged brow presentation may be possible, but this method should be used only when full dilation has been achieved and there is no suspicion of disproportion. The percentage so delivered has fallen, reflecting a general trend in all centres away from difficult vaginal delivery because of the improved prospects of the fetus born by Caesarean section (but see cautionary *Lancet* Editorial 1980).

Craniotomy

This can be used in cases of fetal abnormality. It is otherwise reserved for cases which have passed unrecognized resulting in obstructed labour with a dead fetus under circumstances where Caesarean section is to be avoided if possible. Such conditions should not occur if cases are properly supervised (Lawson & Stewart 1967). In developed countries Caesarean section is usually safer than craniotomy even when the fetus is dead.

Internal podalic or bipolar version have no place in the management of brow presentation.

BREECH PRESENTATION

Among cases in the Perinatal Mortality Survey of 1958 the infant presented as a breech at delivery in 2.11% (Butler & Bonham 1964). A similar incidence was found for singleton pregnancy in the North West London Region (Law 1967) and in the 1970 British Births Survey (Chamberlain *et al.* 1975). In the United States, Hall *et al.* (1965) quoted 3.17% in 190661 deliveries between 1955 and 1959.

Aetiology

Between 30 and 40% of singletons present by the breech between 20–25 weeks and 15% at 32 weeks (Sørensen *et al.* 1979), but by week 34 most have undergone spontaneous version to a head presentation. Subsequent reversion to breech is rare, occurring in 4% (Vartan 1945). It is, therefore, hardly surprising that premature infants comprise up to a quarter of babies born by the breech. In patients who reach term with breech presentation, the cause must be sought among conditions which have prevented spontaneous version. These include multiple pregnancy, oligohydramnios and abnormalities of uterine shape whether congenital or the result of attachment of the placenta in the cornual region or the lower uterine segment (Hall *et al.* 1965, Hay 1959). In 72.6% of a series of 124 full term breech deliveries the placental site was shown to be cornual by ultrasound compared with 4.8% of controls (Fianu & Vaclavinkova 1978). In a multipara with a breech presentation there is a 14% incidence of previous breech delivery. This suggests a persisting abnormality of uterine shape as an aetiological factor. The proportion of frank breech presentations increases markedly towards term, suggesting that extended legs also hinder spontaneous version. Extended legs occur often in the fetus of the primigravida, so possibly accounting for the disproportionately large number of breech presentations noted in these patients (Friedman 1967, Hall *et al.* 1965, Law 1967).

Other conditions which favour breech presentation include hydrocephaly, polyhydramnios, intrauterine fetal death and, very occasionally, pelvic tumours. Opinion is divided over the extent to which breech presentation can be caused by contracted pelvis. Vartan (1945) stated that this was of slight importance in aetiology, though of vital interest when deciding the mode of delivery. Beischer (1966) could demonstrate contracted pelvis clinically in only 3% of his series, though this figure rose sharply in the small group in whom X-ray pelvimetry was performed. Friedman (1967) found disproportion of twice the expected frequency, but commented that with breech presentation this was more carefully sought and evaluated than with head presentations.

Diagnosis

There is no characteristic finding on abdominal inspection. Palpation reveals the hard, round, ballottable head occupying the fundus uteri, with the back on one side and limbs on the other. The rather narrow and softer breech may be mobile above the pelvic brim or may dip through it. When the head is strictly in the mid-line it is probable that the legs are extended, and a frank breech is also suspected if the presenting part is deeply engaged. The fetal heart will be heard best above the umbilicus. On vaginal examination prior to labour the presenting part is usually high, of softer consistency than the head and may be irregular in outline. Confirmation of the diagnosis can be obtained by sonar, which will also exclude placenta praevia and multiple pregnancy, or by radiography which will exclude multiple pregnancy and also reveal major skeletal abnormality. Both methods will show hydrocephalus and will usually exclude major degrees of spina bifida. X-ray examination will reveal the degree of flexion or extension of the head. Sonar will reveal fetal ascites or abdominal tumours.

In labour the presenting part will be high initially, but rapid descent is to be expected and at full dilatation the station should be comparable with that of a vertex presentation. Even when the presenting part is high, a deliberate search must be made to exclude cord presentation. Later, with a frank breech, the tuber ischii, sacrum and anus are palpable and the external genitalia may be identified. During prolonged labour or with slow cervical dilatation, the marked oedema which results may make the distinction difficult between breech and face presentation. Abdominal examination is helpful. On vaginal examination the diagnostic features of face presentation are the maxillae and jaws. Meconium may soil a finger inserted into the fetal anus.

In complete breech presentation the feet may be felt alongside the buttocks, while in foot and knee presentations the appropriate parts are evident. Though

the hard projection of the heel identifies the foot, the examiner should follow the limb in continuity to the buttock before diagnosing a footling breech presentation, as it is possible for a foot to present alongside the head in one form of compound presentation.

Early diagnosis of breech presentation allows time for adequate assessment and delivery under optimal conditions.

Types of breech presentation

EXTENDED OR FRANK BREECH

The lower extremities are fully flexed at the hip and fully extended at the knee (see Fig. 27.5). The feet are thus high in the uterus, leaving a smooth, well-fitting presenting part which tends to engage early, so making external cephalic version less easy. The snug fit results in a low incidence of cord prolapse with a fetus of average size. The frank breech occurs in 60–70% of cases, being more frequent in primigravidas and as term approaches. Difficulty in delivering the aftercoming head would be expected less often than in footling breech, because with a fetus of average size the passage of the combined mass of both thighs and the fetal abdomen is only possible through a fully dilated cervix. It was an unexpected finding in the series of Law (1967) that, except in primiparas in premature labour, the perinatal mortality was uninfluenced by the position of the legs, and that both first and second stages of labour were actually shorter in cases with flexed legs.

FLEXED OR COMPLETE BREECH

Here the hips and knees of the fetus are flexed, the feet being closely applied to the dorsal aspect of the

Fig. 27.5. Types of breech presentation.

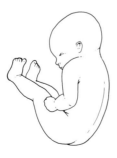   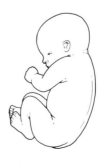   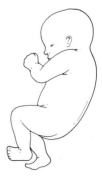

Frank breech   Flexed breech   Footling presentation

thighs (see Fig. 27.5). The presenting part is more irregular and less pointed, so that early engagement is less likely and prolapse of the cord is four times as common as in frank breech (Law 1967), occurring in 4–6.3% of flexed mature breech births; Hay (1959) found prolapse of the cord on 20% of flexed breech and in no case of frank breech. Breech presentation is the commonest association with prolapse of the cord, accounting for 40–50% of cases.

FOOTLING OR KNEE PRESENTATION— INCOMPLETE BREECH

These are self-explanatory, presentation of one or both feet being more common than knee presentation (Fig. 27.5). Not only is there a high risk of presentation or prolapse of the cord but delivery of the infant up to the level of the thorax may occur through an incompletely dilated cervix. This is especially liable to occur if the obstetrician is foolishly tempted to deliver the baby vaginally prior to full dilatation because one or both lower limbs have appeared at the vulva or because of clinical fetal distress or cord prolapse.

The dangers of breech delivery

Risks to the mother include sepsis, tears of vagina, cervix, perineum and uterus, usually due to unwise or unskilled attempts at vaginal delivery. A small increase in postpartum haemorrhage formerly quoted is less obvious when active management of the third stage is employed. The dangers of emergency anaesthesia and emergency Caesarean section must not be forgotten.

The main risks are to the child, but perinatal mortality figures afford only a crude assessment of the efficiency of obstetric management. In considering breech delivery it is usual to correct the figure by excluding antepartum deaths, congenital malformations incompatible with life, cases of haemolytic disease and first week deaths unconnected with the mode of delivery. When this was done in the North West London Region (Law 1967) the figures for multiparas and first labours were 10.5% and 6.6% respectively. Even when cases of low birth weight, placenta praevia and congenital abnormalities were excluded Rovinsky et al. (1973) found the perinatal mortality to be four times that for vertex presentations similarly corrected. There is general agreement that the perinatal loss is greater in multiparous patients (Brenner et al. 1974, Law 1967, Methuen

1958), though Potter et al. (1960) and Wulff et al. (1960) found the converse. Law suggested that increasing maternal age of itself produced increased fetal loss, though Brenner and colleagues disagreed. They found that breech deliveries occurred significantly earlier than non-breech especially in non-white patients and for all parities. Fetal and placental weights were lower than in non-breech cases of comparable gestational age and showed a 6.3% incidence of congenital abnormality compared with 2.4% in non-breech cases. The incidence of placenta praevia and placental abruption in breech cases was another potent cause of fetal loss, being three times that for cephalic presentation.

With careful selection of cases for vaginal breech delivery, full monitoring during labour and ready recourse to Caesarean section for poor progress or fetal distress, perinatal mortality figures should become comparable with those of cephalic presentations of comparable weight and menstrual age.

The long term effects of breech birth in survivors were reviewed by Neligan et al. (1974), wide differences of opinion having been expressed by previous authors. At five years of age they found a lower mean IQ for male breech survivors compared with spontaneous vertex, forceps and Caesarean births, though the difference was relatively small and did not persist at 10 years of age. This compared with previous figures from Greece which suggested that 7.2% of survivors were left with major permanent handicap (Alexopoulos 1973). Neligan concluded that at that time any alteration in obstetric management in breech presentation must be aimed at lowering perinatal mortality rather than attempting to reduce brain damage in survivors. Now, with a much lower perinatal mortality we may need to consider more closely the long term sequelae in determining our plan of delivery. It must be remembered, however, that breech presentation may be the result of abnormal neurological development in utero, in which case the long term outlook is bleak regardless of mode of delivery.

Stillbirth may result from traumatic intracranial haemorrhage if delivery of the aftercoming head is rapid and uncontrolled or from asphyxia if delivery is too slow, and this can also cause intracranial haemorrhage (Wigglesworth et al. 1977). Hypoxia in labour, as shown by abnormal fetal heart records and a lowered mean Apgar score, is three times as common as with cephalic presentation. Prolapse of the cord occurs in 2.3–6% of cases compared with 0.24–0.5% in non-breech labours (Benson et al. 1972).

Medullary coning through the foramen magnum, severance of the cord, brachial plexus injury and transection of the cord may follow forceful traction and abdominal pressure in attempts to deliver the aftercoming head (Tan 1973), especially if it is hyperextended. Other injuries include fractured skull, especially the occipital bone, and fractures of femur, humerus and clavicle (or the more serious epiphyseal separation of these bones). A sternocleidomastoid haematoma and major bruising and tearing of lower lumbar muscles have been reported (*Brit. med. J.* 1975). This last may result in a crush-syndrome effect on the kidneys. Abdominal organs can be injured by rough handling with perforation of bowel or intraperitoneal haemorrhage.

To these one must add any risk inherent in premature rupture of membranes when this occurs.

In 1970 breech delivery was associated with the highest incidence of breathing difficulties in those who died and in survivors, a similar pattern being true for fits and cerebral signs (Chamberlain *et al.* 1975). Much of the increased Respiratory Depression Ratio in breech delivery (24 compared with 4.7 for all the 1970 births surveyed), was associated with the proportion which weighed less than 2500 g, but these facts emphasize the risks of breech presentation even when the baby survives.

Consideration of these hazards in the days before Caesarean section had achieved its present safety led to an attempt to reduce the numbers coming to breech delivery by the use of external cephalic version.

Management

EXTERNAL CEPHALIC VERSION

The fetus is turned to a head presentation by manipulation through the mother's abdominal wall. The presenting part must be disengaged and the uterus neither tense nor irritable. There must be sufficient liquor and the abdominal wall must be thin and relaxed. The last requirement has by some been facilitated by general anaesthesia though this is now not recommended. More recently uterine relaxation by terbutaline infusion later in pregnancy has been reported with 70% success in a series of 53 attempts (Fall & Nilsson 1979). Even advocates of external version do not attempt it in a Rhesus negative mother, in the presence of moderate or severe hypertension, in patients who have experienced antepartum haemorrhage or in those who have placenta praevia,

uterine scars, ruptured membranes or intrauterine growth retardation. It is contraindicated in twin pregnancy, when delivery by Caesarean section is planned for associated reasons, and when major fetal deformity has been demonstrated.

A failure rate of only 3% in 703 cases was claimed by Friedlander (1966) though he found it necessary to use general anaesthesia in 13% after the thirty-third week. The average number of versions per patient after this stage of pregnancy was 2.6, with a rate of reversion to breech of 11.2%. Others have quoted lower success rates even when using general anaesthesia: 72% (Neely 1961) to 85% (Peel & Clayton 1948) with a perinatal mortality due to the version itself of 1 and 1.7% respectively. Spontaneous cephalic version can occur just prior to term of fetuses which have previously defied all attempts at external cephalic version, whilst Vartan (1945) showed that following external version 22% of cases reverted to breech. It has been suggested, therefore, that successful external cephalic version merely anticipates the spontaneous cephalic version which would have occurred naturally. The incidence of breech delivery is similar in clinics where version is avoided and in those where it is routine (Hay 1959).

The complications of general anaesthesia, premature labour with prolapsed cord, placental abruption and ruptured uterus have all followed attempts at external version, whilst the significance of the bradycardia which often follows the procedure is unknown, but fetal death may result.

Considerations such as these led White (1956) to calculate that if one assumed success rates of 70 and 88% in primigravidas and multiparas respectively, with a fetal loss due to version itself of not less than 1%, then the procedure could be justified only in places where the perinatal mortality of breech delivery exceeded that of cephalic presentation by more than 2.5%. In units with skilled obstetric teams and ready recourse to abdominal delivery, corrected perinatal losses which compare with those of cephalic presentation mean that external version is no longer justified. Indeed Husslein (1965) in the survey of European units showed that the perinatal mortality was greater in those units where external version was most practised.

It was well argued by Neely (1961) that external cephalic version, including that under general anaesthesia, might still have a place in areas where facilities are less good, and he claimed to have produced a decrease in the incidence of breech delivery to 1.2% in his small series. The same argument may be applicable also in those countries where Caesarean section is to be avoided because of the risks of a scarred uterus in subsequent pregnancy. Here the suggestion by White (1956) may be relevant, that external cephalic version could be used selectively in cases where minor pelvic contraction was suspected, as the subsequent cephalic presentation would allow of trial labour. The decision to continue or dispense with external version in a unit must be made with particular regard to the facilities available there.

ANTENATAL ASSESSMENT OF CASES

The case of persisting breech presentation must be thoroughly assessed so that the correct route of delivery may be chosen. This is of equal importance in multiparas and primiparas if the perinatal mortality of breech births is to fall.

ELECTIVE CAESAREAN SECTION IN BREECH PRESENTATION

It is a good maxim that delivery by Caesarean section should be considered when the fetus presents by the breech in the presence of another obstetrical problem.

Associated conditions such as diabetes mellitus, moderate or severe hypertension, placenta praevia and fulminating pre-eclampsia may justify elective Caesarean section when major congenital abnormality of the fetus has been excluded. It may be selected in some cases of Rhesus isoimmunization and following placental abruption. Abdominal delivery must also be considered when the fetus is growth retarded. When disproportion is suspected, as with contracted pelvis at any level, the biparietal diameter is large or when the fetus is assessed at 3.75 kg or more elective Caesarean section should be employed. It should be considered whenever footling breech is diagnosed and also in cases where X-ray shows that the fetal head is hyperextended because of the difficulty of delivering the head in such cases (Westgren et al. 1981).

Caesarean section may be performed electively for breech presentation in multiparas with a poor obstetric history, in patients who have experienced difficulty in conceiving and in the primigravida over 35 years of age. In patients with a previous Caesarean section a vaginal breech delivery should be considered only when the malpresentation is the sole complication present. The uterine scar should be sound and previous section performed for a non-recurring indication. The fetus should be of average size and the pelvic capacity should not be in doubt.

A Caesarean section rate of 15–39% in breech presentation is reported in recent series, of which up to 85% have been elective. The vaginal route will be chosen most often in the multipara with a good obstetric history and where the breech has extended legs.

Retrospective studies have shown a poor outcome for preterm infants born by vaginal breech delivery. Routine Caesarean section for impending preterm breech delivery has improved neonatal mortality and morbidity and reduced long term neurological sequelae (Ingemarsson et al. 1978). As neonatal intensive care improves this group of patients becomes even more important, though the high incidence of congenital abnormality demands that a meticulous search be made for detectable abnormality before abdominal delivery. The current position has been reviewed by Crowley and Hawkins (1980) who conclude that for infants weighing less than 1000 g with estimated maturity of less than 28 weeks a policy of Caesarean section is not justified, whilst in infants 1500–2000 g in weight the outcome is independent of the mode of delivery. Between 1000 and 1500 g (average maturity 28–31 weeks). Caesarean section appears to confer advantage. It is also suggested that Caesarean section for all footling breech presentations might be equally profitable, as suggested by Karp et al. (1979) (see also Brit. med. J. 1979).

A study of 127 patients at 36 weeks or more with frank breech presentation, in whom vaginal breech delivery or Caesarean section was randomly selected, revealed a maternal morbidity of 36.4% in the Caesarean group. However, over half the cases randomized to vaginal delivery needed Caesarean section eventually (32 for pelvic contraction; 4 for lack of progress; and 1 for fetal distress in the group of 70) (Collea et al. 1978). This study suggests that there is still a place for vaginal breech delivery in the well chosen case.

SELECTION OF CASES FOR VAGINAL BREECH DELIVERY

Pelvic shape and capacity may be judged by past obstetric history where applicable and by thorough clinical assessment, especially of the shape and size of the outlet. The value of X-ray pelvimetry has been questioned, though Beischer (1966), in a small series, discovered unexpected mid-plane contraction in nearly a quarter of those in whom it was performed. Many obstetricians employ clinical assessment in conjunction with a single upright lateral X-ray pel-

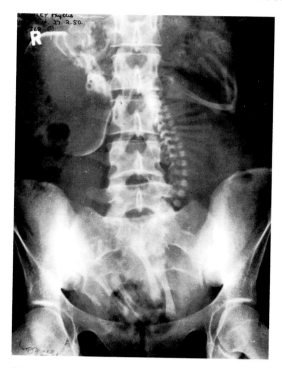

Fig. 27.6. Gross extension of the fetus in a case of breech presentation.

vimetry. In assessing the likelihood of a successful outcome Friedman (1967) stressed the prognostic value of cervical dilatation and station of the presenting part in late pregnancy or early labour.

It has been shown that a large infant is at increased risk. If clinical suspicions are confirmed, by relating ultrasonic measurements of the head, chest and abdomen, an elective Caesarean section is best. Various fetal abnormalities that may have a bearing on the mode of delivery can also be diagnosed by ultrasound, e.g. hydrocephaly, fetal ascites, spina bifida, renal agenesis. X-rays may also reveal skeletal abnormality or give other useful information (Fig. 27.6). In assessing fetal size clinically it must be stressed that there is a consistent tendency to underestimate in both large and small babies. It is important that the most experienced obstetrician available makes this decision on management.

Mechanism of labour

Contrary to older teaching, the first stage of labour is not usually prolonged. It lasted less than 12 hours in 53% of primiparas and 77.2% of mutiparas with mature singleton breech delivery reviewed by Law

(1967). When labour was premature it was even shorter. Friedman (1967) showed that at term there was no difference in the duration of the first stage between flexed and extended breech presentations, and when compared with vertex presentation. A shortening of the latent phase in primiparas was explained by the increased incidence of premature rupture of membranes in this group. There was prolongation of all phases with increasing infant weight. In multiparas all phases of labour were slightly longer. Perinatal mortality rises when the first stage is prolonged.

The presenting part will usually engage with the bitrochanteric diameter occupying an oblique diameter or the transverse diameter and with the sacrum anterior. The anterior hip leads and, on meeting the pelvic floor, is rotated anteriorly beneath the pubic arch. Should the posterior hip reach the pelvic floor first, it usually undergoes long anterior rotation. The hip is now held at the pubic arch, lateral flexion allowing the posterior hip to be born. The child then straightens as the anterior hip is born, the legs and feet following. As the shoulders enter the brim in the oblique or transverse diameter the trunk undergoes external rotation. The shoulders then undergo their own internal rotation to bring them into the anteroposterior diameter of the outlet, the trunk following. The third and final part to enter the pelvis is the head, which rotates until the posterior part of the neck becomes fixed under the subpubic arch and the head is born by flexion, the chin, mouth, nose, forehead, vertex and occiput appearing successively. It is obvious that every attempt must be made to keep the back of the fetus anterior and to maintain flexion of the head by avoiding premature or unwise traction, thus allowing smaller diameters to engage. In general, if the fetal back is kept anterior the head will rotate correctly, but unexpected posterior rotation of the head has been reported occasionally.

The second stage of labour
The length of this is determined largely by the degree of intervention by the obstetrician. Hay (1959) quoted averages of 39 min for primigravidas and 20 for multiparas, whilst Law (1967) found that the stage exceeded 60 min in 45.9% of primigravidas with mature infants, though in only 7.1% of multiparas with mature infants. It is certainly unwise to allow the second stage to continue beyond the time at which satisfactory advance is occurring, and 30 min after full dilatation the case should always be reviewed by an experienced attendant. With epidural

analgesia a little more time may be allowed provided that progress is being made and the fetal heart rate is satisfactory.

The third stage of labour
This is usually managed actively following administration of an oxytoxic drug, but there is still a tendency to excessive blood loss in cases of premature labour and in multiparas (Law 1967).

Conduct of vaginal breech delivery

This should always be in a unit equipped for Caesarean section, and should be attended by an experienced obstetrician and an anaesthetist who is skilled in obstetric anaesthesia. Both must be present at delivery. Fetal heart rate monitoring in breech labour was shown by Wheeler and Greene (1975) to predict all cases (15 of 42 in their series) in which the baby was born with a low Apgar score, though a further 10 which showed abnormal tracings were born in good condition. They suggest that fetal monitoring in this way is more applicable as a routine method than the fetal pH scheme proposed by Eliot and Hill (1972) but that the two methods used together may provide ideal management.

FIRST STAGE

These patients may require general anaesthesia urgently, and should receive adequate fluid and dextrose or fructose intravenously to avoid ketosis. For the same reason, oral intake should be sips of water only, with administration of an antacid 2-hourly to maintain a high pH of the gastric contents. A suggested alternative is the use of cimetidine. Particular care should be taken to observe signs of clinical fetal distress by fetal heart rate monitoring, and in every case at least one vaginal examination should be performed by an experienced attendant prior to rupture of the membranes to seek cord presentation. Incoordinate uterine action, uterine inertia, an unsatisfactory rate of cervical dilatation or a breech which remains high indicates that the case must be reviewed urgently lest previously unsuspected mechanical problems are present. Oxytocin has in some series produced evidence of fetal hypoxia (Benson *et al.* 1972) and should rarely be used in breech presentation, either for induction of labour or for augmentation. When the foot or breech can be seen without a speculum fetal blood sampling has been used in management (Eliot & Hill 1972). Epidural analgesia

has been avoided in many series because of fears that second stage prolongation and increased necessity for breech extraction would result, but in the properly chosen case it is an excellent method of pain relief and eliminates the need for general anaesthesia if assistance or Caesarean section becomes necessary.

SECOND STAGE

Delivery may occur spontaneously, by assisted breech delivery, or by breech extraction.

Spontaneous breech delivery

This occurs rarely except in multiparous patients in premature labour. These cases carry a high perinatal mortality, delivery often occurring rapidly when skilled help is not available.

Assisted breech delivery

The patient should be in lithotomy position with her bladder empty. Full dilatation of the cervix must be confirmed by vaginal examination, which also excludes cord prolapse and detects the rare instances when the child is astride the cord. In this last situation the cord should be displaced over the thigh. If with a tense cord this is not possible then, if the situation allows it, resort may be made to Caesarean section if assessment suggests that the fetus is not distressed and breech extraction would be hazardous. Alternatively, under appropriate anaesthesia the cord may be cut between ligatures and full breech extraction performed without delay.

In most cases the infant's sacrum will be anterior or lateral, but in the few cases where the back is posterior it will usually rotate spontaneously to an anterior position. Especially with a frank breech, the perineum becomes progressively more distended by maternal effort during contractions. Cox (1955) emphasized that delivery should not begin until the fetal anus becomes visible. Latterly, the tendency has been to commence delivery somewhat earlier, but only when the perineum is distended and thinned by a breech which is 'climbing' the perineum. At this time a generous episiotomy is essential, and is easily performed if epidural analgesia has been administered. In other patients, infiltration of the perineum with local anaesthetic may be usefully combined with transvaginal pudendal block anaesthesia. In the Liverpool technique general anaesthesia was rapidly induced when the infant had been born as far as the umbilicus, extended legs being delivered by the Pinard manoeuvre before the shoulders and head were extracted. Conduction analgesia and regional block are being used increasingly with fewer general anaesthetics. This trend is encouraging. Epidural analgesia is most effective. Its potential for eliminating bearing down effects before full dilatation is stressed (Crawford 1974), and the benefits of improved maternal relaxation and reduction of maternal and fetal acidosis produced by the technique (Pearson 1973) were emphasized by Donnai and Nicholas (1975). In both series, together totalling over 380 cases there was, perhaps unexpectedly, no increase in breech extraction though the second stage was longer than in patients managed without epidural. In Donnai and Nicholas' series, 46 of the 108 patients who were not being given oxytocin for induction subsequently needed augmentation of labour, but this seemed to have no ill effect. Whilst 130 delivered vaginally with 1 intrapartum stillbirth, only 10 breech extractions were necessary. Eight patients were delivered by Caesarean section for fetal distress in labour or because the breech remained high at full dilatation.

Unexpected difficulty in delivery in a well chosen case should arouse suspicion of fetal ascites or of tumours of kidneys or other organs though these should have already been identified by a full antenatal ultrasound scan. The arms are usually flexed on the anterior chest wall and will be delivered with the thorax without difficulty. No attempt should be made to deliver an arm until the scapula and one axilla are visible. Extended arms and the rare nuchal displacement usually result from unwise traction by the obstetrician and his failure to keep the fetal back anterior during all manoeuvres. If the baby is unexpectedly large it may be wise to deliver an arm before the shoulders become wedged in the pelvis. For this operation general anaesthesia is necessary. In most instances, however, the Løvset manoeuvre is employed, and only rarely is it necessary to insert a hand into the uterus. If the back has remained anterior and the case is well selected, the head will enter the pelvis and descend without difficulty under the influence of gravity, the attendant merely allowing the body to hang 'for as long as is necessary to rinse the hands'. The processs can be facilitated if an assistant places the palms of his hands above the symphysis pubis and draws up the uterus as in the Brandt–Andrews method for delivery of the placenta.

When the nuchal region is seen, delivery of the head may be conducted by the Burns–Marshall manoeuvre, but more safely with obstetric forceps. Any straight forceps can be used, though the Piper forceps were especially designed for this purpose. The Mauriceau–Smellie–Veit method is not recommended because the traction involved may cause brachial plexus injury. When the head is unexpectedly delayed in the pelvic cavity, adequate vaginal retraction using forceps blades may permit the infant to breathe before the nose and mouth are visible. Once the mouth appears the airway is cleared and extraction of the head proceeds smoothly but without haste. The third stage will be actively managed following administration of an oxytocic, delivery being completed by inspection of vagina and cervix. To facilitate this an assistant should draw the retracted uterus up into the abdomen by suprapubic pressure whilst the forceps blades are used as lateral vaginal wall retractors. This obviates the need for pulling the cervix down with sponge forceps and gives optimal exposure. The episiotomy is then sutured. If by carelessness or accident the head enters the pelvic cavity with the occiput posterior, delivery may be effected by using the Prague grip in reverse, the direction of shoulder traction being downwards and backwards.

One other technique of breech delivery should be mentioned. This, the Bracht manoeuvre, is popular on the Continent and has been described at length by Plentl and Stone (1953).

Breech extraction

The obstetrician delivers the infant with no assistance from the mother. The method has been used to expedite delivery in cases of fetal distress or prolapsed cord, and occasionally when progress ceases in the second stage or for delivering the second twin. Before starting one must know that the cervix is fully dilated and that there is enough liquor to allow intrauterine manipulation. The uterus may be fully relaxed by suitable general anaesthesia. The operator must be confident that there are no mechanical obstacles to delivery, and in particular that progress has not been arrested by unsuspected disproportion. A footling presentation is easier to extract than a breech with extended legs in which the foot must first be delivered by inserting a hand into the uterus and using Pinard's manoeuvre. This should not be attempted before full dilatation. Breech extraction should be avoided with a large infant and should never be performed if a uterine scar is present. It is especially dangerous in the multipara, because of the risk of uterine rupture, with small for dates or premature infants and when there is fetal distress, because of the risks of occipital injury and intracranial damage.

Caesarean section may become necessary in labour for cord prolapse, which occurs in up to 6% of cases, or fetal distress prior to full dilatation, and it should be considered in all cases of incoordinate uterine action, prolongation of the first stage of labour or failure of the breech to descend during the second stage. A most difficult problem is posed by the delivery of the aftercoming head in the presence of asphyxia. It may well be that even if full dilatation has been achieved the baby will be in better condition if Caesarean section rather than breech extraction is performed for fetal asphyxia.

In any form of vaginal breech delivery there is an increased risk of fetal hypoxia and acidosis (Serreyn *et al.* 1973).

TRANSVERSE AND OBLIQUE LIE. SHOULDER PRESENTATION

An incidence of 1 in 322 has been reported at the Mayo Clinic (Johnson 1964), and 1 in 323 by Cruikshank and White (1973).

Aetiology

The majority of the patients are multiparous with a lax pendulous abdomen, but the abnormal lie can occur when engagement of the head is prevented by contracted pelvis, pelvic tumour or placenta praevia. The last is thought to account for 10% of cases (Cruikshank & White 1973, Hall & O'Brien 1961). Prematurity, polyhydramnios and intrauterine fetal death are other possible causes.

Twin pregnancy is an association in between 18 and 40% of various series, usually involving the second twin. The very rare double transverse lie should make one suspicious of conjoined twins.

Abnormal lie can result from abnormal uterine shape, either congenital or peculiar to the current pregnancy by reason of a placenta situated in the fundus or the lower segment (Stevenson 1949).

In transverse and oblique lie the back is usually anterior with the head most often to the mother's left. The fetal attitude is one of flexion. Though dorso-posterior positions are less common they inevitably cause fetal extension with greater risk of arm prolapse and associated twisting of the fetal spine. Rarely the back can be inferior or superior.

Diagnosis

In singleton pregnancy the uterus seems broad and often asymmetrical, the fundus being lower than expected for dates. The long axis of the fetal ovoid lies more often obliquely than transversely with the head in the iliac fossa or flank. In the middle of the abdomen the firm smooth surface of the back or the more irregular prominences of limbs will be felt in dorso-anterior and dorso-posterior positions respectively. There is no fetal pole in the fundus and the pelvic inlet may appear empty or one may feel the prominence of shoulder and arm there.

Vaginal examination is best avoided until placenta praevia has been excluded by ultrasound. It may then reveal an empty pelvis or occasionally a limb presentation. Pelvic contraction or a pelvic tumour may be evident.

In early labour abdominal findings are unchanged; an elongated bag of forewaters can be felt vaginally and may contain a limb or a loop of cord. The presenting part is high, irregular and difficult to define. The membranes rupture early. Later in labour the shoulder descends, and in cases first seen at this stage the landmarks to be identified are the ribs on the medial wall of the axilla, the clavicle and the acromion. They may be obscured by oedema. Where the fetus is very small or macerated the lowest part palpable may be the thorax or back. In other cases a hand or hand and foot together may present, and in all cases prolapse of the cord is likely.

In very late labour abdominal signs are those of obstructed labour, whilst the considerable oedema which ensues may make it hard to differentiate shoulder presentation from breech, face or brow on vaginal examination.

Features of labour and possible outcome

Inertia or incoordinate uterine action may be seen in response to the obstruction which is implicit in transverse lie unless the fetus is very small or macerated. Membranes rupture early, much liquor escapes and infection is a hazard. There may follow a period of inertia. Still later (or more often with no preliminary respite) uterine tone increases, contractions become violent, the lower segment thins and a pathological ring is detected as it ascends in the abdomen (Fig. 27.7). Meanwhile, the bladder becomes thick and is easily felt. Ketosis, dehydration and infection are now evident and the fetus dies of asphyxia. Such an outcome represents obstruction and neglected shoulder

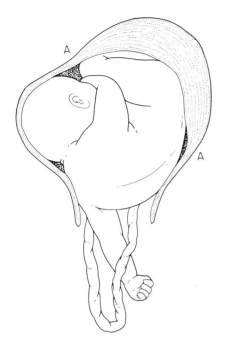

Fig. 27.7. Drawing of a neglected shoulder presentation. The line AA represents the line of the pathological retraction ring.

presentation. It will lead almost inevitably to uterine rupture though, very rarely, secondary inertia has been seen after intrauterine infection with gas forming organisms has occurred.

Other possible outcomes must be mentioned, but their occurrence should never be relied upon: (1) *Spontaneous reversion* to a longitudinal lie can occur only when membranes are intact or very recently ruptured. It is unlikely to occur in established labour; (2) *Spontaneous expulsion* is seen when the fetus is so small or macerated that it can be doubled up by strong uterine action. The first part born is the back, the head and abdomen being expelled together and finally the feet; (3) *Spontaneous evolution* usually involves very small infants (though one of 3300 g has been reported) and violent uterine action. It usually follows prolapse of an arm in dorso-anterior positions. The neck elongates and the presenting shoulder is fixed at the outlet. Continuing contractions result in extreme lateral flexion of the spine. If this occurs with its concavity to the same side as the leading shoulder then the breech will next be born, having been thrust down behind the shoulder. The abdomen, thorax, second shoulder and head follow in order. When the lateral flexion has its convexity

to the side of the leading shoulder then birth of the shoulder is followed by that of thorax, abdomen, breech and legs in sequence, the second shoulder and head appearing last.

It must be emphasized that these are matters of interest only, being rarities and having no part in a properly managed case.

Management

ANTENATAL

When the abnormal lie occurs after 34 weeks' gestation in a multipara, and whenever it is diagnosed in a nullipara, one must first exclude twin pregnancy, fetal abnormality, placenta praevia, contracted pelvis and hydramnios. These conditions having been excluded by radiography or ultrasound, the patient must be told to come to the hospital at once should contractions start or should she lose liquor. Gentle external cephalic version may be followed by engagement of the head. Recurrent 'unstable' lie justifies hospital admission at 37 weeks to await labour, though even earlier admission may be wise in some cases. If the lie is still unstable at the forty-first week it is reasonable to perform external version, and in cases of polyhydramnios perhaps also an amniocentesis, thereafter inducing contractions with carefully monitored oxytocin infusion. One may then rupture the forewaters. In any case with complications, such as pelvic tumour, placenta praevia, contracted pelvis or associated disease, elective Caesarean section will be the best treatment.

IN LABOUR

In singleton pregnancies treatment will vary with the cause and with the stage of labour at which the diagnosis is made. Uterine thinning or rupture, intrauterine infection and fetal death are associated problems in the late case. With a live fetus prolapse of cord, which occurs in 10–15% of cases, may necessitate Caesarean section.

In twin labours transverse lie of the first twin demands Caesarean section. External version, stimulation of contractions and forewater amniotomy are appropriate when the second twin is involved after the first has been born.

External version

This is applicable occasionally in very early labour with weak contractions and intact membranes in cases where there is no indication for rapid delivery and in which pelvic contraction, placenta praevia and pelvic tumour have been excluded. Such patients are rare. External version, rupture of membranes and ventouse delivery are, however, useful for delivering the second twin.

Caesarean section

This should be the most frequent method of delivery. It includes all cases having an associated indication for abdominal delivery, all patients who have borne four children, most primigravidas and all cases of pelvic contraction. The value of a longitudinal lower segment incision, in selected cases and especially when membranes have ruptured, is emphasized because it can be extended upwards if necessary.

In cases of established labour Caesarean section is preferred if the child is alive, and may be safest even when the child is dead, especially in the grande multipara or where uterine thinning is suspected. With severe infection Caesarean hysterectomy may be considered (*see also* p. 436).

Decapitation

Using the Blond-Heidler saw, this is performed for neglected transverse lie with a dead fetus when practising among developing peoples in whom every effort must be made to avoid section. In Western practice it is rarely used.

Internal version

This has little place in the treatment of transverse or oblique lie in labour. It is the commonest cause of ruptured uterus and carries a perinatal mortality of between 40 and 70% (Chapman 1967, Edelstein 1971, Yates 1964). The sole occasional indication for this operation in modern obstetrics has been delivery of the second twin. For this is must be performed immediately if the membranes of the second sac rupture before it has been possible to correct the lie by external manipulation.

RESULTS

Maternal mortality and morbidity rise with the age and multiparity of the patients, their liability to associated conditions such as hypertension, the risks of early membrane rupture and obstructed labour, and finally the frequent need for operative interference.

Fetal mortality and morbidity will rise because of early rupture of membranes, from trauma due to unwise manipulative delivery and hypoxia due to obstructed labour or prolapse of the cord. Hall and O'Brien (1961) quoted a fetal mortality of 28% with vaginal and 7.2% for abdominal delivery.

COMPOUND PRESENTATION

This term includes cases of cephalic presentation when one or more limbs lie alongside and present with the head, and also breech presentation where one or both arms present with the breech.

The causes are similar to those of prolapsed cord which can complicate the compound presentation in 12 to 17% of cases (Cruikshank & White 1973).

Compound presentation can occur if engagement of the head is prevented by contracted pelvis or pelvic tumour. Polyhydramnios, deflexion attitudes of the head and a dead macerated fetus may also predispose to the condition. The most common associations are with prematurity, which was found in 45% of cases reviewed by Sweeney and Knapp (1961), and twin pregnancy which formed 39.7% of their cases.

The incidence of compound presentation is variously given as 1 in 652 (Goplerud & Eastman 1953),

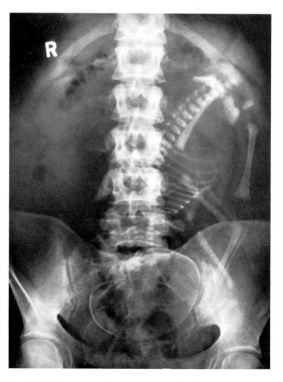

Fig. 27.8. A compound presentation. A hand and a foot, respectively, lie below and alongside the head.

1 in 743 (Fields & Nelson 1959) and 1 In 1293 (Sweeney & Knapp 1961).

Presentation of a hand with the vertex (Fig. 27.8) accounts for about three-quarters of the cases. Next in frequency, a foot presents with the head, or the breech with an arm (11% each), and least common is presentation of arm, foot and vertex (Sweeney & Knapp 1961).

Diagnosis is usually not difficult once the membranes have ruptured and this occurs prematurely in a third of cases. Only 2 of 74 of Sweeney and Knapp's cases were diagnosed when the membranes were intact, and in 62 of the remainder the cervix was over 6 cm dilated, full dilatation having been achieved in 50 patients. The possibility should be considered when there is a slow active phase and the fetal head remains high especially if it is deviated from the mid-line after the membranes rupture.

Treatment

This depends upon the exact presentation, the stage of labour and state of the membranes, the condition and size of infant and whether singleton or twin pregnancy is involved. Efforts are made to exclude congenital abnormality, cephalo-pelvic disproportion and contracted pelvis. Finally, the presence of prolapsed cord takes precedence if the fetus is alive.

In general, expectant treatment is chosen because in most cases the extremity of the limb will recede as the presenting part descends, labour ending with a low instrumental or a normal delivery. Replacement of an arm is rarely necessary, and is superfluous if head and limb engage together. When the arm appears to rise into the uterus with a contraction this is a favourable sign. Active treatment is, of course, necessary in cases of cord prolapse with a live fetus; or if there is brim disproportion, a large fetus or contraction of the pelvis at mid-plane or outlet; Caesarean section is called for. Intrapartum radiography is valuable in assessing these cases. The most dangerous manoeuvre is internal version and breech extraction and it should be abandoned. Even in the case of the second twin, compound presentation is to be treated expectantly unless prolapse of the cord occurs, when the rule invoked is that of immediate delivery by the least traumatic method.

The perinatal mortality in term infants with no prolapse of cord or traumatic operative delivery should not be increased.

PROLAPSE AND PRESENTATION OF THE UMBILICAL CORD

This occurs once in every 200–300 deliveries (Goldthorp 1967, Pathak 1968, Savage et al. 1970). Whilst the membranes remain intact the condition is that of presentation of the cord, which becomes cord prolapse when the sac ruptures. The fetal mortality will be slightly lower with cord presentation, but the problems of presentation and prolapse are similar and must be considered together.

Aetiology

More than one factor may contribute.

The presenting part does not fill the lower segment which is poorly applied to it. Such cases include: transverse lie; breech presentation, especially with flexed legs (Hay 1959) when the risk is trebled (Savage et al. 1970); and face or brow presentation, though Clark et al. (1968) disagree. Occipito-posterior positions, cephalo-pelvic disproportion and, rarely, pelvic tumours predispose to cord prolapse as will excessive fetal mobility in polyhydramnios. In over 53% of cases reported by Clark et al. (1968) a malpresentation was present. Numerically breech presentation is the most common single cause accounting for 40–50% of cases.

Prematurity. This relationship is highly significant because of the small fetus, relatively copious liquor and high incidence of associated malpresentation. Similar considerations apply to multiple pregnancy.

Multiparity. Four-fifths of cases occur in multiparous patients especially in higher parities. The head remains free until labour starts, though the cervix may be somewhat dilated before that time. In one series only was it suggested that primiparas were at increased risk, because of the greater number of operative procedures performed upon them (Mengert & Longwell 1940).

Operative manoeuvres. Forewater amniotomy or manual rotation prior to forceps extraction have been responsible for up to 20% in various series, but in large series the risks of amniotomy appear small (d'Esopo et al. 1964, Keettel et al. 1940). If the cord prolapses at amniotomy, immediate delivery by Caesarean section is possible. Prolapse in labour may be unrecognized for some time unless continuous heart rate monitoring is in progress when cord complications can be suspected from the tracing.

Abnormality of the cord. A long cord or low placental insertion have been thought to contribute by some authors.

Fetal hypotension. It has been suggested that the normally turgid cord will not prolapse and that the occurrence is more likely in cases such as abruptio placentae, in which fetal hypotension ensues (Seligman 1961).

Diagnosis and anticipation

All patients must be told to come to hospital early in labour since the cord prolapse occurs before admission in up to 25% of cases. They must be urged also to come at once if they notice a leak of liquor, even if they feel no contractions. This must be emphasized particularly to women who have malpositions and malpresentations and when minor cephalo-pelvic disproportion exists. Cases of unstable or oblique lie may with advantage be admitted electively in late pregnancy as may all patients with polyhydramnios.

Before amniotomy at surgical induction the level of the presenting part must be assessed. If it is not engaged, it may help to initiate contractions by oxytocin infusion prior to amniotomy. Every patient for amniotomy is a potential candidate for Caesarean section, and must be prepared accordingly. The cord should be sought diligently both before and after amniotomy, especially when fetal heart rate variations follow the procedure. If the cord is thought to be present incision of the forewaters under direct vision through a fetal blood sampling endoscope is a safe technique and will also enable one to see any vasa praevia present.

In every labour, vaginal examination and auscultation should be carried out when the membranes rupture. This is equally important in multiple pregnancy. Even where continuous fetal heart rate monitoring is not available for all labours it should be utilized in cases of breech and compound presentation and in cases where the head is deflexed or high, for in these the risk of prolapse of the cord is great and the recording may give early warning of cord compression. Whenever fetal distress occurs in labour one must suspect cord prolapse either evident or occult. One may feel coils of cord within the forewaters. The distinction from toes may not be easy unless pulsation is evident. The cord may be visible through

an endoscope or may appear within an elongated sac of membranes. In such *cord presentation* it is important to keep the membranes intact whilst preparing for urgent abdominal delivery. Cord compression is possible if liquor is scanty and the head presents. Once the membranes have ruptured the case is one of *cord prolapse.* The strength and frequency of pulsation and any response to uterine contractions must be noted, as well as the degree of cervical dilatation, the nature and station of the presenting part and coexistent pelvic abnormalities. Associated diseases, and the facilities available also influence treatment. Treatment may be withheld if the fetus is known to have a major congenital abnormality incompatible with survival.

Prompt diagnosis at amniotomy and a short diagnosis/delivery interval result in low fetal mortality. When a condition such as breech presentation exists, which carries a high risk of cord prolapse, a strong case can thus be made for early controlled amniotomy in an operating theatre and subsequent continuous monitoring with an internal electrode, rather than awaiting spontaneous rupture of membranes. Even before membranes are ruptured external monitoring may suggest a cord complication.

Treatment

EMERGENCY MANAGEMENT

This is designed to cover the time taken to arrange urgent Caesarean or summon further assistance. It should be stressed that immediate delivery is the ideal if the fetus is alive and sufficiently mature. Cord presentation must be treated as urgently as cord prolapse and the membranes preserved meanwhile.

Postural treatment involves keeping the fingers in the vagina and placing the patient in Sim's or Trendelenburg's position (which are easier than the knee–elbow position). These measures help to keep pressure from the cord. It has been suggested that rapid forceful instillation of 500–700 ml of sterile saline into the bladder via a Foley catheter will produce a similar effect. This could be useful in the rare cases in which the patient needs to be transported some distance. It is of equal importance that the cord should be replaced within the warm, moist vagina, so preventing the vasospasm which results from cold and local irritation.

DEFINITIVE TREATMENT

If the fetus is dead, cord prolapse can be ignored, the problem being the mechanical one of the associated malpresentation. Absence of pulsation in the prolapsed cord is unreliable as evidence of fetal death. When the heart beat is present and the fetus is mature enough to be considered viable the aim is immediate controlled delivery by the appropriate route. An extra delay of only half an hour in cephalic presentations can more than double the corrected perinatal mortality (Bock & Weise 1972). Thus if the cervix is fully dilated instrumental delivery or breech extraction may be optimal. In 110 cases reported by Suraiya and Fernandez (1966), the cervix was fully dilated in 36% at the time of diagnosis.

With a cervix less than 7 cm dilated, Caesarean section is always best, a section rate of 30–35% being usual in recent series. A possible and rare exception would be cord presentation with a longitudinal lie in a multipara where labour is progressing rapidly at 7–8 cm dilatation and the fetus is not distressed. In these circumstances, with the patient in an operating theatre prepared for Caesarean section, and the theatre laid up for surgery, it might be possible to delay intervention in the hope that the membranes remain intact until full dilatation when vaginal delivery might become possible.

The most difficult cases of cord prolapse are those in which the cervix is approaching full dilatation, the fetus is alive and the lie is longitudinal. This group produced the highest mortality in the series of Goldthorp (1967). The choice between Caesarean section on the one hand and manual or vibrator dilatation of cervix with breech extraction or forceps/ventouse delivery on the other has in the past taxed the judgement and skill of the most experienced operator. In virtually all such cases Caesarean section is to be preferred. Internal version and breech extraction produces a damaged or dead baby in up to 40% of cases (Daly & Gibbs 1968) and may injure the mother. It should be abandoned.

Fetal mortality

Various series have shown a corrected mortality of from 10.7% (Goldthorp 1967) to 16.8% (Clark *et al.* 1968). A corrected rate of 1.5% was quoted by Bock and Weise (1972). Prompt diagnosis at amniotomy and a short diagnosis/delivery interval result in low mortality. Among cases reported by Clark *et al.* (1968) the mortality was only 5.5% if delivery was effected within 10 min. Prematurity quadrupled the perinatal mortality in the group described by Daly and Gibbs (1968). Even when the cervix is approaching, but has not attained, full dilatation perinatal mortality is lower in cases delivered by Caesarean section.

REFERENCES

AGÜERO O. & KIZER S. (1972) *Rev. obst. y ginec. Venez.*, **31**, 281.

ALEXOPOULOS K.A. (1973) *Clin. Pediat.*, **12**, 248.

BEISCHER N.A. (1966) *J. Obstet. Gynaec. Brit. Cwlth.*, **73**, 421.

BENSON W.L., BOYCE, D.C. & VAUGH D.L. (1972) *Obstet. Gynec.*, *N.Y.*, **40**, 417.

BERGER M., HEIMANN H. & WICK A. (1967) *Bibl. Gynaec.*, **45**, 1.

BOCK J.E. & WEISE J. (1972) *Acta Obstet. Gynec. Scand.*, **51**, 303.

BORELL U. & FERNSTROM I. (1960) *Acta Obstet. Gynec. Scand.*, **39**, 626.

BRENNER W.E., BRUCE R.D. & HENDRICKS C.H. (1974) *Amer. J. Obstet. Gynec.*, **118**, 700.

BRITISH CONGRESS (Glasgow) (1965) *J. Obstet. Gynaec. Brit. Cwlth.*, **72**, 866.

Brit. med. J. (1975) Editorial, **i**, 158.

Brit. med. J. (1979) Editorial, **i**, 1747.

BUTLER N.R. & BONHAM D.G. (1964) *Perinatal Mortality*. Churchill Livingstone, Edinburgh.

CALKINS L.A. (1953) *Obstet. Gynec.*, *N.Y.*, **1**, 466.

CHALMERS J.A. (1968) *J. Obstet. Gynaec. Brit. Cwlth.*, **75**, 889.

CHAMBERLAIN R., CHAMBERLAIN G., HOWLETT B. & CLAIREAUX A. (1975) *British Births 1970*, vol. 1, Heinemann, London.

CHAPMAN K. (1967) *J. Obstet Gynaec. India*, **17**, 368.

CHISWICK M.L. & JAMES D.K. (1979) *Brit. med. J.*, **i**, 7.

CLARK D.O., COPELAND W. & ULLERY J.C. (1968) *Amer. J. Obstet. Gynec.*, **101**, 84.

COLLEA J.W., RABIN S.C., WEGHORST G.R. & QUILLIGAN E.J. (1978) *Amer. J. Obstet. Gynec.*, **131**, 186.

COX L.W. (1955) *J. Obstet. Gynaec. Brit. Cwlth.*, **62**, 395.

CRAWFORD J.S. (1974) *J. Obstet. Gynaec. Brit. Cwlth.*, **81**, 867.

CROWLEY P. & HAWKINS D.F. (1980) *J. Obstet. Gynaec.*, **1**, 2.

CRUICKSHANK D.P. & WHITE C.A. (1973) *Amer. J. Obstet. Gynec.*, **116**, 1097.

DALY J.W. & GIBBS C.E. (1968) *Amer. J. Obstet. Gynec.*, **100**, 264.

D'ESOPO D.A. (1941) *Amer. J. Obstet. Gynec.*, **42**, 937.

D'ESOPO D.A., MOORE D.B. & LENZI E. (1964) *Amer. J. Obstet. Gynec.*, **89**, 561.

DONNAI P. & NICHOLAS A.D.G. (1975) *Brit. J. Obstet. Gynaec.*, **82**, 360.

EDELSTEIN W. (1971) *Sth. Afr. J. Obst. Gynaec.*, **9**, 18.

ELIOT B.W. & HILL J.G. (1972) *Brit. med. J.*, **iv**, 703.

FALL O. & NILSSON B.A. (1979) *Obstet. Gynec.*, *N.Y.*, **53**, 712.

FIANU S. & VACLAVINKOVA V. (1978) *Acta Obstet. Gynec. Scand.*, **57**, 371.

FIELDS H. & NELSON P.K. (1959) *Amer. J. Obstet. Gynec.*, **78**, 539.

FRIEDLANDER D. (1966) *Amer. J. Obstet. Gynec.*, **95**, 906.

FRIEDMAN E.A. (1967) *Labor. Clinical Evaluation and Management.* Appleton-Century-Crofts, New York.

FRIEDMAN E.A. & KROLL I. (1972) *J. reprod. Med.*, **8**, 117.

GOLDTHORP W.O. (1967) *Brit. J. Clin. Pract.*, **21**, 21.

GOPLERUD J. & EASTMAN N.J. (1953) *Obstet. Gynec., N.Y.*, **1**, 59.

HALL J.E., KOHL S.G., O'BRIEN F. & GINSBERG S. (1965) *Amer. J. Obstet. Gynec.*, **91**, 665.

HALL S.C. & O'BRIEN F.B. (1961) *Amer. J. Obstet. Gynec.*, **82**, 1180.

HAY D. (1959) *J. Obstet. Gynaec. Brit. Cwlth.*, **66**, 529.

HEALEY D.L., QUINN M.A. & PEPPERALL R.J. (1982) *Brit. J. Obstet. Gynaecol.* **89**, 501.

HOLMBERG N.G., LILIEQVIST B., MAGNUSSON S. & SEGERBRAND E. (1977) *Acta Obstet. Gynec. Scand.* (Suppl. 66), 49.

HUGHEY M.J., McELIN T.W. & LUSSKY R. (1978) *J. reprod. Med.*, **20**, 253.

HUSSLEIN H. (1965) *Zlb. Gynäk.*, **87**, 682.

INGEMARSSON I., WESTGREN M. & SVENNINGSEN N.W. (1978) *Lancet*, **ii**, 172.

JOHNSON C.E. (1964) *J. Amer. med. Ass.*, **187**, 642.

KARP L.E., DONEY J.R., McCARTHY T., MEIS P.J. & HALL M. (1979) *Obstet. Gynec., N.Y.*, **53**, 88.

KEETTEL W.C., DIDDLE A.W. & PLASS E.D. (1940) *Amer. J. Obstet. Gynec.*, **40**, 225.

Lancet (1980) Editorial, **i**, 406.

LAW R.G. (1967) *Standards of Obstetric Care.* Livingstone, Edinburgh.

LAWSON J.B. & STEWART D.B. (1967) *Obstetrics & Gynaecology in the Tropics.* Arnold, London.

MADDEN L.H. Jr (1956) *Amer. J. Obstet. Gynec.*, **72**, 31.

METZER R.M., SACHTLEBEN M.R. & FRIEDMAN E.A. (1967) *Amer. J. Obstet. Gynec.*, **100**, 255.

MENGERT W.F. & LONGWELL F.H. (1940) *Amer. J. Obstet. Gynec.*, **40**, 79.

METHUEN D. (1958) *Proc. roy. Soc. Med.*, **51**, 169.

MILLER D. (1930) *Brit. med. J.*, **i**, 1036.

MOSTAR S., AKALTIN E. & BABUNCA C. (1966) *Obstet. Gynec., N.Y.*, **28**, 49.

NEELY M.R. (1961) *J. Obstet. Gynaec. Brit. Cwlth.*, **68**, 490.

NELIGAN G.A., PRUDHAM D. & STEINER H. (1974) *The Formative Years. Birth, Family and Development in Newcastle upon Tyne.* Oxford University Press, London.

O'DRISCOLL K. & MEAGHER D. (1980) *Active Management of Labour.* Saunders, London.

O'DRISCOLL K., MEAGHER D., MacDONALD D. & GEOGHEGAN F. (1981) *Brit. J. Obstet. Gynaec.*, **88**, 577.

PARRY-JONES E. (1968) *J. Obstet. Gynaec. Brit. Cwlth.*, **75**, 892.

PATHAK U.N. (1968) *Amer. J. Obstet. Gynec.*, **101**, 401.

PEARSON J.F. (1973) *J. Obstet. Gynaec. Brit. Cwlth.*, **80**. 218.

PEEL J.H. & CLAYTON S.G. (1948) *J. Obstet. Gynaec. Brit. Cwlth.*, **55**, 614.

PLENTL A.A. & STONE R.E. (1953) *Obstet. Gynec. Surv.*, **8**, 313.

POSNER A.C., FRIEDMAN S. & POSNER L.B. (1957) *Surg. Gynec. Obstet.*, **104**, 485.

POSNER L.B., RUBIN E.J. & POSNER A.C. (1963) *Obstet. and Gynec.*, **21**, 745.

POTTER M.G., HEATON C.U. & DOUGLAS G.W. (1960) *Obstet. Gynec., N.Y.*, **15**, 158.

Report on Confidential Enquiries into Maternal Deaths in England and Wales. 1964–1966 published 1969 HMSO; 1967–1969 published 1972; 1970–72 published 1975 HMSO (edited by Arthur C.H. et al.).

Report on Confidential Enquiries into Maternal Deaths in England and Wales 1973–75 published 1979 HMSO (edited Tomkinson J. et al.).

ROVINSKY J.J., MILLER J.S. & KAPLAN S. (1973) *Amer. J. Obstet. Gynec.*, **115**, 497.

SAVAGE E.W., KOHL S.G. & WYNN R.M. (1970) *Obstet. Gynec., N.Y.*, **36**, 502.

SELIGMAN S.A. (1961) *Brit. med. J.*, **i**, 1369.

SERREYN R., THIERY M., LYBEER E. & DEROM R. (1973) *Int. J. Gynaec. & Obst.*, **11**, 11.

SØRENSEN T., HASCH E. & LANGE A.P. (1979) *Lancet*, **ii**, 477.

STEVENSON C.S. (1949) *Amer. J. Obstet. Gynec.*, **58**, 432.

SURAIYA U. & FERNANDEZ W. (1966) *J. Obstet. Gynaec. India*, **16**, 188.

SWEENEY W.J. & KNAPP R.C. (1961) *Obstet. Gynec., N.Y.*, **17**, 333.

TAN K.L. (1973) *J. Obstet. Gynaec. Brit. Cwlth.*, **80**, 60.

TRAUB A.I., MORROW R.J., RITCHIE J.W.K. & DORNAN K.J. (1984) *Brit. J. Obstet. Gynaec.* (in press).

VARTAN C.K. (1945) *J. Obstet. Gynaec. Brit. Cwlth.*, **52**, 417.

WESTGREN M., GRUNDSELL H., INGEMARSSON I., MÜHLOW A. & SVENNINGSEN N.W. (1981) *Brit. J. Obstet. Gynaec.*, **88**, 101.

WHEELER T. & GREENE K. (1975) *Brit. J. Obstet. Gynaec.*, **82**, 208.

WHITE A.J. (1956) *J. Obstet. Gynaec. Brit. Cwlth.*, **63**, 706.

WIGGLESWORTH J.S., DAVIES P.A., KEITH I.H. & SLADE S.A. (1977) *Arch. Dis. Childh.*, **52**, 447.

WULFF G.J.L., TRUEBLOOD A.C. & HOLLAND R.C. (1960) *Obstet. Gynec., N.Y.*, **16**, 288.

YATES M.J. (1964) *J. Obstet. Gynaec. Brit. Cwlth.*, **71**, 245.

CHAPTER 28
COMPLICATIONS OF THE THIRD STAGE
OF LABOUR

J. M. BEAZLEY

As complications of the third stage of labour, post-partum haemorrhage and retained placenta may occur together. Uterine inversion is much less common but is potentially dangerous; usually it can be avoided by good intrapartum management of the third stage. All three of the complications may occur unexpectedly and retained placenta and uterine invasion are commonly associated with haemorrhage. However, unexpected postpartum collapse may occur without obvious external haemorrhage. This should first raise the suspicion of internal bleeding into either the broad ligament or paravaginal tissues (*see* Chapter 29, p. 423). Otherwise, more uncommon causes such as amniotic fluid embolus, will have to be considered.

POSTPARTUM HAEMORRHAGE

The maternal mortality rate due to primary postpartum haemorrhage has remained virtually unchanged since 1967, despite the fact that death is usually associated with avoidable factors (Maternal Mortality Report 1973–75). The cause may be (a) atony of the uterus or (b) trauma to the genital tract. While the former remains the more common, perhaps for this very reason the latter is the more often neglected in its early stages.

(a) Atony

Atonic haemorrhage is associated with the inability of the uterus to contract and retract effectively and efficiently. The uterus therefore increases in size because of the retained blood and feels soft and 'boggy'. However, it may be very difficult to palpate the uterus and the uterine fundus because it is completely flaccid. The patient has a rapid, thready pulse with a fall in blood pressure and she is pale and apprehensive.

Atony may be associated with any of the following factors:

1 retained products of conception, the placenta itself, a placental cotelydon or fragment, or even a large amount of membranes, may prevent efficient contraction of the uterine muscle;

2 prolonged labour with inertia of the uterus (today's active management of labour, with the ready use of oxytocic infusion to correct ineffective uterine action, has reduced this considerably);

3 operative deliveries, other than simple 'lift out' low forceps or ventouse deliveries, especially if general anaesthesia has been used instead of regional blockade (general anaesthetic agents that relax the myometrium, such as halothane and cyclopropane, have a deservedly bad reputation in this regard);

4 overdistension of the uterus, as associated with polyhydramnios, or possibly multiple pregnancy;

5 a large placental site, as in multiple pregnancy; perhaps overdistension is also present, and there may in addition have been disordered uterine action;

6 placenta praevia, because of the inability of the lower uterine segment to retract;

7 abruptio placentae, where there is interstitial uterine haemorrhage and later hypofibrinogenaemia;

8 multiparity with an increase in the fibrous tissue of the uterus and a decrease in its muscular tissue; the virtual disappearance of the obstetrically notorious 'grand multipara' from many centres and communities has been associated with a significant reduction in the incidence of postpartum haemorrhage, particularly of very large life-threatening losses of blood;

9 multiple fibromyomata, especially of the interstitial type, because of the resulting ineffective uterine contraction and retraction.

PREVENTION

It is important to stress that the prevention of haemorrhage is preferable to measures designed to

deal with this complication. Intramuscular Syntometrine (1.0 ml, containing ergometrine 0.5 mg and
Syntocinon 5 units) should be given with the 'crowning' of the fetal head, except to a patient with a
multiple pregnancy in whom it should be given at
delivery of the last baby only. Intravenous ergometrine in a dose of 0.25 mg or 0.5 mg with the delivery
of the anterior shoulder used to be the standard treatment for 'at risk' patients, but if other measures in
the first and second stages have been taken this is
less necessary and may cause rapid elevation of the
blood pressure. Probably the relative danger of ergometrine has been exaggerated (Dumoulin 1981). Gibbens *et al.* (1972) have shown that intramuscular
Syntometrine is as effective as intravenous oxytocin.
An alternative to ergometrine or Syntometrine that
is equally effective in the prevention of bleeding, but
does not induce transient vasoconstrictive hypertension and also does not have the side effects of
nausea, retching and vomiting (which are common
when ergometrine is used, especially during operative
deliveries under epidural analgesia), is the intravenous injection of oxytocin 10 units (Moir & Amoa
1979, Moodie and Moir 1976). This is, of course,
very easily given if, as is so often the case nowadays
and should always be the case in 'at risk' patients, an
intravenous infusion is already running.

Whichever oxytocic drug is given with crowning
of the the fetal head (some obstetricians prefer the
injection to be made as the anterior shoulder delivers)
its purpose is to promote uterine contraction rather
than to bring about a rushed delivery. Indeed, un-
hurried delivery of the fetal body when the uterus
has responded will keep open the cervix and lower segment until the placenta separates and then, as so often
happens, descends virtually 'on the heels' of the baby.

Uterine inertia as a result of prolonged labour is
much less common if an active approach to the management of labour is practised. Oxytocin is now administered at an earlier stage in labour if progress is
not being made, and this should be continued in reduced dosage until one to two hours after delivery.
This is mandatory if any of the above predisposing
factors are present in order to avoid postpartum
haemorrhage. Kelly *et al.* (1973) referred to the incidence of postpartum haemorrhage after oral prostaglandin or intravenous Syntocinon used for induction. However, there is no increase in blood loss at
and following delivery when an oxytocin infusion,
started during the first stage of labour, is continued
(in decreasing dosage) until an hour after delivery
(Moir & Amoa 1979).

If coagulation disorders are anticipated, as in
abruptio placentae or intrauterine death, the nature
of the disorder should be ascertained as quickly as
possible and expert haematological advice sought if
available (Chapter 36, p. 539). The administration
of fresh frozen plasma is probably the most useful
non-specific resuscitative measure and, with fresh
whole blood, should be given until specific measures
can be employed.

MANAGEMENT

The bleeding must be stopped as rapidly as possible,
oxytocic drugs being given in the first instance.
Whether or not the placenta has been delivered, a
midwife may give an intramuscular injection of Syntometrine or of Ergometrine 0.5 mg, but intravenous
Ergometrine is usually given, although in patients
with hypertension or cardiac disease intravenous
oxytocin is preferable. If not already running, an intravenous drip should be set up without delay and
oxytocin infused. If the placenta is still within the
uterus, an attempt may be made to deliver it when
the uterus contracts, but if this is not successful, it is
important to control the blood loss while resuscitative
measures are taken and arrangements made for
general anaesthesia. When the condition of the
patient permits, the placenta is manually removed,
further oxytocic drugs being given as required, either
by injection or intravenous infusion.

If the complete placenta has been delivered and
traumatic causes have been excluded, the patient is
resuscitated, if necessary by blood transfusion, and
uterine contraction is stimulated by oxytocin in an
intravenous infusion, by Ergometrine, or temporarily
by uterine massage and bimanual compression. If the
uterine fundus is pushed firmly downwards and posteriorly and a pad is placed at the vulva, the blood
loss is restricted to the amount filling the pelvis.
When the uterus is satisfactorily contracted, the vaginal clots can be allowed to escape, and resuscitation
continued. Packing of the uterus and vagina requires
a general anaesthetic to be effective, is probably no
longer indicated with oxytocics available, and many
obstetricians hold the view that this is more likely to
provoke than to prevent further bleeding.

(b) Trauma

Bleeding from a perineal laceration or episiotomy is
likely to be obvious, and prompt ligation of the dam-

aged vessel and repair of the wound is usually sufficient. Vaginal or cervical lacerations may be suspected if there has been any difficulty during the delivery or if it was precipitate. If the bleeding continues when the uterus is well contracted, particularly after an oxytocic drug has been administered, traumatic haemorrhage is confirmed. Immediate exploration is required, and this is best undertaken under general anaesthesia or continued epidural blockade. Vaginal lacerations are readily seen if a good light is available and if the cervix can be grasped and pulled away from the bleeding area. Repair of the laceration with deep sutures will usually control the haemorrhage. When the cervix is being examined, a vaginal speculum is inserted and the anterior lip of the cervix is lightly grasped with sponge-holding forceps. By using two or three pairs of these forceps it is possible to examine the whole of the loose cervix and to identify the bleeding area. This should be sutured, and deep cervical lacerations should be repaired with interrupted catgut sutures.

Haemorrhage from a lacerated or ruptured uterus should be suspected if bleeding persists even when the uterus appears to have responded to oxytocics and when no vaginal or cervical cause can be found. Full exploration under general anaesthesia, with blood available for transfusion, is then required. If a vaginal delivery has followed a previous Caesarean section, exploration of the site of the previous incision is required, particularly if there is excessive bleeding or if the labour and delivery have been complicated. Rupture of the uterus is nearly always treated by hysterectomy, but it may be possible to control the haemorrhage and repair the rupture. Whether a subsequent pregnancy will be possible with safety depends on a number of factors, but generally pregnancy should be avoided.

A haematoma may form in the broad ligament as a result of damage to the uterus, but this can usually be managed conservatively with blood transfusion, and antibiotics to prevent secondary infection. The diagnosis of this complication is not always easy, a progressive anaemia in association with tenderness and swelling in one or other iliac fossa possibly being the only features. Acute symptoms may not be present because of limitation of the haemorrhage by the broad ligament. Concealed bleeding into the very distensible tissues on one or other side of the vagina and vulva can also occur, sometimes very rapidly causing considerable pain and collapse. Unlike a broad ligament haematoma, this tends to be progressive rather than self-limiting so that, in addition to

resuscitation, incision with evacuation of clot and suturing, followed by the application of a firm vulval pad (not a vaginal pack) are needed.

RETAINED PLACENTA

If the placenta cannot be delivered by the methods described, it is 'retained'. With an active policy for the management of the third stage, no time-limit need be exceeded before arriving at this diagnosis. If there is associated non-traumatic bleeding despite the administration of oxytocic drugs, partial separation has certainly occurred, and, therefore, prompt measures to remove the placenta are required. If there is no vaginal bleeding and the uterus is contracted, the placenta has either completely separated or no separation has taken place.

If the placenta has separated, it will descend into the lower segment or vagina, provided it is not caught by the 'retraction ring' at the junction of the upper and lower segments. This is more likely following an Ergometrine injection than when Syntometrine or oxytocin has been given, and most likely with intravenous Ergometrine. The placenta may be wholly or partially trapped by the retraction ring, and if the latter, the lower edge can be felt on vaginal examination. In these circumstances it is advisable to await uterine relaxation before removing the placenta, provided there is no bleeding, and, particularly when there is effective epidural analgesia, this may be assisted digitally through the cervix. If there is excessive bleeding, however, the uterus must be relaxed by a general anaesthetic, and a further oxytocic injection, either intravenously or intramuscularly, will be required after the removal of the placenta.

If the placenta is retained wholly within the uterus, it should be removed under general anaesthesia by digital separation through the spongy layer of the decidua basalis. The other hand should be placed on the uterine fundus to maintain its position in the abdomen and to allow counterpressure to be exerted. After the removal of the placenta, more oxytocin will be required.

There is no place for the use of vigorous fundal compression in an attempt to expel the placenta. This is very painful and may cause complications, including inversion of the uterus, particularly if cord traction is applied at the same time.

If an active policy of management for the third stage is not practised, the indication to remove the placenta manually is vaginal bleeding or intrauterine bleeding with relaxation of the uterus. If there is no bleeding, it is a matter of convenience as to when the placenta should be removed. An intravenous injection of Ergometrine may stimulate a uterine contraction, and an attempt at placental delivery by cord traction may be made at this time. If it is unsuccessful, it is usually advisable to prepare the patient for a general anaesthetic.

A placental cotyledon may occasionally be retained within the uterus. This may not give rise to immediate bleeding but during the puerperium there will be excessive blood loss with the likelihood of uterine infection. It is perhaps surprising how often the placenta is reported as being complete in these patients at the time of delivery. While exploration and curettage are necessary if products are retained, it is distressing and perhaps harmful to explore the uterus and to find no products. Robinson (1972) and Malvern et al. (1973) have shown that ultrasound can be helpful in detecting the presence of retained products.

PLACENTA ACCRETA

When it is impossible to separate the placenta from the uterine wall, placenta accreta may be present. This arises because implantation of the ovum occurred in an area of the uterus in which the endometrium was deficient or damaged, possibly as a result of previous scarring especially after Caesarean section, or a congenital anomaly (Loring 1973). Fox (1972) reviewed this subject and found that placenta praevia and previous Caesarean section were the most common predisposing causes, although curettage was also implicated. Elderly multiparas were the most common group to have this complication. The chorionic villi readily penetrate the endometrium and reach the myometrium. As there is no satisfactory plane of separation, complete or partial placenta accreta is found.

Placenta increta refers to penetration of the myometrium by the chorionic villi, and, when the villi reach the serosal aspect of the uterus, this is *placenta percreta*. Some instances of placenta accreta are associated with placenta praevia, but the condition is rare.

Hysterectomy is the safest method of treatment. If uterine function must be preserved, it is possible to leave the placenta *in situ* and hope that complete autolysis will occur. Further pregnancies have been reported after this form of management, but the risk of uterine infection is considerable. Antibiotic therapy would certainly be required to prevent this. No attempt at 'piecemeal' removal of the placenta should be contemplated, because of the danger of severe haemorrhage.

INVERSION OF THE UTERUS

In this condition, the fundus of the uterus descends through the uterine body and cervix into the vagina, and sometimes protrudes through the vulva. Das (1940), in his review of 391 cases of inverted uterus reported an incidence of 46% spontaneous inversion. Also O'Connor (1977) emphasized the possibility of recurrence of the condition in subsequent deliveries, especially when manual replacement had been used, the overall incidence of recurrence being stated as 33%. Plainly if this figure is correct it calls for extreme caution in the management of the third stage of any subsequent pregnancy. It will not occur if the uterus is contracted, and is most likely when vigorous attempts are made to expel the placenta, or cord traction is used with the uterus in a relaxed state. Whenever acute inversion occurs it is a serious obstetric complication, for despite the availability of blood transfusion and antibiotics, the maternal mortality rate is assessed at about 15%.

It is worthy of emphasis that the use of controlled cord traction to deliver the placenta is likely to result in the occasional case of acute uterine inversion despite efforts to prevent it by counterpressure upwards on the uterine fundus as illustrated in Fig. 24.13 (p. 354). Fell (1966) referred to three such cases occurring in his own hospital within a period of 16 months. More recent reports of inversion of the uterus relate to domiciliary deliveries by less skilled attendants, and death of the patient from septic or haemorrhagic shock still occurs (Massoudnia 1973).

In its mildest form the uterus is 'dimpled', and the ease with which this can occur is demonstrated at Caesarean section when the placenta is removed. Incomplete inversion occurs when the uterine fundus descends through the cervix and comes to lie in the upper part of the vagina. With complete inversion the endometrial aspect of the uterus is seen outside the vulva, sometimes with the placenta still attached. The vagina may be pulled out partially or completely. The abdominal organs, particularly the small bowel, may be found in the funnel produced by the inversion.

The condition may be diagnosed in various ways.

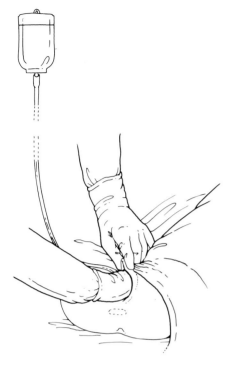

Fig. 28.1. Diagrammatic representation of hydrostatic replacement.

Acute complete inversion resulting from cord traction is immediately obvious. Incomplete inversion should be suspected when a state of shock develops in a patient whose blood loss is insufficient to account for it. If the usual means of resuscitation fail to produce improvement, inversion should always be suspected and a vaginal examination made. Theoretically, incomplete inversion may be recognized by the fundus of the uterus being felt at a lower level in the abdomen; the fundus is also described as feeling 'dimpled'. Neither of these two physical signs is reliable in the diagnosis; the fundus in incomplete inversion is rarely significantly lower in the abdomen than usual perhaps because, as the fundus goes down, the vault of the vagina is drawn up, and characteristic 'dimpling' is frequently masked by lower abdominal guarding.

If the condition is diagnosed immediately it occurs, replacement should be carried out instantly. At this time the pelvic soft tissues will be relaxed and there will be no spasm preventing replacement (Dewhurst & Bevis 1951). Delay by only a few minutes, however, will allow shock to develop and spasms at the neck of the sac will effectively prevent manual re-placement. In this type of case, when the inversion occurs with the attendant present at the bedside, instant replacement can be life-saving.

Once shock has developed it is better to commence resuscitative measures, but it is not likely that real improvement will occur until the uterus has been replaced. Digital replacement under general anaesthetic may be carried out, but the hydrostatic method described by O'Sullivan (1945) is probably more effective and safer. Warm, sterile fluid is gradually instilled into the vagina by means of a douche can and tubing (Fig. 28.1), while attempting the not always easy (perhaps impossible) task of achieving 'hydrostatic occlusion' of the vagina with the closed fist, as much as 4 or 5 litres being required. The fluid pressure reverses the inversion and results in the uterus being distended, so returning to its normal intra-abdominal position. The fluid is then drained off and Ergometrine is given, a hand remaining in the uterus until the fluid has escaped and the uterus is contracting satisfactorily. If the placenta is still adherent, it is probably better to remove it after the uterus has been replaced and conditions are optimal for retraction of the placental site.

HAEMORRHAGE FOLLOWING CAESAREAN SECTION

Secondary haemorrhage is most often the result of retained products of conception and/or infection (Dewhurst 1966). Bleeding some days after Caesarean section is less likely to be due to retained products than to damage to the uterine wound, almost certainly the result of infection. There may be excessive bleeding following the operation if a blood vessel, particularly at a lateral angle of the lower segment incision, has been insecurely ligated, but bleeding some days later may be due to infection lysing a clot in this vessel. This is more likely when the suture material has been absorbed. Severe haemorrhage may result and, if blood replacement is not sufficient to improve the patient's condition, ligation of the anterior division of the internal iliac artery on one or both sides may be effective. The result is dramatic and the function of the uterus including a later pregnancy is not precluded. MacVicar and Graham (1973) reported two cases of secondary haemorrhage following Caesarean section due to rupture of the scar.

UNEXPLAINED COLLAPSE

Collapse may occur at any point during labour if it is due to rupture of the uterus or abruptio placentae or to internal bleeding from some other cause. Collapse late in labour when uterine contractions are very strong may be due to an amniotic fluid infusion; this condition can also present within a short time after delivery when it is to be presumed the infusion preceded delivery but the effects followed a short time later. Postpartum collapse must first be regarded as being due to bleeding which may be external or internal; in the latter case the blood may be retained within the uterus or be paravaginal or intra- or extra-peritoneal. Rupture of the uterus may still be present even though the patient delivers herself *per vaginam* whilst forceps delivery may even have contributed to the rupture. A uterine inversion which is complete is readily recognizable but if it is incomplete it can easily be missed. Adrenal haemorrhage is a rare condition but may occur at any time. Endotoxic shock such as is seen in patients with septic abortions may also be encountered after delivery. Adrenocortical exhaustion may complicate several of the conditions mentioned.

Faced with such a shocked patient the clinical circumstances of the collapse must first of all be rapidly assessed. If the patient is undelivered, do the signs suggest rupture of the uterus or abruptio placentae? Are there pulmonary complications suggesting amniotic infusion? If the patient is postpartum, is the uterus contracted or relaxed? If relaxed, is it full of blood, the fundus palpable high in the abdomen? Was a Créde-type expression of placental delivery undertaken which might aggravate any shock present? Is the postpartum fundus entirely normal to palpation or is uterine inversion a possibility?

An intravenous infusion must be set up at once and if, as will usually be the case, bleeding is the cause of the collapse, the sooner blood can be given the better. A plasma expander may be given in moderate quantity whilst the blood is being cross-matched but more than one litre should not be used; if there is any tendency to a blood clotting defect a plasma expander such as dextran may aggravate it; blood must, moreover, be taken for cross-matching before dextran is set up. If dyspnoea and cyanosis are pronounced features, as in amniotic infusion, mouth-to-mouth respiration, oxygen administration or intubation and mechanical ventilation may be regarded as a matter of urgency.

If, once these measures for resuscitation are begun, the cause of the collapse becomes clear then appropriate treatment as already discussed must be undertaken. If the diagnosis is not clear, a vaginal examination must be done to detect a uterine inversion, and exploration of the uterine cavity under general anaesthesia may be required to locate a rupture. The presence of a paravaginal haematoma or cervical tear will generally be detected at one or other of these examinations. Plasma fibrinogen estimations may be appropriate or measurements of the fibrin degradation products; clinical observation of the speed of clot formation in withdrawn blood may clearly indicate a clotting defect to be present. The investigation of coagulation failure is detailed in Chapter 36 (p. 550).

AMNIOTIC FLUID INFUSION

This condition is sometimes termed 'amniotic fluid embolism'. In some cases the pulmonary embolic aspects are predominant and the patient dies acutely from respiratory failure as in a massive clot embolus. In other cases the pulmonary complications may not be lethal and within a few hours the patient then develops a blood-coagulation disorder initiated by the widespread infusion of amniotic fluid with its thromboplastic qualities into the general circulation.

The 1966–67 Confidential Enquiry into Maternal Deaths in England and Wales gives an excellent account of the clinical picture associated with amniotic fluid infusion.

1   There may be sudden collapse, usually after rupture of the membranes; the collapse may be during labour or within a few hours of delivery. The uterine contractions prior to the collapse are often very strong indeed.

2   In association with the collapse there may be muscular twitching or a convulsion; there is usually dyspnoea and cyanosis and the nose and mouth may be filled with frothy, blood-stained mucus.

3   Blood coagulation disorder later develops which may be associated with postpartum bleeding, intra- or extra-peritoneal haemorrhage and effusions of blood from veni-puncture sites and lacerations.

Other aetiological factors to be mentioned are grand multiparity, a dead or very large fetus and oxytocic administration.

Although precipitate labour or violent uterine action is a factor in some cases of amniotic fluid infusion they are not always encountered. The 1973–75 Confidential Enquiry records that of 14 deaths from such infusion, violent contractions were evident in 5; in 10 cases oxytocins had been used (oxytocin in 8: prostaglandin in 2).

The diagnosis of amniotic fluid infusion may be very difficult and to some extent may be a matter of exclusion of the other conditions mentioned above. Because of the acuteness of the pulmonary embarrassment in many cases, treatment for this must be undertaken at once or the patient will die. Clearing of the air passages, oxygen administration and, if possible, intubation of the patient and positive pressure respiration are to be employed. Until the respiratory embarrassment is under control, little more can be done. Once it is under control it is important to test for the development of a blood coagulation disorder by clinical observation of possible bleeding sites, clotting time of withdrawn blood, the plasma fibrinogen level and that of fibrin degradation products and a platelet count. Obvious bleeding will demand blood transfusion to maintain the circulating blood volume; this is beyond doubt. What is not beyond doubt is what other treatment should then be given. The administration of fibrogen has been advocated or antifibrinolytic agents such as epsilon amniocaproic acid or Trasylol, or indeed both. It seems more logical, however, to suggest heparinization of the patient as advocated by Reid and Weiner (1950); this treatment initiated soon enough, if fibrinogen depletion is recognized, may save a dangerous situation. Heparin therapy for this acute emergency remains controversial, however, 30 years after it was first suggested. A recent recovery in a personal case and a report of a survival in another (Resnik et al. 1976) in which the various measures discussed here were used except for heparin and fibrinogen, etc., indicate that these more questionable measures should be withheld, at least initially, to observe the effect of conventional supporting measures. The mechanisms and management of coagulation failure, following amniotic fluid infusion or other causes, are described in Chapter 36 (p. 539).

Positive confirmation of the diagnosis of an amniotic fluid infusion may be difficult in non-fatal cases. A chest X-ray may or may not give a diffuse picture similar to that of pulmonary oedema, the extent depending upon the extent of the infusion throughout the lung fields. Gregory and Clayton (1973) employed macro-aggregated ^{131}I albumin and a lung scan showed a large perfusion defect in the lower pole of one lung; this could indeed prove to be a helpful technique. These authors advise that the sequence of clinical management in a suspected case should be:

1 immediate administration of heparin when there is a clinical suspicion of amniotic fluid infusion;
2 administration of blood in sufficient quantities to maintain an effective blood volume: fibrinogen may be added if blood fails to clot after heparin therapy;
3 antifibrinolytic agents should be given if the condition continues to deteriorate;
4 confirmation of clinical impression of the diagnosis should be sought by their 131 iodine photoscanning technique.

These authors even go so far as to suggest that, rarely, where poor lung perfusion seems to be the main feature and following confirmation of the clinical impression by a lung scan an extracorporeal circulation should be given prompt consideration.

Unfortunately many cases are still fatal and the final diagnosis is sought at a postmortem examination. It is important for the pathologist to realize that this diagnosis cannot be confirmed by naked eye examination of the lung. Histologically amniotic material may be found in pulmonary vessels if the sections are stained with haematoxylin and eosin; easier identification will be obtained by using the alcian green phloxin method which stains mucus greenish-blue and fetal squames red. Vernix may be demonstrated by using a fat stain. It is unfortunate that careful examination of the lungs as suggested here is not always employed in patients who have died with clinical features suggesting the diagnosis of amniotic fluid infusion. Courtney (1974) has reviewed this difficult subject well.

SHEEHAN'S SYNDROME

In any variety of postpartum collapse with very low blood pressure, especially if sustained for 6–12 hours, there is an urgent need to restore blood pressure to normal not only to save the patient's life but to prevent pituitary necrosis (Sheehan's syndrome). The pituitary, enlarged as a result of pregnancy, is most susceptible to the effects of profound and prolonged hypotension. Sheehan and McLetchie (1943) demonstrated pituitary necrosis, partial or complete, in association with severe cases of postpartum haemorrhage and collapse. In extreme cases the whole anterior lobe may be destroyed. The mechanism is probably arterial spasm (Sheehan & Davies 1968), but disseminated intravascular coagulation may also play a part in some cases.

One early effect of this pituitary damage (though not pathognomonic) is poor or absent lactation. Later there may also be failure of menstruation due to a lack of gonadotrophin secretion. The precise symptomatology depends on the degree of destruction. When widespread destruction occurs, there may be atrophy of breasts and genital organs, weight loss, premature ageing etc.; effects of almost total loss of pituitary function. Early and complete blood replacement is essential to help to prevent this catastrophe.

REFERENCES

COURTNEY L.D. (1974) *Obstet. Gynaec. Surv.*, **29**, 169.

DAS P. (1940) *Obstet. Gynaec. Brit. Emp.*, **47**, 525.

Department of Health and Social Security (1975–1979) *Confidential Enquiries into Maternal Deaths in England and Wales.* HMSO, London.

DEWHURST C.J. (1966) *J. Obstet. Gynaec. Brit. Cwlth.*, **73**, 53.

DEWHURST C.J. & BEVIS D.C.A. (1951) *Lancet*, **i**, 394.

DUMOULIN J.G. (1981) *J. Obstet. Gynaec.*, **1**, 178–181.

FELL M.R. (1966) *Brit. med. J.*, **ii**, 764.

FOX H. (1972) *Obstet. Gynec. Surv.*, **27**, 475.

GREGORY M.G. & CLAYTON E.M. (1973) *Obstet. and Gynaec.*, **42**, 236.

GIBBENS D., BOYD N.R.H., CROCKER S., BAUMBER S. & CHARD T. (1972) *J. Obstet. Gynaec. Brit. Cwlth.*, **79**, 644.

KELLY J., FLYNN A.M. & BERTRAND P.V. (1973) *J. Obstet. Gynaec. Brit. Cwlth.*, **80**, 923.

LORING T.W. (1973) *Amer. J. Obstet. Gynec.*, **116**, 505.

MACVICAR J. & GRAHAM R.M. (1973) *Brit. med. J.*, **ii**, 29.

MALVERN J., CAMPBELL S. & MAY P. (1973) *J. Obstet. Gynaec. Brit. Cwlth.*, **80**, 320.

MASSOUDNIA N. (1973) *Geburtsh. Frauenheilk.*, **33**, 901.

MOIR D.D. & AMOA A.B. (1979) *Brit. J. Anaesth.*, **51**, 113.

MOODIE J.E. & MOIR D.D. (1976) *Brit. J. Anaesth.*, **48**, 571.

O'CONNOR M.C. (1977) *Brit. J. Obstet. Gynaec.*, **84**, 789.

O'SULLIVAN J.V. (1945) *Brit. Med. J.*, **ii**, 282.

REID D.E. & WEINER A.E. (1950) *New Engl. J. Med.*, **243**, 597.

RESNIK R., SWARTZ W.H., PLUMER M.H., BENIRSCHKE K. & STRATTHAUS M.E. (1976) *Obst. Gynec., N.Y..*, **47**, 295.

ROBINSON H.P. (1972) *Scot. med. J.*, **17**, 364.

SHEEHAN H.L. & DAVIES J.C. (1968) *Brit. med. Bull.*, **24**, 59.

SHEEHAN H.L. & McLETCHIE N.G.B. (1943) *J. Obstet. Gynaec. Brit. Emp.*, **50**, 27.

CHAPTER 29
MATERNAL INJURIES AND COMPLICATIONS

J. M. BEAZLEY

Maternal injuries, particularly their avoidance, recognition and management, comprise a fascinating series of acute obstetric events. Moreover, as maternal mortality has diminished, maternal injuries have become increasingly important. Now they contribute significantly towards maternal morbidity.

To include in this chapter such bizarre events as maternal injuries caused by lightning (Rees 1965), or indirect uterine injuries following motor car accidents, seat-belt injuries, or gunshot wounds would be interesting (Christian 1979, Fudge 1912, Johnson 1962, Lawrence & Sherman 1948, Stapleton 1937, Wassenaar 1947). The usual, however, is more interesting and probably more important than the unusual. Therefore only injuries arising directly out of the process of childbirth will be considered here.

Maternal injury predisposes to infection. The vagina is a direct gateway to the peritoneum. Organisms traversing the cervix can cross the uterine cavity, turn right or left at the Fallopian tubes, and emerge at the far end in the peritoneal cavity. Obstetricians are duty bound to prevent such a bacteriological march.

The genital tract from the perineum to the peritoneum resembles a tube. Injuries at each level of the tube may be considered to have arisen within its lumen and inside or outside its walls.

THE VULVA AND VAGINA

Though some attempt is made physiologically and anatomically to prepare the vulva and vagina for parturition, it is hardly surprising, when one considers either the head circumference of a newborn child, or the width of its shoulders, that the mother's genital tract sometimes tears during the passage of these bulky and angular items. In practice, delivery of the fetal head is usually less traumatic to the perineum and lower vagina than delivery of the posterior shoulder. The inexperienced accoucheur will often breathe a sigh of relief following a successful and atraumatic delivery of the fetal head, only to suck his breath in again as he omits to flex the baby laterally and drives its posterior shoulder straight through the perineal floor.

Clinically it is important to recognize the following types of injury in the vulvo-vaginal region. Labial lacerations, which, though painful and tender, are probably of little significance otherwise. Laceration of the remnants of the hymen, the fourchette, the lower part of the vagina and the perineal skin which though common are but minor injuries, and do not involve the perineal body, i.e. a first-degree tear. A more extensive laceration will necessarily involve a variable portion of the posterior vaginal wall and also tears the perineal body, i.e. a second-degree tear. Further extension of such a laceration includes not only more of the vaginal wall, but, in addition, fibres of the external anal sphincter. Sometimes the tear cuts right through the sphincter to open up the mucosa of the anal canal (and perhaps the rectum also), when the situation is indeed serious, i.e. a third-degree tear.

Episiotomy

Buttonholing of the perineal body, which may not necessitate surgical repair, indicates, in my view, that unwarranted separation of the subcuticular tissues has occurred and should have been prevented by the timely execution of an episiotomy.

Devitalized tissue and haematoma formation are probably more significant causes of infection than bacteria. Healthy patients who are niether traumatized unduly nor exhausted can mobilize their defences readily enough, and deal with minor foci of infection. When, however, the bacteria of the vagina and rectum are provided with dead tissue and blood clot in which to multiply excessively, not even the most robust patients can ward off a serious threat from infection without the sophisticated help of medical science.

An episiotomy is a second-degree laceration of the vulva, vagina and perineal body, man-made with scissors, after local infiltration of the tissues with an anaesthetic agent. Older textbooks go to great lengths to enumerate the indications for episiotomy, e.g. occipito-posterior position, breech delivery, forceps delivery, narrow subpubic arch, previous vaginal repairs, shoulder dystocia, or to control the direction of vaginal lacerations, etc. Until recently the modern accoucheur has simply looked for reasons why an episiotomy should not be performed, probably in the belief that a clean surgical incision is more likely to heal by first intention than a bruised tear. However, as Russell (1982) points out there is little objective data to support claims that perineal incision correctly performed 'at the appropriate moment, eases delivery, protects the head of a small baby from trauma, is more quickly repaired than a ragged tear and will heal more quickly and effectively, is less liable to infection than a bruised and torn perineum, and reduces the risk of later complications such as dyspareunia and prolapse.'

In Britain the type of episiotomy incision preferred begins at the midline of the fourchette and runs backwards, tangentially to the pigmented area surrounding the anus, thus avoiding Bartholin's gland and its duct and bypassing any possible injury to the bowel. Midline episiotomies, though now out of favour, are mechanically more sensible. Nevertheless, they are associated with significantly more injuries to the anal sphincter, though, in a comparison of midline and mediolateral episiotomies, Coats *et al.* (1980) found that no recto-vaginal fistulae occurred in a randomized prospective study on 407 primigravid women.

A child's need at the time of delivery is for some increase in the antero-posterior diameter of the pelvic outlet. To achieve this a medio-lateral episiotomy must compensate for the altered angle of the incision and be more generous than a midline episiotomy.

Episiotomies directed laterally are both valueless and contraindicated.

REPAIR

Episiotomies are sutured more easily than lacerations. Where the vagina is lacerated, the apex of the tear needs to be identified so that a suture can be placed in or just above it. Thereafter sutures should be inserted into the edges of the vaginal epithelium down as far as the introitus. The author prefers to use

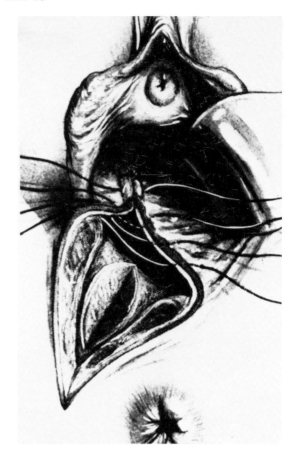

Fig. 29.1. (a) Suture of the vaginal epithelium.

interrupted sutures, which also avoids some possible shortening of the posterior vaginal wall (Fig. 29.1[a]).

Behind the reconstituted vagina there now remains a large 'dead space' which needs to be obliterated by two layers of interrupted sutures, the first layer in the deeper part of the hole, the second in the more superficial structures of the perineal body (Fig. 29.1 [b]). Only the skin now remains to be sutured (Fig. 29.1 [c]).

PROBLEMS

Iatrogenic complications are one of the significant developments of modern surgery. Episiotomy sutures which are tied too tightly will cause oedema and pain and may devitalize tissue. Sutures which are tied too loosely give inaccurate apposition of the tissues and increase scar formation; a matter of some importance to the sexually active couple who have denied them-

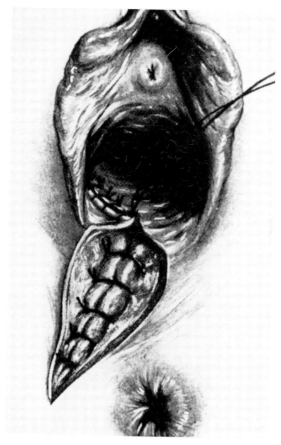

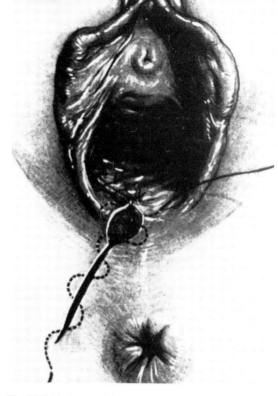

Fig. 29.1 (c) Suture of the perineal skin.

Fig. 29.1 (b) Suture of the perineal body.

selves sexual intercourse during the latter months of pregnancy.

When there is difficulty in reaching the apex of a vaginal tear, it is sometimes helpful to place the first suture at the mid-vaginal point and use it to pull the vaginal epithelium a little downwards. A second suture can then be inserted just above the first; and so on. Using this 'hand over hand' technique the apex is soon reached.

When the laceration is serious and involves the anal, and possibly, the rectal mucosa, the patient requires to be taken to the operating theatre. There, under general anaesthesia, a formal repair of the injury can be undertaken with all the advantages of a good light, good exposure, adequate assistance and a sufficient number of the correct instruments. The apex of the mucosa is first identified and a suture placed above it. The mucosal edges are then correctly aligned and sutured with interrupted sutures down as far as the anal margin. By this time the ends of

the torn sphincter will probably have retracted to make the sphincter 'horseshoe' shaped. One of the easiest ways to retrieve the torn proximal ends from their retracted position is to pick them up with a towel clip, i.e. the type whose two-pronged end is bent almost at right-angles to the main line of the shaft. This particular shape facilitates the probing which is sometimes necessary to locate the torn ends of the sphincter. The torn ends of the sphincter drawn together and united, the repair of the vaginal epithelium and perineal body then continues in the normal way.

Some infection of the area is invariable after this operation. Not only is the site contaminated naturally but it is frequently necessary to insert a finger into the rectum to facilitate suture of the anal mucosa. The use of prophylactic antibiotics may be favoured by some but most prefer to base antibiotic therapy on sensitivity reports when needed.

Bowel action will take care of itself. It seems both

wise and humane, however, to ensure that the first faeces passed have been rendered soft by the judicious use of liquid paraffin, and/or a small olive oil enema introduced into the rectum through a *narrow* and *flexible* cannula.

AFTER-CARE

It is common to observe that postpartum perineal discomfort occurs quite suddenly in patients who have received epidural analgesia for delivery. Perineal injuries may be the source of sufficient discomfort reflexly to cause urinary retention or make defaecation intolerable. Even sitting down might be a problem. The symptoms may persist for days. Sympathetic and sensible after-care can minimize the duration of discomfort. Beard *et al.* (1974) suggested that episiotomies sutured with 2/0 chromic catgut were slightly more uncomfortable than those sutured with polyglycolic acid (Dexon). Both suture materials were found to be easy to use though atraumatic Dexon sutures were more expensive than the corresponding chromic catgut (Ethicon). More recently Roberts and Hart (1983), in a randomly allocated double blind comparison of therapy with proteolytic enzymes (Chymoral) and placebo in 190 patients, reported that the combination of polyglycolic acid sutures and chymoral reduced the level of perineal pain, assessed subjectively, and significantly reduced the analgesic requirements.

In a fresh wound, minor bleeding or oozing and haematoma formation can probably be prevented by the use of ice packs to facilitate vasoconstriction. In an established haematoma, or an oedematous wound, warm applications to the perineum are more comforting and relieve the situation quicker. The author is unimpressed by the use of rubber air rings, proteolytic enzymes by mouth, or infra-red lamps in the treatment of the sore vulva, and finds that the sympathetic use of a mild parenteral analgesic or a night sedative is more appreciated by the patient.

An interesting document published by Baker (1973), a midwife, highlights a number of interesting features of postnatal perineal discomfort. Apparently West Indian women complain less about perineal discomfort than their European or Asian counterparts. There is no significant difference between the discomfort from an episiotomy wound or laceration, and traumatic deliveries, a prolonged second stage of labour, and poor suturing techniques are associated with greater pain than is experienced after short, normal labours and skilled suturing. More provocative

features of the booklet concern the timing of suture, the use of local anaesthetics and the experience of the individuals concerned in the repair. A disturbing report by Reading *et al.* (1982) emphasizes that many women suffer significant perineal pain within 24 hours of episiotomy. (This may be partly related to an increased use of epidural analgesia.) Up to three months after delivery, the incidence of pain at coitus was directly attributed to the episiotomy wound in 88% of women.

THE CERVIX

Lacerations

Minor cervical lacerations are extremely common. Usually they remain undetected. Bleeding which does not appear to be arising from the vagina or perineum and which continues despite a well retracted uterus, is usually the reason for examining the cervix. Cervical bleeding is readily controlled, temporarily, by the broad and even pressure which can be applied with sponge forceps.

Minor symptomless lacerations involving distal portions of the external cervix probably require no surgical treatment. If, however, the apex of the laceration approaches the vaginal vault, or, indeed, if it extends into the vaginal vault, the condition is more serious and warrants special care. Minor cervical lacerations can often be sutured in the labour room. Deep lacerations, however, especially if they appear to involve the vaginal vault, are best treated in theatre. There, examination of the tear, and access to it, are more easily achieved.

General anaesthesia will usually be necessary to determine safely the extent of any cervical tears which have extended forward towards the bladder or laterally towards the ureters, uterine artery, and the base of the broad ligament. Suture of these areas must be undertaken with great care and skill if the vital structures above the vault are to remain uncompromised.

Detachment

Spontaneous annular detachment of the cervix during labour is a rare complication. Most of the information concerning this injury is contained in isolated case reports (e.g. Amatayakul 1964, Burton-Brown 1950, Grant 1955). The most important predisposing factor seems to be cervical dystocia, i.e. failure of the cervix to dilate despite strong normal uterine contractions and close application of the presenting fetal part of the maternal cervix. Increasing pressure, local circulatory arrest and tissue devitalization result finally in tearing and annular detachment of the cervical cap. Because of the pathogenesis of the condition significant haemorrhage does not usually occur with spontaneous annular detachment of the cervix. Puerperal infection is a greater hazard.

As an aetiological factor, fibrosis of the cervix following cone biopsy is more theoretical than real (*Brit. med. J.* 1980, McLaren *et al.* 1974).

The level of cervical detachment varies and it depends chiefly upon the site of the junction between normal and abnormal cervical tissue. Usually detachment occurs just below the vaginal vault. In multiparas the cervix may already have been lacerated throughout a major part of its circumference at a previous delivery, the so-called 'bucket handle' tear. Cervical dystocia is more common in primigravidas.

Active management of labour now results in the early recognition of negligible cervical dilatation. Spontaneous annular cervical detachment is, therefore, likely to become an even rarer condition in England. Should such an unlikely event occur, the probable outcome, without surgical interference, is a cervical stump covered by healthy squamous epithelium which is virtually flush with the vaginal vault.

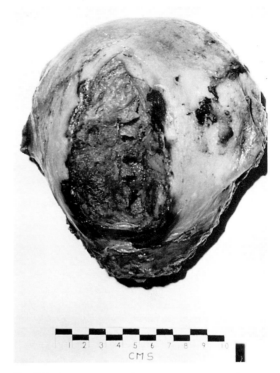

Fig. 29.2. A uterus removed as an emergency procedure following sudden rupture of a classical Caesarean section scar.

THE UTERINE BODY

Rupture of the uterus

Obstetricians who practise in developed countries will appreciate that uterine rupture usually presents in a manner which is quite different from that often seen in less sophisticated regions of the world.

Rupture of the lower segment is the most common form of uterine rupture in Britain. However, in whichever segment of the uterus rupture occurs, the degree of injury sustained is significantly influenced by whether or not the rupture has involved the serosal coat of the uterus, the position of the rupture in relation to the bladder and/or ureter, and the the position of the placenta in relation to the rupture.

Predisposing and precipitating factors
Dehiscence of previous uterine scars is usually quoted as an established cause of uterine rupture. In the Maternal Mortality Report for the years 1973–75 (DHSS 1979), however, only one of the eleven deaths from uterine rupture followed dehiscence of a uterine scar. Three more ruptures resulted from intrauterine manipulation, the remaining seven occurring spon-

taneously. For the first time since 1955–57, the maternal death toll from uterine rupture shows no improvement.

Lower segment scars usually rupture only during labour. Scars from classical Caesarean sections may rupture during the latter part of pregnancy (Fig. 29.2). Rupture of the uterus is not predictable, nor is rupture of a uterine scar.

Perforation of the non-pregnant uterus, caused more frequently by dilatation of the cervix than by endometrial curettage, sometimes results in uterine rupture, especially of the upper segment, in a subsequent pregnancy (Fig. 29.3). Attention has also been drawn recently to the hazard of uterine rupture after hysterotomy (Clow & Crompton 1973). Uterine scars caused by myomectomy rarely result in uterine rupture.

Oxytocic hyperstimulation of the intact uterus has always been considered a potential danger to the integrity of the upper and lower segments. The judicious and controlled use of Syntocinon, however, may be employed without undue anxiety for either

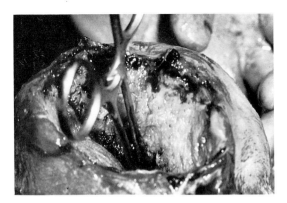

Fig. 29.3. Rupture of the uterus at the fundus through the site of a probable perforation at previous curettage.

the induction of labour or the acceleration of prolonged labour (Chapter 25). Moreover, there is no absolute reason why Syntocinon should not also be used to assist with the planned delivery of a woman with a lower segment Caesarean section scar, so long as her welfare is monitored carefully throughout labour.

Obstetric mismanagement, in particular internal podalic version of a *neglected* transverse lie, may be responsible for rupturing the uterus. Problems of this kind are, fortunately, rare in Britain today.

DIAGNOSIS

Those who perform lower segment Caesarean section regularly cannot fail to have been impressed with the extreme thinness of the lower segment which is sometimes observed at operation. Even unsuspected 'windows' are sometimes found in old scars, and one is left with a sense of wonder that during labour this old injury to the lower segment has not progressed to a disastrous rupture involving the whole uterus and the bladder base to which it is probably adherent. The diagnosis of uterine rupture is indeed difficult. It is the nub of the problem in modern obstetric practice.

It is extremely uncommon for a patient to present during labour with sudden and severe bursting abdominal pain, cessation of progress in labour, fetal death, and all the signs of an internal haemorrhage and an acute abdomen. The dehiscence of a classical Caesarean section scar may result in such a picture, although in modern practice it is more likely to be due to the rupture of a lower vertical midline incision through part of the upper and lower segments. (Incisions of this kind are sometimes necessitated by an uncommon occurrence during a previous operation, such as significant varicosities over the lower segment.)

Of the less dramatic signs of rupture, tenderness in the region of a previous Caesarean section scar, appears to be most unreliable. It is a common finding during labour with or without a Caesarean section scar. Because the sign is unhelpful the author no longer subscribes to the view that epidural analgesia increases the hazard of uterine rupture by removing a valuable sign of impending dehiscence.

Brudenell and Chakravarti (1975) point out that the best chance of detecting uterine rupture now lies in careful and continuous monitoring of uterine contractions and fetal well-being during labour. Thus slowing of the rate of progress of labour for no very obvious reason, as shown by a partograph, associated perhaps with a rise in the maternal pulse rate and a slight trickle of blood per vaginam, with or without the onset of fetal distress, should raise the suspicion of rupture of part of the lower uterine segment. Bleeding is not always a concomitant sign as the lower segment can be relatively avascular at the time of rupture. Indeed, dehiscence of a fibrous scar is attended by virtually no bleeding.

Digital assessment of the lower segment during labour, or of a lower segment scar, is an unsatisfactory procedure and probably dangerous without general anaesthesia. An epidural block may facilitate palpation of the lower segment through the cervix, although the author does not favour this procedure if rupture is suspected. After delivery, palpation of a lower segment scar is recommended by many authors, but in my experience detection of a small dehiscence can be extremely difficult, as it cannot be distinguished from the general substance of the interior aspect of the retracted uterus.

THE MANAGEMENT OF RUPTURE

Should partial rupture of the lower uterine segment be detected after delivery, laparotomy, with formal repair of the injury and examination of the extent of pelvic damage, is advisable. Blood transfusion is usually not required.

Following dramatic rupture of the uterus it is obvious clinically that blood replacement is of primary importance followed by laparotomy under general anaesthesia. The incidence of uterine rupture is now of the order of 1 in 2500 deliveries and the frightening spectacle of gross uterine injury is, therefore, quite rare. Nevertheless, rupture of the lower segment may extend anteriorly into the back of the bladder, or laterally towards the region of the uterine artery or even into the broad ligament plexus of veins, causing extensive haemorrhage and damage.

Whatever the variety of uterine rupture, on entering the abdomen the surgical management will follow one of three courses of action.

Firstly, hysterectomy may be the safest procedure but the hazards should not be minimized. Smith (1980) emphasizes not only the risk of maternal death from emergency obstetric hysterectomy, but, in surviving patients, the complications of ureteric injuries, and pulmonary embolism. When the risks to the bladder and ureter are grave a safe sub-total hysterectomy should not be avoided. Giwa-Osagie et al. (1983) report a series of emergency obstetric hysterectomy in 61 patients of whom 37 had ruptured uterus. The lowest mortality (4%) followed sub-total hysterectomy in booked patients, while the highest mortality (50%) followed total hysterectomy in unbooked patients.

Secondly, if it is desirable, and possible, to preserve the uterus, the surgeon may decide to repair a small rent in the lower uterine segment. Frankly, the author does not favour this limited course of action, although concedes that there may be occasions when it is necessary to assist a patient to achieve her desired family unit, even if it does involve grave anxieties throughout the course of any future pregnancy. Lastly, uterine repair, followed by sterilization, can be performed if significant difficulties with a hysterectomy are anticipated, or, perhaps, the woman wishes to continue to menstruate.

Acute inversion of the uterus

This important accident is considered in Chapter 28, p. 412.

PARAGENITAL HAEMATOMA

Maternal injury to vessels outside the wall of the genital tract may lead to haematoma formation. The damage usually remains undetected until the patient presents as a problem of third stage collapse, with signs of haemorrhage but no obvious uterine or vaginal bleeding. Depending upon the site of formation of the haematoma pain may aggravate the collapsed state and prove misleading.

When trauma has occurred to the walls of the

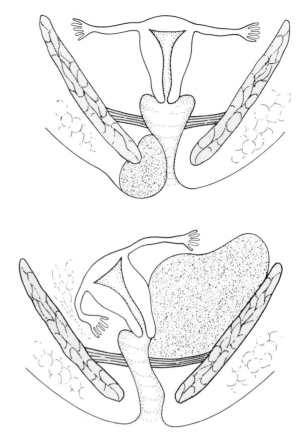

Fig. 29.4. Paravaginal haematoma. In the upper illustration the haematoma lies beneath the levator ani muscle. In the lower illustration the haematoma lies above the levator ani and is spreading upwards into the broad ligament.

genital tract, e.g. an episiotomy, vaginal tear, cervical laceration, or some form of uterine rupture, postpartum haematoma formation, even though it is invisible, is considered early. In the absence of overt genital injury, it is easy to fail to recognize the occult bleeding and this can be a dangerous oversight. The doctor who is not continually awake to the possibility of paragenital haematoma formation is clinically naïve.

A significant distinction should be made between paragenital haematomas which lie above or below the levator ani muscle (Fig. 29.4).

The infralevator haematomas include haematomas of the vulva and perineum, paravaginal haematomas, and bleeding into the ischiorectal fossa. Supralevator haematomas spread upwards and outwards beneath the broad ligament, or partly downwards to bulge into the walls of the upper vagina. (They can impress the vaginal wall sufficiently to close off the upper vagina completely.) A supralevator haematoma which tracks backwards under the base of the posterior leaf of the broad ligament enters the retroperitoneal space.

INFRALEVATOR HAEMATOMAS

The paravaginal plexus of veins is one of the obstetrician's many enemies. Partial disruption of this plexus can follow undue distension of the lower vaginal tract even though the vaginal epithelium remains intact. Imperfect repair of an episiotomy may permit bleeding to continue from the edges of the vaginal wall. If the 'dead space' underlying the vaginal epithelium is not completely obliterated, the paravaginal plexus may continue to ooze into the surrounding tissue. The blood will track downwards into the labial folds and perineal body and result in a very large and painful haematoma of the perineal and labial tissues on one side (Fig. 29.5).

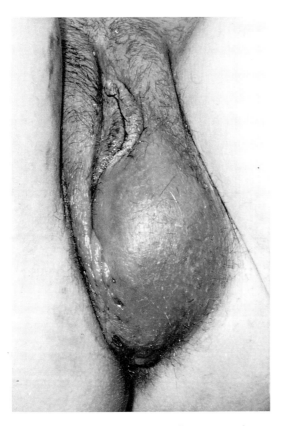

Fig. 29.5. A large vulval haematoma following normal vaginal delivery.

It might be expected that pressure within the injured area would ultimately stop the venous bleeding. No reliance should be put upon such a mechanism. A great quantity of blood can escape laterally into the ischiorectal fossa, or into the paravaginal tissues, bulging the lower vaginal epithelium inwards to the vaginal lumen.

The management of infralevator haematoma formation usually necessitates, in addition to blood transfusion, sedation and/or analgesia, and surgical evacuation of the haematoma in theatre. Exploration of the injured area rarely reveals a definitive haematoma or any obvious bleeding point. Nevertheless clearing the tissue spaces of blood and inserting deep mattress sutures through the injured tissue to firmer tissues beneath, serves to control the haemorrhage and affords the patient relief. If surgery is not undertaken, the patient will usually recover after adequate transfusion and sedation. There is much more pain and illness to be endured, however, and a much longer recovery period to be anticipated.

SUPRALEVATOR HAEMATOMA

Grave anxieties are raised in the mind of the accoucheur who detects the presence of blood in the broad ligament. He must question the possibility of a cervical laceration extending into the vaginal vault, or even the presence of an unsuspected rupture of the lower uterine segment.

Bleeding above the levator ani muscle can be difficult to recognize until the haematoma is large enough to present abdominally. The collection of blood ultimately raises the broad ligament out of the pelvis and a soft mass appears in one or other iliac fossae. Vaginal examination will reveal a 'boggy swelling' in the vaginal fornix of the same side. The uterus is usually pushed contralaterally. As the broad ligament fills, some blood also tracks downwards to the levator ani and pushes the upper vaginal wall inwards to occlude the vaginal lumen.

Because of the large spaces involved pain is not commonly a feature of the early development of supralevator haematomas. Third stage collapse of the patient with signs of internal haemorrhage is a more characteristic form of presentation.

In contrast to infralevator haematomas, those arising above the broad ligament should be managed conservatively whilst such treatment is feasible. A broad ligament filled with haematoma is no place to enter with equanimity, even for an experienced surgeon. Evacuation of the haematoma and firm pack may be all that can be achieved. Certainly the blind insertion of deep sutures is contraindicated, as the position of the ureter is impossible to determine. Hysterectomy too is better avoided unless there is an obvious injury to the substance of the uterus or cervix which cannot easily be repaired.

Faced with a patient deteriorating rapidly, despite attempts to control bleeding by pressure pack, there should be no hesitation in ligating the internal iliac artery on the affected side.

INTERNAL ILIAC ARTERY LIGATION

Ligation of the internal iliac artery was first performed by Kelly in 1894. Few resident gynaecological or obstetric surgeons have seen the operation today, nor are they aware of the important surgical anatomy.

The bifurcation of the common iliac artery will be found at the pelvic brim. At that point the ureter lies on top of the vessels. When the internal iliac artery is identified it will be found to be approximately one-and-a-half inches long. Before surgery is undertaken these landmarks should be identified.

The peritoneum can be cut between the ureter and the internal iliac artery. The ureter will then come up with the leaf of peritoneum, as it is raised to expose the artery beneath. The internal iliac artery is next lifted and the bifurcation re-identified. A ligature is placed under the internal iliac artery and tied without ever cutting that major vessel. It is important to work within the capsule of the artery whenever possible. This should be undertaken as a purposive manoeuvre to avoid damaging veins which may be closely associated with the outside of the arterial capsule. In elderly patients thrombophlebitis, or atherosclerosis may give rise to adhesions which tear veins as the ligature is passed. During the age of childbearing this is not usually a problem.

Burchell (1968) has described the physiology of internal iliac ligation. He points out that, following ligation, three principal collateral circulations can be observed. All involve vessels of smaller diameter than the internal iliac artery. He further points out that the pelvic blood supply is so enormous that, following ligation, there is not even the danger of tissue necrosis, and compensatory growth of the remaining vessels does not occur. Of 45 patients described by Burchell none came to any harm from the procedure.

Why internal iliac artery ligation controls haemorrhage so effectively poses an interesting question. Clinical research has revealed that blood will flow freely from a severed uterine artery, despite bilateral ligation of both internal iliac vessels. Nevertheless, Burchell showed that bilateral ligation reduces arterial pressure and transforms it to a venous-like system by eliminating the trip hammer effect.

The operation is useful when there is a need to anticipate the control of haemorrhage, or as a therapeutic measure, when haemorrhage cannot be controlled by more commonly accepted methods. The author's personal experience of the operation has been favourable. and he believes that postgraduate students should be trained in the technique of internal iliac ligation and made aware of its potential.

PELVIC INJURY

The pubic symphysis

It is well established that the joints of the pelvis increase their mobility during pregnancy. A degree of pelvic 'give' is radiographically manifest during labour.

Movement of the pubic bones in the later part of pregnancy may cause some discomfort about the symphysis. Following a trial of cephalo-pelvic disproportion at the pelvic brim, or, perhaps, difficult Kielland's forceps delivery from pelvic cavity, separation of the fibres of the ligaments surrounding the pubis may occur which gives rise to maternal discomfort. If, during delivery, the degree of pubic separation has been pathological, the pain may seem to occur suddenly in the early puerperium and be extremely severe. Rolling movements of the pelvis, as for example when turning over in bed, can be particularly painful. Minor degrees of discomfort about the symphysis pubis will resolve with adequate rest. The improvement can be facilitated by the judicious use of a corset. More severe injuries may necessitate pelvic support.

Harris (1974) emphasizes that, although rare, features resembling osteitis pubis may be associated with the pubic trauma of repeated pregnancies.

Symphisiotomy is such an uncommon procedure in developed countries that it no longer deserves detailed attention for practitioners working in these areas.

Damage to the symphysis pubis is likely to recur in similar circumstances.

The coccyx

During late pregnancy the sacrococcygeal joint is mobile. During delivery the coccyx is usually displaced backwards, and the coccygeal tip may move as much as 2.5 cm. Because of its mobility, coccygeal damage is unusual during delivery.

The coccyx can be dislocated during parturition or even fractured. Displacement is usually in a backwards direction and the injury is usually non-recurrent.

Forward angulation of the coccyx is sometimes the result of an earlier accident in which the patient unexpectedly fell and injured the base of her spine across the edge of a chair, or on the floor. Fixed forward angulation rarely causes any obstruction to delivery and, if the coccyx will not bend backwards spontaneously, it may be deliberately fractured. The ill effects of this procedure are negligible.

NERVE INJURY

Lumbosacral nerves

Foot drop, often unilateral, may be observed during the first few days after delivery. The condition is usually mild and may pass unnoticed unless the patient specifically draws attention to the disability. Detailed examination of the neurological lesion will reveal a disturbance of the lower motor neuron type in areas served by the femoral nerve or lumbosacral plexus.

Formerly it was considered that dragging the roots of the lumbosacral plexus across the brim of the pelvis during engagement of the fetal head, or direct injury to the nerve roots by the blades of obstetric forceps during rotation procedures, accounted for these injuries. Now it is widely believed that herniation of lumbosacral discs is responsible for the damage.

The joints of the vertebral column share in the increased mobility occasioned by pregnancy. The normal lumbar lordosis of pregnancy serves to exaggerate any potential weakness of the discs in the lumbosacral region. The extent of the herniation of the disc, and the direction of its protrusion, probably determines the degree and distribution of neurological involvement.

Management of damage to the lumbosacral nerve roots is the management of a prolapsed intervertebral disc, namely, rest in bed on a suitable mattress supported by firm boards. Severe degrees of foot drop, which are most uncommon, necessitate consultation with both the orthopaedic and physiotherapy departments to ensure that the patient receives adequate muscle treatment and is fitted with a suitable toe spring to raise the foot during walking.

The peroneal nerve

Clumsy use of the obstetric stirrups when placing a parturient patient in the lithotomy position may result in the bruising of her peroneal nerve against the fibula. The result may be unilateral foot drop. The pathogenesis of this injury is now fully appreciated. As supporting poles are now padded and obstetric stirrups are used with considerable care, peroneal damage after delivery is seen very infrequently.

The pudendal nerve

When it is considered how frequently pudendal nerve blockade is utilized on obstetric practice, it is surprising that the nerve is so rarely injured where it winds about the ischial spine of the pelvis. A reasonable review of the literature has failed to reveal any obvious reports of pudendal nerve damage. The few complications which have been reported after pudendal blockade include vulval bruising, ischiorectal haematoma formation, and perineal oedema or sepsis rather than nerve injury.

GENERAL INJURY

During delivery, the effects of breath-holding and the efforts of 'bearing down' may result in the formation of multiple petechiae over the face, neck and shoulders. Conjunctival haemorrhages may also occur, which sometimes are quite extensive. These minor injuries promote no discomfort to the patient and require no treatment.

REFERENCES

AMATAYAKUL (1964) Brit. med. J., 1, 1613.
BAKER S. (1973) A Survey into Postnatal Perineal Discomfort. S. Maw & Sons, London, with the Royal College of Midwives.
BEARD R., BOYD I. & SIMS C. (1974) Brit. J. clin. Prac., 28, 409.
Brit. med. J. (1980) Editorial, 1, 1393.
BRUDENELL M. & CHAKRAVARTI S. (1975) Brit. med. J., ii, 422.

Burchell R.C. (1968) *J. Obstet. Gynaec. Brit. Cwlth.*, **75**, 642.

Burton-Brown J.R.C. (1950) *Brit. med. J.*, **ii**, 1061.

Christian M.S. (1979) *Brit. med. J.*, **i**, 1411.

Clow W.M. & Crompton A.C. (1973) *Brit. med. J.*, **i**, 321.

Coats P.M., Chan K.K., Wilkins M., Beard R.J. (1980) *Brit. J. Obstet. Gynaec.*, **87**, 408.

Department of Health and Social Security (1975–1979) *Confidential Enquiries into Maternal Deaths in England and Wales.* HMSO, London.

Fudge H.W. (1912) Quoted in *Lancet*, **i**, 1213.

Giwa-Osagie O.F., Uguru V., Akinla O. (1983) *J. Obstet. Gynaec.*, **4**, 94.

Grant F.G. (1955) *Brit. med. J.*, **ii**, 1539.

Harris N.J. (1974) *Brit. med. J.*, **iv**, 209.

Johnson H.A. (1962) *Brit. med. J.*, **ii**, 1660.

Kelly H.A. (1962) *Bull. Johns Hopkins Hosp.*, **5**, 53.

Lawrence R.F. & Sherman D. (1948) *Brit. med. J.*, **ii**, 425.

McLaren H.C., Jordan J.A., Glover M. & Attwood M.E. (1974) *J. Obstet. Gynaec. Brit. Cwlth.*, **81**, 383.

Reading A.W., Sledmere C.M., Cox D.N., Campbell S. (1982) *Brit. med. J.*, **284**, 243.

Rees W.D. (1965) *Brit. med. J.*, **i**, 103.

Roberts A.D.G., Hart D.M. (1983) *Brit. J. Obstet. Gynaec.*, **90**, 650.

Russell J.K. (1982) *Brit. med. J.*, **284**, 220.

Smith A.M. (1982) *J. Obstet. Gynaec.*, **2**, 245.

Stapleton G. (1937) *Brit. med. J.*, **ii**, 367.

Wassenaar J.J.S. (1947) *Brit. med. J.*, **i**, 452.

CHAPTER 30
OBSTETRIC OPERATIONS AND PROCEDURES

J. W. K. RITCHIE

The procedures to be dealt with in this chapter are all practical ones. Practical procedures can be learnt only in action and descriptions are a poor substitute for seeing and doing them. Rather, these discussions will be devoted to the decision to intervene surgically, the choice of procedure, its advantages and disadvantages, risks and consequences. When technical points are relevant to the discussion, however, they will be considered. Destructive operations on the malformed fetus causing dystocia are described in Chapter 26 (p. 382).

FORCEPS DELIVERY

Indications

The reason for intervention with forceps should always be stated clearly in the mother's notes. Often the reason given is imprecise, such as delay in the second stage, when the real need for intervention was poor maternal effort. The common indications are maternal distress, fetal distress, poor maternal effort.

When we consider these, however, it is clear that they are not indications specifically for forceps delivery, although they may be indications for delivery by the most appropriate means. The decision that delivery is required precedes that to use forceps to achieve it, and it will help to avoid the wrong use of forceps to consider things in this way. In this sense, the indications for forceps delivery cannot be separated from the conditions which are necessary before they can be applied. These will now be considered.

Conditions necessary for forceps application

Certain conditions should be fulfilled before forceps are applied:

1 the cervix must be fully dilated;
2 the presentation must be suitable;
3 the position must be known;
4 the head must be engaged;
5 the membranes must be ruptured;
6 the bladder must be empty;
7 there must be no obstruction to delivery at or below the level of the head.

All are excellent rules for the obstetrician in training. Rarely, the expert may consider it wise to break one or more in the best interests of the patient.

CERVIX FULLY DILATED

This is almost, but not quite, an absolute condition. If it is to be ignored, however, the decision to do so must be a deliberate one, once the situation has been fully assessed by an experienced obstetrician.

A tiny rim of cervix remaining undilated will be little barrier to the *application* of forceps for someone experienced in their use. *Delivery* through this rim, however, may give rise to maternal damage of perhaps considerable extent if the conditions permitting easy delivery are absent. Forceps delivery through an incompletely dilated cervix should be attempted only if the largest diameter of the fetal head has passed through the region of the vaginal vault leaving the rim of cervix, and that alone, as the barrier to delivery. If the vault is completely dilated in this way, forceps may be applied and the head gently drawn down through the rim, which is eased upwards over the head at the same time. Delivery with forceps before full dilation of the cervix must be regarded as a serious procedure to be undertaken only in exceptional circumstances and if particular conditions apply. Even if the conditions described above are present the vacuum extractor, if available, will be a preferable instrument to use until the head is drawn through the rim of cervix, when forceps may be substituted.

PRESENTATION

The only suitable presentations for forceps delivery, as a rule, are vertex and face. Only under the most unusual circumstances will it ever be otherwise. Exceptionally, a small baby in a large pelvis may descend almost to the pelvic floor as a brow presentation, when the best treatment may be to apply the forceps as the head presents and exert a little traction. Easy delivery is likely either as a brow or by further flexion or extension of the head at the last moment.

POSITION

Forceps may be applied to a vertex presentation with the head in the anterior, lateral or posterior position, but to a face presentation only when it is in the mento-anterior position. Delivery, however, as distinct from application, will occur with the occiput anterior or posterior or the chin anterior.

In a vertex presentation the head will be delivered more easily as occipito-anterior than occipito-posterior and in most instances of occipito-posterior position rotation to occipito-anterior should precede delivery. If the head is very deep in the pelvis and occipito-posterior, delivery in that position will have much to commend it and may be safer than upward displacement, rotation and delivery as an occipito-anterior. With the head at a high level rotation will almost always be preferable unless there is good reason to believe that the pelvis is predominantly anthropoid in shape.

The occipito-lateral position requires rotation to the occipito-anterior one before delivery. Some years ago, manual rotation under general anaesthesia was the preferred method. More recently, rotation with Kielland's forceps has become the more common one, and appears to have some advantages in modern obstetric practice. Local or epidural analgesia for forceps delivery is now used widely, and manual rotation is more difficult in these circumstances whilst Kielland's forceps can be used with local analgesia perhaps augmented by self-administered gas and oxygen; with epidural analgesia the application of Kielland's forceps is greatly facilitated. Less displacement of the head is needed for forceps rotation, which in many cases can be achieved at the level of arrest or may occur spontaneously on the perineum if the head is drawn downwards to a lower level. The disturbance to the head is also probably less in forceps rotation; a hand grasping the vault for rotation (instead of the face, which is to be preferred) will feel alarming

movements at the suture-lines, suggesting that damage can easily be inflicted if too firm a grasp is employed. Thus, Kielland's forceps appears a preferable method of rotation.

Their application will usually be by the 'wandering method', the anterior blade being manoeuvred gently around the face to its position on the anterior parietal bone; occasionally if the head is very low, direct application of the anterior blade is possible. The 'classical application' of the anterior blade with its cephalic curve forwards, followed by rotation of this blade through 180° after which it is brought downwards into position, should not be employed.

It may be stressed that if the head is in the oblique occipito-anterior position with the occiput pointing to the 2 o'clock or 10 o'clock position, deliberate rotation is unnecessary; the forceps may be applied cephalically or, if this cannot quite be achieved, as close to it as possible, and the head drawn down when 'spontaneous' rotation on the perineum is likely to be observed.

With a face presentation, of course, delivery as a mento-posterior cannot be achieved. Whether delivery can safely be accomplished by forceps with the head in the mento-anterior position is something which can readily be assessed only at the time.

ENGAGEMENT OF THE HEAD

Forceps deliveries have for many years been divided into three categories, called high, mid and low forceps.

High forceps, where the biparietal diameter of the head is just at the pelvic brim, is now seldom employed. The kind of case justifying high forceps delivery is that in which some sudden emergency situation for the child, prolapse of the cord for instance, occurs in a multiparous patient, or there is the need to deliver the second of twins from a high level. The problems of high forceps are concerned partly with the greater difficulty of correct application at a high level, but mainly with the large amount of undilated soft tissue below the head. Virtually the whole of the vagina will be undilated, so that in a primigravid patient or one of low parity there may be considerable resistance to delivery from the soft tissues; damage to the fetal head or laceration to the mother, or both, may result. High forceps delivery, therefore, is only for the experienced obstetrician in particular circumstances; one less experienced is likely to do more harm than good. The vacuum extractor, if available, appears more suitable than high forceps in the situations envisaged above.

With mid forceps extraction the largest diameter of the head is between the brim and the ischial spines, and the presenting part is at or almost at the spines. There should be no more than one-fifth of the head palpable above the pelvic brim. Here also, much of the lower vagina will be undilated and manual stretching to facilitate delivery is advisable before the actual extraction proceeds. In considering mid forceps extraction it must be pointed out that it has become customary to describe the station of a head in a pelvis with reference to its lowest point. If the lowest point of a head is at the ischial spinal level the largest diameter is probably just through the pelvic brim provided there is no marked moulding or caput formation. With both these changes present the largest diameter may be at almost any level. Great care must be taken to ensure that the head is engaged before embarking on forceps delivery. Unless there is an urgent need to interfere, a short wait will often allow the head to descend to a much lower level and the occiput to rotate further forwards. It is a mistake to embark upon forceps delivery for deep transverse arrest when the head is neither deep nor arrested!

Low forceps describes delivery when the biparietal diameter is at or below the level of the ischial spines, and the head should not be palpable above the pelvic brim. It will seldom cause difficulty.

RUPTURE OF MEMBRANES

When advance in the second stage is delayed and the membranes are intact, the correct procedure is to rupture them, after which further interference may be unnecessary.

BLADDER EMPTY

For most forceps deliveries this is an excellent rule. It may be, however, that with the head on the perineum, simple 'lift-out' forceps delivery may be accomplished without the need to catheterize the patient, since there may be little urethral bruising with easy voiding of urine afterwards. The risk of introducing infection into the bladder is then minimized.

NO OBSTRUCTION BELOW THE HEAD

This is an absolute rule. The head should never be pulled past an area of obstruction. Caesarean section is indicated in these circumstances (*see* trial of forceps, below).

Types of forceps

Since forceps were introduced into obstetric practice many designs have been used, only to be superseded by others, which, in their turn, were replaced by better ones. Nowadays, several types of forceps are commonly used in this country. With one exception, the Kielland's forceps, each has a pelvic and cephalic curve. Some have axis traction attachments either to the blades themselves or to the shank. It is debatable if any variety (Kielland's excepted) has a special advantage over its rivals. The instrument is asked to do little more than pull the baby from the relatively low position through the pelvic outlet. Axis traction rods, etc. can be discarded. Indeed, personal preference will generally be the deciding factor between one variety of forceps and another, so that in most situations almost any type will be satisfactory. The very short Wrigley's forceps are useful when delivering the fetal head at Caesarean section but otherwise might with benefit be given up. They may be chosen unwisely for their small size when a larger pair are essential. They are usually too short for controlled delivery of the aftercoming head at a breech delivery.

Kielland's forceps have a real value when rotation is necessary, as has already been discussed.

Failed forceps

This term was applied some years ago to the situation in which an attempt has been made unsuccessfully to deliver a patient with forceps. Happily, it is a rare circumstance in modern obstetrics. It might be thought that the main reason for failure was unrecognized disproportion. In reality, the two most common causes are examples of fundamental errors of technique: the application of forceps before full dilatation of the cervix, and the failure to recognize that the head is in the occipito-posterior position. In either event no progress is achieved when traction is exerted, and the instruments may pull off. Maternal and fetal trauma may be inflicted. These mistakes should not be made since careful examination will disclose the true state of affairs and appropriate treatment can be employed. If the forceps are applied with the head too high, much greater difficulty in delivery may be experienced and the attempt will sometimes fail; this is an important point to which too little attention has been devoted. Other possible causes for failure are other malpresentations, such as brow presentation, unrecognized disproportion, hydrocephalus, etc.

Trial of forceps

The only circumstance when it might be permissible to apply forceps, expecting a vaginal delivery, and later to remove them and deliver the patient by Caesarean section is when such a trial of forceps is employed as a deliberate manoeuvre. The situation will occasionally arise when it is not possible to be certain if there is mild disproportion or not. An experienced obstetrician may apply forceps in the operating theatre and observe progress when reasonable traction is exerted. If advance is not maintained Caesarean section can be carried out immediately. In these circumstances abdominal delivery may be difficult but is facilitated by displacing the head upwards and putting the operating table into a head down tilt.

It is clear that the dividing line between vaginal and abdominal delivery is very narrow. If too great force is exerted the fetus may be damaged, and vaginal delivery may result in a stillborn child or one with a cerebral injury. Even if the decision be made to abandon the attempt at vaginal delivery and deliver the patient by Caesarean section, the result may be the same if traction had been exerted too strongly. Trial of forceps, like much else discussed in this chapter, requires skill and mature judgement to be a safe procedure. With the stress nowadays, quite correctly, upon the birth of a child without any impairment of cerebral function the place of trial of forceps is smaller than it was only a comparatively few years ago. If it is undertaken, attempts to extract the child must be gentle with the fetal heart being carefully auscultated throughout.

VACUUM EXTRACTION

Vacuum extraction, although an old idea, was introduced to obstetrics as a reality by Malmstrom (1954). The instrument has now been used sufficiently long for some assessment to be made of its place in present-day obstetrical practice. The vacuum extractor is a supreme example of the thesis that has pervaded this chapter; that practical procedures can be learnt only in performance. Its wider introduction into obstetrics has undoubtedly been delayed by the fact that it requires an entirely different technique from that of forceps delivery; unless this technique is mastered, poor results will be obtained and the instrument is likely to be blamed rather than the operator.

The vacuum extractor may be used as an alternative to obstetric forceps to deliver a patient whose cervix is fully dilated and on whom forceps would normally be used. Its second use is to expedite dilatation of the cervix when this apparently ceases and labour is becoming prolonged.

As an alternative to forceps delivery it seems likely that there is little to choose between these methods, given uncomplicated cases and operators skilled in their use. The delivery is probably more comfortable for the patient, since the additional distension of the perineum is less with the vacuum extractor. Local analgesia is all that is required in the majority of instances; indeed, in some multiparous patients no anaesthetic may be required at all and the discomfort of the delivery will be comparable with that of a normal birth. There are circumstances in which the instrument has distinct advantages, some of which have already been indicated in the section on forceps delivery. If the fetal head is high, application of the vacuum extractor may be simpler and safer than is the case with forceps. If the head lies occipitoposterior or -transverse, the application of the cup, followed by traction, may permit good advance and easy rotation on the pelvic floor; this rotation may be assisted by pressure on the knob of the cup, but unless this is gentle, and is accompanied by careful traction strictly at right-angles to the plane of the cup, it may pull off. The instrument is ideally suited for application to the high head of a second twin when delay occurs.

With advantages of this kind it is a little surprising that the vacuum extractor has not been more widely received than is the case in Great Britain. The explanation is probably that such a different technique is required that this has not been truly learnt by obstetricians who, after all, need only to take up a pair of forceps to deliver the patients skilfully, easily and safely. The forceps are always available and the vacuum extractor may not be, or perhaps may not be correctly maintained and, therefore, not in proper working condition. The training of the younger obstetrician in the use of the instrument has, therefore, been incomplete, and until this gap is filled it is unlikely that forceps extraction will be replaced by vacuum extraction. Chalmers (Chalmers & Ng 1964, Chalmers & Fothergill 1960) has been one of the chief protagonists of the vacuum extractor in this country and has obtained excellent results with it.

The use of the vacuum extractor in the first stage of labour when progress has ceased has advantages in very special circumstances. When there is delay in labour, with the cervix more than say 8 cm dilated, this delay can sometimes be effectively managed by the vacuum extractor. It is essential, of course, to establish that there is no disproportion before any attempt at extraction is begun. Once the cap has been applied to the head, traction should be exerted gently and intermittently, bringing the head firmly into contact with the undilated portion of the cervix. Initially, little apparent progress may be made, perhaps for 10 or 15 min, but afterwards the cervix will often dilate quite quickly and the remaining rim may be slipped over the head, which is gently drawn down past it.

A few technical points will be mentioned. The largest cup that can be applied is always desirable. It was initially suggested that 6–10 min were essential to build up the necessary vacuum ($0.8\,kg/cm^2$) to fill the cup satisfactorily with the chignon of scalp. This is not always necessary and where speed is essential the vacuum can be taken directly to $0.4\,kg/cm^2$ when the cup has been applied as far back on the occiput as possible. The circumference of the cup is then checked to make sure no cervical or vaginal tissue has been included and the vacuum further increased directly to $0.8\,kg/cm^2$. The whole procedure can be carried out in 1–2 min. The line of traction must be kept within the confines of the circumference of the cup; if excessive lateral traction is applied the cup may slip off causing serious fetal damage. The cup should almost never come off and may be prevented from doing so by applying the thumb of the left hand to the cup while the forefinger is applied to the fetal head. The procedure should be abandoned if there is no descent of the fetal head after three pulls timed to coincide with contractions. Application of the cup should not exceed 30 min in duration, after which the risk of scalp bruising, sloughing or cephalhaematoma is greatly increased.

The maternal risk of the vacuum extractor seems minimal. The fetal results appear comparable with those of forceps delivery, although Malstrom believed the instrument to be superior in this respect (Malmtrom & Lange 1964). The special fetal disadvantage of the instrument is scalp trauma. The 'chignon' usually disappears in a few hours. Occasionally, however, superficial necrosis or more widespread sloughing may be observed. These lesions are more common or more extensive with prolonged application than when the instrument has pulled off and been reapplied. This instrument should not be applied to the head of a preterm infant less than 36 weeks' gestation because of the softness of the skull bones.

CAESAREAN SECTION

Indications

With very few exceptions all the indications for Caesarean section are relative ones. A list of all the conditions that might call for this method of treatment would be very long and quite unhelpful. The indications may be divided into groups, as follows:

IN LABOUR

1 fetal or maternal distress in the first stage of labour;
2 prolongation of the first stage of labour so as to increase the fetal and maternal risk;
3 obstructive labour or disproportion becoming evident during labour.

AS AN ELECTIVE PROCEDURE

1 disproportion or the likelihood of obstructive labour;
2 the need to deliver the patient quickly in the presence of some serious pregnancy disorder such as fulminating pre-eclampsia;
3 when vaginal delivery would cause serious risk to the life or health of the mother, child, or both, such as with placenta praevia or conditions which may be adversely affected by vaginal delivery. Examples are: previous successful repair for a vesico-vaginal fistula, or prolapse, or the existence of a congenital malformation like an ectopic anus;
4 when it is dangerous to allow the uterine contractions of labour because of previous Caesarean section or previous uterine injury or other operation;
5 to minimize the hypoxia associated with labour and the trauma of delivery to the fetus, as in the case of a premature fetus or one affected by growth retardation or maternal diabetes;
6 postmortem, to save the life of the child.

In some circumstances Caesarean section may not be required despite the presence of one or other of the 'indications' mentioned above. A very premature baby, for example, may be so profoundly and quickly affected by fetal distress in labour that it may be decided to withhold Caesarean section as the chances of the child's survival were too slender; maternal distress in labour may be better managed by pain relief such as epidural analgesia might offer; the patient's reaction to a previous Caesarean section may so sway her against its repetition that an attempt at vaginal delivery may be preferred. Many factors must be carefully assessed before deciding on Caesarean section in a particular case.

PREVIOUS CAESAREAN SECTION

The dictum 'once a Caesarean section always a Caesarean section' had few advocates in Britain in the past. The view has generally prevailed that, provided the first operation was carried out for a non-recurrent cause, and provided the obstetrical situation near to term in the succeeding pregnancy was favourable, an attempt, at least, at vaginal delivery was appropriate. In practice, it has even seemed that many obstetricians went further than this, aiming at vaginal delivery following Caesarean section even when the fetal head was high at term, or when borderline disproportion had just failed to be overcome on a previous occasion, or in other circumstances in which it could not be truly said that the obstetrical situation was normal. This tendency to resist Caesarean section arose from the wish not to compromise a patient's obstetric future, for by repeating the operation the obstetrician was making it virtually certain that if there should be another pregnancy a third operation would be required.

A similar view still prevails, although perhaps to a lesser extent. The size of the average family has become smaller, so that to repeat a Caesarean section will, in many instances, have little effect on the patient's obstetric future, which may amount to only one more pregnancy, if that. In the younger patient there still seems to be a place for attempting to achieve vaginal delivery if the obstetrical situation in the next pregnancy is favourable; if it is not, however, or if the patient is older or is towards the end of her childbearing life, repeating the operation may be preferable.

The factors to be weighed in the balance are the risk to the mother of repeating the Caesarean section and the risk to her and her child of rupture of the scar if labour is allowed. A realistic mortality rate for relatively uncomplicated Caesarean section is not easy to determine. In the Confidential Enquiry into Maternal Deaths in England and Wales 1976–1978, the calculated mortality rate for the operation was 0.8 per thousand Caesarean sections, which is the same as the rate reported for 1973–1975. The rates in 1970–1972 and 1967–1969 were 1.0 and 1.2 per thousand respectively. These figures are some ten times that for patients delivering *per vaginam* during a similar period. However, the data almost certainly include cases with serious complications from which

death occurred rather than from the operation. Moreover, the risk to a patient delivered *per vaginam* following Caesarean section is almost certainly greater than that for maternal mortality as a whole.

The risk of rupture of a classical Caesarean section scar was reported by Dewhurst (1957) to be 2.2% for all cases, 4.7% for those in labour and 8.9% for those delivered vaginally; the figures for the lower segment operation were 0.5%, 0.8% and 1.2% respectively. Five out of 100 mothers with a ruptured classical scar died and the fetal mortality was 73%; all 55 mothers with a ruptured lower segment scar survived, the fetal mortality rate being 12.5%.

McGarry (1969) and Peel and Chamberlain (1968) review the position further. Peel and Chamberlain make the important observation that the incidence of scar rupture increases in patients allowed to attempt a vaginal delivery after a previous Caesarean section for disproportion; in this group, moreover, the incidence of successful vaginal delivery fell and perinatal mortality rose compared with attempted vaginal delivery following Caesarean section for other indications. Reducing the number of attempted vaginal deliveries after previous Caesarean section in their own hospital corresponded with a fall in perinatal mortality; when 47% of patients were allowed to go into labour following Caesarean section, perinatal mortality was 71 per 1000, compared with 16 per 1000 when 33% were permitted to labour. McGarry (1969), however, demonstrated that good results are compatible with vaginal delivery following Caesarean section. He reported on 415 women previously delivered by Caesarean section; 242 (58.3%) were delivered vaginally with a perinatal loss of 8 babies (19 per 1000). The deaths of three of the eight babies, however, were in some measure concerned with delivery vaginally. One scar ruptured in the total of 415 patients. A recent report by Merrill and Gibbs (1978) from the United States. shows that 49% of 526 patients with a previous Caesarean section delivered vaginally with low morbidity, short hospital stay and no obvious effect on perinatal mortality. There were three uterine ruptures but none resulted in a serious threat to mother or child.

Other unfavourable factors tending to increase the risk of scar rupture are said to be sepsis following the operation and the implantation of the placenta beneath the scar in a subsequent pregnancy. It seems unlikely that any but gross infection following a Caesarean section would severely affect scar healing. The position of the placenta in the subsequent pregnancy can readily be determined by ultrasound.

Clearly, there are risks to a patient with a previous Caesarean section whatever is done and, as always, many factors will require to be taken into account when deciding what is best for any individual patient. Vaginal delivery after classical Caesarean section can only occasionally be permitted. Adequate precautions must be taken such as establishing an intravenous line, cross-matching blood and monitoring the fetal heart by a scalp clip. If the previous operation has been a lower segment one, the indication non-recurrent and the subsequent obstetrical situation normal, an attempt at vaginal delivery seems reasonable, at any rate in the younger patient or even in one not so young who is anxious to have the emotional satisfaction of experiencing labour. There is much emphasis in the minds of many mothers-to-be nowadays on experiencing the psychological fulfilment of labour and, if possible, vaginal delivery. Whilst this should not override considerations of fetal and maternal safety, it is a point which must be heeded.

A problem that has assumed greater importance in recent years has been that of the patient, often a very young patient, with a *previous hysterotomy scar*. In general one would expect such a procedure to carry a risk of rupture comparable with that of a previous classical Caesarean section and in considering vaginal delivery following hysterotomy this must be borne very firmly in mind. Vaginal delivery is not absolutely contraindicated but great care must be taken during labour. It would be unwise to undertake induction of labour or give epidural analgelsia, as the latter can mask the important signs of rupture, of pain and scar tenderness. There are comparatively few figures available to assess the risk of rupture. Clow and Crompton (1973) reported that the scar was intact in all but one of 31 cases where it was inspected or palpated after a subsequent pregnancy. However the hysterotomy scar was thin in 14 and in 3 of these it was said to be dangerously so. Vlies and Dewhurst (1975) examined 19 scars, of which one had ruptured and four were defective.

Similar caution should be taken when allowing a vaginal delivery to take place *after myomectomy*, though some would recommend elective Caesarean section if the uterine cavity had been entered at previous surgery. Obviously other factors such as infertility need to be considered in each case before making a decision about the correct route of delivery.

A successful pregnancy may follow *uteroplasty* and here too vaginal delivery is not totally contraindicated provided precautions are taken. Spontaneous labour has been permitted when the head is low in the pelvis with no untoward results in five of 23 cases of uteroplasty (Harley, personal communication).

CAESAREAN SECTION IN THE INTERESTS OF THE FETUS

On occasion, Caesarean section is carried out almost entirely in the interests of the fetus. Sometimes the decision is easy and the indication is obvious as in cord prolapse. More often the decision is difficult and made only after assessment of the risks involved to both mother and fetus.

The risk to the mother is small but nevertheless includes those of anaesthesia, Caesarean section itself and its sequelae. The potential risk of labour to the compromised fetus must be considered since spontaneous or induced uterine contractions interfere with uteroplacental blood flow and consequently with gas exchange across the placenta. Prolonged or frequent contractions or protracted labour increase the potential danger. The second stage of labour is normally associated with an acute episode of asphyxia and acidosis which is usually of mild degree but can be unpredictably severe.

Rarely trauma to the fetus may occur during spontaneous vaginal delivery, but is more likely to happen as the result of instrumental or manual manipulation to effect delivery, which may become necessary because of fetal distress.

Such dangers are sufficient to indicate delivery by elective Caesarean section when fetal compromise is known to exist and when conditions suggest a brief easy labour is unlikely. The usual antenatal tests discussed elsewhere should be used to predict fetal well-being. A vaginal examination will reveal the condition of the cervix and station of the presenting part from which an informed judgement may be made concerning the suitability of delivery by the vaginal route.

It is suggested by some that Caesarean section is indicated when the preterm fetus presents by the *breech* (Ingemarsson *et al.* 1978), particularly when the estimated fetal weight is below 1500 g. It seems likely that the degree of asphyxia and trauma associated with vaginal breech delivery may be reduced by this approach, but the evidence is not yet strong enough to advocate this policy universally. It must be remembered that considerable trauma can be inflicted upon the preterm infant during breech extraction through a poorly formed lower segment at Caesarean section. Avoiding this problem by low classical section imparts considerable risk to the mother, both immediate and remote. Furthermore, the outcome of preterm delivery by section has not been accurately compared with vaginal breech delivery by skilled personnel in the presence of expert neonatal assistance. A reasonable compromise has been suggested by Karp *et al.* (1979) that, having excluded anomalies, the footling preterm breech should be delivered by Caesarean section and the remainder vaginally unless there is some complicating factor.

POSTMORTEM CAESAREAN SECTION

Few obstetricians have been required to perform the procedure, but all may be called on to do so at any time. If the mother has died suddenly, there may be little time to weigh the pros and cons, but if maternal death can be foreseen, many of the problems concerned can be considered in advance. The chances of a child surviving will decrease the longer the operation is delayed. Cantoni and Rasini (1960) report the case of a live child born 45 min after the mother's death from subarachnoid haemorrhage, the mother's body having been kept oxygenated by ventilation through an endotracheal tube. In general, however, the fetus will die long before this and, if it is to have a reasonable chance of survival, must be delivered as soon as possible after it is certain that the mother is dead.

It may be difficult to be quite certain that death has occurred, and some attempt to revive the mother will generally be appropriate. An attempt to aerate the lungs and carry out external cardiac massage will often be indicated, but if these attempts are unsuccessful after 10 min or so they should be abandoned and the child extracted.

The relatives' permission should be sought, and in a chronic illness can usually be obtained. Even without it, however, there appears to be little likelihood of a successful legal prosecution of anyone intervening on the infant's behalf (*Brit. med. J.*, 1965).

A classical type of operation is indicated to extract the child with the utmost speed.

Types of operation

The lower-segment Caesarean section should be performed whenever it can safely be done. It will not always be safe, and a few indications for classical Caesarean section remain today.

A lower uterine segment containing fibroids may make entry into the uterine cavity difficult, cause heavy bleeding, and render the lower-segment operation very dangerous. The classical Caesarean section should then be employed, placing the incision away from the tumours. Similarly, if the lower segment is covered by adhesions the increased risk involved in the lower-segment approach may make the classical operation preferable. Postmortem the type of operation should be classical.

Other indications are more debatable. The classical method has been recommended for the patient with carcinoma of the cervix who requires to be delivered before radiotherapy treatment. This seems reasonable if the patient is in labour to avoid interfering with the cervix and its lymph drainage, but seems unnecessary when carried out electively before labour. It has been suggested that transverse lie should be dealt with by the classical approach but the lower-segment procedure may be used if the uterus is relaxed sufficiently by a suitable anaesthetic, and particularly if a lower limb can be felt on vaginal examination.

Classical Caesarean section for central placenta praevia has also been advocated, which is even more debatable still. The bleeding from the lower segment can generally be controlled satisfactorily even though it is necessary to incise the placenta or peel part of it off the uterine wall before extracting the child. Moreover, if very large sinuses bleed heavily they may be directly oversewn to control blood loss. The birth is best accomplished by inserting the hand, grasping a leg and extracting the fetus by the breech.

Timing of elective Caesarean section

When Caesarean section is carried out in the maternal interest one usually has little choice in the timing of the procedure. When the fetal interest is paramount timing of the operation is influenced by two main factors; fetal maturity and fetal condition.

Fetal maturity used to pose a considerable problem but the introduction of the amniotic fluid lecithin/sphingomyelia (L/S) ratio has reduced the risk of inadvertently delivering an infant so preterm that respiratory distress becomes life-threatening. If dates are still in doubt at the time of decision about delivery then amniocentesis should be considered. The traditional X-ray for maturity still has a place in mothers who have booked late, but the wide range of maturity at which the epiphyses around the knee appear must be remembered. Now many obstetricians are accustomed to having every pregnancy under their care dated by ultrasound, which has considerably reduced the need for obtaining the L/S ratio by amniocentesis. This practice is to be recommended, particularly when the indications for elective Caesarean section are obvious in early pregnancy.

The means by which fetal condition can be assessed are becoming more precise and are fully discussed in Chapter 31 (p. 454). Nevertheless clinical skill and experience are still important in making the decision about when the infant is at less risk in the nursery than in the uterus.

Caesarean hysterectomy

Caesarean hysterectomy has become more widely advocated in the United States during the last decade and some consideration of its place in obstetric practice seems appropriate.

It is important at the outset to distinguish between *elective* Caesarean hysterectomy and *emergency* Caesarean hysterectomy. By the latter term is meant that some complication arises during the course of Caesarean section making it necessary to remove the uterus. The principal indication likely to arise during the operation is, of course, haemorrhage for which it may be judged necessary to carry out hysterectomy; the discovery of a paper-thin uterine muscle along the line of a previous classical scar in a patient with several other children is another example of the finding which may be regarded as a firm indication for Caesarean hysterectomy.

Elective Caesarean hysterectomy as a means of sterilization is not justified, though in some patients it may be the only acceptable religious alternative to tubal ligation. Muldoon (1972), in reviewing 374 patients who were followed up for ten years after tubal ligation, reported that 43% required further gynaecological treatment and 25% required further gynaecological surgery, but despite this the balance of risks is against Caesarean hysterectomy. The indications are much stronger when there is a need to remove the uterus due to *existing* disease.

Of the various indications which might call for removal of the uterus following the Caesarean section the most obvious example is probably fibroids. It must be emphasized, however, that the presence of fibroids is not *per se* an indication to remove the uterus. There are two alternatives, Caesarean myomectomy and Caesarean section alone leaving the fibroids to be dealt with later. *Caesarean myomectomy* is a very bloody procedure, and difficulty may be experienced in controlling haemorrhage from the cavity from which the tumours have been enucleated. This is especially so when a fibroid is low down in the uterus or is truly cervical. In these circumstances if the uterus is to be preserved, Caesarean section alone through an incision placed away from the fibroids leaving them untouched will undoubtedly be a safer procedure. Their involution postpartum may be considerable and, if it is not and surgery is still thought to be indicated, it can be undertaken with greater safety at a later date. In some patients with fibroids, however, if further childbearing is not sought, there is clearly every reason to contemplate Caesarean hysterectomy.

Other possible indications for Caesarean hysterectomy might include previous menorrhagia for which hysterectomy was already planned shortly before the pregnancy occurred, or the known presence of an ovarian tumour in an older woman or carcinoma *in situ* complicating the pregnancy. Such conditions may be regarded as reasonable indications for Caesarean hysterectomy in some patients.

If Caesarean hysterectomy is to be considered, however, it must be accepted that the technical difficulties of it are greater than those of Caesarean section. This is not to imply that Caesarean hysterectomy is always a difficult procedure but it is a more difficult procedure than Caesarean section. Greater downward displacement of the bladder is required to perform total hysterectomy than to perform Caesarean section (subtotal hysterectomy seems not to be an acceptable elective procedure although it may be life-saving in an emergency). Similarly, greater displacement of the ureters is necessary than is the case with Caesarean section and clamps are applied close to them; bleeding is greater; tissue planes are more widely opened and deep vein thrombosis must be considered a great risk. All these difficulties are increased when the patient has had one or more previous Caesarean sections (as most patients under consideration for Caesarean hysterectomy will), if there is scarring of the lower segment area and especially if the placenta is low-lying. These difficulties account for the increased rate of urinary tract injury often reported in cases of Caesarean hysterectomy compared with Caesarean section. Barkley (1970) reporting on 689 elective Caesarean hysterectomies described 35 cases in which the bladder was known to have been injured and was repaired at operation, 5 cases in which the bladder was injured but this was not recognized and a fistula developed, whilst in 2 cases the ureter was injured although this was recognized in only 1. Three cases of bowel injury occurred also.

In short, the procedure of Caesarean hysterectomy must be considered a more difficult one than repeat Caesarean section. The surgeon must be skilful; anaesthesia must be of a high order; the risk of deep vein thrombosis must be considered to be raised and prophylactic administration of intravenous dextran or low-dose heparin (*see* p. 549) is indicated. Brenner *et al.* (1970) and Patterson (1970) may be consulted for further reading.

Mortality from Caesarean section

A Caesarean section is a major operation under any circumstances, and maternal mortality figures emphasize this. The number of deaths associated with Caesarean section in the Report on Confidential Inquiries into Maternal Death remained the same in 1976–1978 as in 1973–1975 (0.8 per 1000 Caesarean sections) although it had steadily declined in previous years.

The deaths reported are those associated with Caesarean section and not necessarily due to it, but the precise estimate of the latter number is difficult to obtain. The point must be made that many more deaths are associated with emergency Caesarean section than with the elective procedure. This is not surprising, since the elective operation is usually performed in daylight in the presence of experienced anaesthetic and obstetric staff. Senior staff should be available when operations carrying the most risk are being done such as those for placenta praevia, placental abruption or when the cervix is fully dilated.

A number of the deaths associated with Caesarean section are due to the anaesthetic, and most of these are caused by Mendelson's syndrome. The other major causes are haemorrhage, sepsis and paralytic ileus, and pulmonary embolism. Recently there has been an increase in the number of deaths in which the mother had pre-eclampsia prior to operation, probably reflecting the increasing use of this mode of delivery for the severe form of this condition. The availability of adequate blood, the strict use of aseptic techniques during labour and good surgical practice at Caesarean section, with the seniority of the personnel matching the risk involved, are obvious ways in which deaths can be kept to a minimum.

OBSTETRICAL ANAESTHESIA AND ANALGELSIA

Reference has been made to various forms of analgesia and anaesthesia, in those sections of this book in which different problems requiring pain relief or anaesthetic assistance are discussed. For completeness, a brief consideration will be undertaken of the problem as a whole.

Nowadays, the obstetrical anaesthetist must be a well trained specialist in anaesthesia. No better illustrations can be obtained of the need for a fully competent anaesthetist to administer an obstetrical anaesthetic than the fatalities referred to in the Reports on Confidential Enquiries into Maternal Deaths in England and Wales from 1964 to 1978. It is gratifying to note that the total number of maternal deaths has continued to fall, but the percentage of true maternal deaths due to anaesthesia has risen from 8.2 in 1964 to 13.2 in 1976–78. What is much less satisfying, however, is the fact that an avoidable factor was present in 90% of these deaths. Inhalation of stomach contents was again the most common cause of death; other causes included difficulty with intubation, misuse of drugs, accidents with apparatus and epidural analgesia.

For this reason a detailed account of anaesthetic agents, methods and techniques *by* an obstetrician *for* obstetricians in this increasingly complex field is inappropriate; what is appropriate, however, is how various facets of anaesthesia relate to the obstetrician, and what his position and responsibilities are.

Inhalation of gastric contents

With this, the most important single cause of death due to obstetrical anaesthesia, the obstetrician must do all he can to minimize its likelihood in patients during labour, any of whom may require a general anaesthetic quickly for some unforeseen complication. Gastric emptying time during labour is delayed, so that food taken at the beginning of, or even before, labour, may still be in the stomach when a general anaesthetic is required some hours later. Whilst measures to remove gastric contents are possible, they are seldom completely successful and always unpleasant. The passage of a gastric tube to allow removal of stomach contents is upsetting to most patients and may be accompanied by a degree of hypoxia which could be harmful if, for instance, the complication calling for the anaesthetic were fetal distress.

A better approach is to limit the food taken by mouth during labour to that which is likely to be easily digested and passed through into the duodenum, or is sufficiently fluid or semi-fluid to be removed through a gastric tube in an emergency. Drinks may be taken fairly freely, except for glucose, with which care is required. Crawford (1965) suggests that glucose drinks of greater than 5% concentration increase the delay in gastric emptying; they also have the more important effect of increasing gastric acidity, for it is not only the inhalation of food that causes serious complications of general anaesthesia but the inhalation of acid gastric juices also (Mendelson 1944). Such inhalation, generally referred to as Mendelson's syndrome, causes bronchial and bronchiolar spasm with considerable obstruction to ventilation. Cyanosis develops with rapid respiration, rales, rhonchi, hypoxia and tachycardia. The inhalation may not be evident immediately, general bronchiolar spasm and dyspnoea developing when the effects of the anaesthetic have passed off. Cyanosis, rapid respiration and tachycardia in a patient having just received a general anaesthetic strongly suggests inhalation of gastric contents. Each hospital should have routine instructions to be followed for the prevention of inhalation of stomach contents during anaesthesia.

Level of anaesthesia required

It is out of place for an obstetrician to tell an anaesthetist what anaesthetic agent to use. He should be able to say, however, what conditions he requires for whatever manipulation he has to perform, and it is the duty of the anaesthetist to provide them if at all possible.

In most instances where a general anaesthetic is called for in obstetrics the operator requires a light general anaesthetic with relaxation of the voluntary muscles but not the uterine muscle. The use of nitrous oxide and oxygen, and a muscle relaxant, will produce these conditions, since the uterine muscle will not be affected by the relaxing agent used. If the mother is kept lightly asleep and well oxygenated the infant should be delivered in good condition and the uterus should contract strongly following an injection of syntometrine after delivery.

There are occasions, however, when relaxation of the uterine muscle is essential to permit the appropriate obstetrical manoeuvre to be completed. The presence of a constriction ring will call for it to be relaxed or incised if delivery is to be achieved, and

really deep anaesthesia may be required. Sometimes at Caesarean section, with a baby's head deep in the pelvis, difficulty can be experienced in getting the head out if the uterus remains too irritable; Caesarean section for a transverse lie may be accompanied by difficulty in turning and extracting the child and again, some uterine relaxation may be desirable. The great dangers of internal version in the presence of a transverse lie with ruptured membranes have already been stressed, but there are circumstances when this manoeuvre may have to be attempted; it will be facilitated if some relaxation of the uterine muscle is obtained. During the third stage of labour, hour-glass uterine contraction below the placenta may cause difficulty in manual removal unless the anaesthetist is able to relax the uterine muscle.

Provided the anaesthetist is informed of the conditions required it should not be difficult for him to provide them, except in rare cases. The problem is to obtain sufficient relaxation to permit delivery or other manipulation and yet to allow the uterus to return to a responsive state so that it can contract immediately, or very soon, after delivery. A skilful anaesthetist can usually achieve this with a minimum of risk by employing halothane, but other techniques are available.

Spinal analgesia

The disadvantages of spinal analgesia are more pronounced during pregnancy than at other times, and only under exceptional circumstances should this form of treatment be employed. Alterations to the spinal curvature due to the presence of the full-term pregnant uterus increase the difficulty of controlling the level of analgesia in the spinal cord. The anaesthetic agent may pass to a higher level with maternal respiratory difficulty, paralysis or hypotension. Headache can be troublesome in a high percentage of cases.

Epidural analgesia

Epidural analgesia has deservedly become much more popular in Britain in recent years as its superiority in terms of pain relief over other methods has become recognized. Beazley et al. (1967) attempting an intensive programme to relieve pain by conventional means, achieved a success rate of around 60%. With epidural analgesia, however, Crawford (1972) reported that 84% of primigravida were 'fully satisfied' in the first consecutive 10 000 patients on whom this technique was used in Birmingham, and a figure of 81% was recorded for the second consecutive 1000; 10% and 13% obtained some relief and only 6% and 4% respectively obtained no benefit whatever. The figures for multiparous patients were similar.

For the most part epidural analgesia is undertaken by anaesthetists although a few obstetricians are specially skilful with it or with caudal analgesia. The catheter through which the injections are given at intervals is usually inserted with the patient in the left lateral position (Crawford 1972, Steel 1972) although the sitting position is sometimes employed. Tilting the bed assists the correct distribution of the solution. Steel's account or Crawford's may be consulted for further technical details. Bupivacaine is the drug most commonly used in a strength of 0.25%, although in certain circumstances higher concentrations are used. Other analgesic agents are less satisfactory with the exception of lignocaine which may sometimes be employed for the 'single shot' epidural analgesic for forceps delivery in view of its greater speed of action.

The intention is to relieve the pain of uterine contractions during the first stage of labour and also that of vaginal or perineal distension during the second stage by injecting sufficient volume and strength of analgesic agent to block pain impulses passing along the thin posterior nerve routes but not to block the larger anterior motor fibres. During the first stage the pain of uterine contractions is mediated through T11 and 12 and perhaps L1; the pain experienced by the passage of the head downwards in the second stage is carried through S2, 3 and 4. Modifications are made in amount and strength of anaesthetic solution depending upon the response to a previous injection, the time during labour or the precise purpose for which the block is being used (for example, the normal first stage or a 'single shot' for forceps delivery or for Caesarean section); 5–10 ml of bupivacaine 0.25–0.5% with or without adrenaline is the range from which the choice is usually made.

COMPLICATIONS

There are several possible complications of epidural analgesia. Some concern primarily the anaesthetist and his insertion of the catheter; others concern all the medical and nursing staff attending the labour. Steel (1972) stresses that certain precautions are essential before any attempt is made to administer the analgesic. These are: a control of blood pressure reading; an intravenous line in place; a suitable vasopressor available; a barbiturate immediately available for injection in the remote event of inadvertent injection of the local anaesthetic agent intravenously which might result in central nervous system stimulation; a ready supply of oxygen.

The main complication which may arise from the incorrect insertion of the polythene catheter into the epidural space is a spinal tap which may be recognized without any injection being given or which may result in a spinal anaesthetic perhaps extending to a high level. Crawford (1972) reported a rate of 7.6% of 'dural taps' in the first 1000 cases from Birmingham and 3.2% in the second 1000 cases. Frequency of dural tap is clearly related to the anaesthetist's experience. The direct entry of some of the anaesthetic agent into a vein is another important complication for which the preventive measures must always be on hand. The most important complication of which the obstetric and nursing staff must be aware is hypotension. This is concerned mainly with pressure of the gravid uterus on the inferior vena cava preventing venous return to the heart; this effect is aggravated by the vasodilatory effect of the nerve block. The frequency and severity of hypotensive episodes will depend therefore, more than anything else, upon the correct positioning of the patient by the nursing and medical staff. The patient must spend most of her labour in the right or left lateral position; more than 4–5 minutes at any time in the supine position may be sufficient for significant hypotension to arise. It will be evident that there are many occasions when the patient is at risk of being in such a position for longer: during a vaginal examination, for example, or whenever the abdomen is palpated, especially if instruction in palpation is given to juniors during this time. The delivery itself is the most likely time for the patient to be on her back for a longer time. Hypotension may also follow a period in the upright position such as when the patient is sitting on a bedpan.

Consideration should, therefore, be given to performing as many obstetrical manoeuvres as possible in the lateral position. Vaginal examinations can easily be performed in this way as indeed can normal delivery or forceps delivery, although abdominal palpation is more difficult. If such precautions are taken, the frequency and extent of hypotensive episodes should be small; Crawford reported only 1.4% of such episodes after nearly 6000 'top-up' doses of analgesic had been given. Without good medical and nursing care, however, the percentage will be far higher.

Particular care must be taken to ensure that during 'top-up' injections no untoward complications arise. Such 'top-ups' are frequently undertaken by midwives and it is imperative that, if this is done, the advice laid down by the British Central Midwives Board, based upon the procedure advised by the Obstetric Anaesthetists Association, be followed rigidly. This report stresses that instructions must be clearly written about what is to be done, the dose that is to be given, the position that the patient is to be in and the precautions that are to be taken if any complication does arise, whilst careful check on the dose and amount of the drug to be given must always be made with another person.

The effect of the epidural block on the patient's perineal sensation during the second stage of labour frequently results in her being unaware of the time to push and in her efforts being less successful. Forceps delivery is, therefore, more often required. It is not uncommon for rates of forceps delivery as high as 75% to be experienced in units using epidural analgesia for the first time; as the staff become more expert in dealing with patients under the influence of an epidural analgesic, however, and as they urge her to push more effectively at the correct time a larger percentage of patients can deliver themselves. In this respect, however, it is often forgotten that the type of simple 'lift-out' forceps delivery over a perineum relaxed by an epidural block is different from the forceps delivery required for other indications. A raised forceps rate of this simple kind is little, if any, disadvantage.

SPECIAL CIRCUMSTANCES

Special attention must be made of epidural analgesia in particular circumstances. It is very effective in labours complicated by the occipito-posterior position or when acceleration with oxytocin is required; its hypotensive effects make it applicable to the management of patients with pre-eclampsia or hypertension. The relationship of epidural analgesia to Caesarean section also requires comment. If the patient has previously had a Caesarean section, the complete pain relief obtained from an effective epidural analgesic may mask the abdominal pain and tenderness which could otherwise indicate that the scar was in imminent danger of rupture; this is particularly dangerous in patients with a previous classical Caesarean section or hysterotomy in whom rupture can be catastrophic. It must be admitted that the excellent relaxation obtained from such an analgesic allows

palpation of the scar within the lower uterine segment whenever a vaginal examination is made during the labour. Epidural analgesia for Caesarean section is now proving very popular with patients who wish to be awake and experience the emotional fulfilment of delivery. Sometimes their partners can be present and share the experience with them.

The early postpartum period may be affected by epidural analgesia in several ways. Retention of urine may be more troublesome, especially if the epidural is deliberately prolonged into the first postpartum day to give greater pain relief from the discomfort of an episiotomy, for example. Crawford (1972) reports apparently increased pain sensations in perineal wounds in some patients: the explanation is probably that in these patients the pain-free labour has heightened their awareness of other discomforts when the epidural itself has been stopped and its effect has worn off. Postoperative headache may sometimes be a considerable problem, particularly so if the dura has been tapped; in other circumstances it may not always be directly related to the epidural procedure.

The *caudal route* of administration of the anaesthetic still has its exponents and no doubt can be extremely successful. Steel (1972), however, regards the potential hazards of direct damage to the fetus as greater, and he considers it more likely that there will be an intravascular injection of the analgesic agent. The caudal approach certainly appears less specific since it blocks the sacral roots before it is necessary to do so. The lumbar approach appears to have several advantages over the caudal one.

Local analgesia

Local analgesia, as a *pudendal block*, is employed with considerable benefit in a large proportion of simpler obstetric operations. The technique of pudendal block is easily learnt. The anaesthetic agent should be injected as close to the ischial spines as possible, since the nerve crosses behind the tip of the spine. An additional nerve supply to the vulval area usually comes from the ilio-inguinal and genito-femoral nerves anteriorly, from the posterior cutaneous nerve of the thigh, and sometimes directly from the sacral plexus. These branches can best be anaesthetized by infiltrating locally towards the symphysis pubis, on each side and across the perineum, and in the lateral vulval tissues.

Dangers are involved in *overdosage*. If 1% lignocaine or its equivalent is used, the maximum volume which can safely be injected is 50 ml, if a vasoconstrictor is added, or 20 ml without one. For $\frac{1}{2}\%$ lignocaine, which is usually adequate, double these amounts may be used. If more is given or the injection is given intravenously in error, convulsions, coma or drowsiness may result and death may ultimately occur. These convulsions should be controlled with thiopentone and adequate oxygenation ensured.

REFERENCES

BARKLEY D.L. (1970) *Obstet. Gynec., N.Y.*, **35**, 120.

BEAZLEY J.M., LEAVER E.P., MOREWOOD J.H.M. & BIRCUMSHAW J. (1967) *Lancet*, **i**, 1033.

BRENNER P., SALL S. & SONNENBLICK B. (1970) *Amer. J. Obstet. Gynec.*, **108**, 335.

British Medical Journal (1965) Editorial, **i**, 204.

CANTONI A. & RASINI C. (1960) *Ann. Obstet. Gynec.*, **82**, 31.

CHALMERS J.A. & FOTHERGILL R.J. (1960) *Brit. med. J.*, **i**, 1684.

CHALMERS J.A. & NG J.L. (1964) *Brit. med. J.*, **ii**, 1070.

CLOW W.M. & CROMPTON A.C. (1973) *Brit. med. J.* **i**, 321.

CRAWFORD J.S. (1965) *Principles and Practice of Obstetric Anaesthesia*, 2e., p. 209. Blackwell Scientific Publications, Oxford.

CRAWFORD J.S. (1972) *Brit. J. Anaes.*, **44**, 1277.

DEWHURST C.J. (1957) *J. Obstet. Gynaec. Brit. Cwlth.*, **64**, 113.

INGEMARSSON I., WESTGREN M. & SVENNINGSEN N.W. (1978) *Lancet*, **ii**, 172.

KARP L.E., DOZEY J.R., McCARTHY T., MEIS P.I. & HALL M. (1979) *Obstet. Gynec., N.Y.*, **53**, 88.

McGARRY J.A. (1969) *J. Obstet. Gynaec. Brit. Cwlth.*, **76**, 137.

MALMSTROM, T. (1954) *Acta Obstet. Gynec. Scand.*, **33** (Supplement IV).

MALMSTROM T. & LANGE P. (1964) *Acta Obstet. Gynec. Scand.*, **43** (Supplement I).

MENDELSON C.L. (1944) *Amer. J. Obstet. Gynec.*, **152**, 191.

MERRILL B.S. & GIBBS C.E. (1978) *Obstet. Gynec., N.Y.*, **52**, 50.

MULDOON M.J. (1972) *Brit. med. J.*, **i**, 84.

PATTERSON, S.P. (1970) *Amer. J. Obstet. Gynec.*, **107**, 729.

PEEL J.H. & CHAMBERLAIN G.V.P. (1968) *J. Obstet. Gynaec. Brit. Cwlth.*, **75**, 1282.

Report on Confidential Enquiries into Maternal Deaths in England and Wales 1964–1966 (1969); 1967–1969 (1972); 1970–1972 (1975); 1973–1975 (1979); 1976–1978 (1982). HMSO, London.

STEEL G.C. (1972) *Brit. J. Hosp. Med.*, **November**, p. 595.

VLIES P.R. & DEWHURST C.J. (1975) *Int. J. Gynaec. Obstet.* **13**, 162.

CHAPTER 31
FETAL SURVEILLANCE

J. W. K. RITCHIE

Interest in the fetus during the antepartum period is of comparatively recent origin. In the early years of this century antenatal care was directed mainly to the detection of pre-eclampsia by means of blood pressure measurements and urine testing. Most mothers removed the minimum of clothes on these visits and examination on a couch was uncommon.

In contrast antenatal care now may begin before conception with prepregnancy counselling (e.g. for women with diabetes) but more usually the pregnant woman is advised to seek antenatal care soon after the second missed period. Thus many problems potentially influencing maternal and fetal health can be assessed at an early stage and their effects kept to a minimum. From the third to the fifth month arrangements may be made for confirmation of gestational age by ultrasound and for the diagnosis of potential genetic problems. From the fifth month the obstetrician has an increasing obligation not only to check for complicating factors influencing maternal health but also to assess fetal well-being. The objective of such antenatal supervision is to achieve not only the safe delivery of the mother but also the birth of the infant in optimum condition.

The increased emphasis on careful fetal assessment during the antenatal period has evolved over the past few decades for a number of reasons. Most importantly, the risks of childbearing have become negligible due to improved general health of the population and lower parity, and also as a result of better obstetrical practice and childbirth facilities. These factors have permitted more time and effort to be concentrated on the fetus. Furthermore early delivery for maternal or fetal complications is now feasible because of the excellent results achieved by neonatologists for survival without handicap of the preterm infants. Accurate dating of gestational age and the prediction of lung maturity have both enhanced the rationale upon which intervention is based.

THE FETUS AT RISK

As a result of new information concerning the physiology of the fetus together with major technological advances, it is now possible to identify much more reliably the fetus in jeopardy. Furthermore these recent advances have facilitated the monitoring of day to day changes in fetal condition *in utero*, enabling the timing of intervention to be based on firmer evidence.

Nevertheless it must be recognized that it has become more and more difficult to single out the fetus at risk, because of the substantial fall in perinatal mortality which has occurred over the past two decades. The vast majority of pregnancies are now destined to have a normal outcome and there is only approximately a 1 in 30 chance that the baby will die in the perinatal period or suffer significant handicap. Thus, it is inevitable that many normal pregnancies will be included in the net that in many instances must be cast wide in the hope of identifying the fetus at risk. The attempted prediction of mothers destined to go into preterm labour is a good example of this effect.

There is a further confounding issue concerning the detection of the fetus at risk. It is clear that, even when a complication of pregnancy known to be associated with fetal risk is diagnosed, the effect on the fetus can be very variable, ranging from death to no effect whatsoever. The mother with hypertension illustrates this phenomenon.

Finally, despite the most diligent antenatal care the fetus may still on occasion die *in utero* for no apparent reason. The perinatal death may then be attributed to minor events which are most unlikely to have been the actual cause of death. Also, the appearance of handicap in the newborn may be attributed to events in labour or at delivery which may have had little or nothing to do with the final outcome. Indeed it should be recognized that some infants with inherent developmental neural defects can present with

442

fetal distress in labour or with apparent asphyxia at birth. In such circumstances the obstetrician is left with the suspicion that the forceps used to expedite delivery, or indeed non-intervention, may have caused the damage. It is however of some reassurance that the reserve of the normal fetus to withstand hypoxia is considerable, and there has usually been ample evidence of a prolonged event when death or damage is hypoxic in origin.

The first step in identifying the fetus at risk is to be familiar with the variety of conditions which cause fetal loss and damage and to consider their pathogenesis during pregnancy. Careful perusal of the chapter on perinatal statistics is recommended, particularly the section dealing with factors associated with mortality and morbidity (Chapter 35, p. 530). It is apparent that some causes are difficult to combat. Congenital abnormality is a major cause of death and handicap, but little can be done in the third trimester to reduce this contribution. Preterm birth is another complex and difficult problem to combat, but it accounts for 40% of neonatal deaths.

Many stillbirths still remain unexplained and it is particularly disturbing that the majority of these occur in mature fetuses. Some, on the other hand, are associated with recognized complications of pregnancy and it is in this group of mothers that special investigation is required. Therefore, the major indications for studying fetal health *in utero* are poor fetal growth, antepartum haemorrhage, hypertension and pre-eclampsia or when pregnancy is prolonged.

Often it is too late to wait for evidence of an overt clinical complication of pregnancy to arise; the outcome might well have been improved if the fetus had been identified earlier as being at increased risk. The so-called high risk pregnancy, in which it is implied that the fetus is also at increased risk, is statistically much more likely to occur in easily identified groups of patients. These groups include those mothers at the extremes of the childbearing years, the 'under sixteens' and the 'over forties'. Poor socio-economic circumstances, particularly in association with high parity, alcohol, tobacco or drug abuse, poor diet, illegitimacy and even unplanned pregnancy also increase the chances of a poor pregnancy outcome. Each of these factors may be identified easily when a mother first attends for antenatal care and should be an indication for closer surveillance during pregnancy.

Identification of high risk pregnancies

An experienced specialist should identify pregnancy problems reliably, but the same may not be true of relatively inexperienced hospital obstetrical staff or indeed general practitioners. In recognition that a wide range of experience exists among those looking after pregnant women and, in an attempt to minimize the chances of important factors being overlooked, check lists have been constructed.

One such antenatal card, which contains a checklist for factors identified at booking on the front of the card (Table 31.1) and those developing during pregnancy on the reverse side (Table 31.2), has been designed in Edinburgh. A useful innovation in this system is that the doctor may refer to a plan of management for each complication of pregnancy identified. The card has been used with success in an urban population in that city over the past few years, in the Sighthill Project (K. Boddy, personal communication). The same method has also been applied with similar success in a rural community in Alberta, Canada (J. Parboosingh, personal communication). The relative usefulness of this method of documentation suggests that it might have a wide application where non-specialists are carrying out antenatal care.

In advocating this system Pearson (1982) lists some of its advantages as follows. It ensures that all mothers receive the same thorough assessment during pregnancy and that a high standard of care is encouraged. Also, the card provides the family doctor with immediate information about how serious the problem is and what course of action to take without unnecessary referral to the hospital based specialist. The use of planned protocols for management also allows evaluation of different forms of treatment and permits new methods to be introduced so that all patients may receive the benefit. Finally, the scheme provides a practical means for identifying high risk pregnancies for intensive management during the antenatal period and in labour.

Using another approach, many have attempted to provide scores whereby pregnancy risk may be quantified. Most of these scoring systems are complex and time consuming to complete. One of the simplest systems for the antenatal assessment of fetal risk was put forward by Goodwin *et al.* (1969). It has the advantage of quickly allowing the doctor to assign his own impression of fetal risk at booking and at each subsequent visit. It also provides simple instructions for action to be taken about the level at which

	BOOKING HISTORY
☐	Age less than 18 yrs.
☐	Age over 38 yrs.
☐	Primigravid age 30 yrs or more.
☐	Parity = / more than 5
■	*LMP DETAILS*
☐	LMP uncertain ± 2 weeks
☐	Pill stopped 1 or 2 periods before LMP
☐	Cycle length prior to LMP greater than 30 days
☐	IUCD *in situ*/on Pill after conception
☐	Out of wedlock pregnancy
☐	Vaginal bleeding since LMP
■	*PAST OBSTETRIC HISTORY*
☐	SB/NND
☐	Small for dates (< 10th Centile)
☐	Large for dates (> 90th Centile)
☐	Fetal abnormality ....
☐	Antibodies in previous pregnancy
☐	Hypertension/Eclampsia
☐	Termination of Pregnancy/Spon. Abortion × 2
☐	Premature labour (20–37 weeks)
☐	Previous Cervical Suture
☐	Previous Caesarean Section
☐	PPH/MROP
■	Labour of less than 4 hours
☐	*MATERNAL HEALTH*
☐	Chronic Illness/Drugs ....
☐	Hypertension/Proteinuria
☐	Infertility with Medical Advice
☐	Uterine Anomaly including Fibroids
☐	Smoking 10/day at Conception
☐	Soc. Sec. Benefits
☐	Isolated at Home
☐	Family History of Diabetes/Fetal Abnormality ....
■	Completed by .... Date ....
	BOOKING EXAMINATION
☐	BP = / more than 140/90
☐	Maternal Weight = / more 85 kg
☐	Maternal Weight = / less than 45 kg
☐	Maternal Height = / less than 5 ft
☐	Cardiac Murmur Detected/Referred
☐	Uterus large/small for dates
☐	Other Pelvic Mass Detected
☐	Blood Group Rh Negative
☐	Completed by .... Date ....

Table 31.1. Edinburgh risk assessment card—details at booking visit. (With permission from Dr K. Boddy.)

management should be carried out. The value of the method has been validated in a prospective study (Yeh *et al.* 1977) and the system has been incorporated into a standard record which is now used throughout the Canadian province of Ontario (Goodwin & Chance 1979). The author's modification of this guide to pregnancy risk grading is shown in Table 31.3.

Investigative screening for high risk pregnancies

All fetuses in jeopardy will not be detected by the techniques detailed above. Acute events such as placental abruption or cord prolapse are always difficult to predict, and less acute complications, particularly poor fetal growth, may also escape detection. For these reasons, some have attempted to apply screen-

FACTORS ARISING DURING PREGNANCY

Weeks of Pregnancy																		
FM Not felt																		
Hb < 10 gm %																		
Poor Weight Gain																		
Wt. loss																		
Proteinuria																		
Glycosuria																		
Bacilluria																		
BP Systolic > 155																		
Diastolic > 88																		
Rh Neg/Antibodies																		
Uterus large for dates																		
Uterus small for dates																		
No increase in fundus (Zone)																		
Excess liquor																		
Mal presentation																		
ECV Successful																		
Unsuccessful																		
Head not engaged																		
Any bleeding PV																		
Premature labour																		
Vaginal infection																		
Sign when completed																		
Insert Date																		

Table 31.2. Edinburgh risk assessment card— antenatal complications. (With permission from Dr K. Boddy.)

ing techniques to the whole obstetrical population, aiming to improve the 'pick-up' rate of these problem fetuses.

It is obvious that tests applied in this manner should be inexpensive, simple to carry out and have a good predictive value. There are no tests which currently meet these criteria, but many have been advocated and some are still being evaluated.

BIOCHEMICAL SCREENING TESTS

A number of placental proteins have been measured and their predictive value for the fetus at risk has

---

Grade A   *Pregnancy at no predictable risk*
                      (family doctor able to manage in local community)
No previous perinatal loss or low birth weight infant
No significant maternal medical disease
No pregnancy complications now or in previous pregnancies
Fetal growth seems adequate

Grade B   *Pregnancy at risk*
                      (consultation with specialist and probable continuing collaborative
                         care but with delivery at specialist unit)
Potential diabetes
History of previous stillbirth or neonatal death
History of previous low birth weight infant
History of genetic disease in family
Cervical incompetence
Maternal obesity
Significant tobacco, alcohol or drug intake
Renal disease without hypertension
Rhesus isoimmunization
Grand multipara
Primigravida age 35 or over
Multiple pregnancy
Mild pre-eclampsia
Hypertension without pre-eclampsia
APH
Breech presentation
Anaemia ($<10\,\mathrm{g/1d}$) not responding to iron
Weight gain more than $4.5\,\mathrm{kg}$ (10 lbs) by 30 weeks
Premature painful contractions
Polyhydramnios
Prolonged pregnancy

Grade C   *Pregnancy at high risk*
                      (immediate referral to specialist unit for antenatal care and delivery)
Diabetes
Heart disease
Hypertension with superimposed pre-eclampsia
Renal disease with hypertension
APH continued or repeated
Preterm rupture of membranes
Preterm labour
Fetal growth arrest
Two or more minor risk problems

Table 31.3. Guide to pregnancy risk grading.

been assessed. Even the most promising of these, maternal serum human placental lactogen (a glycoprotein produced by the syncytiotrophoblast), despite closely correlating with placental weight, has not in practice proved accurate enough to be used as a screening test.

Single maternal serum or urinary oestriol estimations have also been advocated as a test of fetal wellbeing between 32 and 36 weeks' gestation but again these have not proved useful in practice. Serial oestriol measurements have limited practical value when a clear trend can be identified.

As a result of antenatal genetic screening programmes it has become apparent that abnormally high maternal serum alphafetoprotein values are also associated with pregnancies in which the fetus is destined to be small for gestational age (Brock *et al.* 1977). The prospective value of this association in identifying pregnancies in which fetal growth should be monitored closely awaits confirmation. It is interesting to note that low values seem to be associated with fetal chromosomal abnormality (Mercatz *et al.* 1984) and may thus provide a screening test to indicate a need for genetic amniocentesis.

BIOPHYSICAL SCREENING METHODS

Since the introduction of ultrasound into clinical practice and the appreciation of its value in measuring fetal growth, the technique has been assessed as a method of screening pregnancies, at approximately 32 weeks' gestation, for poor fetal growth. A number of different fetal measurements, separately and in various combinations, have been evaluated. The most useful of these parameters seems to be that of crown rump length multiplied by abdominal trunk area (Neilson 1980). Although the pick-up rate appears to be quite significant, the procedure is unlikely to be cost-effective when applied as a screening test to low risk pregnancies (Neilson *et al*, 1984).

In recent years as new methods have been introduced in the perinatal field their usefulness has been more carefully evaluated in terms of sensitivity and specificity than was the case with earlier tests such as oestriol measurement. These criteria are now used increasingly in the literature, and the clinician should be aware of their meaning so that the true value of a test may be interpreted (Haynes 1981). The sensitivity of a given test is an index of its reliability in detecting a problem. On the other hand the specificity of a test indicates how accurately the absence of the problem will be predicted. Both terms are usually ex-

pressed as a percentage and the method used to calculate each is given in the standard 'fourfold' format shown in Table 31.4 which has been adapted from Haynes (1981). Leaving aside cost and degree of simplicity none of the currently available tests has the sensitivity or specificity to warrant their recommendation as routine screening procedures.

ASSESSMENT OF FETAL WELL-BEING

Clinical assessment

The first step in the assessment of the fetus at risk is a careful review of the mother's family history and her own medical and social history. If there is a past obstetrical history every detail regarding complications should be recorded. If the mother was delivered in another hospital the relevant information should be obtained from the obstetrician in charge of her care at that time. It may be important to ask specific questions, particularly if a previous infant was of low birth weight. The distinction between prematurity and growth retardation may be made in most cases by knowledge of how the baby behaved after birth with regard to feeding, respiratory problems and weight gain. The preterm infant may require tube feeding and respiratory support and may lose weight after birth, while the growth retarded infant usually feeds well, gains weight immediately and does not require respiratory support.

It is also of vital importance to establish gestational age accurately. In the third trimester one may be in doubt about dates and at this stage it is impossible to resolve this question with any degree of accuracy.

			Eventual diagnosis		
			Problem exists	Problem does not exist	
Test results	Positive—problem detected		**a** True positive	**b** False positive	a+b
	Negative—problem absent		**c** False negative	**d** True negative	c+d
			a+c	b+d	

Table 31.4. The 'fourfold' table demonstrating how the value of a new test may be calculated.

Sensitivity = a/a + c
Specificity = d/b + d
Positive predictive value = a/a + b
Negative predictive value = d/c + d

Needless to say, this makes the assessment of the fetus at risk much more difficult, so it should be routine practice to confirm dates by ultrasonic scans early during pregnancy if gestational age is still in doubt following a careful menstrual history and pelvic examination.

Furthermore, the tests and measurements being done to assess fetal growth and health in the second half of pregnancy, on which decisions may be made about the timing of delivery, can only be interpreted with accuracy if there is also certainty about gestational age. Because of the increased probability of intervention in primigravidas (e.g. pre-eclampsia) an argument could be made for the confirmation of dates by ultrasound in all these patients.

Clinical examination of the patient at each visit should follow careful confirmation of gestational age and checking for all listed potential problems noted. It is surprising how often a diagnosis is missed or a wrong diagnosis made because readily available information has been overlooked.

The mother's weight gain is also assessed, and on abdominal palpation the fundal height is measured in centimetres above the symphysis using a tape measure. The latter may be plotted against an appropriate graph showing the increase in size against gestational age. This simple procedure has been shown to be an excellent guide to growth (Calvert *et al.* 1982). In addition to noting the fetal lie and presentation etc. special attention should be paid to the amount of amniotic fluid surrounding the fetus. When oligohydramnios is present the uterus feels as if it is 'hugging' the fetus tightly. The overall size of the fetus should be assessed and a clinical estimate made of fetal weight; accuracy improves if this is performed every time one examines a patient. During the examination it is useful to ask the mother about fetal activity because it is usual for the normal healthy fetus to 'kick' frequently, particularly in the evening. Mothers may make a daily count of these fetal movements and record them on a chart supplied for the purpose (Pearson & Weaver 1976). They are asked to record the time by which the first ten movements are felt after 0900 hours. If 10 movements have not been felt by 2100 hours then the total number of movements is recorded. The normal fetus usually moves about ten times per hour and even more so in the evening, so that such an inexpensive test has proved useful in some hands as a screening procedure. If ten movements are not felt within the twelve hour period further investigations can be initiated the following day.

The rationale for counting fetal movements is well founded in that the fetus normally passes through rest activity cycles lasting approximately 40 minutes. From animal studies it could seem that one response to chronic hypoxia is a decrease in fetal activity which is presumably a mechanism to conserve oxygen consumption. The time course of these events and the seriousness of the insult necessary to cause a decrease in fetal activity is not certain but it is likely that a cessation of movement is a fairly late event, perhaps occurring 24–48 hours before fetal demise.

The difficulty mothers have in complying with the 'Cardiff count to ten' scheme over a 12 hour period has resulted in shorter time intervals being chosen. It would thus seem more sensible to count fetal movements over a shorter period, perhaps two hours at the same time during each evening when the fetus is known to be most active.

Further investigation

In the absence of reliable screening tests for potential problems the task of surveying the antenatal population must fall to the clinician, and it is therefore at the examination couch that patients must be selected for further investigation. Often help is available from the mother who will volunteer that she is unhappy about the pregnancy for one reason or another. Such remarks always warrant more careful evaluation of the pregnancy.

The investigations which may be undertaken are usually directed to the detection of chronic intrauterine hypoxia which leads to growth retardation and eventually, after a variable period, to intrauterine death. The tests concerned take into account features of fetal growth and health *in utero*. Measurements of growth are useful partly because they are relatively easy to make and also because, as a general rule, the normally growing fetus can also be assumed to be healthy. Measurements of fetal well-being *in utero* on the other hand are not yet as reproducible and they are open to more subjective interpretation.

MEASUREMENTS OF FETAL GROWTH

It is hard to imagine the practice of modern obstetrics without ultrasound. The considerable advances resulting from its use cannot be overestimated, and scanning equipment has now become the extension of the obstetrician's eyes, ears and hands. The detail with which the fetus and its environment may now be viewed is so useful that every doctor providing antenatal care should be aware of its potential. The safety of the equipment should be stressed to patients who may be understandably concerned with this aspect of ultrasound (Royal College of Obstetricians & Gynaecologists, 1984). The number of available parameters of fetal growth has greatly increased in recent years and most are now carried out as routine procedures.

Biparietal diameter

The biparietal diameter (BPD) of the head was the first measurement of fetal growth described (Willocks *et al.* 1964) and it remains the simplest. Provided gestational age is known, fetal head growth may be plotted from serial measurements and a trend determined when two values are obtained a week to 10 days apart.

Two patterns of delayed head growth have been recognized (Campbell 1974). The commonest is shown in Fig. 31.1 where a long period of normal growth is followed by a steady decrease in growth rate. This pattern of intrauterine growth retardation (IUGR) is commonly associated with complications of

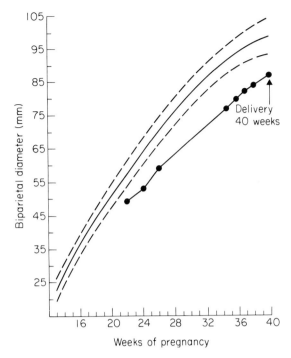

Fig. 31.2. Serial biparietal measurements showing poor growth potential associated with intrinsic factors. After Campbell (1974), with permission from W.B. Saunders, publishers.

pregnancy such as hypertension and pre-eclampsia causing decreased utero-placental blood flow and hence poor fetal growth, and it may be regarded as being due to extrinsic factors.

A less common pattern seen in about a third of all fetuses with IUGR is shown in Fig. 31.2. Here the growth rate of the fetal head is slow over a prolonged period, and the poor growth potential is more likely to be due to intrinsic factors such as fetal chromosomal abnormalities or intrauterine infection. Long term follow-up has shown that the outcome for fetuses exhibiting this pattern is much less favourable (Fancourt *et al.* 1976) than for those in the first group.

Although BPD measurements provide useful information in practice, they have some limitations. Their usefulness is influenced by two main problems. Firstly, the rate of growth normally slows from about 3.5 mm per week between 16 and 26 weeks to 2.0 mm per week between 26 and 36 weeks; secondly, the scatter of normal head diameter increases in the second half of pregnancy, i.e. the 10th and the 90th percentiles become further apart. Thus,

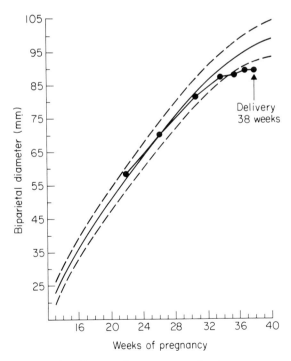

Fig. 31.1. Serial biparietal measurements showing poor growth achievement associated with extrinsic factors. After Campbell (1974), with permission from W.B. Saunders, publishers.

in late pregnancy it is often difficult to be certain of an abnormal delay in head growth. Furthermore two readings at least a week apart are required to show the velocity of growth and the obstetrician may not have this time at his disposal before taking action on clinical grounds. Another disadvantage of BPD measurement in IUGR is that the fetal brain, and hence head growth, is relatively spared because the fetal circulation channels blood preferentially to vital organs. Hence a delay in head growth is not a very sensitive or early index of IUGR.

Abdominal measurements

Normally the accumulation of glycogen in the fetal liver during the last 4–6 weeks of pregnancy results in the diameter of the fetal abdomen outstripping that of the fetal head, but when there is IUGR glycogen deposition and liver size are reduced. Therefore, early evidence of IUGR may be obtained by comparing head and abdominal sizes. When the fetal abdomen is small but the BPD is more or less appropriate for gestational age it can be concluded that the fetus is 'asymmetrically' growth retarded due to an extrinsic cause as discussed above. On the other hand, when both the BPD and abdominal diameter are small 'wrong dates' is a possibility which must be excluded.

The method used to obtain a transverse section of the fetal abdomen at the level of the intra-abdominal portion of the umbilical vein has been described by Campbell and Wilkin (1975). A longitudinal view of the fetal spine, and hence of the longitudinal axis of the aorta, is obtained. The transducer is then rotated through 90° and moved upwards or downwards until the umbilical vein is seen traversing the fetal liver in the anterior third of fetal abdominal antero-posterior diameter.

When this view has been obtained it is usual to measure the antero-posterior and transverse abdominal diameters and to determine the average. This method allows for the oval shape of the abdominal cross section occasionally encountered in the fetus with IUGR as a result of its compression and hyper-flexion due to reduced amniotic fluid volume.

Other useful measurements may also be made in this plane, including abdominal circumference and area. Experience suggests the latter measurement is the most reproducible when the same fetus is measured by different observers. Graphs of both these measurements against gestational age have been produced and are useful in the diagnosis of growth retardation and erroneous dates. In particular the ratio of BPD to abdominal circumference is a sensitive measurement when plotted against gestational age (Campbell & Thoms 1977).

Fetal weight estimation

A number of different methods have been used to calculate fetal weight. Some are very complicated and nearly all incur an error of 8–10%. Perhaps one of the simplest is that of Eik-Nes *et al.* (1982) in which fetal weight may be read from a nomogram using measurements of BPD and abdominal diameter. This method is particularly useful when fetal weight lies between 1.0 and 3.0 kg.

Other suggested methods of detecting fetal growth include total intrauterine volume (Gohari *et al.* 1977). Although this is attractive because all 3 intra-uterine components (fetus, placenta and amniotic fluid) are reduced when there is IUGR, the method has not proved reliable in other hands (Chinn *et al.* 1981).

FETAL PHYSIOLOGIAL CONDITION

Valuable information about fetal growth may be obtained from the measurements of fetal anatomical structures as outlined above. If growth is normal it may be inferred that the condition of the fetus is probably satisfactory. More recently, with the advent of real time ultrasound and new information derived from animal studies, an impression of fetal health may be gained from observing fetal activity, heart rate and amniotic fluid volume.

Fetal activity

The use of fetal activity as assessed by real time ultrasound as a test of well-being depends upon a detailed knowledge of normal events *in utero*. There is a diurnal variation, with increased activity in the evening, which is superimposed on intermittent rest–activity cycles, so it is difficult to assess fetal activity accurately and reproducibly over short periods. Even during normal fetal life there may be periods of up to 75 min without gross fetal body movements taking place.

Fetal activity is reduced or ceases only when the oxygen demands of a quiescent fetus approach the level of oxygen delivered. This would seem to be an effective protection mechanism whereby the fetus can reduce its oxygen consumption and hence oxygen demand. However, its time course is uncertain, and the condition causing the decreased oxygen supply may deteriorate at an unpredictable rate.

Gross *fetal body movements* may be observed with ultrasound. In the normal fetus the chance of seeing no activity in any 5 minute period is 23%. This falls to 7% over 20 mins and 1% over 45 min. A suggested norm is 3 discrete gross body movements and one limb motion during 30 min (Manning *et al.* 1980).

At one time it was hoped that *fetal breathing movements* (FBM) might represent a useful guide to fetal condition because in fetal sheep moderate hypoxia caused FBM to be substantially reduced or to cease altogether (Boddy *et al.* 1974 and *see also* p. 453). It has been shown that in fetal sheep these movements are normally episodic and associated with periods of rapid eye movement sleep. There is also a marked diurnal variation similar to the well recognized pattern of other fetal movements with more activity in the evening and less in the early morning.

In practice it was shown that the period between episodes of FBM can be as long as 60 min in the normal fetus. Thus, it is not surprising that observation of these movements over a short time, such as half an hour, does not correlate well with fetal condition at birth. Nevertheless, the chances of seeing FBM in normal pregnancy are good and a norm of at least one episode lasting 30 seconds during 30 minutes of recording has been suggested (Manning *et al.* 1980).

A combination of counts of gross fetal body movements and FBM has been suggested by Roberts *et al.* (1980) and has been used with some success in assessing fetal compromise. It is suggested that three movements of any combination during 10 min is normal, and if these are not seen with ultrasound further investigation is required.

Fetal heart rate

In recent years the characteristics of the fetal heart rate (FHR) have been used increasingly to predict condition during the antenatal period. The newer generation of cardiotocographic equipment with directional Doppler and autocorrelation has made good continuous recordings easier to obtain.

However, it must be recognized that for a variety of reasons changes in FHR may not be as predictive of fetal health as has been suggested. Firstly, the FHR is influenced by many factors, some of which are transient, such as sleep state, maturity, level of maternal activity or maternal ingestion of drugs. Secondly, the fetal cardiovascular system has considerable reserve so that changes in the FHR pattern often occur only in response to serious deterioration in fetal health.

Some changes in particular are more predictive of abnormal fetal states. If the amniotic fluid volume is decreased cord compression can occur readily, producing reflex decelerations in FHR which do not necessarily indicate serious fetal compromise. The number of methods reported by which the record may be assessed or scored reflects uncertainty underlying the methodology. In summary, there is not yet enough information from which to interpret with confidence the detailed changes in characteristics of a short period of FHR recording.

A simple and reliable method of interpreting the antepartum FHR trace has been reported by Keegan and Paul (1980) and is widely used. Here attention is paid only to accelerations in fetal heart rate in association with fetal movements. These have been taken to indicate fetal 'reactivity', implying that the neural mechanisms controlling FHR are functioning. The criteria used to define the test as reactive are the presence of two or more FHR accelerations, by 15 beats per minute for 15 seconds, associated with fetal movements over a time course of 40 minutes. A 'reactive' test is a good index of fetal health at the time of the test (Keegan *et al.* 1980) and has been used successfully in assessing the high risk fetus. It should be noted that, in one series, decelerations occurred in 5.8% of reactive tests and none of the fetuses came to any harm (Brown & Patrick 1981). This underlines the difficulty in interpreting decelerations which may be normal events in some fetuses.

The predictive value of a test which suggests the fetus is 'non-reactive' is not as precise. This is partly because the normal healthy fetus may remain in a resting phase for up to 75 minutes, making it difficult to distinguish between one that is simply quiescent and one not moving because of hypoxia. A sensible suggestion has been to extend the length of time during which the FHR is recorded. If the test is allowed to run for 120 minutes and is still 'non-reactive' a positive predictive value of 85.7%, for fetal morbidity and mortality, can be achieved (Brown & Patrick 1981). This study also demonstrated that all fetuses which became 'reactive' (at which point the test was terminated) did so by 80 minutes.

The oxytocin challenge test (OCT) or contraction stress test (CST) has been used by some in an attempt to discriminate more accurately between the hypoxic and the healthy quiescent fetus. Even when this test is used as further investigation in those situations where the NST is 'non-reactive', the results have not been easy to interpret and have not made management any more certain. Furthermore it is time consuming to perform (hence expensive) and uncomfortable for the patient.

AMNIOTIC FLUID VOLUME

The amount of fluid present is simple to assess subjectively by ultrasound but quantitative measurement is more difficult. Fluid seen round the fetal buttocks and between the legs when the presentation is cephalic is a good sign. It has been suggested that one pool measuring at least 1 cm in two perpendicular planes (Manning *et al.* 1980) be taken as the lower limit of normal but even this amount represents oligohydramnios. A more reasonable estimate of normality would be at least one pool measuring at least 2 cm in two perpendicular planes.

When oligohydramnios is present fetal abnormality, particularly of the renal tracts, should be considered and this deserves careful study with high resolution ultrasound. Alternatively, oligohydramnios may reflect IUGR, and a recent report records that 83% of growth retarded fetuses were associated with it (Philipsen *et al.* 1983); on the other hand, 8% of such fetuses appeared to have normal amniotic fluid volume.

BIOPHYSICAL PROFILE

It has been argued that the well recognized effects of chronic progressive asphyxia in the neonate should apply to the fetus *in utero*. There is generalized central nervous system depression resulting in diminished or absent movement and muscle tone, poor respiratory drive, poor urine output, and decreased or absent heart rate accelerations. Manning *et al.* (1981) have shown that each of these characteristics may be demonstrated using ultrasound and each scored as shown in Table 31.5.

It should be emphasized that, although this technique has been used with success in clinical practice, the details of the test will require modification in the future. This is partly because each variable has been assigned the same score and each is therefore regarded as being equally sensitive; this may not in fact turn out to be the case. Also the definition of some of the variables may change, for example experience would suggest that the present norm for amniotic fluid volume (less than 1 cm in two perpendicular planes) is too small.

Nevertheless the results reported with this technique have so far been good. After testing over 3000 high risk fetuses, only 12 normal fetuses have been lost (3.5 per 1000), and only 6 of these deaths occurred within one week of a normal test, giving a false negative rate of 0.9 per 1000 (F.A. Manning, personal communication). However, 4 of the 6 'unexpected' deaths occurred in diabetic women, underlining the fact that such pregnancies are still difficult to assess by any presently available means. The mechanism of fetal death in diabetes may involve acute

Parameter	Score 2	Score 0
Amniotic fluid volume	> 1 cm pocket in two perpendicular planes	< 1 cm pocket in two perpendicular planes
Fetal movements	3 or more gross body movements in 30 minutes	2 or less gross body movements in 30 minutes
Fetal breathing movements (FBM)	At least 30 seconds of sustained FBM in 30 minutes	Less than 30 seconds of FBM in 30 minutes
Fetal tone	1 episode of limb motion from flexion to extension to flexion in a rapid motion	No evidence of flexion movements or fetal movement
Fetal reactivity	2 or more FHR accelerations of 15 BPM for 15 seconds with fetal movements in 40 minutes	Less than 2 accelerations in 40 minutes

Table 31.5. Biophysical profile scoring system (from Manning *et al.* 1981).

metabolic or cardiovascular insults which escape detection.

There is little doubt that taking these features of intrauterine life into account, in combination with measurements of fetal growth, allows the clinician much more insight into the obstetric problem with which he is presented. It also gives a sound basis for deciding upon appropriate management.

AMNIOCENTESIS

When IUGR has been diagnosed, particularly early in gestation, there is a place for amniocentesis to check fetal chromosomes; management can then be planned accordingly. The time required to obtain such a result implies this procedure should be considered only when delivery is not being contemplated for some weeks.

Future developments

FETAL BREATHING MOVEMENTS

Reports that intermittent breathing movements during rapid eye movement sleep in fetal sheep are abolished or decreased by hypoxia (Boddy et al. 1974) led to speculation that they may be a useful guide to fetal condition in utero. In clinical practice initial optimism proved unfounded because of the intermittent nature of the breathing movements. The major problem is the length of time required to observe FBM before being certain that the incidence is normal. Because some healthy fetuses have intervals of more than an hour between each episode of FBM, there is difficulty in deciding if their absence is normal or pathological (Patrick et al. 1980).

In view of these difficulties some have examined the effects on FBM of altering the intrauterine environment. For example, raising the maternal arterial PO_2 by breathing 50% oxygen or increasing the maternal arterial PCO_2 by giving the mother 5% carbon dioxide have been used with some success (Ritchie & Lakhani 1978, Dornan & Ritchie 1983). However, the prolonged observation time required precludes the use of these tests in routine clinical practice.

One important aspect of FBM that may eventually be clinically useful is the change in pattern which occurs around 35 weeks' gestation. This change, first noted by Boddy and Dawes (1975), is quite easily seen using real time ultrasound. Before 35 weeks the immature pattern of breathing is evident; it is irregular both in rate and in depth. Thereafter FBMs become much more regular in both these aspects, and a difference in the rate of FBM has been demonstrated between the normal fetus and one with IUGR the rate being slower in the latter (Dornan et al. 1984b). It has also been shown that the regular pattern of FBM occurs earlier in gestation in the presence of IUGR, suggesting that FBM may be associated in some way with lung maturity. This possibility remains to be proven although major differences in lung development have been reported between anencephalic fetuses with normal FBM and those making no FBM whatsoever (Dornan et al. 1984a).

PLACENTAL ARCHITECTURE

Changes in the structure of the placenta are clearly visible using real time ultrasound (Grannum et al. 1979) and include increasing deposition of calcium and fibrin. Progressive cotyledonary formation is represented by indentation of the chorionic plate. Originally these changes were graded and compared with the lecithin/sphingomyelin (L/S) ratio and it was suggested that the appearance of the placenta could be correlated with lung maturity. The reproducibility of this association is open to doubt. Important information may still be obtained by observing the placental architecture. In particular it can help distinguish between the mature and the immature fetus when dates are very uncertain, since it is unusual to see heavy calcification and cotyledonary formation changes before 34 weeks' gestation. On occasion the earlier appearance of these changes has been observed in association with IUGR and when the mother smokes heavily. Further information is required.

FETAL BLOOD FLOW

The speed of red blood cells flowing down fetal vessels can be measured using Doppler ultrasound and when the cross-sectional area of the vessel is known quantitative flow can be calculated. The method used and the rate of flow in the aorta and other fetal vessels have been reported by Griffin et al. (1983).

The method is subject to fairly large errors and is therefore not as potentially useful as it might appear at first sight. On the other hand the characteristics of the flow in the umbilical artery during systole and diastole as gestation advances are now well documented (Erskine & Ritchie 1985). Major changes in the pattern observed during diastole in the growth

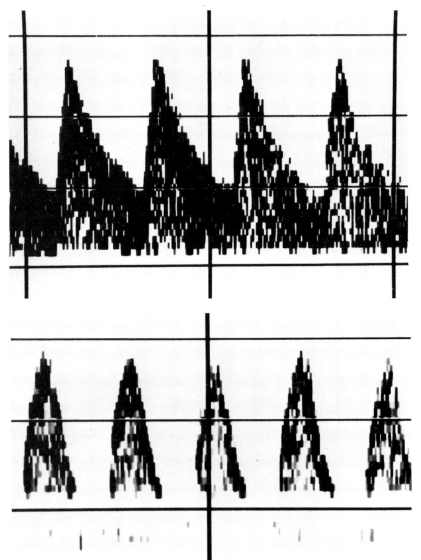

Fig. 31.3. Blood velocity waveforms in the umbilical artery at 32 weeks' gestation. (With permission from the Editor of the *British Journal of Obstetrics and Gynaecology.*) Normal healthy fetus above. Growth retarded fetus beneath.

retarded fetus have been observed and quantified (Fig. 31.3), and this method holds much promise as a measure of fetal compromise. Meticulous study is necessary before such methods can be applied to clinical practice.

UTERINE ARTERY BLOOD FLOW

Using the same Doppler technique, Campbell *et al.* (1983) have shown that flow patterns in the uterine arteries may be recorded. Again, changes in association with pregnancy complications have been observed and this technique also has promising potential, but further study is required before its value can be fully assessed.

DELIVERY

TIMING OF DELIVERY

Timing delivery depends on assessing and balancing between the increasing risk to the fetus if it remains *in utero* and the hazards from neonatal immaturity which decrease with gestational ageing. Failure to demonstrate significant fetal growth is an indication to consider immediate delivery, as is evidence of fetal compromise demonstrated by the tests discussed above. Gestational age is normally established by ultrasound dating in early pregnancy. When in doubt, or when a decision has been made to deliver a mother well before term, it is advisable to take the precaution of determining whether or not hyaline membrane disease is likely to develop. Immaturity of the respiratory system is not the only problem encountered by the premature fetus; immaturity of other systems may also result in serious handicap or even death. However lung function can at least be predicted reasonably accurately by determining the L/S ratio in amniotic fluid obtained by amniocentesis and also whether phosphatidyl glycerol is present (Whittle *et al.* 1981). Both these indices of fetal lung maturity may also be measured on specimens of amniotic fluid collected vaginally after preterm rupture of the membranes.

ROUTE OF DELIVERY

When it is judged that the intrauterine environment will confer no further benefit, the choice of delivery route rests upon several factors. The probable condition of the fetus, as indicated by the investigations described above, must be considered. Evidence of hypoxia in the presence of growth retardation and oligohydramnios indicates that labour may be tolerated poorly. Uterine contractions will usually exacerbate the situation and increase the risk of birth asphyxia and acidosis which is a well recognized hazard of IUGR (Lin *et al.* 1980).

The presentation of the fetus should also be considered. Vaginal breech delivery, which in the normal fetus increases the risk of asphyxia and acidosis, should not be contemplated when fetal health is already compromised.

Finally the state of the cervix should be carefully assessed with a view to estimating the probable response to induction of labour. A relatively short induction–delivery interval may be acceptable when good intrapartum monitoring is available with early recourse to Caesarean section if signs of fetal distress arise.

INTRAPARTUM MONITORING

MATERNAL CONDITION

The traditional maternal observations made during labour are of importance for the safety of both mother and fetus; the maternal temperature, pulse rate and

blood pressure should be recorded regularly throughout its course, urinary output should be measured, and each sample tested for the presence of protein, glucose and ketones.

Maternal pyrexia has important implications for the fetus as it may indicate ascending infection and congenital pneumonia. It may cause tachycardia in a normal uninfected fetus. A maternal tachycardia due to apprehension can also affect the fetal heart rate.

A rise in blood pressure particularly with proteinuria requires careful assessment and may be the first presentation of pre-eclampsia.

Poor urine output may be due to dehydration, which should be corrected by intravenous fluid. Ketonuria leads to maternal acidaemia, and eventually also to fetal acidaemia or an exacerbation of this if it is already present. Ketonuria also impairs uterine contractions, and is best corrected by intravenous fluids using 5% dextrose.

INITIAL ASSESSMENT IN LABOUR

As a result of on-call rotations the personnel managing labour are often different from those who have looked after a woman's antenatal care. It is therefore of paramount importance that the antenatal notes are readily available, that they are legible and that they accurately record the progress of the pregnancy and labour.

The initial vaginal examination in labour also provides important information concerning the fetus as well as about the dilatation and effacement of the cervix which, together with the station of the presenting part, should be recorded on a partogram (*see* Chapter 24). If the membranes are ruptured the degree of caput formation and moulding of the fetal head and the position of the presenting part should be noted as well as the colour of the amniotic fluid. If the membranes are intact and labour has been diagnosed they should be ruptured particularly if the cervix is at least 4 cm dilated. This allows the quantity and colour of the fluid to be determined. The absence of fluid or the presence of meconium demands more intensive assessment and monitoring.

Fetal heart rate monitoring

It is well recognized that the process of labour can result in profound birth asphyxia and acidosis in the newborn. Often there is a good explanation for the hypoxic condition of the newborn at birth, and this is particularly so where acute insults such as prolapse of the cord or placental separation due to eclampsia have occurred. More often, however, the poor condition of the newborn is unexpected. Experience has demonstrated that changes in the FHR are usually present and this change may be used to predict such an outcome.

Birth asphyxia occurs when the cumulative effects of repeated decreases in oxygenation due to uterine contractions are superimposed upon chronic hypoxia which may have already been present before labour starts. Fortunately it would appear, from work in sheep (Peeters *et al.* 1979) and in primates (Adamson & Myers 1977), that there is a wide margin of safety in response to an asphyxial insult. A similar margin of safety would appear to be present in the human fetus since Steiner and Neligan (1975) reported that 18 infants out of 39 with cardiac arrest occurring within 15 minutes of birth survived with no obvious neurological deficit.

In response to intrauterine hypoxia there is a redistribution of blood flow mediated partly by the release of catecholamines. Cardiac output is maintained while blood flow to the brain and heart is increased at the expense of non-vital organs. Brain oedema and necrosis, resulting in permanent and substantial damage, occur only when asphyxia has been prolonged and profound. This helps explain why some infants survive hypoxic insults without long term effects while others incur severe handicap.

The cardiovascular events associated with changes in blood flow in response to asphyxia are associated with changes in the FHR and blood pressure long before there is sufficient hypoxia to result in brain injury. It is on this basis that, traditionally, the FHR has been observed during labour and used as an early warning of hypoxia.

NORMAL PATTERNS

FHR monitoring during labour has a high negative predictive value, that is to say, a normal pattern is reliably associated with a good fetal outcome. However, the technique has a less good positive predictive value, that is to say an abnormal pattern does not reliably predict birth asphyxia in terms of a low Apgar score and low cord artery pH.

The normal FHR pattern associated with a good outcome includes a baseline rate between 120 and 160 beats per minute, with variability of at least 5 beats per minute, and it exhibits no decelerations in association with contractions.

ABNORMAL PATTERNS

Bradycardia (defined as a prolonged episode during which the FHR is persistently below 120 beats per minute) was the main clinical sign traditionally associated with fetal distress. However, in recent years more subtle changes have been described, some of which are associated with fetal hypoxia. The uncertainty associated with FHR monitoring is not so much the recognition of an abnormal change but the degree and duration of hypoxia with which it is associated.

The classification of FHR patterns described by Hon and Quilligan (1968) is based on evidence from animal and human studies. It has stood the test of time, and is based on the following features: changes in baseline heart rate; changes in variability; and periodic or intermittent changes (decelerations or accelerations) in association with contractions.

Changes in baseline FHR
Tachycardia. A *persistent rise* in FHR above 160 beats per minute is termed tachycadia. It is associated with the following conditions: prematurity; maternal or fetal infection; maternal anxiety; maternal hyperthyroidism; drug treatment, e.g. beta-adrenergic agents; fetal anaemia, e.g. haemolytic disease; fetal haemorrhage, e.g. acute bleeding due to placental abruption, vasa praevia or amniocentesis accident.

Fetal tachycardia may occur as a result of prolonged labour when the cause may be a combination of maternal anxiety, exhaustion and dehydration together with possible fetal infection. It should be taken as a warning sign of impending fetal distress and acted upon when seen in association with significant periodic changes (*see* below).

Bradycardia is defined as a persistent FHR of less than 120 beats per minute and is associated with the following:
1 no apparent cause, usually mild between 100 and 120 beats per minute;
2 local anaesthetic drugs, usually mild bradycardia unless drug reaches fetus quickly as for example at cervical block;
3 epidural analgesia, if profound hypotension occurs and is not quickly rectified, bradycardia can result and be severe and prolonged;
4 fetal heart anomaly, often due to a conduction defect and associated with a good fetal outcome; diagnosis may be simplified by recording the fetal electrocardiogram (FECG);
5 post-term fetus: advanced gestational age can be associated with mild bradycardia;

6 umbilical cord compression: tight compression of the cord can lead to prolonged severe bradycardia, in which case severe acidosis may soon result. It is usually seen during the late second stage but it may also occur, as a terminal event, after prolonged episodes of hypoxia. This requires urgent management by expediting delivery.

Variability

Variability in the FHR is controlled by the autonomic nervous system. The sympathetic component continuously influences the heart rate by increasing the rate while the parasympathetic system, acting through the vagus nerve, intermittently modulates the rate by slowing it down. Parasympathetic tone is controlled by a number of factors including information received from the baroreceptors which monitor blood pressure.

FHR variability is sometimes classified as being short term or long term. Short term variability (or beat to beat variation) is a measure of the interval between each R wave of the cardiac cycle (the R-R interval). It can be measured accurately from the FECG and may be analysed by computer using a number of different methods. Long term variability is that which is clearly apparent on the FHR trace when the paper speed is 2 or 3 cm per minute and normally lies between 5 and 15 beats per minute.

The neural control of the fetal heart rate is affected by narcotic and anaesthetic drugs including local agents used in epidural analgesia. All such drugs cross the placenta rapidly and cause depression of the fetal central nervous system, resulting in a loss of variability which appears as a smoothing out or flattening of the FHR trace.

In the preterm fetus variability is normally reduced partly because the FHR is faster and partly because the parasympathetic system is as yet immature. Variability is also reduced in normal circumstances by changes in the cycle of fetal rest and activity which occurs throughout fetal life, the FHR showing less variability during periods of rest.

Finally, pathological loss of variability may occur as a result of central depression due to prolonged fetal hypoxia. A loss of variability for this reason is likely to occur in association with other abnormal changes in FHR. Rarely, when severe fetal anaemia is present, variability may be replaced by regular slow oscillations of 3–5 cycles per minute and this has been called a sinusoidal pattern.

Periodic changes with uterine contractions

Transient decelerations in FHR are not uncommon during labour, and occur in three distinct patterns as shown in Figure 31.4.

Early decelerations have a characteristic uniform 'shape' which is coincident with the uterine contraction. The nadir of the deceleration occurs at the same time as the peak of the contraction and often is in proportion to the intrauterine pressure. This pattern is usually seen in the late first stage of labour and is thought to be due to head compression mediated by pressure of the cervix on the fontanelle. The consequent rise in intracerebral pressure stimulates the vagal nerve causing a slowing of the heart rate. Rarely the pattern may be due to partial cord occlusion (Mendez-Bauer *et al.* 1978) and, if it is persistent, cord presentation or prolapse must be excluded on vaginal examination. The pattern is otherwise often transient and occurs most commonly when the fetus is in the occipito-posterior position with the cervix passing across the anterior fontanelle in the late first stage. When early decelerations become persistent, severe or prolonged, or occur in association with the passage of meconium, delivery should be expedited.

Late decelerations are thought to be due to hypoxia and acidosis resulting from utero-placental insufficiency which is exacerbated by uterine contractions. The effect on the FHR does not reach maximum until after the peak of the contraction has passed and recovery back to the baseline rate does not occur until after the intrauterine pressure has returned to the resting level. In the less severely affected fetus the baseline rate may be exceeded, probably due to catecholamine release, but a tachycardia persisting between contractions or failure of the FHR to return to the baseline indicates progressive deterioration in the fetal condition. On occasion this pattern may be caused by overstimulation of uterine action and can therefore be corrected by immediately stopping the oxytocic infusion. Hypotension in association with epidural anaesthesia may also precipitate this pattern, as may supine hypotension due to inferior vena caval compression. Hypotension should first be corrected by nursing the mother on her side and, in the case of epidural blockade, intravenous infusion of fluids.

If late decelerations are persistent or are found in association with other abnormalities such as poor heart rate variability then delivery should be arranged as soon as possible. This is particularly so if there is clinical evidence of fetal growth retardation or the passage of meconium.

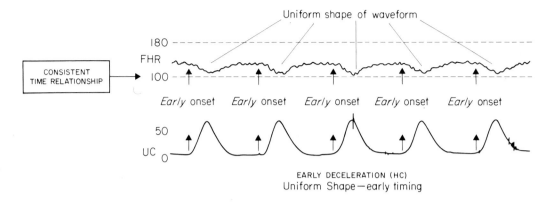

EARLY DECELERATION (HC)
Uniform Shape—early timing

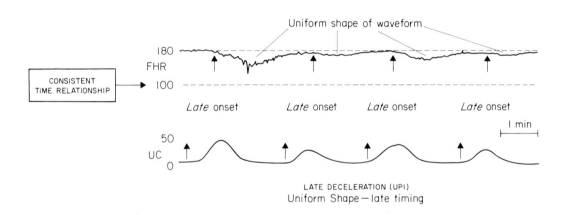

LATE DECELERATION (UPI)
Uniform Shape—late timing

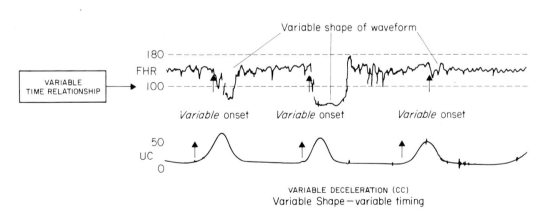

VARIABLE DECELERATION (CC)
Variable Shape—variable timing

Fig. 31.4. Time relationships between fetal heart rate decelerations and uterine contractions (Hon 1968), with permission.

Variable decelerations are variable both in shape and in their timing relative to the onset of contractions. They are thought to be due to umbilical cord compression. The change in FHR is normally abrupt and is due to reflex changes in vagal tone caused by the increase in fetal blood pressure secondary to cord compression. The release of cord compression is also associated with an abrupt return to the baseline rate.

Occasionally a transient increase in rate occurs at the end of the deceleration probably due to release of catecholamines. The possibility that compression is due to cord prolapse should be excluded by vaginal examination.

Transient variable decelerations due to cord compression during labour are common and often disappear when the maternal position is altered. When the pattern persists, or there is loss of variability or a mixed pattern (see below) develops, a scalp blood sample should be obtained for pH measurement (see below). If this cannot be performed arrangements should be made for delivery.

Mixed pattern. When variable decelerations are prolonged, return to the baseline rate may be slow with the recovery features of the late deceleration. It is then referred to as a mixed pattern and is due to significant hypoxia resulting from the cord compression. If persistent it has serious consequences and requires prompt action as suggested above.

Transient accelerations. Brief episodes of increased heart rate or accelerations lasting about 15–45 seconds are commonly associated with fetal movement and are a good prognostic sign. Accelerations demonstrate intact autonomic control of the heart rate capable of responding to fetal activity.

METHODS OF FHR MONITORING

Intermittent auscultation with a Pinard fetal stethoscope has been gradually replaced by more sophisticated methods which allow continuous recordings of the FHR to be made. The most accurate of these is from the FECG obtained by means of a spiral electrode twisted into the fetal scalp or a spring-loaded hook (Fig. 31.5) inserted after the membranes have been ruptured. The disadvantage of both methods is that it requires the mother to be put to bed during her labour, and the electrode occasionally causes infection of the fetal scalp.

There are a number of non-invasive methods which can be used when the membranes are intact. The most reliable of these employs continuous Doppler ultrasound, via the mother's abdomen, to detect movement of the fetal heart, from which the FHR is computed. The most recent equipment incorporates a method of signal improvement termed autocorrelation; this produces a record of the FHR which is almost indistinguishable from that obtained directly from the FECG. The FECG can also be recorded from the surface of the maternal abdomen but the method is not reliable enough for use during labour. Phono-

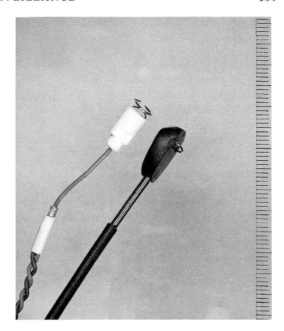

Fig. 31.5. Two types of electrode used to pick up the fetal heart electrical activity directly from the scalp. On the left is a double helix which screws into the scalp tissue, on the right is a spring-loaded hook which can be retracted into the black rubber bed and then released to engage the fetal scalp.

cardiography has also been used to detect the fetal heart and depends upon amplifying the fetal heart sound by means of a microphone. Again this method is impracticable in labour because of a variety of other recorded noises such as maternal muscle movement.

It is clear from the classification of FHR patterns that an accurate measure of uterine activity is essential for interpretation. External measurement of uterine contractions (tocography) is the most common method employed where their strength is measured by a strain gauge placed on the maternal abdomen. Although the method is non-invasive the record of contractions obtained is qualitative rather than quantitative. Using this type of tocography contractions can be timed but their relative strength is uncertain.

The internal method involves measuring amniotic fluid pressure by means of inserting an open-ended fluid-filled catheter past the presenting part and into the uterine cavity. The changes in pressure during uterine contractions are recorded by a pressure transducer. The method is very reliable, providing an accurate quantitative measurement, but carries a small risk of infection, uterine perforation and placental separation.

Internal monitoring of both FHR and uterine contractions is the only reliable technique when abnormalities in the FHR pattern have already been detected or the fetal condition is known to be compromised before labour starts. The external methods of monitoring on the other hand may suffice for routine practice.

INDICATIONS

The place of fetal monitoring during labour is not in doubt where the fetus is deemed to be at *high risk*. Beard *et al.* (1971) originally tabulated such indications and an amended list is shown in Table 31.6.

Another approach is to define *low risk* situations in which electronic fetal monitoring can be withheld as follows: normal antepartum history with no complications significantly affecting the fetus; normal fetal growth; spontaneous labour which progresses normally; normal quantity of amniotic fluid demonstrated.

Currently there is considerable debate about the place of fetal monitoring where the risk to the fetus is estimated to be low. The chance of intrapartum stillbirth occurring in these circumstances is probably of the order of 1 in 1000. Therefore, the consequences of employing invasive monitoring techniques

Table 31.6. Indications for fetal monitoring during labour. Adapted from Beard *et al.* (1971).

Antepartum
   Primigravida aged 35 or more
   Multipara aged 40 or more
   Pre-eclampsia or essential hypertension
   Diabetes
   Rhesus incompatibility with affected fetus
   History of antepartum haemorrhage during present
      pregnancy
   Small-for-dates fetus
   Poor obstetric history
   History of supine hypotension

Intrapartum
   Breech presentation
   Trial of labour
   Clinical signs of fetal distress
   Prolonged labour (12 hours or more)
   Epidural anaesthesia
   Supine hypotension
   Twins
   Oxytocin in use

---

in terms of causing mothers to adopt unnatural positions in labour, an increased risk of infection and operative interference must be considered. The true value of electronic fetal monitoring may lie in the reduction of neonatal morbidity. In an attempt to answer this question, a large randomized trial has been carried out at the National Maternity Hospital, Dublin, in which mothers with low fetal risk were allocated to either intermittent auscultation or electronic fetal monitoring during labour. It would appear that there was a significantly lower incidence of neonatal seizures in the group monitored electronically (MacDonald D., personal communication). Thus, intermittent auscultation cannot be regarded as totally satisfactory in low risk situations.

It is also clear from a number of trials, reviewed by Chalmers (1978), that the Caesarean section rate is increased if FHR monitoring is used alone without recourse to a measure of its effect on fetal acid base status.

Fetal scalp blood sampling

Fetal acidosis occurs in association with significant hypoxia and has two components. Accumulation of carbon dioxide leads to a respiratory acidosis while hypoxia alters cell metabolism from aerobic to anaerobic with resulting formation of lactic acid. The latter causes metabolic acidosis.

The technique of collecting fetal scalp blood to measure pH was first described by Saling (1962). As a result much information has been gained about the significance of abnormal fetal heart rate patterns during labour. The fetal pH associated with various FHR patterns has been reported by Beard *et al.* (1971), showing that some patterns have little effect on pH (Table 31.7). In fact the patterns primarily associated with acidosis are either variable decelerations where the baseline is also abnormal or loss of FHR variability in association with decelerations. The number of fetuses with late decelerations in Beard's series was small but this pattern is now recognized as being predictive of significant fetal acidosis.

In the first stage of labour, during which a gradual mild acidosis normally occurs, the mean fetal scalp blood pH is 7.33. A pH greater than 7.25 or more is therefore considered to be within the normal range. A pH between 7.20 and 7.25 requires careful surveillance and should be repeated within an hour. If the repeat estimation shows a falling trend in pH then delivery should be expedited. In any case when the pH is below 7.20 significant acidosis exists and

	No. of pH estimations	Mean fetal pH ± 1 S.D.
Normal trace	68	7.337 ± 0.0565
Accelerations	20	7.34 ± 0.0328†
Early decelerations	25	7.33 ± 0.0452
Baseline tachycardia (uncomplicated)	43	7.306 ± 0.0426
Baseline bradycardia (uncomplicated)	34	7.326 ± 0.0516
Variable decelerations—normal baseline	30	7.311 ± 0.0478
abnormal baseline	23	7.223 ± 0.0755*
Loss of beat-to-beat variation (uncomplicated)	15	7.301 ± 0.0612
Loss of beat-to-beat variation (complicated)	19	7.242 ± 0.0734†
Late decelerations—abnormal baseline	2	7.28

Table 31.7. Fetal heart rate patterns and mean fetal scalp blood pH in patients who had one or more samples collected. Beard *et al.* (1971).

$^*p < 0.001$
$^†p < 0.005$ ⎫ compared with mean pH of fetuses with normal traces.

delivery is required. During the second stage of labour a value as low as 7.15 may be acceptable provided normal progress is being made.

The usefulness of scalp blood pH estimations depend upon how often they are carried out. When the method is used frequently as an adjunct to FHR monitoring proficiency in carrying it out improves as well as the reliability of its interpretation. On the other hand, when it is performed infrequently, patient discomfort, failure to obtain a sample and poor maintenance of micro-astrup equipment all become major problems.

Management of fetal distress

When fetal distress is diagnosed from examination of the FHR trace a number of procedures should be carried out automatically. Intravenous oxytocin, if in use, should be discontinued and maternal blood pressure checked to exclude supine hypotension. When decelerations due to cord compression occur, maternal position should be altered by rolling her onto one side or another or by tilting the head end of the bed downwards. Oxygen by face mask is also useful and can raise significantly oxygen delivery to the fetus. Finally if the FHR pattern suggests persistent cord occlusion, occult prolapse should be sought by performing a vaginal examination. If the pattern persists preparation should be made to carry out a fetal scalp blood pH.

Future developments

The failure of FHR patterns to predict significant hypoxia and acidosis with certainty has led to a search for other methods. In recent years continuous measurement of fetal scalp tissue pH during labour has been used as a research technique (Flynn & Kelly 1980). Although this may be the most promising of the newer techniques, there are still significant problems with fixation of the electrode and interpretation of results.

Continuous measurement of scalp tissue pO_2 is also possible and has been used to provide information about the physiology of the fetus during labour (Huch *et al.* 1977). There are quite large changes in tissue pO_2 and their interpretation is difficult. It is unlikely that this method will provide information which can be acted upon clinically.

Measurement of lactic acid in a capillary sample of fetal scalp blood during labour has been reported using an electro-chemical enzymatic sensor (Soutter *et al.* 1978). This technique would appear to give as good results, in predicting fetal acidosis, as does pH measurement. This is not unexpected since significant hypoxia is associated with anaerobic glycolysis and the production of lactic acid. The use of the lactate analyser may well become more frequent as technology improves.

It is possible that in the next few years the condition of the fetus in early labour may be screened by a number of methods using ultrasound. An assessment of the fetus in a manner similar to the biophysical profile may prove useful. Certainly the ability to examine blood flow in the major fetal vessels and uterine arteries using Doppler ultrasound will be exploited. These methods may be used also to examine the fetus when distress occurs thus adding to our knowledge of fetal physiology and the unpredictable effects of labour.

REFERENCES

ADAMSON S.K. & MYERS R.E. (1977) *Amer. J. Obstet. Gynec.*, **128**, 893.

BEARD R.W., FILSHIE G.M., KNIGHT C.A. & ROBERTS G.M. (1971) *Brit. J. Obstet. Gynaecol.*, **78**, 865.

BODDY K. & DAWES G.S. (1975) *Brit. Med. Bull.*, **31**.

BODDY K., DAWES G.S., FISHER R. *et al.* (1974) *J. Physiol.* (Lond.), **243**.

BROCK D.J.H., BARROW J., JELEN P., WATT M. & SCRIMGEOUR J.B. (1977) *Lancet*, **2**, 267.

BROWN E. & PATRICK J. (1981) *Amer. J. Obstet. Gynec.*, **141**, 646.

CALVERT J.P., CREAN E.E., NEWCOMBE R.G. & PEARSON J.F. (1982) *Brit. med. J.*, **285**, 846.

CAMPBELL S. (1974) In *Clinics in Obstetrics & Gynaecology* Vol. 1, No. 2, 41.

CAMPBELL S. & THOMS A. (1977) *Brit. J. Obstet. Gynaecol.*, **84**, 165.

CAMPBELL S. & WILKIN D. (1975) *Brit. J. Obstet. Gynaecol.*, **82**, 689.

CAMPBELL S., GRIFFIN D.R., PEARCE J.M., DIAZ-RECASENS J., COHEN-OVERBEEK T.E., WILLSON K. & TEAGUE M.J. (1983) *Lancet*, **i**, 675.

CHALMERS I. (1978) In *Perinatal Medicine, 6th European Congress.* Vienna (Thalhammer O., Baumgarten K. & Pollack A. eds.), 260.

CHINN D.H., FILLY R. & CALLEN P.W. (1981) *J. clin Ultrasound*, **9**, 175.

DORNAN J.C. & RITCHIE J.W.K. (1983) *Brit. J. Obstet. Gynaecol.*, **90**, 210.

DORNAN J.C., RITCHIE J.W.K. & MEBAN C. (1984a) *J. devel. Physiol.* **6 (4)**, 367.

DORNAN J.C., RITCHIE J.W.K., RUFF S. (1984b) *Brit. J. Obstet. Gynaecol.*, **91**, 31.

EIK-NES S.H., GROTTUM P. & ANDERSSON N.J. (1982) *Acta Obstet. Gynecol. Scand.*, **61**, 307.

ERSKINE R.L.A. & RITCHIE J.W.K. (1985) *Brit. J. Obstet. Gynaecol.* **92**, 605.

FANCOURT R., CAMPBELL S., HARVEY D.R. & NORMAN A.P. (1976) *Brit. Med. J.*, **i**, 1435.

FLYNN A.M. & KELLY J. (1980) *Brit. J. Obstet. Gynaecol.*, **87**, 666.

GOHARI P., BERKOWITZ R.L. & HOBBINS J.C. (1977) *Amer. J. Obstet. Gynec.*, **127**, 255.

GOODWIN J.W. & CHANCE G.W. (1979) *Ontario med. Rev.*, 563.

GOODWIN J.W., DUNNE J.T. & THOMAS B.W. (1969) *Can. med. J.*, **101**, 458.

GRANNUM P., BERKOWITZ R.L. & HOBBINS J.C. (1979) *Amer. J. Obstet. Gynec.*, **133**, 915.

GRIFFIN D., COHEN-OVERBEEK T. & CAMPBELL S. (1983) In *Clinics in Obstetrics and Gynaecology*, Vol. 10, **3**, 565. W.B. Saunders, Eastbourne.

HAYNES R.B. (1981) *Can. med. J.*, **124**, 703.

HON E.H. & QUILLIGAN E.J. (1968) *Clin. Obstet. Gynecol.*, **2**, 145.

HUCH A., HUCH R., SCHEIDER H. & ROOTH G. (1977) *Brit. J. Obstet. Gynaec.*, **84** (Suppl 1), 1.

KEEGAN K.A. & PAUL R.H. (1980) *Amer. J. Obstet. Gynecol.*, **136**, 75.

KEEGAN K.A., PAUL R.H., BROUSSARD P.M., McCART D. & SMITH M.A. (1980) *Amer. J. Obstet. Gynec.*, **136**, 81.

LIN C., MOAWADA A.H., ROSENOW P.J. & RIVER P. (1980) *Amer. J. Obstet. Gynec.*, **137**, 553.

MANNING F.A., PLATT L.D. & SIPOS L. (1980) *Amer. J. Obstet. Gynec.*, **136**, 787.

MANNING F.A., BASKETT T.F., MORRISON I. & LANGE I.R. (1981) *Amer. J. Obstet. Gynec.*, **140**, 289.

MENDEZ-BAUER C., RUIZ CANSECO A., ANDUJAR RUIZ M., MENDEL A., ARROYO J., GARDI R.D. *et al.* (1978) *J. perinat. Med.*, **6**, 69.

MERCATZ I.R., NITOWSKY H.M., MACRI J.N. & JOHNSON W.E. (1984) *Amer. J. Obstet. Gynec.*, **148**, 886.

NEILSON J.P., WHITFIELD C.R. & AITCHISON T.C. (1980) *Brit. med. J.*, **i**, 1203.

NEILSON J.P., MUNJANJA S.P. & WHITFIELD C.R. (1984) *Brit. J.*, **289**, 1179.

PATRICK J., CAMPBELL K., CARMICHAEL L., NATALE R. & RICHARDSON B. (1980) *Obstet. and Gynec.*, **56**, 24.

PEARSON J. (1982) In *Recent Advances in Obstetrics and Gynaecology* (Bonnar J. ed.) p 3. Churchill Livingstone, Edinburgh.

PEARSON J.F. & WEAVER J.B. (1976) *Brit. med. J.*, **1**, 1305.

PEETERS L.L., SHELDON R.E. & JONES M.D. *et al.* (1979) *Amer. J. Obstet. Gynec.*, **135**.

PHILIPSEN E.H., SOKOL R.J. & WILLIAMS T. (19783) *Dev. J. Obstet. Gynec.*, **146**, 271.

RITCHIE J.W.K. & LAKHANI K. (1978) *Brit. J. Obstet. Gynaecol.*, **87**, 1084.

ROBERTS A.B., LITTLE D.J., COOPER D. & CAMPBELL S. (1980) In *Real Time Ultrasound in Obstetrics* (Bennett M.J. & Campbell S. eds.), p. 122. Blackwell Scientific Publications, Oxford.

SALING E. (1962) *Arch. Gynäk.*, **197**, 108.

SOUTTER W.P., SHARP F., CLARK D.M. (1978) *Brit. J. Anaesth.*, **50**, 45.

STEINER H. & NELIGAN G. (1975) *Arch. Dis. Child.*, **50**, 696.

WHITTLE M.J., WILSON A.I., WHITFIELD C.R., PATON R.D. & LOGAN R.W. (1981) *Brit. med. J.*, **282**, 428.

WILLOCKS J., DONALD I., DUGGAN T.C. & DAY N. (1964) *J. Obstet. Gynaec. Brit. Cwlth.*, **71**, 11.

YEH S., FORSYTHE A., LOWENSOHN R.I. *et al.* (1977) *Amer. J. Obstet. Gynec.*, **127**, 50.

CHAPTER 32
THE PUERPERIUM AND ITS
COMPLICATIONS

P.W. HOWIE

The puerperium is a time of great importance for both the mother and her baby and yet it is an aspect of maternity care that has received relatively less attention than pregnancy and delivery. During the puerperium, the pelvic organs return to the non-gravid state, the metabolic changes of pregnancy are reversed and lactation is established. If the mother does not breast feed, the potential for fertility may return within a short time and, in the absence of effective contraception, the reproductive cycle may start again within a few weeks.

The puerperium is also a time of psychological adjustment. The mother's joy at the arrival of the new baby may be tempered by anxiety about her child's welfare and her ability to cope. These anxieties may be compounded if she is tired after her labour or if she has any medical complications. Another problem for the new mother may be a plethora of well-meaning, but conflicting, advice from medical and nursing staffs as well as from relatives and friends. It is important that an atmosphere be created where a mother can learn to handle her baby with confidence. In this, the postnatal ward staff play a very important role and a mother's impression of hospital may be coloured more by her experiences in the postnatal wards than by any other part of her maternity care. The objectives of the medical and nursing staffs during the puerperium can be summarized as follows: to monitor the physiological changes of the puerperium; to diagnose and treat any postnatal complications; to establish infant feeding; to give the mother emotional support; to advise about contraception and other measures which will contribute to continuing health.

PHYSIOLOGY OF THE PUERPERIUM

The major physiological event of the puerperium is lactation and this will be discussed in more detail later in the chapter. Following delivery, when the endocrine influences of the placenta are removed, the physiological changes of pregnancy are reversed and the body tissues, especially the pelvic organs, return to their previous state. It is probable that some 6–8 weeks elapse before this return to normal is complete, or as complete as it will ever become; during the first 2 weeks of this time the changes are rapid and become slower thereafter.

THE PELVIC ORGANS

The principal change is uterine involution. After delivery, the uterine fundus is usually palpable in the region of the umbilicus but, 10–14 days later, it will have disappeared behind the symphysis pubis. The process of involution is aided by the release of oxytocin during breast feeding so that the uteri of lactating women tend to be smaller than those of bottle feeding mothers. It is important to monitor fundal height because a delay in involution may indicate infection or retained products of placenta. The uterus weighs about 1 kg at the time of delivery but shrinks to some 50–60 g in weight within a few weeks by autolysis. The excess protein of the uterine muscle and other cells is broken down and excreted in the urine or, to some extent, utilized by the body. The body is in negative nitrogen balance during this time, because more nitrogen is being excreted than is being taken in.

The cervix is very flaccid and curtain-like after delivery but within a few days is returning to its original form and consistency. The external os remains sufficiently dilated to admit a finger for weeks or months (and in some cases permanently) but the internal os becomes closed to a finger during the second week of the puerperium.

The vagina almost always shows some evidence of parity. In the first few days of the puerperium, the vaginal walls are smooth, soft and oedematous. The distension which has resulted from labour remains for a few days but the return to normal capacity is quite quick thereafter. Episiotomies or tears of the vagina and perineum usually heal well, provided adequate suturing has been undertaken. Healing may be impaired in the presence of infection or haematoma formation and the wound may break down. Even if this happens, healing by granulation is usually so satisfactory that it is seldom possible a few weeks later to tell that any difficulty in healing occurred at all.

Within the endometrial cavity, the decidua is cast off as a result of ischaemia and is lost as the lochial flow. The lochia consists of blood, leucocytes, shreds of decidua and organisms. The lochia is initially dusky red but this colour fades after the first week and the flow usually clears completely within 4 weeks of delivery. New endometrium will grow from the basal areas of the decidua but this will be influenced by the method of infant feeding. If lactation is suppressed, the uterine cavity may be covered by new endometrium within 3 weeks and first menstruation may occur at 6 weeks after delivery. In breast feeding mothers, ovarian activity is suppressed and the resumption of menstruation may be delayed for many months. The relationship between breast feeding and ovarian activity is discussed in more detail later in the chapter.

OTHER SYSTEMS

During the first few days the bladder and urethra may show evidence of minor trauma sustained at delivery but they do not usually remain in evidence for long. The changes which occur in the urinary tract during pregnancy disappear in a similar manner to other involutional changes. Within 2–3 weeks the hydro-ureter and calyceal dilatation of pregnancy is much less evident, although a complete return to normal probably does not occur for 6–8 weeks.

There is usually a diuresis during the first day or so of the puerperium when the excess fluid of pregnancy is eliminated. There is a fall in plasma volume during the puerperium and, if blood loss at delivery has been normal, there should be no anaemia and the haemoglobin concentration will rise. Levels of the blood clotting factors and the platelet count rise after delivery (Howie 1979) but the inhibition of systemic fibrinolytic activity which occurs during pregnancy is reversed within 30 minutes of placental delivery (Bonnar et al. 1970, see also Chapter 36, p. 539). The other physiological changes associated with pregnancy also reverse spontaneously during the puerperium and have usually returned to the non-gravid state within six weeks of delivery.

Management of the normal puerperium

The majority of mothers are perfectly well during the puerperium and should be encouraged to establish normal activities as quickly as possible. A major preoccupation is the establishment of infant feeding and this will be discussed in detail later in the chapter.

Immediately following delivery, the mother must remain in the delivery room for close observation until it is clear that all is well. The uterine fundus must be checked at frequent intervals to establish that it remains firmly contracted; the height of the fundus is also important because, if this is rising, it may indicate that the uterus is filling with blood or is being pushed up by a pelvic swelling such as a distended bladder or a pelvic haematoma. Regular checks should be made of the pulse, blood pressure, respiration and external vaginal blood loss. The bladder should be checked, and if this is thought to be full, the mother should be encouraged to pass urine. If she is unable to void and a considerable volume of urine is thought to be in the bladder, catheterization will be required.

The mother should be washed and made comfortable and she should be allowed something to eat and drink, such as tea and toast. Provided that there are no complications, it is highly desirable that the mother and her consort should be allowed some time together with their new baby, with the midwife making the necessary checks as discreetly as possible.

During the remainder of the patient's stay in hospital, she should be asked if she has any complaints and regular checks are made of her pulse, temperature, blood pressure, fundal height and lochial flow. It is also important that the urinary output is satisfactory and that the bladder is being emptied completely. These observations are necessary to give the earliest warning of any possible complications.

The perineum should be inspected every day and great gentleness is required when inspecting or cleansing any episiotomy wound or pelvic laceration. Regular baths, showers or cleaning with bidets are comforting and help to keep the healing wound free from infection. If the perineal wounds are particularly uncomfortable, a heat lamp can help to reduce pain and analgesics, such as paracetamol, may be required. More recently, foam sprays with local anaesthetic agents have come on the market and can be applied directly to the episiotomy wound to give effective but temporary relief from pain.

AMBULATION IN THE PUERPERIUM

Early rising has now, quite properly, become the rule and plays an important role in the prevention of venous thrombosis. If the mother is very tired after her labour, she may wish to sleep for some hours after delivery. After this period of recovery, mobilization should be encouraged under supervision, although the timing of this will be influenced by the mother's sense of well-being. The physiotherapist has an important part to play in returning the patient to normal health during the puerperium. Limb exercises will be particularly important to encourage venous flow in the leg veins of any mother who may be immobilized in bed for any reason. Exercises to the abdominal and pelvic floor muscles are most valuable in restoring normal tone which may have been lost during pregnancy.

TIME OF DISCHARGE FROM HOSPITAL

There used to be fairly rigid rules about the 'ideal' time for a mother to stay in hospital after delivery. It is now realized that the time of postnatal stay should be determined according to the mother's individual needs. When a mother has had an easy labour, feels well and is confident with her baby, she can go home 48 hours after delivery, provided adequate home support is available. In some hospitals, a 'domino' system has been adopted in favourable circumstances when the mother goes home with her midwife six hours after the birth ('domino' is an abbreviation for 'domiciliary, in and out' delivery). This type of arrangement may be particularly welcomed by a mother who wishes to return to her older children as quickly as possible.

On the other hand, there are many mothers who prefer to spend several days in hospital. This is particularly true for primiparous mothers who wish to have time to recover from the labour and to receive help in handling a baby for the first time. In any circumstance where there is a question about the health of the baby, it is better for mother and baby to wait until the paediatric staff are confident that problems have been resolved. Clearly, it is better to adopt a flexible attitude towards postnatal stay than to impose a fixed system on all mothers. Whatever system is adopted, however, all mothers must be under the continuing supervision of a midwife for at least 10 days and the general practitioner should be told of the patient's discharge. It is essential to ensure that the mother has adequate support to cope in the domestic environment.

COMPLICATIONS OF THE PUERPERIUM

Serious, and sometimes fatal, disorders may arise during the puerperium. The most serious complications are thrombo-embolism, infection and haemorrhage although problems from urinary complications, mental disorders and breast infections can cause much morbidity.

Thrombosis and embolism

Therombo-embolism is now one of the main causes of maternal death (*Confidential Enquiry into Maternal Deaths*, 1982) and the majority of deaths occur during the puerperium. Thrombo-embolism presents problems of prevention, diagnosis and treatment and these are discussed fully in Chapter 36.

Puerperal infection

A puerperal pyrexia may have several explanations but it is a clinical sign that always merits careful investigation. The principal sites to be investigated are the chest, the pelvic organs, the urinary tract, any surgical wounds, the legs and the breasts.

RESPIRATORY INFECTION

Respiratory infections are now seen less commonly in the puerperium because the use of general anaesthesia has fallen as epidural anaesthetics have become more widespread. The patients who are most likely to develop a chest infection are those who smoke or have chronic bronchitis and the infection is commonly provoked by a general anaesthetic. The diagnosis of infection is suggested by a productive cough with rales and rhonchi on auscultation and can be confirmed by culture of the infected sputum. It is important, however, not to miss the diagnosis of pulmonary embolism which may masquerade as a chest infection or as wheezing (Windebank *et al.* 1973). If the infection seems particularly severe with much bronchospasm, the possibility of Mendelson's syndrome following inhalation of gastric contents should be considered.

When a respiratory tract infection is present, intensive physiotherapy will encourage the expectoration of mucus from the bronchial tree and is an important part of the treatment. A broad spectrum antibiotic should be prescribed and this may have to be changed once bacteriological sensitivity results are available. In the majority of cases, the infection will respond quickly to treatment but, in occasional cases, an acute infection in a woman with chronic lung disease may require intensive therapy. In such severe cases it is best to seek the help of the respiratory team at an early stage before the patient becomes seriously ill with anoxia and a respiratory acidosis.

PELVIC INFECTION

Before the introduction of antibiotics, pelvic infection was the most important cause of maternal death. Puerperal pelvic infection now rarely results in maternal death, and, although it can still present as an acute life-threatening illness, it more frequently occurs as a low-grade infection which causes both immediate and long-term morbidity. It is important that pelvic infections are diagnosed and treated as expeditiously as possible.

Pathology
At delivery, the normal protective barriers against infection are temporarily broken down, and this gives an opportunity for potential pathogens to pass from the lower genital tract into the normally sterile environment of the uterus. Once the organisms have reached the decidua, they can readily spread to the myometrium, the parametrium and the Fallopian tubes and from there to the peritoneum and the peripheral circulation. If, in virulent infections, the organisms reach the peripheral circulation, the patient may develop signs of septicaemia or endotoxic shock. It is more common, however, for the infection to remain localized in the pelvis and, if treatment is not immediate and effective, there is a danger of chronic pelvic infection with tubal blockage.

Features which predispose to puerperal pelvic infection are a history of prolonged rupture of membranes or a protracted labour with multiple vaginal examinations. If there are retained products of conception or organized blood clot in the uterus these can act as ideal culture media. The most virulent organism which may cause postpartum pelvic infection is a β-haemolytic streptococcus although other streptococci or staphylococci may also cause an acute clinical picture. It is now more common to find the

infective agent to be a coliform, such as *Escherichia coli* or another Gram-negative organism such as *Bacteroides fragilis*. The clostridii may also be involved and, more recently, there has been interest in the role of chlamydia as a cause of pelvic infection (Munday 1983). This organism is difficult to culture but it can cause chronic problems of vaginal discharge and tubal blockage.

Clinical features
The initial clinical picture is usually a puerperal pyrexia associated with offensive lochia and lower abdominal discomfort. On abdominal or bimanual examination the uterus may be tender, especially on moving the cervix. If the infection spreads, a pelvic abscess may form and tender fluctuant swellings may be felt lateral to the uterus or in the Pouch of Douglas. Finally, the infection may spread beyond the pelvis with evidence of peritonitis, septicaemia or bacteraemic shock. By this stage the patient is acutely ill, restless and dyspnoeic with a high swinging temperature and tachycardia; in addition she may show signs of dehydration and have rigors during high spikes of pyrexia. The main objective of management should be to make an early diagnosis and prevent clinical deterioration.

Diagnosis
The diagnosis is initially made on clinical grounds and confirmed by culturing the infecting organism from swabs taken from high in the vagina, from the cervical canal and from the urethra. If there are acute episodes of pyrexia, blood cultures should also be taken. Aerobic and anaerobic cultures are set up but it is sometimes impossible to identify the pathogen with certainty. If the patient fails to respond to treatment, the possibility of some other infective condition, such as acute appendicitis, should be considered and laparotomy may be required. Alternatively, there may be a collection of pus in the pelvis or even under the diaphragm and the patient may not improve until the septic focus has been identified and adequately drained.

Treatment
The mainstay of treatment is appropriate antibiotic therapy. The initial choice of antibiotics will depend on the patterns of antibiotic resistance in any particular hospital and the advice of the bacteriologist may be very valuable. Currently, a popular choice is to combine one of the cephalosporins with metronidazole as this provides a wide range of activity

against Gram-positive and Gram-negative organisms. If the patient is acutely ill, intravenous therapy in the form of cephradine 1 g 6 hourly and metronidazole 500 mg 6 hourly should be given for 24–36 hours until a response has been achieved. When the symptoms are less acute, the oral route is appropriate and treatment should be continued for at least 10 days. Once culture results are available, it may be necessary to change the antibiotic regime according to the sensitivity patterns.

If there is retained placental tissue within the uterine cavity, this can act as a focus of infection and it is best that the uterine cavity is evacuated under anaesthesia. The diagnosis of retained products may be suggested by a dilated internal os of the uterine cervix and confirmed by feeling placental tissue in the cervical canal or by visualizing the tissue on ultrasonic examination.

If the patient becomes acutely ill as a consequence of puerperal pelvic infection, intensive therapy may be required to treat septicaemia or endotoxic shock. The management of acute pelvic infection is discussed in Chapter 41.

URINARY TRACT INFECTION

Urinary tract infections are common during the puerperium and are particularly likely to occur in women with a previous history of urinary infections or in those who required catheterization to relieve urinary retention. Most of the infections take the form of cystitis with the customary symptoms of urinary frequency, urgency and dysuria; the urine may be cloudy and offensive and pus cells can be seen on direct microscopic examination. Less commonly, pyelonephritis may develop when the constitutional upset is much greater, a pyrexia is present and shivering may occur; there may be pain and tenderness in the renal angle which can extend along the line of the ureter.

The diagnosis of a urinary tract infection can be confirmed by culturing the infecting organism on a mid-stream sample of urine. Treatment with a broad spectrum antibiotic should be started and changed at a later date according to the sensitivity results. A good oral intake of fluids should be encouraged and, if vomiting is one of the presenting features, intravenous fluids may be needed to maintain adequate hydration and a good urinary output.

Once the antibiotic course has been completed, a repeat culture should be performed on a mid-stream urine sample to ensure that treatment has been adequate. If there is a history of frequent, recurring urinary tract infections, further investigations of the urinary tract should be undertaken by cystoscopy and intravenous pyelography to exclude any underlying abnormality.

OTHER PUERPERAL INFECTIONS

In the event of a puerperal pyrexia, any surgical wound should be examined for evidence of infection. This is particularly important after Caesarean section, an operation which is being performed with increasing frequency. Wound infection will present as a reddened tender area deep to the incision which may be surrounded by induration. Treatment will depend upon the extent and severity of the infection. If the infection is well localized, it may discharge spontaneously and local irrigation with antiseptic solution may suffice. Until the wound discharges, a kaolin poultice may help to relieve discomfort and encourage localization of the infection. If the infection is more extensive, broad spectrum antibiotic treatment will be required and a swab from the infected wound should be sent for culture. If the abscess cavity is very deep, it is occasionally necessary to resuture the wound after the infection has resolved but, in the majority of cases, the wound will granulate from its base and heal spontaneously.

The legs should be inspected if a puerperal pyrexia is present because thrombophlebitis may be present. This problem is discussed in Chapter 36. A breast abscess can also cause puerperal pyrexia although this is rarely seen in the postnatal wards because it usually occurs after the fourteenth day. The management of a breast abscess is also discussed later in the chapter.

Secondary postpartum haemorrhage

By definition, secondary postpartum haemorrhage may occur at any time after the first 24 hours following delivery until the 6 weeks of the puerperium are completed but the most common time for bleeding is between the eighth and fourteenth day. Dewhurst (1966) reviewed 97 cases of secondary postpartum haemorrhage and found 18 occurring between days 1 and 7, 60 between days 8 and 14, and 19 after the fifteenth day. In the majority of cases the bleeding is not severe enough to threaten the patient's life, although it can occasionally require very energetic treatment.

Clinical features

Secondary postpartum haemorrhage is recognized when the lochial discharge is replaced by fresh red bleeding. The volume of the loss is variable ranging from about 100 ml to heavy bleeding with clotting. There may be cramping abdominal pain and, if the blood loss is heavy, the patient may be pale and eventually develop signs of shock. The uterus may be larger than it should be for the particular stage in the puerperium and, on vaginal examination, blood clot or retained placental tissue may be pouting through the cervical canal. If the bleeding is slight it may resolve spontaneously but it is usually necessary to institute active measures to resolve the problem.

Treatment

The immediate management will usually take place in the patient's own home. If the initial bleeding is relatively slight and eases spontaneously, she can be transferred to hospital; if, on the other hand, bleeding is persisting, 0.5 mg of ergometrine should be given intramuscularly or intravenously, the fundus massaged gently and blood clot or placental tissue removed from the vagina and cervix. These measures will usually serve to control the bleeding but, if not, the services of the obstetric emergency 'flying squad' should be obtained and the patient transferred to hospital under controlled conditions.

If the bleeding is heavy, an intravenous infusion should be commenced and blood transfusion instituted as required. Once the patient's condition has been restored, examination under anaesthesia and surgical evacuation of the uterus is the best method of treatment. This procedure must be carried out with care because it is easy to rupture the soft puerperal uterus. The uterine cavity should be explored initially with the examining finger and as much retained tissue removed as possible. Evacuation should be completed with sponge-holding forceps and by careful blunt curettage and this will usually arrest any bleeding. Although secondary postpartum haemorrhage is usually attributable to retained placental tissue, chorionic villi will often be absent on histological examination. Dewhurst (1966) reported three uterine perforations in the 89 patients treated surgically in his series; he recommends that injury to a recently pregnant uterus calls for immediate operation to establish the extent of the damage and carry out repair. In support of this policy, he reports on a case of uterine rupture in a subsequent confinement which followed probable perforation at previous curettage (Dewhurst 1981).

In rare circumstances bleeding may recur following uterine evacuation and a clotting screen should be carried out to exclude uncommon disorders of haemostasis such as von Willebrand's disease. If the clotting screen is normal, and bleeding persists, the uterus should be re-explored and packed firmly with gauze. If packing fails to control the bleeding, hysterectomy is the ultimate treatment although this should rarely be necessary. On the other hand, it is important not to delay hysterectomy until the patient's condition has deteriorated to the point where surgical intervention becomes a risk to life.

When the secondary postpartum haemorrhage is slight and appears to be resolving spontaneously, conservative management is appropriate. Ergometrine 0.5 mg can be given and the patient observed in hospital. An ultrasonic scan of the uterus should be carried out and if there is retained placental tissue this should be removed surgically. Infection may contribute to secondary postpartum bleeding and if there is any evidence of this, antibiotics should be given. Finally, it should be remembered that choriocarcinoma can occasionally present soon after a normal confinement. If there is a history of persistently increasing red lochial flow, the levels of human chorionic gonadotrophin should be checked in urine or in blood to exclude the possibility of a trophoblastic tumour.

Urinary complications

The commonest urinary complication in the puerperium is infection which has been discussed above but urinary retention or urinary incontinence may also cause problems.

URINARY RETENTION

This is a common complication following delivery, especially if there is bruising and oedema around the bladder base or if there is a painful episiotomy wound. Following epidural anaesthesia, the normal sensory stimuli from the bladder are temporarily interrupted and the bladder can be overdistended without discomfort to the patient. The bladder can hold a litre or more and, as it becomes progressively more distended, retention with overflow may develop. This situation may remain unrecognized, since the unwary attendant may imagine the patient to be passing urine well. The quantities voided will be small, 50–100 ml or so, at frequent intervals and such a pattern calls for an abdominal examination to determine if the bladder is palpable. If the bladder is distended or if there is doubt about the diagnosis, a catheter must be passed to determine the volume of urine retained in the bladder. The treatment of urinary retention is to leave an indwelling catheter on continuous drainage for 48 hours. The patient can be ambulant in the ward during this time and carry the bag with her. After the bladder has been continuously empty for 48 hours, the catheter is removed and a close check kept on the volumes of urine passed. If there is a suspicion of further retention with overflow, the volume of residual urine must be measured. If necessary, the catheter is reinserted for a further 48 hours and the procedure repeated.

INCONTINENCE OF URINE

This is, fortunately, an infrequent symptom following confinement. Stress incontinence may be a late complication of childbirth but is seldom a problem in the early stages. If incontinence is present, it must be established if this is urethral or through a fistula. Careful examination may demonstrate the obvious escape of urine through a fistula or from the urethral orifice.

If there is any doubt, a three-swab test should be performed, placing one swab at the top of the vagina, one in the middle and one at the introitus. Methylene blue is then instilled into the bladder through a catheter and blue staining of the upper or middle swab will indicate the presence of a vesicovaginal fistula. The level of the fistula will be indicated by which swab is stained; if the uppermost swab is stained with urine, but is not blue, a ureteric fistula is present.

Urinary fistulae are uncommon in obstetric practice in Britain, although they are still a major problem in many parts of the developing world. Direct injury with the obstetric forceps or some other instrument may be responsible when the leak of urine will be almost immediate. If the fetal head was pressed on the bladder for too long during a neglected obstructed second stage of labour, necrosis of bladder tissue and subsequent sloughing with fistula formation will occur. Incontinence will develop at about 8–12 days, which is the time necessary for the slough to separate. Alternatively, a ureter may be damaged at a complicated Caesarean section and incontinence will develop after a similar interval.

The management of vesicovaginal and other urinary fistulae is complex and most obstetricians have minimal experience of the problems. Continuous

bladder drainage should be instituted at once, for a very small fistula may close spontaneously. This does not usually happen and, then, surgical repair will be required. Immediate surgery is hardly ever successful and should seldom be attempted unless the injury is a clean hole made at Caesarean section. This, of course, must be repaired at once and bladder drainage instituted.

Specialized treatises, such as those by Moir (1961) and Russell (1962) should be consulted for a more detailed consideration of this subject.

Puerperal mental disorders

The puerperium is frequently associated with feelings of anxiety and depression and the 'fourth day blues' have long been recognized. In addition to these common problems, more serious psychiatric disorders such as a psychotic illness may arise during the puerperium. Although these acute psychiatric disorders are rare they are well recognized and arise with relatively little warning. It is not known whether puerperal psychoses are caused by the endocrine changes which occur during the puerperium or are an uncovering of an underlying psychotic tendency at a vulnerable stage of a woman's life. Nevertheless, psychotic episodes are most distressing not only for the patients themselves but for their relatives and the staff as well. If a mother's mental state is giving cause for concern, the opinion of a psychiatrist should be obtained because the risk of suicide and the safety of the baby are paramount considerations. Warning signs are very variable; features which should be regarded as danger signs are confusion, restlessness, extreme wakefulness, hallucinations and delirium. It is important to bear in mind the possibility of an underlying organic cause, such as acute puerperal infection, because it is very easy for this to be overlooked.

Treatment will depend upon the severity of the condition. In milder forms the mother should be observed closely, encouraged to discuss her anxieties and prescribed appropriate sedative therapy. The partner may play an important role by visiting her more often and helping her to resolve unnecessary fears. In more severe cases, heavy sedation may be required and it may be necessary to transfer the mother to a psychiatric ward. It is desirable to keep mother and baby together, if possible, but separation will sometimes be necessary in the interests of the infant's safety. In the majority of cases, the psychotic illness will settle rapidly and, thereafter, mother and child can be reunited.

The advisability of future childbearing must be considered although, in general, a previous episode of mental disorder does not rule it out. Wilson *et al.* (1972) found that 25% of patients with postpartum mental illness had a recurrence after subsequent pregnancies.

INFANT FEEDING

The establishment of infant feeding is one of the main priorities of the puerperium. Until this century, all babies were breast fed, although some affluent women could hire the services of a wet-nurse. Following the introduction of effective milk substitutes, the mother has a choice of bottle or breast feeding and the factors which influence this decision are complex. Mothers may reject breast feeding because they find the idea of suckling physically unpleasant, because they feel embarrassed at exposing their breasts or because they wish freedom to return to work; also, mothers may feel reassured when they know how much milk the baby is taking. On the other hand, there are several arguments in favour of breast feeding; breast milk is the natural food for the human infant, it is inexpensive and it is always at the right temperature. Breast feeding helps to protect the baby against infection and may contribute to the development of mother–infant attachment. In Britain, the decision to breast or bottle feed is strongly influenced by social class, the incidence of breast feeding being greatest in Social Class I and II and of bottle feeding in the lower social class groups (Martin & Monk 1982). One of the tasks of parentcraft classes is to explain to the mothers the arguments for and against the different methods of infant feeding but once the mother has made her decision this should be accepted. Mothers who choose to bottle feed should not be made to feel guilty because of their decision.

TRENDS IN INFANT FEEDING

The worldwide trends in infant feeding are paradoxical. In the Western world the incidence of bottle feeding reached a peak in the 1960s but since then there has been an increase in the numbers of mothers choosing to breast feed, especially among primigravidas (Martin & Monk 1982). On the other hand, there has been a decline in breast feeding in developing countries, particularly in the urban areas. It is ironic that while mothers in developing countries wish to imitate those in the West by bottle feeding, mothers

in the developed countries are increasingly wanting to return to the natural feeding methods of the developing world.

The rising incidence of bottle feeding in developing countries is a cause for serious concern. In many areas water supplies are infected so that bottle feeding causes gastro-enteritis. In poor areas, mothers may be unable to afford the relatively expensive milk formulae and overdilute the feeds in order to make their supplies last for longer. This practice adds malnutrition to infection. The World Health Organization (1981) have drawn up a recommended code of practice to try help halt or delay the rapid advance of bottle feeding in developing countries. In this Code of Practice it is recommended that breast feeding should be actively promoted and that education programmes should be directed towards mothers and their families as well as towards health professionals. At the same time, steps should be taken to inhibit the advertising and promotion of breast milk substitutes which have the objective of persuading mothers that milk formulae are the best foods for their babies.

ARTIFICIAL FEEDING

If mothers choose to bottle feed, they must be shown how to prepare the feeds correctly and how to sterilize their feeding equipment. There is some evidence that it is the mother who predominantly controls the amount of milk taken at a bottle feed whereas it is the baby who controls the volume of milk taken at a breast feed (Wright 1980); because of this, it is important that mothers are instructed not to overfeed bottle-fed babies.

Mothers who do not breast feed may have some discomfort in the puerperium from breast distension due to milk which is secreted into the breast but not removed. The best treatment, in the majority of cases, is to apply firm support to the breasts and the milk will soon disappear. If there is a great deal of pain from breast engorgement, this can be very effectively treated by bromocriptine in a dose of 5 mg/day for 14 days (Rolland & Schellekens 1973). If this treatment is used, there may be an early return of ovulation so that immediate contraceptive precautions are required to avoid a very early pregnancy (Rolland *et al.* 1975).

Breast feeding

In those mothers who breast feed, lactation is the dominant physiological event of the puerperium. The primary function of breast feeding is to provide continuing nutrition for the new baby but important secondary functions include protection against infant infection, the inhibition of ovarian activity and the encouragement of uterine involution. The lactating breast takes over many of the functions of the placenta and, in a true physiological sense, plays a pivotal role in human reproduction (Short 1976).

PHYSIOLOGY OF LACTATION

The human species is unusual in that the major part of breast development occurs at puberty before the first pregnancy so that the adult breast requires only minimal exposure to the appropriate hormonal stimuli to produce milk (McNeilly 1977). At puberty, the milk ducts which lead from the nipple to the secretory alveoli are stimulated by oestrogen to sprout, branch and form glandular tissue buds from which milk-secreting glands will develop (Fig. 32.1). During pregnancy, this breast tissue is further stimulated so that pre-existing alveolar-lobular structures hypertrophy and new ones are formed. At the same time the milk

collecting ducts also undergo branching and proliferation. Both oestrogens and progesterone are necessary for mammary development in pregnancy but prolactin, growth hormone and adrenal steroids may also be involved. During pregnancy only minimal amounts of milk are formed in the breast despite high levels of the lactogenic hormones, prolactin and placental lactogen. This is because the actions of these lactogenic hormones are inhibited by the secretion of high levels of oestrogens and progesterone from the placenta and it is not until after delivery that copious milk production is induced.

Milk production

Two similar, but independent, mechanisms are involved in the establishment of successful lactation (lactogenesis); the first mechanism causes the release of prolactin which acts upon the glandular cells of the breast to stimulate milk secretion (Fig. 32.2) and the second induces the release of oxytocin which acts upon the myoepithelial cells of the breast to induce the milk ejection reflex (Fig. 32.3). Although these two mechanisms are similar, in that they can both be activated by suckling, they are mediated through two entirely different neuro-endocrinological pathways. As can be seen in Figs. 32.2 and 32.3, the key

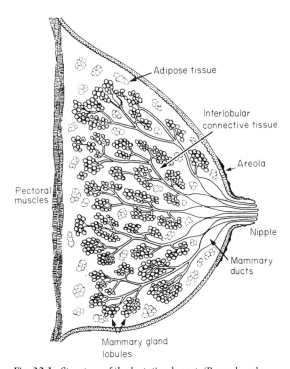

Fig. 32.1. Structure of the lactating breast. (Reproduced from *Human Histology* by D.L. Gardner and T.C. Dodds (eds) Churchill Livingstone, Edinburgh by kind agreement of authors and publisher).

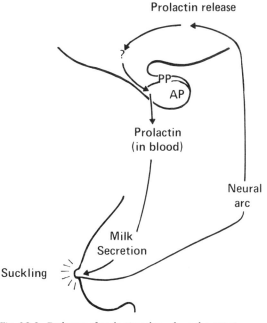

Fig. 32.2. Pathway of prolactin release from the anterior pituitary gland.

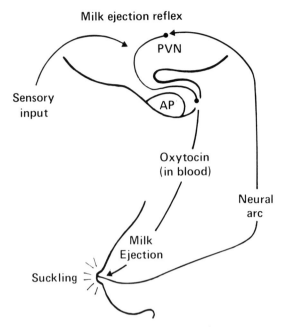

Fig. 32.3. Pathway of oxytocin release from the posterior pituitary gland.

event in lactogenesis is suckling and the sensitivity of the breast accommodates itself to this important activity. During pregnancy the skin of the areola is relatively insensitive to tactile stimuli but becomes much more sensitive immediately after delivery (Robinson & Short 1977). This is an ingenious physiological adaptation which ensures that there is an adequate stream of afferent neurological stimuli from the nipple to the hypothalamus to initiate and maintain the release of prolactin and oxytocin, both of which are required for successful lactation.

Prolactin and milk secretion

Prolactin is a long-chain polypeptide and, although many possible functions have been ascribed to it, the only physiological role that has been established beyond doubt is its action on the lactating breast. Following an episode of nipple stimulation, prolactin is released from the lactotrophs in the anterior pituitary, reaching peak blood levels at 30–45 minutes after suckling and returning to basal levels after two hours. Thus, prolactin levels during lactation are dependent upon the strength, frequency and duration of the suckling stimulus; basal prolactin levels are highest in the immediate puerperium (Fig. 32.4), decline slowly as suckling declines in later lactation and

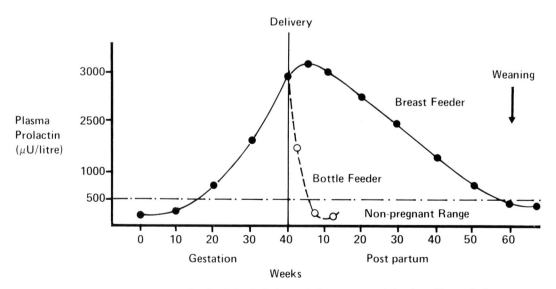

Fig. 32.4. Diagrammatic representation of prolactin levels during and after pregnancy in bottle and breast feeding mothers.

revert to non-pregnant levels immediately after weaning. By contrast, prolactin levels revert to normal immediately after delivery in bottle feeding mothers. Prolactin secretion is under the neuroendocrine control of a prolactin inhibitory factor from the hypothalamus which is generally thought to be dopamine, although the exact mechanisms which control secretion are not clear.

Prolactin appears to be essential for lactation because bromocriptine, a dopamine agonist which selectively inhibits prolactin secretion, will abolish milk production (Roland & Schellekens 1973). Furthermore, lactation fails in Sheehan's syndrome which is associated with pituitary failure and very low levels of prolactin after delivery. The action of prolactin is a direct one on the secretory cells of the breast to stimulate the synthesis of the milk proteins such as casein, lactoglobulin, lactalbumin, lactose and lipids. The main activity of the prolactin molecule is to bind to specific receptor sites on the cell membrane but prolactin may also have some action within the alveolar cell itself (Robyn & Meuris 1982). In addition to the action of prolactin, milk secretion is dependent upon adequate emptying of the milk-secreting glands, because accumulation of milk in the alveoli will cause distension and mechanical atrophy of the glandular epithelium. Thus, adequate milk secretion requires both the correct endocrine stimulus to the breast and satisfactory stripping of the milk from the stimulated gland.

Milk-ejection reflex

Successful breast feeding depends as much upon effective milk transfer from the breast to the baby as upon adequate milk secretion. The milk-ejection reflex is mediated by the release of oxytocin from the posterior pituitary gland (Fig. 32.3). Oxytocin causes contraction of the sensitive myoepithelial cells which are situated round the milk-secreting glands and also dilates the ducts by acting upon the muscle cells which lie longitudinally in the duct walls. Contraction of these cells, therefore, has the dual effect of expelling milk from the glands and of encouraging free flow of milk along dilated ducts. This is recognized by the mother as the milk 'let-down' and she may be aware of milk being ejected from the opposite breast from which the baby is suckling. In contrast to prolactin, which is secreted only in response to suckling, oxytocin can be released in response to sensory inputs such as the mother seeing the baby or hearing its cry. Indeed, one study reported that milk let down occurred regularly at about 90 minute intervals, irrespective of whether feeding took place or not (McNeilly & McNeilly 1978). Oxytocin has a very short half-life in the circulation and is released from the posterior pituitary in a pulsatile manner. As shown in Fig. 32.5, the highest levels of oxytocin may be released prior to suckling in response to the baby's cry while prolactin is released only after suckling commences. The milk ejection reflex is readily inhibited by emotional stress and this may explain

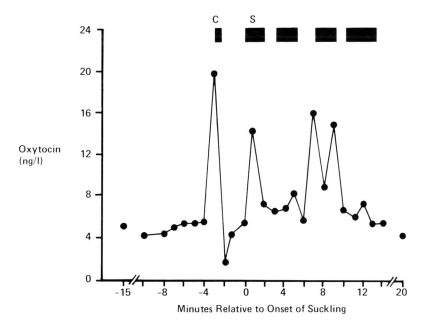

Fig. 32.5. Pattern of oxytocin release in response to the infant's cry (C) and to suckling (S). (From McNeilly *et al.* 1982, reproduced by kind permission of the authors and the Editor of the *British Medical Journal*.)

Oxytocin (ng/l)

Minutes Relative to Onset of Suckling

why maternal anxiety frequently leads to a failure of lactation. Successful breast feeding depends upon engendering confidence in the mother and ensuring correct fixing and sucking at the breast.

FUNCTIONS OF BREAST FEEDING

The primary function of breast feeding is nutritional and in order to provide for the baby's needs the milk must be adequate in both quality and quantity.

Composition of breast milk
Human breast milk is not a constant substance because colostrum differs from mature milk, and the milk of the early puerperium differs from the milk of late lactation. Furthermore the composition of the milk will differ between two feeds on the same day and, even within a single feed, the content varies because the fat concentration rises towards the end of the feed. Claims by milk manufacturers that they have produced a 'natural' milk should not be taken too seriously because it is impossible to characterize human milk in a single static formula. Nevertheless, when the approximate compositions of human and cow's milk are compared, obvious differences can be seen and some of these are summarized in Table 32.1. It can be seen that the energy value of human

Table 32.1. Comparison of the constituents of human and cow's milk.

Constituent	Human milk	Cow's milk
Energy (kcal/100 ml)	75	66
Protein (g/100 ml)	1.1	3.5
Fat (g/100 ml)	4.5	3.7
Lactose (g/100 ml)	6.8	4.9
Sodium (mEq/litre)	7	22

milk is higher than cow's milk and, although the total solid content is similar, human milk contains less protein but more fat and lactose than cow's milk. This makes human milk more digestible than cow's milk for the human baby. Human milk contains fewer of the major minerals and the lower sodium content is of particular importance because excessive sodium can be dangerous to a baby who is dehydrated following vomiting and diarrhoea.

It would seem that human milk is a complex substance which is capable of being finely adapted to meet the requirements of the human infant. There appear to be subtle interactions between the mother and her baby, and although these are incompletely understood, it is probable that milk content can be modified by the intensity and frequency of infant sucking. This is an important area for future research.

Volumes of breast milk
During the first 24 hours of the puerperium, the human breast usually secretes small volumes of milk but with regular suckling, milk volumes steadily increase and, by the sixth day of the puerperium, an average volume of 500 ml will be taken by the baby. Once lactation is fully established, an average daily milk volume is about 800 ml, although under optimal conditions, volumes of well over a litre per day can be achieved (Rattigan *et al.* 1980). The time at which it is necessary to introduce supplementary food is a contentious issue and many authorities recommend that supplements should be introduced at four months. Ahn and McLean (1980), however, found that fully breast-fed infants of well-nourished mothers could continue to grow at normal rates at least until 8 months of life suggesting that breast feeding can be adequate for the baby for longer than has been previously realized.

Protection against infection
One of the most important secondary functions of breast feeding is to protect the infant against infection. This is particularly important in developing countries where, it has been estimated, that in each year there are 500 million cases of diarrhoea in infants and children and about 20 million of these are fatal (*Lancet* 1981). Even in developed countries, breast feeding appears to have a protective effect not only against gastro-enteritis but against respiratory infections and otitis media as well (Chandra 1979).

A number of mechanisms contribute to the anti-infective properties of breast milk (*Lancet* 1981). Breast milk contains lactoferrin which binds iron, and because *E. coli* requires iron for growth, the multiplication of this organism is inhibited. Breast feeding also encourages colonization of the gut by a non-pathogenic flora which will competitively inhibit pathogenic strains. In addition, there are bacteriocidal enzymes, such as lysozyme, present in breast milk which will contribute to its protective effect.

The most specific anti-infective mechanism, however, is an immunological one. If a mother ingests a pathogen which she has previously encountered, the gut associated lymphoid tissue situated in the Peyer's patches of the small intestine will respond by producing specific immunoglobulin A which is transferred to the breast milk via the thoracic duct (Fig. 32.6). This immunoglobulin, which is present in large amounts in breast milk, is not absorbed from the infant's gastro-intestinal tract but remains in the gut to attack the specific offending pathogen against which it is directed. In this way the breast-fed infant

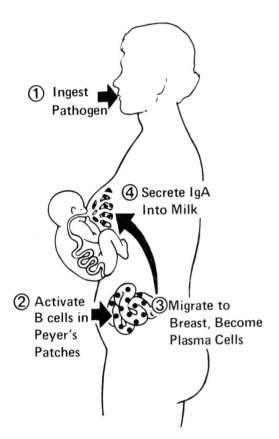

Fig. 32.6. Diagram of pathways involved in secretion of IgA in breast milk by the entero-mammary circulation. (Kindly provided by Professor R. V. Short, Melbourne, Australia.)

is given protection from the endemic infections in the environment against which the mother will already have immunity. Breast milk contains living cells, such as polymorphs, lymphocytes and plasma cells, and although their functions are not yet fully understood, they may also be active against invading pathogens.

Breast feeding and atopic illness

There are a number of reports that show lower incidences of atopic illness such as eczema and asthma in breast-fed babies (Chandra 1979). This effect is particularly important when there is a family history of atopic illnesses (Fergusson *et al.* 1981). When the atopic illness is present, it is commonly associated with raised levels of IgE, especially to cow's milk protein.

Fergusson *et al.* (1981) suggest that, apart from a positive family history, the most important predisposing factor for atopic illness is the early introduction of weaning foods. The protective effect of breast feeding against atopic illness, therefore, may be secondary, rather than primary, because breast feeding mothers tend to introduce supplements at a later stage. Nevertheless, mothers with a family history of atopic illness should be informed of the advantages of breast feeding and of the dangers of introducing supplements too quickly.

Breast feeding and fertility

The natural contraceptive effect of breast feeding has received scant attention in the Western world because it is not a reliable method of family planning in all cases. Nevertheless, on a population basis, the anti-fertility effect of breast feeding is large and of major importance in the developing world. It has to be remembered that the majority of women in the Third World do not use artificial contraception and rely on natural checks to their fertility (Howie & McNeilly 1982). By far the most important of these natural checks is the inhibition of fertility by breast feeding. In many developing countries mothers breast feed for 2 years or more with the effect that their babies are spaced at about 3 yearly intervals. In the mid-1970s Rosa calculated that, in the developing world, more pregnancies were prevented by breast feeding than by all other methods of family planning combined. The current decline in breast feeding in the Third World is a cause for great concern because, without a sharp rise in contraceptive usage, the loss of its anti-fertility effect will aggravate population increase in these countries. For example, Lesthaege (1982) has calculated that if, in Bangladesh, the duration of lactational amenorrhoea fell from its current average of 21 months to 3 months, contraceptive usage would have to rise from the current rate of 9% to 52% to keep fertility rates at the same level. The potential benefits of family planning programmes in the Third World will be neutralized if the anti-fertility effects of breast feeding are neglected. For fuller information about these issues, the reader is referred to the several discussions of this subject (e.g. Short 1976, Howie & McNeilly 1982, McCann *et al.* 1981).

Mechanisms of lactational amenorrhoea

The mechanisms of lactational amenorrhoea are complex and incompletely understood. The key event is a suckling induced change in the hypothalamic sensitivity to the feedback effects of ovarian steroids (Baird *et al.* 1979). During lactation, the hypothalamus becomes more sensitive to the negative feedback effects and less sensitive to the positive feedback effects of oestrogen. This means that if the pituitary secretes enough FSH and LH to initiate the development of an ovarian follicle, the consequent

oestrogen secretion will inhibit gonadotrophin production and the follicle will fail to mature. Glasier *et al.* (1983) have shown that there is inhibition of the normal pulsatile release of LH from the anterior pituitary gland during lactation which is consistent with this hypothesis.

From a clinical standpoint, the major factor is the frequency and duration of the suckling stimulus. In Fig. 32.7 the postpartum endocrine events in a bottle feeding mother are shown. Immediately after delivery, prolactin levels return to the non-pregnant range, and thereafter there is follicular development (total urinary oestrogens > 10 μg/24 hours) ovulation (urinary pregnanediol > 1 mg/24 hrs) and menstruation by 14 weeks post-delivery. This pattern is

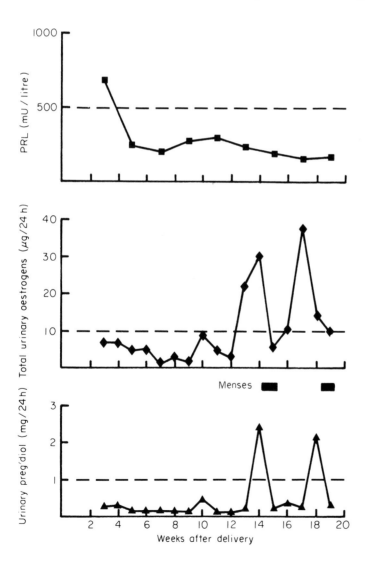

Fig. 32.7. Return of postpartum ovarian follicular activity (urinary total oestrogens > 10 μg/24 h) and ovulation (urinary pregnanediol > 1 mg/24 h) in a bottle feeding mother.

typical for bottle feeding mothers who have normal ovarian activity and the potential for fertility restored within a few weeks of delivery. In Fig. 32.8 the contrasting pattern in a breast feeder is shown. During the first weeks of suckling, ovarian activity is inhibited and menstruation suppressed. At 32 weeks, when suckling has fallen to 25 minutes per day, follicular activity returns although the first cycle is anovular. The next four cycles are also characterized by follicular development with either absent or defective luteal phases. It is not until 52 weeks' postpartum that a normal ovulatory cycle occurs (urinary pregnanediol > 1 mg/24 hrs).

Although breast feeding has an important contraceptive effect it is not absolutely reliable especially after menstruation returns. Between 1 and 10% of women will conceive during the period of lactational amenorrhoea and most women in developed countries seek extra protection from a contraceptive method (McCann *et al.* 1981). This is discussed later in the chapter.

MANAGEMENT OF BREAST FEEDING

Despite the fact that it is a physiological event, many women experience difficulties in establishing breast feeding. The greatest asset that a nursing mother can have is the support of an experienced and sympath-

etic counsellor. This counsellor may be a midwife, a health visitor or a lay person but the creation of a relaxed and confident environment is vital for successful breast feeding. Babies are individuals, so that there is no simple formula that works in every case; mothers should be encouraged to learn to respond to their own babies but all too often well-meaning but dogmatic and conflicting advice is given. The best approach is to give mothers options and let them make their own decisions; they will soon learn by trial and error what is best for their own babies.

It is, however, possible to outline a few general principles which are conducive to successful breast feeding.

1 Mothers should be encouraged to suckle for the first time as soon after delivery as possible because there is some evidence that this policy is associated with higher success rates (Salariya *et al.* 1978). The timing of the first feed will, however, be dictated by the health of the mother and baby at the time of delivery and successful breast feeding can be established even if the first feed is delayed for several hours.

2 The baby should be fed 'freely' or 'on demand' when he or she indicates that the time is right. Rigid schedules have no physiological basis and should be avoided (Illingworth & Stone 1952). In the early days

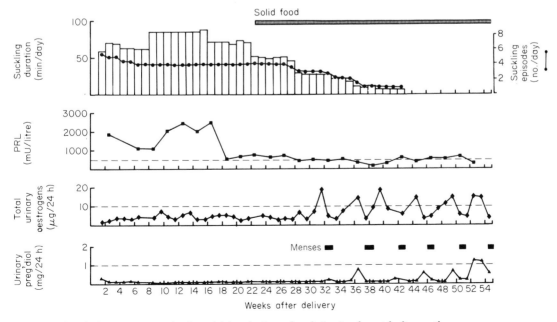

Fig. 32.8. Infant feeding patterns, prolactin and delayed return of ovulation in a breast feeding mother.

of the puerperium, frequent suckling helps to establish the milk flow.

3   Mothers should be shown how to fix the baby properly at the breast. If the baby sucks on the end of the nipple, this will cause cracked nipples which are very painful and make feeding difficult. The baby must take the nipple well into its mouth so that it milks the collecting sinuses behind the nipple itself.

4   The mother and the baby should not be separated unnecessarily and rooming-in should be encouraged. Close contact helps the mother to learn how to interpret her baby's behaviour and develops her confidence.

5   The use of supplements should be reduced to an absolute minimum. Most babies should be able to establish breast feeding without additional water, dextrose or, worse still, formula milk.

Additional fluids should be advised only if medically indicated; if a supplement is required banked human milk may be the best choice. The more a baby relies upon its mother the more quickly milk flow will be established.

6   Test-weighing should be abandoned as a routine procedure because it is threatening to the mother's confidence; furthermore, feeds should last as long as is dictated by the baby because there is great individual variation in feeding patterns (Drewitt & Woolridge 1979, Howie *et al.* 1981). Many infants are able to take their full feed within a few minutes while others may spend more than 20 minutes before taking a similar volume. There is no evidence that prolonged sucking causes sore nipples; incorrect fixing is much more likely to be the cause.

The success of breast feeding is greatly influenced by the support which the mother receives both in hospital and at home (Houston *et al.* 1981), but probably the most important factors are the mother's own enthusiasm and the attitude of her partner. The importance of the partner's role is something which should be emphasized during the antenatal parentcraft classes.

PROBLEMS DURING BREAST FEEDING

Mothers may experience a variety of problems during breast feeding such as anxieties about her milk supply, sore or cracked nipples, tiredness, breast engorgement or a breast abscess and these will be discussed briefly.

Stimulation of milk supply

Many mothers worry about having 'insufficient milk' and this is the commonest reason for early discontinuation of breast feeding. In most cases reassurance and increased suckling will overcome this problem. More recently, there have been a number of papers which have shown that drugs, such as metoclopramide or sulpiride, which raise prolactin levels have a beneficial effect on a failing milk supply (Ylikorkala *et al.* 1982). There is no case for the routine use of these drugs but the early reports suggest that they may prove to have a place in the management of a mother in whom the milk supply is drying up. This approach to treatment requires further assessment.

Absence of the milk-ejection reflex can also lead to breast feeding failure and some controlled studies have suggested that nasal oxytocin can be of value. As with drugs to stimulate prolactin production, the place of nasal oxytocin will probably prove to be a small one in selected cases although there is evidence that it is helpful, particularly in mothers whose babies were delivered pre-term (Ruis *et al.* 1981).

Sore or cracked nipples

If a mother develops a cracked nipple, the most important question to ask is whether the baby is fixing correctly. In the majority of cases this will be the problem but it may be necessary to rest the affected breast until the crack has healed and to manually express the breast milk until this has happened.

Tiredness

Many mothers feel tired while breast feeding and it is important that they are given sufficient domestic support to enable them to cope. There are times when the baby demands the breast more frequently than usual and this has the dual effect of aggravating tiredness and making the mother conclude that she has insufficient milk. In most cases it is the natural way by which the baby increases milk supply to meet growing demand and the phase of increased sucking usually settles within a day or two. It is wise to warn mothers of the possibility of these episodes in advance so that they do not reach the incorrect conclusion about their milk supply and unnecessarily stop breast feeding.

Breast engorgement

Breast engorgement can be extremely painful and distressing and is most common about the fourth day while the milk is 'coming in'. The breasts must be given firm support and compresses may be comforting. In severe cases analgesia will be required. If the breast is very hard, the baby will have difficulty fixing. It is helpful to express some milk initially to soften the breast sufficiently to allow suckling to commence. Usually, engorgement settles within a day or so, when the milk flow adjusts to supply and demand, but the mother will require much help until this happens.

Breast abscess

Breast abscesses usually develop after the mother has left hospital because they are rarely encountered before the fourteenth day. There will be a red, painful fluctuant swelling and the patient will feel feverish and unwell. Although antibiotics are commonly prescribed, it is often better to allow the abscess to localize and to incise it under general anaesthesia. In many cases the mother wishes to stop breast feeding when an abscess develops, but it is possible to sustain the baby on the unaffected breast and to express the affected side until the abscess has settled down. Once the infection has cleared, the baby can resume sucking on both breasts.

Breast feeding is a skill which is not instinctive but has to be learned. Many mothers of the present generation have never seen a baby being breast fed and it is an important task for medical and nursing attendants to support mothers as this important activity is relearned in the community.

SUPPORT DURING THE PUERPERIUM

As mentioned in the discussion on breast feeding, mothers require emotional support during the puerperium. The need for support applies to bottle feeding mothers as well as to breast feeders because all mothers share the same anxieties. Much has been written about 'bonding' between the mother and her child although similar emotional adjustments are occurring between the father and the child as well.

The emotional aspects of the puerperium are less scientific than the technological but are just as important (Reading 1983). Points that have been stressed as important by psychologists are early skin-to-skin contact (Klaus & Kennell 1976) and the avoidance of unnecessary separation (de Chateau 1979). The puerperium is a time of adjustment for new parents, and staff must be aware of their needs. Special handling is required for the management of patients who have lost a baby or who have had a baby with a congenital malformation.

COUNSELLING OF PARENTS AFTER PERINATAL DEATH

There has been much recent discussion on the appropriate management of parents after a perinatal bereavement. In the past it has been common practice to remove the dead baby quickly, to say little to the parents and to send the mother home as quickly as possible. These steps were taken on the grounds that these measures would avoid causing distress. It is now clear that if parents do not grieve for the lost child, problems may be created at a later stage. Some of the potential long-term problems are mothering difficulties with subsequent babies, marital problems, severe disturbances at anniversaries, puerperal psychosis in the next pregnancy and fracturing of the doctor–patient relationship (Bourne & Lewis 1983). Some of these problems may be prevented if the parents are encouraged to grieve. This process can be helped if they are encouraged to see, touch and name their dead baby, have a photograph of the child and hold a funeral. The mother's discharge from hospital should not be hurried, allowing contact with medical staff, community midwife, social worker and general practitioner (Forrest *et al.* 1982). Help can also come from contact with members of Stillbirth and Perinatal Death Association. Clearly, individual reactions will vary but time should be spent with bereaved parents to help them to come to terms with their loss.

Problems can also be encountered when a child is mentally or physically handicapped or separated from the parents because of a prolonged stay in the special care baby unit. The appropriate management will depend upon the specific problem but staff at all levels must be aware of the special needs of such parents.

Contraceptive and other advice

During the puerperium, mothers should be given advice about contraception and given an opportunity to discuss any anxieties about themselves or their babies.

CONTRACEPTIVE ADVICE

If the mother is bottle feeding, contraceptive advice is essential if she is not going to be pregnant again in the immediate future because ovulation may resume as early as 6 weeks postpartum. The bottle feeding mother can use any of the available methods and, if she is going to use the combined oestrogen–progestogen pill, this should be commenced within 4 weeks of delivery. It is unwise to advise waiting until first menstruation as conception can occur before then. If an intrauterine contraceptive device (IUCD) is to be fitted, it is best to wait for 4 weeks until uterine involution is complete.

Breast feeding mothers are best to avoid the combined oestrogen–progestogen pill because several studies have shown an adverse effect of the pill on the milk supply. If a breast feeding mother wishes to use an oral method, the progestogen-only pill is to be preferred as it does not diminish the milk supply and is effective in the lactating woman. (For a fuller discussion *see* McCann *et al.* 1891.) The barrier methods and IUCDs are also suitable for the breast feeding mother, but care has to be taken with fitting devices because there have been reports of uterine perforation during insertion in breast feeders. If the couple feel that their family is complete, sterilization may be appropriate but it is best to delay this for a few weeks.

At the postnatal clinic mothers should be asked if they have any complaints and a general physical examination carried out. If a cervical smear was not done antenatally, this is a convenient opportunity to have the cervical cytology checked. If there were any problems during pregnancy or delivery, these should be discussed especially if they have any implications for subsequent pregnancies. Finally, the puerperium is a time which gives an opportunity to the health visitor or general practitioner to explain about immunzation and continuing infant care. In this way, the puerperium can be seen as a bridge between the birth of a child and his or her subsequent integration into the community.

DRUGS DURING LACTATION

Drugs which are taken by a breast-feeding mother may pass to the child and it is important to consider whether or not the particular drug will have any effect. This is often a difficult problem to decide upon because many factors can influence the potential effects of the drug. The passage of a drug into milk will depend on the size of the molecule, its binding to protein and its solubility in lipid and water. In addition to these factors, the effect of the drug will depend upon whether it appears in the milk in its active form or as an inactive metabolite; also, the route of administration to the mother, the drug's half-life and the drug dissociation constants have to be considered. Even after considering all these factors, it has to be determined whether the infant can absorb the drug

from the gastrointestinal tract and, if so, can the baby excrete it or detoxify it normally.

From the consideration of all these factors, it is clearly difficult to predict, on purely theoretical grounds, the effect of any particular drug on a breast-fed infant. There are a number of sources such as the British National Formulary or Lawrence (1980), which can be consulted for information about the advisability of individual drugs in nursing mothers. In general, the potential effects of maternal medication on the infant can be minimized by a number of practical steps. The long-acting form of any drug should be avoided whenever possible because infants may have difficulty in excreting them, leading to tissue accumulation. If the drug is given immediately after a breast feed, peak maternal blood levels will usually have subsided by the next feed. In this way scheduling of doses may be helpful. It is also wise to choose the drug which produces the lowest levels in the milk. Finally, the infant should be carefully observed for any possible adverse effects such as a change in feeding habits, sleeping pattern, skin rash or other unusual signs (Lawrence 1980). In general, it is best to avoid the use of drugs during lactation, whenever possible, and their need should be carefully considered before they are prescribed.

REFERENCES

AHN C.H. & MCLEAN W.C. (1980). *Amer. J. clin. Nutr.*, **33**, 183.

BAIRD D.J., MCNEILLY A.S., SAWERS R.S. & SHARPE R.M. (1979). *J. clin. Endocrinol. Metab.*, **49**, 500.

BONNAR J., MCNICOL G.P. & DOUGLAS A.S. (1970). *Brit. med. J.*, **2**, 200.

BOURNE S., LEWIS E. (1983). *Brit. med. J.*, **286**, 145.

CHANDRA R.K. (1979). *Acta Pediatr. Scand.*, **68**, 691.

Confidential Enquiry into Maternal Deaths 1976–1978 (1982). HMSO, London.

DE CHATEAU P. (1979). *Sem. Perinatal*, **3**, 45.

DEWHURST C.J. (1966). *J. Obstet. Gynaec. Brit. Cwlth.*, **73**, 53.

DEWHURST C.J. (1981). *Integrated Obstetrics and Gynaecology for Postgraduates*, Third Edition, p. 443. Blackwell Scientific Publications, Oxford.

DREWETT R.F. & WOOLRIDGE M. (1979). *Early Hum. Dev.*, **34**, 315.

FERGUSSON D.M., HORWOOD L.J., BEAUTRAIS A.L., SHANNON F.T. & TAYLOR B. (1981). *Clin. Allerg.*, **11**, 325.

FORREST G.C., STANDISH E. & BAUM J. (1982). *Brit. med. J.*, **285**, 1475.

GLASIER A., MCNEILLY A.S. & HOWIE P.W. (1983). *Clin. Endocrinol.*, **19**, 493.

HOWIE P.W. (1979). *Postgrad. med. J.*, **55**, 362.

Howie P.W. & McNeilly A.S. (1982). *J. reprod. Fertil.*, **65**, 545.

Howie P.W., Houston M.J., Cook A., Smart L., McArdle T. & McNeilly A.S. (1981). *Early Hum. Dev.*, **5**, 71.

Houston M.J., Howie P.W., Cook A. & McNeilly A.S. (1981). *Health Bull.*, **3913**, p. 166.

Illingworth R.S. & Stone D.G.H. (1952). *Lancet*, **i**, 683.

Jelliffe D.B. & Jelliffe E.F.P. (1978). *Human Milk in the Modern World*. Oxford University Press, New York.

Klaus M.H. & Kennell J.H. (1976). *Maternal–Infant Bonding*. C.V. Mosby, St. Louis.

Lancet (1981). Editorial, **i**, 1192.

Lawrence R.A. (1980). In *Breast-Feeding, A Guide for the Medical Profession*. C.V. Mosby Company, St. Louis.

Lesthaege R.J. (1982). Paper presented at *WNO/NRC Workshop on Breast Feeding and Fertility Regulation*, Geneva, February 1982.

McCann M.F., Listin L.S., Piotrow P.T., Rinehart W. & Fox G. (1981). *Population Reports Series J*. **9(5)**, 525–75.

McNeilly A.S. (1977). *J. Biosoc. Sci., Suppl.*, **4**, 5.

McNeilly A.S. & McNeilly J.R. (1978). *Brit. med. J.*, **2**, 466.

McNeilly A.S., Robinson I.C.A.F., Houston M.J. & Howie P.W. (1982). *Brit. med. J.*, **286**, 257.

Martin J. & Monk J. (1982). *Infant Feeding 1980*. Published by OPCS.

Moir J.C. (1961). *The Vesico-Vaginal Fistula*. Ballière, Tindall & Cassell, London.

Munday P.E. (1983). In *Progress in Obstetrics and Gynaecology* (Ed. Studd, J.) p. 231. Churchill Livingstone.

Rattigan S., Ghisalberti A.V. & Hartmann P.E. (1981). *Brit. J. Nutr.*, **45**, 243.

Reading A.E. (1983). In *Progress in Obstetrics and Gynaecology*, Vol. 3, Ed. J. Studd, Churchill Livingstone.

Robinson J. & Short R.V. (1977). *Brit. med. J.*, **1**, 1188.

Robyn C. & Meuris S. (1982). *Sem. Perinatal*, **6**, 254.

Rolland R. & Schellkens L.A. (1973). *J. Obstet. Gynaecol. Brit. Cwlth.*, **80**, 945.

Rolland R., Lequin R.M., Schellekens L.A. & de Jong F.H. (1975). *Clin. Endocrinol. (Oxf.)* **4**, 15.

Rosa F.W. (1975). *WHO Protein Advisory Group Bulletin*, **5**, (3) 10.

Ruis H., Rolland R., Doesburg W., Broeders G. & Corbey R. (1981). *Brit. med. J.*, **283**, 340.

Russell C. (1962). *Vesico-Vaginal Fistulas and Related Matters*. Thomas, Springfield, Illinois.

Salariya E., Easton P.M. & Cater J.I. (1978). *Lancet*, **ii**, 1141.

Short R.V. (1976). In *Breast Feeding and the Mother*, CIBA Foundation Symposium, **45**, 73–80. Elsevier, Amsterdam.

WHO (1981). *International Code of Marketing of Breast Milk Substitutes*, Office of Publications, WHO, Geneva.

Wilson J.E., Barglow P. & Shipman W. (1972). *Comprehensive Psychiatry*, **13**, 305.

Windebank W.J., Boyd G. & Moran F. (1973). *Brit. med. J.* **(i)**, 90.

Wright P. (1980). *Scot. Health Bull.*, **39**, 197.

Ylikorkala O., Kaupilla A., Kivinen S. & Viinikka L. (1982). *Brit. med. J.*, **285**, 249.

CHAPTER 33
MULTIPLE PREGNANCY

C.R. WHITFIELD

IMPORTANCE AND INCIDENCE

Many obstetric complications occur with increased frequency in multiple pregnancies. Maternal risks are greater and, in particular, perinatal mortality and morbidity are increased several times over that of single pregnancies. For example, for multiple births in Scotland during 1984, a perinatal mortality rate almost 7 times that among singletons (64.7 compared with 9.8 per 1000 births) was reported (Scottish Home and Health Department, 1985), and during the years 1977–81 almost 10% of all perinatal deaths in Scotland related to multiple pregnancies (McIlwaine *et al.* 1985). Nor is increased wastage confined to the perinatal period, for in addition to a probably increased incidence of first and second trimester abortions, the occasional retention of a dead twin as a fetus papyraceus while gestation continues as a 'single' pregnancy is well recognized, and more recently ultrasound has revealed how often one twin 'disappears' in early pregnancy. Also, due mainly to very low birthweight and very early preterm delivery, increased wastage persists beyond the first week of life.

Multiple pregnancies must therefore be identified and managed as 'very high risk' from early in pregnancy to delivery, and the offspring will often remain at high risk during the whole neonatal period and sometimes for even longer.

There are considerable ethnic and geographic variations in the frequency of multiple pregnancy. The highest rates occur in Africa, with up to 45 twin pairs per 1000 births in Nigeria, compared with rates of less than 5 per 1000 births in some Far Eastern countries and intermediate rates of about 10 or 12 per 1000 births among Caucasians (Nylander 1975).

These variations in frequency are due almost entirely to very different rates for dizygotic (DZ) twinning, with the proportion of twin pairs that are DZ varying from about 70% in Europeans to 90% or more among some African populations. Also, since the incidence of many complications is generally believed to be higher in monozygotic (MZ) than DZ twin pregnancies, and this is certainly so to a considerable degree for fetal malformations and the hazards arising from the shared placental circulation of most MZ twins, the mechanisms of twinning and the determination of zygosity will be considered first.

MECHANISMS OF TWINNING

Fig. 33.1 is a diagramatic representation of DZ and MZ twinning.

Dizygotic twinning

DZ twinning represents duplication of the normal process of conception, implantation and further development of the embryo, arising from fertilization of two ova from the same or opposite ovaries. Each fetus will have its own membranes, both chorion and amnion, and its own placenta. When the implantation sites happen to be close together the placentas may become fused, but separate placental circulations will be maintained. The duplication of the membranes is described as dichorionic diamniotic. The fetuses may be like or unlike in sex, and will have differences in genetic constitution detectable by genetic marker studies and usually becoming obvious later as different physical characteristics develop.

Little time need be wasted in considering the possibilities of superfecundation and superfetation. The former is the fertilization by separate acts of coitus of two ova released during the same menstrual cycle, and is almost certainly extremely rare; the latter is the theoretical possibility that DZ twinning might arise from coitus during different cycles, and is probably impossible; neither is of practical importance to the obstetrician.

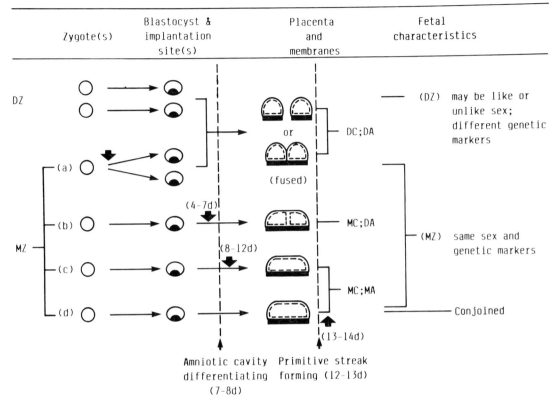

Fig. 33.1. Diagramatic representation of the mechanism of dizygotic (DZ) and monozygotic (MZ) twinning, showing zygote and blastocyst/implantation stages, placentation/membranes and fetal genetic characteristics. The types of MZ twinning (a,b,c,d) depend on the time of splitting (indicated by broad arrows, in days after fertilization). In the diagrams of the placenta and membranes the unbroken line represents the chorion and the broken line represents the amnion.

Monozygotic twinning

Unlike DZ twinning, which is the duplication of normal development, MZ twinning is a gross departure from the normal process. Its several varieties are determined by the time (days after fertilization) when splitting occurs in the embryo, giving rise to different structural arrangements of the membranes. It should be realized, however, that this is not a precisely established timetable of rigid stages, but a continuum of development is occurring in which there is overlap between the differentiation of some tissues and there may be small variations of timing between different embryos (Benirschke & Kim 1973).

If splitting occurs no later than the 8-cell stage (3 days after fertilization; [a] in Fig. 33.1) while cells remain unspecialized and thus retain their full potentiality, two separate normal blastocysts form and if both implant successfully a twin pregnancy results. There are separate implantation sites, which may or may not be close together, and the structural arrangements of the membranes and placentas (dichorionic diamniotic) are exactly the same as in DZ twinning. However, unlike DZ twins, the fetuses will be identical. This early splitting at the blastomere stage accounts for one-third of MZ twins.

If splitting is delayed until the inner cell mass is forming (4–7 days; [b] in Fig. 33.1) a single blastocyst will implant with a single chorion giving rise to one placenta in which there are anastomoses between the two fetal circulations, but if the amnion has not yet differentiated each embryo will develop its own amniotic membrane and cavity (monochorionic diamniotic). This intermediate form of splitting occurs between 4 and 7 days after fertilization, and the offspring will of course be identical. It accounts for two-thirds of MZ twins.

When later splitting of the inner cell mass occurs, after differentiation of the amnion but before the appearance of the primitive streak (8–12 days; [c] in

Fig. 33.1), two identical fetuses will develop with a single amniotic cavity as well as sharing a single chorion and placenta with communications between the two circulations (monochorionic monoamniotic). This accounts for about one per cent of MZ twins.

Still later, after the primitive streak has appeared (from about 13 days; [d] in Fig. 33.1), incomplete splitting of the germinal disc is an extremely rare aberration that gives rise to conjoined twins.

Determination of zygosity at birth

Twins of unlike sex are DZ, and careful examination of the placenta and membranes will identify the majority (two-thirds) of MZ twin pairs that share a single chorionic membrane.

Dichorionic twins of like sex may be DZ or MZ (due to early splitting) and tests for genetically determined markers in the blood and in the placenta are required to determine if the twins have an identical genetic constitution (MZ) or there are differences (DZ). As much blood as possible should be drawn from a vessel on the fetal surface of the placenta, and a slice taken from the centre of each placenta and deep-frozen for dispatch to a specialized laboratory if tissue marker studies become necessary. The demonstration of only one genetic difference between co-twins suffices to establish dizygosity, and this may be achieved by red cell antigen testing (blood group and genotyping). If not, other useful marker systems are histocompatibility antigens, red cell enzymes and serum proteins, and placental enzymes.

Triplets and higher multiple births

Triplets, which occur once in about 6000 births in Europe, most often originate in 3 separate zygotes (trizygotic), particularly in populations with high rates for DZ twinning (e.g. in Africa); each fetus is surrounded by its own membranes (trichorionic triamniotic) and has its own placenta with an independent circulation even when there is placental fusion. Less commonly a triplet pregnancy is DZ, one of the embryos having split in the same way and with one of the same variations in the membranes as in MZ twinning; the other embryo develops its own membranes and placenta in the usual way. MZ triplets are very rare, occurring when one of the two embryos formed by the initial separation splits again; this is the only form of triplet pregnancy with a single chorion and intercommunicating circulations through vascular anastomoses in a common placenta.

Various combinations of multizygosity and repeated splitting explain the still rarer quadruplet and higher multiple pregnancies. Most reports of naturally occurring multiple pregnancies resulting in more than five births are probably not authentic, but the use of gonadotrophins and other ovulation inducing agents in the treatment of infertility has been followed by such high multiple births, even of octuplets (Prokop & Herrmann 1973). It is to be hoped that the overenthusiastic transfer of multiple embryos following *in vitro* fertilization will be kept within the bounds of good practice.

Factors influencing twinning rates

Ethnic and geographic variations in the frequency of twin births have already been noted. DZ twinning occurs more frequently with rising maternal age, rising to a peak between 35 and 39 years following which there is a decline, and also with increasing parity independently of maternal age. It has also been suggested that women who conceive very easily, e.g. within three months of marriage, are also more likely to conceive twins. A nutritional influence is suggested by a higher incidence of DZ twinning in tall women, and a reduced rate in underweight mothers. These factors have no influence on MZ twinning.

Women who have had twins previously are more likely to conceive twins than are other women, and the belief that twinning rates are influenced by hereditary factors, maternal and perhaps also paternal, is a long established one. Many studies have confirmed that this is so for DZ but not for MZ twinning (e.g. Bulmer 1958 and 1980), with a majority view that it is inherited on the maternal side only. These conclusions were confirmed by Nylander (1970) in a study of almost 1000 twin pairs in Western Nigeria, in which more than 90% were DZ pairs.

MATERNAL PHYSIOLOGICAL CHANGES

The maternal response to twin pregnancy, which may be summarised as an increased adaptation of all the systems and especially the cardiovascular system, has been investigated intensively, notably in Aberdeen, where many normal values for twin pregnancy have been documented and were described by Mac-Gillivray (1984). Apart from increased pressure effects caused by excessive uterine enlargement, such as the exacerbation of varicose veins, haemorrhoids and dependent oedema, all the changes seem to be brought about by the increased production of placental hormones. They are further augmented in triplet and higher multiple pregnancies, although normal values for these are less well documented because few cases are available for study and complications are very common. In twin pregnancy, higher plasma and urine values for oestrogen and progesterone are well documented, and the placental protein hormones are also increased (Towler *et al.* 1976) although their possible role in bringing about maternal changes remains uncertain.

Cardiovascular changes

Cardiac output is much higher in the presence of twins, and the normal increase in plasma volume during pregnancy is also much greater. The normal increase in total circulating red cell mass shows an additional increment of about 250 ml in twin pregnancies, but because this is not in proportion to the increment in plasma volume, haematocrit and haemoglobin values are even lower than in single pregnancies. The total intravascular protein mass is greater with twins, but plasma protein values are also lower because of the disproportionate increase in plasma volume.

Apart from a small increase in fibrinogen, plasma values for coagulation factors are the same as in single pregnancies (Condie & Campbell 1978).

Other maternal changes

The healthy mother's dietary intake, including protein, trace elements and energy, is the same in twin and single pregnancies (Campbell *et al.* 1982) despite the greater (combined) birthweight and a greater maternal weight gain with twins. Plasma iron concentration is lower in the presence of twins, and this reduction will be greater still should the mother begin her pregnancy with reduced iron stores and also, of course, with the extra demands of three or more fetuses.

Other maternal differences, in twin compared with single pregnancies, are a greater increase in respiratory tidal volume, a higher glomerular filtration rate, and higher maternal serum alphafetoprotein levels (*see* p. 490).

COMPLICATIONS OF MULTIPLE PREGNANCY

Traditionally most or all complications of pregnancy have been considered to occur with increased frequency in the presence of twins, and with even greater incidences in triplet and higher multiple pregnancies. However, careful reviews show that this is not true of many complications, and it has also become clear that the incidence of some is related to zygosity.

Fetal abnormalities

An increased incidence of fetal malformation in multiple pregnancies is almost certainly confined to MZ fetuses, and rates for concordance (i.e. both twins affected) may be as high as about 30% for some abnormalities such as congenital dislocation of the hips. The relatively high incidence, but low concordance, of malformations of the heart and of the central nervous system (hydrocephaly and neural tube defects) in MZ twins (Carter 1965) suggests that a 'local' environmental factor, perhaps placental vascular anastamoses (Hay & Wehrung 1970), may have a causal role.

Two very rare malformations in MZ twins are the acardiac monster and conjoined twins. The former occurs only in one of a pair of monochorionic MZ twins, probably as a result of cardiac atrophy brought about by some early disturbance in the shared placental circulation. The various types of conjoined twins (most commonly thoracopagus), which may or may not share incompletely duplicated organs, result from late embryonic splitting.

Although a rather higher than usual incidence of Down's syndrome and other chromosomal anomalies might be expected because of the increased twinning rate in older mothers, these aberrations are apparently no more common in twins than in singletons.

Abortion

Threatened abortion is probably no more frequent in multiple than in single pregnancies (Nylander & MacGillivray 1975), but it is generally believed that spontaneous abortion is more likely to occur in the former, and there are two good reasons why this should be so. Firstly, there is the increased incidence of fetal abnormalities. Secondly, whatever factors cause the considerably increased incidence of very early spontaneous preterm labour must surely also predispose to late spontaneous abortion.

Hyperemesis

The frequency and severity of nausea and vomiting during the first trimester are increased in multiple pregnancy, and these symptoms not infrequently persist beyond this phase. Severe hyperemesis, with dehydration, electrolyte disturbances and nutritional effects, has become an uncommon problem in pregnant mothers, but it remains more frequent in multiple than in single pregnancies; so much so that its occurrence during the early months should suggest the possibility that more than one fetus is present.

Anaemia

It has become fashionable to attribute the lower haematocrit and haemoglobin values found in multiple pregnancy entirely to the much greater increase in plasma volume that occurs in comparison with single pregnancy. However, megaloblasts and reduced iron stores are often found in the bone marrow, and two and more decades ago, when anaemia was a common complication of pregnancy, its increased incidence and severity in women with multiple pregnancies was well documented. It is likely that its present reduced incidence in multiple pregnancy merely reflects the steady reduction in pregnancy anaemia in general due to improved nutrition, reduced demands through fewer and better spaced pregnancies and the effect of hormonal contraception in controlling menstrual loss. The diminished iron stores in 40% of women carrying twins (Hall *et al.* 1979) does represent iron deficiency, and makes the case for routine iron supplementation whenever multiple pregnancy has been diagnosed. Since there is megaloblastic erythropoiesis in a significant proportion of these mothers prophylactic folic acid supplementation is indicated as well.

Polyhydramnios

It is generally agreed that polyhydramnios is several times more common in multiple than in single pregnancies, although reported incidences vary considerably largely because it is a subjective clinical diagnosis. Except for acute polyhydramnios, this complication is probably no more common with MZ than DZ twins (Nylander & MacGillivray 1975) and

in most cases it is not associated with a fetal abnormality.

Antepartum haemorrhage

Although a few studies have not shown an unusually high incidence of antepartum haemorrhage in twin pregnancies (Nylander & MacGillivray 1975), the general impression and many other studies support the view that placenta praevia is more common. It seems probable that in multiple pregnancy an increased incidence of bleeding from placenta praevia is obscured when all instances and causes of antepartum haemorrhage are considered together.

Hypertensive complications

Pre-eclampsia is second only in importance to preterm labour as a complication of multiple pregnancy, with a reported incidence between 3 and 5 times greater than in single pregnancies, and with a tendency to take a more fulminant course that is more likely to lead to eclampsia. It also tends to occur earlier in pregnancy, and the occurrence of severe pre-eclampsia by about 28 weeks should suggest the likelihood of multiple pregnancy when this has not already been excluded by ultrasound. As in single pregnancy, pre-eclampsia is principally a disease of primigravidas. Late pregnancy hypertension, which must include mothers in the earliest premonitory stage of pre-eclampsia without fulfilling its defined criteria, is to a lesser degree also more common in multiple than single pregnancy and in primigravidas than parous mothers.

The incidences of proteinuric pre-eclampsia and late pregnancy hypertension, and their relationship to gravidity and zygosity, in 1206 twin pregnancies were reported by MacGillivray (1983). His findings, summarized in Table 33.1, besides showing no differences in the incidence between DZ and MZ twin pregnancies, confirm the higher incidences in primigravidas, especially of proteinuric pre-eclampsia (18.3% compared with 8% in multigravidas). There were 3 cases of eclampsia among the primigravidas in this series.

Rhesus disease

There is no reason to suppose that the incidence of pre-existing Rhesus (Rh) immunization is any different in multiple than in single pregnancies. However, when Rh sensitization occurs in a multiple preg-

Table 33.1 Incidences of proteinuric pre-eclampsia and late pregnancy hypertension in primigravidas and multiparas subdivided by zygosity (MZ = monozygotic; DZ = dizygotic): adapted from data reported by MacGillivray (1983).

	Zygosity	No.	Proteinuric pre-eclampsia		Late pregnancy hypertension	
			No.	%	No.	%
Primigravidas	MZ	119	21	17.6	32	26.9
	DZ	236	44	18.6	57	24.2
		355	65	18.3	89	25.1
Multiparas	MZ	223	16	7.2	30	13.5
	DZ	628	52	8.3	108	17.2
		851	68	8.0	138	16.2
Total		1206	133	11.0	227	18.8

nancy, it is often unusually severe, leading to critical or fatal haemolytic disease in the next Rh-positive pregnancy; this is because in multiple pregnancies the sensitizing feto-maternal haemorrhage is much more likely to be a large one, very often due to considerable placental separation during the interval between the first birth and eventual completion of the third stage of labour.

Assessment of the haemolytic process in the fetus of a Rh-immunized mother, from amniotic fluid bilirubin estimations, has been described in Chapter 18 (p. 271). The same principles apply when more than one fetus is present, but an individual prediction of severity must always be made for each fetus. Even before the introduction of ultrasound it was usually possible, using marker dyes (e.g. methylene blue) or radio-opaque contrast (amniography), to obtain amniotic fluid samples from each fetus. With ultrasound guidance it should always be possible to do so.

When the twin fetuses of a Rh-negative woman are DZ and their father is heterozygous Rh-positive, then it is possible for one fetus to be Rh-positive but the other Rh-negative. In such cases, when the mother is already Rh-immunized a fetus severely affected by haemolytic disease may co-exist with one that is unaffected. Even when both fetuses are Rh-positive, there can be a significant difference in the severity of haemolysis and in prognosis. The most difficult decisions arise when the amniotic fluid bilirubin estimations indicate that very early intervention, by either intrauterine blood transfusion or rescue to intensive neonatal management, is required for one fetus but not for the other which is predicted to be more mildly affected or possibly unaffected. Other factors must be taken into account, but as a general rule the less affected (or unaffected) fetus should not be compromised in the interests of a fetus that might in any case be fatally affected. However, with skilled ultrasound guidance, an experienced operator can usually give an intrauterine transfusion without difficulty to one of twins, or indeed to both if necessary. Before real time ultrasound became available, but instead by using fluoroscopy and both amniography and colour markers, the author had the experience of giving two intrauterine transfusions to the worst affected of triplets and transfusing the other Rh-positive fetus of the trio on the second of these occasions, without interfering with the third fetus which had been predicted to be no more than mildly affected (following birth this baby was found to be Rh-negative; all three survived).

Twin-to-twin transfusion syndrome

The presence of anastomoses between the two placental circulations of all monochorial MZ twins pairs leads to twin-to-twin transfusion in some of them. It seems probable that the two types of anastomoses described (superficial and deep) are responsible for different forms of the twin-to-twin transfusion syndrome (Cameron 1968). Thus, on the fetal surface of the placenta there are artery-to-artery and less frequently vein-to-vein connections which may be quite small and usually cause no problem before labour because of similar pressures in each circulation, but as a result of some haemodynamic disturbance during parturition the acute form of the twin-to-twin transfusion syndrome occasionally occurs (Klebe and Ingomar, 1972). The donor fetus is pale and the recipient plethoric, but there are no inequalities in development, and a discrepancy in haemoglobin and haematocritic values between them is not demonstrable until a few hours after their births.

The more common twin-to-twin transfusion, occurring probably over weeks or months, results from arteriovenous anastomoses in the depth of the placenta (Benirschke and Driscoll 1967). In this chronic form of the syndrome, there is often polyhydramnios in relation to the plethoric recipient twin, possibly due to increased glomerular filtration resulting from the augmented blood volume, and the heart is usually enlarged. The pale donor twin is growth-retarded, and significant haemoglobin and haematocrit differences are present at birth. That part of the placenta relating to the donor twin is pale and oedematous, resembling the placenta associated with hydrops fetalis due to haemolytic disease, and this twin's blood contains nucleated erythrocytes as evidence of compensatory marrow overactivity. The recipient's placental territory is small and congested.

Frank evidence of the twin-to-twin transfusion syndrome in liveborn MZ twins, defined by Rausen *et al.* (1965) as a difference in haemoglobin concentration at birth of more than 5 g/dl, or probable evidence in the form of polyhydramnios in one sac and a marked discrepancy in birthweight and organ size, was present in 19 of their series of 130 monochorial twin pregnancies (15%) and this was also the incidence of the syndrome reported from the Birmingham Twin Study (Cameron 1968). It seems likely that mild examples of the syndrome go unrecognized, so that its true incidence is probably much higher as would be expected from the presence of at least small anastomoses in all monochorial placentas. The dangers to the fetuses are intrauterine distress and death, resulting from anaemia and hypoxia in the growth retarded donor twin, or from cardiac failure and possible thromboses due to hyperviscosity of the blood in the recipient. In the series of Rausen and his colleagues, 25 of the 38 fetuses (66%) died, 12 of them having birthweights below 500 g (i.e. the donor twins), and in only 4 of the 19 pregnancies did both eventually survive.

The twin-to-twin transfusion syndrome is usually only suspected from the appearance of the babies at or soon after birth, and it is usually the anaemic fetus that first attracts attention. Either baby may need intensive care. The anaemic baby is best treated by exchange blood transfusion, while digitalization and exchange transfusion with plasma or albumin may be needed for the recipient twin. During labour the possibility of twin-to-twin transfusion should be suspected when the monitored heart rate of one twin shows changes suggesting hypoxic distress. During pregnancy repeated ultrasound imaging and measurement may reveal that one of a pair of twins sharing one placental mass is becoming growth retarded while the other shows an unexpected increase in growth rate with cardiac enlargement accompanied by the development of polyhydramnios. The syndrome has been diagnosed in this way in an unusual example of acute twin-to-twin transfusion occurring at only 18 weeks' gestation and soon resulting in miscarriage; this resulted from an anastomosis of a placental artery of the donor twin with a vein in the placental territory of the recipient (Elejalde *et al.* 1983). Distress in either fetus may be reflected in abnormal cardiotocographic tracings, and it seems likely that further developments in ultrasound Doppler studies of blood flow in the fetus and umbilical cord, together with improved placental imaging and fetal echocardiography, will be helpful in the early detection of chronic twin-to-twin transfusion.

Intrauterine growth retardation

Retarded fetal growth is common in multiple pregnancy, affecting either or both of twins and occurring most often when the placenta is monochorionic. One-third or more of twin fetuses have birthweights below the tenth percentile for gestational age using singleton standards, with almost one quarter below the fifth percentile. However, although they are often used for this purpose, either of these percentile limits is an imperfect definition of intrauterine growth retardation that probably underestimates the real incidence of this complication; it includes some fetuses which have achieved their genetically endowed low growth potentials, but it almost certainly excludes a larger number which have failed to sustain greater genetic growth profiles but still achieve birthweights above the chosen percentile. Recent experience in Glasgow, where the stillbirth rate among twins was 36 per 1000 births and where ultrasound measurements are used routinely in early pregnancy to establish gestational age as accurately as possible, suggests that there is severe growth retardation in almost half of all non-malformed stillborn twins, without evidence of any alternative cause of death. The liveborn growth retarded baby remains at risk of neonatal complications and this is especially so when the baby is premature as well.

Unexplained intrauterine death

Even with postmortem examinations by expert perinatal pathologists, and when fetal deaths are attributed to twin-to-twin transfusion if there is evidence to suggest that this has occurred, or to severe growth retardation if birthweight is less than the fifth percentile for the gestational age at which the fetus died, there will remain a few quite unexplained intrauterine deaths. These are most likely to have occurred in one or both of monochorionic MZ twins and/or when autopsy is uninformative because of maceration of a fetus retained *in utero* for some time after it has died.

Prematurity

At birth rather more than half of the babies of multiple pregnancies are of low birthweight (< 2.5 kg) compared with about 6% of singletons, and one-tenth weigh less than 1.5 kg compared with only 1% of singletons. In the great majority of cases this is due to preterm birth rather than to retarded growth *in utero* or to a combination of both factors. Thus, in a recent survey of twin pregnancies in Scotland (Patel *et al.* 1985) delivery occurred before 37 weeks of gestation in 44%, compared with 5.5% of singletons; it was before 32 weeks in almost 10% of twin pregnancies, compared with only 1% of single pregnancies, and it is of course in this excess of very premature babies that the considerably increased neonatal mortality and morbidity from multiple pregnancy is concentrated, although survival rates at corresponding birthweights are generally no worse among twins than singletons. A small number of the babies born before 32 weeks are delivered electively because of an acute obstetric complication (usually antepartum haemorrhage or severe pre-eclampsia) but in the majority preterm labour occurs spontaneously or it follows spontaneous rupture of the membranes.

Preterm labour, especially when preceded by spontaneous membrane rupture, is more likely to occur in MZ than in DZ twin pregnancies (MacGillivray 1982), perhaps partly due to the more frequent development of polyhydramnios in the former. Uterine overdistension, leading to cervical dilatation and perhaps myometrial overactivity, may also predispose to preterm labour even when there is no obvious polyhydramnios, but early and increased ripening of the cervix due to augmented hormonal activity is likely to be a contributory factor. Otherwise, little or no more is known about the causes of spontaneous preterm labour in multiple pregnancies than is understood about its aetiology in general. The hazards faced by the very premature infant are well recognized, and, despite steadily improving results of intensive neonatal care, they still represent the main factor in the increased wastage associated with multiple pregnancies.

ANTENATAL MANAGEMENT

The particular hazards of twin and other multiple pregnancies, described above, must be kept in mind in planning the intensified programme of antenatal care required for the optimal management of these high risk pregnancies. The obvious first step is to make the diagnosis of multiple pregnancy as early as possible during gestation.

Diagnosis

When the diagnosis of multiple pregnancy depended on a high degree of clinical suspicion followed by careful abdominal palpation, usually then confirmed by X-ray, in about one-fifth of cases the presence of two or more fetuses remained undetected until delivery, and sometimes the diagnosis was not made or suspected until after the first baby had been delivered. Nowadays proficient ultrasound scanning provides a

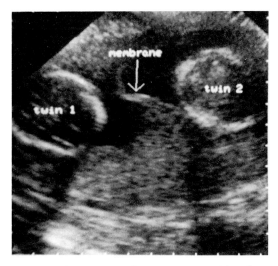

Fig. 33.2. Ultrasonogram of twin pregnancy at 16 weeks, showing membrane separating the gestation sacs.

sure method of diagnosing multiple pregnancy as early as the 8th week of pregnancy, and sometimes even earlier, and of counting the number of fetuses present. Clearly the detection rate is best when an ultrasound examination is a routine procedure, either at booking or, as seems to be the more frequent policy, at about 16–18 weeks' gestation (e.g. Fig. 33.2). Thus, at the Queen Mother's Hospital in Glasgow, where a routine booking scan is carried out and many mothers have additional scans for a variety of reasons during the second trimester, all 115 pairs of twins during 3 years were detected, including 87% at the booking scan.

Where ultrasound is not readily available or is not used as a routine procedure, there is need for a high degree of watchfulness for any circumstances suggesting that the pregnancy may be a multiple one. Occasionally excessive pressure symptoms, unusually persistent hyperemesis or very early severe pre-eclampsia, may direct attention to this possibility, as should the knowledge that pregnancy followed therapeutic induction of ovulation. The usual clinical pointer to the diagnosis is overdistension of the uterus, with a multiplicity of palpable fetal parts which usually include three identifiable fetal poles. Polyhydramnios may be present and should suggest the possibility of multiple pregnancy, but it may make the clinical diagnosis by palpation difficult or impossible. The diagnosis, and the number of fetuses, should always be confirmed by ultrasound (or, less preferably, by X-ray) and each fetus should be inspected carefully by this means to exclude (or detect) structural abnormality.

Routine care

Because of the more frequent incidence of complications, most of which tend to occur earlier and often become more severe than in single pregnancies, antenatal care should be based on more frequent attendances. To limit inconvenience to the mother and thus encourage her full participation in this intensive supervision, shared responsibility between the hospital obstetric team and a general practitioner experienced in antenatal care has obvious advantages; a valuable working link between the two is provided by a hospital-based midwife attached to the general practitioner's health centre in the community. By limiting the number of time consuming visits to the hospital, shared care does much to reconcile the requirement for frequent assessments with the important need for extra rest throughout a multiple pregnancy. Adequate rest will reduce tiredness and pressure symptoms, it should improve utero-placental blood flow, and it may sometimes avoid or at least postpone the onset and perhaps limit the severity of pre-eclampsia. It is suggested that the mother carrying twins should be seen as frequently as fortnightly between 20 and 30 weeks, and weekly thereafter. There may also be a policy of routine admission to hospital (see below), and prolonged admission is certainly the rule when she carries triplets or more.

Good nutrition, with expert advice by a trained dietitian when necessary, is of particular importance, as is routine supplementation with iron and folic acid (see p. 254). All the routine antenatal investigations are carried out in the usual way, and the measurement of maternal serum alphafetoprotein (MSAFP) is especially useful in multiple pregnancy. Not only may there be abnormally high levels of this fetal protein in the mother's blood simply because more than one fetus is present, or there may be a neural tube defect or other deformity in one or very occasionally both of twins, but it has become clear that high MSAFP values provide a useful indicator that there are increased risks of late abortion or preterm labour and of the fetus dying *in utero*. In the West of Scotland MSAFP screening programme, using 5 multiples of the median (MOM) singleton value (at 16–20 weeks) as the critical limit (i.e. twice the 2.5 MOM cut-off used for single pregnancies; *see* p. 311) 59% of twin pregnancies identified in this way, and with both fetuses normally formed, ended with the loss of one twin or more commonly both of them (Ghosh *et al.* 1982). Using an even lower cut-off at 4 MOM, it was also shown that 50% of twin pregnancies with raised MSAFP terminated before 34 weeks, and there was an extended mortality rate (combining perinatal and later prematurity-attributable deaths) of 40% (Redford & Whitfield 1985).

Prenatal diagnosis of fetal abnormality

For screening for fetal neural tube defects and other anomalies associated with raised MSAFP the 5 MOM cut-off used in twin pregnancies is as effective as the 2.5 MOM critical value for singletons (Ghosh *et al.* 1982). When values above 5 MOM are obtained a detailed inspection of each fetus by ultrasound is the preferred next diagnostic step, which will usually reveal or exclude a relevant fetal abnormality. Amniocentesis can usually be performed from each sac without difficulty, although it is probably associated with a higher subsequent abortion rate than is am-

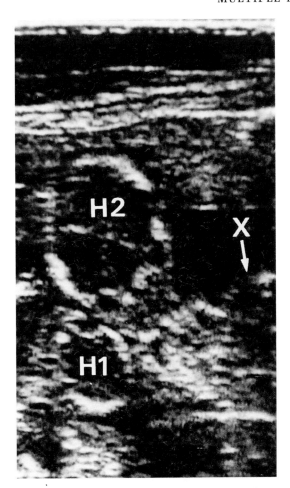

Fig. 33.3. Ultrasonogram of twin pregnancy at 18 weeks, showing collapsed head of dead twin (H1) beside normal head (H2) of malformed twin with a body stalk anomaly (X); pregnancy terminated after diagnosis.

niocentesis in single pregnancies. This risk is in any case significantly increased when the indication is a high MSAFP level, but, if detailed ultrasound examination of both fetuses leaves some doubt about a neural tube defect or other relevant deformity, double amniocentesis for estimation of alphafetoprotein in each sac is indicated. Other structural anomalies in a twin fetus, that are not associated with raised MSAFP, are also detectable by ultrasound (e.g. Fig. 33.3).

Amniocentesis for fetal karyotyping should in any case be offered at the same maternal age (35–37 years) as in single pregnancy, but very careful counselling is required and double genetic amniocentesis

should always be carried out by obstetricians experienced in this field.

Thorough counselling is also important when a severely handicapping abnormality has been detected in one twin but the other is normal. In this circumstance, some parents will choose to continue the pregnancy, while others will opt for termination. Selective 'feticide', by which the abnormal twin is killed by fetoscopic air embolization via an umbilical cord vessel, seems usually to be followed by continuation of the pregnancy with survival of the normal fetus (Rodeck *et al.* 1982) and will be acceptable to many parents in this difficult situation, although there is as yet insufficient experience to provide an assessment of its likely complication rate.

Ultrasound and cardiotocography

Intrauterine growth retardation in one or both of twins can be identified by ultrasound measurement of the fetal trunk alone or in combination with other dimensions (Neilson 1981) and its severity and further course followed by repeated measurements. Repeated fetal inspection and measurement by ultrasound will sometimes reveal signs suggesting twin-to-twin transfusion which may be chronic or acute (*see* p. 487). In either case, and also when growth retardation has been demonstrated, the state of each fetus should be followed by frequent external cardiotocography which may allow impending intrauterine death to be detected and anticipated by timely elective delivery (Bailey *et al.* 1980). With non-stress cardiotocography repeated weekly, the predictive value of reactive tracings is particularly good, as shown in a 3-centre American study of 94 multiple pregnancies (193 fetuses) reported by Blake *et al.* (1984); in 168 fetuses with reactive final tracings there were only 2 perinatal deaths (1.2%) and intrapartum distress occurred in only 3 of 79 that were not delivered by elective Caesarean section (3.8%); while in the 25 fetuses with non-reactive last tracings, there were 2 perinatal deaths (8%) and 7 of 9 exposed to labour showed evidence of distress (78%), the usual indication for immediate elective Caesarean section in this group being a 'positive' contraction stress test.

Because each fetus of a multiple pregnancy can be monitored separately, ultrasound and cardiotocography are much superior to biochemical testing which cannot assess each feto-placental unit individually, and the relative usefulness of which even in single pregnancies is being questioned increasingly. Indeed, a combination of repeated skilled ultrasound examinations, frequent cardiotocography whenever retarded growth or twin-to-twin transfusion is suspected or some other complication supervenes, and immediate delivery (usually by Caesarean section) when the tracings suggest that fetal death may be imminent, provides the best available means at present of reducing the high perinatal mortality associated with twins and other multiple pregnancies. If resources permit, routine biophysical monitoring in this way is easily justified. It seems very likely that measurement of blood flow in the uterus, umbilical cords and each fetus, using Doppler ultrasound, will provide a valuable addition to the biophysical surveillance of multiple pregnancies, not only in assessing the state of a growth retarded fetus (Giles *et al.* 1985, Erskine & Ritchie 1985), but especially in detecting and measuring the effect of twin-to-twin transfusion.

A further use of ultrasound is to estimate the size (i.e. weight) of each fetus when preterm labour has not occurred. This information is of particular importance in labour if the second twin is significantly larger than the first one.

Prevention of preterm labour

The establishment of effective means to prevent preterm labour, or at least to postpone it until the fetuses are sufficiently grown and mature to survive without intensive care, would represent by far the most important possible advance in the antenatal management of multiple pregnancy. Three main approaches that have been tried, but so far have not been shown conclusively to be of value as routine prophylactic measures, are hospitalization during a specified time in late pregnancy, the insertion of cervical sutures, and tocolysis using beta-sympathomimetic drugs.

HOSPITALIZATION

It was once quite common routine practice to admit mothers with twin pregnancies to hospital for extra bed rest from 32 or 34 weeks until 36 or 37 weeks when it was considered that the babies would have achieved sufficient maturity. Doubts about its efficacy, together with improving survival rates following birth within this period of gestation, led some obstetricians to abandon this policy and others to advance the time for hospitalization to a gestational age range during which delivery was still associated with very significant neonatal and later mortality, e.g. from 30 to 34 weeks. Further improvements in

methods and results of intensive care of very premature infants suggest that, if admission is still to be advised as a routine or preferably for its value to be assessed by adequate controlled trials, the time should be brought forward still further to the month between 28 and 32 weeks. Thereafter, continued inpatient rest and supervision would be indicated if very early labour had already threatened to occur, as shown by sustained or repeated uterine hyperactivity, significant cervical dilatation detected by vaginal examinations, or of course if the membranes have ruptured.

When the likelihood of very early labour has been revealed in some of these or other ways, including perhaps repeated measurements of MSAFP as a marker indicating that some placental separation leading to feto-maternal bleeding has occurred, there would be ample justification for selective (as opposed to routine) admission to hospital.

Apart from possibly bringing about a worthwhile postponement of labour in some mothers, routine or selective admission for extra bed rest should improve utero-placental blood flow and would guarantee that if very early delivery does occur, perhaps after a rapid labour, it will be under optimal conditions in hospital and not at home or on the way between the two.

In addition, there should always be an increased readiness to advise admission to mothers with twin pregnancies and in whom there is some elevation of the blood pressure, reduced fetal movements, evidence suggesting intrauterine growth retardation or other departures from normal progress. For all the reasons stated in relation to twins, and because of the increased frequency of other complications, mothers with multiple pregnancies in excess of twins will usually be supervised in hospital throughout the third trimester, and sometimes for much of the second trimester as well.

CERVICAL SUTURE

As an alternative or an addition to extra rest in hospital, some obstetricians have inserted cervical sutures when twin pregnancy has been diagnosed. As a routine measure, this has been subjected to fewer trials and reviews than has routine hospital admission, and with the same lack of consensus so far. It also ignores the fact that in twin pregnancy there is usually some effacement and dilatation of the cervix throughout, or sometimes beginning before the third trimester; an artificial resistance to this expected 'give' may well stimulate excessive uterine activity in some cases, and thus actually contribute to the occurrence of early labour.

One of the most useful evaluations of these routine policies to reduce the risk of preterm twin births was a 3-way trial, conducted in Liverpool, in which a comparison of routine bed rest in hospital, routine cervical suture, and non-interventional (control) management showed no differences in prolongation of pregnancy, birth weight or wastage (Weekes *et al.* 1977).

TOCOLYSIS

More recently there have been reports suggesting that oral prophylactic treatment with beta-sympathomimetic drugs, e.g. ritodrine and salbutamol, may postpone very early labour significantly in a useful proportion of twin pregnancies and that this may lead to improved perinatal survival (Tambyrajah *et al.* 1978). This was not confirmed in other studies (O'Connor *et al.* 1979). Also, the much increased maternal blood volume in the presence of twins would predispose the mother to the potentially dangerous cardiovascular side effects of sympathomimetic drugs. For such reasons there has been a general reluctance to use these tocolytics in multiple pregnancy, especially over a long period of treatment. Nevertheless it may well be that they are more effective in preventing very early labour than in suppressing it once it threatens, and their careful use to prevent excessive uterine activity and to limit early cervical dilatation in twin pregnancies remains to be evaluated properly.

LABOUR IN MULTIPLE PREGNANCY

In 70% of twin pregnancies the first fetus presents by the vertex, and in 40% both will be born by this presentation. Malpresentations are common, especially of the second twin, but mechanical difficulty is rare as the fetuses tend to be small. The second twin is also at more risk than the first from intrapartum hypoxia.

Labour should be conducted in a well equipped hospital under the supervision of an experienced obstetrician, with an expert obstetric anaesthetist and a paediatrician in attendance, or two paediatricians if the labour is preterm or there are other complications. In early labour an intravenous infusion should be set up to which oxytocin may later be added if necessary. Continuous recording of the heart rate of both twins, the first by scalp electrode and the second by external recording, is required. Whenever possible an intra-amniotic catheter should be used to record the uterine contractions, and this recording can be transmitted from the output of the first monitor to be displayed also on the write-out of the second one.

The first stage is usually not prolonged, and with small fetuses may be very rapid. The indications for oxytocic stimulation or other intervention are the same as those for a singleton with the same presentation. Epidural analgesia is ideal if there is time to establish it, but pudendal block with perineal infiltration is also usually satisfactory for delivery. General anaesthesia may become necessary at any time. Episiotomy is usually advisable.

The first cord is divided between an artery forceps on the fetal side and ligature or Hollister type clamp on the placental side to eliminate any risk of haemorrhage from the second fetus through communicating placental circulations.

Immediately the first twin is delivered, a transverse or oblique lie of the second fetus is sought and corrected by external version through the lax abdominal wall. If this proves difficult to effect or to maintain, the second bag of membranes should be ruptured, and internal version and breech extraction performed. Vaginal examination is also required to identify an uncertain presentation, or to exclude prolapse of the cord of the second twin when its membranes rupture. Fetal heart monitoring must be continued because some degree of uterine retraction is inevitable once the first twin, its liquor and possibly the liquor from the second sac have been expelled, and utero-placental blood flow may well be jeopardized.

With the presenting part fixed in the pelvic brim (and oxytocin may be added to the infusion to aid this) the membranes of the second sac are ruptured to reduce to a minimum the time interval between births. A conscious mother can push with contractions, and it matters little whether the second baby is delivered by the vertex or the breech because the birth canal has been already stretched, an episiotomy has been made, and there is in any case little opportunity for the head to mould. Where a general anaesthetic has already been administered or the second presenting part remains high, the ventouse is ideal when the head presents, or rupture of membranes and bringing down a leg enables breech extraction to be performed if the presentation is podalic; but these manoeuvres are not often required in properly conducted twin deliveries and, although they are usually carried out without difficulty, they are associated with increased risks of trauma and morbidity in the baby, or even its subsequent death particularly if there was already serious intrapartum hypoxia.

In some cases the second twin is the larger and, especially if instrumental delivery of the first has been needed, it is important to exclude disproportion before attempting vaginal delivery, and it is in such cases that prior estimation of the weight of each fetus by ultrasound is so useful. Rarely Caesarean section for the second twin may be necessary because of its size. Its requirement simply because the cervix has been allowed to close down by undue delay in effecting the second delivery should not be allowed to arise.

Twins predispose to postpartum haemorrhage, a risk that is minimized by continuous oxytocin infusion through and for some time after the third stage of labour, reinforced if there is any subsequent uterine relaxation or undue bleeding by the intravenous injection of 0.5 mg of ergometrine.

Occasionally, twins may remain undiagnosed until the birth of the first infant, and if syntometrine or ergometrine have been administered the ensuing vigorous uterine action may expel the second twin too rapidly, or produce death of the fetus from anoxia. Tocolytic drugs may be given at once by intravenous injection, and if necessary general anaesthesia is rapidly induced with halothane in an attempt to relax the uterus. If the fetus is retained the membranes are then ruptured and the fetus delivered by forceps, ventouse or breech extraction. Immediate action in this way will usually effect delivery, but with an increased risk of hypoxia and/or trauma to the baby, and Caesarean section is sometimes the better course. Internal version should not be attempted because of the risk of uterine rupture.

With triplets or a greater number of fetuses, pregnancy is often complicated by severe pre-eclampsia and placental insufficiency. Because it is important to avoid fetal hypoxia, Caesarean section should usually be the preferred method of delivery if sufficient maturity has been reached and if labour has not been so rapid that vaginal delivery is about to occur when the mother presents. In a review of 59 triplet pregnancies Itzkowic (1979) showed that all babies lost were born by vaginal delivery and that, as with twins, perinatal loss increased with birth order.

The greater risk to the second than to the first twin has been noted. This is in part due to the inevitable uterine retraction which follows expulsion of the first but also because of the greater incidence of malpresentation, internal manipulation, placental insufficiency and perhaps also congenital abnormality.

Difficult cases of twins

Interlocking is extremely rare, and is most likely when the first fetus is delivered by the breech but the head of the second enters the pelvis alongside the neck of the first. It may be possible to push the head of the second twin upwards out of the pelvis so permitting delivery of the first. Should this fail the first baby will die from cord occlusion, and then decapitation of this fetus allows delivery of the surviving twin followed by the free head of the first. Very occasionally, when the fetuses are very small the two heads of a double vertex presentation may lock in the pelvic brim, but under general anaesthesia the higher head can usually be dislodged upwards until it is freed.

The other rarity of conjoined twins may be diagnosed by ultrasound, or suspected if X-ray shows two heads lying at the same level in the uterus or if the fetuses maintain a constant and corresponding relationship to each other. Oblique films usually clarify the diagnosis. The incidence has been estimated at less than one in 60 000 deliveries. Since conjoined twins can often be separated surgically, the mother should be delivered at or near term by Caesarean section in a perinatal referral centre. Prior detailed ultrasonic imaging to assess the extent of the union, including its involvement of internal organs, is helpful in such cases, and early consultation with the neonatal and paediatric surgical teams is of course essential.

REFERENCES

BAILEY D., FLYNN M., KELLY J. & O'CONOR M. (1980) *Brit. J. Obstet. Gynaec.*, **87**, 561.

BENIRSCHKE K. & DRISCOLL S.G. (1967) *The Pathology of the Human Placenta.* Springer Verlag, Berlin.

BENIRSCHKE K. & KIM C.K. (1973) *New Engl. J. Med.*, **288**, 1276.

BLAKE G.D., KNUPPEL R.A., INGARDIA C.J., LAKE M., AUMANN G. & HANSON M. (1984) *Obstet. and Gynec.*, **63**, 528.

BULMER M.G. (1958) *Annals of Human Genetics*, **22**, 158.

BULMER M.G. (1960) *Annals of Human Genetics*, **24**, 121.

CAMERON A.H. (1968) *Pro. roy. Soc. Med.*, **61**, 229.

CAMPBELL D.M., MacGILLIVRAY I. & TUTTLE S. (1982) *Acta Genet. med.*, **31**, 221.

CARTER C.O. (1965) *Progress med. Genetics*, **4**, 59.

CONDIE R.G. & CAMPBELL D.M. (1978) *Brit. J. Obstet. Gynaec.*, **85**, 37.

ELEJALDE B.R., DE ELEJALDE M.M., WAGNER A.M. & LEBEL R.R. (1983) *J. clin. Ultrasound*, **11**, 442.

ERSKINE R.L.A. & RITCHIE J.W.K. (1985) *Brit. J. Obstet. Gynaec.*, **92**, 605.

GHOSH A., WOO J.S.K., RAWLINSON H.A. & FERGUSON-SMITH M.A. (1982) *Brit. J. Obstet. Gynaec.*, **89**, 817.

GILES W.B., TRUDINGER B.J. & COOK C.M. (1985) *Brit. J. Obstet. Gynaec.*, **92**, 490.

HALL M.M., CAMPBELL D.M. & DAVIDSON R.J.L. (1979) *Acta Genet. med.*, **28**, 279.

HAY S. & WEHRUNG D.A. (1970) *Amer. J. hum. Genet.*, **22**, 662.

ITZKOWIC D. (1979) *Brit. J. Obstet. Gynaec.*, **86**, 23.

KLEBE J.G. & INGOMAR C.J. (1972) *Pediatrics*, **49**, 112.

MACGILLIVRAY I. (1982) *Europ. J. Obstet. Gynaec. reprod. Biol.*, **15**, 263.

MACGILLIVRAY I. (1983) In *Pre-eclampsia: the Hypertensive Disease of Pregnancy.* (MacGillivray I. ed.). Holt-Saunders, Eastbourne.

MACGILLIVRAY I. (1984) In *Progress in Obstetrics and Gynaecology.* (Studd J. ed.), **4**, p. 139. Churchill Livingstone, Edinburgh.

MCILWAINE G.M., DUNN F., HOWAT R.C., SMALLS M., WYLLIE M.M. & MACNAUGHTON M.C. (1985) *Brit. J. Obstet. Gynaec.*, **92**, 9.

NEILSON J.P. (1981) *Brit. J. Obstet. Gynaec.*, **88**, 27.

NYLANDER P.P.S. (1970) *Acta Genet. med.*, **19**, 457.

NYLANDER P.P.S. (1975) In *Human Multiple Reproduction.* (MacGillivray I., Nylander P.P.S. & Corney G. eds.), p. 87. W.B. Saunders, London.

NYLANDER P.P.S. & MACGILLIVRAY I. (1975) In *Human Multiple Reproduction.* (MacGillivray I., Nylander P.P.S. & Corney G. eds.), p. 137. W.B. Saunders, London.

O'CONNOR M.C., MURPHY H. & DALRYMPLE I.J. (1979) *Brit. J. Obstet. Gynaec.*, **86**, 706.

PATEL N., BARRIE W., CAMPBELL D., HOWAT R., MELROSE E., REDFORD D., MCILWAINE G.M. & SMALLS M. (1985) *Scottish Twin Survey 1983: Preliminary Report.* University of Glasgow.

PROKOP VON O. & HERRMANN U. (1973) *Zbl. Gynäk.*, **95**, 1497.

RAUSEN I.R., SEKI M. & STRAUSS L. (1965) *J. Pediat.*, **66**, 613.

REDFORD D.H.A. & WHITFIELD C.R. (1985) *Amer. J. Obstet. Gynec.*, **152**, 550.

RODECK C.H., MIBASHAN R.S., ABRAMOWICZ J. & CAMPBELL S. (1982) *Prenatal Diagnosis*, **2**, 189.

SCOTTISH HOME AND HEALTH DEPARTMENT (1985) *Perinatal Mortality Survey Scotland 1984.* Information Services Division of Common Services Agency, Edinburgh.

TAMBYRAJAH R.L., ATPUTHARAJAH V. & SALMON Y. (1978) *Aust. ZN.Z. J. Obstet. Gynaec.*, **18**, 179.

TOWLER C.M., HORNE C.H.W., JANDIAL V., CAMPBELL D.M. & MACGILLIVRAY I. (1976) *Brit. J. Obstet. Gynaec.*, **83**, 775.

WEEKES A.R.L., MENZIES D.N. & DE BOER C.H. (1977) *Brit. J. Obstet. Gynaec.*, **84**, 161.

CHAPTER 34
NEONATAL CARE FOR OBSTETRICIANS

F. COCKBURN

Birth marks an important and critical stage of maturation for the new human in his progress towards an independent existence. Full independence from parental care normally takes many years to attain and there is evidence that the quality of parenting during pregnancy, birth, infancy and childhood has a marked influence on the quality of that child's subsequent behaviour and life style. The good obstetrician understands the rational and irrational fears, anxieties and expectations of the mother and father of the birth process itself and can help allay them. Improved understanding of the integrated physiological processes surrounding pregnancy, birth, delivery and early nurture has not only played a part in reducing maternal, perinatal and infant mortality but also is revealing the dangers to normal physical, mental and emotional development of the child when these processes are interrupted.

CARDIOVASCULAR ADAPTATION AND THE INITIATION OF RESPIRATION

The structure of the placenta and the fetoplacental circulation are described on pages 104 and 98. Reduced oxygen supply to the fetus, whether due to maternal hypoxia, hypotension or placental insufficiency, results in a range of compensatory fetal responses. These responses are coordinated by an elaborate system of homeostatic mechanisms which safeguard the fetal tissue oxygenation.

FETAL CIRCULATION

A variable proportion of oxygenated fetal blood from the placenta travels from the umbilical vein where the Po_2 is 4.0 kPa (30 mmHg) directly to the inferior vena cava via the ductus venosus. A smaller proportion enters the left lobe of the liver where there is some admixture with portal venous blood (Fig. 34.1).

Most of the inferior vena caval blood is directed through the foramen ovale into the left atrium where it mixes with pulmonary venous blood, enters the left ventricle and from there is pumped towards the head and upper limbs. A smaller flow of inferior vena caval blood enters the right atrium, mixes with poorly oxygenated blood returning from the superior vena cava and enters the right ventricle. From the right ventricle this blood mainly enters the ductus arteriosus, bypasses the lungs and enters the descending aorta. This relatively less oxygenated mixture of blood in the descending aorta supplies the trunk, lungs through the bronchial arteries, abdominal organs, lower limbs and placenta through umbilical arteries. This pattern of circulation is maintained largely through the muscle tone in fetal vessel walls. Pulmonary arterial pressure is higher than left ventricular and aortic pressure because of a higher resistance in the pulmonary arterioles than in the ductus arteriosus and aorta. The muscle tone in fetal blood vessels depends largely on the oxygen content of the blood perfusing them, mediated locally through prostaglandins and also on autonomic activity predominantly affecting the smaller vessels.

LABOUR

The vascular changes associated with gas exchange being transferred from placenta to lungs take place quite abruptly with cessation of umbilical arterial and venous flow and removal of the low resistance placental circuit. Pulmonary arterial blood flow increases dramatically when the infant lungs expand and is the result of a reduced pulmonary arteriolar resistance and functional closure of the ductus arteriosus, ductus venosus, foramen ovale and umbilical vessels. The foramen ovale and ductus venosus close mainly as a result of mechanical pressure changes, but the constriction of the ductus arteriosus and dilatation of the pulmonary arterioles is mediated through the increased oxygen content of blood perfusing these vessels and vasoactive substances. In

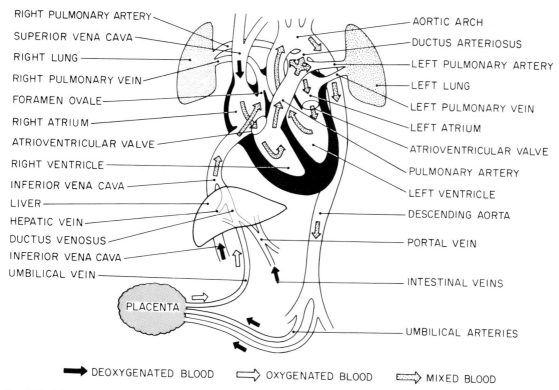

Fig. 34.1 Schematic representation of the fetal circulation.

RIGHT PULMONARY ARTERY
SUPERIOR VENA CAVA
RIGHT LUNG
RIGHT PULMONARY VEIN
FORAMEN OVALE
RIGHT ATRIUM
ATRIOVENTRICULAR VALVE
RIGHT VENTRICLE
INFERIOR VENA CAVA
LIVER
HEPATIC VEIN
DUCTUS VENOSUS
INFERIOR VENA CAVA
UMBILICAL VEIN

AORTIC ARCH
DUCTUS ARTERIOSUS
LEFT PULMONARY ARTERY
LEFT LUNG
LEFT PULMONARY VEIN
LEFT ATRIUM
ATRIOVENTRICULAR VALVE
PULMONARY ARTERY
LEFT VENTRICLE
DESCENDING AORTA
PORTAL VEIN
INTESTINAL VEINS
UMBILICAL ARTERIES

PLACENTA

➡ DEOXYGENATED BLOOD   ⇨ OXYGENATED BLOOD   ⇨ MIXED BLOOD

studies of the isolated ductus arteriosus, prostaglandin (PGF$_2\alpha$) thromboxane A2 (TXA2), acetylcholine, bradykinin, angiotensin, adrenaline and noradrenaline produce constriction. Inhibition of the dilator prostaglandins PGE2 and PGI2, which maintain ductal patency during fetal life, might also contribute to ductal closure. It is the balance between pulmonary vasodilatation and ductus arteriosus constriction which determines the effectiveness of vascular adaptation to birth. Asphyxia of the infant after birth can allow the ductus arteriosus to re-open and the pulmonary vascular resistance to increase, thus restoring the fetal situation and causing profound hypoxia.

FIRST BREATH

There are intermittent fetal breathing movements associated with the electroencephalographic changes of rapid eye movement (REM) sleep throughout pregnancy. The physiological basis for the change to the continuous breathing pattern seen after birth is not known. Within the intra-alveolar spaces and tracheo-bronchial tree of the fetus there is a substantial volume of fluid, some of which is expressed during the normal birth process but most of which is absorbed into pulmonary lymphatics. Table 34.1 summarizes the stimuli which contribute to the initiation and maintenance of postnatal ventilation. None of these factors is essential for the initiation of ventilation, but the stimulation of carotid and aortic body chemoreceptors by low arterial Po$_2$ is a very powerful stimulus. In the normal infant sensory stimuli initiate a first breath of some 30–40 ml air, and this requires the creation of a negative intrathoracic pressure of between -4 and -10 kPa (-40 and -100 cmH$_2$O). This negative pressure opens the terminal airways and expands the stiff (low-compliance) fluid filled lungs. Lung compliance (volume for unit pressure change) increases from about 1.5 ml/cm H$_2$O to about 6 ml/cm H$_2$O, whilst the negative intrathoracic pressures required fall to -5 cm H$_2$O. Infants born at term have an average tidal volume of 20 ml and a breathing frequency of about 30 breaths per minute creating a minute ventilation of about 600 ml/min. Preterm infants may have tidal volumes as low as 5–10 ml. During the first few days of life there may be minor degrees of right to left shunting through the

Table 34.1. Stimuli which may contribute to the initiation and maintenance of respiration in the newborn, assuming intact nerve pathways between receptors and functional respiratory centres and from these centres through the spinal cord and lower motor neurones to the respiratory muscles

Thermal	Chilling through loss of heat at about 2.5 kJ/min
Pain	Skin, muscle and tendon receptors
Pressure	Gravity (departure from liquid environment)
	Increased intrathoracic pressures during delivery
	Increased intracranial pressures during delivery
	Changes in intratracheal and intrathoracic pressure
Tactile	Trigeminal area particularly important
Receptors in lungs and pleura	Hering–Breuer reflex
Receptors in muscle, tendon and joints of limbs, spine and chest wall	Stimulated by alterations in posture during and after delivery
Auditory	
Visual	
Olfactory	
Cord clamping:	
Increased arterial pressure	Carotid barorecptors
Decreased aterial Po_2	Aortic and carotid body chemoreceptors
Increased arterial Pco_2	Direct effect on respiratory centre
Increased arterial [H^+]	

foramen ovale and ductus arteriosus, and because of an inadequate ventilation perfusion balance some blood is not fully oxygenated during passage through the lungs. The ventilation perfusion balance can be aggravated by an absence or deficiency of alveolar surfactant material produced by type 2 alveolar lining cells or pneumocytes. The lipoprotein-surfactant complex lowers surface tension in the fluid film lining the alveolus, and this film can lower surface tension further as alveolar surface area falls during expiration and increase it as alveolar surface area increases during inspiration. Prematurely born infants develop the respiratory distress syndrome when surfactant production is inadequate.

At term the fetal blood haemoglobin (Hb) concentration is between 16 and 18 g/dl and is predominantly (60–80 per cent) fetal haemoglobin (HbF). The Po_2 at which blood is 50 per cent saturated with oxygen in the term fetus is only about 2.6 kPa (20 mmHg) but in the mother about 4.0 kPa (30 mmHg). This difference enables the fetal blood to take up oxygen readily from maternal blood and is due to the greater affinity of HbF for oxygen. Although fetal red cells are avid for oxygen, fetal tissues have a very low Po_2 (approximately 2.0 kPa). The fetus is able to unload more of this oxygen to the fetal tissues because of a higher level of 2,3-diphosphoglycerate in the fetal blood.

ASYPHXIA

The responses of the fetus to asphyxia and haemorrhage during delivery are prompted by chemoreceptor and baroreceptor activity causing release of catecholamines. After an initial period of tachycardia there is a vagal bradycardia so that there is a combined autonomic response when hypoxaemia is severe, similar to those responses found in submerging mammals. In the 'diving reflex' there is a sympathetic discharge with noradrenaline release causing a redistribution of blood flow to increase cardiac, cerebral and adrenal flow and to diminish flow to the skin of the trunk and limbs, skeletal muscle, liver, kidneys and intestine. There is also a vagally mediated bradycardia. Vascular responses to asphyxia and haemorrhage in the newborn infant can be thought of as protective in that they maintain essential blood flow to the heart and central nervous system. During delivery fetal noradrenaline values exceed maternal and this ratio is markedly increased in asphyxial states. Figure 34.2 shows the pattern of events associated with acute asphyxia in the newborn monkey immediately after birth where after a period of hyperpnoea there is a period of initial or primary apnoea. Regular gasping follows the initial apnoea and, after a terminal acceleration in rate but diminution in depth, gasping ceases about 8 minutes after birth. The apnoeic period which follows the last spontaneous gasp is called secondary or terminal apnoea and death will ensue unless resuscitation is

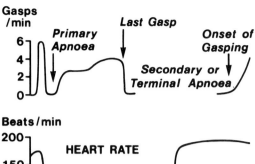

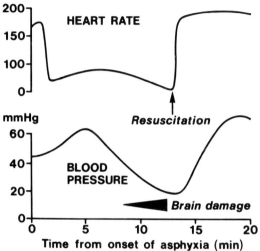

Fig. 34.2 Acute asphyxia in the fetal rhesus monkey (Dawes 1958).

successfully performed. Acute asphyxia of the fetus may occur with sudden complete placental separation or umbilical cord obstruction, but more commonly the hypoxic insult is intermittent or subacute and can be detected with fetal heart monitoring and fetal blood sampling.

RESUSCITATION

Inadequate or delayed resuscitation may lead to permanent brain damage and death. It is preferable to have someone skilled in tracheal intubation present at all high risk deliveries. Most normal newborn infants (75%) respire within a minute of delivery. Most of the rest have breathed before 3 minutes and only about 5% take longer than this.

Assessment

Where possible, it is helpful to commence a time clock at the time of the infant's delivery. It is customary to aspirate the nasal and oral passages carefully immediately after delivery using a sterile, plastic-tipped catheter. This removes the amniotic and lung fluid in the oropharynx and stops the aspiration of blood, meconium and other debris into the upper airway. Excess fluid is normally dried from the infant's skin with a warm towel and the infant checked briefly for

Table 34.2. Clinical evaluation of the newborn infant (Apgar scoring method). Sixty seconds after complete birth of the infant (disregarding the cord and placenta) the five objective signs are evaluated and each given a score of 0, 1 or 2. A score of 10 indicates an infant in the best possible condition

Sign	0	1	2
Heart rate	Absent	Slow (below 100)	Over 100
Respiratory effort	Absent	Weak cry; hypoventilation	Good: strong cry
Muscle tone	Limp	Some flexion of extremities	Active motion: extremities well flexed
Reflex irritability (response to stimulation of sole of foot)	No response	Grimace	Cry
Colour	Blue; pale	Body pink; extremities blue	Completely pink

Apgar score

A clinical score based on heart rate, respiratory effort, muscle tone, responses to stimuli and skin colour was described by Apgar (1953) and has been found valuable in the assessment of the newborn. The Apgar score is usually made at 1 minute after birth and repeated at 5 minutes. A time interval of 1 minute was chosen by Apgar because at this time most infants in her large series had achieved their lowest score. The 5-minute score has been shown to have some correlation with subsequent brain damage whereas the 1-minute score gives some index of the need for active resuscitation, correlates well with biochemical assessment of acidosis and is inversely proportional to the neonatal death rate.

the presence of severe congenital abnormalities such as spina bifida and microcephalus. The Apgar score (Apgar 1953, see Table 34.2) is assessed at one minute and if the infant is apnoeic, gentle sensory stimuli e.g. flicking feet or blowing cold air/oxygen over the infant's face through a face mask should be given. If these stimuli fail to initiate breathing movements, tracheal intubation should commence at two minutes. A heart rate of less than 80/min would be an indication for intubation and ventilation before two minutes of age.

Ventilation

Figure 34.3 shows the technique of tracheal intubation and the appearance of the larynx. Lung inflation at a rate of 20–30 times per minute, maintaining inflation for approximately one second at inflation pressures limited to 30 cm H$_2$O should be instituted. Chest movement should be observed and the chest auscultated to ensure adequate air entry on both sides of the chest. If there is no air entry, the tube is likely to be in the oesophagus and it should be withdrawn and the infant reintubated. Air entry to the right lung alone indicates that the endotracheal tube has entered the right main bronchus and air entry to the left lung usually improves if the endotracheal tube is withdrawn slowly while listening over the unventilated lung. Occasionally a pneumothorax or diaphragmatic hernia can confuse the picture which may be resolved only by chest X-ray. Should the heart rate fail to increase in spite of adequate venti-

lation, it is likely that the infant has a severe metabolic acidaemia and the injection of sodium bicarbonate 8.4% intravenously over 3–5 minutes, 10 ml to a normal term infant and 5 ml to a preterm infant, should be given. If the heart rate remains less than 100, external cardiac massage at 100–120 beats per minute should be instituted. Seven to 10 cardiac compressions should be alternated with 3–4 ventilations. If opiates have been given to the mother in the six hours prior to delivery and the infant fails to establish respiratory efforts, naloxone 0.01 mg/kg can be given by intravenous or intramuscular injection. Even when the respiratory depression is thought to be due to maternal opiates, the same indications for intubation and intermittent positive pressure ventilation (IPPV) should be used. Extubation should be carried out as soon as regular respiration and good colour are observed. When an infant is born without pulsation or heart sounds (Apgar 0–1) but a fetal heart was recorded up to 20 minutes before delivery, intubation, external cardiac massage, intravenous sodium bicarbonate and intracardiac adrenaline 1 ml of 1:10000 iu should be given. If there is no respiratory effort by 30 minutes after institution of resuscitation these attempts should be abandoned. If intermittent but inadequate respiratory movements occur it is then reasonable to ventilate the infant continuously for 24–48 hours, assess the neurological status and make a decision whether to withdraw or continue support.

There is advantage in having a resuscitation unit with overhead heating, a time clock, an oxygen supply and 30 cm H$_2$O pressure valve close to the delivery area. It is most important to maintain the infant's temperature and prevent cooling during resuscitation. It is essential that an appropriate func-

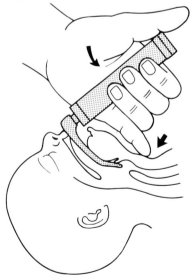

Fig. 34.3 Intubation technique.

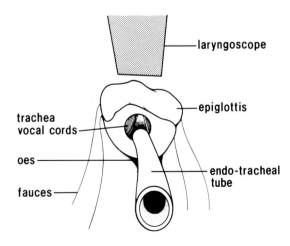

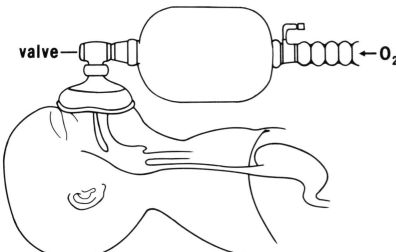

Fig. 34.4 Bag and mask ventilation.

tioning laryngoscope and endotracheal tubes be immediately available in any delivery area, also that suction catheters, intravenous catheters and the required drugs mentioned be immediately available. The initial resuscitation can conveniently be carried out with the infant in a 30° head-down position, but after spontaneous respiration is occurring, the infant should be placed horizontal or in the 30° head-up position.

The majority of infants who require resuscitation can be extubated within 1–2 minutes and are probably not at significant risk and can be nursed with their mothers given adequate nursing supervision. Those requiring longer resuscitation should be admitted to a special or intensive care nursery for subsequent observation for apnoea, convulsions and neurological status. These infants require a check of Hb, blood glucose and blood gas determinations and any abnormalities corrected. If the term infant has no convulsions and is feeding normally within 48 hours, the long term prognosis is usually good.

When there is no one available to perform endotracheal intubation, infants can be resuscitated using a bag and a face mask. Available systems include the Ambu-Oa mask (Ambu International, Copenhagen, Denmark), and the Laerdal mask (Laerdal, Stavanger, Norway). After the airway has been adequately cleared with gentle suction (-5 cm H_2O) the mask is positioned to ensure an adequate face seal and the bag with a 30 cm H_2O leak-valve inflated at a rate of 20–30 per minute (Fig. 34.4). A complication can be gaseous distension of the stomach. Where prolonged bag and mask ventilation is required the insertion of a nasogastric tube can help.

BLOOD LOSS, ANAEMIA AND JAUNDICE

Anaemia

Severe anaemia present at birth is due to haemorrhage or intrauterine haemolysis. When it develops after birth it may be due to internal, external or occult bleeding, to haemolytic disease or to a failure of red cell production.

Haemorrhage

The physical signs of haemorrhage will depend on the rapidity and size of the bleed. Causes are shown in Table 34.3. A rapid bleed of 30–50 ml can cause severe peripheral circulatory failure with tachycardia, tachypnoea, pallor and poor capillary refill on blanching of the skin with finger tip pressure. The Hb concentration can be normal for an hour or so after an acute bleed, but the central venous pressure (CVP) will be low and immediate whole blood replacement is essential.

Anaemia of slower onset results in severe pallor, but less evidence of cardiopulmonary upset; the Hb will be low but the CVP normal or increased. Extreme degrees of anaemia cause hydrops fetalis with enlarged liver and spleen from extra-medullary erythropoiesis.

INVESTIGATIONS AND TREATMENT

Treatment of acute blood loss should not await precise diagnosis. Immediately the airways have been cleared and spontaneous respiration or ventilation

Table 34.3. Blood loss in newborn infants.

Before and during delivery
Fetomaternal transfusion
Fetofetal transfusion in twins
Rupture of umbilical cord vessels
    abnormal vessels—varices or aneurysm
    normal vessels—precipitate delivery
Rupture or incision of placental vessels
    placenta praevia, abruptio placenta and at
    Caesarean section

After delivery
External blood loss
    Cord stump
    Gastrointestinal—haematemesis and melaena
    Skin injury—bruising and incisions
    Oro- and naso-pharyngeal
    Uterine and circumcision loss

Internal blood loss
    Subgaleal and cephalhaematoma
    Intraventricular, subarachnoid and subdural
    Pulmonary
    Adrenal and renal
    Liver and spleen—rupture and subcapsular
    Muscles

established, the umbilical vein should be catheterized and a blood sample withdrawn for measurements of Hb and haematocrit, platelet and reticulocyte counts, blood grouping, Coombs' testing, cross-matching and coagulation defect screen where relevant.

Blood volume expansion with 20 ml/kg body weight group O Rh negative blood should be given immediately into the umbilical vein catheter. If blood is not immediately available, plasma or plasma expander could be used. Dependent upon clinical response, a further 10–20 ml/kg can be given. If circulatory failure has been prolonged, the resulting metabolic acidaemia can be corrected with sodium bicarbonate 8.4% as for asphyxia. Vitamin K1 (2 mg) should be given by intravenous injection. Subsequent management will depend on the origin of the bleeding.

When one monovular twin bleeds into the other, so that one is anaemic and the other plethoric with a high haematocrit, the anaemic one may require a transfusion and the plethoric an exchange transfusion with plasma (20–30 ml/kg) to correct heart failure and the vascular thromboses which occur when the haematocrit exceeds 70%.

When bleeding is not external and the source not clinically evident, the blood loss may be occult into the maternal circulation. Maternal blood should be examined by the Kleihauer technique (p. 265).

Treatment of severe chronic anaemia with increased CVP and heart failure is exchange transfusion with packed red blood cells until the anaemia is corrected.

Haemolytic anaemias

In the haemolytic anaemias the essential feature is a reduced red cell survival time which may be due either to exogenous agents such as maternal antibodies, infections (viral, bacterial and protozoal), hypoxia, drugs or nutritional deficiency (vitamin E) acting on normal red cells, or to genetically determined abnormalities of red cell metabolism (G–6PD deficiency and pyruvate kinase deficiency: galactosaemia) and morphology (e.g. congenital spherocytosis, hereditary elliptocytosis and the haemoglobinopathies).

An increase in unconjugated bilirubin is another common feature of haemolysis when the hepatic glucuronyl transferase enzyme system is unable to conjugate fat-soluble bilirubin released during Hb breakdown into water-soluble conjugated bilirubin which can be readily excreted in stool and urine. Unconjugated bilirubin can penetrate and damage neurones, particularly those of the basal ganglia and brain stem resulting in kernicterus. Children and infants who develop kernicterus may die or be severely handicapped with athetoid cerebral palsy and deafness. The preterm infant brain is more susceptible to such damage. Table 34.4 gives a guide to the investigation of unconjugated hyperbilirubinaemias. It is evident that specific treatments will be required for some aetiologies such as antibiotics for bacterial septicaemias, but the aim otherwise is to keep the concentrations of unconjugated bilirubin below values which are likely to cause brain damage. Fig. 34.5 gives a guide to the use of phototherapy and exchange transfusion in term and preterm infants.

TREATMENT

Exchange transfusion with cross-matched blood is required when severe haemolysis reduces the Hb in cord blood to 10 g/dl or when the unconjugated bilirubin values exceed those shown in Fig. 34.5.

Light energy at a wavelength of 410–460 mmu (i.e. blue light) enhances the degradation of unconjugated bilirubin in the skin to water-soluble, nontoxic products. Important practical aspects of photo-

Table 34.4. Investigation of unconjugated (indirect) hyperbilirubinaemia

Diagnosis	Screen	Investigations
All	General	Family and maternal drug history Plasma concentrations of unconjugated (indirect) and conjugated (direct) bilirubin.
Haemolytic disease Rh (D) ABO, minor groups	Immune	Maternal and infant blood grouping. Maternal serum and infant red cell antibodies.

Viral
Bacterial
Congenital:
  rubella
  cytomegalovirus
  toxoplasma
	Infection	*Infant* Blood, urine, stool and CSF cultures, umbilical swab, nasopharyngeal secretions, chest and long bone X-rays, virology culture and serum antibodies, toxoplasma fluorescent antibody test.
		Maternal Bacteriology and virology, samples and serology, toxoplasma fluorescent antibody test.

Blood resorption
Red cell disorders:
  spherocytosis
  elliptocytosis
  G-6PD deficiency
  pyruvate kinase
Drugs: Heinz body anaemia
Disseminated intravascular coagulation
	Haematological	Hb, PCV, reticulocyte count, blood film, rbc fragility, rbc enzymes, methaemoglobin, coagulation screen, film, degradation products.

Galactosaemia Tyrosinosis Hereditary fructose intolerance Glycogen storage disease	Metabolic	Red cell galactose 1-phosphate uridyl transferase. Urinary reducing sugars. Plasma and urine amino acid concentrations. Liver function tests. White cell glycolytic enzymes.
Respiratory distress syndrome Asphyxia Hypoglycaemia Dehydration	Substrate	Blood glucose, pH, gases, urea and electrolytes.
Prematurity Physiological	Glucuronyl Transferase a) Immaturity	Gestational age assessment.
Breast milk jaundice Crigler–Najjar syndrome Familial transient Hypothyroidism	b) Inhibition or abnormality	Family and drug history. Blood TSH and T4.

therapy are to cover the eyes with a cotton mask to protect against the intense light and to ensure that body temperatures and fluid intakes are maintained.

The early clinical signs of developing kernicterus are increasing lethargy, poor feeding, a weak cry and diminished reflexes which progress to convulsions, apnoea, opisthotonos and death if untreated with exchange transfusion.

Albumin binds unconjugated bilirubin and holds bilirubin in the plasma compartment where it cannot readily diffuse into the tissues and cause kernicteric damage. Acidaemia, low plasma albumin, drugs including sulphonamides and increased plasma free fatty acid concentrations allow free unconjugated bilirubin more readily to enter and damage tissues.

Jaundice which persists beyond the first week in an otherwise mature infant may be due to liver disease or anomaly. If there are increasing concentrations of conjugated bilirubin in plasma, intrahepatic biliary atresia and neonatal hepatitis must be differentiated from extrahepatic atresia and choledochal cysts which are surgically correctable. Open liver

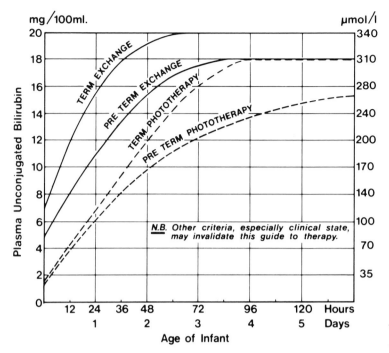

Fig. 34.5 Criteria for exchange transfusion and phototherapy.

biopsy and operative cholangiogram may be necessary to identify the cause of the obstructive jaundice.

Bleeding disorders

The most common causes of bleeding in the newborn are clotting deficiencies (particularly vitamin K dependent factors), thrombocytopenia and disseminated intravascular coagulation. Blood loss from vascular accidents can precipitate a bleeding disorder.

HAEMORRHAGIC DISEASE OF THE NEWBORN

The vitamin K dependent clotting factors (II, VII, IX, X) are normal in term infants at birth but decrease within two to three days. In vitamin K deficient infants there is prolonged bleeding time and bleeding may occur into the skin or gastrointestinal tract at the sites of injections or surgical incisions (circumcision) or internally. Small amounts of vitamin K given orally or by intramuscular injection are sufficient to correct the clotting factor defects unless liver function is immature in a sick or preterm infant. Table 34.5 gives a summary of the differentiation of haemorrhagic disease, consumption coagulopathy and neonatal thrombocytopenia.

HAEMATEMESIS AND MELAENA

Maternal blood may be swallowed during delivery and thereafter vomited. The vomitus may be of bright red or altered blood. Swallowed maternal blood may pass to the stool relatively fresh or altered depending on how long the blood has been in the upper gastrointestinal tract. Clinical evidence of acute blood loss is lacking and blood of maternal origin may be identified in the vomitus or stool by mixing a small amount of red bloody stool or vomitus with 10 ml of water and centrifuging. To 5 parts of the pink supernatant 1 part 0.25 M sodium hydroxide is added. If HbF is present the solution will remain pink, but if maternal (adult) Hb is present it becomes brown.

The newborn infant may bleed into the gastrointestinal tract from local trauma caused by passage of oral and nasal tubes, peptic ulceration, duplication of bowel, Meckel's diverticulum, intussusception, volvulus, haemangioma or telangiectasis of the bowel, rectal prolapse, anal fissure, enteric infections systemic bleeding disorders such as haemorrhagic disease and rarely tumours.

CONSUMPTION COAGULOPATHY

The phenomenon of disseminated intravascular coagulation (DIC) is an important disorder in neonatal

Table 34.5. Neonatal bleeding disorders.

	Haemorrhagic disease	Thrombocytopenia	Consumption coagulopathy
History	Breast feeding	Maternal disease, drugs platelet antibodies	Asphyxia infection and haemolytic disease
Blood film	Normal	Platelet deficiencies and abnormalities	Red cell fragmentation
Platelet count	Normal	Reduced	Reduced
PT	Prolonged	Normal	Prolonged
PT after vit K	Improved	Normal	Unchanged
PTT	Prolonged	Normal	Prolonged
TT	Normal	Normal	Prolonged usually
FDP	Normal	Normal	High

PT	Prothrombin Time
PTT	Partial Thromboplastin Time
TT	Thrombin Time
FDP	Fibrin Degradation Products.

practice. The induction of the coagulation cascade can result in deposition of fibrin throughout the smaller vessels and consumption of coagulation factors, particularly fibrinogen and factors V and VIII, can result in a bleeding problem. Aggregation of platelets involved in the process can produce thrombocytopenia and red blood cells are damaged causing the characteristic fragmentation seen on the blood film. The coagulation disorder can be triggered by Gram-negative bacterial infections, intrauterine and postnatal viral infections, polycythaemia, acute haemolysis, exposure to placental thromboplastins, asphyxia, acidosis and hypothermia. In twin pregnancies the maceration of one may release thromboplastins into the circulation of the other and produce DIC. Purpura and bruising of the skin is a common manifestation and there may also be gastrointestinal bleeding, pulmonary haemorrhage and bleeding into internal organs. In the preterm infant with respiratory distress, intraventricular and periventricular haemorrhage is a feature.

Infants with clinical and laboratory evidence of DIC are best treated by correction of the underlying precipitating cause and judicious replacement of clotting factors with fresh frozen plasma (10 ml/kg), platelet concentrates, cryoprecipitates rich in fibrinogen and prothrombin complex concentrate.

THROMBOCYTOPENIA

In neonatal thrombocytopenia platelet antibodies can sometimes be demonstrated in maternal serum.

Clinical manifestations are variable and depend on the degree of depression of the platelet count. Mild cases have only cutaneous manifestations such as petechiae and purpura, whereas severe bleeding into the gastrointestinal tract, from the nose and umbilical stump and into the brain can occur when the platelet count falls below $20000/mm^3$. Systemic maternal disease such as idiopathic thrombocytopenic purpura (ITP) and systemic lupus erythematosus are associated with thrombocytopenia in mother and infant. Maternal drug induced thrombocytopenia e.g. with quinine or thiazides is rarely associated with neonatal thrombocytopenia and when it does occur the condition is transient. There are disorders where there is inherent platelet abnormality or defective platelet synthesis and more rarely where there is marrow replacement e.g. with leukaemia and neuroblastoma. In the immune thrombocytopenias, treatment for severe haemorrhage can be achieved with compatible screened platelet transfusions.

MAINTENANCE OF BODY TEMPERATURE

The highly metabolically active human fetus generates heat which is removed by placental heat exchange to maternal tissues which are about $0.5°C$ cooler than fetal. Mothers are often uncomfortably aware of their need to lose more heat during later pregnancy. Heat balance in the homeothermic infant after birth has to ensure a deep body temperature of $37°C$. In spite of large variations in ambient ture, the newborn infant is, because of a large surface area and wet skin, susceptible to heat loss and also to excessive heat gain. Whereas in other homeothermic animals, changes in fur and feathers, body position and posture, huddling with others in a nest or against mother, and sprinkling water over their bodies are methods used to maintain thermal regulation, in man clothing, air conditioning and heat systems reduce the extremes of temperature to which newborn infants are exposed.

At lower environmental temperatures more energy has to be expended and more oxygen consumed to maintain the infant's body temperature. The environmental temperature range at which oxygen consumption and metabolic rates are basal is described as the thermoneutral range, and in the first 24 hours of age in the term infant this is 34–36°C and by the end of the first week 30–32°C. Heat loss from the body core to surface is increased by cutaneous vasodilatation and reduced by vasoconstriction. Heat loss from surface to environment is achieved by evaporation from the skin, convection, conduction and radiation. A major factor in the infant's body heat loss is its relatively large surface area to weight ratio. Modern incubators for nursing sick and preterm infants are designed largely to reduce heat loss and can supply warmed humidified air/oxygen mixtures, reduce evaporative and radiant heat losses and maintain a thermoneutral temperature range, thus reducing oxygen requirements to a minimum.

Heat production in the newborn infant may be from skeletal muscle movement, but non-shivering thermogenesis is more important in infants and takes place predominantly in liver, brain and adipose tissues. The average brain weight of a normal 3.5 kg infant is about 400 g and it has been estimated that at rest in a thermoneutral environment the infant brain creates 70% of the total body heat production. At birth there is about 530 g of fat in an average 3.5 kg infant of which 40–50 g is brown adipose tissue. Release of heat from brown fat in response to cooling is mediated by the sympathetic nervous system and release of noradrenaline. Oxygen consumption may double with an environmental temperature change from 32°C to 28°C and most of this increase is related to increased blood flow to and heat production in brown adipose tissue. The white (subcutaneous) fat of infants has proportionately more active cytosol and mitochondria than adult fat but less than brown fat and, apart from its role as a subcutaneous insulator, can release fatty acids to heat producing brown fat and liver cells and can produce some local

heat. Glucose can act as a fuel for cold-induced thermogenesis, but probably contributes less than 20% of the total body heat. Preterm and light for date infants do not have reserves of brown adipose tissue or subcutaneous fat to maintain heat production and are therefore more susceptible to hypothermia. The presence of a hypoxic state will inhibit heat production, and thus a preterm infant with respiratory problems is at increased risk from hypothermia and hypoglycaemia.

The normal infant's body heat is best conserved by nursing the infant clothed in a cot with sides which protect from draughts. The small infant weighing less than 1200 g and larger infants requiring frequent observation and medical attention are most conveniently nursed naked or partially clothed in incubators.

The very preterm infant (less than 30 weeks' gestation) may lose up to 120 ml/kg/day water from transcutaneous water loss which is associated with further massive evaporative heat loss. In order to overcome the evaporative and radiant heat losses of these very small infants environmental temperatures of 38°C or higher may be required and cannot be achieved in standard incubators. Newer double-walled incubators can reduce radiant heat loss and evaporative water loss can be reduced by raising the relative humidity. Overhead radiant heaters unfortunately exacerbate transcutaneous water loss and fluid requirements may need to be increased by up to 30%. Such heaters must only be used with a servo-control from the infant's skin temperature. When the core temperature of an infant falls to less than 35°C the infant should be gradually warmed by placing in an incubator with an environmental temperature kept 1°C above skin temperature until normal body temperature is achieved. The temperature increase usually is instituted at hourly intervals until the core temperature reaches 37°C. It is important to monitor blood sugar by capillary blood Dextrostix estimations four-hourly during the period of rewarming and for at least 24 hours thereafter. Use of translucent bubble thermal blankets can help maintain body temperatures of the very small, immature infants.

EXAMINATION OF THE NEWBORN INFANT

Once the infant has been delivered and respiration established, mother's chief concern will be 'is my baby all right?' In a normal infant the cord is clamped twice at 5 and 6 cm from the umbilicus usually after cord pulsation has ceased, and the cord divided between the two forceps. The infant may then be held closely by the mother. Some obstetricians prefer not to clamp the cord until after the infant has been in skin to skin contact with the mother and the 'bonding process' initiated. Warmth and freedom from draughts are critical to the welfare of the infant at this time. Sterile disposable cord clamps are applied about 1 cm from the umbilical skin and closed by pressure with the fingers. The cord is then cut approximately 1 cm beyond the clamp to prevent it slipping. This clamp may be removed after 24–48 hours. When plastic cord clamps are unavailable, sterile tape ties or rubber bands may be used.

A preliminary examination of the baby should be carried out in the delivery room to establish sex and look for any congenital abnormality of form and to assess any abnormality of function requiring immediate treatment. It is most important that an entirely dependable system of identification should operate for each infant born and the most commonly used method is to write the infant's surname and date and time of birth on a tape or bracelet which is attached to the infant's wrist or ankle in the presence of the infant's mother. After mother has had the opportunity to cuddle her infant and to put him to the breast should she wish to do so, the infant should be placed in a cot previously prepared and kept warm. A suitable environmental temperature for cot and infant is 30°C. The umbilical cord should be checked carefully for bleeding during the first 12 hours and the rectal temperature checked. Weight, length and head circumference should be carefully recorded and daily observations thereafter would include general well being, i.e. skin colour, muscle tone, crying, movement and feeding. Rectal temperature should be recorded daily with low reading thermometers (scale to 25°C); weight daily or at birth, third and fifth days; passage of meconium within 24 hours and passage of urine, again normally within 24 hours. Daily care should involve careful examination of the eyes for infection, the mouth for signs of thrush infection, the skin and particularly the umbilical cord area for infection.

The length, weight and head circumference measurements should be compared with standard charts and those prepared by Gairdner and Pearson (1971) showing 10th, 50th and 90th percentiles for head circumference, length and weight from 28 weeks' gestation to 100 weeks after birth are widely used.

Posture and movement of the infant should be observed. Asymmetry of facial and limb movement, unusual movements or a lack of movement should be noted. Irritability and undue apathy should be looked for. The skin should be carefully examined to note pallor, cyanosis, haemorrhage, jaundice, rashes or birth marks. Careful recording of all observations is essential. If there is considerable moulding or caput, head circumference measurements should be delayed until the 3rd day. Cephalhaematoma do not normally appear until after 24 hours of age. Facial features should be noted and may indicate a diagnosis (e.g. Down's syndrome, fetal alcohol syndrome). Checking patency of the nasal airways should be part of the routine neonatal examination. This can be done by ensuring that the mouth is closed and then occluding each side of the nostrils in turn. Gross distress and indrawing of the chest wall indicates choanal atresia. Examination of the mouth will begin with an assessment of lower jaw development, the size and position of the tongue will be noted and the palate carefully examined for defect. Occasionally one or more teeth, generally lower incisors, are present at birth and are often loose and readily removed.

Examination of the eyes is difficult but with patience and a slow rocking movement from supine to erect posture the eyes will open to allow examination. Detection of cataracts can be difficult. Eye movements are not fully coordinated and momentary squinting is common.

Respiratory movements should not exceed 60 per minute, chest movement should be symmetrical with no indrawing and auscultation should reveal good bilateral air entry. Breast engorgement may occur normally in both male and female infants, reaching a maximum between the 3rd and 5th days postnatally with occasional secretion of colostrum.

Cyanosis indicates hypoxaemia and in the absence of respiratory or haematological problems, this is most likely to be due to shunting of venous blood from the pulmonary to systemic circulation. Radial and femoral pulses should be palpated and compared for both volume and timing. High volume femoral pulses with a cardiac murmur may be an indication of a persistent ductus arteriosus. Murmurs do not in themselves indicate cardiac abnormality unless they persist or are accompanied by other evidence of cardiac defect. Conversely no murmur may be heard in an infant with a major cardiac defect.

Abdominal distension with or without marked peristalsis is abnormal and may indicate the need for immediate investigation, especially if no meconium is evident. There should be three vessels in the umbilical cord; absence of an artery may indicate a congenital skeletal or renal abnormality. Genitalia should be carefully examined as should the limbs, hands and feet.

Assessments of the range of movement at each joint should conclude with examination for the stability of the hip joints. With the infant lying supine, the pelvis is held with the left hand while the right hand holds the left femur between the thumb and forefinger with the end of the finger lying over the greater trochanter. With the femur held vertically, pressure is applied downward and outward and then the femur is lifted forward and pressed inward. The head of the femur will be felt to ride forward and inward as it re-enters the acetabulum if the hip joint is unstable. This movement may be accompanied by a low-pitched clunk. High-pitched clicks without the sensation of the head of the femur leaving or re-entering the acetabulum are not significant. The hand positions should be reversed and the right hip examined. Many unstable joints, particularly following breech delivery, become stable within a few days. The demonstration of instability of one or both hips is an indication for re-examination after an interval of about 4 days. If the hips at the original examination are found to be dislocated without pressure being applied, treatment in an abduction splint should be instituted immediately. In true dislocation, abduction at the affected hip joint is limited and difficulty in abducting either hip to $80°$ should always raise suspicion of congenital dislocation.

Examination of the vertebral bodies and auscultation of the thorax is next performed with the infant in the prone position. Throughout the handling a good assessment of muscle tone can be obtained. The normal term infant should, when left supine, return to a posture in which the limbs are flexed and adducted.

There are a series of reflexes, including: the grasp reflex in both hands and feet elicited by pressing a finger lightly against the palm or sole; the crossed-extension response, elicited by extending one leg and stimulating the sole of the foot which normally should produce a movement of extension and adduction of the other leg; the Moro reflex in which gentle but abrupt neck extension normally results in sudden extension and abduction of the limbs followed by a slower adduction and flexion to the resting position; the rooting response in which the normal infant, when touched on the cheek, turns eagerly to the stimulus and eye movements in which the infant's eyes move in a direction opposite to that of a rota-

tional movement of the infant's head (doll's-eye phenomenon). The responsiveness of an individual infant to these tests depends on a number of factors including the degree of alertness, hunger and well-being. A further important observation is the feeding vigour of the infant and the normality of his or her cry.

At the end of the first week of life, routine capillary blood tests for the presence of hyperaminoacidaemia (phenylketonuria, maple syrup urine disease and homocystinuria), galactosaemia, hypothyroidism and cystic fibrosis are tests for metabolic disorders carried out in some centres. Where abnormalities are found in these examinations a consultant paediatric opinion should be sought.

FLUID AND ELECTROLYTE METABOLISM

After oxygen requirements have been met, the next immediate need for survival in the newborn is an adequate supply of water. It has been calculated that the 28-week-gestation infant might survive for three to four days, the 40- week infant for 30 days and a well nourished adult for 90 days if supplied with water alone. This difference in survival is related to body reserves.

BODY COMPOSITION

Infants are not born nutritionally equal. Some have starved *in utero* because of maternal or placental dysfunction and some are born prematurely without the reserves of nutrient normally laid down in the third trimester of pregnancy. Table 34.6 shows the body compositions of preterm infants who have grown appropriately *in utero*, but delivered at 22, 26, 29 and 40 weeks. As cell division proceeds, the relative amount of extracellular water diminishes. At term, water comprises 69% of total body weight, and about 40% of the total body water is extracellular. Of the total energy in a 1 kg preterm infant, 1.47 MJ (350 kcal) are contained in protein and 0.47 MJ (110 kcal) in fat and carbohydrate. In term infants

Table 34.6. Infantile body compositions.

Gestational age (wk)	22	26	29	40
Weight (g)	500	1000	1500	3500
Water (g)	433	850	1240	2380
Fat (g)	6	23	60	525
CHO (g)	2	5	15	34
Protein (g)	36	85	125	390

the total non-protein energy reserves are approximately 21.0 MJ (5000 kcal). The fat and carbohydrate content of the preterm infant is almost entirely structural and, in the absence of a fresh nutrient supply, tissue breakdown must commence within hours of birth and growth must cease. Growth cannot take place until a minimum balanced fluid and nutrient intake supplying at least 0.47 MJ (110 kcal)/kg/day is achieved. In starvation a minimal catabolic energy release of 0.32 MJ (75 kcal)/kg/day is necessary to maintain life. A further important factor in any consideration of fluid and electrolyte balance is the blood volume. During the first year of life this is about 85 ml/kg and thus the 1 kg preterm infant has a total blood volume of about 85 ml and a plasma volume of about 45 ml. Plasma water in the term infant accounts for 7% of the total body water.

Losses of water from skin and lungs account for the greater part of fluid requirement in the unstressed infant (30–70 ml/kg/day) but this may double when the environmental temperature is increased.

Water tolerance in the immature infant is reduced because of renal immaturity and can be markedly influenced by dietary osmotic load. During the first three days of life the newborn infant has very little response to a water load, but by the fifth day can begin to dilute and concentrate urine. By three months of age a urinary osmolality of 750–1000 mosmol/kg can be reached. Together with the lungs the kidneys play an essential role in the maintenance of acid base balance.

Maintenance of good renal, gut and hepatic perfusion and oxygenation is a vital factor in promoting anabolism and tissue growth. The blood pressure in infancy is around 80/50 mmHg and this lower perfusion pressure may influence renal blood flow and glomerular filtration rate which are dependent on arterial pressure and renal vascular resistance. When an infant is growing satisfactorily there is sufficient renal concentrating capacity and hepatic function to cope with minor disturbance of fluid and electrolyte intake. When growth fails and there is tissue catabolism, such disturbances in intake can be disastrous.

INFANT FEEDING

Successful establishment of breast feeding is essential to the survival of all mammals except when man intervenes. The processes ensuring adequate lactation in the mother, maternal identification of and bonding with her infant and co-ordination of reflex feeding activities by the infant are complex. Colostrum provided during the first few feeds has a greater concentration of protein and minerals than later mature milk and also provides large numbers of leucocytes. Ingestion of colostrum and mature milk provides the infant with passive humoral and cellular immunity through the presence of specific antibodies (particularly secretory IgA), humoral factors (lactoferrin, peroxidase, complement and lysozyme), bifido bacteria and nutrients for these bacteria. Colostrum contains approximately 3×10^6 cells/ml of which 40% are macrophages, 50% polymorphonuclear leucocytes and 7% lymphocytes, with the remainder colostral and epithelial cells. There is an entero-mammary axis whereby secretory IgA antibodies against the various food and microbial antigens, to which the mother's intestinal mucosa has been exposed, are produced in her milk. Consequently the breast fed infant is provided with intestinal mucosal secretory IgA protection against most antigens he is likely to meet in his and his mother's environment. There are in human colostrum significant but smaller quantities of IgG, IgM and IgE. Most, if not all, of the circulating immunoglobulin in the human infant is normally acquired transplacentally. The potential for absorption of antigenically intact food proteins in man exists, but as the gut matures there occurs functional gut closure to these proteins. There are higher concentrations of antibodies to food proteins in preterm infants at 3 to 6 months after birth than in term infants.

Ingestion of human colostrum and milk is gradually established in the first week after birth and the milk intake, together with the utilization of reserves, results in a limited (5%) body weight loss which is regained towards the end of the first week in the normal term infant. Human milk normally provides a balanced nutrient intake of water, carbohydrate, fat, protein, minerals and vitamins. After birth digestion and absorption of human milk is very efficient with about 80% and 90% absorption of proteins and fats respectively.

Hepatic function in the fetus is geared to fetal growth, haematopoiesis and to a certain extent storage of glycogen, minerals and vitamins. After birth enzyme systems such as glucuronyl transferase are switched on and this enzyme enables the infant to excrete bilirubin into the gut and bladder instead of clearing it through the placenta. Degrees of 'physiological' jaundice may occur during the first few days of extrauterine life before this enzyme is fully active.

More severe degrees of jaundice can occur in infants born preterm.

Most mothers find infant feeding, whether by breast or bottle, enjoyable. If a mother sees her baby thriving and contented she will be satisfied and not interested in theoretical calculations as to what her baby should be having. The healthy infant has the appropriate anatomy, strength and neurological maturity to perform the complicated manoeuvre of rooting, fixing and suckling at his mother's breast. The infant normally draws the nipple well into his mouth so that the areola of the nipple lies at the level of his gums. By closing the gums and elevating the tongue, milk is squeezed from the mammary ducts. This milk then enters the pharynx where neuromuscular coordination ensures that the milk enters the oesophagus and stomach and not the lungs. A let-down reflex involving an oxytocic response in the mother will project milk into the back of the infant's pharynx and aid feeding. Infants of less than 34 weeks' gestation or older infants with depression of central nervous system function from whatever cause are unable to coordinate sucking and swallowing and will require to be tube fed. In addition to neurological immaturity, nasal obstruction can cause feeding difficulties.

Healthy term infants breast fed on demand will attain an intake of approximately 150 ml/kg/day by about the 4th–5th day of life. Sick term infants unable to obtain breast milk or modified cow's milk should be fed approximately 40–70 ml/kg/day for the first 48 hours increasing to 150 ml/kg by the 5th day via a 5 French gauge nasogastric tube 4 hourly. The first feed should be given within 6 hours of birth. Preterm or small infants should receive at least 60 ml/kg/day during the first 24 hours, 90 ml/kg/day in the second, 120 ml/kg/day in the third, 150 ml/kg/day in the fourth and 180 ml/kg/day in the fifth 24 hours continuously via a nasogastric tube. Feeding should commence, particularly in the light for date infant, within 1–2 hours of birth. Failure to achieve an intake of 90 ml/kg/day by the third day of life might be an indication for parenteral nutrition to prevent tissue breakdown and tissue damage. When continuous feeding is indicated, an appropriate syringe or roller pump should be used to provide accurate flow rates.

Light for date and preterm infants have limited vitamin reserves and should be placed on vitamin supplements by the tenth day of life if fed enterally and earlier if fed parenterally. An iron containing preparation (6 mg Fe/day) should be introduced by the fourth week of age. All preterm and sick infants should receive 1 mg of vitamin K by intramuscular injection soon after birth. It is important that preterm infants have an early adequate intake of the fat soluble vitamins A, D, E and K. Newer premature infant milk formulae contain higher concentrations of protein, minerals and vitamins to meet their increased requirements for these materials.

The best indicator of appropriate nutrient intake is a good weight gain best judged by plotting the weights on a centile chart, given that there is no evidence of fluid retention (oedema, hepatomegaly, hydrocephalus).

For infants who are unable, because of immaturity or other reasons, to take milk directly from their own mother's breasts it is possible for them to have the nutritional and immunological advantages of breast milk if they are fed on their mother's expressed breast milk (EBM). Direct feeding using mother's EBM is ideal when the milk can be fed fresh. For mothers who have returned to homes at a distance, milk can be collected, pasteurized and stored. Such milk loses some of the potentially protective elements, but retains many not present in artificial milks or sterilized breast milk.

Both breast and bottle fed infants will thrive if receiving a satisfactory intake. Differences in relationships between mothers and infants fed by breast or bottle can be measured, but the long term importance of these feeding patterns on behaviour and emotion is as yet unknown. The establishment of a satisfactory feeding pattern and a happy relationship between mother and infant is more important than theoretical considerations of the relative advantage of one feed over another. This said, every encouragement must be given to mothers to feed their own infants.

CONTRAINDICATIONS TO BREAST FEEDING

There are very few circumstances in which mothers should be advised against breast feeding. Even in conditions such as phenylketonuria, breast feeding can be given as a complement to the low phenylalanine milk diet which is essential. Mothers with chronic respiratory, renal or cardiac disease may be unable to maintain the additional metabolic load of up to 4200 kj (1000 kcal/day). Mothers with potentially infective diseases may be a source of risk to their infants and consideration has to be given as to whether it is safe for the mother to handle the child until the infection has been brought under control (e.g. tuberculosis). Drugs which may be excreted by

Table 34.7. Drugs and breast feeding (with permission from Pitman Medical).

	Anti-inflammatory	Antibacterial agents	Cardiovascular	Endocrine drugs	Nervous system drugs	Other drugs
Not advised	Indomethacin Phenylbutazone	Chloramphenicol Isoniazid Nalidixic acid Tetracyclines	Phenindione Reserpine	Carbimazole Iodides Oestrogens	Lithium Meprobamate	Anthraquinone Antineoplastics Atropine Ergotamine Senna
Doubtful	High-dose salicylates	Aminoglycosides Co-trimoxazole Ethambutol Sulphonamides Nitrofurantoin	Beta-blockers Nicoumalone Thiazide diuretics Warfarin	Oral hypoglycaemics Progestogens Thyroxine High-dose corticosteroids	Carbamazepine Phenytoin Primidone Sodium valproate High doses of: barbiturates benzodiazepines phenothiazines	Propantheline
Advised	Codeine Dextropropoxyphene Flufenamic acid Ketoprofen Paracetamol Pethidine Low-dose salicylates	Cephalosporins Clindamycin Erythromycin Lincomycin Metronidazole Penicillins Rifampicin	Clonidine Digoxin Heparin Methyldopa	Insulins Low-dose corticosteroids	Barbiturates Benzodiazepines Chloral Dichloralphenazone MAOI Phenothiazines Tricyclics	Antacids Antihistamines Bisacodyl Bulk laxatives Recommended doses of iron and vitamins

the mother in her milk in small concentrations are shown in Table 34.7.

A term infant sleeps an average of 15–18 hours a day with periods of sleep lasting 3–5 hours and wakefulness 2–3 hours, usually coincident with feeding behaviour. There is a gradual postnatal reduction in the total duration of sleep to 13 hours by six months of postnatal age.

RESPIRATORY DISORDERS

Intermittent or periodic breathing is common in newborn infants and is usually not clinically significant. In some infants, particularly those born preterm, prolonged respiratory pauses (> than 20 seconds) may be associated with cyanosis and bradycardia. These are called apnoeic attacks and may be a sign of septicaemia, meningitis or intracranial haemorrhage but in the majority of instances in preterm infants are unassociated with any obvious metabolic problem or illness. Neonatal convulsions may present as apnoeic episodes. Careful investigation of the infant for infection, hypoglycaemia, hypocalcaemia and intracranial haemorrhage should be undertaken and oxygen administered if the infant is hypoxic. When no trigger

for the apnoea is found, oral theophylline given in an initial dose of 5 mg/kg and thereafter maintained on the basis of blood concentration measurements (8–15 µg/ml) with a dose of theophylline between 1 and 2 mg/kg 12 hourly may reduce the frequency of the apnoeic episodes.

Respiratory distress

Respiratory difficulties may occur in infants asphyxiated during delivery. This may be from primary atelectasis with failure to expand lungs normally or may be secondary to aspiration of meconium and meconium stained amniotic fluid into the lungs. Postnatal aspiration of gastric contents, particularly in tube fed preterm infants, may give rise to respiratory difficulties. The aspiration of foreign material such as meconium or gastric contents leads to severe irritation of the lungs with congestion, oedema and haemorrhage and with radiological evidence of patchy emphysema, secondary atelectasis and pulmonary oedema. There is usually tachypnoea, costal recession and crepitations on auscultation. The infant usually requires incubator nursing with extra oxygen as necessary and antibiotics given to prevent *E. coli* pneumonia. Some infants with severe meconium aspiration develop pneumomediastinum and/or pneumothorax which may require the insertion of a chest drain.

Transient tachypnoea of the newborn is a condition in which the infant has a moderate degree of intercostal retraction and respiratory difficulty is related to poor or delayed clearing of normal lung fluid. Chest X-ray shows a slightly enlarged heart with streaky infiltrates radiating from the hilum of the lung. Persistent fetal circulation can aggravate this condition as can congenital heart defects with inadequate pulmonary blood flow. Treatment with supplemental oxygen is required for those infants whose arterial oxygen tensions fall below 50–60 mmHg (6.7–8.0 kPa). If blood gas measurements are not available, oxygen supplementation may be administered in concentrations just high enough to relieve cyanosis. When arterial blood gas determinations are available, the arterial Po_2 should be maintained at 70 mmHg (9.3 kPa).

HYALINE MEMBRANE DISEASE

The respiratory distress syndrome associated with hyaline membrane and inadequate surfactant activity may require treatment with continuous positive airways pressure (CPAP) at a pressure of 4–6 cm H_2O. The concentrations of inspired oxygen are adjusted to maintain the arterial Po_2 above 55 mmHg (7.3 kPa). If intermittent positive pressure ventilation (IPPV) is required the lowest peak inspiratory pressures and respiratory rates required to maintain the arterial Po_2 are given. Peak inspiratory pressures rarely should exceed 26 cm H_2O or the rate 30/minute. High frequency ventilatory rates are presently being evaluated. Usually such infants require intensive care management. It is important to ensure that such infants do not have a congenital bacterial pneumonia, particularly with group B streptococcus and to maintain adequate hydration and nutrition. Bronchopulmonary dysplasia may be a long term problem in ventilated infants.

CARDIAC DISORDERS

Early cardiac failure presents usually with tachycardia and tachypnoea and with evidence of fluid retention (peripheral oedema, pulmonary oedema, hepatomegaly and increased CVP).

In the preterm infant a *persistent ductus arteriosus* is the most common cause of congestive heart failure and is associated with full femoral pulses. In the term infant, hypoplastic left heart is the most common cause of congestive failure and differential diagnosis may be quickly clarified by echocardiography.

In *cyanotic congenital heart disease* transposition of the great arteries, severe pulmonary stenosis, large atrial and ventricular septal defects and total anomalous pulmonary venous drainage are to be considered. In transposition of the great arteries it may be critical to maintain a patent ductus arteriosus and this requires infusion of prostaglandin (PGE2).

The treatment of congestive failure requires restriction of fluid intake to 70 ml/kg/day and with a diuretic such as frusemide (1–2 mg/kg/day). If this treatment fails then for a persistent patent ductus arteriosus, indomethacin (2 mg/kg IV on 3 occasions at 12 hour intervals) can be given if there is no thrombocytopenia or increased blood urea. If this management fails or there are contraindications to the use of indomethacin, surgical closure of the ductus is required.

GASTROINTESTINAL DISORDERS

Oesophageal atresia with or without tracheo-oesophageal fistula should be suspected when there has been polyhydramnios. After birth the infant may show the immediate onset of respiratory distress, cyanosis, excessive mucus in the oro-pharynx and choking with feeds. The condition may be diagnosed by failure to place a radio-opaque catheter in the stomach. Frequent or continuous gentle suctioning of the oesophageal upper pouch must be instituted with the infant nursed propped upright until surgical evaluation is made and the type of associated tracheo-oesophageal fistula, if present, ascertained.

The infant with abdominal distension and vomiting must be suspected of having an *intestinal obstruction*. A plain X-ray film of abdomen can frequently confirm the presence of the obstruction which may be a high intestinal one such as duodenal atresia or a mid-gut volvulus where the X-ray will show the level of obstruction. Hypertrophic pyloric stenosis does not usually present with gastric distension and projectile vomiting until the age of 2–6 weeks. Lower intestinal obstruction may be associated with meconium ileus due to cystic fibrosis, Hirschsprung's disease, intussuception, meconium plug syndrome, hypoplastic left colon and imperforate anus. With multiple bowel atresias there are decreased bowel sounds, vomiting and air-fluid levels on abdominal X-ray. Paralytic ileus and necrotizing enterocolitis associated with infectious necrosis of an ischaemic bowel wall may present similar clinical findings. Nutritional support, parenteral if necessary, and early surgical opinion is required.

Omphalocele, in which part or all of the intestine and sometimes the liver and spleen may be visible through a peritoneal sac in relation to the umbilical cord, and *gastroschisis*, in which there is a congenital defect of the abdominal wall with herniation of all or part of the abdominal organs, require early surgical consultation. With omphalocele other congenital anomalies are common and should be sought and assessed before consideration of surgical correction. The defect, if large, should be covered with sterile moist swabs until a surgical opinion is obtained.

In *diaphragmatic hernia* there is herniation of abdominal contents into a hemithorax (usually the left) because of a defect in the diaphragmatic muscle. Infants may present at birth with severe respiratory difficulties, cyanosis and failure to respond to ventilation. There may be hypoplasia of one or both lungs and pneumothorax is a not infrequent complication. Early surgical repair can give good results. The initial management is to insert a large bore open-ended, nasogastric tube into the stomach to prevent gaseous distension of the bowel further embarrassing lung movement.

RENAL DISORDERS

Renal failure may occur in infants who have been asphyxiated and hypotensive during the neonatal period. It may be two to three days before renal flow is restored and the urine will contain protein and red cells if there has been glomerular damage. Fluid restriction will prevent pulmonary and peripheral oedema. Early correction of the hypoxia and hypotension and management of hyperkalaemia will usually allow normal renal function to return.

The incidence of urinary tract anomalies is about 8/1000 births. Abdominal masses in a newborn infant may be due to hydronephrosis, cystic kidneys, renal artery or renal vein thrombosis and rarely due to neuroblastoma and Wilms' tumour. In infants with oligohydramnios and squashed features (Potter syndrome) renal agenesis should be suspected.

Infants with prolonged jaundice, failure to thrive and vomiting may have urinary tract infections and may indicate an underlying anomaly of the urinary tract.

NEUROLOGICAL DISORDERS

Structural defects may be detected by ultrasound prenatally and include microcephalus and hydrocephalus with and without spinal cord defect and spina bifida. Early paediatric opinion is best sought as to whether surgical or other intervention should be advised.

Brain damage in the term infant may be due to perinatal asphyxia, trauma, congenital abnormalities or central nervous system infections. Severe hypoxia may result in severe central nervous system depression immediately after birth and the infant is slow to make spontaneous respiratory efforts, has a high-pitched irritable cry, absent or poor Moro reflex, diminished phasic reflexes, diminished muscle tone and retinal haemorrhages. Over the first 24–48 hours the reflexes become extremely brisk, there is a failure to develop the feeding reflexes and the infant may remain hypotonic or alternatively develop increased tone with opisthotonos and spasticity. If the infant recovers normal tone and develops feeding reflexes quickly, a good prognosis can be given. If the infant fails to develop cough, feeding and gag reflexes, has cranial nerve palsies, disorders of muscle tone, breathing and temperature control after 24–48 hours, the chance of permanent neurological deficit and/or death is high.

Subarachnoid or subdural haemorrhage related to a difficult or precipitate delivery may result in an infant who appears well at birth but who may develop irritability, increased muscle tone, high-pitched cry and convulsions within the first 24 hours. The asphyxiated and the injured infant require careful observation, early correction of hypoxia, hypoglycaemia, hypocalcaemia and blood loss. Ventilatory and circulatory support may be required for a varying length of time. Ultrasound, computerized tomography (CT) and magnetic resonance scans can help the differential diagnosis.

Convulsions occurring soon after delivery in term infants are more likely to be due to intracranial haemorrhage, hypoxia and more rarely to metabolic disorders such as pyridoxine dependency. Infections such as meningitis and encephalitis more commonly produce convulsions after 3–4 days. Hypoglycaemia can cause convulsions and may occur in the infant with intrauterine growth retardation or in the asphyxiated infant and may be associated with lethargy, poor feeding, jitteriness and apnoea. Blood glucose concentrations should be measured frequently during the first few days of life in all infants at risk of hypoglycaemia, particularly light for date infants, infants with rhesus haemolytic disease, infants of diabetic mothers and those asphyxiated at birth, particularly if born preterm. Early institution of feeding should prevent hypoglycaemia in most infants but if this fails, intravenous infusions of 10% dextrose can correct most hypoglycaemic episodes although higher concentrations occasionally may be required.

Hypocalcaemia may occur shortly after birth in association with asphyxia, maternal hyperparathyroidism, infants of diabetic mothers and intrauterine infection. Late onset hypocalcaemia may appear towards the end of the first week of life in infants fed milks with a high phosphorus content. Such infants may be twitchy or tremulous or may have convulsions and administration of intravenous calcium gluconate will stop the convulsions. Occasionally hypomagnesaemia may cause convulsions and can be corrected with intramuscular magnesium sulphate.

Infants of mothers addicted to narcotics may have tremors, irritability, hyperactivity, increased muscle tone and appear excessively hungry and may occasionally have seizures.

When there is no obvious underlying correctable metabolic disorder, control of neonatal convulsions can be achieved by giving phenobarbitone in a dose of 5–10 mg/kg intravenously. Maintenance oral phenobarbitone can be given subsequently at a dose of 5–10 mg/kg/day. If convulsions are not controlled with phenobarbitone, diazepam may be given in a dose of 0.1–0.3 mg/kg by intravenous injection but the half life is short (15 minutes) and respiratory depression may result.

In the preterm infant *periventricular and intraventricular bleeding* from subependymal haemorrhage may present with apnoea or seizures. The extent of the haemorrhage can be assessed by ultrasound. If ventricular dilatation with blood is present, serial ultrasound examinations are required. At present the best management for intraventricular haemorrhage is uncertain. Rapidly increasing ventricular size is an indication for ventricular drainage either intermittent with a needle or by insertion of an appropriate drainage system.

NEONATAL INFECTIONS

Micro-organisms can infect infants *in utero* through haematogenous spread from the placenta, by aspiration from infected amniotic fluid after premature membrane rupture, by colonization during delivery and through damage to the skin and mucous membranes during and after birth. The newborn infant, particularly the preterm infant, is susceptible from immature cellular and humoral immune systems.

Particular attention must be paid to hand washing with a germicidal soap for everyone involved in handling the newborn infant. Great care must be taken to prevent cross-infection and contamination of equipment involved in neonatal nurseries.

A diagnosis of infection may depend on the maternal and obstetric history. Maternal illnesses including urinary tract infection, amnionitis, prolonged rupture of the membranes, genital herpes, syphilis, gonorrhoea, chlamydia, and group B streptococcal infections can help diagnose the cause of the infant's illness. It is helpful to know the results of maternal cultures for the antibiotic sensitivities of the organisms concerned.

An infected infant may be irritable or lethargic, have feeding difficulties, apnoea, peripheral circulatory problems resulting in skin mottling and have difficulty in maintaining body temperature. These signs are non-specific and may result from infections of any part of the body such as meningitis, urinary tract and septicaemia. There may be elevation of the white count, but diagnosis depends on a high index of suspicion and cultures of blood, urine and cerebrospinal fluid together with peripheral swabs of skin and secretions.

In addition to the specific treatment for individual infections, the infant requires careful management of cardio-respiratory failure, fluid and electrolyte balance and nutrition.

SEPTICAEMIA

Escherichia coli and group B *β*-haemolytic streptococci are the two organisms presently responsible for most cases of neonatal septicaemia in the UK. Other organisms which are usually non-pathogenic in older children and adults such as *Staphylococcus albus*, non-haemolytic streptococci and candida may cause severe problems in immature newborn infants. Preterm infants requiring ventilatory support and parenteral nutrition are particularly susceptible and early treatment with appropriate antibiotics and antifungal agents is necessary to ensure undamaged survival. Mortality rates vary between units but even in well staffed and equipped units the mortality may be 20–30% and the subsequent morbidity including mental retardation, deafness and development delay may also be 20–30%.

PNEUMONIA

The lungs may be infected *in utero* as a result of aspiration of infected amniotic fluid before or during birth and tachypnoea, cyanosis and intercostal recession is an indication for tracheal aspirate and blood cultures. A chest X-ray may reveal atelectasis and pneumonia. Treatment includes ventilatory support and antibiotics which will deal with the organisms known to be in the infant's environment. In most nurseries this means the use of antibiotics which will deal with group B streptococcus, *Escherichia coli* and *Staphlococcus aureus*. Early treatment will usually allow complete recovery.

MENINGITIS

Clinical diagnosis of meningitis in the newborn infant is difficult. Although occasionally there may be a bulging fontanelle and signs of meningeal irritation with opisthotonos and seizures, more commonly the infant is found to be apathetic, disinterested and with poor peripheral circulation. Unexplained metabolic acidaemia may be the result of meningitis and/or septicaemia. Lumbar puncture will help identify the organism which may again be *E. coli* or group B streptococcus. The mortality and morbidity rates are similar to those for septicaemia. Complications include cerebral oedema and the later complications of leukomalacia, hydrocephalus, brain abscess and deafness.

URINARY TRACT INFECTION

As part of the screen for any suspected neonatal infection, urine should be obtained for microscopy and culture. If there is albumin and an increased cell count in a bag sample of urine, a further sample of urine should be obtained by suprapubic aspiration for examination and culture. Jaundice may be a presenting feature in an infant with a urinary tract infection. Every neonatal urinary tract infection requires aggressive antibiotic therapy and subsequent investigation of the urinary tract to exclude anomalies.

DIARRHOEA

Acute diarrhoea in newborn infants in a hospital nursery is of major concern. Many such cases are associated with viral enteritis but *E. coli*, klebsiella and salmonella may be involved. In some parts of the world salmonella and shigella cause epidemic diarrhoea in nurseries. Necrotizing enterocolitis may be associated with clostridial organisms. Treatment involves prompt fluid and electrolyte replacement with intravenous therapy if oral therapy is inadequate to maintain circulation and hydration. Specific antibiotic therapy used systemically will depend on the organisms isolated and their antibiotic sensitivities.

OMPHALITIS

Periumbilical redness and oedema indicating cellulitis is an indication for culture of the skin around the cord base and blood culture together with initial treatment with antibiotics for Gram-positive and Gram-negative organisms. When the cultures are available, the treatment can be modified in the light of findings. *E. coli*, streptococci and staphylococci are the common organisms and a major hazard of umbilical cord infection is retrograde progression to cause septic thrombophelebitis, hepatic abscesses, septicaemia and portal vein thrombosis. Such problems are aggravated when umbilical vessels have been catheterized.

SKIN INFECTIONS

The preterm infant's skin is particularly susceptible to minor trauma and is early colonized by organisms in the environment. Severe cellulitis may be due to staphylococci or streptococci and requires systemic antibiotic therapy after culture. Careful skin care using a soap containing an appropriate antiseptic such as Irgasan can help minimize the risks of local and deep infections.

Other specific site infections such as osteomyelitis and otitis media are found in newborn infants and require early diagnosis and treatment, if long term problems such as joint immobility and deafness are to be avoided.

CONGENITAL INFECTIONS

Congenital cytomegalovirus infection usually occurs in an asymptomatic mother and in most instances the infant appears normal. In severe infections the infant may be acutely ill, small for gestational age, have signs of meningoencephalitis, jaundice, petechiae, hepatosplenomegaly and feeding difficulties. The virus may be cultured from urine, upper respiratory tract secretions and cerebrospinal fluid. In milder cases in which there is no clinical evidence of the disease, there are sometimes late sequelae such as hearing loss and learning disorders.

Congenital rubella infection occurs as a result of rubella infection in the mother during pregnancy. This can be associated with major anomalies including microcephalus, congenital heart disease, light for gestational age, cataracts, hepatosplenomegaly, pneumonia, myocarditis, hepatitis and thrombocytopenia with petechiae and purpura. X-rays of the infant's long bones may show characteristic radiolucent areas in the distal metaphyses of long bones. No specific treatment for rubella or cytomegalovirus infection is presently available.

Congenital or neonatal infections with herpesvirus hominis type 2 may cause defects in the brain, eye and liver with jaundice and convulsions. Prevention may be attempted by Caesarean section delivery when maternal genital lesions are present and is best done before membrane rupture. If diagnosed early, in addition to management of cerebral oedema with fluid restriction and mannitol, systemic treatment with acylovir should be given.

Other viral infections. Coxsackie, ECHO, mixo, parvo, varicella and hepatitis B are amongst the viruses to be considered when meningoencephalitis, hepatitis, myocarditis, pneumonias, diarrhoea, jaundice and cataract formation are unexplained. Chlamydial infections may cause severe ophthalmia in the newborn and occasionally are associated with pneumonitis. Treatment with systemic erythromycin and local tetracycline to the eyes is effective.

Toxoplasmosis. Toxoplasma gondii is a protozoon transmitted to the fetus from the placenta *in utero* and is associated with intrauterine growth retardation, cerebral damage and microcephaly or hydrocephaly, choroido-retinitis, microphthalmia, thrombocytopenia and jaundice. The organism may be cultured and the diagnosis confirmed by the indirect fluorescent antibody test in maternal and infant serum. A combination of pyrimethamine given orally in a dose of 0.5 mg/kg twice daily and sulphadiazine given orally in a dose of 100 mg/kg/day is recommended for three to four weeks.

Congenital syphilis can present in the newborn with hepatosplenomegaly, anaemia, thrombocytopenia, jaundice and oedema. There may be characteristic bone changes on X-ray. After three to four weeks a maculopapular skin rash with mucocutaneous lesions, snuffles and pseudoparalyses may develop. Most newborn infants with congenital syphilis are well and the disease does not become manifest for several weeks. At this time jaundice, anaemia, hepatosplenomegaly, oedema and signs of meningitis may develop. This is comparable to secondary disease in the adult.

Adequate treatment of mothers with secondary syphilis detected by routine serological testing should reduce the incidence of congenital syphilis in a community. Prompt treatment of the affected infant with penicillin is indicated if there is clinical or X-ray evidence of the disease, or if cord blood serology is positive and the mother has not been adequately treated. If uncertain, the infant should be given protective penicillin therapy and quantitative serological measurements and physical examinations made at monthly intervals. Infants with congenital syphilis require lumbar puncture and abnormal cerebrospinal fluid is an indication to give crystalline penicillin G, 50000 units/kg by intramuscular or intravenous injection daily in two divided doses for a minimum of 10 days. Infants with normal cerebrospinal fluid should be given benzathine penicillin G, 50000 units/kg by intramuscular injection in a single dose.

Gonococcal infection due to *Neisseria gonorrhoea*, a Gram-negative diplococcus, is a sexually transmitted disease in adults picked up by the infant delivered through an infected vulva. If the diagnosis in mother is known from serum testing or the detection of Neisseria in swabs, a cord blood serum sample should be tested for specific antibody and the test repeated again at 6–12 weeks. Conjunctivitis and keratitis can be prevented with local antibiotic treatment but if a systemic infection with rising titre is present then systemic antibiotic therapy with penicillin is necessary.

If a mother has active *tuberculosis* with positive sputum at the time of delivery, she and her infant can be kept together while both receive treatment. Alternatively the infant can be kept separated until the mother has had at least three weeks active therapy. If isoniazid (INH) resistant BCG is available 0.1 ml of this can be given to the infant together with 20 mg/kg INH per day. The infant should have a tuberculin test at 6–8 weeks; if negative he should be revaccinated and retested 6–8 weeks later. The prophylactic INH should continue until the mother's sputum is negative and the infant has become tuberculin positive. If isoniazid-resistant BCG is unavailable, INH 20 mg/kg/day should be given in a daily single dose starting immediately after birth with isolation for 48 hours from mother. Breast feeding should then be instituted with the infant isolated between times as much as possible from the mother until she is non-infective. BCG does not confer absolute immunity to tuberculosis and occasionally vaccinated infants develop the disease later. Regular supervision and follow-up of mother and infant with adjustment of INH dosage as the infant increases in size should continue for six months when the INH can be discontinued.

Neonatal tetanus can result from the introduction of spores of *Clostridium tetani* to the umbilical cord stump during the cutting or dressing of the cord in conditions where hygiene is poor. Intense muscle spasms of jaw, face, trunk and limbs and convulsions are presenting features occurring two hours or more after birth. Treatment is with penicillin G i.v.– 150000 i.u./kg/day, sedation with i.v. diazepam 1 mg/kg/day in 4 divided doses, tetanus immune globulin 500 i.u. by i.m.i. Tracheal intubation and ventilation with pancuronium paralysis may be required if ventilation and diazepam are ineffective. Active immunization of the population with tetanus toxoid and of the pregnant woman during pregnancy would greatly reduce the risk to the newborn in areas of the world where this problem is common.

Congenital malaria is rare except in non-immune mothers who, during pregnancy, have received inadequate protection or none. The degree of immunity to malaria possessed by an infant at birth is directly related to that of the mother, so that in spite of heavy or massive parasitization of the placenta found in the highly immune indigenous dwellers of endemic areas, the incidence of congenital malaria is rare. When it does occur, fever, convulsions and severe haemolytic anaemia with jaundice, hepatosplenomegaly and brain damage and a high mortality is the result. In the partially immune child less severe infections occur and present with signs similar to that of a bacterial septicaemia. In endemic areas, transfused blood may be an important source of acquired infection in the newborn, which should be treated with a full therapeutic course of chloroquine or other relevant antimalarial drug for that area. Treatment of the infected newborn is usually with chloroquine 5 ml/kg by injection or 75 mg chloroquine base orally followed by 37.5 mg twice daily for two days.

Neonatal hepatitis B (HB) infections are more common in some populations than others, but world wide they are a major public health problem. Neonatal liver disease due to HB viraemia is very variable and can present as fulminant hepatic necrosis, chronic persistent hepatitis, mild focal necrosis or may be asymptomatic. Portal hypertension and primary liver cancers are later complications. The infant is most at risk when the mother has acute HB hepatitis during the third trimester and at delivery. Chronic HB surface antigen (HBs Ag) positive carrier mothers, particularly if they are also HBe Ag positive, HBe antibody negative or have high serum HBc Ab values are highly infective to their infants. In endemic areas, infants act as carriers and excretors of the virus. Protective immunization of susceptible women of childbearing age and of infants within 48 hours of birth, particularly infants born to carrier mothers should be instituted in populations or sub-populations with high rates of HB virus infection.

REFERENCES

APGAR V. (1953) *Anesth. Analg.* **32**, 260.

COCKBURN F. & DRILLIEN C.M. (1974) *Neonatal Medicine.* Blackwell Scientific Publications, Oxford.

DAWES G. (1958) *Fetal and Neonatal Physiology.* Yearbook Medical Publishers, Chicago.

FORFAR J.O. & ARNEIL G.C. (1984) *Textbook of Paediatrics.* Churchill Livingstone, Edinburgh.

GAIRDNER D. & PEARSON J. (1971) *Arch. Dis. Child.*, **46**, 783.

CHAPTER 35
VITAL STATISTICS FOR OBSTETRICIANS

G. V. P. CHAMBERLAIN

Obstetricians, like most doctors, dislike statistics. They try to disguise their distrust but their antipathy stems from two sources: teaching in hospital is aimed at a one-to-one doctor–patient relationship so that the patient with a complaint becomes the conventional modular unit of medical practice and less thought is given to groups of patients with illnesses. Secondly, the basic mathematical processes are poorly developed during medical education. All obstetricians are literate and can read and write; few are numerate so that they can handle data. Innumerate doctors do not try to use collective numerical facts. They condemn all figures in Disraelian terms—'Lies, Damn Lies and Statistics'; in so doing they put to one side a valuable measuring tool which can help evaluate current practice and predict future trends.

In obstetrics vital statistics are related to the data about births and deaths. In this the obstetrician is more fortunate than many other doctors for he has firm measures of outcome to assess. A birth and a death are finite events, usually recognizable by many grades of doctor with low false positive and false negative rates. In consequence, the data are valid, different from statistics derived from morbidity when the interpretation of clinical signs and symptoms varies greatly from one observer to another.

Vital statistics are concerned with birth rates, maternal deaths and deaths of the fetus or newborn (stillbirths, neonatal and perinatal deaths). When any such statistics are quoted, the obstetrician should know their background and from where the data are collected so that the region or country of origin can be identified and the population at risk can be known. This is particularly important when dealing with vital statistics from the British Isles when at different times data are presented for the United Kingdom (England, Wales, Scotland and Northern Ireland), for Great Britain (England, Wales and Scotland), for England and Wales as one unit until 1973 or, more recently, separately for any of the kingdoms of England, Wales, Scotland or Northern Ireland. There are large population differences between the Celtic areas and England, and considerable variations in results exist depending upon which country is studied.

The period of time over which the data are collected should be known. Usually in vital statistics this is a year but it might be a quinquennium. Which year is important for data collection and processing takes time yet the current vital statistics commonly quoted often are three or four years out of date. This matters when there are rapid changes occurring in the population.

It is wise also to know who has dealt with the data. Most vital statistics in England and Wales come through the Office of Population, Censuses and Surveys which used to be the Registrar General's Office. Those for Scotland and Northern Ireland are published by their respective General Register Offices. The information is collected from statutory certification of births and deaths. Some of the material about perinatal deaths comes from non-governmental sources collected by research workers, such as the Perinatal Mortality Survey (1958) or the British Births Survey (1970). The obstetrician looking at vital statistics would do well to check their background. He would want to know where information came from, when and who dealt with it.

Most vital statistics are not expressed in absolute figures but as rates. Since the number of happenings is often small, quoting the rate per 100 would produce figures with many decimal places and so percentages are rarely used and the ratios are more commonly expressed per thousand of the total population. In certain areas, such as maternal mortality, even the number of happenings per thousand is small and this too is becoming a difficult figure to conceive. Such comparatively rare events are now better expressed in ratios per 100 000 of the population or even per million. This is more than just a mathematical trick for it allows the observer to work in whole numbers and even the most numerate prefer numbers to the left of the decimal point than to the right.

BIRTH RATE

In the United Kingdom the number of births is determined from both the registrations and the notifications made in the country. These are probably accurate for there is a statutory obligation to register and the data come from two sources which cross-check each other. There is a legal responsibility for parents to register the birth of a child with the local registrar within 42 days of delivery. That registrar is then responsible to the Registrar General. In addition it is mandatory that any midwife attending a birth informs the prescribed medical officer of the area within 36 hours. This medical officer then notifies the local registrar so that he can check his records and thus contact any parents who may have forgotten to register their child.

The *birth rate* can be calculated from the number of viable births (both live and dead) occurring and the census returns of the population.

$$\text{Birth rate} = \frac{\text{Number of births in the year} \times 1000}{\text{Mid-year population}}$$

The birth rate should perhaps be related to the number of women in the reproductive age group present in a population rather than the total, for no men, and few women below 15 and over 44 years, have children (Fig. 35.1)

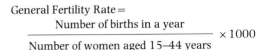

$$\text{General Fertility Rate} = \frac{\text{Number of births in a year}}{\text{Number of women aged 15–44 years}} \times 1000$$

A contraction of this is the *total period fertility rate* (TPFR), the average number of children who would be born per woman assuming those women experienced the age specific fertility rate, in the time considered, throughout their fertile life span (15–44 years) (Fig. 35.2). This is a more precise measure than *completed family size*, a concept which has to be used well after the time and in retrospect.

Figure 35.3 shows in more detail the births in England and Wales of the last 30 years. The rate in 1955 was low having fallen steadily since the post-war boom. It then started to rise for no very well understood reason reaching a peak in 1964. About this time several extrapolations were made about the need for maternity services. These were frustrated by the drop in birth rate which followed so that the birth rate of 11.6 in 1977 is the lowest recorded since the 1930s. After this it has risen slightly until 1980 whence it has returned to 12.1 per 1000 in 1984. Having been misled before, obsteticians should place no certainty on these trends in birth rate when planning future obstetrical or childhealth services. Whilst the overall impression has been downward for over a decade, it is now increasing for a short while but

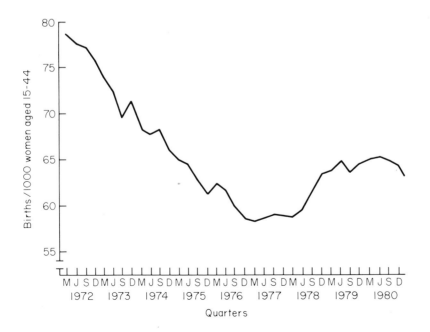

Fig. 35.1. Seasonally adjusted general fertility rates, 1972–1981, England and Wales.

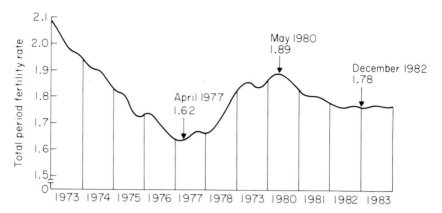

Fig. 35.2. Trend in total period fertility rate, 1973–1983.

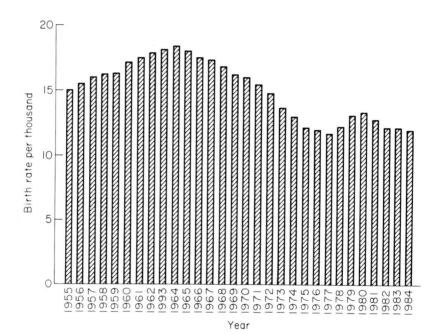

Fig. 35.3. Birth rate (1955–1984) England and Wales.

the variation in birth rate varies in different parts of the country. In the big towns it declines faster than in the countryside and is undoubtedly correlated with the economic situation of the country. Poorer sections of the community have a higher birth rate than the wealthier ones.

Figure 35.4 shows the figures for England and Wales in the last century. When the country is prosperous births boom, and all the contraceptive programmes are put a little to one side. Economic depression is accompanied by a fall of conceptions.

Figure 35.5 shows the population size in the United Kingdom over the last 400 years with a projection for the rest of the century. These are statistical guesses and they have been very inaccurate in the past but they seem to show a continuation of the upward trend.

Underdeveloped countries have a higher birth rate but tend to lose more of their population earlier. Pakistan in the last decade had an average birth rate of 50 per thousand when most European countries, rates were below 20. The highest in Europe was Albania with a birth rate of 35 and in many African countries it is between 35 and 50.

If the birth rate data are properly set against mortality statistics in each age group, a very accurate idea of population trends can be seen. Population projections depend upon four factors: the birth rates

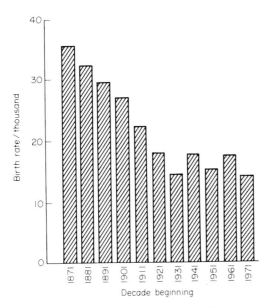

Fig. 35.4. Birth rate (1871–1980) England and Wales.

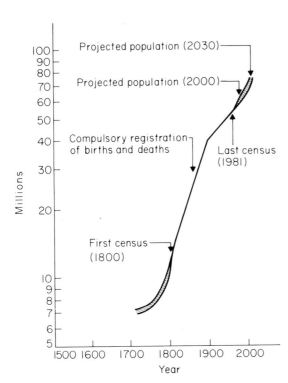

Fig. 35.5. The population of the United Kingdom (1580–2000). (Redrawn from *The Otimum Population of Britain*, Ed. R.I. Taylor, 1969.)

and the death rates obviously act against each other but in addition the number of persons moving into or out of an area by migration must be considered.

Figure 35.6 shows the trend in a developing country—Costa Rica. Here the population structure tapers for the young grossly outnumber the old. As conditions improve in such a society the younger people will live to become older and a more rectangular pattern will follow.

Figure 35.7 outlines the demographic trends for a stable population like Sweden. The birth rate is 14 per thousand and this is matched by deaths at the other end of life. There is little migration in or out so that the trend is roughly rectangular until the late fifties and approximately equal groups are found in each age group until death by ageing removes numbers so that the demogram tapers.

The effects of a major change in birth rates can be seen by examining demograms in a longitudinal fashion. Figure 35.8 shows the effects in the Hong Kong population over 20 years. The bulge in births of the 1960s is working its way through the school years to those of employment.

United Kingdom data are shown in Fig. 35.9. Better nutrition, better health and improved obstetrical services have all contributed to many more lives being saved in the first year of life. This has led to a cohort of ageing people who will eventually overweight the upper end of the demogram. Thus there is a top-heavy structure filling the geriatric wards

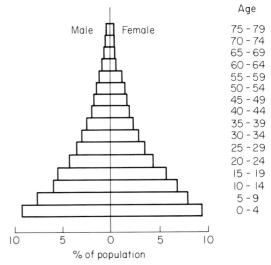

Fig. 35.6. Smoothed-off population demogram from Costa Rica relating percentage of male and female population in each quinquennium to the total population.

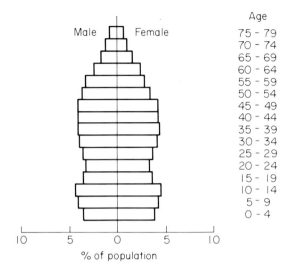

Fig. 35.7. Smoothed off population demogram for Sweden relating percentage of male and female population in each quinquennium to the total population.

now and for the next twenty years. The effects of the reduction in birth rate since 1966 are also seen as a narrowing down at the foot of the diagram.

MATERNAL MORTALITY

A maternal death is one that can be attributed to pregnancy or childbirth. Definitions vary from one country to another but it is considered generally that the death occurs in association with pregnancy, childbearing or in the 6 weeks of the puerperium (the definition used by Fédération International Gynaecologique et Obstetrique—FIGO). Some of the mortalities

relate strongly to the obstetrical event, such as a death after a postpartum haemorrhage, but others have a more tenuous relationship. For instance a suicide occurring at 20 weeks of pregnancy may have been provoked by the pregnancy itself and perhaps would not have happened if the woman had not been pregnant. In Great Britain, deaths up to one year after a birth or an abortion are considered.

International agreement divides maternal deaths into direct and associated. The former result directly from obstetical complications such as bleeding, fitting or infection. The later associated causes are now divided into indirect and fortuitous. The former of these are deaths resulting from a previous existing disease aggravated by the physiological effects of pregnancy. An example would be mitral stenosis. Fortuitous deaths are those among well women who were pregnant at the time of death (or were within a year of it) but the death was apparently not related to the pregnancy, for example a road traffic accident. Differentiation often depends upon the opinion of the clinical advisers. Data put out by different countries should be examined carefully to see what is included in maternal deaths. One major cause of maternal death is abortion and this is not included in all national statistics. Anyone studying international figures should check what is included in the data and, perhaps more important, what is excluded.

Maternal mortality rates (MMR) are expressed relating the number of maternal deaths (MD) to births occurring in the same period of time.

$$MMR = \frac{MD}{Total\ Births} \times 1000.$$

As well as the problem of defining maternal death, there is also a source of error in the denominator.

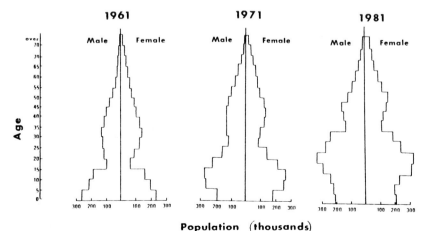

Fig. 35.8. Population demogram for Hong Kong over 20 year period.

Population (thousands)

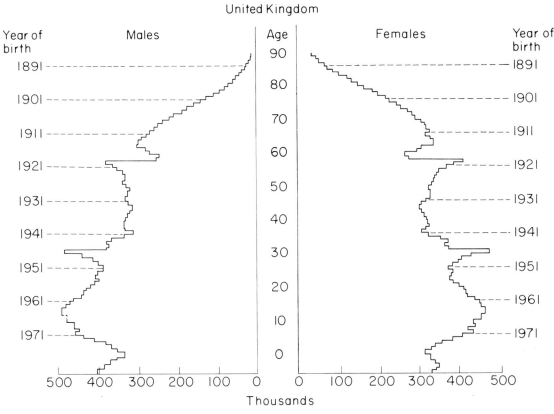

Fig. 35.9. Population demogram for the United Kingdom (1982 data) drawn in annual steps compared with quinquennia used in the previous demograms. This shows changes in finer detail. (Redrawn from *Social Trends*, 1983, HMSO.)

Only births are statutorily registered in this country and not pregnancies; hence the number of pregnancies which finish spontaneously before 28 weeks can be only guessed at, so that the maternal mortality rates in relation to events in the first two-thirds of pregnancy are only approximate.

The maternal mortality rate has been dropping over the last century and Fig. 35.10 shows the steep fall in the last 40 years. In 1980 it was 0.11 per thousand total births in England and Wales or 11 in every hundred thousand births. Much of this improvement is associated with the better health of the population and improved nutrition. Better obstetrical training, the increased use of blood transfusion and antibiotics have had their part to play in this, but the obstetrician should not try to claim all the credit for the improvement in maternal mortality over the century.

The data on maternal mortality are particularly interesting in England and Wales for as well as the

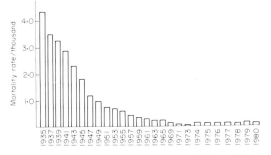

Fig. 35.10. Maternity mortality rates in England and Wales (1935–1980).

statutory returns to the Registrar General, there is a mechanism for examining all maternal deaths in more detail through the Confidential Enquiry into Maternal Deaths, a self-auditing system run by the profession with the help of the Department of Health. The district medical officer, learning of a maternal death in a local hospital or under the care of one of the community midwives, initiates an enquiry by sending a comprehensive form to the obstetrician or, more rarely, the general practitioner involved. Full details of clinical care and, if available, a post-mortem report are added. The form then goes to a regional assessor, a senior obstetrician who assesses the records and adds his views about the cause of death. He further uses his judgement to see if there was any avoidable factor in care, looking for some departure from the accepted standards of care which may have played a part in the ensuing death. If necessary, the assessor can refer again to the clinical or administrative doctors originally dealing with the case. If there are pathological features (e.g. an autopsy) the regional pathology advisor gives an opinion and if anaesthetic procedures have to be considered, a senior anaesthetist is involved at this stage. When the regional obstetrical assessor is satisfied, his report and comments go to a central committee at the Department of Health and Social Security. A small central group of obstetricians, community physicians and anaesthetists collate all these maternal deaths and every three years publish a report on the confidential inquiries into maternal deaths. These reports are a unique form of medical auditing and are no judicial inquiry; efforts are made to prevent identification of individual patients or their attendants. The confidential inquiry team consider maternal deaths reported up to a year after pregnancy or childbirth, thus enlarging on the six weeks limit recommended by the

Fédération International of Gynæcologique et Obstetrique (FIGO).

The last published Report of the Confidential Inquiry into Maternal Deaths (1976–1978) recovered 99% of all known cases, and the major causes of death were pulmonary embolism, toxaemia and haemorrhage, while those associated with abortion were only 8% of the total.

Figure 35.11 shows the main causes of maternal deaths over the previous fifteen years and the proportional drop in each group can be seen. The other major causes of maternal death were ectopic pregnancy (10%), sepsis (7%) and amniotic fluid embolism (5%).

ABORTION

Deaths associated with abortion were usually after procured or illegal interference and the actual cause of death was haemorrhage, sepsis or renal failure. The risks of therapeutic abortion are increased if a concomitant sterilization takes place and the risks of Utus paste in the endocervix has been emphasized for a number of deaths have followed this ineffectual and dangerous medicament. The latest report showed a continued reduction in legal abortion deaths following the Abortion Act (1967). The hope of supporters of that bill that deaths from illegal abortion would be reduced considerably seems to have been justified for they too have been drastically reduced from 51 per million to 7.4 per million. Perhaps even more effec-

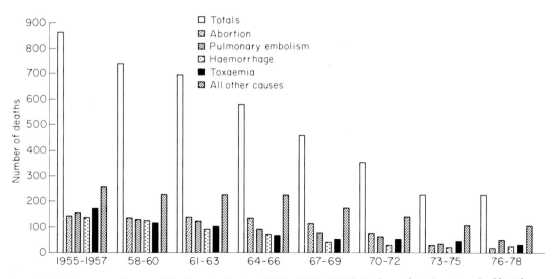

Fig. 35.11. Main causes of maternal deaths in England and Wales (1952–1978). (Redrawn from *Reports on Confidential Inquries into Maternal Deaths.*)

tive than this will be the proper prevention of unwanted pregnancies by the wider use of contraception. The removal of the financial barrier in 1975
has helped patients who would otherwise not have
used an effective contraceptive method.

PULMONARY EMBOLISM

Fatal pulmonary embolism is one of the biggest
causes of maternal death (Fig. 35.12). Two-thirds of
such deaths occur after delivery and about a third in
the antenatal period. All these deaths are secondary
to venous thrombosis but commonly the death is sudden without any warning signs of the predisposing
clotting. In the most recent Report on the Confidential Inquiries (1976–78), 47 women died from pulmonary embolism; 45 had a post-mortem examination and in 16 of these it was considered that the
embolus had come from the leg veins and in 12 from
the pelvic veins, while in a few cases there was
evidence of both pelvic and femoral vein thrombosis.
More commonly in the pelvic veins there is a

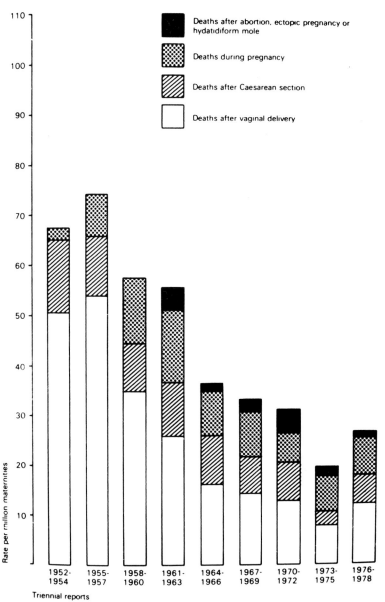

Deaths after abortion, ectopic pregnancy or
hydatidiform mole

Deaths during pregnancy

Deaths after Caesarean section

Deaths after vaginal delivery

Rate per million maternities

1952-   1955-   1958-   1961-   1964-   1967-   1970-   1973-   1976-
1954   1957   1960   1963   1966   1969   1972   1975   1978

Triennial reports

Fig. 35.12. Death rate per
million maternities from
pulmonary embolism,
1952–1978. (With
permission from HMSO.)

thrombophlebitis which is infective in origin producing an unstable and friable clot. In the leg veins there is more usually a phlebothrombosis caused by blood stasis and so a more stable clot is formed but, presumably, there are more leg vein thromboses than pelvic vein ones. Because of the often unexpected nature of the embolism only about a quarter of the maternal deaths were considered to be avoidable. Factors that increased the risk of the pulmonary embolism were a previous episode of thrombosis, an operative delivery (particularly Caesarean section), obesity and the age of the patient.

There is an association of thrombosis, but not necessarily pulmonary embolism, with suppression of lactation by exogenous oestrogens, particularly in the older patient (Jeffcoate et al. 1968). There is also a strong association of embolic disease amongst women of certain blood groups. Jick et al. (1969) showed a significant deficit of Group O patients among women developing thrombosis. However, the Report on Confidential Inquiries into Maternal Deaths shows this deficiency to be less marked (Table 35.1).

Table 35.1. Relation between blood groups and maternal deaths from pulmonary embolism.

Blood group	All Confidential Inquiries 1963–75 (Distribution %)	Expected frequency of blood groups in general population
O	38	46
A	41	42
B	12	9
AB	9	3

Since over half the deaths occur after little warning, preventive measures might be applied trying to detect early thrombosis in the legs or the pelvis, the former being easier for the veins are more available for examination. Each time the midwives make a patient's bed they should squeeze the back of both calves and check for any tenderness. Minor rises of temperature should be noted and investigated accordingly in case they are low-grade pelvic infection which could lead to a thrombophlebitis in the pelvic veins. If there is clinical evidence of a thrombosis, anticoagulation should begin immediately at any time in pregnancy or the puerperium. There is very little risk to a patient in pregnancy from anticoagulation and she can labour with no increased blood loss provided she is properly supervised. There is only slight risk in the puerperium of secondary haemor-

rhage in an anticoagulated patient, so this therapy should be more widely used. Possibly, prophylactic anticoagulation should also be used more (see p. 549). Any woman who has had previous thrombosis in pregnancy should be anticoagulated throughout any later pregnancy, labour and puerperium. This might be extended to treating prophylactically all women having operative deliveries, the over-40-year-olds or the obese. Scanning aids for the diagnosis of peripheral thrombosis may be more widely used in hospitals in this country. Hull et al. (1977) correlated the clinical findings with the use of radioactive fibrinogen scanning of the legs after surgery. Bonnar (1981) reviewed the tests available for the diagnosis of pulmonary thrombosis itself and concluded that arterial blood oxygen estimation and a lung scan provided the best sustantiation to clinical data. The use of Trendelenburg's operation of pulmonary embolectomy should be confined to the occasional occurrence of a pulmonary embolus in a woman who is actually within a hospital which has a cardiothoracic surgical team on site and which is ready for bypass surgery. Transferring such patients to other hospitals has not significantly improved results.

HAEMORRHAGE

Postpartum haemorrhage
Deaths from this cause were reduced at a steady rate until 1966. For the past 20 years however they have not improved, there being 16, 15, 13 and 18 such deaths respectively in the last four triennia reported (Fig. 35.13). Bleeding can follow poor contractions of an atonic uterus after delivery or trauma to the genital tract. Undoubtedly the reduction in deaths following postpartum haemorrhage has been associated with the giving of routine oxytocic drugs. Martin and Dumoulin (1953) were among the first to show that a routine oxytocic given at the end of the second stage could reduce primary postpartum haemorrhage rates to a tenth. Unfortunately a small group of women in the United Kingdom and U.S.A. are rejecting such therapy as a part of naturalistic philosophy of giving birth. They should be watched. Further improvements have followed the delivery of patients in hospitals where blood is readily available. Should a patient who has to deliver in a less well-equipped unit or in her home have a postpartum haemorrhage, the Flying Squad is called; one of the primary functions of this unit is to carry blood so that replacement can be given before transfer to the hospital for such a patient is at grave risk during the time of transport.

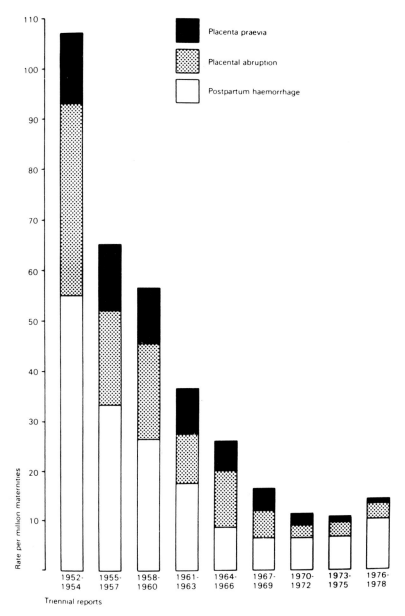

Fig. 35.13. Death rate per million maternities from haemorrhage, 1952–1978. (With permission from HMSO.)

Abruptio placentae

Deaths from this cause are generally reducing. This may be a factor of the lower incidence of this condition but probably also stems from better understanding and management. Early and adequate blood transfusion is now mandatory and central venous pressure recording should be set up. Blood is given until the venous pressure returns to the normal level for by this means serious after-effects, such as renal shutdown, are avoided.

Placenta praevia

This condition is now associated with few deaths, 2 in the three years 1976–1978. Any patient who has bled vaginally in later pregnancy must be referred to a specialist unit quickly and without any vaginal examination having been performed. Diagnostic tests, such as ultrasound or radioisotope scanning, can be applied to check the position of the placenta. If a placenta praevia is present, Caesarean section should be performed at the appropriate time by the most senior person available, for it can be a difficult and bloody operation.

In all the deaths from haemorrhage, increase occurs with age and higher parity—aetiological factors in all three groups. Avoidable factors are thought to be present in over half these deaths and might be due to a poorer standard of antenatal care, too junior staff looking after the patient, or refusal by the patient to accept medical advice about the safest place for treatment or delivery.

TOXAEMIA

In the past it was almost impossible to avoid the use of this antiquated term when both pre-eclamptic women and patients with pre-existing hypertension were grouped together. As well as these, the Confidential Inquiries into Maternal Deaths used to group other conditions into toxaemia such as jaundice and liver disease. In the latest report for 1976–78, hypertensive diseases of pregnancy are considered as a distinct entity although this heading includes all hyper-

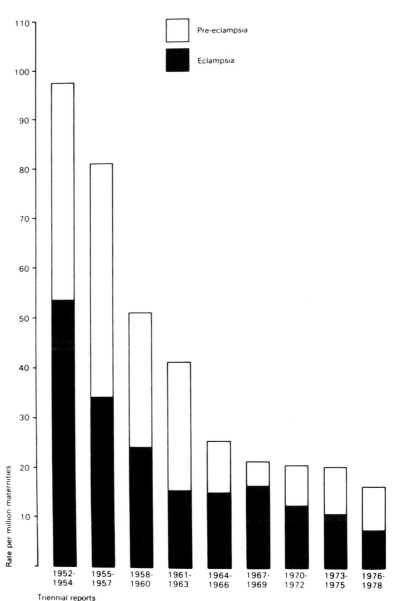

Fig. 35.14. Death rate per million maternities from hypertensive diseases of pregnancy, 1952–1978. (With permission from HMSO.)

tensive conditions irrespective of aetiology. Figure 35.14 shows that the deaths following eclampsia alone have been reduced until the last twenty years when they have stayed steady as have those after all toxaemias. The actual causes of death are mostly cerebral haemorrhage, hepatic failure, cardiac or renal failure. While eclampsia is now being seen proportionately more in the postpartum period, the deaths associated with hypertension are highest in the ante- and intrapartum periods. The earlier in pregnancy eclampsia occurs, the more likely it is to be severe, leading possibly to fulmination and death.

The increased health of the population has reduced pre-eclampsia but this cause of maternal death could be further reduced by frequent checking of blood pressure in pregnancy and, equally important, dealing with patients who show any elevation. It is sometimes hard to persuade a patient who feels well to accept treatment which may mean hospitalization and leaving other members of the family, but by such preventive measures eclampsia and deaths from this cause may be reduced. The reports of the Confidential Inquiries delineate two kinds of temperament seen in patients who refuse treatment. One is the woman who is unable to understand the possible consequences of refusal to act on the advice offered, and the other is the patient who is so utterly devoted to her husband and children that she will not leave them when she feels well.

ANAESTHESIA

Despite the reduction in the number of obstetrical general anaesthetics given in this country, there has been no recent reduction in the number of deaths associated with anaesthesia (Fig. 35.15). Over half of these are due to aspiration of regurgitated stomach contents during the induction of, or recovery from, the anaesthetic. While the need for endotracheal intubation is widely accepted, the skills of those passing the tube may not yet be of sufficient standard. In the Report of the Confidential Enquiry 1976–78 difficulty with intubation accounted for a half of the anaesthesia-associated deaths. The majority were considered unavoidable but were performed by anaesthetists of registrar level or below. General anaesthesia for a woman in labour is a high-risk situation and senior anaesthetists should be available constantly for obstetrical emergencies. As well as death following Mendelson's Syndrome, a high risk is shown in the giving of an anaesthetic to an ill-prepared patient who is already suffering from an

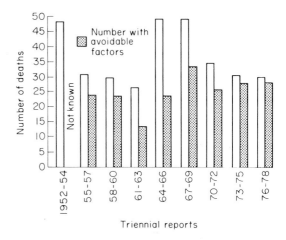

Fig. 35.15. Maternal deaths associated with anaesthesia in England and Wales (1952–1978). (Redrawn from *Report on Confidential Inquiries into Maternal Deaths.*)

obstetrical complication even though she may have been given conventional antacid therapy.

In this section as well as the vital statistics available from the Office of Population Studies and Censuses, the Reports on Confidential Inquiries into Maternal Deaths have been valuable to obstetricians as a further analysis of factors associated with maternal death. These Reports should be read by every obstetrician when they come out, approximately every 3 years, for they are an established example of the medical profession's self-examination of its own actions, and to learn from others' mistakes is less painful than to learn from one's own.

FETAL AND NEONATAL MORTALITY

The number of babies who are born dead and the number born alive but who die in the neonatal period are well recorded for many years. Since the number of total births is also reasonably accurately known, the neonatal death rate and stillbirth rate can be accepted as valid figures. Unfortunately, the first 28 weeks of pregnancy are not so well covered statistically. The number of spontaneous abortions can only be guessed at because the certification of pregnancy itself, as opposed to birth, is not statutory. Hence there are no accurate vital statistics for the first two-thirds of pregnancy, only for the last third. The difficulty of collecting data on the former period is well known to the obstetrician for both the diagnosis of pregnancy itself and that of a spontaneous abortion is sometimes in doubt and both are much more vague than the diagnosis of the birth of a child—a precise, well-observed event. In the past health authorities have been so concerned with the data on viable babies that it has rather put the non-viable to one side. However, as the standard of living improves and fewer babies die, it may be important to seek further back into pregnancy for many of the causes of neonatal and perinatal morbidity and mortality lie there.

If data from conception are treated in a life table, the relative mortality of the perinatal period is well shown (Fig. 35.16). Starting from fertilization, an unknown number of embryos die in the first nine days before implantation (and before the woman can even miss a period). Miller *et al.* (1980) showed this to be 40% in a selected group. Another fifth of known pregnancies in Great Britain are removed by legal termination of pregnancy. Those still surviving have a perinatal mortality rate of about 12 per thousand and infant mortality of those alive after one week accounts for another six per thousand. Thus of 1000 conceptions, over a half are never considered in perinatal or infant mortality figures.

come the time difficulty by imposing a weight standard of 500 g, below which the case is categorized as an abortion. A case can be made for standardizing perinatal mortality rates by birth weight, so eliminating many anomalies of definition and clinical practice.

A neonatal death is a baby born alive but who dies within 28 days of birth. It does not matter whether the baby was born before or after the time of viability at 28th week of pregnancy. This may be changed in the next few years.

Perinatal death is a term used for a total of all the stillbirths and the first week neonatal deaths. There is no statistical grouping of all the stillbirths and all the neonatal deaths (i.e. for the first 28 days). In some European countries the perinatal death period goes as far as ten days and not seven as it is in Great Britain and America. Since the majority of neonatal deaths do occur in fact in the first week of life, the perinatal death group includes the vast majority of all stillbirths and neonatal deaths and probably embraces all for which an obstetrical association may reasonably be sought. However, with greater paediatric skills, more babies are living until the second and

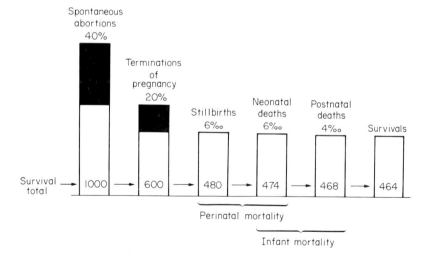

Fig. 36.16. Life table of 1000 conceptions in the United Kingdom in 1981, showing that only 464 survived the first postnatal year.

Figure 35.17 illustrates the definitions of the three major time-groups of death around birth. A stillbirth is a baby born after 28 weeks gestation who shows no signs of life after separation from the mother. This definition can be vague both in the timing of the 28th week, for some women are uncertain of their dates, and in the signs of life after separation. A feeble heart beat might not be recorded or recordable. In other countries some attempt has been made to over-

third weeks of life and so some are doubting the usefulness of perinatal mortality data and are requesting a return to stillbirth and neonatal death rates.

An abortion implies the expulsion prior to the 28th week of gestation of a fetus which showed no signs of life after separation from the mother. Should there be any signs of life, then the fetus should be registered as a live birth and when it dies a few minutes later

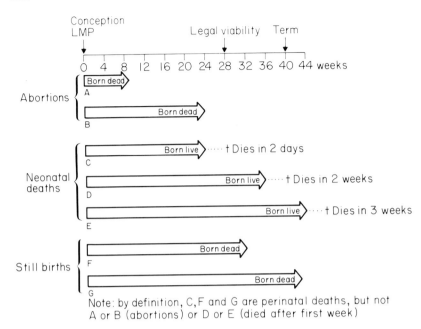

Note: by definition, C,F and G are perinatal deaths, but not
A or B (abortions) or D or E (died after first week)

Fig. 35.17. The time relationship of deaths around birth (see text).

it becomes a neonatal death. There is an obvious anomaly here for while data definition is strict, observers' interpretations vary.

The perinatal mortality rate (PNMR) is the number of perinatal deaths, stillbirths (SB) and first week neonatal deaths (NND), expressed as a proportion of a 1000 total births occurring in the same area at the same time.

$$PNMR = \frac{SB + \text{one week NND}}{\text{Total Births}} \times 1000$$

In the United Kingdom the rate has been dropping steadily for 40 years (see Fig. 35.18).

The perinatal mortality rate in England in 1979 was 14.8 per thousand but since 1973 when the figures have been published separately for England, Wales and Scotland, the wide differences between the three countries which make up Great Britain have been emphasized.

Figure 35.19 shows the perinatal mortality rate in this country in comparison with other European states in 1975. No nationalistic pride should be taken

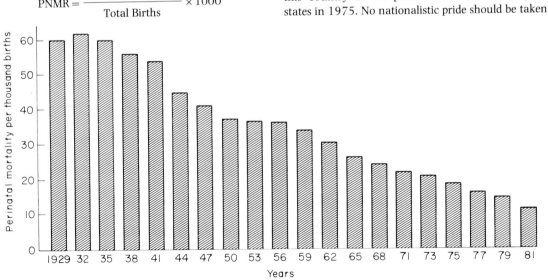

Fig. 35.18. Perinatal death rates in England and Wales (1929–1983).

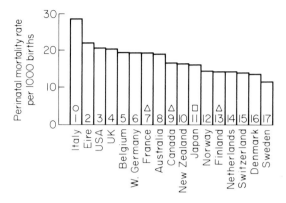

Fig. 35.19. Perinatal mortality rates in various countries for 1975. △ 1974 data; ○ 26 weeks' gestation and above only; □ 28 weeks gestation and above only. From *On the State of the Public Health*, HMSO (1977).

in the position being better than other countries, nor need it be assumed obstetrical services here are that much worse than countries with a lower perinatal mortality rate than our own. Each country has a different population with different nutritional and morphological characteristics. Some are small countries with a uniform population of large women where there has been little poverty in the past. Perinatal mortality rates should be compared only between similar populations. Unfortunately, such rates are not available for all states. In some countries both the biological background of the population and the maternity services might be a lower standard than the western world and perinatal mortality data may be helpful to examine the needs of that society. Such countries, however, do not have a sufficiently sensitive recording system so that the deaths and the births are not known nationally, the information about the perinatal mortality being meagre and coming from a few big centres only.

Many analyses of fetal and neonatal deaths now concentrate on perinatal death rates only. The neonatal and stillbirth rates can be dealt with separately but the combination of these figures does give a guide to the hazards occurring around the time of childbirth. These may be endogenous to the pregnancy and the mother's health or imposed by the care given to that mother and baby. Fuller analyses of perinatal mortality rates try to sort this out but their deficiencies, as pointed out previously, highlight the limitations of these data in sophisticated perinatal units. Most western countries are now examining their data at regular intervals.

Perinatal mortality rates can be calculated for any group of the population and most large maternity units do reckon their own for their annual report. Obviously such data concern a comparatively small number of deliveries and the population attending any one hospital does not reflect accurately the make-up of that region for hospitals tend to have selective programmes of accepting patients. However, hospital data are usually correlated by one person from a set of uniform notes that are kept in a standard way and referral back about doubtful cases can be done readily. Further, examination of yearly trends may indicate the value of some specific obstetrical procedures. Population changes are slow and rapid alterations of perinatal mortality following a change in policy of a hospital may demonstrate the merit of that alteration in management. As an example, Tipton and Lewis (1975) considered that the conjunction of an active abortion policy to reduce the number of congenital abnormalities, a more intensive induction and a wide fetal monitoring policy in labour was associated with a drop in perinatal mortality from 22.2 to 10.6 per thousand in 2 years. Similarly, Edington *et al.* (1975) considered that the drop in perinatal mortality rate from 15.8 to 11.7 per thousand in a year was due to the elimination of intrapartum stillbirths and a significant reduction of neonatal mortality following a widespread continuous fetal monitoring programme in labour. Such changes could be seen only in a limited population, intensively observed and all subjected to the alterations under examination.

At a national level, perinatal mortality rates are estimated from death certification, correlating this with birth notifications. This has the advantage of using large numbers and covering the whole country but obviously it is difficult to investigate restrospectively any doubtful cases. Since changes in management take time to introduce and are patchily implemented, the effects of improvements which follow would be blurred.

There is much debate in the United Kingdom about the use of perinatal mortality rates as a measure of obstetric care. As well as the variations imposed by socio-economic and biological backgrounds there is another feature to be considered. As in other branches of medicine crude death rates are recognized as being too blunt a measure of medical intervention in a disease process. Hence adjusted rates are calculated and standardized mortality rates produced. In the perinatal field birthweight-specific mortality rates would probably be more useful as a monitor of care. A good review of this is presented by MacFarlane *et al.* (1980).

Factors influencing perinatal mortality

The background of the mother and the community in which she lives have a large influence on perinatal mortality rates. Health of the whole community and its nutritional state are important while the efficiency of the health care service and the cooperation between the mother and her doctors are also factors. Running through the whole is the continuing thread of the biological background of age, parity and social class.

Figure 35.20 shows the effect of age on perinatal

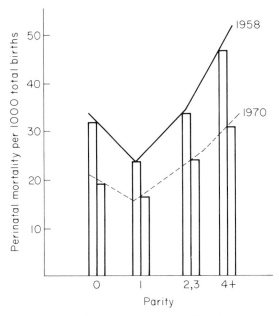

Fig. 35.21. The effect of parity in 1958 and 1970. (Taken from the NBT surveys of those years.)

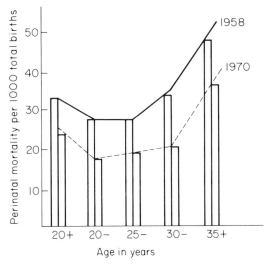

Fig. 35.20. Effect of age on perinatal mortality rates, 1958 and 1970. (Taken from the NBT surveys of those years.)

mortality. Undoubtedly in this country the age at lowest risk in any parity is between 20 and 29 with a higher risk for the very young or old mothers. In the former group, there tends to be a lack of antenatal care, whilst in the latter there is an increased incidence of hypertension and incidental diseases such as diabetes and renal problems. There is possibly also an ageing process of uterine blood vessels.

Higher parity seems to carry an increased risk of perinatal mortality also. It is hard completely to dissociate this from age, for with increasing parity is bound to go an older mother. Figure 35.21 shows this but at all ages, the lowest perinatal mortality appears in the second pregnancy. The first baby may be at greater risk for there is an increased incidence

of pre-eclampsia and more difficult deliveries. It may also be that the uterine vessels are not yet open to their full capacity. Babies delivered after a fourth pregnancy may suffer because there is some maternal rejection of antenatal care and the increased incidence of twinning and malpresentations. Further there may be recurrent thrombosis of the uterine vessels.

A married woman's social class is determined by her husband's occupation, not a chauvinistic ploy but a reasonable way of dividing a population. If the woman's own occupation were to be examined, the vast majority of the married would be housewives, and before marriage they would occupy variations of secretarial, shop assistant and other posts. This would make a meaningless classification.

All occupations have been analysed by the Registrar General and coded into five groups depending on a series of factors of training and managerial capacities (Table 35.2). Such an index should be referred to every time the social class is needed rather than guessing. The unclassified group contains the wives of students, those in the Armed Forces and those for whom no adequate description of the job is available.

The social class of the married women gives a guide to several factors. As well as telling about the present socio-economic state of the family, it gives a good guide to the socio-economic background, the nutritional and the educational development. It is an

Table 35.2

Class	Description	% of total population	% of women having babies
I	Professional workers	3	4
II	Intermediate non-manual workers	15	12
III	Skilled and clerical workers	50	58
IV	Intermediate manual workers	20	11
V	Unskilled workers	8	9
Not Classified		5	6

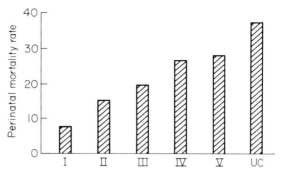

Fig. 35.22. Perinatal mortality rate according to socio-economic status; UC = unclassified. (From *British Births* 1978.)

index compounded from factors arising from parental background, education, early diet, housing, age of marriage and age of childbirth. As shown in Fig. 35.22 social class V has a perinatal mortality four times that of social class I. This is undoubtedly related to past development of the mother. Even worse are the rates for the unsupported mother (the single, the divorced and the widowed).

Another major background variable is the mother's ethnic origin. Some large hospitals in the United Kingdom have up to a quarter of their deliveries among women from non-European races, mostly from the Caribbean zone and the Indian sub-continent. Such women carry with them their past medical history and their background of childhood,

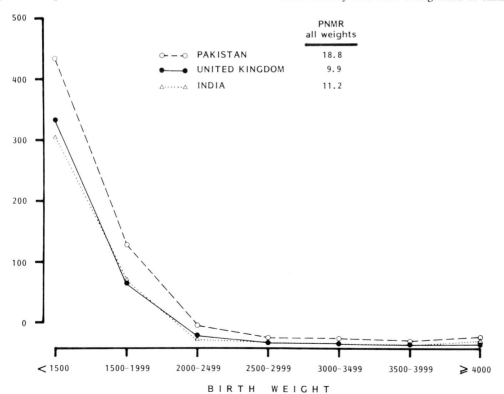

Fig. 35.23. Perinatal mortality in England and Wales by mothers' country of birth.

nutrition and education acquired earlier in life. In addition, even though they live in a United Kingdom environment, they stay in groups of their own sort and so perpetuate dietary and social customs. An example of the effects is seen in Fig. 35.23 where the PNMR for 1983 by birth weight is plotted in the women delivering in England and Wales who were themselves born in India, Pakistan or the United Kingdom. While the U.K. and Indian groups show very similar PNMR at all weight groups, the Pakistani population is consistently worse off, considerably so below 2500 g birth weight.

Associated obstetrical factors in perinatal mortality

Analysis of perinatal deaths shows that they may be associated with maternal conditions in pregnancy and labour and with the management of patients. Antepartum perinatal deaths have a high proportion of toxaemias and abruptio placentae in the current pregnancy. Those occurring during labour are often related to obstetrical care and the place in which the mother is delivered. First day deaths are strongly related to maturity at delivery, although babies with certain congenital abnormalities do die at this time. In the rest of the neonatal period, the second to the seventh day, the commonest causes of death are low birth weight and its associated respiratory distress syndrome. Lesser causes in this time are congenital abnormalities and infection.

Pathological causes for perinatal mortality

The pathological causes of perinatal mortality are those attributed by death and stillbirth certification. The cause written down has to satisfy the registrar of deaths but may not be the real underlying pathology. For example, a baby weighing 900 g when born at 28 weeks' gestation dies 2 days later. The

cause of death might be recorded as Respiratory Distress syndrome and therefore thought to be respiratory but the immaturity of the whole child is the real cause of demise. The specific cause is reported and so is coded and provides information for analysis. It might not truly represent the whole picture.

Usually, the major causes of PNM are low birth weight, congenital abnormalities and asphyxia. Data from England and Wales are shown in Table 35.3.

LOW BIRTH WEIGHT

About 40% of stillbirths and 80% of early neonatal deaths were associated with low birth weight. The definition is one of birth weight less than 2500 g and the problems of sorting out the immature baby from the small-for-dates infant are dealt with elsewhere. Low birth weight is associated with a series of other pathological conditions, such as respiratory distress syndrome and problems of the maintenance of blood pressure, temperature regulation and feeding. The condition could best be treated by prevention of such deliveries. A small number are iatrogenic for inductions are performed to avoid complications to the mother of fetus, e.g. in severe pre-eclampsia. Better understanding and management of such conditions would reduce the need to induce early. More accurate assessment of gestational age before induction reduces incorrectly timed premature deliveries. A major part of the problem of low birth weight follows spontaneous preterm labour. If a mother is going to deliver a preterm baby, she should be in a proper obstetrical unit close to an intensive care baby unit where full care can be given to that child as soon as it is delivered. If such a delivery is inevitable, a labouring woman with a baby *in utero* travels better than an immature child in an incubator.

CONGENITAL ABNORMALITIES

A fifth of stillbirths and a similar proportion of early neonatal deaths had a major abnormality, those of the central nervous system being the most common and accounting for a half of the serious abnormalities (anencephaly and spina bifida).

The treatment of this cause of perinatal mortality is difficult. Obvious teratogens such as thalidomide or X-rays can be avoided in early pregnancy and the worse effects of infections such as rubella guarded against. Genetic counselling of those who have a past or family history of abnormalities may prevent preg-

Table 35.3. Some principal causes of PNMR (percentage of causes that year).

	1971	1976	1983
PNMR (per thousand)	22.3	17.7	10.4
Congenital abnormality	20	21	20
Low birth weight	7	7	6
Asphyxia	17	9	9
Birth trauma	13	10	1

nancies with another abnormality. Amniocentesis done at the correct time may give warning of chromosomal defects or the excessive presence of markers like alphafetoprotein in the liquor in maternal blood may indicate anencephaly or spina bifida. These pregnancies can then be terminated appropriately to prevent congenitally abnormal babies being born. Since abnormalities of the nervous system often have no familial or past history associations, some obstetricians recommend a serum alphafetoprotein test for all pregnant women about 16 weeks of gestation. The implementation of such a programme has great financial implications. Before being introduced in any area, its value must be assessed locally. For example while it would be cost effective in the west side of Scotland and north of England, it would not be so in the southern counties of the United Kingdom where abnormalities of the central nervous system are so much less common (Report of Working Party on Neural Tube Defects 1979).

ASPHYXIA

Post-mortem evidence of asphyxia is found in a half of stillbirths and a tenth of early neonatal deaths. Before labour, this may happen acutely at an abruptio placentae. More probably poor placental exchange will be diagnosed because of poor fetal growth in the last weeks of pregnancy. In labour, uterine contractions may cut off the venous return from the placental bed and later its arterial supply. Such babies at risk for poor placental exchange of oxygen in labour can be pinpointed in the antenatal period because of poor growth in the last weeks of pregnancy. This cause of death might be prevented by selecting the correct groups and seeing that they are delivered in the correct place with fetal monitoring. However, Edington et al. (1975) have indicated that the prediction of high risk groups is not good enough; they showed an improvement in perinatal mortality rates, particularly for intrapartum hypoxia, by monitoring all fetuses during labour, for they consider that prediction of risk is not fine enough. A compromise between what might be ideal and resources available will have to occur here. A rare cause of hypoxia in labour is cord prolapse. At delivery there may be depression of respiration of the newborn baby from analgesic drugs given to the mother in late labour; this may need reversing.

National perinatal mortality rates from different communities have been used to indicate a postpartum cause of hypoxia. Cross and Bolton (1974) pro-

duced a hypothesis that the limitation of oxygen therapy, because of the risks of retrolenal fibroplasia, is responsible for many deaths in preterm infants from lack of oxygen.

BIRTH INJURY

As a cause of perinatal death, this is rapidly reducing so that in 1983 in only 1% was there evidence at post mortem of birth injury. This may be associated with too fast a delivery because of rapid contractions or an immature fetus; a breech presentation with insufficient time for moulding of the fetal head may also be associated with birth trauma. There may be too difficult a delivery because of the misdiagnosis of the degree of disproportion or a malperformed operative delivery with forceps. Prevention of birth injury is very much a factor of obstetrical care and has been reduced considerably in the last decade.

HAEMOLYTIC DISEASE

This accounted for only 0.45% of perinatal mortality in 1983. It has been reduced considerably in this country due to the active programme of rhesus antibody detection and the giving of gammaglobulin to prevent immunization after delivery. Where such programmes are not available, perinatal deaths do occur from hydrops fetalis, which usually results in a stillbirth, or after delivery from kernicterus or anaemia in the newborn.

RESPIRATORY DISTRESS SYNDROME

This is associated with immature babies and with the reduction of that, the incidence of respiratory distress will also decline. In 1983, 7.6% of perinatal deaths were attributed to this cause. Its treatment has improved particularly by having the child in an intensive neonatal care unit; intermittent positive pressure oxygen and biochemical monitoring have contributed to the cure rates.

INFECTIONS

These may occur either during intrauterine life, particularly after prolonged rupture of the membranes, or in the neonatal period. The latter is often associated with overcrowding of the babies and infection from staff or mothers. Infections that may be associated with a high mortality rate are of the alimentary tract (gastroenteritis) or the respiratory tract (pneumonia). Infections are not a common cause of peri-natal death in this country (0.7% in 1983) but may be so in those where there are poorer standards of hygiene or maternity care.

Factors that may reduce perinatal mortallity

A better standard of living of the whole population is one of the surest ways to reduce perinatal mortality. Both improved nutrition and prevention of disease are important; education of the mother to explain why antenatal care is important and equally how to space families to healthy intervals with contraception will improve results. The Health Services might provide more acceptable antenatal care and concentrate on moving mothers into intensive care units at the time of maximum need so that they and their babies may have the best facilities. The antenatal detection of high risk groups could lead to effective monitoring of those who need it during labour when it can be shown to be associated with some reduction in peri-natal deaths from hypoxic causes.

If modern knowledge and resources of perinatal care were made generally available throughout the country, mortality might be reduced by a further third. All these factors should be the aim of the obstetrical services in order to provide a healthier population. Reduction of perinatal mortality carries with it a proportional but much greater reduction in morbidity and thus produces a population better con-ditioned to deal with the future.

REFERENCES

BONNAR J. (1981) *Clin. Obstet. Gynaec.*, **8**, 455–73.

BUTLER N.R. & ALBERMAN E.D. (1969) *Perinatal Problems*. E. & S. Livingstone, Edinburgh and London.

CHAMBERLAIN G., PHILIPP E.E., HOWLETT B. & MASTERS K. (1978) *British Births 1970*. Vol II. William Heinemann Ltd., London.

CROSS K.W. & BOLTON G. (1974) *Lancet*, **i**, 445.

DANIEL D.G. (1969) *Amer. Heart. J.*, **78**, 720.

EDINGTON P.T., SIBANDA J. & BEARD R.J. (1975) *Brit. Med. J.*, **3**, 241.

HULL R., HIRSCH J., SACKETT D.L., POWERS P., TURPLE A. & WALKER I. (1977) *New Engl. J. Med.*, **296**, 1469.

JEFFCOATE T.N.A., MILLER J., ROOS R.F. & TINDALL V.R. (1968) *Brit. med. J.*, **4**, 19.

JICK H., WESTERHOLM B., VESSEY M.P., LEWIS G.P., SLONE D., INMAN W.H.W., SHAPIRO S. & WORCESTER J. (1969) *Lancet*, **i**, 539.

MACFARLANE A., CHALMERS I. & ADELSTEIN A. (1980) *Health Trends*, **12**, 45.

MARTIN J.D. & DUMOULIN J.G. (1953) *Brit. med. J.*, **2**, 643.

Reports on Confidential Inquiries into Maternal Deaths in England and Wales (1952–4, 1955–7, 1958–60, 1961–3, 1964–6, 1967–9, 1970–2, 1973–5). HMSO, London.

Report of Working Party on Neural Tube Defects (1979) DHSS.

MILLER J., WILLIAMSON E., GLUE J., GORDON Y., GRUDZINSLAAS J. & SYKES A. (1980) *Lancet*, **ii**, 556.

TIPTON R.H. & LEWIS B.V. (1975) *Brit. med. J.*, **i**, 391.

CHAPTER 36
THE COAGULATION AND FIBRINOLYTIC SYSTEMS, AND THEIR DISORDERS IN OBSTETRICS AND GYNAECOLOGY

P.W. HOWIE

There are a number of clinical problems in both obstetrics and gynaecology which involve the coagulation and fibrinolytic systems and these will be discussed in this chapter. In order to understand the pathophysiology of these disorders, it is first necessary to consider the mechanisms responsible for normal haemostasis.

Normal haemostasis and the vascular tree

The normal function of the coagulation and fibrinolytic systems is to maintain an intact but patent vascular tree. Three main components play a part in normal haemostasis: vascular constriction; the formation of a platelet plug; and fibrin generation. The fibrinolytic system is complementary to these activities and is responsible for the removal of fibrin and the restoration of vascular patency (Sherry *et al.* 1959).

Vascular constriction and the formation of a platelet plug are not by themselves sufficient to maintain adequate haemostasis. In haemophilia, haemorrhage may be initially arrested by a platelet plug but, if this is not stabilized by fibrin, haemostasis is deficient and subsequent bleeding will take place. Under normal circumstances, the aggregation of platelets and the formation of fibrin take place simultaneously at the site of blood vessel injury. Although the steps leading to platelet aggregation and fibrin formation will be discussed separately, they are interdependent processes which have a common function to seal deficiencies in a damaged vascular tree.

PLATELET FUNCTION

Platelets play an important role in maintaining the integrity of the vascular tree by sealing microscopic defects in vascular endothelium with microthrombi. These microthrombi are either digested by fibrinolysis or washed away by the blood stream. Prostacyclin (PGI_2) is a potent antiplatelet agent released by vas-

cular endothelium which limits the size of these microthrombi and prevents overt thrombus formation. It has been suggested that there is a balance between the actions of prostacyclin and the powerful platelet aggregating properties of thromboxane which is released by the platelet itself (Moncada & Vane 1979). If there is any imbalance between these two, the end result can be a predisposition to either bleeding or thrombosis.

If a large injury occurs in a blood vessel, the exposure of collagen in the basement membrane stimulates a very rapid adhesion of platelets to seal the defect. Following the initial phase of adhesion, platelets change shape from discs to spheroids and form pseudopodia. This shape change stimulates the platelet reaction in which ADP, ATP, serotonin and other active agents are released to stimulate further platelet release aggregation and the formation of a platelet plug. Without adequate numbers of normally functioning platelets, the initial phase of haemostasis is abnormal and petechial haemorrhages will be the clinical result.

FIBRIN FORMATION—THE COAGULATION SYSTEM

To secure haemostasis, it is necessary for fibrin to bind and stabilize the platelet plug. In large blood vessels platelets may be unable to seal a defect on their own and haemostasis will depend largely upon effective vasoconstriction and fibrin formation (Letsky 1984).

The formation of fibrin from fibrinogen (factor I) is the end product of a complex cascade of enzymatic reactions (McFarlane 1964, Davie & Ratnoff 1964) the product of each reaction being an active enzyme which initiates the next stage of the sequence. The introduction of Roman numerals to describe each clotting factor by international agreement has helped to clarify confusions of nomenclature. Plasma coagulation factors and their corresponding Roman numerals are listed in Table 36.1, and the range of values found in normal pregnancy in Table 36.2. The letter 'a' is added to the Roman numeral to indicate the activated form of the enzyme which is ready to catalyse the next reaction of the sequence.

As can be seen from Fig. 36.1, prothrombin (factor II) is split enzymatically by the prothrombin converting principle to release biologically active thrombin (factor IIa). The prothrombin converting principle, which consists of activated factor X and factor V with phospholipid, can be formed by two different pathways. The first pathway, the extrinsic pathway, is activated when blood comes in contact with injured tissues. The tissue factor activates factor VII which in turn activates factor X. Phospholipid, which is supplied by platelets, will combine with Xa and Va to form the prothrombin converting principle and this

reaction will lead to the formation of fibrin within a few seconds. The second pathway is the intrinsic pathway, which is activated when abnormal vascular endothelium or sub-endothelial substances such as collagen stimulate factor XII, the 'contact' factor, to initiate the cascade series of reactions. The formation of prothrombin converting principle by this pathway is much slower, and is the mechanism whereby fibrin can be formed within an intact vascular tree.

ACTION OF THROMBIN

When thrombin is formed, the first traces convert factors V and VIII into their activated forms to potentiate the intrinsic pathway and create a second more explosive burst of thrombin formation within a few seconds (Rapaport *et al.* 1963). In this way, a

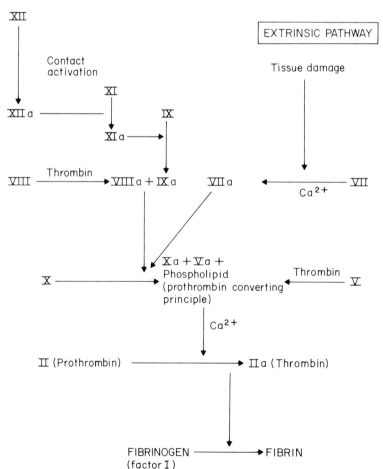

Fig. 36.1 Components of the coagulation system

Table 36.1. Nomenclature of the coagulation factors by international agreement

Factor Number	Name
I	Fibrinogen
II	Prothrombin
III	Tissue factor
IV	Calcium
V	Labile Factor
	AC-globulin
VI	Proconvertin
VIII	Anti-haemophilic factor
	Anti-haemophilic globulin
XI	Christmas factor
	Plasma thromboplastin component
X	Stuart Prower factor
XI	Plasma thromboplastin antecedent
XII	Hageman factor
XIII	Fibrin stabilizing factor

Table 36.2. Comparison of coagulation factors and inhibitors between non-pregnancy and late pregnancy. (From W.E. Hathaway & J. Bonnar (1978) *Perinatal Coagulation*, with permission from the authors and Grune & Stratton, New York.)

Factor	Non-Pregnant	Late Pregnant
Fibrinogen	2–4.5 g/litre	4.0–6.5 g/litre
Factor II	75–125%	100–125%
Factor V	75–125%	100–150%
Factor VII	75–125%	150–250%
Factor VIII	75–150%	200–500%
Factor IX	75–125%	100–150%
Factor X	75–125%	150–200%
Factor XI	75–125%	50–100%
Factor XII	75–125%	100–200%
Factor XIII	75–125%	35–75%
Antithrombin III	85–110%	75–100%
Antifactor Xa	85–110%	75–100%

relatively minor stimulus to the coagulation system can generate highly efficient fibrin formation within a short time. The main action of thrombin, however, is to split fibrinopeptides A and B from fibrinogen to form fibrin monomer; fibrin monomers can combine to form long chain fibrin polymers which are unstable forms of fibrin. Factor XIII, the fibrin stabilizing enzyme, transglutaminase, is also activated by thrombin to stimulate the formation of chemical bonds between fibrin polymer chains and this stabilizes the fibrin molecule.

A failure of normal fibrin formation, which is a cause of bleeding problems, may result from a number of factors. There may be insufficient fibrinogen for conversion to fibrin, but, if this is the only abnormality, fibrinogen levels have to be very low before a clinical problem is apparent. There may also be deficiencies in one or more of the clotting factors, leading to defective thrombin generation. If this occurs, the response to a haemostatic challenge may be insufficient and bleeding will be the end result. Finally, a failure of normal fibrin stabilization leads to the formation of loose clot formation which may be unable to secure effective haemostasis. Fibrin degradation products can interfere with fibrin stabilization and add to the problems of coagulation failure. When there is a clinical bleeding problem in obstetrics, it is usual to find that there are multiple factors operating to interfere with the haemostatic mechanisms.

COAGULATION INHIBITORS

In order to limit the action of thrombin *in vivo* to the site where fibrin formation is required, there are a number of coagulation inhibitors circulating in the blood. The most important of these factors is antithrombin III which is an α_2 globulin, and an inhibitor of both thrombin and activated factor X (Biggs *et al.* 1970). When the generation of thrombin is very high, near the site of vessel injury, the neutralizing action of antithrombin is insufficient and fibrin formation results. As the distance from vessel injury increases, antithrombin levels become sufficient to neutralize the diminishing thrombin activity and thrombus formation is inhibited. The potential clinical importance of antithrombin activity is illustrated by those people who have congenital antithrombin III deficiency because they have a very high risk of fatal thromboembolic disease early in life (Egeberg 1965).

FIBRINOLYSIS

Fibrin is broken down by the action of the proteolytic enzyme plasmin, which is derived from its inactive plasma precursor, plasminogen (Fig. 36.2). Fibrinolytic activity is dependent upon fibrinolytic activators which can be extracted from most human organs, except the placenta. Plasminogen activator activity is mainly centred round the walls of blood vessels and is greater in veins than in arteries (Todd 1964). When plasmin acts upon fibrin, or fibrinogen, fibrin degradation products are formed; the larger molecular weight products are called X and Y and the smaller fragments are termed A, B, C, D and E.

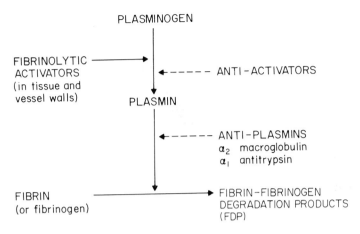

Fig. 36.2. Components of the fibrinolytic system

Because these fragments are not thrombin clottable, they can be measured in serum or in urine and are an index of active fibrinolysis having taken place.

Because plasmin can digest a variety of substrates, it is essential that its activity should be restricted to the dissolution of fibrin clots. There are powerful inhibitors of plasmin and plasminogen activators in the circulation and these are able to prevent and neutralize free plasmin activity. The two main anti-plasmins are alpha$_2$ macroglobulin which reacts quickly but reversibly with plasmin, and alpha$_1$ antitrypsin which reacts more slowly but firmly to produce an inactive complex. When fibrin is formed plasminogen is adsorbed onto the substance of the deposit but antiplasmins are excluded so that blood clots carry within themselves the seeds of their own destruction. When plasminogen activator diffuses into the clot from the vessel wall, plasmin is generated and digests fibrin in an environment free from inhibitors. If plasmin spills into the circulation, it will be immediately neutralized by antiplasmin. If there is an explosive generation of plasmin, antiplasmins may be overwhelmed and free plasmin may appear in the circulation, leading to a 'plasminaemic' state. It is important, therefore, to distinguish between localized and systemic fibrinolytic activity, the former being a physiological response to fibrin deposition and the latter being a highly dangerous pathological process.

COAGULATION AND FIBRINOLYSIS SYSTEMS IN PREGNANCY

Placental separation during the third stage of labour represents a major haemostatic challenge to the mother. Although myometrial contraction is of major importance in constricting the blood vessels in the placental bed, adequate fibrin generation is also required. Physiological adaptations occur during pregnancy to help the mother to meet this haemostatic challenge, and, taken together, the change in coagulation and fibrinolysis in pregnancy represents a 'hypercoagulable' state.

COAGULATION SYSTEM DURING PREGNANCY

Plasma fibrinogen concentrations rise during pregnancy by about 50% and, taking the increase in circulating plasma volume, this means that double the amount of fibrinogen is available to the pregnant woman at delivery compared to the non-pregnant state. Concentrations of many of the other clotting factors also rise during pregnancy, especially prothrombin and factors V, VII, VIII, IX, X and XII (see Table 36.2). Notable exceptions are factors XI and XIII whose concentrations fall during pregnancy.

Despite the increased potential to form thrombin in pregnancy, there is no compensatory rise in antithrombin III (Howie et al. 1971). Because antithrombin III is probably identical to heparin cofactor, this may, in part, account for the relative resistance to heparin during pregnancy (Bonnar 1976).

The platelet count shows little, if any, change during the course of normal pregnancy and most studies have reported that tests of platelet function and platelet lifespan during pregnancy do not differ from the non-pregnant state (Shaper et al. 1968, Rakoczi et al. 1979).

Thrombin activity during pregnancy
The raised levels of clotting factors do not automatically mean that there is increased clotting activity

during normal pregnancy. There are two tests, however, which suggest that there is an increase of thrombin activity during normal pregnancy. Fibrin polymer complexes are generated by thrombin activity and, using fibrinogen chromatography (*see* Fig. 36.3), a small rise of these complexes has been shown

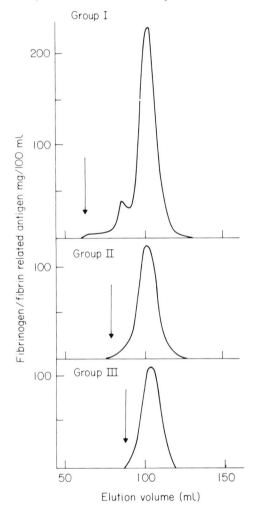

Fig. 36.3. Representative fibrinogen/fibrin related elution curves from a pre-eclamptic patient (group I), a normal pregnant control (group II) and a normal, non-pregnant control (group III). The curve indicates the volume at which FR antigen was first eluted. Compared to non-pregnancy the shift to the left in normal pregnancy indicates an increased concentration of fibrin polymers. The even greater shift to the left, together with a separate peak, in pre-eclampsia indicates a very high concentration of circulating fibrin polymers in this condition. From McKillop *et al.* (1976) with permission from the authors and the Editor of *Lancet*.

during normal pregnancy (McKillop *et al.* 1976). The second test is the factor VIII antigen-activity ratio; when factor VIII is activated by thrombin, it loses its coagulant activity but retains its antigenic potential so that increase in antigen relative to coagulation activity is a sign of thrombin action. A rise of factor VIII antigen-activity ratio has been described in normal pregnancy, suggesting that an increase of thrombin-like activity is a protective mechanism for the normal pregnant woman (Thornton & Bonnar 1977).

Fibrinolysis during pregnancy

Plasma plasminogen levels rise during pregnancy in tandem with the rise of fibrinogen so that there is an increased potential to generate plasmin (Bonnar *et al.* 1969). By contrast, the euglobulin lysis time, which essentially measures plasminogen activator activity, is markedly prolonged suggesting a sharp reduction in the immediate availability of plasminogen activator in the blood (Bonnar *et al.* 1969). Antiplasmins also rise during pregnancy (Howie *et al.* 1971) so that the capacity to generate plasmin may be reduced; nevertheless, there is good evidence that, if the stimulus to fibrinolysis is sufficiently strong, the pregnant woman is able to generate plasmin in adequate amounts and clear the circulation of unwanted fibrin clots.

COAGULATION AND FIBRINOLYSIS DURING THE PUERPERIUM

Following delivery, major changes occur in the coagulation and fibrinolytic systems. The most dramatic change is the rise in plasminogen activator activity (as measured by the euglobulin lysis time) which returns to the non-pregnant range within 30 minutes of delivery (Bonnar *et al.* 1969). On the other hand, fibrinogen levels and the platelet count rise during the early puerperium and these changes may contribute to an increased risk of thrombosis at this time. Antithrombin activity, however, rises as well and this may be a compensatory mechanism to balance those changes which predispose to thrombosis. Following the initial phase of increased clotting factors in the puerperium, the coagulation and fibrinolytic systems gradually revert to normal and all tests are within the normal non-pregnant range six weeks after delivery (Howie *et al.* 1971).

EFFECT OF OESTROGENS ON COAGULATION AND
FIBRINOLYSIS

There is now a well established link between high-
dose oestrogen–progestogen oral contraceptives and
thrombo-embolic disorders (Inman & Vessey 1968).
The high-dose oestrogen pills induce some but not all
of the changes in coagulation and fibrinolysis which
are observed during pregnancy. The pill increases levels of fibrinogen and factors II, VII and X (Poller &
Thomson 1966). In addition, antithrombin III activity falls and antiplasmin rises, both effects being
related to the oestrogen but not to the progestogen
component of the pill (Howie *et al.* 1970). Although
plasminogen levels rise in response to oral contraception, the prolongation of the euglobulin lysis time,
which is characteristic of pregnancy, does not occur.
It has been reported, however, that women who developed thrombosis during oral contraception had deficient release of fibrinolytic activator from vessel
walls in response to venous stasis (Astedt *et al.* 1973).

Similar changes in the coagulation and fibrinolytic
systems have been reported following the use of oestrogens to suppress lactation in the puerperium (Daniel *et al.* 1968, Howie *et al.* 1975). Because of the
epidemiological evidence implicating oestrogens in
puerperal thrombosis (Jeffcoate 1968), this form of
therapy to suppress lactation should no longer be
used.

There is less agreement about the extent of the
changes in coagulation and fibrinolysis associated
with hormone replacement therapy. Although some
studies have reported changes in clotting factors and
antithrombin III similar to those induced by oral contraceptives, others have not found such effects (for
summary of results see Notelovitz & Ware 1982). In
general, it would seem that the lower oestrogen doses
of hormone replacement therapy induce quite small
changes in the haemostatic mechanisms and their
clinical importance has yet to be established.

Venous thrombo-embolism

There are three factors which can influence the formation of thrombin within the vascular tree, namely
the condition of the vessel wall, blood flow and the
constituents of the blood. All of these factors may be
altered during pregnancy to predispose towards
thrombus formation. Blood vessels may be damaged
by hypertensive disease, by operative surgery in the
pelvis or by pelvic infection. Blood flow, particularly
in the veins of the lower limbs and pelvis, may be

reduced by pressure from the pregnant uterus and
bed rest, for any reason, will aggravate venous stasis.
Finally, the constituents of the blood are changed in
a hypercoagulable direction, so that it is not surprising that venous thrombo-embolism is a potential
complication of pregnancy and the puerperium. In
gynaecology, the post-operative period is the major
time of potential danger as is the case after all surgical procedures.

Venous thrombo-embolism can exist in three
forms, namely superficial thrombophlebitis, deep venous thrombosis and pulmonary embolism. Although
it is convenient to discuss them as separate clinical
entities, they represent a spectrum of the same
clinical problem, with increasingly severe implications for the patient as one form of the disease progresses to the next.

INCIDENCE OF THROMBO-EMBOLISM IN
PREGNANCY

The reported incidences of thrombo-embolism in
pregnancy have varied widely, but the risk in pregnant or puerperal patients is about five times greater
than in normal non-pregnant women of the same
age (Siegel 1972). Because diagnosis is difficult, the
incidence of thrombo-embolism may be seriously underestimated but the range of estimates extends from
0.18 to 2.9 per thousand (Villasanta 1965). If superficial thrombophlebitis is considered as well, the incidence of thrombo-embolism rises to 14 per thousand (Aaro *et al.* 1966). Maternal deaths due to
pulmonary embolism have fallen less rapidly than
deaths from other causes and retain an important
place in the league of maternal mortality. The figures
from the Confidential Enquiry into Maternal Deaths
in England and Wales are shown in Table 36.3. The
majority of deaths occur in the puerperium and are
more common after Caesarean section than after vaginal delivery. It is important to remember, however,
that many of the Caesarean sections have associated
complicating factors, and these antecedent events
may be the major explanation for the increased risk
of pulmonary embolism after abdominal delivery
(Aaro & Juergens 1974). Nevertheless, it is a matter
for concern that the most recent confidential report
on maternal deaths has described a rise in maternal
deaths from pulmonary embolism after a succession
of years which reported progressive falls. The increase
was due to more deaths in the puerperium after both
Caesarean section and vaginal delivery. When avoidable factors were considered to be present, the most

Table 36.3. Maternal deaths due to pulmonary embolism in England and Wales (1961–78). (From *Reports on Confidential Enquiries into Maternal Deaths in England and Wales.*)

	During pregnancy No.	After vaginal delivery No. (rate/million)	After Caesarean section No. (rate/million)	Total No.
1961–63	47	66 (40)	27 (360)	140
1964–66	27	43 (20)	25 (270)	95
1967–69	28	36 (20)	18 (180)	82
1970–72	25	30 (10)	17 (160)	72
1973–75	17	15 (10)	6 (70)	38
1976–78	16	22 (15)	9 (77)	47

frequent problem was a failure to recognize and treat the clinical signs of deep vein thrombosis or pulmonary embolism. It is clear that continuous clinical vigilance is required to reduce the tragedies associated with postpartum thrombo-embolism. On the other hand, 19 of the 31 deaths in the puerperium occurred without warning. Improvement in these figures will be achieved only by methods of prevention and prophylaxis.

A number of other factors are associated with an increased risk of thrombo-embolism in pregnancy and these include maternal age, parity and obesity. Prolonged bed rest during pregnancy or any other factor leading to venous stasis will predispose to thrombosis in the deep veins of the legs or pelvis. Patients at particular risk are mothers with severe pre-eclampsia who are rested in bed prior to delivery by Caesarean section (de Swiet 1984).

In addition, any mother who has had a previous episode of deep vein thrombosis or pulmonary embolism, whether it be during the existing pregnancy, a previous pregnancy or during oral contraception, must be considered 'at risk'. The concept of the 'at risk' mother is important because it is used to determine those mothers in whom it is appropriate to consider preventive measures.

CLINICAL FEATURES

Superficial thrombophlebitis
The clinical features of superficial thrombophlebitis are easily recognized. There is a reddened, tender area in relation to a superficial vein with surrounding oedema and inflammation. If the thrombosis is limited to the superficial veins, there is no immediate hazard to the patient. If extension to a deep vein occurs, then the potential risk of pulmonary embolus increases greatly. When superficial phlebitis is present, active mobilization of the affected limb

should be encouraged and the local application of a kaolin poultice may be comforting. The condition will usually resolve spontaneously within a few days.

Deep venous thrombosis
The clinical signs of deep venous thrombosis vary widely. At one end of the clinical spectrum, the patient may have severe pain and develop an oedematous white leg due to extensive iliofemoral thrombosis. The old name given to this syndrome was phlegmasia alba dolens but the full blown clinical picture is now seen infrequently. At the other end of the spectrum there may be no abnormal clinical signs and pulmonary embolism may be the first evidence of thrombo-embolic disease. Modern methods of investigation have shown that asymptomatic deep vein thrombosis is relatively common, particularly after gynaecological surgery (Friend & Kakkar 1972). Many cases fall between these two extremes and clinical signs may be very difficult to interpret. The classical signs of deep vein thrombosis are oedema, calf tenderness and a positive Homans sign, which is calf pain on dorsiflexion of the foot. Clinical signs alone are unreliable and if ascending phlebography, or some other confirmatory test, is not used, it has been estimated that two out of three patients will be treated unnecessarily (Ramsay 1983). Because anticoagulants carry risks in pregnancy, it is important that their use should be restricted only to those who require them. In addition, a diagnosis of deep vein thrombosis has implications for advice about the wisdom of future pregnancies, the use of oestrogens for contraception and the need for anticoagulation at future operations. It is clearly important, therefore, that confirmatory investigations should be undertaken when the diagnosis is in doubt.

PULMONARY EMBOLISM

Major pulmonary emboli are associated with acute respiratory and cardiovascular symptoms. Acute chest pain, breathlessness, cyanosis and haemoptysis may be accompanied by hypotension and collapse. There may be a third heart sound, parasternal heave and a raised jugular venous pressure. The patient is acutely ill and may die within an hour of the onset of symptoms.

The clinical signs of smaller pulmonary emboli are not always obvious and may easily be ignored. There may be transitory dyspnoea, a tinge of cyanosis or some pleuritic chest pain. During the puerperium, an unproductive cough, an unexplained pyrexia, a tachycardia or a leukocytosis can be signs of pulmonary embolism and may merit detailed investigation. In other cases, pulmonary embolism may precipitate wheezing and be diagnosed as asthma (Windebank *et al.* 1973).

It is important to diagnose small pulmonary emboli because they may be followed by larger, and possibly fatal, embolic events. A high index of clinical suspicion is required on the part of the obstetricians, especially during the puerperium.

INVESTIGATION OF THROMBO-EMBOLISM

A number of techniques are now available for the investigation of thrombo-embolism; there is sometimes reluctance to use these investigations in pregnancy, but the hazards of the investigations have to be balanced against the potential risks of unnecessary anticoagulation or of untreated thrombo-embolism.

Ascending phlebography
This method involves the injection of radio-opaque dye into a vein in the dorsum of the foot and enables visualization of the veins of the leg. The presence of venous thrombi will be shown by filling defects in the major veins and, in addition, a collateral circulation may bypass the obstructed portion of the deep venous system. To obtain satisfactory views of the soleal veins, lateral views are required and the most accurate results are obtained by an experienced radiologist. In good hands the technique is very reliable and will visualize 95% of peripheral thrombi (Browse 1978).

If phlebography is used during pregnancy, the fetus should be shielded from radiation by a lead apron; provided that the shielding is adequate, the direct radiation dose to the fetus is small, although some scattered radiation will occur (Laros & Alger 1979). Except in patients where the clinical diagnosis is made with certainty there is a strong case for undertaking ascending phlebography prior to anticoagulation.

Isotope venography
An alternative to ascending phlebography is the use of microspheres or macroaggregates of albumin labelled with radioactive technetium ($^{99}Tc^m$). The biological half-life is short and most of the macroaggregates are trapped in the lung, so that the radiation passing to the placenta and the fetus is very low. The method is also suitable for breast feeding mothers because the quantities of technetium in breast milk are negligible (Tribukait & Swedjemark 1978).

A gamma camera is used to record the flow of radioactive particles and a concentration of radioactivity may indicate the presence of a thrombus. Care has to be taken to avoid false positive results because 'hot spots' can occur even in the absence of a thrombus. One advantage of this test is that scanning of the deep veins of the legs and the pelvis can be combined with investigation of the lung fields at the same time. The test, however, requires specialized equipment and expertise and is usually available only in specialized centres.

Ultrasonic scanning
A useful non-invasive test is to place a Doppler ultrasonic probe over the femoral vein and gently compress the veins in the calf. If the deep veins are patent, a rushing sound will be heard as the blood passes beneath the probe. One problem of this test in pregnancy is that the fetal head may interfere with venous return and cause a false positive result. This problem can be overcome to some extent by carrying out the test with the patient in the left lateral position. A great advantage of this test is that it can be carried out with the Doppler equipment which is readily available in nearly all obstetric units and gives immediate results. It has been claimed to have a diagnostic accuracy of about 85% in major cases of venous thrombosis (Jacques *et al.* 1977).

Radioactive fibrinogen (^{125}I) test
Radioactive iodine should not be used in pregnancy because it is readily passed to the fetus where it is trapped in the fetal thyroid and can cause hypothyroidism. Similarly, the test should not be used in breast feeding mothers because the isotope is transferred to the nursing infant through the breast milk.

The test is, however, a valuable one and may be appropriate in gynaecological patients or non-lactating puerperal mothers who have a clinical suspicion of deep vein thrombosis.

Pulmonary embolism
A chest X-ray may be helpful in establishing the diagnosis of pulmonary embolism, although in some cases the appearances may be normal. The diagnosis can be confirmed in doubtful cases by either pulmonary angiography (Mills & Sutton 1970) or by a lung scan. If there is evidence of pulmonary embolism, a respiratory physician should be consulted because the condition is highly dangerous and early treatment is required.

TREATMENT OF THROMBO-EMBOLISM

The mainstay of therapy in the management of thrombo-embolism is anticoagulation and this should be started without delay.

Anticoagulants in pregnancy
All anticoagulants carry some degree of risk but there are special problems associated with the use of anticoagulants in pregnancy.

Oral anticoagulants, of which warfarin is the most commonly used, exert their effect by lowering the activity of the vitamin K dependent clotting factors II, VII, IX, and X. Oral anticoagulants have a molecular weight of about 1000 and readily cross the placenta into the fetus. The fetus already has low concentrations of the vitamin K dependent clotting factors (Bonnar et al. 1971) which fall dangerously in the fetus in response to warfarin even when the levels are in the therapeutic range in the mother. Warfarin, especially in late pregnancy, is a recognized cause of retroplacental or intracerebral bleeding, and a fetal mortality of 15–30% has been reported in association with its use (Villasanta 1965, Filmore & McDevitt 1970, Henderson et al. 1972). If warfarin is used in pregnancy, it should be stopped at 36 weeks and replaced by heparin for the remainder of the pregnancy (Hirsh et al. 1970).

There is also evidence of a low risk of embryopathy following the use of warfarin in the first trimester of pregnancy. The most commonly reported abnormality is chondrodysplasia punctata which is characterized by abnormal bone and cartilage formation (Shaul et al. 1975). There have also been sporadic reports of microcephaly which is thought to be due to repeated small cerebral haemorrhages in the baby.

The teratogenic risks of warfarin should not be overstated, however, because the majority of women deliver normal babies even when the drug is taken in early pregnancy (Chen et al. 1982).

Patients who are on warfarin can be allowed to breast feed because there is no detectable secretion of the drug in breast milk (Orme et al. 1977); by contrast phenindione can be transferred to the baby in sufficient amounts to cause bleeding problems and should not be given to nursing mothers (Eckstein & Jack 1970).

Heparin acts by inhibiting a number of clotting factors including thrombin and factors IX, X, XI and XII. Heparin also potentiates the action of antithrombin III and, in small amounts, will inhibit factor Xa. It is this effect which is its rationale in the use of low-dose heparin therapy. A major advantage of heparin in pregnancy is that its high molecular weight of 10000–40000 stops it from crossing the placental barrier. The main risk of heparin is bleeding, and bruising can be a problem when it is administered subcutaneously. It is wrong to assume that heparin is entirely safe during pregnancy because Hall et al. (1980) have reported increased fetal wastage associated with its use. One further problem of long term heparin therapy is osteopenia (de Swiet 1984) especially when it has been used for six months or more. Even in asymptomatic women, a degree of bone demineralization may occur. Clearly, all anticoagulants carry some degree of risk and they should be used only after careful consideration of the risk–benefit ratio in individual cases.

Acute phase treatment
During the acute phase of deep vein thrombosis or pulmonary embolism, anticoagulation is required and a continuous intravenous infusion of heparin is usually the treatment of choice. This method of administration will anticoagulate the patient quickly and can be reversed rapidly by protamine sulphate in the event of bleeding problems. The objective of heparin therapy is to limit the extent of any thrombus formation and reduce the risks of pulmonary embolism. Villasanta (1965) reviewed the literature on thrombo-embolism in pregnancy and reported that anticoagulants improved maternal survival. In 163 women with antepartum thrombo-embolism who were not given anticoagulants, pulmonary embolism occurred in 26 (15.9%) and there were 21 maternal deaths (12.8%). By contrast, there were 134 women with antenatal thrombo-embolism who were given

anticoagulants and, in this group, there were 26 (19.4%) with pulmonary emboli but only one (0.7%) maternal death. Even allowing for the fact that this was not a controlled series, the results show two things; first, there was a high risk of pulmonary embolism in established antenatal deep vein thrombosis and secondly, anticoagulants were associated with lower maternal mortality.

The initial dose of intravenous heparin is of the order of 40000 units per day and should be administered in saline through an infusion pump. Intermittent injections of heparin have the disadvantage of producing unpredictable swings between hyper- and hypocoagulability (Sasahara 1974). The partial thromboplastin test is commonly used to monitor heparin anticoagulants and the objective should be to prolong the test to $1\frac{1}{2}$ times (Bonnar 1981). During pregnancy there may be some resistance to heparin and higher doses may be needed to achieve satisfactory anticoagulation as compared with the non-pregnant state. Adequate doses of intravenous heparin should be maintained until the acute clinical signs have resolved.

Alternative treatment
During the acute phase of thrombo-embolism in the non-pregnant patient, thrombolytic agents, such as streptokinase or urokinase, can be used effectively to help resolve large thrombi. During pregnancy, however, there is a risk of severe haemorrhage, especially if delivery is imminent, so that these drugs will rarely be indicated. Likewise, in the postoperative patient, thrombolytic therapy may precipitate bleeding from the operative site. In exceptional circumstances their use may be appropriate if fatal thrombo-embolism seems probable without their use (Bonnar 1981).

The place of surgery in the management of thrombo-embolism is controversial. In cases of massive iliofemoral thrombosis thrombectomy may be indicated and caval ligation may be considered in cases of recurrent pulmonary embolism. When anticoagulation is adequate, however, surgery will rarely be required (Silver & Sabistan 1975). Following massive pulmonary embolism, pulmonary embolectomy under cardiopulmonary bypass may give the best hope for survival and has been used in selected cases. All these alternative forms of treatment are highly specialized and require management teams with particular experience in their use.

Chronic phase treatment
Following the acute phase of thrombo-embolism, it is

necessary to maintain anticoagulation until the period of risk has passed. The duration of anticoagulation will depend upon the timing and severity of the thrombotic episode; in puerperal patients anticoagulants should be continued for 6 weeks, because recurrent thrombo-embolism can occur if treatment is stopped too soon (Bonnar 1981). In many puerperal and postoperative patients the most suitable longterm anticoagulant is warfarin because it is administered orally and can be easily controlled by the prothrombin time. Patients can be discharged home on warfarin once the clinical signs of thrombosis have resolved and have their anticoagulant control monitored at an outpatient clinic. When the thrombosis occurs during pregnancy, warfarin is less suitable because of the reasons already discussed. Alternative treatment is subcutaneous low-dosage heparin therapy which can be maintained for several months. The heparin is administered as either calcium or sodium heparin and an initial dose of 10000 i.v. 12 hourly may be reduced to 5000 i.v. 12 hourly depending on the plasma heparin levels. Bonnar (1981) reported that sodium heparin induced higher plasma heparin levels than calcium heparin in pregnancy and recommended that an 8 hourly regime of calcium heparin would be more appropriate.

The subcutaneous heparin should be administered in concentrated solution through a short 25 gauge needle to minimize the problem of bruising. A fold of skin, usually in the abdominal wall or thigh, is gently raised and the injection made at right-angles to the skin surface after the area has been cleansed. After the injection, the needle should be removed slowly and the injection site should not be rubbed or massaged. Correct technique is important to avoid unnecessary bruising or acceleration of the rate of heparin absorption. Most patients can be taught to administer the subcutaneous heparin to themselves and can be managed on an outpatient basis.

Because heparin does not cross to the fetus, the subcutaneous regime is the method which is most commonly used when chronic phase anticoagulation is required during pregnancy. If the mother is maintained on subcutaneous heparin until delivery, the heparin can either be stopped or reduced during labour to avoid the risk of haemorrhage at the time of placental separation. If heparin is continued during labour, epidural anaesthesia should be avoided, because there is a danger of epidural haematoma formation (Crawford 1978). An alternative to heparin is the use of intravenous dextran (Bonnar & Walsh 1972) but if dextran is used blood must be taken for cross-matching before the infusion is started because dextran interferes with cross-matching methods in the laboratory. Dextran and heparin should not be given together because the two drugs have a synergistic effect which can increase the risk of bleeding (Bonnar 1981).

Prophylaxis of thrombo-embolism

The most important measure in the prevention of thrombo-embolism is early mobilization in the post-operative and puerperal periods. Physiotherapy to encourage good venous flow in the lower limbs reinforces the advantages of early mobilization.

If a woman is taking the combined oestrogen–progestogen oral contraceptive pill, it may be wise to discontinue this if she is to be admitted for major surgery. If this advice is given, however, it is essential to ensure that an effective alternative method of contraception is used, because an inadvertent pregnancy may cause even greater problems. In some women the pill is the only form of contraception which they will accept and, if this is the case, it may be better to allow them to continue the pill until the time of surgery; a judgement has to be balanced between the degree of risk of thrombo-embolism and the possibility of an unwanted pregnancy.

In addition to these general preventive measures, there are circumstances in which it is necessary to consider the use of prophylactic anticoagulants; the three main groups are those who have had major gynaecological surgery, pregnant women with a previous history of thrombo-embolism and women with artificial heart valves.

Anticoagulants after gynaecological surgery

Research studies using radiolabelled fibrinogen have shown that occult deep vein thrombosis is a common feature after major surgery reaching incidences of between 10 and 20% after gynaecological procedures (Bonnar & Walsh 1972). Although only a small proportion of these thrombi will cause clinical problems, it is important to take all practical measures to reduce the risk of pulmonary embolism.

Because anticoagulants increase the risk of bleeding during surgery, very few gynaecologists are prepared to use prophylactic anticoagulants on a routine basis. It is more common for a selective approach to be used, when a number of factors are employed to identify patients who have a particularly high risk of thrombosis. High risk factors include increasing age, obesity, varicose veins, malignant disease and cigarette smoking (Clayton *et al.* 1976). In patients who

have one or more of these high risk factors, the potential benefits of prophylactic subcutaneous heparin may outweigh the dangers and should be used in the postoperative period. If longer anticoagulation is required because of particularly high risk features, warfarin will be a more suitable alternative.

Prophylactic anticoagulants in pregnancy

In a retrospective study, Badaracco & Vessey (1974) estimated that a woman with a previous history of thrombo-embolism had about a 12% risk of recurrence during pregnancy. This risk was unaffected by whether it occurred during a previous pregnancy, after previous surgery or in association with oral contraception. In an assessment of current practice, de Swiet *et al.* (1980) found that 88% of British obstetricians would use prophylactic anticoagulants if the previous thrombo-embolism had occurred in pregnancy, 79% if it had occurred during oral contraception and 50% if it had occurred ten years previously outwith pregnancy or oral contraception. Most of the obstetricians preferred to use warfarin in the regime recommended by Hirsh *et al.* (1970) changing to heparin at 36 weeks' gestation, a regime with potential risks to the pregnancy (*see* discussion above).

In his analysis of this problem de Swiet (1984) points out that all methods of anticoagulation, including subcutaneous heparin, carry some risk in pregnancy. He also considers that the 12% estimate of risk of recurrence by Badaracco and Vessey (1970) is likely to be an exaggeration because their study was based on a postal survey and the diagnosis of thrombo-embolism may have been based on flimsy evidence in many cases. Because of the risk of long term anticoagulants, he suggests that a previous history of thrombo-embolism should not be an automatic indication for anticoagulants throughout pregnancy. The first task is to review the evidence which was used to make the previous diagnosis of thrombo-embolism, because, in many cases, the diagnosis will be based on rather vague clinical signs without confirmation from a reliable diagnostic test. The policy suggested by de Swiet is to avoid anticoagulants during pregnancy unless there is a feature of particularly high risk. High risk features include bed rest in hospital, a history of two previous episodes of thrombo-embolism or a family history of antithrombin III deficiency. When there is a history of previous thrombo-embolism, de Swiet recommends that dextran should be used during labour to allow epidural anaesthesia and that subcutaneous heparin should be given for six weeks after delivery. This policy obviously represents a compromise but is a good attempt to achieve a balance between the risks and benefits of prophylactic anticoagulants in pregnancy.

Pregnancy in patients with artificial heart valves
A particularly difficult problem arises in those patients with artificial heart valves who wish to become pregnant. The normal anticoagulant which is used in such patients is warfarin but the alternative of subcutaneous heparin may be insufficient to prevent embolic problems in pregnancy (Limet & Crondin 1977). In their study, Limet and Crondin (1977) estimated that the risk of an embolic episode was 1 per 100 months of exposure if no anticoagulants were used in the presence of an artificial heart valve. In pregnancy, the risk rose to 25% per pregnancy but was reduced to 5% by effective anticoagulation. Despite the risks of warfarin in pregnancy, it is probably better for women with artificial heart valves to take warfarin until 36 weeks; at this time, patients should be admitted to hospital and given continuous intravenous heparin until delivery. If the mother goes into labour prematurely warfarin should be stopped, vitamin K should be given and intravenous heparin commenced (de Swiet 1984). After delivery, intravenous heparin should be continued until warfarin can be recommenced.

In this clinical situation, as in the others described in this chapter, there is no regime of anticoagulants that is both completely safe and fully efficient and the plan of treatment must reflect the balance between risk and benefit in individual cases.

Problems of coagulation and fibrinolysis in obstetrics

A number of specific clinical obstetric conditions can lead to coagulation failure with bleeding problems. The coagulation failure is usually initiated by either localized fibrin formation or disseminated intravascular coagulation which stimulates a secondary fibrinolytic response. The clinical features depend upon the pace of events and upon the relative balance between the coagulation and fibrinolytic processes.

ABRUPTIO PLACENTAE

The most common cause of coagulation failure in obstetrics is abruptio placentae. Although minor degrees of defibrination can be demonstrated after moderate degrees of abruptio placentae, they are rarely of clinical importance. The haemostatic problems are nearly always seen after a major placental separation, when a large retroplacental bleed is associated with the classical signs of concealed abruptio placenta. The mother complains of severe abdominal pain, the uterus becomes wooden hard and tender and the fetal heart is absent. There are clinical signs of shock and there may be evidence of bleeding from venepuncture sites or from mucous membranes. An acute coagulation problem of this kind requires urgent and determined management.

The coagulation defect in abruptio placentae is brought about by several mechanisms which operate in such close succession that their effects may overlap. The first mechanism of coagulation failure is the deposition of large amounts of fibrin, platelets and other clotting factors in the retroplacental clot which may consume up to 5 litres of blood. In some cases, the huge size of the retroplacental clot may, by itself, explain the sharply reduced levels of circulating fibrinogen, platelets and clotting factors. The defibrination is, however, aggravated in most cases by a widespread intravascular coagulation which is stimulated by the release of thromboplastins from the site of placental damage into the blood stream. If the patient is shocked, the hypotension itself is a further stimulus to the process of disseminated intravascular coagulation and may lead to renal shutdown. In response to the intravascular coagulation, local fibrinolytic activity is stimulated and high levels of fibrin degradation products appear in the circulation. The fibrin degradation products themselves add to the haemostatic difficulties because they have anticoagulant activity and interfere with the stabilization of fibrin clots. It is possible for the locally generated plasmin to lyse fibrinogen as well as fibrin but it is unusual for the fibrinolytic activation in abruptio placentae to be sufficiently severe to cause a plasminaemic state.

The investigation of the haemostatic defect in abruptio placentae must use tests which give rapid results to the clinician. The most helpful tests are fibrinogen titre, platelet count, thrombin time, prothrombin time, partial thromboplastin time and estimation of fibrin degradation products (FDPs). In the thrombin time, thrombin is added to citrated plasma, the clotting time is measured and the result is compared to a control; the thrombin time is prolonged if severe fibrinogen depletion has occurred and is a valuable overall screen of haemostatic competence. By performing the thrombin time in serial dilutions of the patient's plasma a rapid, although crude, estimate of fibrinogen level can be obtained. If a clot forms and then subsequently dissolves, this is an indication of active systemic fibrinolytic activity. The one stage prothrombin time is a test of the extrinsic coagulation system and the partial thromboplastin time is prolonged if the intrinsic system is defective. The measurement of FDPs is not critical to the management of haemostatic failure, but values will be grossly elevated after abruptio placentae. From the results of these tests and the clinical picture of the patient, it can be judged whether active treatment of any coagulation defect is required or not.

Management

The most urgent requirement in the management of abruptio placentae is the correction of hypovolaemic shock. Not only will this restore the patient's circulation but it will prevent a deterioration of the intravascular coagulation. Banked blood should be transfused as soon as suitably cross-matched blood is available. Until blood is available, an intravenous line should be set up and the appropriate initial therapy will depend upon the urgency of the circumstances. If the patient's condition is reasonably stable, Hartmann's solution may be sufficient until cross-matched blood becomes available for transfusion. If the patient is more severely ill, fresh frozen plasma can be used to expand the intravascular compartment. Fresh frozen plasma is much superior to fibrinogen because, in addition to fibrinogen, it contains other clotting factors, such as factors V and VIII, which are also depleted. The coagulation inhibitor antithrombin III is also present and may help to limit disseminated intravascular clotting. Other plasma substitutes have been used but all have various problems; dextrans, for example, adversely affect platelet function, can cause anaphylactoid reactions and interfere with subsequent cross-matching tests (Letsky 1984). There is no substitute for adequate blood transfusion and it is easy to underestimate the amount of blood which is required to treat abruptio placenta adequately. A central venous pressure line should be set up and this will indicate if there has been overloading with excess fluid replacement.

In the majority of cases, early and adequate blood transfusion will be sufficient to correct hypovolaemia and restore adequate haemostatic competence after abrupio placentae. If a coagulation problem persists after the transfusion of banked blood, it may be necessary to replace some of the haemostatic components which are absent. Fresh blood has been advocated for this purpose because it contains all the elements required for haemostasis, including platelets (Bonnar & Hathaway 1981). Whole fresh blood is now rarely used because there is insufficient time to complete hepatitis surface antigen and blood grouping tests before the blood can be released from the Transfusion Centre (Letsky 1984). The alternative is to transfuse a combination of fresh frozen plasma, banked red cells and platelet concentrates, if required. This combination contains all the elements necessary for haemostasis and does not have the risks of fresh blood. Correction of the coagulation defect should be followed by delivery of the fetus, placenta and retroplacental clot which is the underlying pathological problem. The appropriate obstetric management will depend upon the fetal condition and the uterine response to induction of labour.

In recent years heparin has been used to treat disseminated intravascular coagulation caused by many factors; in abruptio placentae, however, it would take great courage to anticoagulate an actively bleeding patient and there is no documented evidence to support such a policy. The great majority of patients will respond well to blood transfusion, replacement of haemostatic components and uterine evacuation.

RETAINED DEAD FETUS

Following intrauterine death, thromboplastic substances may be released into the maternal circulation and intravascular coagulation can be precipitated. This is a slow process but after 3–4 weeks there is a risk that circulating clotting factors may be depleted to dangerously low levels. If the clotting defect is unrecognized, bruising may occur and there may be severe haemorrhage at the time of placental separation. Patients with a retained dead fetus should have a clotting screen carried out prior to induction of labour, particularly if the intrauterine death is of long standing. If there is evidence of defective haemostasis, the coagulation defect should be corrected prior to delivery. This can usually be achieved by infusing 1000 units of heparin per hour intravenously over a 48 hour period during which time the levels of fibrinogen, platelets and clotting factors will return to normal. When the clotting factors are restored, heparin should be discontinued and labour induced, usually with prostaglandins. It is prudent to have an adequate supply of fresh frozen plasma, compatible red cells and platelets available to treat any haemorrhage that may arise at placental separation. Coagulation problems associated with a retained dead fetus are now seen very rarely because, in the great majority of cases, the diagnosis is made and delivery achieved long before a clinical problem has developed.

The most acute form of coagulation failure in obstetrics occurs as a consequence of amniotic fluid embolism. After the amniotic fluid enters the maternal circulation, platelet-fibrin thrombi are formed and are trapped within the pulmonary vascular tree. The response of the fibrinolytic system may be so intense that the amounts of plasmin overwhelm the circulating antiplasmins and a 'plasminaemic' state is established. Free plasmin will digest fibrinogen and, together with the effects of massive intravascular coagulation, there is total consumption of coagulation factors. The clinical picture is one of profound shock, respiratory distress and cyanosis. The patient will cough up blood-stained sputum and severe bleeding may occur from many sites.

In severe cases the outcome is usually fatal but, even when the diagnosis of amniotic fluid embolism is suspected in association with a less florid clinical picture, the management of the coagulation defect presents major problems. The priorities in the management of amniotic fluid embolism are to support the circulation and to maintain adequate oxygenation and any treatment of the coagulation defect will be secondary to these aims. The most logical treatment is to anticoagulate the patient to prevent further intravascular coagulation but, as with abruptio placenta (discussed above), it takes great courage to anticoagulate a bleeding patient. In the case of active systemic fibrinolysis, it is tempting to use antifibrinolytic agents but their use may further aggravate the widespread intravascular clotting in the lungs and make oxygenation of the patient more difficult. The best management policy may be to sustain respiratory and circulatory function while leaving the natural fibrinolytic response of the mother to clear the vascular tree. If bleeding is severe, replacement therapy on a large scale may be required using whole blood, fresh frozen plasma, red cells and platelet concentrations as required. Because this syndrome is uncommon, it is impossible for any single group to establish sufficient experience of its management to evaluate different approaches to treatment. Those readers who wish a more detailed discussion of the problem are referred to the review by Morgan (1979).

PRE-ECLAMPSIA

It is now well established that a low-grade form of intravascular coagulation occurs in pre-eclampsia (for reviews *see* Howie 1977, MacGillivray 1983). The intravascular coagulation bears a relationship to the severity of the disease, being greatest in patients with severe pre-eclampsia and eclampsia. This process is secondary to the microvascular damage which is characteristic of pre-eclampsia, and histological and electron microscope studies have shown that platelets and fibrin are deposited in the microvasculature of the kidney (Vassalli *et al.* 1963), the placental bed (Sheppard & Bonnar 1976) and the liver (Arias & Mancilla-Jiminez 1976). These pathological features are associated with a number of changes in the coagulation and fibrinolytic systems.

One of the most characteristic changes in severe pre-eclampsia is a fall in the platelet count (Howie *et al.* 1971), which may start from early in the disease process (Redman *et al.* 1978) and is probably explained by platelet consumption during low-grade intravascular coagulation. This conclusion is supported by the finding of increased platelet turnover in pre-eclampsia (Rakoczi *et al.* 1979). In addition to the changes in platelet count, there is evidence of thrombin activation in pre-eclampsia. Cryofibrinogen describes fibrinogen which is precipitated by exposure to cold and it is not usually present in healthy non-pregnant women. Cryofibrinogen is thought to represent circulating fibrin polymers produced as a result of thrombin activity, and cryofibrinogen is present in large amounts in pre-eclampsia (McKay & Corey 1964, Howie *et al.* 1971). Circulating fibrin polymers can also be demonstrated by the more sophisticated technique of fibrinogen chromatography, and this method has been applied to the study of thrombin activity in pre-eclampsia (McKillop *et al.* 1976). As illustrated in Fig. 36.3, fibrin polymer complexes were higher in normal pregnant women than in non-pregnant controls but the levels were much higher in severe pre-eclampsia than in either of the control groups. Another index of increased thrombin activity is the factor VIII antigen-activity ratio (see above) and this is also raised in pre-eclampsia confirming the hypercoagulability associated with the disease (Thornton & Bonnar 1977).

In response to the fibrin platelet deposition in pre-eclampsia there is some activation of the fibrinolytic system because FDPs appear in raised amounts both in the serum and in the urine. Fibrinolytic activity is decreased in normal pregnancy but is even more suppressed in pre-eclampsia; there is increased resistance to fibrinolytic activators and fibrinolysis does not recover to normal levels immediately after delivery as occurs in normal women (Howie *et al.* 1971). Because of the partial inhibition of fibrinolytic activity during pre-eclampsia, clearance of the fibrin is not fully effective until after delivery when there is a rapid rise of FDPs during the recovery period. Taken together, these changes suggest that, in pre-eclampsia, intravascular platelet-fibrin deposition is precipitated by increased thrombin activity and that clearance of the vascular tree does not occur until fibrinolytic activity returns to normal after delivery. The major question is whether the coagulation changes are of primary or secondary importance in the aetiology of pre-eclampsia. At present, it seems most likely that the intravascular coagulation is secondary to some other pathological mechanism operating at the microvascular level. On the other hand, the coagulation changes are characteristic of pre-eclampsia and do not merely reflect hypertension, because there are no abnormalities of coagulation, fibrinolysis or platelet function in essential hypertension during pregnancy (Howie *et al.* 1971).

The coagulation changes in pre-eclampsia do not usually constitute a haemostatic problem. In some cases of severe pre-eclampsia, however, the disseminated intravascular coagulation can be sufficiently severe to precipitate microangiopathic haemolytic anaemia (Brain *et al.* 1967). In this process, red cells are damaged and undergo lysis as they pass through the blood vessels which are lined by intravascular fibrin. The red cells have a characteristic appearance under the microscope showing the effects of damage sustained in the small blood vessels. The patient develops haemoglobinaemia and will have dark urine as a result of haemoglobinuria. This syndrome is almost always associated with severely deteriorating pre-eclampsia, and early delivery will be required in the maternal interest. It is interesting to note that thrombo-embolism is relatively common in pre-eclamptic women who have been rested in bed, and it may be that the increased thrombin activity of the pre-eclamptic process contributes to this problem.

Attempts have been made to influence the course of pre-eclampsia with anticoagulants but, despite isolated reports which have claimed success (for review *see* Howie 1977), there is no well-documented evidence to suggest that anticoagulants are of value. There has been a suggestion that antiplatelet drugs might improve placental function but more evidence is required to substantiate this possibility (Howie *et al.* 1975). One of the risks of severe hypertension in pregnancy is cerebral haemorrhage, so that, in the absence of any evidence of benefit, anticoagulants should not be used in the management of pre-eclampsia.

THERAPEUTIC ABORTION USING HYPERTONIC SOLUTIONS

There have now been a number of reports showing that the use of intra-amniotic hypertonic solutions to induce therapeutic abortion can precipitate changes in the coagulation and fibrinolytic systems consistent with intravascular coagulation. The cause of the intravascular coagulation is probably the release of tissue factors from the damaged placenta. In some cases the process has been sufficiently severe to result in massive haemorrhage and maternal death. The danger of hypertonic solutions is one of the main reasons why prostaglandins are preferred for the induction of mid-trimester abortion. The treatment is blood transfusion with replacement of clotting factors by fresh frozen plasma and red cells as required (Letsky 1984).

HYDATIDIFORM MOLE

A coagulation defect, similar to that encountered after a missed abortion, can be associated with hydatidiform mole. This is discussed in Chapter 37, which deals with the complications of molar pregnancy.

Inherited defects of haemostasis

The most common inherited defects of haemostasis in women are von Willebrand's disease and Christmas disease and both conditions can present problems in obstetrics and gynaecology.

Von Willebrand's disease

The defect in von Willebrand's disease is a combination of reduced factor VIII activity and a defect in platelet function. The condition is passed on as an autosomal dominant so that it can present in both men and women. The extent of the clinical bleeding problem in von Willebrand's disease is variable but both third stage haemorrhage and menorrhagia can occur. During pregnancy factor VIII levels should be monitored and, in most cases, there will be a progressive increase towards term. If levels of factor VIII remain low at term or if a bleeding problem develops, the clotting defect can be treated by infusion of cryoprecipitate which has high concentrations of factor VIII. This treatment will also improve the platelet function. After delivery, factor VIII levels will fall to non-pregnant values and secondary postpartum haemorrhage can occur. If this happens, cryoprecipitate should be given and, if this is insufficient, a fibrinolytic inhibitor such as epsilon amino caproic acid (EACA) may help to stabilize the fibrin which is formed at the placental site. This is one of the rare indications for the use of fibrinolytic inhibitors in pregnant women. If menorrhagia is a problem, the use of EACA to reduce menstrual loss is a logical treatment and may be helpful. Alternatively, the combined oestrogen–progestogen oral contraceptive may be valuable both by its local effect on the endometrium and by increasing factor VIII activity.

Christmas disease and haemophilia carriers

Christmas disease, or factor IX deficiency, is a rare disease which may occur during pregnancy. The principles of treatment are the same as those described for von Willebrand's disease. Although women to not suffer from haemophilia (factor VIII deficiency), they may be carriers and have factor VIII levels which are about 50% of normal. Usually, there is sufficient factor VIII to ensure normal haemostasis and the levels will rise during pregnancy. It is wise, nevertheless, to monitor the level in pregnancy and consider cryoprecipitate if the level is low. Patients with these rare clotting defects should be managed in centres where there are physicians who are experienced in their management.

Thrombocytopenia

This is an acquired haemostatic disease which is characterized by a low platelet count, petechial haemorrhages and a potential risk of bleeding. In a small number of cases, the disease is secondary to diseases such as systemic lupus erythematosus, lymphoma or even neoplastic infiltration but, in the majority, it is usually of the idiopathic type. In the idiopathic type, antiplatelet antibodies are present which may be bound to platelets or, if they are free in the circulation as IgG antibodies, may cross the placenta and affect the fetus. If the fetus becomes thrombocytopenic, there is a risk of intracranial haemorrhage and perinatal mortality rates as high as 20% have been reported (Carloss et al. 1980). Idiopathic thrombocytopenia is commonest in the reproductive age group so that its appearance not infrequently coincides with pregnancy. The choice of therapy lies between corticosteroids and splenectomy. Splenectomy is associated with an appreciable maternal and fetal mortality in pregnancy, especially if it is performed late in gestation, and should be avoided, if possible (Carloss et al. 1980). The majority

of patients will respond well to steroids and the splenectomy can be delayed until after delivery when the mortality associated with surgery is almost nil. If there is no response to corticosteroids, there may be no alternative to surgery but it should only be undertaken with expert haematological support to deal with any bleeding problems which may arise.

There has been some controversy about the optimum mode of delivery because an affected baby has a risk of cerebral haemorrhage. On the other hand, there may be bleeding difficulties associated with Caesarean section and, in the majority of cases it is better to aim for vaginal delivery. On the other hand, it is important to avoid any fetal trauma and, if any difficulty at vaginal delivery is anticipated, Caesarean section may be advisable.

Thrombocytopenia is discussed in more detail in Chapter 21.

REFERENCES

AARO L.A., JOHNSON M.R. & JUERGENS J.L. (1966) *Obstet. Gynecol.*, **28**, 553.

AARO L.A. & JUERGENS J.L. (1974) *Med. Clin. North Amer.* **58**. 829.

ARIAS F. & MANCILLA-JIMINEZ R. (1976) *New Engl. J. Med.*, **295**, 578.

ASTEDT B., ISACSON S., NILSSON I.M. & PANDOLFI (1973) *Brit. med. J.*, **IV**, 631.

BADARACCO M.A. & VESSEY M.P. (1974) *Brit. med. J.*, **1**, 215.

BIGGS R., DENSON K.W.E., AKMAN N., BORRETT R. & HADDEN M.E. (1970) *Brit. J. Haematol.*, **19**, 283–305.

BONNAR J. (1976) In Kakkar V.V. and Thomas D.P. (eds) *Heparin Chemistry and Clinical Usage*. Academic Press, New York.

BONNAR J. (1981) *Clin. Obstet. Gynaecol.*, **8**, 455.

BONNAR J. & HATHAWAY W.E. (1981) In *Perinatal Coagulation* (eds. Hathaway W.E. & Bonnar J.) Monographs in Neonatology. Grune & Stratton, New York.

BONNAR J. McNICOL G.P. & DOUGLAS A.S. (1969) *Brit. med. J.*, **3**, 387.

BONNAR J., McNICOL G.P. & DOUGLAS A.S. (1971) *J. Obstet. Gynaec. Brit. Cwlth.*, **78**, 355.

BONNAR J. & WALSH J.J. (1972) *Lancet*, **i**, 614.

BRAIN M.C., KUAH K.B. & DIXON H.G. (1967) *J. Obstet. Gynaec. Brit Cwlth.*, **74**, 702.

BROWSE N.L. (1978) *Brit. med. Bull.*, **34**, 163.

CARLOSS H.W., McMILLAN R. & CROSBY W.N. (1980) *J. Amer. med. Ass.*, **244**, 2756.

CHEN W.W.C., CHAN C.S., LEE P.R., WANG R.Y.R. & WONG V.C.W. (1982) *Quart. J. Med.*, **51**, 358.

CLAYTON J.K., ANDERSEN J.A. & McNICOL G.P. (1976) *Brit. med. J.*, **2**, 910.

CRAWFORD J.S. (1978) In *Principles and Practice of Obstetric*

Anaesthesia, 4th Ed. p. 182. Blackwell Scientific Publications, Oxford.

DANIEL D.G., BLOOM A.L., GIDELINGS J.C., CAMPBELL H. & TURNBULL A.C. (1968) *Brit. med. J.*, **1**, 801.

DAVIE E.W. & RATNOFF O.D. (1964) *Science*, **145**, 1310.

DE SWIET M. (1984) In *Medical Disorders in Medical Practice* (ed. de Swiet M.) p. 95. Blackwell Scientific Publications, Oxford.

DE SWIET M., BULPITT C.J. & LEWIS P.J. (1980) *J. Obstet. Gynaecol.*, **1**, 29.

ECKSTEIN H. & JACK B. (1970) *Lancet*, **i**, 672.

EGEBERG O. (1965) *Thromb. Diath. Haemorr.*, **13**, 516.

FILLMORE S.J. & McDEVITT E. (1970) *Ann. intern. Med.*, **73**, 731.

FRIEND J.R. & KAKKAR V.V. (1972) In *Thromboembolism* (Eds. Kakkar V.V. & Jouhan A.J.) pp. 131. Churchill Livingstone, London.

HALL J.G., PAULI R.M. & WILSON K.M. (1980) *Amer. J. Med.*, **68**, 122.

HENDERSON S.R., LUND C.J. & GREASMAN W.T. (1972) *Amer. J. Obstet. Gynec.*, **112**, 476.

HIRST J., CADE J.F. & O'SULLIVAN E.F. (1970) *Brit. med. J.*, **i**, 270.

HOWIE P.W. (1977) *Clin. Obstet. Gynaecol.*, **4**, 595.

HOWIE P.W., PRENTICE C.R.M., MALLINSON A.C., HORNE C.H.W. & McNICOL G.P. (1970) *Lancet*, **ii**, 1329.

HOWIE P.W., PRENTICE C.R.M. & McNICOL G.P. (1971) *J. Obstet. Gynaec. Brit. Cwlth.*, **78**, 992.

HOWIE P.W., PRENTICE C.R. & FORBES C.D. (1975) *Brit. J. Obstet. Gynaecol.*, **82**, 711.

HOWIE P.W., EVANS K., FORBES C.D. & PRENTICE C.R.M. (1975) *Brit. J. Obstet. Gynaecol.*, **82**, 968

INMAN W.H.W. & VESSEY M.P. (1968) *Brit. med. J.*, **ii**, 193.

JACQUES P.F., RICHEY W.A., ELY C.A. & JOHNSON G. (1977) *Amer. J. Roentgenol.*, **15**, 539.

JEFFCOATE T.N.A., MILLER J., ROOS R.F. & TINDALL V.R. (1968) *Brit. med. J.*, **4**, 19.

LAROS R.K. & ALGER L.S. (1979) *Clin. Obstet. Gynecol.*, **22**, 871.

LETSKY E. (1984) In *Medical Disorders in Obstetric Practice* (Ed. M. de Swiet) p. 70. Blackwell Scientific Publications, Oxford.

LIMET R. & CRONDIN C.M. (1977) *Ann. Thorac. Surg.*, **23**, 337.

McFARLANE R.G. (1964) *Nature* (London), **202**, 498.

MacGILLIVRAY I. (1983) In *Pre-eclampsia* (Ed. McGillivray I.) W.B. Saunders Co. Ltd, London.

McKAY D.G. & COREY A.E. (1964) *Obstet. Gynecol.*, **23**, 508.

McKILLOP C., HOWIE P.W., FORBES C.D. & PRENTICE C.R.M. (1976) *Lancet*, **i**, 56.

MILLER G.A.H. & SUTTON G.C. (1970) *Brit. Heart. J.*, **32**, 518.

MONCADA M.D. & VANE J.R. (1979) *New Eng. J. Med.*, **300**, 1142.

MORGAN M. (1979) *Anaesthesia*, **34**, 20.

NOTELOVITZ M. & WARE M. (1982) In *Progress in Obstetrics and Gynaecology*, **Vol. 2** (Ed. J. Studd) p. 228.

ORME M.L'E., LEWIS P.J., DE SWIET M., SERLIN M.J., SIBEON R., BATY J.D. & BRECKENRIDGE A.M. (1977) *Brit. med. J.*, **1**, 1564.

POLLER L. & THOMSON J.M. (1966) *Brit. med. J.*, **2**, 23.

RAKOCZI I., TALLIAN F., BAGDANY S. & GATI I. (1979). *Thrombin. Res.*, **15**, 533–6.

RAMSAY L.E. (1983) *Brit. med. J.*, **286**, 698.

RAPAPORT S.I., SCHIFFMAN S., PATCH M.J. & AMES S.B. (1963) *Blood*, **21**, 221.

REDMAN C.W.G., BONNAR J. & BEILIN L.J. (1978) *Brit. med. J.*, **i**, 467.

SASAHARA A.A. (1974) *J. Amer. med. Ass.*, **229**, 1795.

SHAPER A.G., KEAR J., MacINTOSH D.M., KYOBE J. & NJAMA D. (1968) *J. Obstet. Gynaec. Brit. Cwlth.*, **75**, 433–41.

SHAUL W.L., EMERY H. & HALL J.G. (1975) *Amer. J. Dis. Childh.*, **129**, 360.

SHEPPARD B.L. & BONNAR J. (1976) *Brit. J. Obstet. Gynaecol.*, **81**, 497.

SHERRY S., FLETCHER A.P. & ALKJAERSIG N. (1959) *Physiol. Rev.*, **39**, 343.

SIEGEL D.G. (1972) In *The Epidemiology of Venous Thrombosis* (Ed. Foster C. *et al.*) **50**, 15, Milbank Memorial Fund Quarterly.

SILVER D. & SABISTON D.C. (1975) *Surgery*, **77**, 3.

THORNTON C.A., BONNAR J. (1977) *Brit. J. Obstet. Gynaecol.*, **84**, 919.

TODD A.S. (1964) *Brit. Med. Bull.*, **20**, 210.

TRIBUKAIT B. & SWEDJEMARK G.A. (1978) *Acta Radio (Oncol.)*, **17**, 379.

VASSALLI P., MORRIS R.H. & McCLUSKY R.T. (1963) *J. Exp. Med.*, **118**, 467.

VILLASANTA V. (1965) *Amer. J. Obstet. Gynecol.*, **93**, 142.

WINDEBANK W.J., BOYD G. & MORAN F. (1973) *Brit. med. J.*, **i**, 90.

CHAPTER 37
TROPHOBLASTIC DISEASE

P.W. HOWIE

One of the great mysteries of placentate reproduction is the mechanism whereby the trophoblastic invasion of the maternal host is halted. On the occasions when this process is disrupted, the consequences may be trophoblastic disease in the form of a hydatidiform mole or choriocarcinoma, the latter frequently developing as a sequel to the former. In considering trophoblastic disease, the usual yardsticks of malignancy are hard to apply because there is no basement membrane, violation of which can be interpreted as indicating an invading neoplasm. Pathological classification becomes very difficult and categorization is more appropriate on the basis of the clinical behaviour than on the histological findings. A further problem is that, in normal pregnancy, trophoblast is commonly found to have embolized to the maternal lungs (Attwood & Park 1961) so that the presence of 'metastases' may not always signify invasive malignant disease. Despite the problems of classification, however, it is normal to regard hydatidiform mole as the benign form of trophoblastic disease, which as a potentially malignant condition may progress to the frankly malignant disorder of choriocarcinoma. While the division into hydatidiform mole and choriocarcinoma is convenient, it must be remembered that there is a spectrum of disease and many individual cases are borderline and do not fall unequivocally into one or other category.

In recent years the understanding and management of trophoblastic disease has advanced over a number of fronts. The most significant development has been the introduction of effective chemotherapy for choriocarcinoma which has transformed an almost invariably fatal condition into one which carries a favourable prognosis. The advent of effective therapy heralded the need for an effective tumour marker which could demonstrate malignant degeneration of hydatidiform mole at a very early stage. Such a tumour marker became available in the form of human chorionic gonadotrophin (HCG) and, when an accurate radioimmunoassay was developed, large

scale monitoring became feasible because it was possible to carry out large numbers of assays. The tumour marker has become indispensable not just for early diagnosis but also for monitoring the progress of therapy.

Tumour registers and regional follow-up centres have been established and these have made an important contribution by ensuring effective monitoring for all patients who have been delivered of a hydatidiform mole. Early diagnosis of the primary disease has also become an important consideration, because any delay in diagnosis increases the risk of complications and worsens the long term prognosis. Ultrasonic examination, by making it possible to visualize the uterine contents directly, has greatly assisted the cause of early and accurate diagnosis.

The understanding of the pathogenesis of hydatidiform mole took a great leap forward following the demonstration that molar tissue contained a double contribution of paternal chromosomes, indicating that the underlying problem was established at the time of conception. It has also made it clear that hydatidiform mole is appropriately subclassified into two types, its complete and partial forms. These advances have made the management of trophoblastic disease one of the great success stories of gynaecological oncology and the new developments will be discussed in more detail in the chapter.

HYDATIDIFORM MOLE

EPIDEMIOLOGY

The most striking feature of the epidemiology of hydatidiform mole is the wide difference in incidences in different parts of the world. The incidence is much higher in Asiatic countries than in the Western world although the reasons for this are not known. In order to achieve as much comparability as possible, the incidence of mole is usually expressed in relation to the total number of pregnancies rather than as a proportion of the total population. In this way, the effect of differing birth rates on the incidence is removed. The most accurate incidence is the one expressed as a ratio to the total number of pregnancies in a complete population, but many studies have reported on the incidences in hospital populations. In countries where many normal births take place outside hospital, a figure expressed as the ratio to total hospital births will overestimate the true incidence and this will often be the case in developing countries. The reported incidences of hydatidiform mole are shown in Fig. 37.1 with the rates based on studies of total populations in shaded bars and of hospital populations in open bars. Despite the difficulties of achieving an exact definition of incidence in many countries, there seems to be no doubt that the incidence in Asiatic countries is higher than in the West.

It is a point of some interest to determine whether the high incidence in Asiatic women is due to geographic or racial factors. In the multiracial population of Hawaii, Jacobs et al. (1982) reported an increased incidence of complete moles amongst the most recent immigrants, the Filipinos, but only an average incidence among the Asiatic peoples who had lived in Hawaii for some time. These data suggest that Asian racial groups can lose their high risk of hydatidiform mole once they adjust to an alternative way of life and would support the view that the differences in incidence are geographical or environmental rather than racial. Jacobs et al. (1982) found that women with partial moles had the same ethnic distribution as the general population.

Maternal age influences the risk of hydatidiform mole, the incidence being increased in women under the age of 20 years and rising sharply after the age of 40 years and especially after the age of 45 (Buckley 1984). From a consideration of published studies, the risk of a mole in the 45–49-year age group is 24 times greater than that of the 25–29-year age group. This risk may be related to genetic factors because the processes of normal fertilization are more frequently disturbed in older women (see below). There is also evidence of an increased risk in women who have had a previous molar pregnancy compared with those who have no such history. Despite this increased risk, the overall chance of recurrence remains small and is only of the order of 0.5–2% so that most women are subsequently able to have a normal family. It is frequently suggested that poor nutrition and adverse socio-economic factors

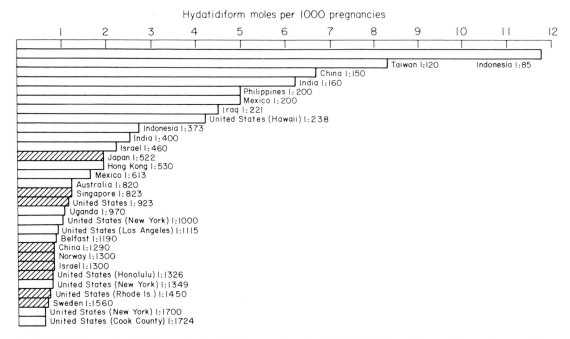

Fig. 37.1 Incidence of hydatidiform mole; in shaded bars, results of studies in defined populations and in open bars, results from studies in hospital populations. (From Buckley et al (1984) with permission from author, Editor of *Clinical Obstetrics and Gynecology*, and Lippincott, Harper & Row, Philadelphia.)

increase the risk of hydatidiform mole, but detailed consideration of the literature finds little direct evidence to support this contention. Much of the epidemiological information has been based on all cases of hydatidiform mole. Now that a clear distinction can be made between complete and partial mole, some of the epidemiological findings may be found, on further exploration, to apply only to one form of the disease and not to the other.

GENETIC FEATURES OF HYDATIDIFORM MOLE

One of the most remarkable discoveries about hydatidiform mole has been the demonstration that complete moles have chromosomes exclusively derived from the paternal side (Kajii & Ohama 1977). This discovery came from the use of banding techniques which were able to determine whether chromosomes were maternally or paternally derived. In complete hydatidiform mole, the karyotype is nearly always 46,XX and only rarely is 46,XY observed. The normal mechanism is for a haploid sperm, 23X, to fertilize an 'empty egg' and to duplicate itself to form a 46,XX complement (Fig. 37.2). Much less commonly, by the process of dispermy, two spermatozoa, one being 23,X and the other 23,Y, can fertilize an 'empty egg' to give a 46,XY karyotype. Presumably, a small number of 46,XX karyotypes are also produced by dispermy, but a 46,YY complement is never seen because at least one X chromosome is essential for cell survival.

It is of some interest how the loss of the female haploid contribution occurs because it seems impossible that the chromosomes are absent at the completion of ovum maturation. This means that the maternal chromosomes are lost just before or at the time of 'fertilization' (in this context, entry of the sperm) or are driven out by the double set of male chromosomes prior to first mitotic cell division. The exact mechanisms responsible for the loss of the female haploid contribution remain unknown.

In partial mole, the normal finding is a triploid karyotype which means that they possess 69 chromosomes instead of the normal 46 (Szulman & Surti 1984). The most common mechanism appears to be the fertilization of a normal egg by two sperm giving a complement of 69,XXY with two of the chromosomes being of paternal origin. The alternative mechanism is for a sperm which has failed to undergo normal meiosis to fertilize a normal egg. The sperm carries a paternal load of 46,XY so that the end result is again a complement of 69,XXY with a

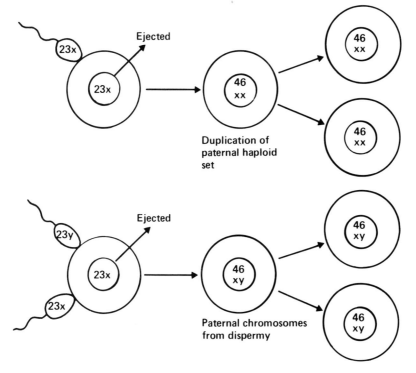

Fig. 37.2 Potential chromosomal mechanisms leading to complete hydatidiform mole by either duplication of paternal haploid set or by dispermy. Note that dispermy could also lead to a 46. XX karyotype.

double contribution from the paternal side. Not all triploid conceptuses lead to the formation of a partial mole, but, in these circumstances, the double contribution is from the maternal side. Although the majority of partial moles have triploid contributions as described above, there are exceptions to the rule and a variety of other abnormal chromosomal patterns have been described (Jacobs *et al.* 1982).

In summary, a complete mole is a pathenogenome of total paternal origin and is usually homozygous XX or rarely heterozygous XY; a partial mole is usually triploid with the extra sets of chromosomes being paternally derived. Because of this new understanding of the genetic origin of hydatidiform mole, it is appropriate to compare the pathological and clinical features of the two types, namely the complete and the partial mole.

PATHOLOGICAL FEATURES

In the classical picture of complete hydatidiform mole there are numerous oedematous vesicles, which on naked eye examination look like a bunch of small clear grapes. Usually a fetus cannot be identified and no membranes are present although a diligent search may yield embryonic fragments. On microscopic examination, the large oedematous villi tend to be avascular and there is a variable degree of trophoblastic hyperplasia. By contrast, a partial hydatidiform mole shows a less clear-cut picture; the formation of vesicles is usually focal and a fetus with membranes may be present. On histological examination, the appearances of molar degeneration are less obvious, the extent of trophoblastic hyperplasia is variable, and the vesicles have a degree of vascularity.

From a practical point of view, the histological examination presents the pathologist with a number of problems. It can be difficult to differentiate hydropic degeneration in an abortus from a partial mole; this distinction is an important one because the abortus has no important sequelae whereas the patient with a partial mole requires follow-up with all the anxiety, inconvenience and expense that this entails. It is also necessary to distinguish partial mole from complete mole because complete mole carries a greater risk of maligant degeneration and requires longer follow-up. The pathologist may also try to predict the malignant potential of a hydatidiform mole on the basis of the histological appearances; in general terms, the more active the trophoblast appears, the greater the risk of malignancy but agreement on this, even amongst expert pathologists, can be very diffi-

cult. In individual cases, however, the subsequent management depends more on the HCG results than the histological reports or even the clinical behaviour.

CLINICAL FEATURES

The symptoms of hydatidiform mole are those of pregnancy, commonly occurring in an exaggerated form, and the clinician needs to have a high index of clinical awareness to suspect the diagnosis. The most common features of hydatidiform mole are bleeding in early pregnancy, hyperemesis gravidarum, a large-for-dates uterus and, in some cases, the signs of pre-eclampsia. In complete mole the signs usually appear by 6–8 weeks of gestation and, if untreated, spontaneous abortion occurs by about 16–18 weeks (Kohorn 1984). In partial mole, the clinical features of mole may be less obvious, particularly when the hydatidiform change in the placenta is relatively small.

Bleeding
Bleeding in early pregnancy after a variable period of amenorrhoea is the most common clinical sign of mole, occurring in over 90% of cases (Goldstein & Berkowitz 1983, Curry *et al.* 1975). The bleeding is of variable amount and may be interspersed with a dark brown vaginal discharge. In rare cases the bleeding may be very severe and life threatening (Chun *et al.* 1964). There may be associated anaemia and a haemoglobin of less than 10 g/dl has been reported in over 50% of cases in some series (Goldstein & Berkowitz 1983) although the frequency of anaemia will be reduced by early diagnosis.

Hyperemesis gravidarum
Excessive vomiting occurs in about 25% of molar pregnancies (Goldstein & Berkowitz 1983) and the possibility of hydatidiform mole should be looked for in all patients with hyperemesis gravidarum. Excessive vomiting appears to be more common when the uterus is much enlarged and the HCG levels are very high. Ultrasound examination will help to distinguish hydatidiform mole from other causes of excessive vomiting such as multiple pregnancy.

Uterine enlargement
The uterus is commonly 'large-for-dates' when hydatidiform mole is present although, in a small proportion of cases, the uterus may be the correct size for gestational age or even small for dates. In a classical hydatidiform mole, the uterus is described as hav-

ing a doughy consistency, fetal parts are not palpable and the fetal heart is absent. In some cases, however, hydatidiform degeneration can co-exist with a fetus so that the presence of a fetal heart does not rule out the possibility of a partial mole. The clinical picture of a large-for-dates uterus may be exaggerated if large theca lutein cysts of the ovary are present. These cysts are a manifestation of excessive HCG stimulation and are present in about 20% of hydatidiform moles.

Pre-eclampsia

Pre-eclampsia can occur in association with hydatidiform mole; the reported frequencies range widely from 12% to 54% (Curry *et al.* 1975, Chun 1984). This variation is probably explained by differing times of diagnosis because the longer the pregnancy progresses the greater is the chance of pre-eclampsia developing. This risk of pre-eclampsia is an important argument in favour of early diagnosis and evacuation of the mole. If the signs of pre-eclampsia appear early in pregnancy, the possibility of hydatidiform mole should be looked for without delay.

Other clinical manifestations

Signs of hyperthyroidism develop in a small proportion of women with hydatidiform mole (Herschman & Higgins 1971) and this may be due to the thyrotrophic effects brought about by the high levels of human chorionic thyrotrophin (Twiggs 1984). In severe cases there may be goitre, fine tremor, supra-

ventricular tachycardia and weight loss (Herschman & Higgins 1971). Usually, the thyroid changes are of little clinical importance despite the elevated thyroid function tests on laboratory investigation. Invariably, the features of hyperthyroidism will resolve after evacuation of the mole.

Disseminated intravascular coagulation can develop in long-standing hydatidiform mole when there is embolization of trophoblastic tissue to the lung. The trophoblast leads to the release of thromboplastic substances which stimulate fibrin and platelet deposition within the vascular tree and may lead to coagulation failure. The best management is to correct the platelet and fibrinogen depletion using fresh frozen plasma, platelet transfusion and, rarely, cryoprecipitates, before proceeding to evacuate the hydatidiform mole.

DIAGNOSIS OF HYDATIDIFORM MOLE

Ultimate confirmation of hydatidiform mole comes when the characteristic vesicles are passed vaginally. It is, however, desirable that moles are diagnosed before this confirmatory sign. The mainstay of early diagnosis is ultrasonic examination, supported by serum HCG estimation. The advent of ultrasound has been a major advance because the diagnosis of mole can be made with confidence, even in the first trimester of pregnancy. The characteristic appearance on ultrasound is the 'snowstorm' appearance, resulting from the many echoes from the vesicular tissue (Fig.

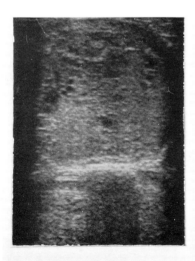

Transverse Section

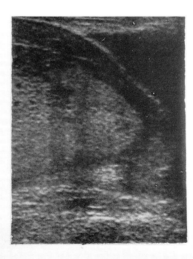

Longitudinal Section

Fig. 37.3 Ultrasonic picture of hydatidiform mole showing 'snowstorm' appearances of uterine contents. (Kindly supplied by Dr A.D. Christie, Ninewells Hospital, Dundee.)

37.3). In addition, fetal echoes and the fetal heart will not be present. The precision of diagnosis by ultrasound depends on the experience of the operator, but in skilled hands the diagnosis can usually be made with confidence. There can be occasional diagnostic difficulties due to conditions such as a degenerating fibroid, which give a similar ultrasonic picture; another uncommon problem which can give rise to diagnostic difficulty is the co-existence of a normal fetus with a hydatidiform mole, although the normal fetus will rarely survive under these circumstances (Jones & Laverson 1975).

If the diagnosis of hydatidiform mole is suspected clinically or suggested by ultrasonic examination, serum HCG estimation should be carried out although the results must be interpreted with care. In normal pregnancy HCG levels will rise, so an exact knowledge of gestational age is important. In normal singleton pregnancy, serum HCG levels are unlikely to rise above 500 000 international units/litre but may do so in twin pregnancy, which is the main diagnostic difficulty. Even in multiple pregnancy HCG levels will fall, so that a sustained rise of HCG may be of more value than a single elevated reading.

Further methods of diagnosis include amniography, pelvic arteriography and, even, X-ray. These methods all pose varying degrees of risk to a normally developing fetus and have now been largely abandoned in favour of ultrasound.

PROGNOSIS

The risks of hydatidiform mole are in three categories: 1 immediate, from haemorrhage, sepsis or pre-eclampsia; 2 from the occurrence of molar metastases; 3 from subsequent choriocarcinoma.

Haemorrhage, sepsis and pre-eclampsia

Treatment of all these conditions has vastly improved recently so that too much reliance should not be placed on retrospective data. In Hong Kong, Chun et al. (1964) recorded massive haemorrhage in 19 cases (7%) and one patient died. Access to appropriate blood transfusion services is essential for all who are responsible for treating hydatidiform mole. Sepsis is now not often a serious problem with the range of antibiotic and chemotherapeutic agents available. Pre-eclampsia is rarely severe enough to cause convulsions although it may occasionally prove fatal (Acosta-Sison 1955).

Molar metastases

Molar metastases of a non-proliferative type can occur in association with hydatidiform mole. In the series of Chun and her colleagues 11 out of 235 cases developed metastases which were not choriocarcinoma and this incidence of approximately 5% is in accord with other figures (Coppleson 1958, Park & Lees 1950). In some cases, embolization of trophoblastic tissue to the lung can lead to respiratory compromise and hypoxaemia with pulmonary oedema can occur, especially after evacuation of a large mole (Twiggs 1984). Early diagnosis may help to reduce the incidence of such 'benign' metastatic lesions. Even when they occur and persist after evacuation of the mole, the prognosis with methotrexate therapy is good.

Choriocarcinoma

The most important danger associated with hydatidiform mole is the development of choriocarcinoma and about 10% of cases require further treatment because of persistent post-molar trophoblastic disease (Bagshawe & Lawler 1982). After hydatidiform mole careful follow-up with serial HCG estimations is essential to give the earliest possible warning of malignant degeneration so that intensive chemotherapy is started without delay. This is discussed below.

MANAGEMENT OF HYDATIDIFORM MOLE

The aim of treatment is to eliminate all trophoblastic tissue from the maternal system. In those cases where the mole aborts spontaneously, all that may be required is gentle curettage of the uterine cavity. Evacuation of the uterus, whether spontaneous or surgical, may be complicated by haemorrhage, so that compatible blood should be cross-matched and oxytocics administered.

Prior to evacuation of the uterus, the patient's general condition should be assessed so that any metabolic upset can be corrected as necessary. Blood should be taken for a full blood count, a coagulation screen and an electrolyte check. If there is any dehydration as a result of hyperemesis, this should be corrected by intravenous fluid replacement. A chest X-ray should be carried out to exclude pulmonary metastases and, if they are present, blood gas analysis should be requested. If pre-eclampsia or thyrotoxicosis are present, they may require treatment depending upon their severity. In general terms, however, the bigger the mole the greater are the chances of complications so that it is desirable to evacuate the uterus without undue delay.

If hydatidiform mole is diagnosed before any sign of spontaneous abortion, steps should be taken to evacuate the uterus. This can be achieved by one of three main methods, namely suction curettage, uterine stimulation or surgical evacuation.

Suction curettage

The method of uterine evacuation influences the number of patients who require subsequent chemotherapy (Stone & Bagshawe 1979) and, for this reason, suction curettage is recommended by many authorities as the method of choice even when evacuating a large hydatidiform mole (Schlaerth 1984). Evacuation is usually carried out under general anaesthesia, although a paracervical block may be sufficient. The cervix is dilated carefully to avoid traumatic damage until a 12 mm diameter suction curette can be introduced. An intravenous oxytocin infusion is started and the suction curette is introduced into the uterine cavity using a negative pressure of about 60–70 cmHg. The curette is gently rotated in place and the majority of the molar tissue is evacuated rapidly. As the uterine size decreases, the curette is moved more liberally but care must be taken to avoid rupture of the soft uterus.

Following evacuation of the mole, gentle evacuation with a curette can be carried out. Over-zealous use of the sharp curette can cause Asherman's syndrome so that care is required and it may be safer to use blunt curettage. If the uterus is less than 10 weeks' size, curettage can be used as the primary method of evacuation.

Uterine stimulation

Intravenous oxytocin is not effective as a primary method to evacuate hydatidiform mole although it is of value when used to minimize haemorrhage during spontaneous abortion or suction evacuation of a mole.

Prostaglandin E_2 offers a more effective method of uterine stimulation. The preferred method is to introduce a Foley catheter through the cervix into the 'extra-amniotic' space and to infuse the prostaglandin E_2 by means of a continuous infusion pump. The prostaglandin E_2 is made up in saline in a concentration of 5 μg/ml and the infusion increased from 1 to 5 μg/minute (Calder et al. 1976). Prostaglandin E_2 appears to be a safe and effective method of treating hydatidiform mole and is particularly valuable when there is a co-existing fetus. With this method, as with

all methods, there is a risk of haemorrhage at the time of abortion of the mole and steps should be taken to prepare for the eventuality.

Surgical evacuation

Hysterectomy has been recommended as a suitable method of treating hydatidiform mole in the older woman who has completed her family. The risk of post-molar trophoblastic disease increases with maternal age and by removing the uterus, this risk may be reduced. Care must be taken to carry out the hysterectomy with as little manipulation as possible to avoid precipitating embolization of trophoblastic tissue. The utero-ovarian and uterine vessels should be clamped as quickly as possible and, in some cases, it may be necessary to puncture large theca lutein ovarian cysts to gain adequate access to the pelvis. In rare cases, hysterectomy may be required to control haemorrhage in emergency circumstances. In general, however, the place of hysterectomy in the management of hydatidiform mole is decreasing because of the effectiveness of the alternative forms of management. Similarly, hysterotomy, which was previously used to treat hydatidiform mole, is very rarely indicated.

FOLLOW-UP OF HYDATIDIFORM MOLE

It is important that women who have had a hydatidiform mole should have close surveillance of serum human chorionic gonadotrophin (HCG) levels after evacuation of the uterus to ensure early recognition of persistent trophoblastic disease. In about 90% of patients who have had a hydatidiform mole, the trophoblastic tissue dies out spontaneously after the uterus has been evacuated. In the remaining 10% the trophoblastic tissue does not die out completely and may persist or recur either as an invasive mole or as choriocarcinoma. Such patients will require chemotherapy and, to aid the completeness of follow-up, in the United Kingdom all patients who have had a hydatidiform mole should be registered through the Royal College of Obstetricians and Gynaecologists. Three units in Britain offer a postal follow-up service and they are centred at Charing Cross Hospital, London, the Jessop Hospital, Sheffield, and Ninewells Hospital, Dundee. The follow-up is by urinary HCG monitoring and, at the appropriate intervals, containers for the urine specimens are sent to the patients at their own homes. The patient sends her specimen to the regional centre and the results are transmitted to the clinician concerned. Registration forms are obtained from the three units who will endeavour to ensure that no patient is lost to follow-up. Continuing surveillance is recommended for 2 years after a complete hydatidiform mole and for 6 months following a partial mole (Newlands 1983).

After a molar pregnancy, the HCG levels will usually have returned to non-pregnant levels by 4–6 weeks after uterine evacuation and the task of the monitoring units is to identify those patients in whom the HCG regression curve is abnormal. The indications for chemotherapy after molar pregnancy are listed in Table 37.1. Abnormal HCG levels may be

Table 37.1 Indications for chemotherapy for patients who have had a hydatidiform mole (modified from Bagshawe *et al.* 1973 with permission from Professor Bagshawe and the *British Journal of Obstetrics and Gynaecology.*)

Urinary HCG values > 30000 i.u. 24 h or serum HCG
  > 20000 i.u./1 at 4–6 weeks after evacuation of the mole
Progressively rising HCG at any time post-evacuation of
  mole
Raised HCG values at 5–6 months after evacuation of the
  mole
Evidence of intracranial, hepatic, gastrointestinal
  metastases
Pulmonary metastases with persisting or rising HCG
  values
Persistent uterine haemorrhage with a raised HCG value

---

identified by a failure of urinary HCG levels to fall to normal within 6–8 weeks of evacuation, by a rise in HCG levels at any time or by a plateau of HCG levels over a period of three weeks or more. If any of these patterns are detected, the patient should be referred to a specialist centre for consideration of appropriate chemotherapy. In the United Kingdom chemotherapy is carried out by Professor Bagshawe's Unit at Charing Cross Hospital in London.

If HCG levels rise during the period of surveillance, it is possible that this indicates a new pregnancy. Patients are advised to avoid pregnancy during the period of follow-up and effective contraception is recommended. Oral contraception, which is the most reliable method available, can be used although some authorities recommend that it is better that it should not be started until HCG levels have returned to normal after delivery. The reason for advising this delay is that it has been shown that the molar trophoblast may die out more slowly in patients on the pill and more of them require chemotherapy (Stone & Bagshawe 1979).

The traditional pregnancy test is not sufficiently accurate to be a satisfactory method of monitoring the progression of trophoblastic disease and follow-up should use a reliable radioimmunoassay for HCG. The normal radioimmunoassay for HCG cross-reacts with luteinizing hormone (LH) but a more specific assay for the β subunit of HCG is available which cross-reacts with LH to only a minimal extent. The more specific assay is not necessary for patients who are undergoing routine follow-up but it is essential as a means of monitoring those who are undergoing chemotherapy.

Early diagnosis of persistent trophoblastic disease ensures a good prognosis and an effective system of follow-up is essential to achieve this objective.

CHORIOCARCINOMA

Malignant trophoblastic disease can exist in two forms, namely in a non-metastatic form, invasive mole, or in a metastatic form, choriocarcinoma. The distinction between the two conditions is somewhat artificial because both are treated with chemotherapy and monitored by the levels of that reliable tumour marker HCG. It is now becoming more important to subdivide choriocarcinoma into good-prognosis and poor-prognosis disease because such a distinction has implications for the most appropriate method of treatment.

EPIDEMIOLOGY

The incidence of choriocarcinoma is difficult to establish with certainty but has been estimated as lying between 1 : 10000 and 1 : 70000 pregnancies in the West and between 1 : 250 and 1 : 6000 pregnancies in Asia (Buckley 1984). The antecedent pregnancy is a hydatidiform mole in about 57% of cases of choriocarcinoma, a normal pregnancy in about 26% and an abortion or ectopic pregnancy in about 17% (Buckley 1984). The risk of choriocarcinoma after a hydatidiform mole is about 2–4% which is a thousand times greater than after a normal pregnancy. Choriocarcinoma is more likely to occur after a complete mole although a small number of cases of choriocarcinoma after partial mole have been described.

The maternal blood group influences the incidence, because a deficit of choriocarcinoma has been reported in association with group O and an excess with group A. In addition, choriocarcinoma is more likely to occur after matings between individuals of group A and group O than after matings in which both partners are group O or both are group A. The prognosis is also affected by blood groups, being less favourable in women with blood groups B or AB (Bagshawe 1976). The explanation for these findings is unknown.

PATHOLOGICAL FEATURES

Choriocarcinoma is a malignant neoplasm composed entirely of active chorionic epithelium which is avillous, necrotic and haemorrhagic. The tumour invades into the myometrium and metastasizes readily to the lung, the brain, the liver and other organs. Confirmation of the diagnosis may come from the histological examination of uterine curettings although it must be remembered that curettage carries the risks of uterine rupture and of dissemination of the tumour tissue. The critical factors in the diagnosis are clinical suspicion and measurement of the HCG levels.

CLINICAL FEATURES

One of the most striking features of choriocarcinoma is its diverse clinical features. Vaginal haemorrhage is the commonest presenting symptom and is a consequence of the tumour invading the uterine cavity. A complaint of abdominal or vaginal swelling may develop and there may also be amenorrhoea due to the production of HCG from distant tumour metastases. Dyspnoea and haemoptysis may occur as a result of pulmonary metastases and neurological abnormalities may indicate the presence of metastatic disease in the brain. The chest signs may be confused with pulmonary tuberculosis and this impression may be supported by the chest X-ray appearances. A high index of clinical awareness is required to make the diagnosis when the antecedent pregnancy has been an abortion or a normal pregnancy but will be relatively easy after a mole when routine monitoring of the HCG levels will be underway. The important practical problem is to identify those patients who require chemotherapy; in addition to those with abnormal HCG levels after molar pregnancy, this will be necessary in those women who have radiological or clinical evidence of choriocarcinoma, radiological or clinical evidence of metastases or persistent uterine haemorrhage with raised HCG values.

PROGNOSIS

A number of factors have been identified which influ-ence the prognosis in patients with malignant trophoblastic disease. These factors appear to operate in an additive way, the greater the number of adverse factors, the poorer the prognosis. A score can be calculated from the various factors as shown in Table 37.2 and the patient allocated to a low, medium or high risk category depending upon the result.

A high level of pretreatment HCG is a poor prognostic factor and this may reflect a large mass of tumour tissue. The number and size of metastases are important features, the poorest prognosis being associated with large masses and with brain, liver and gastrointestinal metastases. A long interval between the antecedent pregnancy and the onset of chemotherapy is an adverse prognostic factor, and delay in diagnosis may explain the poorer outcome in choriocarcinoma following term pregnancy or abortion. Changes in immune response during normal pregnancy may also have an effect on outcome because those patients who are relatively unreactive immunologically to the tumour have a less favourable outcome. A history of previous unsuccessful chemotherapy is a poor prognostic factor; this may be related to drug-resistant tumour, to accumulated toxicity from the drug therapy or to impermeability to chemotherapeutic agents because of scarring and fibrosis (Hammond & Soper 1984). A large number of deaths in choriocarcinoma can be attributed to drug resistance. Finally, increased maternal age and parity as well as maternal blood groups B and AB adversely affect the outcome.

If, however, the diagnosis is made at an early stage the prognosis is favourable for the great majority of patients and a survival rate of 97% is expected when the interval between the antecedent pregnancy and the onset of chemotherapy is less than 4 months (Bagshawe 1976).

TREATMENT OF CHORIOCARCINOMA

The management of choriocarcinoma is highly specialized and optimum results will be achieved only in units with special expertise in this field. There have been a number of detailed descriptions of the management of choriocarcinoma (e.g. Bagshawe & Begent 1981, Newlands 1983, Hammond & Soper 1984) and only the general principles of management will be discussed here. The mainstay of treatment is chemotherapy, because, before its introduction, the prognosis was very poor with only a small number of women surviving after hysterectomy alone (Ober 1971). The first drug to be used was the folic acid antagonist methotrexate (Li *et al.* 1956) and it remains one of the most valuable therapeutic agents. A variety of other cytotoxic drugs have been introduced such as actinomycin D, cyclophosphamide, VP 16–213, vincristine and vinblastine and, in addition, drugs with limited single-agent activity are adriamycin, cis-platinum, mustine, 6-mercaptopurine and 6-azauridine (Newlands 1983). By the use of these agents in appropriate combined regimes, the prognosis has been transformed and the prospect of complete cure can be offered to the great majority of patients.

Staging of choriocarcinoma

The first task of management in the regime used in Charing Cross Hospital is to stage the disease according to the scheme indicated in Table 37.2. The obstetric history, the findings at clinical examination, the HCG results and the histology reports are considered with a number of investigations; the patient has an ultrasonic assessment of the pelvis, a chest X-ray, a liver scan and a lumbar puncture for measurement of HCG in the cerebro-spinal fluid. On the basis of these investigations the patient is allocated to a low risk, medium risk or high risk category and treated accordingly. Details of the regimes are given in Newlands (1983).

Chemotherapy

Patients in the low risk category are treated for eight days receiving methotrexate and folinic acid on alternate days. Courses of therapy are repeated at seven day intervals and serum HCG levels are monitored twice weekly. It usually takes 4–8 weeks' treatment to reduce HCG levels to normal and treatment is then continued for a further 8 weeks. The advantage of this regime is that methotrexate is relatively non-toxic and is associated with minimal alopecia. The folinic acid is added to reduce the risk of stomatitis. The majority of patients in the low risk category are successfully treated with this regime and, although about 20% may require further chemotherapy with an alternative regime because of drug resistance, the outcome is very favourable.

The medium risk category of patients receive a more complicated regime than the low risk patients because single dose treatment leads to a high incidence of drug resistance. Three combinations of treatment are used in rotation, these being: 1. VP 16-213; 2. a combination of hydroxyurea, 6-mercaptopurine and methotrexate/folinic acid; 3. actinomycin-D.

If drug resistance develops to any of these, a combination of vincristine and cyclophosphamide is substituted. This regime is more toxic than the one used for the low risk patients and reversible alopecia

Table 37.2 Categorization of patients with gestational trophoblastic tumours. Scores for individual risk factors are added and risk group determined by the total score as follows: Low risk 50 or less; Medium risk 55–95; High risk > 95. (From Newlands (1983) in *Progress in Obstetrics & Gynaecology* (Ed. Studd J.) Churchill Livingstone, with permission.)

Risk factors	0	10	20	40
Age	< 39	> 39		
Parity	1,2, > 4	3 or 4		
Antecedent pregnancy	Mole	Abortion	Term	
Interval (AP-chemotherapy in months)	< 4	4–7	7–12	> 12
HCG (plasma miu/ml or urine iu/day)	< 10^3	10^3–10^4	10^4–10^5	10^5
ABO ♀ × ♂	A × A	O × O	B ×	
	× B	A × O	AB ×	
	× AB			
No. of metastases	Nil	1–4	4–8	> 8
Site of metastases	Not detected	Spleen	GI tract	Brain
	Lungs	Kidney	Liver	
	Vagina			
Largest tumour mass	< 3 cm	3–5 cm	> 5 cm	
Lymphocytic infiltration	Marked	Moderate	Slight	
		Unknown		
Immune status	Reactive		Unreactive	
Previous chemotherapy	Nil		Single drug	Two drugs or more

usually occurs. The level of bone marrow depression is monitored by the white cell and platelet counts but it is necessary to depress these haemopoietic factors severely to achieve the required therapeutic effect. The introduction of VP 16-213 has appeared to have reduced the incidence of drug resistance in this group of medium risk patients so that they now have a favourable overall prognosis which is similar to that of the low risk patients (Newlands 1983).

The patients in the high risk category present by far the biggest therapeutic challenge. Drug resistance is common in this group of patients and a variety of combinations of the drugs used for the medium risk category are employed. Treatment is continued until the white cell count drops below 1000 or the platelet count below 50000 per cu mm. Because of the low white cell and platelet counts, there are dangers from infection and haemorrhage. If infection is a problem, patients may require to be isolated and have prolonged antibiotic therapy. If there is evidence of septic shock this may require separate management in its own right. If haemorrhage occurs in the presence of a low platelet count, blood replacement and platelet transfusion may be required. In addition, the nausea, vomiting and mucositis caused by the cytotoxic drugs may lead to severe dehydration and nutritional depletion and require appropriate replacement therapy. Such intensive therapy requires great fortitude on the part of both the patients and the staff and the psychological impact of the management should not be forgotten. The patient will be separated from her family for long spells and family counselling is an important part of the management. Although the overall prognosis in the high risk group is reasonable, with a complete remission rate of about 67%, a number of patients die, usually as a result of drug resistance. Even when patients have cerebral metastases, the outcome can be favourable if the tumour is sensitive to the drugs; if, however, cerebral metastases develop during chemotherapy, the prognosis becomes extremely poor. The successful management of the formidable problems caused by intensive chemotherapy requires the multidisciplinary skills of a highly specialized team.

Surgery

Before the introduction of chemotherapy, hysterectomy was the only treatment to offer the patient any chance of survival. Many of the women who have choriocarcinoma are able to have pregnancies after successful chemotherapy, so that it is desirable to avoid hysterectomy and retain reproductive function.

Although there is some evidence that hysterectomy at the time of commencing chemotherapy can reduce the duration of treatment (Hammond *et al.* 1980), the use of surgery in the management of choriocarcinoma has been greatly reduced and is usually reserved for those who have completed their families.

Radiotherapy

The use of radiotherapy in the management of choriocarcinoma is limited and its value uncertain. Following the introduction of CT scanning, it may be possible to identify tumour areas more exactly and direct irradiation to the target site with more precision. In the light of the success of chemotherapy, the use of radiotherapy will be limited to a small number of drug-resistant cases.

Further management

After the successful treatment of choriocarcinoma, most women are able to have further pregnancies with an outcome which is closely similar to that of the normal population (Goldstein *et al.* 1984). Following the completion of treatment, however, patients are advised to avoid pregnancy for at least 12 months so that the cytotoxic drugs can be fully metabolized and excreted because they are potentially teratogenic. The interval of 12 months is also the time when there is the greatest risk of relapse and the need for further chemotherapy, although relapse occurs in less than 5% of cases (Newlands 1983).

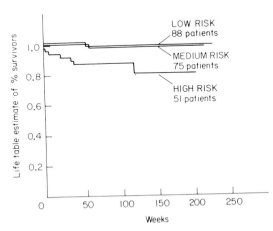

Fig. 37.4 Life Table Analysis of 214 patients treated between 1974 and 1979 according to their prognostic score. The overall survival of the 3 groups = 94%. (From Newlands, 1983 with permission of the author, and Editor of *Progress in Obstetrics and Gynaecology*, Churchill Livingstone, Edinburgh.)

Following treatment for choriocarcinoma, patients are followed up with HCG monitoring for life and this will permit the construction of Life Table Analysis. The results for patients treated in Charing Cross Hospital between 1974 and 1979 are shown in Fig. 37.4, according to their prognostic classification. As can be seen from the results, the overall prognosis is good even for the patients in the high risk category. Clearly, the good results which are dependent upon a combination of early diagnosis and appropriate management, are achieved only by good cooperation between the local gynaecologists and the specialist team.

REFERENCES

ACOSTA-SISON H. (1955). *Philipp. J. Surg. Obstet. Gynec.*, **10**, 61.

ATTWOOD H.D. & PARK W.W. (1961). *J. Obstet. Gynaec. Brit. Cwlth.*, **68**, 611.

BAGSHAWE K.D. (1976). *Cancer*, **38**, 1373.

BAGSHAWE K.D. & LAWLER S.D. (1982). *Brit. J. Obstet. Gynaec.*, **89**, 255.

BAGSHAWE K.D., WILSON H., DUBLON P., SMITH A., BALDWIN M. & KARDANA A. (1973). *J. Obstet. Gynaec.*, **80**, 461.

BAGSHAWE K.D. & BEGENT R.H.J. (1981). In *Gynecologic Oncology*. (Ed. Coppleson M.) Vol. 2, p. 757. Churchill Livingstone, Edinburgh.

BUCKLEY J.D. (1984). *Clin. Obstet. Gynecol.*, **27**, 153.

CALDER A.A., McKENZIE T.Z. & EMBREY M.P. (1976). *J. reprod. Med.*, **16**, 271.

CHUN D., BRAGA C., CHOW C. & LOK L. (1964). *J. Obstet. Gynaec. Brit. Cwlth.*, **71**, 180.

COPPLESON M. (1958). *J. Obstet. Gynaec. Brit. Cwlth.*, **65**, 238.

CURRY S.L., HAMMOND C.B., TYREY L., CREASMAN W.T. & PARKER R.T. (1975). *Obstet. Gynecol.*, **45**, 1.

GOLDSTEIN D.P. & BERKOWITZ R.S. (1983). In *Major Problems in Obstetrics and Gynecology*, Vol. 14, W.B. Saunders, Philadelphia.

GOLDSTEIN D.P., BERKOWITZ R.S. & BERNSTEIN M.R. (1984). *Clin. Obstet. Gynecol.*, **27**, 221.

HAMMOND C.B. & SOPER J.T. (1984). *Clin. Obstet. Gynecol.*, **27**, 228.

HAMMOND C.B., WEED J.C., CURRIE J.L. (1980). *Amer. J. Obstet. Gynecol.*, **136**, 844.

HERSCHMANN J.M. & HIGGINS H.P. (1971). *New Engl. J. Med.*, **284**, 573.

JACOBS P.A., HUNT P.A., MATSUURA J.S., WILSON C.C., SZULMAN A.E. (1982). *Brit. J. Obstet. Gynaec.*, **89**, 258.

JONES W.B. & LAVERSON N.H. (1975). *Amer. J. Obstet. Gynecol.*, **122**, 267.

KAJII J. & OHAMA K. (1977). *Nature*, **268**, 633.

KOHORN E.I. (1984). *Clin. Obstet. Gynecol.*, **27**, 181.

LI M.C., HERTZ R. & SPENCER D.B. (1956). *Proc. Soc. exp. Biol. (N.Y.).*, **43**, 361.

NEWLANDS E.S. (1983). In *Progress in Obstetrics and Gynaecology* (Ed. Studd J.) Vol. 3, p. 158. Churchill Livingstone, Edinburgh.

OBER W.B., EDGCOMBE J.H. & PRICE E.B. (1971). *Ann. N.Y. Acad. Sci.*, **1972**, 299.

PARK W.W. & LEES J.C. (1950). *Archs. Path.*, **49**, 205.

SCHLAERTH J.B. (1984). *Clin. Obstet. Gynecol.*, **27**, 192.

STONE M. & BAGSHAWE K.D. (1979). *Brit. J. Obstet. Gynaecol.*, **86**, 782.

SZULMAN A.E. & SURTI V. (1984). *Clin. Obstet. Gynecol.*, **27**, 172.

TWIGGS L.B. (1984). *Clin. Obstet. Gynecol.*, **27**, 199.

CHAPTER 38
CONTRACEPTION AND STERILIZATION

RODNEY. P. SHEARMAN

Contraception and sterilization are subjects that can be almost guaranteed to generate controversy. Because this book is designed for clinical gynaecologists and obstetricians, not demographers, sociologists, moralists, theologians or politicians, the approach chosen here will therefore be clinical.

The ideal form of contraception would be 100% effective, completely reversible, totally acceptable and absolutely free of side effects. No such method exists.

Assessment of effectiveness

One of the first methods used to describe effectiveness was that developed by Raymond Pearl (1932), hence called the Pearl Index. This is the number of pregnancies per hundred woman years (HWY) in those women at risk of pregnancy. A woman year is 12 menstrual cycles. The Pearl Index is a good summary statistic mirroring the incidence rate in a population but the rate can be biased by a disproportionate number of women in a study who have extremely long contraceptive use without failure. To overcome this bias a life table technique to assess 'use effectiveness' was introduced. This method estimates the probability of pregnancy while using any method during a fixed time interval, the pregnancy rate being expresses as x per 100 women per year. It should be evident that neither of these figures takes into account women who become pregnant because they give up a method not in order to become pregnant but because of method dissatisfaction. Tietze and Lewit (1968) introduced the term 'extended use effectiveness' to estimate the chances of an unwanted pregnancy occurring within a fixed interval after the initiation of contraceptive use, whether or not the contraceptive had been abandoned.

Two further types of effectiveness are also often noted: method failure and patient failure. Method failure is failure attributable to a method if it is used perfectly and reliably under ideal circumstances. Patient failure is attributed to less than ideal use of that particular method. For example sexual abstinence has a theoretical effectiveness of 100%. If, however, the couple do not observe continued sexual abstinence pregnancies will occur and these could be seen as patient rather than method failures. In the real world use effectiveness is the most useful index.

The range of pregnancies expressed as the Pearl Index in a group of women using well established methods of contraception is shown in Fig. 38.1.

Measurement of risk

The first indication of risk usually starts with anecdotal case reports. While these may be a valuable early warning, they provide no statistical assessment. Two methods are used to assess risk: case control and cohort studies. In the former, groups of patients suffering from a disease thought to be attributed to a method of contraception are compared with matched controls who have no such disease. The differential use of the particular method of contraception is then assessed. Cohort studies take two groups of subjects. These are then followed longitudinally over an appropriate number of years. One group uses a method of contraception under study while another group (control) does not use that method of contraception. The incidence of complications ('events') is then compared in the two groups. While confounding variables such as age, parity, reproductive history are usually considered, other variables that might ultimately emerge to be of great significance such as sexual history, smoking habits, hypertension or obesity have not always been recorded. The *relative risk* of the contraceptive is the ratio of the rates observed for contraceptive users to the rates of the same event observed among a control group. It may be less than unity. The difference in the rates may be considered as the *excess* or *attributable* risk of the contraceptive regime.

'The interpretation of relative or excess risk is not always straightforward. If one compares the risk of cervical dysplasia among users of oral contraception

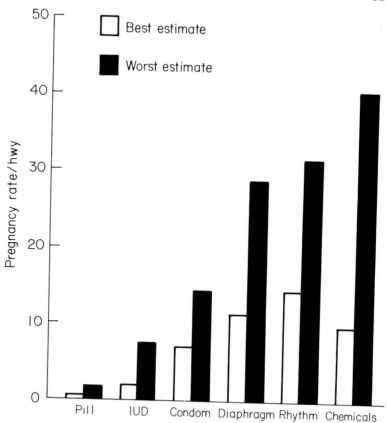

Fig. 38.1. Failure rates of contraceptive methods. From Peel and Potts (1969).

to that of users of the diaphragm the relative risk may reflect no excess risk among the pill users but a depressed risk (a benefit) among users of the diaphragm. The risk ratio may be greatly in excess of unity simply because the diaphragm may protect, while the pill may not protect, although it does not exacerbate the condition' (Sivin 1979).

METHODS AVAILABLE

NATURAL METHODS

All of these are based on the relatively short time when the ovum can be fertilized and the slightly longer time that sperm are capable of surviving with fertilizing potential in the female genital tract. Each of these depends on the ability to predict the time of ovulation. The calendar method relies on an analysis of the woman's menstrual data over the preceding twelve months and from these data the earliest and latest time of ovulation in future cycles is predicted. Failures from this method, if assembled, would form legions. The sympto-thermal method restricts intercourse until 48 hours after the basal body tempera-

ture has risen. For those couples who find any method of 'artificial' contraception unacceptable, the ovulation method is used most widely and has been the subject of carefully controlled studies. Use effectiveness shows a pregnancy rate of about 25/HWY. Keen supporters of this method take the attitude that the theoretical effectiveness is 100% and that pregnancy will occur only if the couple do not follow the advice they are given. These supporters do not accept the concept of use effectiveness or extended use effectiveness. The method relies on a woman being trained to determine changes in her own cervical mucus secretion, the fundamental observation being based on the increased secretion of clear, slippery vaginal mucin which can be detected in the vagina on the days preceding ovulation.

The World Health Organization and other international agencies have attempted to develop 'kitchen methods' to predict ovulation such as a 'dip-stick' to determine changes in urinary steroid production. None of these has found acceptance. A careful analysis of methods of ovulation prediction will be found in Brown and Gronow (1985).

COITUS INTERRUPTUS

This method is far more widely used than many people recognize. For many years an extraordinary number of side effects including insomnia, anxiety and suicide were attributed to the method but these attributions are not based on fact. For well motivated couples who mutually determine that this is the best method this is an acceptable form of contraception with a failure rate of about 18/HWY. Whatever its failures it is certainly safe. There is only one documented death—Onan.

CONDOMS

This is one of the oldest and also the most widely used methods of birth control. The condom has the advantage that it is readily available in most societies, does not need medical supervision, provides substantial protection against sexually transmitted disease and as long as it is used properly gives a reasonable degree of protection, the best estimates indicating a Pearl Index of 5.

SPERMICIDES AND DIAPHRAGMS

Spermicides share with condoms the advantage that they can be used without any medical advice or supervision. However, when used alone they are relatively ineffective and are usually combined with a vaginal diaphragm. This method has the disadvantage that it is coitally related. Apart from personal choice the only contraindication to the use of a diaphragm and spermicide is the concurrence of substantial uterine prolapse. Cervical caps are not as widely used as the diaphragm. Spermicides are available as suppositories, foams or creams. The cream is most suitable for use in conjunction with the diaphragm. The most widely used are ricinoleic acid and nonylphenoxypolyethoxyethanol (nonoxynol-9), alone or in combination. More recently, in a remarkable piece of serendipity, Zupper et al. (1983) have shown that the well known beta blocker propranolol is an effective spermicide used vaginally as an 80 mg tablet. One development, utilizing a combination of mechanical and spermicidal methods, has been the introduction of the 'sponge', a polyurethane device impregnated with nonoxynol-9. Reported pregnancy rate is between 9–27/HWY making it comparable to other barrier methods.

INTRAUTERINE CONTRACEPTIVE DEVICES (IUD)

Intrauterine contraceptive devices have proved to be a fertile field for those gynaecologists who want eponymic immortality. From Grafenberg and Ota through Margulies and Birnberg to Lippes and Tatum the breed has proliferated. With the exception of Tatum and Lippes most eponymic devices have been decently interred. It would be counter-productive and certainly inaccurate to attempt a complete list of intrauterine devices available throughout the world. Essentially they are of three types: 'inert' devices such as the Lippes loop; devices with various applications of copper designed to increase effectiveness and reduce surface area (Copper T, Copper 7, Multiload); and medicated intrauterine devices releasing low concentrations of progesterone or norgestrel (for example the Progestasert). If adequate attention is paid to contraindications many of the difficulties seen with IUDs relate more to the skill and experience of the inserter than to the actual device.

The Lippes loop, in its various sizes, remains the bench-mark against which other devices are assessed. It has the great advantage that there is no need for it to be replaced whereas the copper devices, although perhaps having slightly greater effectiveness and, because of their lower surface area, some reduction in bleeding, all require removal and reinsertion at intervals recommended by the manufacturer.

Progestin releasing devices are not widely available. They have the advantage that menstrual blood loss is very substantially reduced but the disadvantage that removal and reinsertion may be required frequently (with the Progestasert once a year). The need for adequate follow-up so that devices can be removed and replaced makes these relatively unsuitable in many parts of the world. Because of their lack of general availability, the medicated devices will not be considered further.

Mechanism of action
This is still not fully understood and is probably multifactorial. The major action appears to be interference with endometrial implantation of the blastocyst. Because of its action in preventing implantation, orthodox Roman Catholics will regard IUDs as abortifacient. In addition, copper releasing devices undoubtedly interfere with endometrial enzymes such as carbonic anhydrase and probably also reduce the rate of sperm ascent to the Fallopian tube.

Contraindications

Intrauterine devices should not be used in the presence of: pregnancy; multiple fibroids, especially if they impinge upon and distort the uterine cavity; congenital uterine abnormality affecting the shape of the uterine cavity, for example bicornuate, septate or unicornuate uterus; acute or subacute pelvic inflammatory disease (PID) or active vaginal inflammation; carcinoma of the cervix or body of the uterus; valvular heart disease; abnormal uterine bleeding; known allergy to copper if a copper IUD is being chosen.

Those who doubt the risk of bacterial endocarditis in women with valvular heart disease should read a short but sharp reminder from Sparks (1984).

Choice of device

The copper devices have a lower surface area and therefore cause less uterine bleeding. They seem to be better tolerated in nulliparous patients than larger inert devices. However a nulliparous patient may not be the best subject in whom to use an IUD. An inert device, such as a Lippes loop, should be used if you cannot be certain of patient compliance for follow up. The smallest device (A) should be used for nulliparous patients while in most parous patients size C is appropriate.

Insertion

The critically important factor here is adequate training. There is ample evidence from many developing countries that appropriately trained paramedical personnel can achieve results as acceptable as those achieved by medical graduates. In most developed countries insertion of IUDs will remain the prerogative of medical practitioners. However there is nothing magical about having a medical degree after one's name. A practitioner, whether he be general or consultant, should not insert intrauterine devices without appropriate training. Discussion of techniques will be found in Kleinman (1980).

Follow-up

Since expulsion (*see* below) occurs most frequently around the time of the first menstruation after insertion, the patient should either be trained to assess the presence of the thread of the device or she should be examined to determine that the device is still *in situ* soon after her first post-insertion period. Apart from this and in the absence of complicating symptoms, no more than routine follow-up applicable to any sexually active woman is indicated, but the patient must be advised of the need for removal and reinsertion of copper bearing devices.

Effectiveness

During the first year after insertion between 2 and 3% of women will conceive. This includes those in whom pregnancy has occurred because the device has either been expelled or translocated to the peritoneal cavity or cervical canal, as well as those who conceive with the device *in situ*. After the first year there is a decline in pregnancy rate leading to a cumulative annual failure rate of less than 1% after 6 years.

Benefits

Having been inserted and provided it is not expelled or removed, there is no longer any need for continuing motivation to practise this method of contraception. In addition it lacks any systemic metabolic effects and has an effectiveness only slightly less than that seen with oral contraceptives. The risks must be weighed against the benefits.

Risks

Increased blood loss. Although some vaginal bleeding is the rule immediately after insertion most of the problems with blood loss relate to an increase in the volume of menstrual bleeding. The mean normal blood loss of about 35 ml in the cycle increases to about 80 ml in patients wearing Lippes loop and 50–60 ml in those wearing the smaller copper bearing devices. This increased blood loss may be sufficient to cause or compound iron deficiency anaemia. In addition to those women who experience increased but regular bleeding there is a small group who have irregular and unpredictable bleeding often associated with pain.

Pain. Many women will experience some cramping pain for a few days after the device is inserted. Many will suffer dysmenorrhoea during menstruation and this is particularly common in nulliparous women. If crampy pain is the only side effect, substantial relief may be obtained by the use of prostaglandin synthetase inhibitors such as mefenamic acid in a dose of 500 mg three times daily on days 1 and 2 of the cycle.

Perforation. This usually occurs at the time of insertion and most frequently is through the uterine fundus. In large series of insertions the perforation rate is about 1:1000. Perforation should be suspected if the patient states at follow-up that she cannot feel the tail. While this often means that the device has rotated within the uterine cavity it also often means that it has become translocated. Pelvic ultrasound will help to localize the device whether it is within or without the uterus. Intraperitoneal devices can usually be recovered through a laparoscope. Because of the tendency for copper to promote intraperitoneal adhesions removal is mandatory if a copper device perforates. Those devices with a straight vertical arm such as the copper T or the copper 7 may perforate the cervical canal. This complication is rarely associated with symptoms but contraceptive effectiveness is reduced. The first follow-up visit should therefore include inspection of the cervix to determine that the thread is *in situ* and palpation of the cervical canal with a uterine sound.

Infection. Insertion of an intrauterine device can never be a sterile procedure and transient colonization of the endometrium is the norm for a few days after insertion (Mishell 1979). More recently there has been increasing concern about an excess incidence of pelvic inflammatory disease in women bearing intrauterine devices compared with those of similar sexual activity using other methods of contraception, in particular oral contraceptives or barrier methods. There is some evidence that this risk is even higher in nulliparous than parous women. For this reason the author is very reluctant to employ an intrauterine device in a woman who has not previously had children. The full spectrum of expected organisms may be found including chlamydia, gonococcus, anaerobes and rarely infection with *Actinomycoses israelii*. If PID does occur, while awaiting bacteriological confirmation, treatment to cover aerobes and anaerobes should be started. Most gynaecologists believe that the device should be removed when treatment is initiated. If a further device is to be used, and the author has very grave doubts whether this is ever wise in a person who has had PID with an intrauterine device *in situ*, at least two months should be allowed for complete resolution of the inflammatory response before reinsertion.

It is a mistake to believe that only those women with fever and peritonism have PID with an IUD *in situ*. A substantial number of those women with irregular bleeding and intermenstrual and menstrual pain will, on laparoscopy, be shown to have active pelvic inflammatory disease. In addition a proportion of patients rendered infertile by peritubal adhesions

have no risk factor in their previous history apart from the use of an IUD.

The very serious problem of infection associated with spontaneous abortion and an IUD will be discussed below.

Ectopic pregnancy. Because of the increased risks of PID with an IUD, it might be expected that long term follow-up of patients who have used this method will show an increased incidence of ectopic pregnancy as well as infertility. Relevant data are not yet available. In a very large study from the Population Council it is clear that both intrauterine and tubal pregnancies are reduced by an IUD, the reduction of the former being 99.5%, and the latter 95%. There is no reduction in the incidence of ovarian pregnancy (Mishell 1979).

Spontaneous abortion. Pregnancy occurring with an IUD *in situ* is associated with a spontaneous abortion rate of about 55%, an increase of about threefold compared with women not using an intrauterine device. By definition, any pregnancy with an intrauterine device *in situ* is unplanned but it is a mistake to assume that every unplanned pregnancy is unwanted. If the patient elects to proceed with the pregnancy removal of the IUD (if the tail is still visible at the external os) reduces the risk of abortion.

Infected abortion. In the mid 1970s it became apparent that some spontaneous abortions associated with an IUD were accompanied by severe, sometimes overwhelming and indeed lethal infection. Although described more commonly with the Dalkon shield (now discontinued) this unnerving and catastrophic complication may occur with any intrauterine device complicated by intrauterine pregnancy. If the patient elects to continue with pregnancy the IUD should be removed. If the tail of the IUD cannot be seen then the risks should be discussed with the patient and her partner. The final decision whether to terminate or proceed with the pregnancy should be left to them.

Prematurity. If a patient with an IUD and concurrent uterine pregnancy does not abort she still faces a substantial (fourfold) increase in the risk of spontaneous prematurity. It is possible that there is also an increased risk of intrauterine death due to fetoplacental transfusion.

Putting this into perspective the majority of women who do not abort go to term. The IUD is expelled with the placenta, usually lying nicely behind it.

ORAL CONTRACEPTION IN THE FEMALE

On best estimates, about 60 million women throughout the world are currently taking oral contraceptives. It is a widely accepted, effective, usually reversible method of contraception. An adequate substitute for the present generation of low dose pills cannot be seen even on a distant horizon. The original oral contraceptives developed in the late 1950s contained far more of both components, the oestrogen and the progestogen, than were needed for their pharmacological action. The history of pill development has been a progressive reduction in dosage to what is now probably the lowest dosage compatible with therapeutic effect, that is to inhibit ovulation.

Although combined oral contraceptives have multiple effects, the dominant action for contraception is inhibition of the midcycle LH peak and therefore inhibition of ovulation. Progestogen only pills (the 'minipill') probably have important additional actions such as effects on cervical mucin; ovulation will occur in a substantial minority of patients taking these pills.

It would be an exercise in futility to attempt to draw up a table of all commercially available oral contraceptives, as these differ widely from country to country. Sequential oral contraceptives have been withdrawn from the market in many countries, but where they are available there are only three generic types:

1 Progestogen only (mini) pills. These consist of either norgestrel or norethisterone given each and every day and contain either $30 \mu g$ of levonorgestrel or $350 \mu g$ of norethisterone;
2 Combined oral contraception;
3 Sequential oral contraception.

Only two oestrogens are used (mestranol or ethinyl oestradiol) but there is a greater variety of progestins.

(a) *Oestrogens.* Ethinyl oestradiol is used in most preparations. A small minority contain mestranol, the 3 methyl ether of ethinyl oestradiol.

(b) *Progestogens.* Fundamentally there are two groups of progestogens: those containing, or metabolized to, norethisterone; and those containing norgestrel or its close relative desogestrel. As first introduced, norgestrel was a mixture of the d and l isomers. It became evident that the pharmacological activity rested entirely with the laevo form. Consideration of the other family of progestogens is much simpler if it is recog-

nized that, with the exception of norgestrel and desogestrel, all other progestins, including of course norethisterone itself, are effective *in vivo* after metabolism to norethisterone. Therefore norethisterone, its acetate, ethynodiol diacetate and lynestrenol should be considered in the family of norethisterone.

Potency
This is a vexed question and a great deal of nonsense has been written about it.

(a) *Oestrogens.* Mestranol is effective in the human after demethylation to ethinyl oestradiol. Strictly speaking mestranol is very slightly less potent than the same microgram weight of ethinyl oestradiol. However, the difference is so small that for practical purposes they may be considered equally potent. It is obvious that $30 \mu g$ of ethinyl oestradiol is substantially less potent than $100 \mu g$ of ethinyl oestradiol or mestranol.

(b) *Progestogens.* In the norgestrel group, accepting that d-norgestrel is endocrinologically inert, $250 \mu g$ of levenorgestrel is equipotent to $500 \mu g$ of dl-norgestrel. Levenorgestrel and desogestrel are of approximately equal potency.

Since all of the other progestins are either norethisterone *de novo* or metabolized to that compound before pharmacological activity occurs, comparison within that group becomes much easier. In clinical practice it is probably reasonable to say that any of the 'norethisterone group' are equipotent microgram for microgram.

Most difficulties have arisen in attempting to compare the biological potency of the norethisterone group with the norgestrel group. There is no scientific consensus about the best method of measuring progestational potency. The problem is compounded further when it is recognized that for such important metabolic effects as those seen on lipid metabolism, the effect of a given dose of a particular progestin is modified substantially by the amount of oestrogen administered. Therefore, although it is easy to look at differential potency of one dose of oestrogens compared with another dose of the same oestrogen or one dose of laevo norgestrel compared with a different dose of that drug, there are very real difficulties in comparing the potency of norgestrel with the potency of a progestogen from the norethisterone group. If one accepts the pharmacological fundamental that no more of any drug should be prescribed than is needed to secure the biological effect that is being sought, much of the heat engendered in arguments about potency becomes meaningless. This will be discussed more fully when dealing with initial therapy.

Side effects and other concerns

Minor. These side effects, which are mainly of nuisance value, consist of disturbances of the menstrual cycle, changes in weight and change in mood.

If a large number of women taking oral contraceptives are studied then there is no doubt that, statistically, menstrual (or withdrawal) bleeding is far more regular and predictable than in women who are cycling spontaneously. Irrespective of the combined preparation used, menstrual blood loss is almost invariably less than that experienced by the patient before or after treatment with the pill. Within that general statement there are, however, some disturbances of menstrual loss that might cause concern to individuals.

Breakthrough bleeding may occur, particularly in early treatment cycles. This may be one of two types, either midcycle spotting or frank breakthrough like an early and badly timed period. Midcycle spotting is far more common in early treatment cycles and is more common with the new lower dose pills than it was with the older tablets. If midcycle spotting alone is present then treatment should continue as this usually settles after the second or third cycle. If it does not, a higher dose pill may be needed. If frank and heavier breakthrough bleeding occurs, the patient should be instructed to stop treatment, throw away the partially used pack of pills and start a new packet seven days later. If this occurs on more than two occasions a different method or a higher dose pill should be considered. These episodes are common and pill-related in early treatment months. If midcycle bleeding occurs in a woman who has previously had regular control on the pill it should be investigated as midcycle bleeding would be in any other patient.

Amenorrhoea during treatment was relatively common during the 1960s when high dose pills were the rule. In some women failure to have withdrawal bleeding occurs repeatedly. This is very rare with low dose pills and, provided steps are taken to exclude pregnancy, is no contraindication to continuing whatever oral contraceptive the patient is taking.

Weight change, particularly an increase, is more common with high dose pills. When large numbers of women taking the more modern pills are studied, weight change, either up or down, is not significantly different from the rest of the population.

Mood changes do occur in some women taking oral contraceptives. If depression develops for the first time in a woman taking the pill it is good therapeutics to stop treatment and determine what effect, if any, this has. Appropriate advice should be given about alternative methods of contraception while this is being done.

Major. These relate to four areas:—future fertility; the cardiovascular system; carbohydrate metabolism; and malignancy.

Future fertility. There is no doubt that a small proportion of women remain anovulatory for a substantial length of time after they stop the pill (Shearman 1966), about 6 women in 1000 having amenorrhoea for more than 12 months. What is not yet resolved is whether this 'post-pill' amenorrhoea is causal or casual. It seems to be more common in women who have a history of irregular cycles before starting treatment, women who have substantial weight *loss* on the pill and women who enter very heavy exercise programmes while they are taking oral contraceptives. Even if this is a casual relationship, it is usually relatively easily treated by induction of ovulation and thus quite different from infertility related to tubal damage that may be seen after the use of an IUD. However, just as in any other woman with secondary amenorrhoea, organic disease such as pituitary tumour must be excluded (Chapter 7).

Cardiovascular system. The first serious side effects attributed to oral contraceptives relate to the cardiovascular system. On the venous side oral contraceptives increase the risk of venous thrombosis and pulmonary embolism in a dose dependent fashion related to the amount of oestrogen in the pill. When the early data of this relationship were collected in the 1960s many of the pills contained $100\,\mu g$ or more of oestrogen. Most of the pills in current use contain $50\,\mu g$ or less. So it is not surprising that this problem is seen very much less frequently now. There are not yet sufficient data to say that there is no increased risk with doses of 30–$35\,\mu g$ of ethinyl oestradiol but if there is a risk it must, indeed, be very small.

In the 1970s concerns surfaced about side effects on the arterial side of the vascular tree, side effects relating to hypertension and/or cerebrovascular accidents and coronary heart disease (CHD). Earlier and somewhat conflicting case controlled studies did show a relationship between current or previous use of oral contraceptives and an increased risk of all of the conditions mentioned in this section (Vessey 1980). But large and comprehensive prospective (cohort) studies, such as the Walnut Creek study in the United States of America could not confirm this, any excess risk being seen only in women on the pill who smoked. In Australia these types of side effects leading to death have never been noted in our national mortality statistics. In fact there has been a progressive decline in the death rate from cerebrovascular accidents and myocardial infarction in women since the 1960s (Shearman 1981). However it would be idle to believe that there *may* not be a problem and this needs to be considered.

The effects of oral contraceptives on the cardiovascular system are complex and present a nice illustration of the interaction between the dose of oestrogen and the dose of progestin. For example, while there is no very good evidence that either oestrogens or progestogens alone increase the risk of hypertension, there is good evidence that in women exposed to oestrogens, synthetic progestogens increase the risk of hypertension in a dose dependent fashion. There are two corollaries to this statement: one is that the amount of oestrogen and progestin should be the lowest possible to obtain the desired pharmacological effect; secondly that measurement of blood pressure should be part of the routine follow-up of any woman on the pill.

The problems are even more difficult as far as thrombosis is concerned. High doses of oestrogens are known to increase the risk of platelet thrombosis. But oestrogens increase high density lipid (HDL) cholesterol and reduce low density lipid (LDL) cholesterol and therefore are almost certainly protective against atherosclerotic disease of arteries. The position is quite different with progestins which in a dose dependent fashion decrease HDL cholesterol and increase LDL cholesterol. They should, therefore, if given alone in large quantities, increase the risk of CHD and possibly cerebral thrombosis. When given together the action of one steroid is balanced by the other, a balance that varies with the relative dose of each. Theoretically one is therefore in the difficult position that, in a desire to give the lowest effective dose of oestrogen, this may be so low that it does not block the action of a particular dose of the progestogen on lipid metabolism.

There is evidence that on balance the older high progestin tablets changed lipid metabolism in the direction of greater risk of CHD. Studies with the lowest dose compounds (the tri-phasic preparations)

seem to show no significant effect. But, insufficient large longitudinal studies have been done comparing women so treated with matched untreated controls and it is possible that even with low dose formulations, the pill may further compound the risk of arterial disease in those women already at risk because of hypertension, obesity, smoking or pre-existing hyperlipidaemia.

Carbohydrate metabolism. Most data on the older pills showed that oral contraceptives diminished carbohydrate tolerance in apparently normal women and caused further diminution in established diabetes. The data with lower dose pills are not conclusive but nevertheless reassuring. Any effects observed are of minor degree and probably clinically insignificant. Given adequate supervision low dose oral contraceptives may be used safely in insulin dependent diabetics. For many of these women this is the most desirable form of reversible contraception.

Malignancy. Adequate studies have now shown that combined oral contraceptives reduce the incidence of endometrial malignancy and ovarian malignancy (Mishell 1985).

Breast cancer remains the commonest malignancy in women (rapidly being overtaken by lung) and, not surprisingly, one of the most feared. There was until recently no study showing any relationship between oral contraceptives and increased risk of breast cancer. That statement remains true for adequate prospective studies. Very recently one case controlled study from the United States of America has presented data suggesting that there may be a relationship between intake of oral contraceptives in young women and the development of breast cancer under the age of 35. Reanalysis of some prospective English data has shown that this effect may be evident if the pill is taken before the first pregnancy. If true, this is a matter of serious concern. Present information does not indicate the need to change oral contraceptive practice in young or old women with regard to breast cancer; sufficient additional information should be soon available to clarify this important problem.

Since the 1960s there have been several epidemiologically inadequate studies indicating that oral contraceptives might increase the risk of developing cervical dysplasia or even intraepithelial neoplasia. Some of those studies were felt to be inadequate because the important confounding variables of age at first intercourse and number of sexual partners were not considered. A recent study from Oxford, where sexual patterns were available for analysis in a small subset of patients did, however, show an increased risk both of intraepithelial neoplasia and an increased rate of transformation from carcinoma-*in-situ* to invasive carcinoma in women who had been on oral contraceptives for more than 8 years. This is another important and potentially disturbing problem. However, unlike breast cancer, adequate screening techniques with exfoliative cytology are available to detect this risk if, in fact, it proves to be true. A reasoned discussion of these problems will be found in Drife (1983).

Interaction with other drugs
Barbiturates, sulphonamides, and rifampicin cause accelerated biotransformation of steroids in the human. There are anecdotal reports of oral contraceptive failure with other antibiotics such as penicillin and ampicillin as well as phenytoin, an anticonvulsant. However in pharmacological practice the only clinical circumstance which appears to prohibit the use of oral contraceptives is the concurrent use of rifampicin. Even with that drug evidence is inconclusive but there is sufficient uncertainty to suggest that a woman taking rifampicin should use some other method of contraception.

Contraindications
These are shown in Table 38.1. The absolute contraindications are clear and just that: absolute. The relative ones are a little more difficult. There is not the slightest doubt that a woman who is over 35 years old, who smokes, who is obese and hypertensive should not use the pill. Given the option it might be much safer for her to stop smoking, lose weight and continue the pill; but in practice that is often unrealistic or unacceptable advice. The author does not hesitate to continue low dose oral contraceptives until

Table 38.1. Contraindications to the use of oral contraceptives (from Shearman 1984).

Absolute	Relative
Breast cancer	Smoking
History of DVT or pulmonary embolism	Age > 35
	Obesity
Active liver disease (congenital or acquired)	Hypertension
Concurrent treatment with rifampicin	Breast feeding
Familial hyperlipidaemia (pending further study)	Irregular spontaneous menstruation
Previous arterial thrombosis	
Pregnancy	

the age of 50 in women who do not smoke, who are of normal weight and who are normotensive.

The older combined oral contraceptives reduced the amount of milk and this is important in those women for whom breast feeding is critically important. There are no adequate data on this question with low dose pills. The amount of steroid and metabolite in breast milk is so tiny that it would have no pharmacological activity in a breast fed baby.

The young woman with irregular cycles should recognize that there may be an increased chance of subsequent amenorrhoea if she uses the pill. However, this may be an acceptable risk for a particular patients; if she has acne or mild hirsutism, then the benefits she might obtain from oral contraceptives (in addition to contraception) may make that the most acceptable treatment.

What pill to prescribe
Progestogen minipill. These have a higher failure rate and a greater incidence of irregular bleeding than combined oral contraceptives. They have little place in women who need effective hormonal contraception. My own view is that the main indication for the minipill is in a patient who wishes to breast feed but have contraceptive protection additional to that endowed by the act of demand feeding itself. The minipill may also have a place in a patient who finds other methods of contraception unacceptable and in whom oestrogens specifically are contraindicated. For all practical purposes this means a patient who has had a history of deep venous thrombosis or pulmonary embolism.

Combined pills. The lower limit of age at which the pill may be used is an issue that is partly legal and partly medical. The problems created by differences in the age of consent and in its interpretation between countries obscures the present legal position. From a strictly medical point of view there is no reason why oral contraceptives may not be used in any girl exposed to the risk of pregnancy who wants contraceptive advice and who has regular periods.

The pill of first choice should be that containing the lowest total steroid load compatible with the desired effect and that, by 1984 in many countries, meant one of the tri-phasic preparations. Where this is not available a formulation containing not more than 30 or 35 μg of oestrogen should be used. Higher dose preparations containing, for example, 50 μg of ethinyl oestradiol should probably be restricted to those women who have poor cycle control on the lower dose pills or in whom there is an additional therapeutic objective such as the control of acne. It is difficult to see any reason, other than habit, for the continued use of tablets with more than 50 μg of ethinyl oestradiol or mestranol or for those containing more than 1 mg of norethisterone or 150 μg of laevonorgestrel or desogestrel.

Follow-up
Even if a patient is happily established on an older high dose pill you should discuss with her the benefits of changing to a lower dose.

Blood pressure should be checked at 6 and 12 months and then annually. Cervical cytology should be taken annually initially; after 2 normal smears, in the absence of symptoms, biannual smears are sufficient. You should examine the patient's breasts each year.

LONG-ACTING STEROID CONTRACEPTION

A very full review of this subject will be found in Mishell (1983). If contraception in general can be a controversial subject the use of injectable preparations and, in particular, Depo-provera, seems able to cause almost hysterical levels of controversy. Two injectable long-acting preparations are available although either or both of these is still unavailable in many countries.

Medroxyprogesterone acetate (Depo-provera)
This compound was first used for 'pregnancy support' in threatened or recurrent abortion. After it was found to cause subsequent amenorrhoea it was then developed as a systemic contraceptive and the literature on this subject is enormous. Argument continues and an exhaustive review will be found in Fraser and Weisberg (1981). It is used most frequently by deep intramuscular injection into the gluteal region every three calendar months in a dose of 150 mg, the first injection commencing within 3 days of the previous menstrual period. In use effectiveness it compares well with oral contraceptives and it does not inhibit lactation. Common side effects are irregular and unpredictable uterine bleeding in early cycles while most women develop complete amenorrhoea if they persist with it. Although there may be a delay of up to 18 months in restoration of ovulation, within two years of discontinuance pregnancy rates are the same as achieved after other methods of contraception. However, because of this delay in restoration of

fertility it is not a good preparation to use in a woman who may want a child in the near future.

Most of the reasons for the failure of this drug to secure approval for contraception in the United States of America, Australia, and until recently in the United Kingdom appear to be emotionally rather than intellectually determined. The author's view is that it has a very real place in contraceptive practice, particularly for women who cannot or should not take oestrogens.

Norethisterone oenanthate
This drug has also been available for almost 20 years but despite this has still not secured widespread acceptance for contraception. If given every 3 calendar months the pregnancy rate is higher than that seen with Depo-provera but if given every 60 days that disadvantage disappears. It is now evident that after six months the 60 day interval may be increased to 84 days (Annus *et al.* 1983).

Implants
Efforts to develop biodegradable implants with zero-order kinetics have, to date, been unsuccessful. However using non-biodegradable polysiloxane (silastic) effective and apparently acceptable method of contraception has been developed. The most widely used of these is the NORPLANT system which utilizes six implanted capsules containing norgestrel (*Studies in Family Planning* 1983). Field trials have shown a high degree of acceptability and effectiveness.

Medicated vaginal rings
These were first developed by Mishell and have been discussed by him in detail (Mishell 1985). These are hollow silastic rings inserted into the vagina by the patient for a period of 3 weeks beginning on the fifth day of a menstrual cycle and removed for a period of one week to allow withdrawal bleeding. Steroids are released at a relatively constant rate and absorbed through the vaginal epithelium. The rings currently in use employ oestradiol and because of the transvaginal absorption first liver bypass is avoided. Laevenorgestrel is used as the progestin and the rings contain sufficient steroid for six months of recurrent use. In trials to date, patient and partner acceptance has been good.

PREGNANCY INTERCEPTION

These methods are aimed at preventing implantation in women who have been exposed to unprotected unpremeditated intercourse during the fertile time of the cycle. The oral preparations used to be called 'the morning after pill'. For hormonal treatment the most widespread regime is that described by Yuzpe *et al.* (1982). Two tablets containing 0.05 mg ethinyl oestradiol and 0.5 mg of dl-norgestrel should be taken within 72 hours of exposure and repeated in 12 hours. Pregnancy rate is about 1%, and nausea is a common side effect. This method is not suitable for recurrent use because of the high dose of steroids given. For those patients who require ongoing contraception in addition to pregnancy interception, a copper containing intrauterine device has proved to be effective if inserted within 48 hours of intercourse.

MALE CONTRACEPTION

Women who complain that the male is insufficiently involved in contraception should recognize that the two most widely used methods of contraception in the world, coitus interruptus and condoms, are totally dependent on male compliance. It is not through lack of trying that systemic methods of contraception have not been developed. To date no really effective acceptable and reversible method of contraception employing either steroids, plant extracts such as gossypol or gonadotrophin release factor analogues have yet been developed.

STERILIZATION

It would be difficult to detail absolute contraindications to this operation. Although organic complications are rare, emotionally determined complications do occur and seem to be more common in the following circumstances: where sterilization is carried out in an effort to save a rocky marriage; where tubal ligation is carried out in the immediate puerperium; in women or men under the age of 30; in women or men with only one child. Requests for reversal come commonly from these groups.

Any method of sterilization will have failures. In the female the highest failure rates are seen when tubal ligation is done in association with Caesarean section or in the immediate puerperium. For interval sterilization the failure rates depend more on the experience of the operator than the type of procedure used. Because of its higher complication rate laparoscopic sterilization using unipolar or bipolar diathermy should be replaced by one or other of the tubal rings or clips. In neither the female nor the male is there any evidence of subsequent endocrine disturbance. Suggestions that tubal ligation may be followed by an increased incidence of menorrhagia have not been borne out in the very few studies where menstrual loss has been actually measured nor is there any evidence of significant autoimmune development in men after vasectomy. Earlier fears that vasectomy increased the risk of coronary artery disease have also been dispelled.

Although the patient should always have such an operation on the assumption that it is irreversible, with careful microsurgery more than 50% of these procedures may be reversed provided that in the female rings or clips are used to minimize tubal destruction and that in the male not more than 1 cm of the vas is devascularized.

OTHER METHODS

Other forms of contraception such as an anti-pregnancy vaccine have been awaited with varying degrees of enthusiasm for more than 15 years. No practising gynaecologist should hold his breath waiting for these to turn up on the shelves of his friendly pharmacy.

REFERENCES

ANNUS J., BENAGIANO G., DIETHELM P., GRAY R., HALL P.E. & HOLCK S.E. (1983) *Contraception*, **28**, 1.
BROWN J.B. & GRONOW M.J. (1985) in *Clinical Reproductive Endocrinology* (Shearman R.P. ed.) Churchill Livingstone, London.
DRIFE J. (1983) *Brit. med. J.* **287**, 1397.
FRASER I.S. & WEISBERG E. (1981) *Med. J. Aust.* (Suppl.) **1**, 1.
KLEINMAN R.L. (1980) (ed.) *Family Planning Handbook for Doctors*, International Planned Parenthood Federation, London.
MISHELL D.R. (1979) *Int. J. Obstet. Gynec.*, **16**, 482.
MISHELL D.R. (1983) (ed.) *Long Acting Steroid Contraception*, Raven Press, New York.
MISHELL D.R. (1985) in *Clinical Reproductive Endocrinology* (Shearman R.P. ed.), Churchill Livingstone, London.
PEARL R. (1932) *Human Biology*, **4**, 363.
PEEL J. & POTTS M. (1969) *Textbook of Contraceptive Practice*, Cambridge University Press.
SHEARMAN R.P. (1966) *Lancet*, ii, 1110.
SHEARMAN R.P. (1981) *Med. J. Aust.*, **1**, 698.
SHEARMAN R.P. (1984) *Australian Family Physician*, **13**, 685.
SIVIN I. (1979) *Int. J. Obstet. Gynec.*, **16**, 460.
SPARKS R.A. (1984) *Lancet*, i, 957.
STUDIES IN FAMILY PLANNING (1983), **14**, No. 617.

TIETZE C. & LEWIT S. (1968) *Demography*, **5**, 931.

VESSEY M.P. (1980) *Brit. J. Fam. Plann.*, **6**, Suppl. 1.

YUZPE A.A., SMITH R.P. & RADEMAKER A.W. (1982) *Fertil. Steril.*, **37**, 508.

ZIPPER J., WHEELER R.C., POTTS D.M. & RIVERA M. (1983) *Brit. med. J.*, **287**, 1245.

CHAPTER 39
MAKING A GYNAECOLOGICAL DIAGNOSIS

G. V. P. CHAMBERLAIN

The most favourable treatment depends upon a correct diagnosis. Without this, the gynaecologist is left treating symptomatic complaints without any scientific foundation. Often in the past, practitioners have done this and, in some parts of the world, symptomatic complaints are still dealt with by empirical therapy. This may work just as infusions of foxgloves slowed a fast heart in William Whitteridge's day, but we have moved forwards a little since the 18th century and in this chapter we would urge the gynaecologist to determine a firm diagnosis before starting treatment.

All diagnoses in medicine depend upon the triad of history, examination and investigations. In the human, different diseases present in different ways so that various facets of the classical triad are of most use. For example in general medicine, the diagnosis of pulmonary tuberculosis depends little on the history or examination but the investigation of chest X-rays gives a more precise diagnosis and, in consequence, radiological investigations become the best means of diagnosing pulmonary tuberculosis while history and examination are less useful. Similarly, in gynaecology, the diagnoses of dysplasia and carcinoma-*in-situ* of the cervix depend upon investigations for history and examination are not discriminating enough, although they can produce confirmatory and supporting aetiological factors from the past. It is the skilled examination of the cervical smear or the colposcopic directed biopsy that make the real diagnosis of dysplasia or carcinoma-*in-situ* of the cervix. Again, investigations have taken over from the rest of the triad.

In much of clinical gynaecology however this is not so. In internal medicine, some physicians turn away from the clinical skills of the history and examination relying on sweeps of laboratory and imaging investigations. In gynaecology still the clinical methods are essential for making a diagnosis and probably in the majority of gynaecological problems, the history is the major agent which leads the

gynaecologist towards the correct diagnosis. The examination of the abdomen and the pelvis are usually confirmatory to this and investigations have little or often no place in helping to establish the diagnosis. Frequently it is the ultimate examination, the surgical exploration of the pelvis, that is needed to clinch the diagnosis finally.

THE ANATOMY OF MAKING A DIAGNOSIS

The skeleton of the diagnostic process starts with taking a history, performing the relevant examinations and asking for the germane investigations. All these need interpretation derived from knowledge and experience to produce the full process.

The first essential is to gain the confidence of the woman who presents in the outpatient clinic, consulting room or ward. Rapport must be established between the examiner and the patient or nothing will be achieved. Assuming she speaks English as fluently as the examiner, obviously words can help make this bridge. If, as happens so often in the United Kingdom now, the examiner is of a different race from the patient, words cannot be used to their full advantage and here all the skills of the examiner are required. He must obviously be seen to be friendly. A smile, shaking the woman's hand and making her comfortable on the couch will transcend language.

HISTORY

The examiner needs to learn something about the woman's background and some information about the disease process of which she has symptoms. Far the best is to allow her to tell the story in her own words, letting her lead towards her principal symptom. This often differs from that referred to in the General Practitioner letter. This does not mean that the examiner has to take down verbatim all the statements made. However, he can after a few minutes start to guide the interview towards the principal symptoms which he may then state in his history sheet. By gentle but relevant questions, he may lead the woman to elaborate on that aspect of her history which he considers the most important. In a postgraduate volume of this nature, we need not enter into details of the branching questions that should follow a woman complaining of lower abdominal pain, heavy periods or vaginal discharge; they should be well known to the reader but he must be prepared to pursue them down such ramifications so that he has all the information he can get about the presenting symptoms.

In the history, it is also important to garner information about the background of the woman. We need to know about her present health, appetite, well-being, any fatigue and how her urinary tract and bowels are behaving. Informed ideas are required about the essence of her and her husband's occupations thus fitting them into their socio-economic background. One needs to know something about any past history of admissions to hospital for serious illnesses and in some cases any past obstetrical history in some detail. The personal history should be perused including the taking of any drugs, indulgences in alcohol and cigarettes and the aspects of any family history that may be recurring.

Details of the menstrual pattern are usually helpful. The history of menstruation in recent months gives the gynaecologist much information. Many women say they menstruate to a 28 day cycle but if asked directly will admit to the variations which come inside normal distributions. Pay particular attention to the story and if possible ask the woman if she has kept a record of her menses in her personal diary.

The best guide to any increased menstrual blood loss is to ask the woman herself about the pads she uses. Whilst she may become more fastidious and use more pads for personal hygiene reasons, the commonest reason for any increase in the number of pads or tampons used each day is heavier blood loss.

Another good guide to increased loss is the passing of clots now which did not occur previously. This indicates an overwhelming of the inborn fibrinolytic systems that usually exist during normal menstruation.

Try to distinguish between days of menstruation and other bleeding in the course of the menstrual cycle. Commonly, the other bleeding will not be

heavy or liquid blood but smears or spotting of blood, whereas menstruation will be liquid blood.

Enquire into the association of pain with menstruation and be careful to distinguish between pain that occurs with menstruation and that which occurs before, for they are of different prognostic significance.

Sexual activity is a sensitive area of the history which should not be embarked upon at the beginning of the interview. However, there is often valuable information particularly if the discussion relates to a fertility problem. If the question 'do you have intercourse regularly?' is unthinkingly asked, the answer may be 'yes' but the frequency may be rare, as in the woman who attended the fertility clinic and accepted that she had regular intercourse 'on my husband's birthday each year'.

All these will help the gynaecologist fit his patient into a background of biology and health which is so important in making a diagnosis.

EXAMINATION

Only after collecting the data he needs to make a tentative diagnosis should the gynaecologist proceed to examine the woman although occasionally some questions are better answered if asked through the curtains while the woman is undressing preparatory to the examination. The lack of visual contact often adds a security to answers about matters of embarrassment such as sexual contacts. Obviously examination starts with the whole woman. Her apparent age and relation to the biological information she has given about her age and skin, her face, its lines and marks of stress. The gynaecologist examines the tongue for anaemia and for signs of dehydration.

How the woman holds herself on the couch is important, whether she is relaxed and moving easily or is to some degree restricting her movements by guarding any part of her abdomen.

Examination of cardiovascular, respiratory and nervous systems is usually unnecessary in a gynaecological examination, but occasionally one meets a woman who has symptoms in one of these areas. Then the gynaecologist should be able to perform the basic examination although he may not be adept at some of the details. More important, he has probably forgotten the interpretation of relevant findings; should he feel that there is anything important to be gained from examination of these other systems of the body, he should seek the opinion of an expert. This is not denigrating the body into organ systems but the subtle changes in reduction of power in an elbow jerk or sensation of one hand may be lost on the amateur neurological examiner, for this is what the gynaecologist is. Such changes will be appreciated by the professional neurologist and may help towards making a diagnosis at a much earlier stage than would be made otherwise.

Examination of the abdomen

Basic principles of abdominal examination will not be reiterated here for they are well known. However, certain aspects deserve emphasis. The classical quadrad of inspection, palpation, auscultation and percussion are a good frame but are only a frame and the gynaecologist need not follow all parts of it. It is over-zealous to auscultate an abdomen unless one expects to detect a condition which has an acoustic element in it so that it would sound different. Thus in gynaecology it might be sensible to auscultate the abdomen if you thought there was a fetus present for a fetal heart signal would help to make the diagnosis, otherwise only the very rare highly vascular tumours or those with variations in their blood vessels such as renal tumours would produce vascular noises. To listen for gut sounds in the normal woman is a waste of time.

Similarly with percussion, one should percuss if one feels a mass or suspects ascites; to percuss what has already been palpated and considered as normal, is time consuming and does not aid diagnosis.

The patient should be comfortable. This is such an obvious remark as almost not needing reiteration but she should be lying with one pillow under her head. To lie flat on a doctor's couch is never comfortable and the single pillow allows a degree of relaxation of the anterior abdominal wall. The gynaecologist can then learn more when he comes to palpation.

Inspection of the abdomen should not be neglected, looking for scars of previous operations, changes in the distribution of pubic hair and any swellings. Visible masses should be divided in the gynaecologist's mind into central or on one side and their symmetry inspected from the bottom of the bed. Never forget to check for hernias in the groins.

When palpating, the experienced gynaecologist will always ask again if there is any pain or tenderness in the abdominal area before starting. The hands should be warm. This is a courtesy which should not need restating; it is important to wash your hands before examining a patient and this can be done under a warm tap in virtually all situations where the gynaecologist will be examining a woman. The abdomen is palpated gently to gather superficial signs; if there is no tenderness, then it is assessed more deeply. It is wise to learn to use the left hand to examine the lower abdomen for it leads one down more sensitively to likely sites of pathology arising from the pelvis. Tenderness, and more importantly rebound tenderness, should be checked. Guarding, if found, should not be overcome by firmer palpation for this will lead to a spasm of the anterior abdominal wall. The gynaecologist will learn no more physical signs from that patient.

Percussion should be performed if masses are found or ascites expected. Auscultation of the abdomen is needed if sound producing tumours are expected, e.g. a 20-week fetus or a vascular tumour of the ovary.

Examination of the breasts

The gynaecologist should be capable of examining the breasts and indeed, in many countries of the world, breast treatment is in the hands of a woman's gynaecologist. If one considers that gynaecology cares for the diseases of the genital organs then the breast is one of these, but in the United Kingdom it is conventional for the gynaecologist not to treat breast disease.

During examination, the breasts should be inspected briefly and palpated both in the sitting and the lying position. Inspection assesses symmetry and scrutinizes for inverted nipples, any obvious lumps or skin changes in either breast. Palpation is best done by examining each of the four quadrants discretely and a separate examination of the anterior upper axilla. It is important to press down to the chest wall, thus spreading the soft breast tissue out between the examining fingers and pressing on to the pectoralis major muscle. Any pathological lumps will be felt; pea or bean size masses will spring from the fingers, slipping sideways as one examines. Obviously a more advanced malignant tumour may be tethered; such a mass will be fixed and this is a most sinister sign.

It must be stressed however that most examinations of the breast do not detect any mass and that the woman should be assured that all is normal in the breast and there are no masses to be found. Should a lump be detected, it should be checked that it is only in one quadrant to the breast and whether it is attached to either the skin overlying it or the pectoralis major muscle below it. Formal biopsy or needle biopsy are indicated and discussion with a surgeon dealing with this area should be sought.

Assuming the examination to be normal, this is an opportunity for the gynaecologist to instruct his patient in self-palpation of breasts. It is well worth while. She is told to do this a day or two after the end of each menstrual period while in the bath. A remarkable number of women have detected lumps about which they are unhappy and which have driven them to the gynaecologist for assessment. Usually these are benign fibroadenomata and not serious. The lymph nodes in the axilla should be pursued and supra-clavicular lymph nodes should also be checked.

Examination of the pelvis

No woman likes a pelvic examination; no one enjoys being examined vaginally and few doctors wish to do it. Yet despite this bilateral antipathy, a pelvic examination is one of the more valuable assessments for without it one is ignorant about some 500 ml of the abdominal cavity. Further, it assists the bimanual process by pushing up pelvic organs from below into the abdomen to allow fuller examination. A bimanual examination requires both hands. The finger or fingers in the vagina steady and elevate the uterus and adnexa so the abdominal palpating hand has a greater chance to feel the organs in the pelvis. An experienced gynaecologist builds up a three-dimensional space picture of the pelvis in his mind from the signals of both hands simultaneously; the examiner would be hard pressed to say whether it was the abdominal or vaginal examining fingers which gave him the most information. Both sets of fingers are moving over the genital organs and they will give a three-dimensional image.

As in examination of other parts of the body, inspection comes first. The pudenda may show pathological changes and gentle parting of the labia allows inspection of the clitoris and the urethral orifice. Now is the time to check for stress incontinence but remember the woman will probably have been instructed to empty her bladder recently so it does not always show and the woman may have to be re-checked later.

During pelvic examination it is conventional to wear a protective glove on the vaginal hand although it is not necessary to so do on the other hand. Many gynaecologists would find that a glove on the abdominal hand (nearly always the left hand of the examiner) will interfere with the sensitivity of palpation.

Many gynaecologists examine the pelvis with two fingers, hoping that the middle finger of the right hand will gain them about a centimetre in length. However, using both fingers may give them a slight linear advantage but it increases the diameter of probe in the vagina by at least a centimetre in width. Some gynaecologists examine with a single finger in the vagina using that to steady and manoeuvre the pelvic organs to help the left hand palpate from the abdomen. It is a matter of choice and no gynaecologist should be imposed upon by others about how he performs a pelvic examination. A pelvic examination is judged by the information it gives the doctor without being uncomfortable for the woman.

There is dichotomy among gynaecologists whether a pelvic assessment is best performed with the patient in the dorsal or the lateral position. The dorsal position has been used traditionally because it is familiar from examination of the abdomen, so the pelvis becomes an extension in the abdomen in the examiner's mind. It also allows better inspection of the external genitalia. For some women the dorsal position however was considered more embarrassing while if she lies on her side with her back towards the examiner, a left lateral examination may be performed without eye to eye contact. Many gynaecologists find the left lateral difficult to orientate, particularly in examination of the right adnexa. Using a Simm's speculum the lateral position does give an excellent view of the anterior wall of the vagina; hence it is commonly used when assessing a prolapse or looking for vesico-vaginal fistulae.

There is no great merit in making too strong a case for one or the other method of examination. Most commonly, gynaecologists stick to what they started with in their early training but it is wise to try both methods and use the one which produces results of the findings of the examination without hurting the patient.

Rectal examination

Rectal examination is not commonly required in a pelvic assessment but has a special use if the gynaecologist is seeking problems at the back of the uterus in the pouch of Douglas, for example in ovarian cancer or endometriosis. If he is going to do it, the woman should be turned to the left side and warned of the approaching examination. Inspect the anus by spreading the buttocks slightly and then with a little lubrication, put the pulp of the gloved index finger on the anal sphincter. Allow the finger to sink gently in and, once it has been inserted up to two phalanges, turn it round so that the palm of the hand is facing the front of the woman. If the rectal examination is performed this way the most nervous of people can be persuaded into the examination.

Sigmoidoscopy

An extension of the rectal examination is proctoscopy and sigmoidoscopy. According to the level in the large bowel that the gynaecologist suspects problems, either or both examinations may be performed in the outpatient clinic. The latter, however, is better done after bowel preparation or faeces may obscure the vision.

INVESTIGATIONS

With the full range of biophysical, biochemical and biological investigations available for him, the gynaecologist should have a provisional clinical diagnosis in his mind after assuming the relevant findings of the history and examination. Only if he does this will investigations be of use. It may well be that there are still several conditions which need excluding but one diagnosis should be more favoured. Investigations should then be ordered to confirm or exclude this rather than just blindly ask for a battery of tests and performing a fishing expedition hoping that some unthought of condition will be in the net at the end.

In an attempt to rank the frequency of tests done in our gynaecological department, we asked our pathology and X-ray departments for an analysis of tests commonly requested. It was not very helpful for it reflected the tests that were done before giving an anaesthetic rather than those required in gynaecology. Many of the women who come to the gynaecological department receive anaesthesia. A haemoglobin estimation and chest X-ray were the two most commonly performed investigations. These do not help make a diagnosis but assist the gynaecologist's colleagues in giving a safe anaesthetic.

HAEMATOLOGICAL TESTS

Confirmation of anaemia is the major test used in gynaecology. The haemoglobin level is conventionally used but packed cell volume, or the examination of a film by an experienced haematologist are probably better guides. Further indices such as bone marrow counts and serum ferritin are required to sort out the less common anaemias.

The leucocyte count and differential is useful in assessing infections particularly if used in a longitudinal fashion.

The examination of a thick blood film often will help sort out a pyrexia of difficult origin, revealing malarial parasites, an infestation seen more commonly with the wider travel of populations around the world.

URINE ANALYSIS

Simple ward tests on the urine may reveal the presence of sugar or protein, both of which have their relevance. If indicated, the presence of human chorionic gonadotrophins can be estimated (*see* p. 585) in checking for pregnancy or its sequalae.

MICROBIOLOGICAL TESTS

When infection or infestation with pathogens is suspected, the appropriate samples should be taken for examination and culturing. In gynaecology, swabs may be taken from the posterior fornix of the vagina (high vaginal swab) or from the cervical canal. These should not be allowed to dry or cool and are best taken into special transport media (e.g. Stuart's medium for suspect trichomonas). Similarly urethral and vulval swabs may be taken. This should always be done before starting specific antibiotic therapy in case the clinical diagnosis or the presumed sensitivity of the organisms is incorrect and we have to restart with another antibiotic. If urinary infection is contemplated, a midstream catch sample should be centrifuged, examined microscopically and cultured before therapy starts.

Some viruses require especial techniques of sample gathering, e.g. herpes genitalis is best detected by a blunt scraping of the suspect ulcer's base. Enquire about each one and do not expect the laboratory to do a blind sweep for you.

HORMONE TESTS

All the hormones involved in gynaecological investigations are carried in the blood and laboratory measurement of these has become more precise in the last decade. However, it should be remembered that one is measuring these hormones only during their transport. The tests measure the total amount of hormone present in the blood but this is usually bound to proteins by a variable amount and only the fraction of hormone which is unbound has any biological effect. Further, the state and speed of activity of hormone receptors on cell membranes varies greatly from one hormone to another and in different phases of health. Ideally, the hormone levels in tissues should be estimated but this would be impractical in most investigations.

A full account of the chemistry and actions of hormones involved in gynaecology appears in Chapter 5. The tests most useful in gynaecological investigation only will be outlined.

PITUITARY HORMONES

Both luteinizing hormone (LH) and follicular stimulating hormone (FSH) are released from the anterior pituitary gland controlled by a negative feedback in oestrogen from the ovary. Measurement of FSH can be useful in sorting out the causes of anovulation.

Prolactin, similar to growth hormone, comes also from the anterior pituitary gland. High blood levels are associated with inhibition of oestrogen secretion of the ovary and so with anovulation. Whilst many laboratories would consider the upper limit of normal to be about $350\,\mu g/l$, most clinicians would not take action until a very much higher level of hyperprolactinaemia were detected, e.g. over $1000\,\mu g/l$.

OESTROGENS

Oestrogens are mostly produced in the ovary although a significant amount are made by the adrenal glands and from androstenedione precursors in the fat and skin. They may be measured easily in the plasma or in the urine whence their conjugated end products pass. Their varying levels of production in relation to ovulation can be useful for checking on that function, particularly in fertility work when a precise knowledge of the time of ovulation is required.

PROGESTERONE

Progesterone is mostly derived in the non-pregnant woman from the corpus luteum in the ovary. It can be estimated in the plasma or as its secretory product pregnanediol in the urine. In the second half of the menstrual cycle, a raised progesterone level indicates that a corpus luteum has been formed and so ovulation has occurred.

CHORIONIC GONADOTROPHINS

These hormones are produced only by trophoblast cells; in a vast majority of cases this means a pregnancy is present and elevated levels of human chorionic gonodotrophic (hCG) are the basis of the pregnancy test, a commonly performed investigation in gynaecology. While hCG can be detected in blood or urine, for most diagnostic tests, the latter suffices if the concentration of hormones is high enough (i.e. if the specimen is the first in the day and pregnancy has advanced far enough). Over two and a quarter million such tests were done in the United Kingdom in 1983, a figure to be set against 700 000 pregnancies, 150 000 terminations of pregnancy and perhaps an equal number of spontaneous abortions occurring each year. Allowing for the fact that some women have multiple tests, this is approximately two tests for each pregnancy that happened, or three for every birth.

The commonly used immunoagglutination test on the urine will allow diagnosis by detection of a sufficient concentration of hCG at about 20–24 days from the development of the embryo (that is 35–40 days after the last normal menstrual period). The newer monoclonal antibody testing kits will reduce this delay to about 14–18 days from conception (about the time of the missed period). Even more sensitive is the detection of the specific beta-unit hCG in the plasma by radioimmunassay. This can be done by about eight or nine days after conception, that is four or five days before the missed period. According to facilities available and the urgency of the test, the gynaecologist can order this from his laboratory and get a result the same day.

There are many other hormone tests that might be of use in obscure cases such as the products of the thyroid or adrenal gland. Most can be done in the ordinary laboratory of the District General Hospital, but a few require the Supraregional Assay Service. These and some of the tests used in early pregnancy, such as the pregnancy associated placental proteins (PAPP-A), are very rarely used.

X-rays

The use of X-rays in gynaecology has always been limited for the best images are obtained when there are greater differences in densities in the tissue to be examined. When bony abnormalities might be expected (e.g. a dermoid tumour which in 20% of cases contains abnormal bone formation) an X-ray would be helpful. For excluding bowel and urinary problems, special X-rays are of great assistance. An X-ray will help locate a missing intrauterine device, particularly if it is a copper bearing one.

The major use of X-rays in gynaecology lies in hysterosalpingography which provides a simple means of checking patency of the uterus and Fallopian tubes and showing up lesions which would appear in silhouette. Whilst commonly done as an outpatient procedure, the gynaecologist should remember that a hysterosalpingogram can be painful, and it is probably best if instrumentation in X-ray departments is done by someone who is gynaecologically rather than only radiologically trained. The use of screening at the same time will reduce radiation and allow the woman herself to see what is going on, thus relieving much anxiety and discomfort.

Ultrasound

Ultrasound estimations can help particularly when there is greater acoustical density in the tissues being looked for. However, to ask thoughtlessly for an ultrasound on every woman who comes in with an incomplete abortions or a mass on the side of the pelvis, does not really aid diagnosis; it merely puts off the time when the gynaecologist must think of specific treatment. Beware using ultrasound as an excuse for not making the diagnosis of an ectopic pregnancy.

Other imaging methods

In the last five years more imaging methods are becoming available. Magnetic imaging can show tumours very precisely and is already showing its worth in ovarian carcinoma, assessing spread by non-invasive methods. Radioisotope methods are not so useful in gynaecology for they depend upon a precise pick-up of a specific labelled element by a given tissue.

Laparoscopy

This investigation is more commonly used in the last decade. Table 39.1 shows a breakdown of the indications for some 21 000 diagnostic laparoscopies performed in the United Kingdom during the course of the year in which the Royal College of Obstetricians and Gynaecologists Confidential Enquiry into gynaecological laparoscopy was performed.

The greatest indication for diagnostic laparoscopy is for pain. Most gynaecologists would use the test for those who have a specific site of pain, well localized to one area of the pelvis. Such an investigation can be as a day case, usually under general anaesthesia, and it yields valuable information about the pelvis. The causes of chronic pain can be more precisely diagnosed and some of them, such as small patches of endometriosis, can be treated through the laparoscope. Even if nothing is found, it often helps the woman to be told that there is no serious pathology present and the pain will usually go. Should a specific cause be found this investigation can obviously lead to correct surgical treatment. A good example is the diagnosis of the leaking ectopic pregnancy which has not ruptured. Previously women could stay in the ward for many days awaiting a diagnosis which then depends upon a laparotomy, a much larger operation. Now a laparoscopy can exclude or confirm the diagnosis promptly and the woman may either return home or be dealt with.

Table 39.1 shows that the second largest diagnostic indication for laparoscopy is the investigation of infertility, when not just tubal blockage but the whole pelvis can be assessed through the laparoscope. Salpingography gives silhouettes of the lumen of the Fallopian tube but laparoscopy allows a much wider examination in the tube. Kinking or adhesions

Table 39.1. Indication for diagnostic laparoscopy among 20 971 women. (From *Confidential Enquiry into Laparoscopy*, RCOG 1978.)

Major indication	Numbers	Percentage
Infertility	9048	43.1
Pain	10825	51.7
Infertility and pain	186	0.9
Menorrhagia	84	0.4
Ovarian enlargement	389	1.9
Lost IUD or other foreign body	156	0.7
Other	283	1.3
Total	20971	100.0

Includes 385 cases where diagnostic and sterilizing indicated.

can be examined, the fimbrial end can be assessed and the mobility of the tube can be checked. In addition, a corpus luteum may be seen in the ovary and the capacity of the tube to service the ovary is important. Anyone contemplating tubal reconstruction or reversal of sterilization should always do a preliminary laparoscopy himself in order to assess the pelvis and the chances of benefit from the surgery. The passage of dye indicates tubal patency.

Ovarian biopsy may be performed through a laparoscope although it is often those ovaries from which a biopsy is most needed that are the hardest to actually grasp. The smooth billiard ball ovary is the one that is least likely to be ovulating and is the one from which the biopsy is hardest to obtain. In order to give the pathologist a reasonable bite of tissue, it is useless to use the small crocodile bladed forceps so often provided by the manufacturers in the laparoscopy kits; the gynaecologist will need the screw punch biopsy forceps devised by Raoul Palmier.

A small number of laparoscopies are done to help refine the diagnosis of ovarian enlargement. Most gynaecologists would consider that if the ovarian tumour is bigger than about 6 cm in diameter, the mass should be removed surgically and so a laparotomy will be the right way to deal with this and thus save theatre time. However some smaller tumours may be worth inspecting by laparoscopy.

A new area for diagnostic laparoscopy is the second look for women treated for ovarian cancer; details of this do not enter into this chapter.

Cystoscopy

Examination of the lining of the urethra and bladder is an easy outpatient procedure which is not often done by the regular gynaecologist. However, if he has a lot of urodynamic work referred, it may be easier to perform this investigation in the outpatient clinic grouping women into a fortnightly session or doing it at the same time as their outpatient urodynamic flow studies. A little local anaesthetic gel on the cystoscope and a gentle manner allow full cystocopy on the conscious and help make or exclude bladder and urethral diagnosis.

Curettage

This biopsy of the endometrium is really an investigation rather than an operation. Previously, an anaesthetic was required to perform a preliminary dilatation of the cervix to get at the endometrial cavity. Now narrow tubes (3 mm) can be introduced (Vabra) with minimum discomfort and, by vacuum, a strip of endometrium be removed. This investigation is of most use when histology of the endometrium would give an indication of the hormonal state of the women, e.g. in anovular dysfunction uterine bleeding.

CONCLUSIONS

Gynaecology is very much a clinical subject. In it we make our diagnoses using the physical senses and logical thought. Occasionally investigations are helpful but this is much less than in modern internal medicine. Some junior doctors coming to the subject from other branches feel more vulnerable without the laboratory test to protect their diagnostic ability, but they soon recover their clinical skills.

CHAPTER 40
INFERTILITY

RODNEY P. SHEARMAN

Inability to conceive may, for some couples, be an absolute disaster; for others it is a matter of relative indifference. The couple's attitude to this problem may also change with the passage of time. Many who, at least in the first instance, are obsessed with their infertility ultimately accommodate to that situation quite well. In determining those investigations to be carried out, the patients' attitude must remain of paramount importance.

Many textbooks describe the prevalence of infertility at about 10% of all unions. This figure seems to have attained an inbuilt momentum as it is repeated frequently from book to book without very much documentation concerning the validity of the figure. There is increasing pressure to investigate and treat infertility. At least part of this is due to the increased difficulty in securing babies for adoption in most developed countries. There is no doubt that this patient pressure may lead to unnecessary or repetitive investigations. This does not help the couple to adjust to or accept their infertility.

More recently efforts have been made to determine the true incidence of infertility. Two terms need to be understood. *Fecundability* is the monthly probability of pregnancy (when the opportunity for pregnancy exists) and is the reciprocal of the mean time required for conception expressed in months (Jansen 1984). The *Pearl Index* is the number of pregnancies per 100 woman years excluding time spent pregnant, a woman year being equivalent to 12 menstrual cycles. Table 40.1 shows the cumulative probability of conception (F) in normal populations based on data from the United Kingdom and the United States of America. In the United Kingdom 82% of the population will have achieved pregnancy after 12 months'

Table 40.1 Cumulative probability of conception (F) in a normal population. Calculated using the formula $F = 1 - (1-f)^n$, where f is the monthly fecundability, and n the number of months. From Cooke *et al.* (1981).

Months	UK (monthly rate = 0.12)	US (monthly rate = 0.20)
3	0.32	0.50
6	0.54	0.74
9	0.68	0.87
12	0.82	0.93
15	0.85	0.96
18	0.90	0.98
21	0.93	0.99
24	0.95	0.99

Table 40.2 The approximate relationship between fecundability (monthly probability of conception) and the Pearl Index (pregnancies per 100 woman years) over a range from normal fertility to infertility or adequate contraception. From Jansen (1984).

Fecundability	Pearl Index	Type of woman	Mean time to pregnancy
0.4	480	age 25, fertile, attempting first pregnancy	2–3 months
0.158	190	all ages, attempting first pregnancy	6 months
0.11	132	AID frozen semen: 25 years	9 months
0.07	84	treated endometriosis (danazol + surgery)	16 months
0.065	78	AID frozen semen: 35 years	15 months
0.027	32	mucus awareness for contraception	2.5 years
0.011	13.2	treated endometriosis + AID: 35 years	7.3 years
0.0083	9.9	unexplained primary infertility, 2 years	10 years
0.0025	3	intrauterine contraception (IUD)	33 years
0.00017	0.2	combined oral contraceptive	500 years

exposure and 95% after 2 years. It should be noted that the rise in the cumulative probability of conception is very sharp during the first 12 months and then flattens off. Inability to conceive for a period of 12 months is probably, therefore, a reasonable time to determine that investigation should be undertaken.

The probability of different groups of women becoming pregnant is shown in Table 40.2

Aetiology of infertility

It should be stated at once that there is a great deal to be learnt about infertility. It should also be recognized that there is no uniformity of opinions about the proportion of various factors to which infertility is attributed. Coital problems are probably related in about 3–4% of couples. At one extreme this may be due to impotence in the male or such severe dyspareunia in the female that coitus occurs rarely, if ever. If one assumes that a normal ovum can only be fertilized for 12–24 hours and that normal sperm survival in terms of fertility is up to 72 hours in the Fallopian tubes, coital frequency of less than 3 times a week may in its own right contribute to difficulty in conception.

Substantial reduction in sperm numbers or motility, including azoospermia, occurs in up to 30% of infertile unions. Disorders of ovulation account for another 20–30% of cases while tubal disease may be present in between 15–30% of couples. Endometriosis will be found in about 10–15% of women. Cervical factors, including immunological incompatibility, may be present in about 5%. In many couples more than one factor may be operative. Finally it must be recognized that in a substantial minority of couples (somewhere between 4 and 10%) complete investigation shows no reason for their infertility. The rather grim prognosis of unexplained infertility of more than 2 years' duration will be seen in Table 40.2.

CLINICAL APPROACH TO INVESTIGATION

The history and physical examination

Since infertility is a problem affecting two people, every effort should be made to see both partners at the initial interview and at appropriate stages during follow-up. A full medical history is needed. The male should also be asked whether there has been any history of testicular injury, urinary infection (pointing to sexually transmitted disease), relevant surgery such as herniorrhaphy or operation for undescended testis. The man's occupation is probably only relevant if this takes him away from his home for prolonged intervals.

For the woman a complete menstrual history is needed. If she has regular periods with an interval of 24–36 days and particularly if these are associated with some degree of dysmenorrhoea and premenstrual disturbances such as breast soreness or premenstrual tension, ovulatory cycles are very likely. A history of a ruptured appendix with peritonitis in childhood would point very clearly towards potential peritubal problems, while a history of pelvic inflammatory disease or post-abortal sepsis suggests that there may be tubal problems. An excess of tubal factors will be seen in those women who have used an intrauterine device for contraception.

You should also determine if there have been previous pregnancies, particularly in earlier unions. Whether this information is sought in the presence of both partners or from each independently is a matter of judgement which will usually emerge during the consultation.

Each partner should have a full physical examination. It is difficult to understand the reluctance of some gynaecologists to examine the male. Apart from a general physical examination, inspection of the external genitals is obviously relevant as is assessment of testicular volume. For this purpose an orchidometer is very useful. Normal testicular volume is 20 ml or more. A testicular volume of less than 10 ml is compatible with a primary testicular problem. The presence of a varicocoele should be noted but there is no consensus on whether such a finding is relevant to infertility.

Full examination of the female must include estimation of blood pressure. It is catastrophic to see a patient who has been investigated and treated successfully for infertility only to find that she has severe hypertension and/or renal disease that in their own right prejudice a successful outcome to the pregnancy. Vaginal examination will take note of any abnormalities. In this context, nodules in the Pouch of Douglas, with or without a fixed painful retroversion, would suggest the possibility of endometriosis or previous pelvic inflammatory disease.

The investigations needed should be discussed fully. These will determine whether the male has a potentially fertile semen analysis, that the woman ovulates, that she has normal tubal patency, that there is no evidence of other pelvic disease which might reduce the prospects of pregnancy and that there are no cervical (including immunological) factors present.

Semen analysis

It is unwise to rely on less than three separate semen analyses in any individual male. The specimens are best collected by masturbation after abstinence for between 3 and 5 days. Examination should be prompt, within 2 hours of collection, and ideally done in a laboratory that has substantial experience in this assessment.

There is no uniformly accepted definition of a normal, potentially fertile semen analysis. A reasonable series of criteria are that the volume should be between 2–5 ml, sperm density more than 20 million per ml, sperm motility more than 60% and sperm morphology showing less than 40% abnormal forms (Hudson *et al.* 1980). Peroxidase positive round cells

are normally absent. In a very long follow-up of patients, Bostofte *et al.* (1982) have shown a clear relationship between a high number of abnormal sperm and reduced fertility.

Tests for ovulation

The only proof of ovulation is pregnancy or the recovery of an ovum. If the patient was pregnant she would hardly complain of infertility while ovum recovery in the human is not usually technically, medically or ethically desirable, apart from its place in *in vitro* fertilization. All other evidence of ovulation is inferential.

Apart from the historical assistance that will be obtained when talking to the patient three methods of determining ovulation are in widespread use and any or all of these indices may be needed in each couple.

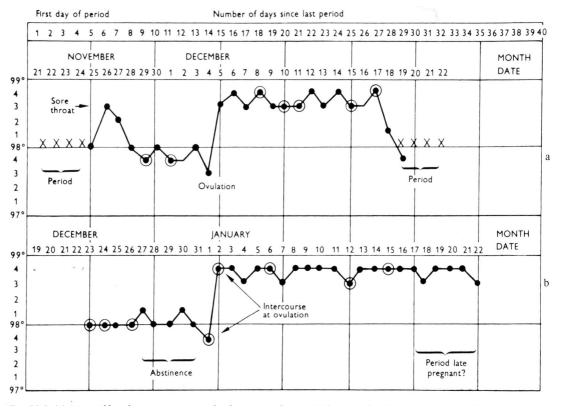

Fig. 40.1. (a) A typical basal temperature record indicating ovulation. At the time of ovulation there is a brief fall in temperature of a few hours' duration, followed by a rise which is maintained until the next period. An ovulatory chart, therefore, has the biphasic pattern shown here. (b) An ovulatory temperature chart followed by pregnancy. The rise in temperature is maintained. (By courtesy of John Sherratt & Son and Ortho Pharmaceuticals Ltd.)

BASAL BODY TEMPERATURE

Progesterone is thermogenic and an adequately recorded basal body temperature chart will often confirm ovulation. The temperature should be recorded either rectally or vaginally, it should be done first thing in the morning before the patient gets out of bed or has morning tea and the temperature should then be graphed as shown in Fig. 40.1. Intercurrent illness, a very late night, or irregular sleeping hours associated with shift work may make such a temperature chart difficult to interpret. In those women who have an irregular menstrual interval, the basal body temperature chart will usually show that the irregularity is in the follicular phase of the cycle rather than the luteal phase.

ENDOMETRIAL BIOPSY

While this procedure is widely used in the investigation of infertility it is doubtful that it has a major place in the assessment of ovulation where other indices, such as the progesterone index (see below), can be measured. There is no doubt that an endometrial biopsy performed in the second half of the cycle will confirm ovulation or otherwise. The time of the following period is more important in endometrial assessment than the time of the biopsy related to the previous period. In those societies where endometrial tuberculosis is common, full dilatation and curettage is justified.

PROGESTERONE ASSAY

Since all of the tests to confirm ovulation are based on the production of progesterone in the corpus luteum measurement of this hormone is the most reasonable way of determining ovulation. The differences between ovulatory and anovulatory levels are quite large (see Chapter 5). In the follicular phase of the cycle levels of less than 2 nmol/l are usual while after ovulation levels well in excess of 10 nmol/l are seen. Progesterone values may also help to unravel the very vexed area of the 'inadequate corpus luteum'. Assessment of this problem by endometrial histology is fraught with difficulty. Lenton and Langren (1985) have shown a high degree of consistency in progesterone levels in the same woman from the one cycle to the next. They have also shown two populations in those women who ovulate. Those with normal luteal progesterone levels show a very high fertility rate in the absence of any other factors. There

is a sub-population of women who clearly ovulate but are of low fertility with a low progesterone index.

Assessment of tubal factors

There are several methods of assessing tubal patency. One of these, the Rubin's test using carbon dioxide insufflation, is of historical interest only and has no place in modern gynaecology. Two other methods, hysterosalpingography and laparoscopy, are widely used but there is no consensus about the relative place of either. The disadvantage of hysterosalpingography is that this permits only the examination of 'shadows'. If tubal patency is established it does not allow an assessment of other intrapelvic problems such as peritubal adhesions or endometriosis that might relate to infertility but do not cause tubal blockage. However, hysterosalpingography has the advantage that anaesthesia is not required and the additional advantage that if it is normal, there is a clear therapeutic effect, more notable if oily contrast is used rather than a water-soluble medium (de Cherney et al. 1980). If hysterosalpingography is to be done, it should be performed in the follicular phase of the cycle to avoid exposing an undiagnosed early pregnancy to radiation.

Major tubal disease shown by hysterosalpingography is seen in Fig. 40.2.

LAPAROSCOPY

There is no doubt that the introduction of laparoscopy has transformed the ability to investigate longstanding infertility. It has the advantage over hysterosalpingography that the uterus, tubes and ovaries are visualized directly and that full information can be obtained about concurrent pelvic disease. For this reason, many gynaecologists use it as the primary method of assessing tubal patency. However, because it requires general anaesthesia and entry into the peritoneal cavity it is not free from complication.

My own view is that it should be done in any couple with more than two years' infertility where all other investigations have been normal. If, however, the history, physical examination or hysterosalpingogram point to pelvic pathology then laparoscopy may be done much sooner. In general terms, if a group of couples with more than 2 years' infertility are assessed, laparoscopy will show significant and related pathology in about 20% of women where investigations, including hysterosalpingography, have, to date, been normal. Overwhelmingly the two most

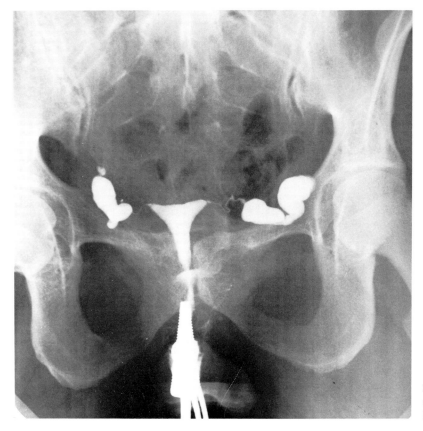

Fig. 40.2. Hysterosalpingogram showing bilateral hydrosalpinx.

likely related conditions are varying degrees of endometriosis (*see* Chapter 42) and peritubal adhesions.

If a laparoscopy is to be done, then it should be done properly. Only rarely can an adequate view of the whole of the pelvis be obtained unless a probe is inserted through a second incision just above the pubic hair line. Retrograde injection of methylene blue through the cervix will help to determine tubal patency and normality.

Assessment of cervical factors

It is notoriously difficult to assess the presence of true cervical factors relating to infertility. Direct examination of cervical mucin will, in most women, show the days preceding ovulation very clearly and if a post coital test is to be done it should be timed to coincide with that type of clear and elastic mucus. A further index of cervical receptivity may be obtained *in vitro* by the Kremer test (Kremer & Jaeger 1976). This test, although tedious, is very reproducible and has the advantage that control mucin and semen is used.

The role of immunological factors in infertility remains to be determined. Tests for sperm agglutinating and, more importantly, sperm immobilizing antibodies may be of assistance. A full discussion will be found in Jones (1980).

Hysteroscopy

The place of hysteroscopy in the assessment of some patients with secondary amenorrhoea and in others with recurrent abortion is discussed elsewhere in this volume.

TREATMENT

Coital problems

When deep dyspareunia is due to organic disease such as endometriosis or pelvic inflammatory disease, corrective surgery may help. The vast majority of coital problems, whether they relate to vaginismus in the female or absolute or relative impotence in the male are more likely to be behaviourally determined. Few gynaecologists have the appropriate skills to treat these patients, while psychiatric care has little to offer. We have found that specific counselling clinics for those with psychosexual problems has been of some assistance. Appropriately trained clinical psychologists sometimes help. If there is no abnormality except impotence this may be one of the very few circumstances where artificial insemination using the husband's semen would be appropriate.

Treatment of male factors

Infertility with azoospermia or severe oligospermia is, as a rule, therapeutically unrewarding. The only real exception to this statement is the male with hypogonadotrophic hypogonadism. With this particular problem, secondary sexual characteristics will not have developed spontaneously and the diagnosis will always have been made before that man presents as part of an infertile union. Under these circumstances treatment with human pituitary gonadotrophins and hCG produces satisfactory results.

There are many anecdotal reports about the use of androgens, clomid, surgery for varicocoele, suggesting that these regimes improve semen analysis and prospects of fertility but almost without exception adequately controlled studies have not been done. Similarly in men with epididymo-orchitis as evidenced by persistent increase in leucocytes in seminal plasma, while it might be expected that appropriate antibiotic treatment such as Doxycycline would help there are no adequately controlled studies to show that it does.

There is a ray of hope for the oligospermic male. Kerin et al. (1974) have shown that intrauterine insemination of a washed motile fraction of the spermatozoa is associated with an increase in conception rate.

Anovulation and inadequate corpus luteum

The investigation and treatment of anovulation have been discussed fully in Chapter 7 and will not be referred to here. The relationship between corpus luteum inadequacy and infertility remains vexed and controversial. The frequency of infertility associated with alleged corpus luteum deficiency varies widely between clinics, even when the same population is studied and for this reason many gynaecologists doubt the true relevance of this in practice. However, the work of Lenton and Langdren referred to above does seem to indicate that some women do have persistently inadequate progesterone production after

ovulation. If confirmed this appears to be a scientifically acceptable way of making such a diagnosis. Having made the diagnosis treatment is then a problem. There are good reasons to believe that an inadequate corpus luteum is founded on an inadequate follicle. Treatments directed specifically at corpus luteum inadequacy after ovulation such as progesterone suppositories or injections, or the administration of hCG to utilize its luteotrophic effect cannot be assessed properly because of poor control in most of the studies. Similarly, efforts to produce a better follicle with either clomid or pituitary gonadotrophins have not been done often enough nor sufficiently well controlled to reach any logical conclusion.

Tubal difficulties

While many of these relate to pelvic inflammatory disease arising de novo, in association with an intrauterine device or from peritonitis in children from a ruptured appendix, a regrettably large amount of tubal infertility is iatrogenic resulting from postoperative adhesions incurred during surgery on the ovary.

In young women where retention of reproductive potential is important all intrapelvic surgery should be approached with the perceptions and skills of a microsurgeon. Recognizing that this book is not about 'how to do it' it would be irrelevant to go into details of the microsurgical approach to the Fallopian tubes whether this is for tubal obstruction or peritubal adhesions. However it must be stressed that 'orthodox' surgery in this area has no place in modern gynaecology. Those who would like further details should refer to Wood and Paterson (1980) or Winston (1981).

Cervical factors, including sperm antibodies

Any gynaecologist with a heavy commitment to the investigation of infertility must see a large number of patients where a diagnosis of 'cervical hostility' has been made by either the family doctor or other consultants. In most instances that the author has seen the diagnosis is usually based on post-coital or Kremer tests done at an inappropriate time of the cycle. In the absence of immunological factors to be discussed shortly, impenetrability of normal preovulatory cervical mucin by sperm is really very rare. When it does occur it has been customary to treat this with low doses of oestrogens but in my own experience this frequently results either in delay of ovulation or even ovulatory suppression. This is one of the very many grey areas of infertility needing further investigation.

The patient with a high titre of sperm immobilizing antibodies in cervical mucus unequivocally has a reduced potential to become pregnant. There is some evidence that occlusive therapy (such as the use of condoms by the husband) is associated with a fall in the level of these antibodies and then an increased conception rate. However, information is still too meagre for firm conclusions to be drawn. Similarly, in the male who has a high and significant titre of autoantibodies, there is suggestive evidence that immunosuppression might help his potential fertility. But this is not trivial therapy and in the state of present knowledge this type of treatment should be regarded as 'on trial' and restricted to ultraspecialist units before being applied generally.

Endometriosis

This common and ill understood problem is discussed in Chapter 42 and will not be dealt with further here.

Unexplained infertility

This monument to medical ignorance is, or should be, a cause of major concern. As already indicated this diagnosis applies to couples who have had more than two years' infertility and in whom appropriate investigations have shown absolutely no cause. In the absence of a determined cause there is, in logical sequence, no specific treatment. This is one of the groups where *in vitro* fertilization and embryo transfer (*see* below) may well have a role.

Artificial insemination by donor (AID)

Although to some couples this treatment is not acceptable for ethical, religious, cultural or legal reasons, it is now in very widespread use throughout most developed countries where the commonest technology is to keep sperm under cryostorage in a sperm bank. In some countries and in some of the states of Australia, recent legislation has clarified the legal status of offspring resulting from this treatment. This removes one of the main impediments to its more widespread use. There is no doubt that with appropriate care and technology, where the male is azoospermic and there are no identifiable factors relating to infertility in the female, this technique produces extremely good results. It also has a place in the treatment of the couple where the only problem is

persistent oligospermia or persistent low motility (Kovacs *et al.* 1982).

In vitro fertilization and embryo transfer (IVF & ET)

This technology has been called a 'two-edged sword' (Mudge 1983). It is a programme only for the best motivated couples served by a dedicated group whose commitment is almost total to this technology. It should be recognized that the 'take home baby rate' is still relatively low and for those who do not ultimately achieve pregnancy, disappointment is profound and often difficult to deal with. Despite that, IVF and ET have become well established techniques in many parts of the world. It is used in three groups of women. First, those who have either irretrievable tubal damage or have previously had bilateral salpingectomy, for example for tubal pregnancy. The second group are those in whom no reason has been established for infertility (unexplained infertility), while a third is a selected group of patients with endometriosis that has not responded to surgery or medical management (Chapter 42).

This particular approach to artificial conception has caused, and continues to cause, soul-searching in the medical profession and some segments of the public. It is a very clear example of an increasing problem of medicine, where technology has outstripped full community, ethical and legal discussion. It would be foolish, however, to pretend that the technique was not here to stay and for those couples who do achieve a successful pregnancy, the reward outweighs all the many and substantial difficulties that must be passed to reach that objective.

Details of the technique and selection of patients are beyond the scope of a general text but a full review will be found in Kovacs *et al.* (1985).

Age

Ageing is an inevitability of life. While age seems to have little impact on potential male fertility, at least up to the end of the seventh decade, the data relating advanced female age to reduced fertility are very clear although not widely recognized. Bongaarts (1982) and Schwartz and Mayaux (1982) have both shown a substantial reduction in fecundity in women over the age of 35 compared with those under the age of 25. No single reason has emerged to explain this differential of almost 60%, and the possible contributing reasons are discussed in some detail by Jansen (1984). Whatever other substantial contributions medical science can make to the investigation and treatment of infertility it cannot change a patient's age.

REFERENCES

BONGAARTS J. (1982) *Family Planning Perspectives*, **14**, 75.

BOSTOFTE E., SERUP J. & REBBE H. (1982) *Int. J. Androl.*, **5**, 379.

COOKE I. D., SULAIMAN, R. A., LENTON, E. A. & PARSONS, R. J. (1981) in *Clinics in Obstetrics and Gynaecology* (Hull M. G. ed.) p. 531, Saunders, London.

DE CHERNEY A. H., KORT H., BARNEY J. B. & DE VORE G. R. (1980) *Fertil. Steril.*, **33**, 407.

HUDSON B., BAKER H. W. G. & DE KRETSER D. M. (1980) in *The Infertile Couple* (Pepperell R. J., Hudson B., Wood C. eds.) p. 70. Churchill Livingstone, London.

JANSEN R. P. S. (1984) *IPPF Med. Bull.*, **18**, No. 2, 4.

JONES W. R. (1980) in *The Infertile Couple* (Pepperell R. J., Hudson B. & Wood C. eds.) p. 126. Churchill Livingstone, London.

KERIN J. F. P., KIRBY C., PEEK J., JEFFREY R., WARNES G. M., MATTHEWS C. D. & COX L. W. (1984) *Lancet*, **i**, 533.

KOVACS G. T., LEETON J. F., MATTHEWS C. D., STEIGRAD S. J., SAUNDERS D. M., JONES W. R., LYNEHAM R. & MCMASTER R. (1982) *Clin. Reprod. Fertil.*, **1**, 295.

KOVACS G. T., TROUNSON A. O. & WOOD C. (1985) in 'Clinical Reproductive Endocrinology' (Shearman R. P. ed.) Churchill Livingstone, London.

KREMER J. & JAGER S. (1976) *Fertil. Steril.*, **27**, 335.

LENTON E. A. & LANGDREN B.M. (1985) in 'Clinical Reproductive Endocrinology' (Shearman, R. P. ed.) Churchill Livingstone, London.

SCHWARTZ D. & MAYAUX M. J. (1982) *New Engl. J. Med.*, **306**, 404.

WINSTON R. M. L. (1981) in *Progress in Obstetrics and Gynaecology* vol. 1 (Studd J. ed.) p. 291. Churchill Livingstone, London.

WOOD C. & PATERSON P. J. (1980) in *The Infertile Couple* (Pepperell R. J., Hudson B., & Wood C. eds.) p. 43. Churchill Livingstone, London.

CHAPTER 41
PELVIC INFECTION

C. R. WHITFIELD

Despite the availability of many powerful antibiotic drugs, pelvic inflammatory disease remains a common reason for emergency admission to gynaecological wards. Although acute pelvic infection should be more easily treated, chronic inflammatory conditions are still found in women attending infertility and general gynaecological clinics, and some of these patients have repeated admissions to hospital with acute exacerbations of chronic pelvic infection.

A variety of organisms cause pelvic sepsis, and secondary infection readily occurs so that the primary pathogen is often not identified, especially when sought in cultures from high in the genital tract. Gonococci, coliforms and other Gram-negative organisms including anaerobes (principally bacteroides, Gram-positive pyogens, gas-forming organisms, or mycoplasmas) may be responsible, and on recent evidence chlamydial infection may cause a significant proportion of pelvic inflammatory disease as well as infection of the lower genito-urinary tract. Occasionally pelvic infection is tuberculous or actinomycotic.

Although in some cases no source of infection is apparent, the route of infection is most commonly ascending from the vagina and cervix to the uterus, and parametrial tissues, Fallopian tubes, ovaries and the pelvic peritoneum; but salpingitis may also occur as a result of spread from the pelvic peritoneum, e.g. following appendicitis or diverticulitis, and it is by blood-borne infection that tuberculosis of the female genital tract usually occurs. There may be an obvious aetiological factor such as a recent abortion, delivery, gynaecological surgical procedure or insertion of an intrauterine contraceptive device.

ACUTE INFECTION

Infection following abortion, delivery or gynaecological procedures

After pregnancy the uterus, particularly the placental site, is an excellent culture medium for infecting organisms. There is little local resistance to the infection which soon spreads from the endometrium (decidua) to involve the myometrium. Organisms may then reach the peritoneum and parametrial tissues, with involvement of the broad ligaments, the Fallopian tubes and the surface of the ovaries. After abortion, particularly when this was induced criminally, but now also not uncommonly after legal termination, especially in the second trimester when there may well be some cervical or uterine trauma and perhaps also a delay in completing the process of abortion, infection is likely and may spread rapidly to the parametrial tissues with early involvement of the adnexae. In these circumstances the most common infecting organisms are the *Escherichia coli*, other Gram-negative bacilli including *Bacteroides fragilis*, the clostridii, streptococci and staphylococci. Bacteraemia and toxaemia occur, and in the most serious cases this results in 'septic shock', sometimes even in the death of the patient if treatment is not prompt and effective.

Postoperative sepsis, usually polymicrobial, is a relatively common complication of gynaecological surgery, particularly abdominal or vaginal hysterectomy, when pathogens present in the normal vaginal flora gain access to traumatized tissues and haematomas readily become infected. It begins as an extraperitoneal cellulitis, but peritonitis and abscess formation may occur.

PATHOLOGY

Acute inflammation is found in the endometrium, with hyperaemia and necrotic areas. Acute salpingitis is of the interstitial type, with cellular infiltration of the mesosalpinx and muscle but usually with only minimal involvement of the endosalpinx. Oophoritis or the formation of a tubo-ovarian abscess results from spread of the infection to the ovary. Congestive thickening with thrombophlebitis occurs in the parametrial tissue, and peritonitis leads to the formation of adhesions. Usually the peritonitis is localized to the Pouch of Douglas where a pelvic abscess may point into the vagina or rectum; but generalized peritonitis may occur, particularly if a tubo-ovarian abscess ruptures.

With early and effective antibiotic treatment there may be complete resolution, although usually at least a few adhesions form, but chronic changes often do develop despite treatment. The fimbrial ends of the Fallopian tubes usually remain open, but adhesions on the serosal surfaces of the tubes may kink and occlude them, or infertility may also result from ovarian adhesions.

CLINICAL FEATURES

The patient looks ill and is generally restless, usually lying on her back with flexed legs, her temperature is high and her pulse rapid, she has fetid breath, and may have had rigors and sometimes vomiting. She will usually admit to vaginal discharge and frequency of micturition with some dysuria. There is severe lower abdominal and pelvic pain. The lower abdomen is distended, held rigid, and acutely tender with rebound tenderness. Bowel sounds are usually present on admission, but ileus may develop. On vaginal examination there is acute tenderness, exacerbated by movement of the cervix, and parametrial thickening or acutely tender bilateral swellings may be felt beside the uterus or in the Pouch of Douglas, although unilateral pelvic inflammatory masses are probably a more common finding than traditional teaching would have us believe. The tender uterus feels enlarged and often seems to be fixed in position. The vaginal discharge may be seen to be purulent or bloodstained, it is often offensive, but is sometimes quite scanty.

With Gram-negative infection there may be septicaemia and septic shock, and this may also follow infection with other organisms when a tubo-ovarian abscess or pyosalpinx ruptures. Three phases of septic shock have been described (Cavanagh & Rao 1973). In the initial phase of 'warm hypotension', the patient is alert but apprehensive, she is feverish and flushed, with rapid pulse and breathing, the arterial blood pressure is low but pulse pressure is usually maintained and oliguria has not yet developed. In the second phase of 'cold hypotension', the patient becomes less anxious and less alert, tachycardia persists but the temperature is often subnormal and the skin is cold and clammy, pulse pressure is no longer maintained and oliguria develops. In the final phase of 'irreversible shock', there is acidosis due to cellular hypoxia, there is anuria, and ultimately the patient dies from cardiorespiratory, adrenal or hepatic failure.

Another life threatening complication of acute pelvic infection is pulmonary embolism from thrombosed pelvic and iliac veins. Pelvic thrombophlebitis may also cause leg oedema.

In patients who recover, residual effects include infertility, intestinal adhesions with the risk of obstruction, and the manifestations of chronic pelvic inflammatory disease with the likelihood of subacute or acute recurrences. Sinus and fistula formation may complicate bacteroides infection or actinomycosis, or may result when pelvic infection has originated in bowel injury. A more common tragic consequence is the 'pelvic cripple', with her chronic general ill-health and anxiety, and whose persistent pain includes dyspareunia leading to marital disharmony or breakdown.

DIFFERENTIAL DIAGNOSIS

A history of a recent abortion, delivery or pelvic operation is highly suggestive, but is not always obtained. In acute appendicitis with perforation the pain usually begins centrally and moves to the right iliac fossa, and the temperature is usually lower than in acute pelvic infection. With a disturbed ectopic pregnancy or accidents to an ovarian cyst, fever is much lower, the patient is not toxic and abdominal signs are mainly unilateral (at least initially). If there is doubt about the diagnosis, laparotomy may be an obvious requirement, but in less severe cases laparoscopy may reveal the diagnosis and show if further surgery is required.

TREATMENT

Initial identification of the infecting organism should always be attempted by obtaining 'triple swabs' for aerobic and anaerobic culture from high in the vagina, from the cervical canal, and from the urethra, and blood culture is occasionally successful, but often the pathogen can be grown and identified only from swabs taken at laparotomy or when an abscess is drained into the vagina. It may be that there should be more ready resort to culdocentesis to obtain fluid for culture (Brown 1982). In any case, antibiotic treatment should be started at once, but may then be changed if the response is unsatisfactory, by which time the bacteriological culture and sensitivity reports will be available. Antibiotics with broad spectrum bacteriocidal effects should be selected, awareness of drug resistance trends and recognition of the importance of infection by bacteroides usually dictating the choice. In the acutely ill patient, a combination of a cephalosporin, such as cephradine 1G 6-hourly intravenously, and metronidazole 500 mg 6-hourly intravenously is suitable, changing to oral administration when there has been some response (usually within 24–36 hours) with doses of 500 mg of cephradine 6-hourly and 200 mg of metronidazole 6-hourly. Treatment should be continued for at least ten days. The extended spectrum and greater potency of a 'third generation' cephalosporin, e.g. cefotaxine, may be preferred to cephradine, but when a response has occurred intramuscular (not oral) injection is necessary and metronidazole is needed to deal with the bacteroides. An alternative and usually effective parenteral therapy is provided by gentamycin in a daily dosage of up to 5 mg per kg of body weight intramuscularly or intravenously, but this should also be combined with metronidazole. Advice from a medical microbiologist aware of the current hospital infection and antibiotic resistance trends is very useful, especially when an optimal response to the antibiotics of first choice is not occurring. With the bewildering and ever lengthening list of marketed antibiotic preparations and the constant emergence of resistant strains of bacteria, a hospital antibiotic policy would seem essential but is all too often opposed by 'clinical freedom fighters'. Such a policy must be flexible to take into account exceptional circumstances, and it must follow guidelines that are scientifically rational, clinically useful and, whenever possible, inexpensive (Williams 1984).

Prompt resuscitation is important, blood loss being replaced by transfusion, and fluid and electrolyte balance being carefully controlled. Anuria or marked oliguria dictate the need for the advice of a renal physician, and appropriate treatment may include dialysis. Ileus is treated in the usual way by gastrointestinal suction, together with intravenous fluids and electrolytes.

If it is likely that there are still products of conception in the uterus, these should be removed following resuscitation and after antibiotic therapy for several hours, by which time effective blood levels of the antibiotics will have been obtained. It is certainly preferable that this should be carried out within 12 hours of the commencement of treatment (Cavanagh et al. 1973). Retained products of conception can usually be removed easily with ring forceps so that curettage may not be necessary, and in any case should never be performed vigorously in these circumstances.

Laparotomy may be necessary when there is doubt about the diagnosis, for example when appendicitis is suspected, but a grid iron incision with its limited access should not be made. If bowel injury is suspected, it should be sought and repaired, and operation jointly by surgeon and gynaecologist is sensible. Rupture of a tubo-ovarian abscess is an acute surgical emergency that sometimes proves fatal, and if it seems that an abscess is likely to rupture, prompt surgical intervention with drainage is required. If feasible, the infected organs may be removed, but drainage of the abscess and the peritoneal cavity is the essential procedure. Abscesses may be multiple and multilocular, and all pockets must be drained. Adequate exposure is essential, and thorough peritoneal cleansing with lavage before closure, e.g. using povidone-iodine solution (Brown 1982), is probably as effective as continuous postoperative peritoneal lavage with an antibiotic solution (Shweni et al. 1980). Surgery also becomes necessary when there is no response to antibiotic and supportive treatment, but timing operation in such cases can be one of the most difficult decisions in clinical gynaecology. Basing his view on practice in Africa, where dangerously acute pelvic inflammatory disease is a common emergency, Brown (1982) recommends surgical intervention if there is no obvious response to conservative treatment within 24 hours, or no reduction in pelvic masses within 48 hours. In British practice conservative management is often persisted with a little longer, and this is probably justified but very careful observation for any signs of deterioration is essential. Acutely infected tubes should not be removed, nor should the uterus in this circumstance, but collections of pus should be drained and material obtained for cultures.

A pelvic abscess obviously pointing into the vagina should be evacuated by posterior colpotomy, followed by insertion of a wide bore drain. This is often curative for posthysterectomy abscesses, but it is less likely to be effective in the case of tubo-ovarian abscesses which are frequently multilocular (Rubinstein et al. 1976). After a tubo-ovarian abscess has been treated initially by intensive antibiotic therapy, with some improvement in symptoms and signs including control of the systemic upset, persistence of the mass unchanged or the development of more local signs (e.g. pointing) calls for surgical removal or drainage.

Following surgery in any of these circumstances,

if continued resolution of a mass is not then maintained, removal of the affected organs under antibiotic cover will usually become advisable.

The treatment of septic shock merits special mention. It must be both prompt and vigorous, and, because of both the complexity of the mechanisms involved and the need for uninterrupted sophisticated monitoring, it is best carried out in a central intensive care unit. Until this can be effected, management is along the following lines: maintenance of the airway with administration of oxygen in high concentration; restoration and maintenance of circulatory blood volume by administration of blood or plasma, together with electrolyte monitoring and replacement; appropriate intravenous antibiotic therapy as already described; glucocorticoids given early and in high dosage; insertion of an indwelling catheter into the bladder to measure urinary output, and usually a central venous pressure line if this can be achieved easily. Subsequently, and preferably in an intensive care unit, respiration may be maintained by endotracheal intubation and assisted ventilation, and the circulation is maintained by carefully controlled intravenous infusion of crystalloids and colloids; while vasopressor drugs may be of value in the warm hypotensive phase, subsequently there is vasoconstriction and a vasodilator such as chlorpromazine may be given to assist perfusion; digoxin and diuretics such as mannitol and frusemide are sometimes required, and the development of coagulopathy will require expert haematological advice and perhaps the use of heparin. If there is renal failure, antibiotics or other drugs that are nephrotoxic (e.g. gentamycin and other aminoglycosides) should be avoided, and dialysis may become necessary. Retained products of conception should be removed gently as soon as effective antibiotic cover and resuscitation have been established, and collections of pus that are already present or which develop subsequently should of course be evacuated and drained.

The intensive biophysical and biochemical monitoring possible in an intensive care unit includes continuous electrocardiography, continuous measurement of arterial and central venous pressure and of peripheral temperature gradients; pulmonary ventilation is monitored, and measurements made of blood pH, base, and gases; the indwelling catheter permits continuous measurement of urinary output, and frequent measurements are made of blood electrolytes. While the supportive and monitoring measures listed are of great value, it must be emphasized that the three main features leading to irreversible shock and death are prolonged duration of the shock, failure to remove surgically accessible sepsis including retained products of conception, and inappropriate antibiotic therapy (Willocks 1978).

Postoperative infection—treatment and prophylaxis

Treatment of established postoperative infection follows the same principles, and must take into account the likely pathogens and their sensitivity patterns. However, the use of prophylactic antibodies in patients undergoing hysterectomy (Ohm & Galask 1976) remains controversial. If such chemoprophylaxis is to be used it should be a standard regimen as part of an agreed and updated antibiotic policy based on effective infection monitoring by the hospital's microbiology service; this is more likely to succeed than is 'blind' chemoprophylaxis (Geddes 1982). Therapeutic serum concentrations to control contamination during surgery can be achieved by single-dose parenteral treatment, by intramuscular injection shortly beforehand or preferably by intravenous infusion during the operation, and this is the method least likely to result in development of antibiotic resistance or to lead to superinfection. Intravenous cotrimoxazole has been used successfully in this way to 'cover' hysterectomy performed through the abdomen (Mathews et al. 1977) or by the vaginal route (Mathews et al. 1979); alternatives include cefotoxin, a parenteral cephalosporin effective against anaerobes including bacteroides, broad spectrum ureidopenicillins (e.g. mezlocillin or piperacillin) which are antipseudomonal but may be unstable to B-lactamases in some strains of Bacteroides fragilis, and combinations of penicillins with B-lactamases inhibitors (e.g. amoxycillin with clavulanic acid, in 'Augmentin'). Nevertheless, many gynaecologists perform 'cold' surgery, including hysterectomy but excluding patients known to have chronic or recent acute pelvic inflammatory disease, without chemoprophylaxis, and this perhaps is presently the wisest course if local postoperative infection rates are not unusually high or rising.

Infection associated with intrauterine contraceptive devices

Special mention must be made of pelvic infection (including actinomycosis, *see* p. 606) associated with intrauterine contraceptive devices. It seems clear that the route of infection is from the vagina through the cervix, the thread tail of most devices probably acting as a 'wick'. *In vitro* tests have shown that pathogens, including *B-haemolytic streptococci* and *Bacteroides fragilis*, will colonize cervical mucus coating the tail of a device (Purrier *et al.* 1979), and, following hysterectomy bacteria can usually be grown from the uterine cavity when a tailed device is *in situ* but not when there is an intrauterine device without a tail (Sparks *et al.* 1981).

A three- or four-fold increased incidence of pelvic inflammatory disease in intrauterine contraceptive device users was reported from Britain (Vessey *et al.* 1976), Sweden (Westrom *et al.* 1976) and America (Eschenbach *et al.* 1977). More recently, in a cohort study of 17000 married women attending Family Planning Association clinics (Vessey *et al.* 1981) the hospital admission rates for acute and chronic pelvic infections were, respectively, two and a half and ten times as common in intrauterine contraceptive device users than in non-users, acute infection was most likely to occur soon after insertion or re-insertion of a device, and an increased risk of chronic (although not acute) infection was maintained following its removal. In this study, there was no very firm evidence that any one type of intrauterine contraceptive was more likely than others to be associated with infection. In Britain, five deaths from sepsis associated with intrauterine devices of different types have been described (Smith *et al.* 1983; Gruer *et al.* 1983, Roberts 1983), and there have been reports from elsewhere of fatal septicaemia in women wearing devices and without any other predisposing factors (Scott 1968, Marshall *et al.* 1973).

In addition to the antibiotic and supportive treatment already described, when pelvic infection occurs in the presence of an intrauterine contraceptive, the device should be removed. Removal of this foreign body assists the response to treatment, and the device should be submitted for culture. Following recovery an alternative method of contraception, oral or barrier, is advisable.

Toxic shock syndrome associated with vaginal tampons

The recently recognized association between an acute and potentially lethal shock syndrome, caused by staphylococcal exotoxin, and the use of vaginal tampons during menstruation (Shrock 1980, Shands *et al.* 1980) quickly achieved notoriety in the United States where, at its peak during 1980, it was estimated to have occurred in about 10 per 100000 menstruating women per year. Its incidence decreased when one

particular superabsorbent tampon (Rely) was withdrawn from sale, but it occurs with other brands, although few cases have been reported elsewhere than in the United States. The same toxic shock syndrome also occurs occasionally in children, in women not wearing tampons or not menstruating, and indeed also in men.

Staphylococcus aureus is usually isolated from the vagina and the tampon, presumably having been introduced on the inserting fingers; it multiplies in the retained menstrual blood where it produces its exotoxin, which is absorbed through the vaginal epithelium into the circulation and may also ascend into the uterus to be carried, by retrograde menstrual flow, into the peritoneal cavity.

Fever and hypotension are accompanied by erythema and subsequently desquamation of the skin, muscle pains, abdominal and gastrointestinal symptoms, and by disturbances of electrolytes and liver function. Further complications may include respiratory distress due to shock lung, thrombocytopenia and sometimes disseminated intravascular coagulation, and renal failure.

Management consists of removal of the tampon, taking cultures from it and from the vagina and blood culture (usually negative), vaginal lavage, broad spectrum antibiotic therapy, resuscitation and support of vital functions, and the treatment of whichever complications may develop. This is best carried out in an intensive care unit.

Gonococcal infection

The reported incidence of Neisserian pelvic inflammatory disease varies considerably, and in some communities gonococci may be isolated in almost half of the women presenting with pelvic infection. Although it may sometimes be coincidental, Cunningham *et al.* (1978) reported the culture of gonococci from Pouch of Douglas aspirates in more than half of their patients with both pelvic inflammatory disease and gonorrhoeal infection of the lower genital tract. The initial site of infection is usually the cervix, but there may also be the infection of the urethra or occasionally Bartholinitis. By direct spread across mucosal surfaces, infection ascends quickly from the cervix to the endometrium, and thence often to the endosalpinx. The Fallopian tubes quickly become oedematous and hyperaemic with the risk of exudation of pus into the pelvic cavity to cause peritonitis, sometimes an abscess, and subsequently adhesions. The fimbrial end of the tube may close so that a pyosalpinx results. Because damage to the tubal epithelium is quite often severe, and because pelvic adhesions are also likely, tubal occlusion and infertility frequently result. This risk may be minimized, but cannot always be avoided, by prompt and effective antibiotic treatment.

CLINICAL FEATURES

Pelvic inflammatory disease due to gonoccocal infection often presents just after menstruation, but the patient may admit to an earlier purulent vaginal discharge and perhaps to a sexual contact with a suspected infected partner. Lower abdominal pain and tenderness is accompanied by elevation of the temperature and by tachycardia, and sometimes there is nausea and vomiting. There is usually bilateral pelvic tenderness on vaginal examination, and this is exacerbated by moving the cervix. Thickening or enlargement of the uterine adnexae may be felt. The pelvic findings are in other words similar to those present in acute pyogenic infection, but the fever and systemic upset are usually much less. Appendicitis with peritonitis, ectopic pregnancy, torsion of or haemorrhage into an ovarian cyst, and occasionally even urinary tract infection are the main conditions to be differentiated. The history and the usually bilateral nature of the pelvic signs and symptoms are often helpful in making the right diagnosis. When an abdominal surgical emergency cannot be excluded, diagnostic laparoscopy is called for, following which a bacterial culture can often be obtained from the tip of the instrument, or sometimes laparotomy without prior laparoscopy may be preferred. Cervical, vaginal and urethral swabs should of course also be taken.

TREATMENT

Although the usual treatment of gonorrhoea is by single intramuscular injection of procaine penicillin, with probenecid to retard the excretion of the penicillin, if it is thought that an acute pelvic infection is gonorrhoeal large doses of penicillin should be given for 10 days. Often the bacteriological diagnosis will be in doubt and initial broad spectrum therapy will have been started before the presence of Gram-negative diplococci is reported from direct examination of the swabs or gonococci are identified by culture. Resistant infection by penicillinase-producing strains will respond to parenteral treatment with cephalosporins, co-trimoxazole or spectinomycin. Although the systemic upset is less severe than in acute py-

ogenic infection, attention should be paid to fluid and electrolyte balance, and the patient should be nursed in a sitting position to localize any peritonitis.

As with pyogenic infection, careful follow-up is necessary as there may be residual (often secondary) infection, tubal patency tests may be called for after complete remission for six months, re-infection is of course possible and indeed likely in some patients, and contact tracing should be carried out from the sexually transmitted diseases clinic.

Chlamydial infection

With improved tissue culture methods it has become apparent that certain serotypes of the obligate intracellular parasite *Chlamydia tracomatis*, the organism that causes lymphogranuloma venereum, trachoma and ocular infection, may be isolated with surprising frequency from the lower and upper genital tracts. This is particularly so from the lower genital tracts of women attending clinics for sexually transmitted disease (up to 30% may be chlamydia-positive, with the highest rates in those who also harbour the gonococcus or who are known contacts of men with nongonococcal or proven chlamydial urethritis), but much lower rates are found in family planning, infertility and antenatal clinics (Munday 1983). There is also little doubt that a significant amount of pelvic inflammatory disease is chlamydial in origin, perhaps a majority of cases in Scandinavia as shown by chlamydial antibody levels and positive cultures from the cervix and from the Fallopian tubes at laparoscopy (Mardh *et al.* 1977). In some of these cases, of course, the chlamydiae are present as secondary invaders. Tetracycline or erythromycin should be prescribed when chlamydia have been isolated from salpingitis, and should be added to the antibiotic regimen when it is thought that chlamydia might be the cause of pelvic infection, e.g. when the organism has been isolated from the cervix or urethra, or when the patient's recent sexual history suggests this possibility.

Chronic pelvic infection

Chronic pelvic infection is an important cause of pelvic pain, with dyspareunia and secondary dysmenorrhoea, infertility due to tubal obstruction and menstrual upsets usually in the form of menorrhagia with polymenorrhoea. It may become a most distressing disorder for the patient, its long course marked by repeated admissions to hospital during acute or subacute relapses. Management of the 'pelvic cripple' represents one of the most trying, and all too often unrewarding, problems for the gynaecologist. Chronic pelvic infection usually follows an episode of acute infection, initial treatment of which may have been delayed or otherwise inadequate. Sometimes there is no such history and presumably a low grade infection has become chronic; indeed, in a few patients quite unsuspected pelvic inflammatory disease with tubal obstruction is found in an infertile woman without other symptoms. The initial infection may be pyogenic or gonococcal, but very occasionally it is tuberculous.

Regular menstrual shedding of the endometrium usually eliminates local infection so that, unless there are retained products of conception and except when the infection is tuberculous (*see* p. 604), the uterus is not usually actively involved in the infective process, although accompanying mild chronic inflammatory changes in the myometrium, with congestion and fibrin deposition, may result in recognizable enlargement of the uterus.

PATHOLOGY

Tubal infection provides the main pathological feature. Gonococcal infection may have destroyed the endosalpinx, with subsequent formation of intraluminal adhesions, but more often the tube is bound down and kinked by peritubal adhesions. It may have become blocked at either or both the isthmic and fimbrial ends, and if both ends are occluded a pyo- (or hydro-) salpinx forms, in which case the wall of the tube is thinned and its lining mucosa has lost its many plicae. The ovary is likely to be involved in the process, showing chronic inflammatory changes and perhaps becoming imbedded in the wall of a pyosalpinx. Sometimes a tubo-ovarian abscess forms, but very rarely is there abscess formation in the ovary itself. Eventually dense fibrous adhesions may form, effectively 'loculating' the ovary from the tube, or binding together the adnexae, uterus, bowel and occasionally even involving the bladder in a 'frozen pelvis'. The pelvic veins may show septic thrombophlebitis.

CLINICAL FEATURES

A known history of previous pelvic infection is obviously helpful, or a history suggesting such infection may be obtained. However, previous gonorrhoea, or a septic abortion may not be admitted, and some-

times a pyrexial illness following delivery or spontaneous abortion may not be recalled. In other cases, there has been no obvious primary infecting event, but the presence (or recent presence) of an intrauterine device should always bring the possibility of pelvic infection to mind.

Pelvic pain, perhaps severe, is the main complaint and it is exacerbated by coitus and by menstruation. Dyspareunia, which is deep, may be bilateral or localized to one side; it may also be felt towards the back, and some patients will localize it as in the rectum. Dysmenorrhoea is of the secondary congestive type, often increasing in severity during the few days preceding each period and becoming less marked towards the end of menstruation. Mittelschmerz is also quite common in these patients, and some may complain of pelvic pain on defaecation. Others will complain of pelvic pain and a lower abdominal ache virtually all the time, frequently with low backache in addition, but careful questioning will usually confirm exacerbation by intercourse and menstruation. Menorrhagia is common and, because one or both of the ovaries are so often involved in the inflammatory process, this may be accompanied by some menstrual irregularity or, more typically, polymenorrhoea. Chronic cervicitis, with a history of an excessive yellow vaginal discharge, is often present, but, as already described, some patients will present complaining of infertility only, and this is often secondary infertility. In long-standing cases with at least moderately severe symptoms, patients may be demoralized and debilitated, there may be weight loss, and marital disharmony becomes all too likely as a result of persistent dyspareunia, menstrual irregularity and general lack of physical and mental vigour.

On examination there is tenderness in both iliac fossae, or right across the lower abdomen, and it is sometimes possible to feel the upper part of a pelvic swelling on one or both sides. On pelvic examination, besides usually confirming the presence of chronic cervicitis, the uterus is usually fixed in retroversion, it usually feels a little enlarged, and attempts to move it cause pain. There is almost always tenderness on each side of the pelvis, usually with obvious adnexal thickening or a pelvic mass, which in some cases may be large enough to displace the uterus to the other side. Tenderness may prevent a very useful vaginal examination, but it is generally possible to elicit at least some of these signs; in a few patients it is not really possible to distinguish separate organs, but the frozen nature of the pelvic contents is apparent. Rectal examination should not be omitted, adnexal thickening and the extent of small adnexal swellings often being more apparent by this means that by vaginal examination; exclusion of a rectal lesion is obviously also important in itself.

DIFFERENTIAL DIAGNOSIS

This is mainly from endometriosis which may give a closely similar clinical picture but without the history of acute initiating infection and also one without any cervicitis. Occasionally nodular thickening in the parametria may suggest endometriosis rather than inflammatory disease, but certain differentiation is not possible on pelvic examination. Laparoscopy, or occasionally laparotomy, will make correct diagnosis possible and it may be useful at the same time to check tubal patency. Conditions giving rise to tender pelvic swellings include acute complications in an ovarian cyst (e.g. torsion or haemorrhage), appendix abscess, and occasionally diverticulitis or Crohn's disease, but the unilateral nature of these and the history and other clinical features will usually suggest the right diagnosis.

TREATMENT

Management is usually conservative including appropriate antibiotic therapy, but surgery is called for in certain circumstances and, in such cases, it should not be delayed. Apart from the patient's age, parity and reproductive intentions, choice of treatment depends on the patient's general condition, the nature and severity of her symptoms, the nature and extent of the pelvic inflammatory lesions, and the course of the disease, particularly its response so far to treatment.

Conservative management includes attention to general nutrition and treatment of anaemia, analgesics as required, and antibiotics when indicated. While not as effective as in acute pelvic infection, antibiotic therapy is called for when an exacerbation of symptoms and signs suggests that an acute or subacute 'flare-up' is about to occur, and another possible indication is when previous gradual improvement with reduction in the size of pelvic masses has halted and the patient is perhaps occasionally pyrexial. Without an operative procedure, it is not usually possible to obtain material for bacterial culture, but broad spectrum treatment (e.g. a cephalosporin and metronidazole) should be chosen. Patients responding to conservative management, but with persistence of pelvic pain, were in the past frequently treated by means of pelvic shortwave diathermy, but many gynaecologists now doubt the efficacy of such treatment, it has never been (and possibly could not be) evaluated in a controlled manner, and considerable exacerbation of pain during the course of treatment is a very frequent occurrence. Likewise, the use of electrodiathermy or cryocautery to the cervix when chronic cervicitis is present is almost certainly a therapeutic irrelevance, and is sometimes indeed followed by an exacerbation of the pelvic infection.

Surgery, which should usually be radical with removal of the uterus, tubes and often also the ovaries, is indicated if: (1) there is general deterioration in health despite intensive conservative management (including at least one empirical change in the choice of antibiotics); (2) there are repeated acute exacerbations of the chronic pelvic infection (except perhaps if these are becoming clearly less frequent and less severe); (3) there is persistence unchanged, or an increase in size, of pelvic masses (adnexal or in the Pouch of Douglas) despite conservative management including antibiotic therapy; (4) there is persistence unchanged, or an increase in, pain including dyspareunia despite continued conservative management including antibiotic therapy; (5) there is persistence of menorrhagia that is incapacitating and/or causing anaemia; (6) laparotomy is required for differential diagnosis from cancer (bowel or pelvic).

Although laparoscopy may be used to determine the nature of the condition, particularly for the differential diagnosis from endometriosis or for assessment when infertility continues despite good clinical resolution, it should be used with caution. Particularly in the most long-standing cases, dense adhesions may make intestinal damage a very real possibility, and they may in any case prevent a satisfactory view of the pelvic and lower abdominal contents. If exploration is required but laparoscopy seems likely to be difficult or hazardous, then laparotomy should be chosen without hesitation. When laparotomy is required for any of the indications listed, it should usually be undertaken during antibiotic treatment, perhaps by a single-dose intravenous infusion (*see* p. 599). Material for bacterial culture should always be obtained at operation although this often proves sterile. The surgical procedure required depends on the listed (above) features governing the choice of management, particularly the extent of the inflammatory process, and the age and reproductive intentions of the patient. In the younger patient, some apparently healthy ovarian tissue should, and can almost always, be preserved; but if this is not feasible without difficulty and the patient does not wish further pregnancies, then there need be no hesitation in removing both ovaries completely and prescribing hormone replacement therapy later. Unless it seems technically very difficult or dangerous, hysterectomy would usually be performed in the older patient, and in the younger woman who has completed her family but has intractable menorrhagia and/or severe dysmenorrhoea it is also usually called for. In other cases it may often be feasible to separate and remove hydrosalpinges without removing the uterus. Surgery, both decisions on the procedures to be undertaken and the performance of the operation itself, may be difficult and even dangerous in these patients; it should therefore be performed by, or under the immediate supervision of, an experienced operator, and blood should always be available for transfusion. It is occasionally better in these circumstances to resort to subtotal hysterectomy than persist with an attempted total hysterectomy that endangers either bowel or bladder. Pelvic abscesses may develop when there is a flare-up of chronic pelvic infection, and their drainage has already been described. The investigation and operative treatment of tubal infertility following resolution of chronic infection is not dealt with in this chapter; any tubal restorative operation should be deferred until well after the inflammatory process has settled, but when laparotomy is undertaken in patients with active inflammation it may well be wise to carry out a ventrosuspension procedure to prevent fixation of the uterus in retroversion, with possible persistent dyspareunia, and to minimize the chance of further tubal adhesions.

Pelvic tuberculosis

Tuberculosis of the female genital tract, once common enough to be found in 1% of women with dysfunctional uterine bleeding (Sutherland 1949) and in 4% of adolescents with excessive menstrual loss (Sutherland 1953), has shared in a general dramatic decline in the incidence of tuberculous disease that has followed introduction of anti-tuberculosis drug therapy. This is well illustrated by the reduction in incidence of endometrial tuberculosis in infertile women investigated in Glasgow from 5% before 1951 (Sharman 1952) to 1% during recent years (Black 1978). A continued decline in incidence may be anticipated, but particularly in areas such as the West of Scotland where there has always been a comparatively high incidence of tuberculosis, and also in some sections of the immigrant population, it will remain an occasional but important cause of gynaecological disorder especially infertility.

Almost invariably tuberculosis of the genital tract is secondary to a primary lesion elsewhere, and the latter is usually quiescent by the time pelvic involvement is diagnosed. Sexual transmission from a male with tuberculous epididymitis is possible but is extremely rare. In a minority of cases the tubes, ovaries and the serosal surface of the uterus are involved in the peritoneal spread from an intra-abdominal lesion, but generally infection reaches the genital tract (the tubes in most cases) by blood spread, usually from a pulmonary lesion. A vulval lesion, secondary to intestinal infection by the bovine or human *Mycobacterium tuberculosis*, is a rarity; otherwise, the infecting mycobacterium is the human type. From the tubes, infection reaches the endometrium where either it persists in the basal layer that is not shed at menstruation or re-infection occurs from the tube following menstruation. It may also spread from the tube to the peritoneal cavity and ovaries, and before the introduction of effective drug treatment caseating peritonitis with fistula formation sometimes followed but this is very exceptional today.

Tuberculosis of the female genital tract may produce no symptoms apart from infertility; or there may be the symptoms and signs of pelvic infection, more often simulating chronic rather than acute ,pyogenic infection.

PATHOLOGY

The Fallopian tubes are not only the usual site at which tuberculous infection reaches the genital tract but both tubes become involved almost invariably. Infection begins in the mucosa, and then spreads through the tubal wall to the peritoneal surface. The macroscopic appearances are similar to those of non-tuberculous chronic salpingitis with tubal thickening, fibrosis and adhesions. Miliary nodules may form on the surfaces of the tubes, although not every example of *salpingitis isthmica nodosa* is due to tuberculosis. The ends of the tube may be closed, and a pyosalpinx may form. Not infrequently the fimbrial end is open and everted, but, although the tube may be patent in such cases, it is rigid and narrow; the muscle becomes replaced by fibrous tissue, and the mucosal folds are destroyed and sometimes artificial diverticulae and crypts develop. These changes cause failure of tubal function and thus infertility. The ovary may be involved, with adhesions and perhaps miliary nodules, and miliary spread to the uterine and other peritoneal surfaces may be seen.

Histological examination shows typical tubercles with giant epithelioid and round cells. Caseation is prominent in advanced cases, especially in a pyosalpinx or a tuberculous tubo-ovarian abscess. Endometrial infection is demonstrable in 80% of cases, but this probably represents an underestimate since histological features are not usually prominent (or may be absent) in curettings not obtained towards the end of the menstrual cycle. Re-infection from the tube may perhaps not occur during every cycle, or with patchy infection curettage may remove only normal tissue. In advanced cases there may be complete destruction of the endometrium with formation of a caseous pyometra. Tuberculous cervicitis, either an ulcer resembling ectopy, or a proliferative lesion resembling carcinoma, is uncommon.

CLINICAL FEATURES

Symptoms vary considerably with the severity and stage of the disease. At one extreme, many patients have no symptoms and often almost no abnormal physical signs, but tuberculous endometritis is diagnosed during the investigation of infertility. At the other extreme, and much less infrequently since the advent of antituberculosis drugs, quite large pelvic or even abdomino-pelvic masses may form and there are the symptoms of chronic pelvic inflammatory disease. There may be excessive and perhaps irregular menstruation, while ovarian involvement is usually associated with an accelerated menstrual cycle. Sometimes, however, menstruation is scanty, and amenorrhoea may result when there is extensive endometrial destruction and/or general debility. Excessive vaginal discharge is frequent. General symptoms that may be present include weight loss, anorexia, occasionally night sweats and pyrexia, and there may be anaemia. Reporting a very large personal series of 638 patients, Sutherland (1979) noted that 44% of them complained of infertility, 25% of pelvic pain, 18% of excessive menstrual loss, and there were palpable pelvic masses in 46%.

DIAGNOSIS

Endometrial curettings are examined microscopically for the presence of tubercles, but diagnosis depends on the identification of *Mycobacteria tuberculosis*. These may be seen after Ziehl–Neelsen staining, but whenever tuberculosis is suspected clinically or his-

tologically (and in any patient complaining of infertility) endometrium should always be cultured specifically for tubercle bacilli. Cultured organisms should be submitted to sensitivity tests to the drugs in current use for the treatment of tuberculosis.

Very occasionally infection is confined to the tubes, or for the reasons already stated it may be missed in curettings, in which case investigation may be continued by hysterosalpinography or nowadays more often by laparoscopy. Radiological findings that should suggest tuberculous salpingitis include rigid 'pipe stem' narrowing of the isthmus, punctate opacification of crypts and diverticulae in the lumen of this part of the tube, a 'clubbed' ampulla, and calcification in the tubes and/or ovaries. Laparoscopy or laparotomy may show the tubal and other appearances already described, but macroscopic differentiation between tuberculosis and other infections is not possible. When surgery is undertaken, drained pus or caseous material in any tissue excised should be examined histologically and bacteriologically.

TREATMENT

The first line of treatment is with drugs effective against *Mycobacterium tuberculosis*, and all proven cases of gynaecological tuberculosis should be treated. Sutherland (1979) has told how, soon after the introduction of the first antituberculosis drugs, all of 33 control patients followed up for at least a year showed positive evidence of persistent infection or had already required treatment for clinically obvious deterioration. Treatment should be started as soon as the diagnosis has been made, and should not await bacteriological confirmation when a positive diagnosis has been made from histology. However, a careful general physical assessment, including blood count and sedimentation rate, search for active tuberculosis elsewhere, including particularly the respiratory and urinary tracts, should first be made.

Various regimens using antituberculosis drugs singly, or more often in combination, have been used since this form of therapy became available, but it is important to follow current therapeutic practice as for the treatment of pulmonary lesions. Close joint supervision of treatment by a chest physician in addition to the gynaecologist is therefore advisable, although regrettably this does not obtain everywhere with the result that some women with pelvic tuberculosis are treated less effectively than need be (Crofton 1979). Currently, the most usual drug programme is rifampicin and isoniazid, which are available in a combined tablet (Rifinah), with etham-butol in addition during the first 60–90 days. Because of effects on vision, the last mentioned drug must not be continued for a longer period, and initial examination by an ophthalmologist is advisable, as is the performance of liver function tests. Ethambutol is given in a single daily dose after breakfast, 15 mg/kg body weight. Rifampicin and isoniazid are given to-gether in a single oral dose before breakfast; patients weighing less than 50 kg should receive 450 mg of rifampicin daily, and heavier patients should have 600 mg per day. Two varieties of the combined tablet are available so that, whichever dose of rifampicin is called for, a standard daily dose of 300 mg of isoniazid is taken.

Except when there are other extensive lesions or marked constitutional effects, or when a flare-up has occurred following initial curettage or other operative procedure, drug treatment is carried out on an out-patient basis, with the patient re-attending for review at monthly and then three-monthly intervals. At the end of the course, or earlier if steady subjective or objective improvement has not been maintained, en-dometrial curettage and bacteriological examination is carried out to confirm 'cure'. Persistence of pelvic masses or of tuberculous infection in the endo-metrium would of course necessitate the continua-tion of antituberculosis drugs in accordance with sensitivity testing. Recurrences subsequent to apparent cure are not exceptional and follow-up should be continued for at least five years with an-nual endometrial curettage as an outpatient. Suth-erland (1979) holds that indefinite follow-up, includ-ing repeated curettage, is always necessary, but recurrences after more than five years relate to treat-ment before the introduction of rifampicin. Therefore, most gynaecologists will discontinue follow-up after five years in remission, although it is wise to arrange for subsequent reassessment if general or gynaeco-logical symptoms recur.

Surgery for pelvic clearance is occasionally called for. Indications include persistent active or recurrent disease following adequate drug treatment, persistent pain or severe menorrhagia, the persistence or de-velopment of substantial pelvic masses, the occa-sional co-existence of an ovarian cyst or fibroid, or the suspicion of malignant disease. Hysterectomy with removal of both tubes and ovaries should be performed, although dense adhesions may make the operation difficult. Antituberculosis drug therapy should be continued for six months after operation and, with this precaution and careful surgical tech-

nique, fistula formation is no longer a likely compli-cation.

PREGNANCY FOLLOWING TREATMENT

The prospect of successful pregnancy is remote if tuberculosis of the tubes has been proved, although occasional cases of successful intrauterine pregnancy have been reported (Francis 1964). There is a very considerable risk of ectopic pregnancy, which is further increased after salpingostomy or other tubal surgery, and in such cases the necessary emergency surgery may be technically difficult. The patient who seeks a pregnancy following an apparent cure of proven pelvic tuberculosis should be advised of these risks, and the gynaecologist is probably wise to de-cline to perform restorative tubal surgery in such patients.

Pelvic actinomycosis

Infection of the female genital tract by the Gram-positive (non-acid-fast) mycelium-bearing anaerobic fungus *Actinomyces israelii* was considered rare until recently. This organism is a normal commensal of the mouth and gut, and pelvic actinomycosis was formerly almost always secondary to an intestinal lesion, usually a ruptured appendix or sometimes traumatic perforation of the colon (McCarthy 1955), but now it is more often associated with the presence of an intrauterine contraceptive device. In these cases the route of infection is from the anus, across the perineum and upward through the vagina and cer-vix, and there is often co-existent infection by other anaerobes; the combination of a foreign body, caus-ing chronic trauma, and the adjacent heavy anaero-bic flora of the vagina provides ideal conditions for opportunistic colonization and occasionally frank in-fection by actinomyces (Lomax *et al.* 1976). The first reports concerned metallic contraceptive devices (Draper & Studdiford 1926, Stevenson 1957), the traumatic effect of spring devices seeming to carry a particular risk (Schiffer *et al.* 1975), but a variety of modern plastic devices, including the Copper 7 gravi-gard, have now been implicated (Dische *et al.* 1974, Charnock & Chambers 1979, Hager & Majudar 1979).

Gupta *et al.* (1978) identified colonies of *Actino-myces israelii* in cervical smears from more than 500 women wearing intrauterine contraceptive devices, and Duguid *et al.* (1980) demonstrated this in 31% of women wearing plastic devices not containing copper, compared with only two out of 165 women with copper-containing devices, and in none of 300 controls using oral contraception. These findings suggest that, although pelvic actinomycosis will probably be diagnosed with greater frequency in future, the copper in certain devices may have a relative protective bacteriostatic effect against this organism. Cervical colonization is most likely when the device has been in place for more than two years, it correlates with clinical and cytological evidence of local vaginal and cervical infection, and occasionally results in an ascending infection of the uterus and pelvic tissues.

Some cases of pelvic actinomycosis present as acute, or more often acute-on-chronic pelvic inflammatory disease requiring major surgery. Multilocular granulomatous pelvi-abdominal masses form, some such abscesses may rupture (Purdie et al. 1977) to cause generalized peritonitis and perhaps subphrenic abscess formation; a fatal case of abscess formation and rupture, two years-after insertion of a plastic device, has been reported (Hagar & Majmudar 1979). In other cases, there is only local endometrial infection, usually causing some pain, an offensive vaginal discharge and irregular bleeding. Actinomyces may be difficult to culture, but microscopic tissue diagnosis can be made by recognizing typical sulphur-body colonies surrounded by pus containing lipid histiocytes, and then confirming the presence of actinomyces by special staining.

The principle of treatment of actinomycosis is wide surgical excision combined with a long course of an antibiotic effective against this fungus and also against other anaerobes that are likely to be present, and this policy should be applied to the treatment of pelvic lesions (Charles 1980). Penicillin in very high dosage to obtain an effective concentration in the relatively avascular lesions will provide effective cover for surgery which is usually pelvic clearance. Tetracycline, erythromycin and clindamycin are alternatives.

REFERENCES

BLACK W.P. (1978): personal communication to Sutherland A.M. (1979) Brit. J. Hosp. Med., 22, 569.

BRON I. (1982) In Progress in Obstetrics and Gynaecology, Volume 2 (Studd J. ed.) p. 274. Churchill Livingstone.

CAVANAGH D., DAHM C.H. & RAO P.A. (1973) Int. J. Gynaec. Obstet., 11, 61.

CAVANAGH D. & RAO P.S. (1973) Clin. Obstet. Gynec., 16, 25.

CHARLES D. (1980) Major Problems in Obstetrics and Gynecology, 12, 80.

CHARNOCK M. & CHAMBERS T.J. (1979) Lancet, i, 1239.

CROFTON J. (1979) Brit. med. J., i, 52.

CUNNINGHAM F.G., HAUTH J.C., GILSTRAP I.C., HERBERT W.N.P. & KAPPUS S.S. (1978) Obstet. Gynec., 52, 161.

DISCHE F.E., BURT J.M., DAVIDSON N.J.H. & PUNTAMBEKER S. (1974) J. Obstet. Gynaec. Brit. Cwlth., 81, 724.

DRAPER J.W. & STUDDIFORD W.E. (1926) Amer. J. Obstet. Gynec., 11, 603.

DUGUID H.L.D., PARRATT D. & TRAYNOR R. (1980) Brit. med. J., ii, 534.

ESCHENBACH D.A., HARNISCH J.P. & HOLMES K.K. (1977) Amer. J. Obstet. Gynec., 128, 838.

FRANCIS W.J.A. (1964) J. Obstet. Gynaec. Brit. Cwlth., 71, 418.

GEDDES A.M. (1982) In Good Antimicrobial Prescribing, Lancet Review, p. 8.

GRUER L.D., COLLINGHAM K.E. & EDWARDS C.W. (1983) Lancet ii, 677.

GUPTA P.K., ERAZAN Y.S. & FROST J.K. (1978) Acta Cytol., 22, 281.

HAGER W.D. & MAJMUDAR B. (1979) Amer. J. Obstet. Gynec., 133, 60.

LOMAX C.W., HARBERT G.M. & THORNSTON W.N. (1976) Obstet. Gynec. 48, 341.

McCARTHY J. (1955) J. Path. Bact., 69, 175.

MARDH P.A., RIPA T., SVENSON L. & WESTROM L. (1977) New Engl. J. Med., 296, 2377.

MARSHALL B.M., HEPLER J.K. & JINGUJI M.S. (1973) Obstet. Gynec., 41, 83.

MATHEWS D.D., ROSS H. & COOPER J. (1977) Brit. J. Obstet. Gynaec., 84, 894.

MATHEWS D.D., AGARWAL V., GORDON A.M. & COOPER J. (1979) Brit. J. Obstet. Gynec., 86, 737.

MUNDAY P.E. (1983) In Progress in Obstetrics and Gynaecology, Volume 3 (Studd J. ed.) p. 231. Churchill Livingstone.

OHM, M.J. & GALASK R.P. (1976) Amer. J. Obstet. Gynec., 125, 442.

PURDIE D.W., CARTY M.J. & McLEOD T.I.F. (1977) Brit. med. J., ii, 1392.

PURRIER B.G.A., SPARKS R.A., WATT P.J. & ELSTEIN M. (1979) Brit. J. Obstet. Gynaec., 86, 374.

ROBERTS G. (1983) Brit. med. J., 287, 1880.

RUBENSTEIN P.R., MISHELL D.R. & LEDGER W.J. (1976) Obstet. Gynec., 142, 145.

SCOTT R.B. (1968) Obstet. Gynec., 31, 322.

SHANDS K.N., SCHMID G.P., DAN B.B., BLUM D., GUIDOTTI R.J., HARGRETT N.T., ANDERSON R.L., HILL D.L., BROOME C.V., BAND J.D. & FRASER D.W. (1980) New Engl. J. Med., 303, 1436.

SHARMAN A. (1952) Fertil. Steril., 3, 144.

SCHIFFER M.A., ELQUEZABAL A., SULTANA M. & ALLAN K. (1975) Obstet. Gynec., 45, 67.

SCHROCK C.G. (1980) J. Amer. Med. Assoc., 243, 1231.

SHWENI P.M., PITSOE S.B. & MOKOKONG E.T. (1980) S. Afr. Med. J., 57, 117.

SMITH P.A., ELLIS C.J., SPARKS R.A. & GUILLEBAUD J. (1983) Brit. med. J., 287, 1537.

SPARKS R.A., PURRIER B.G.A., WATT P.J. & ELSTEIN M. (1981) *Brit. md. J.,* **282,** 1189.

STEVENSON A.E. (1957) *J. Obstet. Gynaec. Brit. Cwlth.,* **64,** 345.

SUTHERLAND A.M. (1949) *Glasgow med. J.,* **30,** 1.

SUTHERLAND A.M. (1953) *Glasgow med J.,* **34,** 496.

SUTHERLAND A.M. (1979) *Brit. J. Hosp. Med.,* **22,** 569.

VESSEY M.P., DOLL R., PETO R., JOHNSON B. & WIGGINS P. (1976) *J. Biosoc. Sci.,* **8,** 373.

VESSEY M.P., YEATES D., FLAVEL R. & McPHERSON K. (1981) *Brit. med. J.,* **282,** 855.

WESTRO L., BENGTSSON L.P. & MARDH P.A. (1976) *Lancet,* **ii,** 21.

WILLIAMS J.D. (1984) *Brit. med. J.,* **288,** 343.

WILLOCKS J. (1978) In *Essentials of Obstetrics and Gynaecology.* p. 179. Churchill Livingstone, Edinburgh.

CHAPTER 42
ENDOMETRIOSIS

C. R. WHITFIELD

In endometriosis tissue similar to normal endometrium in structure and function is found in sites other than the lining of the uterine cavity. This tissue, consisting of both glands and stroma, may be in the myometrium of the uterus, in which case it has been known as endometriosis interna, but is better referred to as adenomyosis. More commonly the aberrant tissue is found outside the uterus, and is then called endometriosis externa or true endometriosis; it may be in the pelvis, or abdomen, or in more remote sites.

Although the two conditions are histologically similar, they are probably of different origin, they appear in different types of patient, and they will be described separately.

Malignant change in an endometriotic lesion occurs very occasionally, but the extremely rare uterine tumour termed stromal endometriosis or stromatosis, in which the cells resemble normal endometrial stromal cells, is unrelated to endometriosis or adenomyosis; it behaves, is best regarded, and should be managed as a sarcoma of low grade malignancy, and it will not be considered further in this chapter.

ADENOMYOSIS

In this condition, first described by Rokitansky in 1860, ingrowths of endometrium occur into the myometrium, and glandular and stromal tissue are to be found among the uterine muscle fibres. The lesion is surrounded by muscle, but as it is thought to arise by direct growth from the endometrium it is likely that a connection exists to the endometrium.

Aetiology and pathogenesis

The condition is usually found in multiparous women, and it is thought that repeated pregnancies may predispose to the extension of the endometrium into the myometrium. Vigorous curettage may perhaps lead to damage to the uterine wall, thus allowing access to the endometrium (Ringrose 1962). Cystic glandular hyperplasia of the endometrium may be present in patients with adenomyosis, and it can be postulated from this that hormonal imbalance, particularly with oestrogen in excess, may be a contributory aetiological factor (Emge 1958).

Pathology

The uterus is usually enlarged in this condition, but the enlargement is most often symmetrical. The lesion may be localized or diffuse throughout the uterine wall. Localized lesions are not encapsulated as are fibromyomata, but they may be multiple.

If the uterus is incised, small pale areas with central 'blood spots' within the myometrium may be seen, but sometimes there are quite large cystic spaces filled with blood. On histological examination areas of glandular tissue resembling endometrium are found, and each is associated with stromal cells and surrounded by muscle fibres (Fig. 42.1). The columnar epithelium and the stromal cells of the glandular tissue respond to a variable extent to the cyclical hormonal changes in the menstrual cycle. The major response is to oestrogen. Secretory endometrium may be seen, or even decidual changes in pregnancy, but these are uncommon because the invading basal layer of the endometrium is not very responsive. Menstrual discharge from the adenomyoma may reach the uterine cavity if a patent connection is present, but more often blood collects in the gland 'lumina' in the uterine wall.

Clinical features

The condition is found in women near the end of their reproductive lives, nearly always in multiparas and more commonly in the higher socio-economic groups. The lesions and symptoms may be minimal, but the principal features are menorrhagia, perhaps

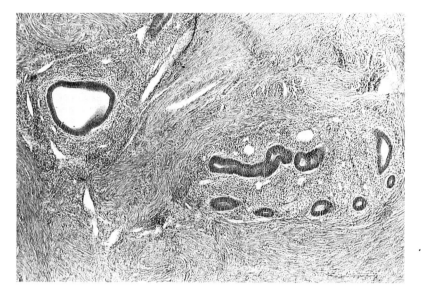

Fig. 42.1. Adenomyosis, showing endometrial glands and stroma within uterine muscle. (This and the next photomicrograph in this chapter are reproduced by kind permission of the Department of Obstetrics and Gynaecology, University of Edinburgh.)

because of interference with the normal uterine haemostatic mechanism, progressive secondary dysmenorrhoea, and sometimes pelvic discomfort and dyspareunia. There may also be bladder and bowel discomfort, but these symptoms, and also any dyspareunia, may be due to co-existent pelvic endometriosis.

The uterus is 'bulky' or frankly enlarged, and it may be tender. The enlargement is occasionally irregular, and the diagnosis of fibromyomata is usually made.

Treatment

If the lesion is localized and further childbearing is desired, an attempt may be made to resect the adenomyoma, but this is not the usual circumstance. Total hysterectomy is almost always the better operative treatment, but the ovaries may be retained in premenopausal women provided there is not associated pelvic endometriosis.

ENDOMETRIOSIS

Although isolated reports of endometriotic deposits in the pelvis had appeared earlier, Sampson (1921) described in some detail perforating chocolate cysts of the ovaries, and Blair-Bell coined the terms 'endometriosis' and 'endometrioma' in the following year. Wherever it occurs, the ectopic endometrium re-

sponds to the cyclic changes in circulating ovarian hormones in the same way as does the normally situated endometrium. Thus, with each menstruation it proliferates and then breaks down and bleeds, causing a localized inflammatory reaction followed by fibrosis. Once established, cyclic repetition of this process disrupts and distorts the affected tissue, and typically dense scar tissue and adhesions eventually form.

Aetiology and pathogenesis

While numerous theories have been propounded to explain the occurrence of the condition, it seems certain that no one theory will explain all forms of endometriosis.

Implantation theory

Sampson (1921 and 1940) suggested that menstrual blood containing fragments of endometrium might pass along the Fallopian tubes in a retrograde manner and thus reach the peritoneal cavity. The endometrium would then implant on the peritoneal surface of organs or tissues in the abdomen and pelvis, where in subsequent menstrual cycles it would undergo the sequence of proliferation and bleeding, each time with the possibility of seeding further endometrial implants. In support of this theory, there is experimental evidence that degenerated endometrium can implant, and that endometriosis may develop following intraperitoneal injection of menstrual blood (Ridley & Edward 1958, Ridley 1961). Hughesdon

(1958) not only confirmed that retrograde menstruation does occur but he also found evidence of endometriosis in patients who persistently showed it. That it is a common occurrence is now well established by, for example, the frequent observation of blood in the Fallopian tubes when laparoscopy is performed at the time of menstruation. Further support for the retrograde menstrual implantation theory comes from the increased incidence in women with lower genital tract atresia (Schifrin et al. 1973) and a reduced incidence when there is tubal occlusion (Scott 1966).

The iatrogenic implantation of viable endometrial cells may occur in abdominal incisions at Caesaerean section or other operations when the uterus is opened (Szlachter et al. 1980) or in episiotomy scars.

While retrograde menstruation and implantation explains endometriosis occurring at its most common sites, on the ovaries and uterosacral ligaments and in the Pouch of Douglas, and in other less commonly involved intraperitoneal structures, it does not explain its occasional occurrence in sites away from the peritoneal cavity, e.g. in the mediastinum, pleura, or a limb, nor can it explain the occasional occurrence of endometriosis in women who do not menstruate because of Müllerian agenesis or endometrial aplasia (Scott 1960).

Coelomic metaplasia theory

Ivanoff (1898) and Meyer (1903) independently suggested that endometriosis might result from metaplasia of immature groups of cells derived from the primitive coelomic epithelium. As well as giving rise to the epithelial cells lining the Müllerian duct, this primitive coelomic epithelium is also differentiated into peritoneal and pleural epithelium and the cells on the surface of the ovaries. If these peritoneal or pleural or 'ovarian' cells return to their original embryological function of forming Müllerian epithelium, they could differentiate into ectopic endometrium, with the surrounding cytogenic tissue forming the endometrial stroma. This theory can explain the occurrence of endometriosis in nearly all its sites, including thorax, kidney and rectovaginal septum, and even in the limbs, because coelomic epithelium may become isolated in unusual sites during development. Why this metaplasia of endometrial epithelium occurs remains unknown, although repeated stimulation by hormones or inflammatory irritation may cause the transformation.

Steck and Helwig (1966) suggested that endometrial cells themselves might stimulate imitative metaplasia (cellular replication) when they are transported by any means, most probably by retrograde menstruation in the majority of cases, to a susceptible tissue. This concept therefore combines those of retrograde menstruation and coelomic metaplasia. It is supported by the work of Merrill (1963) who buried millipore chambers containing endometrium beneath the peritoneum of rabbits. Histological evidence of endometriosis developed adjacent to the chambers within eight weeks although there was no cellular transfer across the filter.

Lymphatic and vascular dissemination

Sampson (1922) demonstrated the presence of endometrial cells within both lymphatics and blood vessels, and this was confirmed by Halban (1924) who postulated that, during menstruation, viable endometrial cells enter open basal lymph and blood vessels and are embolized to ectopic sites. Similar embolization might occur during curettage. Javert (1951) also found endometrium in lymph nodes and blood vessels. Yah (1967) in reviewing reports of intrathoracic endometriosis found eight cases arising as blood-borne 'metastases' rather than by spread from the pleura, and Abdel-Shahid et al. (1974) found endometrium within the lumen of a vein in relation to an isolated endometrioma of the ureter. It seems unlikely that vascular or lymphatic dissemination is common, but it may well be responsible for some of the rare lesions especially those that are deep seated.

PREDISPOSING FACTORS

While there is now general acceptance that most examples of endometriosis arise by peritoneal implantation following retrograde menstruation, the latter is a common event and it remains uncertain why viable implants occur only occasionally. Also, it is likely that only some of the lymphatic and blood-borne endometrial emboli become established and proliferate. It seems, therefore, that only a minority of women are predisposed to develop endometriosis.

Age, reproductive history and social class

There are three well established predisposing factors. The peak incidence, in the fourth decade of life, a close association of endometriosis with infertility, and the particular vulnerability of women who delay their first pregnancies and of those in the higher social classes, are probably all inter-related factors, with delay and continued failure to gain the relative protection afforded by pregnancy being probably the most important. Thus, endometriosis has been de-scribed as 'the scourge of the private patient' (Scott & Te Linde 1950), but these women and others in the higher social groupings are also those most likely to postpone childbearing, to present with early or mild symptoms of endometriosis, and to be offered diagnostic laparoscopy without delay.

Genetic predisposition

Family studies by Simpson *et al.* (1980) showed that 7% of first-degree relatives of women with endome-triosis are themselves also affected by the disease, compared with only 1% of unrelated controls, and the disease tended to be more severe in the familial group.

An unusually high incidence of endometriosis in Japanese women has been reported (Miyazawa 1976), but the traditional view that coloured women have a low incidence is contradicted by the recent observation, based mainly on increased use of lapa-roscopy, that coloured women in Britain are at equal risk as white women with the same reproductive his-tories (Noble 1983).

Auto-immune mechanisms

Such mechanisms have been proposed, both for the development of endometriosis in predisposed women and for the non-susceptibility of the majority. Weed and Arquembourg (1980) demonstrated local peri-tonitis, tissue damage and fibrosis occurring as an immune response to an antigen released by endo-metrial degradation products, whereas Dmowski *et al.* (1981) found evidence of increased cell-mediated im-munological tolerance to autologous endometrial tissue in control monkeys compared with those de-veloping endometriosis.

Pathology

The macroscopic appearance of the lesions depends to a large extent on the organ or tissue involved, and the secondary response elicited in the surrounding tissues. They vary in size from very small black dots, the so-called 'powder burns', seen typically on the uterosacral ligaments and peritoneum of the recto-vaginal pouch, to large cystic masses filled with dark, rather viscous 'chocolate' material in the ovaries. If there is haemorrhage from the endometriotic tissue or a cystic lesion ruptures into the peritoneal cavity, peritonitis follows with a fibrotic reaction around the lesions. Dense adhesions may result from this. The absorption of the fluid content of the blood in the cyst gives rise to the tarry material found in these lesions, but it is important to appreciate that an ovarian chocolate cyst may be due to follicular or corpus lu-teum cyst haemorrhage or to bleeding into a cystad-enoma after torsion.

Microscopically, endometrial glands, endometrial stroma and, usually, evidence of either recent or old haemorrhage, can be seen (Fig. 42.2). Red cells may be found in the gland lumina, or haemosiderin pig-ment may be present in the glands or in macro-phages. Because of the pressure within a cyst, the wall may be denuded of epithelium in some areas. During pregnancy, or as a result of combined oestro-gen–progestogen therapy for contraception or for

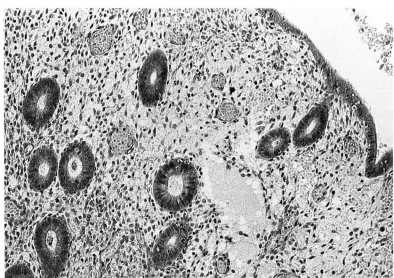

Fig. 42.2. Endometriosis. Endometrial glands and stroma outside the uterus.

pseudopregnancy treatment, the endometrium undergoes a characteristic decidual reaction.

Clinical features

Endometriosis is found during the active reproductive era, although the consequences of adhesive disease in the pelvis, bowel or ureter may still be evident in postmenopausal women. It tends to occur in women between 30 and 45 years of age, although it is found in younger women, and Schrifrin *et al.* (1973) described it in four girls aged between 12 and 14 years. The patients are characteristically nulliparous or have had one or two children some years prior to the onset of symptoms. It would seem that the condition is becoming more common, but the increasing use of laparoscopy, for sterilization as well as for diagnostic purposes, has led to the recognition of endometriosis in many more women, some of whom have no referable symptoms. In other instances, it is a coincidental finding at operation or autopsy. The size of the lesion may bear no relation to the severity of the symptoms, the site of the disease and its ability to respond to hormones being of more importance.

Pain is the most common symptom. Its nature depends largely on the site and extent of the ectopic endometrial lesions (*see* below), but frequently there is pelvic discomfort, lower abdominal pain and backache, secondary dysmenorrhoea and deep dyspareunia. It may be felt in the rectum, perineum or vagina. Typically it starts at the time of onset of menstruation, or perhaps one or two days before, and it continues throughout the period. Sometimes it occurs at the end of menstruation, presumably because the ectopic endometrium does not respond to the ovarian hormones as readily as does the normal endometrium so that shedding and bleeding occurs later than in the uterus. If the lesion is not confined by fibrosis, there may be minimal discomfort. Often there is menorrhagia, and if ovarian function is altered by bilateral endometriosis irregular menstruation or polymenorrhoea may also result.

Rupture of an ovarian endometriotic cyst, or more rarely of an endometrioma elsewhere in the abdominal or pelvic cavity leads to peritonitis, but this is an unusual acute abdominal emergency requiring laparotomy.

Patients with or without these symptoms frequently present for the investigation of infertility (*see* below). They may have had no pregnancies previously or perhaps one child followed by involuntary infertility.

In young patients endometriosis may be found in the presence of an anomaly of the Müllerian duct such as cervical stenosis or vaginal atresia. Even 'congenital retroversion' has been thought to impede menstruation and predispose to a retrograde flow (Schifrin *et al.* 1973).

On examination, hard, fixed nodules of variable size may be detected in the uterosacral ligaments, the Pouch of Douglas, on the posterior surface of the cervix or uterine wall, or in the rectovaginal septum. These nodules can be felt on vaginal, or often more easily on rectal or combined rectovaginal, examination. Other suspicious findings include obliteration of the Pouch of Douglas and a fixed retroversion of the uterus. Palpably enlarged ovaries are often found, and are usually bilateral and fixed to surrounding structures.

Speculum examination may reveal a bluish nodule in the posterior fornix if the vaginal wall is involved. Movement of the cervix results in pain and pelvic tenderness is present, particularly when nodules of endometriosis are palpated during menstruation.

Examination under anaesthesia, including combined vaginal and rectal palpation, may be more informative when there is much tenderness, but the diagnosis of endometriosis is made by visual recognition of the lesions, or much less commonly by biopsy. Laparoscopy, which permits visualization of the whole pelvis and aids in determining the most appropriate treatment, has replaced culdoscopy and is mainly responsible for the increasing frequency with which endometriosis is now being diagnosed. Laparotomy may be required if the pelvis contains dense adhesions, and it is followed by definitive surgery if necessary. In certain circumstances barium enema, intravenous pyelography and cystoscopy may also be indicated if endometriosis of the bowel or urinary tract is suspected.

DIFFERENTIAL DIAGNOSIS

Depending on the site of the endometriosis, the differential diagnosis is from adenomyosis, pelvic inflammatory disease, carcinoma of the colon or rectum, and the 'pelvic congestion syndrome' must sometimes be considered.

Rupture of an endometriotic cyst presents as an acute abdominal emergency, with features similar to those found with a ruptured ectopic pregnancy, haemorrhage into, or torsion of, an ovarian cyst, or acute salpingitis.

Staging

Since the extent of pelvic endometriosis is a determinant of the patient's symptomatology, and particularly for her prognosis for fertility following treatment, and because laparoscopic re-evaluation is used increasingly to monitor such treatment, a standardized practical classification to stage laparoscopic and operative findings is needed.

Dmowski and Cohen (1978) used a modification of the simple system devised by Acosta *et al.* (1973) to grade initial laparoscopic appearances as mild, moderate or severe, and then to re-evaluate these after treatment with Danazol. Kistner *et al.* (1977) introduced a detailed five-stage classification based on the presence and extent of lesions on the broad ligaments, tubes and ovaries, in the Pouch of Douglas, and in the bowel, appendix and bladder. Because these and other classifications have not been adopted generally, the comparison of results reported from different centres and following different methods of treatment is often of limited value. However, a committee of the American Fertility Society (1979), which included some of the originators of the earlier staging classifications, has now devised and recommended a standardized systematic point-scoring method (Table 42.1), based on the extent of endometriosis and associated adhesions on the peritoneum and on each ovary and tube. It is to be hoped that the system will find general acceptance internationally.

Sites of endometriosis

Ovarian endometriosis
The ovary is the most usual site for endometriosis, and the lesions may be either superficial or deep. The small, superficial, dark bluish cysts contain altered blood, and from these the escape of small quantities of blood results in the formation of adhesions to the surrounding structures, with subsequent fibrosis. When the adhesions are broken down, the cysts are damaged and chocolate material escapes. The Fallopian tube may also be involved.

The features include pelvic pain, backache, dysmenorrhoea, menorrhagia, dyspareunia and infertility. It is often difficult to distinguish the condition from chronic salpingitis.

Pelvic peritoneal endometriosis
There may be few, or numerous, bluish areas of endometriosis involving most frequently the rectovaginal pouch and septum, and the uterosacral ligaments, as well as the posterior and sometimes the

Table 42.1. The American Fertility Society's scoring system to classify endometriosis.

PERITONEUM	Endometriosis	< 1 cm	1–3 cm	> 3 cm
	score	1	2	3
	Adhesions	Filmy	Dense with partial obliteration of Pouch of Douglas	Dense with complete obliteration of Pouch of Douglas
	score	1	2	3
OVARY	**Endometriosis**	< 1 cm	1–3 cm	> 3 cm or ruptured endometrioma
	Right-score	2	4	6
	Left-score	2	4	6
	Adhesions	Filmy	Dense with partial enclosure of ovary	Dense with complete enclosure of ovary
	Right-score	2	4	6
	Left-score	2	4	6
TUBE	**Endometriosis**	< 1 cm	> 1 cm	Tube occluded
	Right-score	2	4	6
	Left-score	2	4	6
	Adhesions	Filmy	Dense with tube distorted	Dense with tube occluded
	Right-score	2	4	6
	Left-score	2	4	6

Stage I (mild) = 1–5   Stage II (moderate) = 6–15
Stage III (severe) = 16–30   Stage IV (extensive) = 31–54

anterior layers of the broad ligament, and the surface of the uterus. Adhesions may obliterate the rectovaginal pouch, fix the uterus in retroversion and distort the pelvic colon. They cause a variety of symptoms, including dysmenorrhoea, pelvic pain, dyspareunia and bowel discomfort. The involvement of the rectovaginal septum causes rectal and perineal pain and tenesmus.

Bowel endometriosis

The bowel may be involved in endometriosis along with other sites in the pelvis, but sometimes it alone has deposits on its surface. The rectum is involved when there are deposits in the rectovaginal septum, most obvious on rectovaginal palpation during menstruation, while peritoneal endometriosis may spread to the bowel. The pelvic colon and rectum are most frequently affected, the lesion being on the peritoneal surface and in the muscular layers, but rarely involving the mucosa.

Macafee and Greer (1960) drew attention to the symptomatology and diagnostic features. If there is no obstruction, there may be no symptoms unless there is associated pelvic endometriosis, or perhaps vague abdominal pain during menstruation. Rectal pain or bleeding is present in about 25% of cases (Schneider 1983). If there is obstruction it may be partial or complete, due to fibrosis affecting the wall of the bowel, and this is most commonly seen in the ileal region and the pelvic colon. Although the endometriotic deposits will atrophy and become quiescent after removal of the ovaries or after the menopause, the stenosis due to fibrosis will not disappear and surgical relief may be required. This may entail a colostomy or resection with end-to-end anastomosis, often followed by hormone therapy. Gray (1966 and 1973) gave good accounts of the management of this problem; recurrences occurred in at least 20% of patients, and he concluded that the best method of treatment was complete excision of the lesion if possible.

The most important alternative diagnosis is carcinoma of the colon or rectum, and the conditions must be differentiated because of the different management and prognosis. In endometriosis there is a periodicity of symptoms associated with menstruation, diarrhoea, pain in the rectum, blood in the stools and obstructive symptoms. There may also be an unexplained infertility; there is no loss of weight in the presence of symptoms suggestive of carcinoma, and there is dysmenorrhoea. Barium enema may show a long, constant, filling defect, intact bowel mucosa and fixation of the bowel with tenderness on palpation. On sigmoidoscopic examination during and after menstruation, an intact mucosa with reddening and puckering may be seen.

Obstruction of the ileum by endometriosis is uncommon but Venable (1972) reported four cases. Involvement of the appendix may give rise to symptoms of acute appendicitis at the time of menstruation. While the diagnosis may be incorrect, appendicectomy is the appropriate treatment, but it is essential to determine if there are other endometriotic deposits in the pelvic region before anticipating complete cure by this means.

Lower genital tract endometriosis

Cervical and vaginal endometriomas are bluish in colour and their cystic consistency is readily recognized, and there may be tenderness on palpation especially during menstruation. The referable symptoms are dyspareunia, dysmenorrhoea, and perhaps bleeding which is not usually recognized separately from menstruation. Perineal deposits may be found in episiotomy scars, but these are not common.

Urinary tract endometriosis

This was well reviewed by Kerr (1966). Involvement of the bladder mucosa is much less common than small implants on its peritoneal surface. Blue areas may be seen at cystoscopy if the mucosa is involved, and frequency, dysuria, haematuria and abdominal pain are characteristic.

Endometriosis may give rise to ureteric obstruction (Reddy & Evans 1974, Klein & Cattolica 1979), and the recent report that a ureteric endometrioma may arise by intravascular deposition has already been noted (Abdel-Shahid *et al.* 1974). In premenopausal women the possibility of endometriosis should be considered whenever ureteric obstruction is detected. Dick *et al.* (1973) reviewed the published accounts, and they described ureteric obstruction in a postmenopausal woman. Greenhalf and de Vere (1973) presented an interesting report on a patient with unilateral ureteric obstruction with hypertension treated by surgery. A diagnosis of carcinoma is the more likely and can be excluded only by histological examination of the mass after operative removal.

Umbilical endometriosis

Steck and Helwig (1966) found that 21 out of 82 reported cutaneous lesions of endometriosis involved the umbilicus. The lesion is a blue swelling at the umbilicus which may bleed at menstruation. Treatment is by excision.

Endometriosis in scars

A swelling in a laparotomy or Caesarean section scar which is painful and tender, especially or sometimes only during menstruation, is highly suggestive of endometriosis. It may follow operation on the uterus or on an abdomen in which there is widespread endometriosis. An endometrioma in an amniocentesis needle tract has also been reported (Kaunitz & Di Sant' Agnese 1979).

Other sites

Spread to the inguinal region by means of the round ligament has been reported, but it must be distinguished from hernia and lymphadenitis.

Deposits have been found in the limbs when painful swellings have been excised. Haemoptysis may be the first sign of pulmonary endometriosis, probably as a result of blood spread, although spread from the peritoneum to the pleura may be the explanation.

Endometriosis and infertility

Not only does absolute or relative infertility predispose to the development of endometriosis but this disease is itself an important cause of subfertility. Although it may be found in 15% of infertile women, and some 40–60% of women with endometriosis may suffer from infertility (Jones & Jones 1981) the relationship between the two is complex and imperfectly understood.

The protective effect of pregnancy is probably related to the absence of menstruation, including retrograde bleeding, and possibly to the altered hormonal milieu which may prevent the secure establishment of recently seeded endometrial implants and may sometimes bring about decidualization and resorption of well established endometriomata.

Extensive adhesive disease in the pelvis that damages or distorts and occasionally obstructs the tubes, or may bury the ovaries, is an obvious cause of infertility. Lesser adhesions and fibrosis may interfere with ovum acceptance by the fimbriae (Kistner 1979), but very often there is only mild endometriosis without apparent tubal involvement. In such patients it is possible that tubal motility, ovarian steroidogenesis and ovum release may be disturbed by prostaglandins and their metabolites produced in larger amounts by ovarian endometrial tissue than by either normal ovaries or normally situated endometrium (Moore *et al.* 1981). The peritoneal fluid in patients with endometriosis has been shown to be more copious and richer in prostinoid compounds than it is in normal women (Drake *et al.* 1981, Schneider 1983).

Brosens *et al.* (1978) claimed that at laparoscopy luteinized, unruptured follicles are often seen in the ovaries of women with endometriosis, and they suggested that this may explain subfertility when the tubes are patent and the hormonal changes normally associated with ovulation are occurring. However, the laparoscopic recognition of the follicular stigmata of ovulation is sometimes uncertain, and Dmowski *et al.* (1980) found ovulatory stigmata in infertile women with endometriosis as often as they did in those without evidence of the disease. There is an obvious need for more information on the possible importance of luteinized unruptured follicles, and also about the composition and related effects of the peritoneal fluid, in patients with endometriosis.

Treatment

Treatment may be surgical, or by hormones, or a combination of both; while in a few patients with mild disease and minimal symptoms observation, reinforced as necessary by analgesics, may be appropriate. The choice of treatment must be tailored to the patient's particular needs, taking into account her age and reproductive wishes, the severity of her symptoms, and the site and extent of her endometriosis. The therapeutic aims are to relieve pain and permit satisfactory coitus, to control abnormal bleeding, to promote the possibility of pregnancy if the patient wishes it, and to achieve these purposes without unacceptable therapeutic side effects. Preventive management perhaps receives too little attention (see below).

The efficacy of treatment is often expressed as percentage rates of symptom relief, pregnancy and recurrence, but comparisons of reported results are of little value unless a reliable diagnosis of endometriosis has been made, usually by laparoscopy but occasionally by laparotomy and/or biopsy, and unless a standardized classification of the findings is used (see above). Also, the fact that some women in a 'surgical' series have also had pre-operative or postoperative treatment with hormones, and that some in a 'medical' series have already undergone conservative surgery, is not always made entirely clear or it is ignored. Instead, surgery and hormone therapy should be regarded as complementary methods, and often both will be used in a management plan that may be altered as time passes and the patient's reproductive hopes are fulfilled, alter or have to be abandoned.

PROPHYLAXIS

To reduce the chance of viable endometrial fragments being carried through the Fallopian tube, tests of tubal patency should not be performed immediately after curettage or at around the time of menstruation. Kistner (1979) has also suggested that if pelvic examination is required during or just after menstruation, forcible manipulation should be avoided. Because of the beneficial effects of pregnancy, married women known to have a close family history of endometriosis should be encouraged not to delay starting and completing their planned families; the same advice obviously applies to those already known or suspected to have developed the disease. When contraception is required, Kistner has suggested that a low oestrogen-strong progestogen oral preparation may be prophylactic by causing endometrial atrophy or by reducing menstrual flow and thus the likelihood of retrograde bleeding; he has observed at hysterectomy during withdrawal bleeding related to oral contraception that the tubes do not contain blood as they do during normal menstruation.

HORMONE THERAPY

To reproduce the beneficial effects of pregnancy on endometriotic deposits, and to prevent menstruation including retrograde flow, the use of sex hormones to induce anovulation and amenorrhoea is theoretically sound. Oestrogens, androgens, progestogens, and combinations of oestrogens and progestogens have all been used.

Oestrogens in large doses have been used, but most patients are unable to tolerate the doses given and the side effects are considerable, including severe uterine bleeding. The thrombotic effect of prolonged oestrogen therapy may also be a disadvantage.

Androgen therapy has been used in the past with some success, but especially with doses sufficient to suppress ovulation, virilizing side effects are distressing; some women develop these even on low dosage.

Treatment of endometriosis with oestrogens alone or with androgens is now obsolete.

Pseudopregnancy

Because of the side effects of treatment with oestrogens alone, and because such therapy brings about hyperplasia instead of decidualization of the endometrium, Kistner (1958) introduced combined oestrogen–progestogen treatment. This is given continuously and in increasing dosage for up to nine months

to induce a state of 'pseudopregnancy', with anovulation and amenorrhoea, and with decidual transformation of both normal and ectopic endometrium followed by gradual necrosis and absorption of the decidualized cells. The preparations most commonly used have been norgestrel with ethinyloestradiol or norethynodrel with mestranol (Enavid), but other combined oral contraceptives may be used, generally starting with the usual contraceptive dose of one tablet daily and increasing as necessary to control breakthrough bleeding and provide continuous amenorrhoea. Apart from breakthrough bleeding, which can be heavy, other oestrogen-induced side effects include nausea and vomiting, breast enlargement and discomfort, weight gain which may be considerable, and sometimes psychological upsets. These symptoms often resemble those frequently experienced during early pregnancy and, like them, may improve after two months or so of treatment. Pseudopregnancy treatment has the virtue of being cheap.

The early promise shown by this form of treatment has not generally been fulfilled in the largest series reported. Following pseudopregnancy, significant symptomatic relief may be obtained, but it may not continue for long, and there may be some delay in the resumption of ovulation. If success is assessed by non-recurrence and by fertility subsequent to treatment, Andrews and Larsen (1974) found that surgery alone achieved better results than hormonal pseudopregnancy with or without surgery. However, Kistner (1979) reported a pregnancy rate of 50.8% following treatment by pseudopregnancy alone in 186 women in whom endoscopy had revealed surface ovarian endometriosis without adhesions. He also recommended prolonged pseudopregnancy therapy for unmarried patients with maximal symptoms but minimal palpable findings. A short oestrogen–progestogen course pre-operatively may help the identification and excision of multiple small endometriotic deposits, and postoperatively four to six months of treatment may be useful when it has not been possible to remove all the areas of endometriosis.

A variant of pseudopregnancy is the intermittent use of any of the common oestrogen–progestogen contraceptives, taken continuously for up to four months at a time and without increasing dosage. In this way, as recommended by Noble (1983), the patient with mild disease, and who is unmarried or unwilling to start a pregnancy soon, may have her symptoms relieved and her endometriosis held in check while having only occasional withdrawal bleeds which are unlikely to cause bleeding into the tubes (*see* above).

Pseudopregnancy induced by progestogen alone seems to be less satisfactory than administration of oestrogen and progestogen together, and it has been suggested that it may occasionally be complicated by spontaneous rupture of an endometrioma (Ranney 1974). However, when oestrogen-induced side effects are severe and persistent, treatment with intramuscular injections of medroxyprogesterone acetate (Depo-provera) is an alternative. A disadvantage, when pregnancy is hoped for, is that ovulation may be delayed for as long as six to twelve months after ceasing this form of treatment. For this reason, and for simplicity of administration, oral treatment with Danazol would now be preferable (*see* below).

Danazol

An orally effective synthetic isoxazol derivative of 17-α-ethinyl testosterone, Danazol, is now very often used in preference to the much cheaper combined oestrogen–progestogen pseudopregnancy regimes, or it may be used when the latter fail to bring about acceptable and lasting benefit. It is readily absorbed when taken by mouth and has a circulating half-life of almost five hours (Davison *et al.* 1976). It causes anovulation, amenorrhoea and endometrial atrophy, and is also mildly androgenic and anabolic. It may act at four levels (hypothalamus, pituitary, the ovarian follicle, and the target tissues) but its complex effects (Barbieri & Ryan 1981, Luciano *et al.* 1981, Meldrum *et al.* 1983) are not yet understood fully. There is less evidence for reduced gonadotrophin release, or inhibition at hypothalamic or pituitary level, in premenopausal women than in those beyond the menopause or in castrated animals, but follicle stimulating hormone and luteinizing hormone surges are probably suppressed. Most studies confirm significantly low circulating oestrogen, although Danazol also seems to displace oestrogen and other hormones from sex hormone-binding globulin. It inhibits development of the ovarian follicle, interfering with steroidogenesis, and it binds to steroid receptors in several tissues.

First used in the United States by Greenblatt, who reported symptomatic improvement and reduction in pelvic deposits in 22 of 40 patients (Greenblatt *et al.* 1971), Danazol therapy was soon reported to lead to pregnancy in about half of two small groups of previously infertile women (Friedlander 1973, Greenblatt *et al.* 1974), and Dmowski and Cohen (1975) reported significant control of endometriosis, eval-

uated by laparoscopy and histology before and after treatment with active endometriosis persisting in only 15% of patients. They went on to describe 99 women treated with 800 mg of Danazol daily for an average of six months and re-evaluated clinically an average of three years later, when 39% symptomatic and 33% objective recurrence rates were noted; and 39 of 84 women desiring pregnancy had conceived, a rate of 46% corrected to 72% by excluding those with other cause of infertility (Dmowski & Cohen 1978). Using this recommended standard dosage, comparable rates for improvement, recurrence and subsequent pregnancy were reported from other centres in North America, e.g. Greenblatt and Tzingounis (1979) who followed up 49 patients for between four and five and a half years, Henriques *et al.* (1982) who re-evaluated 50 after a mean post-treatment interval of five and a half years (a few of their patients received 600 mg of Danazol daily) and Puleo and Hammond (1983) who followed 39 treated patients for shorter periods. In another series (Barbieri *et al.* 1982) all 100 women studied had laparoscopic re-evaluation on completion of full dosage treatment (of 17 weeks' mean duration), more than half then underwent laparotomy for conservative surgery, and 10 eventually had 'third-look' laparoscopy; as would be expected, recurrence rates reflected the initial staging of the disease, and 85% of the patients had significant side effects which, however, led to only one of them discontinuing Danazol. One of these reports noted a high incidence of second or third trimester fetal deaths in women conceiving within the first three post-treatment cycles (Dmowski & Cohen 1978), but this was not observed in the other series.

In reviewing 370 women with clinical evidence of endometriosis treated (usually for five to seven months) at 10 different centres, Young and Blackmore (1977) claimed that therapeutic efficacy is dose-related. Thus, there was partial or complete amelioration of dyspareunia in 84% of women treated with 800 mg daily compared with 75% of those receiving 200–400 mg daily, and resolution of induration in the Pouch of Douglas in 82% taking 800 mg daily compared with 73% having the smaller doses; but these are small differences, and only one-quarter of the patients in these collected series had both pretreatment and post-treatment laparoscopy.

In three subsequently reported studies a combined total of 97 women with pelvic endometriosis had a repeat laparoscopy after six months' treatment with different 'low' doses of Danazol (100, 200, 400 and 600 mg daily, in double blind fashion). In one of these studies (Biberoglu & Behrman 1981) small differences in dose-related improvement rates, similar to those in Young and Blackmore's collected series (above) were observed, but endometriomas of at least one cm size did not regress and side effects were not reduced by the low doses. At post-treatment laparoscopy Moore et al. (1981) found that mild and moderate endometriosis responded well to less than 400 mg Danazol daily, but they concluded that severe endometriosis required treatment with at least 600 mg daily, often combined with conservative surgery, and that endometriomas more than 2 cm in diameter required full dosage. In the third of these series Dmowski et al. (1982) found that laparoscopic improvement was dose-related, but this and clinical response was less than can be obtained with full dosage although at two-year follow-up recurrence rates (29%) were no worse with low than with full dosage. They also found that regression of endometriosis was greatest in patients who remained amenorrhoeic throughout treatment, suggesting that sustained amenorrhoea might be a good indicator of clinical improvement. A better opinion of low dosage Danazol was expressed by Barbieri and Ryan (1981), who found 200 mg two or three times daily as effective as the recommended full dosage of 400 mg twice daily, noting significant subjective improvement in 70–100% of patients, objective improvement at laparoscopy in about 90% and an uncorrected fertility of about 45%.

In Britain, where doses of less than 800 mg daily are more usual, the most extensively reported experience is from Worcester, and it supports the view that 200 mg of Danazol daily may be adequate for most cases of endometriosis (Chalmers 1982). In 40 patients treated in this way for six months there was prompt relief of symptoms in more than 90%, only one patient needing a higher dosage (400 mg daily); the only side effect noted was breakthrough bleeding in three cases, but this was subsequently avoided by starting Danazol no later than the fifth day of a cycle. Although the importance of precise diagnosis, usually by laparoscopy, was emphasized, no staging of the severity of endometriosis in these patients, or in earlier groups treated with higher dosage, was described. Chalmers' indications for Danazol therapy are young women needing to keep reproductive capacity, residual endometriosis after conservative surgery, and extragenital lesions inaccessible or not readily accessible to surgery. Support for treatment of mild endometriosis with this low dosage (given as 100 mg of Danazol twice daily), but doubling to 400 mg daily if amenorrhoea is not achieved by two months, comes from a comparative dosage trial in Glasgow, in which laparoscopy or laparotomy was performed before and after six months' treatment, and a scoring system was used to document its effect on pelvic endometriosis (Low et al. 1984).

The most important side effects from treatment with Danazol result from either gonadotrophin inhibition, including breast changes (usually reduced breast size), flushes and sweating, with occasionally atrophic vaginitis, or from its androgenic activity including acne (particularly in oily skinned brunettes with a previous history of this complaint), slight hirsutism and occasionally voice changes. Some patients complain of headaches, fatigue, anxiety or depression, while a few report muscle cramps or mild intestinal symptoms such as nausea and vomiting. Generally, and particularly with low dosage treatment, any side effects are usually mild, and they are readily accepted by patients experiencing significant pain relief or hoping for pregnancy.

Danazol sometimes causes minor changes in liver function, and also induces insulin resistance with mild impairment of glucose tolerance, but these metabolic effects are temporary and they do not preclude its use for up to a year for a valid indication (e.g. severe endometriosis), although a significant incidence of the side effects mentioned, and perhaps temporary aggravation of diabetes if present, should be anticipated, but there must be reservations about longer treatment particularly in combination with other steroids (Wynn 1977).

Luteinizing hormone releasing hormone

Simultaneous reports from Edinburgh (Shaw et al. 1983) and London (Pring et al. 1983) have introduced a possible alternative hormone therapy free, or virtually so, from side effects. A superactive analogue of luteinizing hormone releasing hormone, taken as an intranasal 'snuff', was used to render the pituitary's gonadotrophin-secreting cells insensitive to endogenous releasing hormone with consequent suppression of ovarian steroidogenesis, anovulation and amenorrhoea (apart from occasional breakthrough bleeding early during treatment). Pain was relieved except in one woman with very severe endometriosis and treated in smaller dosage than the others. In these other eight patients post-treatment laparoscopy revealed reduction or resolution of all endometriotic lesions. One previously infertile woman conceived within two months of completing the six months of treatment.

SURGICAL TREATMENT

The surgical cure of endometriosis requires that all the ovarian tissue or all the endometriotic deposits be removed. The form of treatment employed, therefore, depends on the age of the patient and her desire regarding further pregnancy, as well as the extent of the disease, the symptoms it is causing and any secondary changes which have resulted from it.

In a young woman removal of the ovaries is to be avoided so local endometriotic deposits are removed and pregnancy is encouraged in the hope that any remaining lesions will undergo atrophy. Pre-operative and post-operative hormonal treatment may be helpful (above). This form of conservative treatment consists of the division of pelvic adhesions, mobilization of the appendages and sometimes fimbrioplasty or salpingostomy. Ovarian and other accessible endometriomas are excised. After adhesions in the rectovaginal pouch have been divided, some form of ventrosuspension of the uterus is beneficial at least temporarily, and fertility might be improved by this. It may be useful to cover raw areas, especially in the Pouch of Douglas, by omental grafts (Kistner 1979). Small implants in the pelvis are excised if possible, or fulgurated with diathermy. If pain is a prominent feature, presacral neurectomy is very occasionally performed, but hormonal therapy has, perhaps, superseded this operation. It is advisable to remove large endometriomata prior to hormone therapy because of the risk of a rupture, with the development of an acute abdominal emergency.

As more cases of endometriosis, often in young women, come to light through the increasing use of diagnostic laparoscopy, and with the availability of effective medical treatment, there has been a marked and welcome trend towards conservative rather than radical surgery. However, many gynaecologists still believe that, in young women, endometriosis is best treated by careful surgery with or without additional therapy. If, later, unbearable symptoms develop and are not controllable by hormone therapy, a second operation of a more radical nature may be carried out. This is better than performing radical surgery in the relatively young before other methods are tried.

Surgical laparoscopy now has its advocates (Daniell & Christianson 1981, Cohen 1982). By this means thermocoagulation can be used to fulgurate implants and small endometriomas and for lysis of tubo-ovarian adhesions. It is possible to perform salpingostomy by this means, and the pregnancy rate following correction of distal tubal obstruction has been claimed to be as good (30%) as with microsurgery at laparotomy (Mettler *et al.* 1979). Biopsy can be performed if wished. As with diagnostic laparoscopy for suspected endometriosis, chromotubation can be carried out to check tubal patency, and timing the procedure for the postovulatory phase enables an early corpus luteum and its ovulatory stigma to be recognized. It seems likely that, with careful selection, this approach may become more widely used as an alternative method for performing conservative surgery at the same time as confirming and staging endometriosis and assessing the need for combined treatment with hormones.

Radical surgery involves the removal of both ovaries and, usually, the uterus, and its use is usually restricted to women near the menopause who are having distressing symptoms. A more radical approach may be permissible in young women if further pregnancies are definitely not desired. If there is encirclement of the bowel or ureter, surgical treatment must be radical, and even then some form of decompression procedure may be necessary. It may not be technically easy to remove the uterus completely, and in such patients preoperative hormone therapy possibly has a place for a short time in order to control symptoms and soften the pelvic adhesions.

Schifrin *et al.* (1973) believe that endometriosis might be prevented, in some patients at least, if any obstruction to the menstrual flow is removed before retrograde flow occurs. This applies obviously to congenital anomalies, but can equally well apply to acquired lesions such as cervical stenosis.

RADIOTHERAPY

The production of an artificial menopause may be indicated in certain patients in whom operation is contraindicated, but these are now extremely rare and X-ray castration can be regarded as a virtually obsolete method.

CHOICE OF TREATMENT

Management will usually follow the general strategy outlined below, but as noted already it should be individualized to suit each patient, principally the nature and severity of her symptoms and her reproductive wishes, and of course it also depends on the extent of her endometriosis.

Mild endometriosis

Should this be diagnosed or suspected in an unmarried woman with dysmenorrhoea controlled by analgesics, and who does not need contraception, observation without active medical or surgical treatment may well be the appropriate course to take. This would also be appropriate initial management when the patient is trying to conceive. In either case, review after six months is important. A different viewpoint is that, since endometriosis is a progressive condition, even mild disease confirmed at laparoscopy or laparotomy should be treated surgically (Cohen 1982). Women in clinical remission after treatment should also be reviewed six monthly to detect recurrence early, in which case laparoscopic re-evaluation might be appropriate before deciding about further treatment.

With more severe symptoms despite only mild disease in unmarried patients, or in married women wishing to defer pregnancy, treatment by pseudopregnancy or Danazol is indicated. A trial of pseudopregnancy may be worthwhile before deciding to use the more costly Danazol in low dosage. However, because conception is more likely to occur soon after discontinuing Danazol, this would be the better initial choice when a patient wishes to defer pregnancy for only a short period. When there is dyspareunia associated with fixed uterine retroversion, laparotomy is called for to mobilize and ventrosuspend the uterus as well as to excise or fulgurate endometrial implants.

Moderately severe endometriosis
(E.g. well established broad ligament and tubo-ovarian adhesions that distort the tubes and partially enclose the ovaries, approximating to the American Fertility Society stage III on the basis of adhesions alone, or endometriomas measuring at least 1 cm.)

When the patient's family is complete surgery is usually indicated; this will include hysterectomy and often bilateral salpingo-oophorectomy, but if the patient is young it may be feasible to conserve some healthy ovarian tissue. Sometimes, despite moderately severe disease, symptoms may be mild and a trial of Danazol therapy may lead to clinical remission without recourse to surgery, although there is always the risk of recurrence later on. Sizeable endometriomas and chocolate cysts should be resected. Conservative surgery, followed by Danazol, is the treatment of choice for those whose families are not yet complete. The superiority of Danazol, in terms of symptom control, side effects and subsequent fertility, was shown in possibly the only reported randomized trial comparing it, in low dosage, with pseudopreg-

nancy (Noble & Letchworth 1980). Even Kistner's team, so experienced in management by pseudopregnancy, has confirmed that in the presence of well established adhesions and endometriomas measuring more than 0.5 cm there is usually much less residual endometriosis after Danazol (Barbieri *et al.* 1982).

Severe endometriosis
When there is dense pelvic fibrosis and large endometriomas or chocolate cysts surgery is obviously required, and in the patient with a completed family it should take the form of hysterectomy with bilateral salpingo-oophorectomy, followed by Danazol for any residual endometriosis that could not be excised. Before potentially difficult surgery, a short course of preoperative Danazol may be helpful. With such severe disease those wishing further fertility are likely to be disappointed, but conservative surgery, including careful mobilization of the tubes and ovaries and tubal reconstruction if necessary, followed by Danazol, will sometimes allow pregnancy to occur. It goes without saying that the partner's fertility should be confirmed. In the future, *in vitro* fertilization procedures, with the partner's or donor sperm, will have a role in managing this problem.

Extrapelvic endometriosis
Superficial lesions, in scars or at the umbilicus, are excised. Inaccessible lesions distant from the pelvis should respond to castrating surgery, but Danazol may be effective, e.g. in recently reported cases of ureteric obstruction due to endometriosis (Gardner & Whitaker 1981) and of a pulmonary lesion (Ronnberg *et al.* 1981).

Additional hormone treatment
There is no contraindication to repeating Danazol courses for recurrent endometriosis when this seems to be the appropriate treatment. When an infertile patient has been managed by conservative surgery and Danazol, continued infertility should suggest the possibility of defective ovulation, e.g. poor luteal phase or luteinized unruptured follicle syndrome. There is no contraindication to properly indicated and monitored use of ovulation-inducing drugs.

Especially in young patients, severe menopausal symptoms following radical surgery may require hormone replacement therapy. It has been suggested that if conjugated oestrogens are used it is very unlikely that residual lesions of endometriosis will be reactivated (Hammond & Haney 1978). An alternative would be one of the common oral contraceptives taken continuously (Noble 1983).

Malignant change in endometriosis

Malignant change in an endometriotic lesion is very uncommon, and when it occurs ovarian endometriosis is usually involved. Schneider (1983) estimated that at least 150 cases of malignancy arising in ovarian endometriosis had been reported under various headings, whereas only 45 reported cases of malignant change in endometriosis elsewhere than in the ovaries were identified by Brooks and Wheeler (1977). There must be both benign and malignant endometriosis present and the malignant tissue must not have invaded the benign tissue to permit this diagnosis to be made, although late tumours will certainly have invaded the surrounding tissue. Histologically, the tumour is either an adeno-acanthoma or an endometrioid carcinoma (Scully *et al.* 1966). Fathalla (1967) reviewed 637 specimens of ovarian endometriosis and found only four with malignant features.

Malignant change in adenomyosis is extremely rare, but adenomyosis and adenocarcinoma may coexist in the same uterus.

The possibility of malignant change occurring in endometriosis need not influence the proposed management of a patient. The presence of ovarian malignancy, however, must be considered when an alternative diagnosis is an endometrioma or chocolate cyst of the ovary. Removal of the lesion is the only certain method of establishing the diagnosis.

REFERENCES

ABDEL-SHAHID R.B., BERESFORD J.M. & CURRY (1974) *Obstet. Gynec.*, **43**, 113.

ACOSTA A.A., BUTTRAM V.C., BESCH P.K., MALINAK L.R., FRANKLIN R.R. & VANDERHEYDEN J.D. (1973) *Obstet. Gynec.*, **42**, 19.

AMERICAN FERTILITY SOCIETY (1979) *Fertil. Steril.*, **32**, 633.

ANDREWS W.C. & LARSEN C.D. (1974) *Amer. J. Obstet. Gynec.*, **118**, 643.

BARBIERI R.L. & RYAN K.J. (1981) *Amer. J. Obstet. Gynec.*, **141**, 453.

BARBIERI R.L., EVANS S. & KISTNER R.W. (1982) *Fertil. Steril.*, **37**, 737.

BIBEROGLU K.O. & BEHRMAN S.J. (1981) *Amer. J. Obstet. Gynec.*, **139**, 645.

BROOKS J.J. & WHEELER J.E. (1977) *Cancer*, **40**, 3065.

BROSENS I.A., KONINCKX P.R. & CORVELEYN P.A. (1978) *Brit. J. Obstet. Gynaec.*, **85**, 246.

CHALMERS J.A. (1982) *Scot. med. J.*, **27**, 143.

COHEN M.R. (1982) *J. reprod. Med.*, **27**, 240.

DANIELL J.F. & CHRISTIANSON C. (1981) *Fertil. Steril.*, **32**, 384.

DAVISON C., BANKS W. & FRITZ A. (1976) *Arch. int. Pharmacol. Ther.*, **221**, 294.

DICK A.L., LANG D.W., BERGMAN R.T., BHATNAGAR B.N.S. & SELVACCI F.P. (1973) *Brit. J. Urology*, **45**, 153.

DMOWSKI W.P. & COHEN M.R. (1973) *Obstet. Gynec.*, **46**, 147.

DMOWSKI W.P. & COHEN M.R. (1978) *Amer. J. Obstet. Gynec.*, **130**, 41.

DMOWSKI W.P., RAO R. & SCOMMEGNA A. (1980) *Fertil. Steril.*, **33**, 30.

DMOWSKI W.P., STEELE W.R. & BAKER (1981) *Amer. J. Obstet. Gynec.*, **141**, 377.

DMOWSKI W.P., KEPETANAKIS E. & SCOMMEGNA A. (1982) *Obstet. Gynec.*, **59**, 408.

DRAKE T.S., O'BRIEN W.F., RAMWELL P.W. & METZ S.A. (1981) *Amer. J. Obstet. Gynec.*, **140**, 401.

EMGE L.A. (1958) *Amer. J. Obstet. Gynec.*, **76**, 1059.

FATHALLA M.F. (1967) *J. Obstet. Gynaec. Brit. Cwlth.*, **74**, 85.

FRIEDLANDER R.L. (1973) *J. reprod. Med.*, **10**, 197.

GARDNER B. & WHITTAKER R.H. (1981) *J. Urol.*, **125**, 117.

GRAY L.A. (1966) *Clin. Obstet. Gynec.*, **9**, 309.

GRAY L.A. (1973) *Ann. Surg.*, **177**, 580.

GREENBLATT R.B. & TZINGOUNIS V. (1979) *Fertil. Steril.*, **32**, 518.

GREENBLATT R.B., DMOWSKI W.P., MAHESH V.B. & SCHOLER H.F.L. (1971) *Fertil. Steril.*, **22**, 102.

GREENBLATT R.B., BORENSTEIN R. & HERNANDEZ-AYUB S. (1974) *Amer. J. Obstet. Gynec.*, **118**, 783.

GREENHALF J.O. & DE VERE R.D. (1973) *J. Obstet. Gynaec. Brit. Cwlth.*, **80**, 754.

HALBAN J. (1924) *Wien Klin. Wschr.*, **37**, 1205.

HAMMOND C.B. & HANEY A.F. (1978) *Fertil. Steril.* **30**, 497.

HENRIQUES E.S., JOFE M.H., FRIEDLANDER R.L. & SWARTZ D.P. (1982) In *Genital Endometriosis in Infertility* (Semm K., Greenblatt R.B. & Mettler L. eds), p. 55. Georg Thieme Verlag, New York.

HUGHESDON P.E. (1958) *J. Obstet. Gynaec. Brit. Cwlth.*, **65**, 944.

IVANOFF N.S. (1898) *Wschr. Geburtsh. Gynak.*, **7**, 295.

JAVERT C.T. (1951) *Amer. J. Obstet. Gynec.*, **62**, 477.

JONES H.W. & JONES G.S. (1981) In *Novak's Textbook of Gynecology*, 10th Ed., p. 609. Williams & Wilkins, Baltimore.

KAUNITZ A. & DI SANT'AGNESE P.A. (1979) *Obstet. Gynec.*, **54**, 753.

KERR W.S. (1966) *Clin. Obstet. Gynec.*, **9**, 331.

KISTNER R.W. (1958) *Amer. J. Obstet. Gynec.*, **75**, 264.

KISTNER R.W. (1979) *Clin. Obstet. Gynec.*, **22**, 101.

KISTNER R.W., SIEGLER A.M. & BEHRMAN S.J. (1977) *Fertil. Steril.*, **28**, 1008.

KLEIN R.S. & CATTOLICA E.V. (1979) *Urology*, **13**, 479.

LOW R.A., ROBERTS A.D.G. & LEES D.A.R. (1984) *Brit. J. Obstet. Gynaec.*, **91**, 167.

LUCIANO A.A., HANSEN K.S., CHAPLER F.K. (1981) *Amer. J. Obstet. Gynec.*, **141**, 723.

MACAFEE C.H.G. & GREER H.L.H. (1960) *J. Obstet. Gynaec. Brit. Cwlth.*, **67**, 539.

MELDRUM D.R., PARTRIDGE W.M., KAROW W.G., RIVIER J., VALE W. & JUDD H. (1983) *Obstet. Gynec.*, **62**, 480.

MERRILL J.A. (1963) *Surg. Forum*, **14**, 397.

METTLER L., GIESEL H. & SEMM K. (1979) *Fertil. Steril.*, **32**, 384.

MEYER R. (1903) *Virchows Arch. path. Anat.*, **171**, 443.

MIYAZAMA K. (1976) *Amer. J. Obstet. Gynec.*, **48**, 407.

MOORE E.E., HARGER J.H., ROCK J.A. & ARCHER D.F. (1981) *Fertil. Steril.*, **36**, 15.

NOBLE A.D. (1983) *Drugs*, **26**, 440.

NOBLE A.D. & LETCHWORTH A.T. (1980) *Brit. J. Obstet. Gynaec.*, **87**, 726.

PRING D.W., MARESH M. & FRASER A.C. (1983) *Brit. med. J.*, **2**, 1718.

PULEO J.G. & HAMMOND C.B. (1983) *Fertil. Steril.*, **40**, 164.

RANNEY B. (1974) In *Controversy in Obstetrics and Gynecology*, 2nd Ed., (Reid D.E. & Christian C.D., eds). W.B. Saunders, Philadelphia.

REDDY A.N. & EVANS J. (1974) *J. Urol. Baltimore*, **111**, 474.

RIDLEY J.H. (1961) *Amer. J. Obstet. Gynec.*, **82**, 777.

RIDLEY J.H. & EDWARD I.K. (1958) *Amer. J. Obstet. Gynec.*, **76**, 783.

RINGROSE C.A.C. (1962) *Can. Med. Ass. J.*, **83**, 1541.

RONNBERG L., YLOSTALO P. & JARVINEN P.A. (1981) *Acta Obstet. Gynaec. Scand.*, **60**, 77.

SAMPSON J.A. (1921) *Arch. Surg.*, **3**, 245.

SAMPSON J.A. (1922) *Arch. Surg.*, **4**, 217.

SAMPSON J.A. (1940) *Amer. J. Obstet. Gynec.*, **40**, 549.

SCHIFRIN B.S., EREZ S. & MOORE J.G. (1973) *Amer. J. Obstet. Gynec.*, **116**, 973.

SHAW R.W., FRASER H.M. & BOYLE H. (1983) *Brit. med. J.*, **2**, 1667.

SCHNEIDER G.T. (1983) In *Progress in Obstetrics and Gynaecology*, No. 3, **2**, 246 (Studd J.W.W., ed). Churchill Livingstone, Edinburgh.

SCOTT R.B. (1960) *Clin. Obstet. Gynecol.*, **3**, 429.

SCOTT R.B. (1966) *Postgraduate Medicine*, **39**, 295.

SCOTT R.B. & TE LINDE R.W. (1950) *Ann. Surg.*, **131**, 697.

SCULLY R.E., RICHARDSON G.S. & BARLOW J.F. (1966) *Clin. Obstet. Gynec.*, **9**, 384.

SIMPSON J.L., ELIAS S., MALINAK L.R. & BUTTRAM V.C. (1980) *Amer. J. Obstet. Gynec.*, **137**, 327.

STECK W.D. & HELWIG E.B. (1966) *Clin. Obstet. Gynec.*, **9**, 373.

SZLACHTER N.B., MOSKOWITZ J., BIGELOW B. & WEISS G. (1980) *Obstet. Gynec.*, **55 (Suppl. 52)**, 3.

VENABLE J.H. (1972) *Amer. J. Obstet. Gynec.*, **113**, 1054.

WEED J.C. & ARQUEMBOURG P. (1980) *Clin. Obstet. Gynec.*, **23**, 885.

WYNN V. (1977) *J. int. med. Res.*, **5 (Suppl. 3)**, 25.

YEH T.J. (1967) *J. thorac. cardiovasc. Surg.*, **53**, 201.

YOUNG M.D. & BLACKMORE W.P. (1977) *J. int. med. Res.*, **5 (Suppl. 3)**, 72.

CHAPTER 43
DYSFUNCTIONAL UTERINE BLEEDING

D. A. DAVEY

Dysfunctional uterine bleeding (DUB) is defined as 'abnormal bleeding from the uterus in the absence of organic disease of the genital tract' or, in the words of Novak *et al.* (1971) 'abnormal bleeding from the uterus unassociated with tumour, inflammation or pregnancy'. The term dysfunctional uterine bleeding may be applied to any abnormal pattern of uterine bleeding, though it is most commonly applied to bleeding which is excessive either in amount, duration or frequency. Dysfunctional uterine bleeding is not a single disease entity with one aetiology but is a group of disorders of differing aetiologies which result in abnormal uterine bleeding or menstruation. The most common dysfunction is some disorder of the endocrine or vascular mechanisms which results in menstruation, and the dysfunction may arise in the endometrium, ovary, pituitary, hypothalamus or higher centres. In theory the nature of the underlying dysfunction should be determined in each case but in practice the diagnosis of DUB is usually made by excluding organic disease of the genital tract.

CLASSIFICATION

DUB may be usefully classified into primary, iatrogenic and secondary (Table 43.1).

Primary DUB is diagnosed when there is no detectable disease in the genital tract or elsewhere in the body, there is no intrauterine contraceptive device present and there has been no prior administration of sex steroids or other hormones.

Iatrogenic DUB is diagnosed when the abnormal uterine bleeding is associated with some contraceptive or therapeutic agent, e.g. an intrauterine contraceptive device (IUCD), the injection of depot medroxyprogesterone acetate (Depo-provera: Upjohn) or administration of oestrogens at the menopause.

Secondary DUB is diagnosed when there is no detectable disease of the genital tract but where there is a known disorder outside the genital tract which

Table 43.1 Classification of dysfunctional uterine bleeding (DUB)

Primary	DUB due to dysfunction arising within the genital tract and reproductive system including the pituitary, hypothalamus and higher centres
Iatrogenic	DUB secondary to the administration of sex hormones or to various forms of contraception including a) *Oestrogens or Oestrogen–Progestogen Combination* in perimenopausal women b) *Progestogens* as depot injection c) *Intrauterine contraceptive device*
Secondary	DUB secondary to an organic disease or a functional disorder in any organ or system outside the genital tract or reproductive system.

is responsible for the abnormal uterine bleeding e.g. myxoedema, leukaemia, thrombocytopenic purpura.

DIFFICULTIES IN DIAGNOSIS BY EXCLUSION

The diagnosis of DUB by exclusion of organic disease of the genital tract is not entirely satisfactory and presents some real practical difficulties. The diagnosis thus depends upon: what is regarded as 'disease of the genital tract'; what is regarded as 'organic disease'; the extent of the investigation performed to exclude organic disease of the genital tract in any case.

Definition of 'disease of the genital tract'
By definition any disease of the vulva, vagina, cervix, uterus, Fallopian tubes or ovaries is regarded as disease of the genital tract. This means that any uterine bleeding associated for example with hormone producing tumours of the ovary, is regarded as organic disease of the genital tract, even though the bleeding may have resulted from endometrial hyperplasia

secondary to the secretion of oestrogens produced by the ovarian tumour. Such cases are regarded as organic disease of the genital tract and are not regarded as cases of DUB.

Definition of organic disease of the genital tract

The definition of organic disease or an organic lesion in relation to DUB may also present a problem, particularly with regard to endometrial conditions, many of which are secondary to dysfunction in the ovary or hypothalamic–pituitary axis. Such conditions, which include benign endometrial hyperplasia, completely regress when the original endocrine disorder is reversed and are therefore best regarded as primary dysfunctional changes. Other endometrial conditions such as pseudodecidual reaction or Arias Stella phenomenon which are also reversible should similarly be regarded as dysfunctional. Once, however, some irreversible change is present the condition should be regarded as organic. Carcinoma *in situ* or invasive carcinoma of the endometrium and endometrial polyps should thus be regarded as organic lesions. In the same way chronic endometritis should, in the absence of a detectable aetiological organism, also be regarded as dysfunctional. Once, however, causative micro-organisms are demonstrated or the histological picture is pathognomonic of a particular type of infection, such as tuberculosis, the condition should then be regarded as organic.

Extent of investigations to be performed to exclude organic disease

The extent of the investigations which should be performed to exclude organic disease of the genital tract so that a diagnosis of DUB can be made is a further problem. It is generally accepted that an abdominal and pelvic examination and a curettage or endometrial sampling must be performed in every case. If under these circumstances no organic disease of the genital tract has been discovered, then the condition is diagnosed as DUB. It must be recognized that in any series of women diagnosed as having DUB there will inevitably be a small number of patients who have organic disease of the genital tract which was missed at the first examination.

INCIDENCE AND AGE DISTRIBUTION

DUB is one of the most frequently encountered conditions in gynaecology, being the principal diagnosis in at least 10% of all new outpatients in both hospital and private practice. The bleeding may be abnormal in frequency, duration or amount, or any combination of these three.

The age distribution of DUB is difficult to establish as most investigators have limited their studies to patients admitted to hospital. Teenage girls with DUB however are usually treated as outpatients and not admitted and are usually excluded from such series. On the other hand, most cases of perimenopausal bleeding are admitted for curettage even though the menstrual disturbance may be minor. Oral contraception also produces a reduction in menstrual loss. The incidence of DUB by age groups in a series of 861 women reported by Sutherland (1949) before the advent of oral contraception is shown in Table 43.2. It will be noted that contrary to the frequently made statement that DUB occurs only at the extremes of reproductive life, over 50% of the women admitted for curettage were in the 20–40-year age group, 39% were aged 40 years or more and only 11% of patients were under 20 years. DUB therefore does occur in the 20–40-year-old age group, both spontaneously and secondary to steroidal contraception (Gray 1980), and it constitutes a frequent clinical gynaecological problem in this age group as well as in both younger teenage and older perimenopausal women.

BLOOD LOSS IN NORMAL AND ABNORMAL MENSTRUATION

The variation in cycle length between different women not using any contraceptive is considerable, the 5th and 95th percentile of cycle length being from 23 to 39.4 days with a mean of 29.6 days (Vollman 1977). The duration of a menstrual period similarly varies from 2–8 days with a mean of 5 days (Guillebaud & Bonnar 1978). The best measure of excessive uterine bleeding however is provided by the total menstrual blood loss (MBL) or the total blood loss in any cycle or month. In a Swedish population Hallberg *et al.* (1966) found a definite decrease in haemoglobin concentration and plasma iron concentration when the MBL exceeded 80 ml and this is generally accepted as the upper limit of normal range. The number of women in any population whose loss exceeds 80 ml varies but has been reported as 11% in a random group of Swedish women (Hallberg *et al.* 1966) and 14% in a group of apparently normal women requesting IUCDs (Guillebaud *et al.* 1976). Haynes *et al.* (1977) studied 50 women with unexplained MBL exceeding 80 ml, including 12 women whose loss exceeded 200 ml and 5 women whose loss exceeded 450 ml and found no

Table 43.2. Age incidence in patients with dysfunctional uterine bleeding (Sutherland 1949).

Age group	No. of cases	%	%
20 and under	33	3.9	
21–30	194	22.5 ⎫	56.8
31–40	295	34.3 ⎭	
41–50	325	37.7 ⎫	39.3
Over 50	14	1.6 ⎭	

change in duration of menstruation or the distribution of the blood loss. Ninety-two-percent of the total menses was lost in the first 3 days and women with menorrhagia tend to have the greatest increase in blood flow in the first 2–3 days of menstruation. In the same study of women attending a gynaecology clinic because of menorrhagia it was found that 76% had objective evidence of heavy menstrual blood loss but 24% had normal blood loss. In a further study from the same hospital Chimbira *et al.* (1980a) found no correlation between the true measured blood loss and the number of days of bleeding, the number of sanitary pads or tampons the patients used and the patients' subjective assessment of the blood loss. Unless the total blood loss is measured (which is not practical clinically) the diagnosis of DUB normally depends upon the patient's subjective assessment and implies a subjective increase or change in menstrual bleeding pattern and not always a truly excessive loss.

MECHANISM OF NORMAL MENSTRUATION

In normal menstruation a half to threequarters of the menstrual discharge is blood, the rest being fragments of endometrial tissue, desquamated vaginal epithelium and mucus. Menstrual blood does not clot readily as the endometrium normally produces a lytic substance that causes any clots that do form in the uterine cavity to disintegrate. When menstrual loss is excessive, the flow of blood is too great for the amount of lysin available, resulting in the passage of blood clots typical of menorrhagia. Menstrual clots are not however true clots as they do not contain fibrin but are 'red cell aggregations of mucoid substances, mucoproteins and/or glycogen' (Beller 1971). The clots moreover are usually formed not in the uterus but in the vagina.

The unique feature of primate females who menstruate is the presence of spiral arterioles in the uter-

us. In the proliferative phase of the cycle these blood vessels grow upwards from the basal layer of the endometrium to the more superficial layers, where a capillary network develops. During this phase the vessels appear to be in spasm. Following ovulation and the formation of the corpus luteum the spiral arterioles are more dilated. There is also a marked increase in the coiling and length of the arterioles. If pregnancy does not occur the corpus luteum starts to atrophy and about two days before menstruation the blood flow through the spiral arterioles decreases. At the same time the endometrial glands empty of secretion and buckle and the whole endometrium shrinks, causing the spiral arterioles to become even more coiled, and to kink. This is followed by spasmodic contraction of the spiral arterioles, focal necrosis and rupture of their walls and local extravasation of blood into the endometrium. Numerous venous and capillary lakes appear in the spongiosa and areas of haemorrhage finally coalesce to lift off islands of devitalized tissue. Bleeding occurs from the coalesced blood lakes, from the superficial venules which have been torn open and from the open ends of the remaining parts of the spiral arterioles in the basal layer of the endometrium. In normal menstruation most of the endometrial tissue in fact involutes or is reabsorbed and only about one-quarter is shed. Regeneration then begins immediately with the occlusion of the tips of the spiral arterioles within a few hours. New capillaries grow from the basal part of the arteries and repair and resurfacing of the denuded areas is normally completed in 4–7 days.

This description of menstruation is based on observations of ocular transplants of endometrium by Markee (1950) who described four different types of bleeding at menstruation: passage of blood through the capillary walls by diapedesis; escape of blood from a breakage in the capillary wall, with formation of haematoma in the stroma; confluence and enlargement of venous haematomas causing separation of superficial layers of the endometrium and bleeding from ruptured venules; surface bleeding from exposed superficial anteriolar branches.

More recently Christiaens *et al.* (1982) have described the changes in the uteri of patients in whom a hysterectomy was performed either premenstrually or during early menstruation which they compare with haemostasis in a normal skin wound. These authors emphasize several new features determining the nature and amount of menstrual blood loss.

Spiral arterioles as end arteries

Spiral arterioles supply separate narrow longitudinal segments of mucosa varying in size from 4–9 mm without anastomoses, making the superficial layer of the endometrium much more vulnerable to vascular alterations than the basal layer. In the immediate premenstrual phase another important feature is the appearance of gaps between the endothelial cells lining some of the vessels, with open communications between the vascular layer and the subendothelial collagen but without new platelet aggregation or other haemostatic reaction.

Venous lakes and sinusoids

In the secretory phase the venous plexus is drained by numerous large venous channels running parallel to the glands. The different veins join with frequent anastomoses and form sinusoidal dilatations or venous lakes. These vessels which are near the surface are common in both hyperplastic and atrophic endometrium and may be responsible for breakthrough bleeding and bleeding from atrophic endometrium. Bleeding from veins and venules also appears to last longer than bleeding from spiral arterioles and capillaries and some authors believe menstruation is primarily of venous origin.

Haemostatic plug formation

Primary haemostasis is achieved by platelet plugs which form within 10 s of a transection of a vessel. The plugs grow in size and protrude from the vessel ends. Fibrin appears after 30 min and recognizable fibres with infiltration of leucocytes are present after 2 hr. If the endometrial haemostatic plug formation is less than expected, the plugs do not protrude from the ends of the vessels and may not occlude the lumen. Moreover the plugs are shed as the tissue layers are shed and new plugs are progressively formed 'upstream'. Approximately 20 hr after onset of bleeding most of the functional layer of the endometrium has been shed but no more thrombi are found, the absence of thrombi in damaged vessels being a striking feature of human placentation. This suggests that anti-aggregatory substances such as prostacyclin are formed in normal endometrium, particularly in the basal layers.

Vasoconstriction and occlusion of the spiral arterioles by endothelial proliferation

The main mechanism ensuring haemostasis after 20–24 hr when the endometrium has been shed is constriction of the spiral arterioles together with swelling of the arteriolar endothelial cells which produces a complete occlusion of the vessel lumen.

Heparin-like activity, plasminogen and fibrinolysis in uterine fluid

The endometrium and cervix are the site of marked fibrinolytic activity and plasminogen activators have been demonstrated in myometrium, endometrium and menstrual blood, being maximal on the first day of bleeding and increased in women with IUCD. The high fibrinolytic activity of the endometrium and the cervix promote emptying of the uterus by liquefaction of the fibrin and shed tissue. Plasminogen activators are in much higher concentration in uterine than in vaginal collected discharge, indicating consumption during the passage from the uterine cavity to the vagina and explaining why menstrual blood clots usually occur in the vagina and not in the uterus. Heparin-like activity which increases towards the end of the menstrual cycle and decreases during menstruation has also recently been found in uterine fluid. Any increase in fibrinolytic or heparin-like activity will cause a disturbance of the equilibrium between the formation of the haemostatic plugs in the spiral arterioles and their lysis and may result in excessive menstrual loss.

The role of prostaglandins

The role of prostaglandins in menstruation and DUB has recently been reviewed by Granestrom et al. (1983). It seems established that the human endometrium is able to synthesize relatively large amounts of $PGF2\alpha$ and PGE2. These prostanoids increase during the secretory phase, reach a maximum premenstrually and are then released into menstrual blood. Significantly higher amounts of these prostaglandins have been found in patients with menorrhagia, endometriosis, endometrial carcinoma and dysmenorrhoea. Guillebaud et al. (1978) also showed that excessive bleeding with intrauterine contraceptive devices is associated with abnormally high concentrations of prostaglandins in the endometrium. Willman et al. (1976) reported a disproportionate increase in PGE2 (which is vasodilator) as compared with $PGF2\alpha$ (which is vasoconstrictor) in patients with menorrhagia (but not dysmenorrhoea). Smith et al. 981) have demonstrated an inverse correlation between $PGF2\alpha$ and PGE2 in secretory endometrium and in menstrual blood loss. The efficacy of prostaglandin inhibitors in reducing menstrual blood loss is also testimony to the role of prostaglandins. It is tempting to postulate that it is the effect of the relative excess of the vasodilatory PGE2 on the spiral arterioles which causes the excessive blood loss in women with DUB.

Few measurements have been made of the newly discovered prostanoids prostacyclin (which prevents platelet aggregation and causes vasodilatation) and thromboxane (which is a powerful platelet aggregator and vasoconstrictor). Samples of myometrial and endometrial homogenates, however, have been reported to show a significant increase in 6-keto PGF1α (the main metabolite of prostacyclin) whereas thromboxane and other arachidonic metabolites remained unchanged. It is once again tempting to postulate that it is the disturbed ratio of prostacyclin to thromboxane which prevents the formation of adequate thrombotic plugs and contributes to the excessive menstrual blood loss in DUB. It is noteworthy that at the onset of menstruation the walls of the spiral arterioles normally lose their continuity with resulting holes in the endothelium and the basal membrane. The circulating platelets are then exposed to the subendothelial collagen but there is no adhesion or accumulation of platelets, suggesting that a powerful antiplatelet aggregatory factor must be secreted at this time. Once menstruation starts however the vessel becomes filled with intravascular plugs of degranulated platelets and fibrin as described above.

A third class of prostanoids are the leukotrienes formed by lipoxygenase from arachidonic acid. These are potent vasoconstrictors in many different vascular beds as well as being powerful chemotactic agents for leucocytes. Their presence in the endometrium would explain many of the phenomena seen at menstruation, such as cellular infiltration. The role of leukotrienes in normal and abnormal menstruation, however, awaits elucidation.

Prostanoids are intimately involved in the premenstrual and menstrual phases of the menstrual cycle and abnormalities in prostanoid metabolism, whether primary endometrial or secondary to hormonal changes, play a significant part in the aetiology of DUB.

THE IMMEDIATE CAUSE OF MENSTRUATION AND ABNORMAL BLOOD LOSS

Oestrogen and progestogen withdrawal

Markee (1950) showed that abrupt changes in sex hormone concentrations are needed to cause menstrual bleeding. Daily hormone assays have shown that on the first day of menstruation plasma oestradiol levels fall from approximately 250–750 pmol/l to 100–300 pmol/l and plasma progesterone levels fall from levels of 20–100 pmol/l to 0.25–5 m mol/l. The fall in oestrogens following bilateral oophorectomy, destruction of mature ovarian follicles or discontinuation of oestrogen therapy in oophorectomized women similarly results in 'withdrawal bleeding'. Oestrogen administration however need not be discontinued completely for bleeding to occur, since halving of the oestrogen dose is also followed by menstrual loss. Continuous administration of small doses of oestrogen furthermore not uncommonly results in 'breakthrough bleeding.'

Endometrial shedding also occurs following a fall in progesterone when the corpus luteum regresses, on surgical removal of the corpus luteum, and on discontinuing progestogen therapy. Progesterone withdrawal bleeding however occurs only in an endometrium primed by oestrogens, and this observation forms the basis for the diagnostic use of progesterone in amenorrhoea. Endometrial withdrawal bleeding also occurs in the absence of progesterone (e.g. in anovulatory cycles) so that progesterone withdrawal is not essential for endometrial shedding and menstruation though the bleeding pattern is often abnormal.

Normal menstruation depends upon the combined cyclical secretion of oestrogen/progesterone during the proliferative and secretory phases and the withdrawal of both oestrogen and progesterone just before the onset of the menses. There is much to suggest that the effects of oestrogens and progestogens on the endometrium are mediated by the various prostanoids. The tissue concentrations of prostaglandins PGF2$_\alpha$ and PGE2 and the prostanoids thromboxane and prostacyclin are determined not only by the rate of synthesis but also by the rate of degradation of the compounds and by the pathway into which the endoperoxide intermediates are directed (Fig. 43.1). It has been shown that oestrogen depresses and progesterone stimulates the activity of the enzyme 15-hydroxyprostaglandin dehydrogenase (PGDH), a main enzyme catalysing the initial step in the degradation of PGE2 and PGF2$_\alpha$ (Flower 1977). An increase in oestrogen and a decrease in progesterone will thus not only stimulate the formation of prostaglandins before and during menstruation but may also increase their concentration and prolong their action by inhibiting their degradation. Dysfunctional uterine bleeding can thus result from some abnormality in prostaglandin metabolism which may occur primarily in the endometrium, or may be secondary to ab-

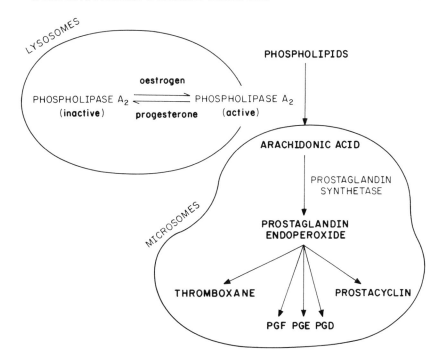

Fig. 43.1. The arachidonic acid 'cascade' is shown in bold capital letters and bold arrows. The main rate-limiting step is the activation of phospholipase A_2 shown at the top left of the diagram.

normalities in oestrogen or progesterone secretion by the ovary.

Endometrial lysosomes and relaxin

The breakdown of the endometrium at menstruation may also be due to the acyl hydrolase enzymes which are stored in the Golgi-lysomal complex of the endometrial cells (Schultz *et al.* 1975, Grieves & Liggins 1976). One of the main acyl hydrolases is the enzyme phospholipase -A_2 which controls the release of arachidonic acid from glycerophospholipids. Arachidonic acid is the obligatory precursor of $PGF2_\alpha$, prostacyclin and thromboxane -A_2, and the amount of the enzyme phospholipase -A_2 is the rate-limiting step in the formation of all these compounds. Prostaglandins, unlike other hormones, such as catecholamines, are not stored in the tissues, but are synthesized and released as soon as arachidonic acid is liberated from its ester.

Progesterone has been shown to promote the formation of lysosomes in the endometrium (Henzl *et al.* 1972), and ultrastructure studies have furthermore shown that progesterones have a stabilizing effect and oestrogens a labilizing effect on these lysosomes (Boshier & Liggins 1974). Progesterone will thus not only promote the formation of lysosomes but its withdrawal at menstruation will allow the release of the phospholipase -A_2 from the lysosomes into the cyto-

plasmic cell. This will initiate the arachidonic acid cascade and the formation and release of prostaglandins, prostacyclin and thromboxane. The release of lysosomes may be the initiating cause of breakthrough or intermenstrual bleeding particularly in cases of unopposed oestrogen secretion.

Lysosomes may be responsible for the premenstrual and menstrual regression of the endometrium. In animal species which do not menstruate, macrophages with phagocytosed material migrate through the glandular epithelium at the end of the cycle towards the uterine cavity. The uterine secretions at this time are rich in acid phosphatase which is a marker for lysosomal enzymes. The importance of premenstrual and menstrual endometrial regression as compared with endometrial shedding has probably been underestimated in the past. Relaxin which is a polypeptide hormone whose amino acid sequence has now been identified is primarily associated with its action on pelvic joints and the cervix in pregnancy. It is however present in endometrial granulocytes which become degranulated premenstrually. It has also been shown to cause premenstrual stromal disintegration and hypertrophy of the endothelium of spiral and basal arteries. It is noteworthy that plasma immunoreactive levels of relaxin are depressed in women using a progesterone releasing IUCD, the only device that decreases menstrual loss suggesting that lack of relaxin may also play a role in DUB.

Tissue regeneration and epithelialization

After shedding of the superficial layers the basal layer of the endometrium rapidly becomes re-epithelialized, normally commencing from the basal glandular trunks and intact areas on the 2nd or 3rd day of menstruation and being completed by the 4th or 5th day. The re-epithelialization coincides with the decrease and cessation of menstrual flow and is probably dependent on the growth of new ovarian follicles and the increase in secretion of oestrogen. The regeneration of the endometrium is normally an important factor in curtailing menstruation, and delay in re-epithelialization (perhaps due to delay in development of a new ovarian follicle) may result in prolonged and excessive periods. Delayed regeneration of the endometrium also occurs in the presence of an IUCD and is accompanied by menorrhagia and prolongation of menses.

FACTORS DETERMINING THE AMOUNT OF
BLOOD LOSS IN MENSTRUATION AND
DYSFUNCTIONAL UTERINE BLEEDING

The amount of blood loss during menstruation and during episodes of DUB is determined by a number of factors including: the total area of the endometrial cavity; the vascularity of the uterus and myometrium and the number and calibre of the endometrial vessels and the presence of any structural changes in the vessel walls; the amount of haemorrhage into the endometrium and of necrosis of the endometrial tissue; the nature, potency and amount of vasoconstrictor and vasodilator substances released during menstruation and the responsiveness and functional state of the spiral arterioles; the potency and balance of effects of the various coagulation and lytic factors liberated from the endometrium and the coagulability of the blood in the spiral arterioles; the rate of regeneration of the endometrium.

One or all these factors may be involved in the excessive or abnormal blood loss in DUB.

Aetiology of dysfunctional bleeding

PRIMARY DYSFUNCTIONAL UTERINE BLEEDING

Primary DUB is usually assumed to be due to failure in ovulation or corpus luteum formation but may result from a dysfunction in the endometrium. Some of the theories which have been offered to explain primary DUB include various endocrine dysfunctions, coagulation disorders, increased capillary fragility, defects in the spiral arterioles, failure in endometrial regeneration, alterations in the formation and secretion of prostaglandins and increased fibrinolysis, secretion of a heparin-like substance and lysosomal defects in the endometrium. Zondek (1954) noted that 'since bleeding can take place in such widely varying phases in the development of the endometrium, with such different degrees of vascularization, and with either decreasing or constant hormonal levels, the mechanisms cannot be the same in every case of bleeding'. The finding of secretory endometrium in 88% of women with dysfunctional bleeding suggests that anovulation is the exception rather than the rule. More recently Haynes *et al.* (1980a) have challenged the whole concept of endocrine dysfunction and anovulation as a common cause for primary DUB. These workers performed daily hormonal assays throughout the menstrual cycle in 29 women with an average menstrual loss of 80 ml or more who were not receiving treatment and who had no obvious pelvic abnormality. They compared the results with a control group who had a menstrual loss within the normal range and found that 26 out of 29 patients with DUB had normal hormone profiles and that only 3 had abnormal results. They concluded that no pituitary ovarian abnormality is present in the majority of women with menorrhagia and that bleeding is most likely to be due to local causes within the uterus. Whatever the underlying primary aetiology DUB must arise from some disturbance of normal endometrial function and the final common pathway must include some abnormality of the endometrial blood vessels and capillaries and the coagulation of blood in and round these vessels.

The postulated mechanisms are:
1   Failure in vasoconstriction due to excessive secretion of PGE2 and increase in PGE2/PGF2α ratio.
2   Failure in formation of adequate thrombotic plugs, perhaps due to prostacyclin excess or to increase in PGI2/TXA ratio.
3   Excessive fibrinolysis with failure in formation of secondary thrombotic plugs.
4   Increase in endometrial lysosomal enzymes with excessive formation of prostanoids.
5   Failure in vascular endothelial proliferation due to decreased relaxin.
6   Delay in endometrial regeneration.

All these changes may occur as a primary defect in the endometrium, or secondary to changes in the ovary, pituitary, hypothalamus and high centres. A classification of DUB based on the presumed dysfunction of the ovarian, pituitary, hypothalamic axis has been put forward by Vorys and Neri (1968) (Table 43.3) and represents the classical approach to DUB.

Table 43.3. Classification of dysfunctional uterine bleeding according to aetiology and common symptoms (after Vorys & Neri 1968).

Ovulatory	(a) Long proliferative or secretory phases	Oligomenorrhoea
	(b) Short proliferative or secretory phases	Polymenorrhoea
Corpus luteum abnormality	(a) Insufficiency	Premenstrual spotting Menorrhagia Polymenorrhoea
	(b) Prolonged	Menorrhagia Oligomenorrhoea
Anovulatory	(a) Cyclical	Oligomenorrhoea Menorrhagia
	(b) Acyclical	Metrorrhagia

Ovulatory dysfunctional uterine bleeding

Disorders of menstruation associated with normal ovulation more commonly cause a disturbance of the cycle or amenorrhoea rather than excess menstrual loss.

Ovulatory oligomenorrhoea is usually due to a prolonged proliferative phase. It most commonly occurs in adolescence and may be a normal feature of the menarche. It may, however, be a forerunner of the Stein–Leventhal or polycystic ovary syndrome. Ovulatory oligomenorrhoea also occurs (but less commonly) in older women when it may precede the menopause. The secretory phases of these menstrual cycles are usually normal.

Ovulatory polymenorrhoea is commonly due to a shortening of the proliferative phase, particularly in adolescence when it is thought to be due to hypersensitivity of the ovary. Ovulation is normal and there is an abnormality in the amount of mentrual blood loss. Polymenorrhoea with a shortened secretory phase may occur in older women and may progress to oligomenorrhoea and amenorrhoea of ovarian failure. It is due to premature degeneration of the corpus luteum and is really a form of corpus luteum insufficiency.

Dysfunctional bleeding with corpus luteum abnormalities

This is said to occur most commonly in the adult reproductive years.

Corpus luteum insufficiency is due to failure in the development of the corpus luteum with a decreased secretion of progesterone and oestrogen in the second half of the cycle. Endometrial biopsy at the time of menstruation may show 'irregular ripening' of the endometrium (Traut & Kuder 1935). The condition is typically associated with hypermenorrhoea and premenstrual spotting. Early involution of the corpus luteum may result in a shortening of the menstrual cycle and polymenorrhoea.

Corpus luteum prolonged activity. In some cycles regression of the corpus luteum may be delayed. In a group of cases of dysfunctional uterine bleeding McKelvey and Samuels (1947) have demonstrated an 'irregular shedding of the endometrium' associated with the secretion of pregnanediol persisting throughout the bleeding period. This abnormality is comparatively rare and may be associated with the development of a corpus luteum cyst. It results in prolonged and excessive menstruation and possibly in oligomenorrhoea due to the prolonged cycles.

Anovulatory dysfunctional uterine bleeding

Failure of ovulation is the most common abnormality of the menstrual cycle. It may result in: normal regular cycles with apparently normal periods; regular cycles with excessive loss (anovulatory hypermenorrhoea); irregular menstruation in which periods of amenorrhoea are followed by excessive loss (metropathia haemorrhagica).

Anovular menstruation occurs at the extremes of reproductive life, i.e. at the menarche and preceding the menopause. Anovulatory menstruation is the rule rather than the exception at these times and should be regarded as normal provided there is no abnormal uterine bleeding.

Irregular shedding of the endometrium. In this condition there is a progressive rise of oestrogen secretion to comparatively high levels of 100 μg or more per day, which is then followed by a sudden fall in secretion due to feedback inhibition of the pituitary and of FSH secretion. With the fall in oestrogen secretion the endometrium which is proliferative does not undergo the generalized ischaemic process as normally occurs at menstruation. The shedding of the endometrium is in consequence often irregular, incomplete and prolonged, resulting in excessive blood loss. The cycles in these cases are nevertheless regular or only slightly irregular.

Threshold bleeding. A second type of anovulatory abnormality is when the oestrogen secretion does not increase but 'teeters' about a critical threshold below which the endometrium cannot be maintained. This results in so-called 'threshold' bleeding which is often completely irregular and acyclical.

Metropathia haemorrhagica. This is the classical form of dysfunctional uterine bleeding. There is a slowly increasing secretion of oestrogen but no secondary feedback inhibition of the pituitary. The cycle is therefore prolonged, resulting in a period of amenorrhoea, and the prolonged stimulation of the endometrium by oestrogen causes a hyperplasia of the endometrium. The hyperplasia continues until such time as there is a fall in oestrogen secretion or until particular areas of the endometrium outgrow their blood supply and slough. The hyperplastic endometrium may be shed and a normal menstrual cycle may follow though the episodes of metropathia haemorrhagica tend to recur. Alternatively the endometrium may not be completely shed and this results in continuous or acyclical bleeding. This type of anovulatory bleeding is often associated with the formation of multiple cysts of the ovary. The Graafian follicles presumably fail to rupture and continue to produce oestrogen until such time as the granulosa and theca cells degenerate.

Table 43.4. Histology of endometrium in dysfunctional uterine bleeding.

Diagnosis	Sutherland (1949)		Kistner (1964a)	
	No.	%	No.	%
Normal	547	63.5	230	57.5
Hyperplasia	265	30.8	123	30.8
Irregular ripening	26	3.0	—	—
Chronic menstrual	—	—	31	7.8
Irregular shedding	13	1.5	9	2.2
Atrophy	10	1.2	7	1.7
Total	861	100	400	100

IATROGENIC DYSFUNCTIONAL UTERINE BLEEDING SECONDARY TO STEROIDAL CONTRACEPTION AND INTRAUTERINE CONTRACEPTIVE DEVICES

This subject has been reviewed by Diczfalusy, Fraser and Webb (1980) in their book *Endometrial Bleeding and Steroidal Contraception* based on a symposium organized by the WHO in 1979. It was found that excessive and irregular bleeding occurs most commonly with IUCDs, continuous oral administration of low dose progestogen or injectable depot progestogen.

Steroidal contraceptives cause important vascular changes in the endometrium, including underdevelopment of the arterioles and degenerative changes in the venules and, in a small number of cases, lesions of the vascular endothelium or vessel wall (Maqueo 1980) (Fig. 43.2).

Large doses of progestogens commonly produce dilated venules with suppression of spiral arterioles in the endometrium (Ober 1966, Ober 1970). The dilated venules are often quite large and are found very superficially in the endometrium. They are found very frequently in atrophic endometrium and may occur, but much less commonly, in hyperplastic endometrium (Ober & Labay 1972).

Contraceptive agents induce structural changes in endometrial vessels and these contribute to the bleeding irregularities (Dallenbach-Hellweg 1980).

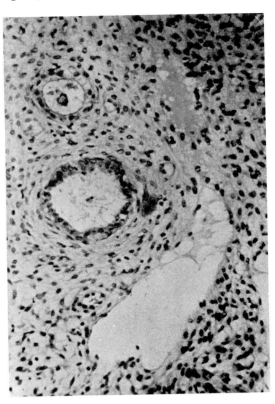

Fig. 43.2. Suppressed endometrium with involuted glands and loose stroma. Notice the large dilated venules with very thin walls (× 107) (Maqueo 1980).

SECONDARY DYSFUNCTIONAL UTERINE BLEEDING ARISING FROM DISEASE OUTSIDE THE GENITAL TRACT

Secondary DUB is commonly seen in thrombocytopenia, thrombocytopathia such as von Willebrand's disease, afibrinogenaemia and other coagulation disorders as well as in thyroid disorders sudch as myxoedema.

Haematological disorders

Abnormal uterine bleeding is characteristic of several but not all of the hereditary bleeding disorders (Simpson & Christakos 1969). Excessive menstrual bleeding is common in thrombocytopenic purpura and in Minot–von Willebrand syndrome and may be the first sign of these diseases. This may be due to the diminution in platelets and increasing capillary fragility normally seen in the luteal phase of the cycle. Quick (1966) stated 'Because normal menstruation is observed in afibrinogenaemia, severe hypothrombinaemia, marked reduction of factor VII and hyperheparinaemia, it can be concluded that the control and termination of the cyclic uterine bleeding depends upon a mechanism other than the clotting of blood. Menorrhagia is associated with lack of blood clotting factors V, VII and X and is common in platelet deficiency as well as in the Minot–von Willebrand syndrome.' More recent information suggests that menorrhagia does occur in congenital afibrinogenaemia and in factor II, V, VII, X and XI deficiency, and it is concluded that the increased frequency of menorrhagia in patients with platelet and coagulation disorders confirms that haemostatic plug formation plays an important role in uterine haemastasis during menstruation (Christiaens *et al.* 1982).

Thyroid disease

Women with myxoedema frequently have menstrual disorders characterized by excessive bleeding which may be the presenting complaint (Goldsmith *et al.* 1952, Scott & Mussey 1964). The abnormal menstruation responds promptly to therapy and often to doses of thyroxine insufficient to correct all other stigmata of hypothyroidism. Hyperthyroidism in contrast is associated with amenorrhoea and oligomenorrhoea and the decrease in flow is proportional to the severity of the thyroidoxicosis (Benson & Dailey 1955).

Anaemia and iron deficiency

Though anaemia is common in DUB the precise relationship between anaemia and abnormal menstruation is difficult to establish. Many gynaecologists regard the haemoglobin level in peripheral venous blood as a measure of the amount of menstrual blood loss and maintain that if uterine bleeding is excessive it will produce anaemia and that a patient with a normal haemoglobin concentration

cannot have excessive blood loss. There may be some truth in these widely held beliefs but they ignore the fact that women blood donors can lose relatively large amounts of blood over long periods without any persisting effect on the haemoglobin levels. Fowler and Barer (1942) thus found that women blood donors can lose on an average 555 ml or 2.2 g haemoglobin in addition to the normal menstrual blood loss and that the haemoglobin will return to normal in an average of 52 days (range 43–73 days).

Some women can therefore lose excessive amounts of blood at menstruation (up to 300 ml) and still maintain a normal haemoglobin. The development of anaemia probably depends upon a number of factors, such as the iron intake and the efficiency of the erythropoietic system, as well as upon the amount of menstrual blood loss.

Some investigators maintain that iron deficiency and anaemia are causative factors in DUB (Taymor *et al.* 1964). Others hold that anaemia may cause a reduction in menstrual blood loss. Jacobs and Butler (1965) measured the blood loss in 17 normal women and in 15 women with iron deficiency anaemia. When the blood loss was measured after the anaemia had been fully treated, many of the anaemic women had a considerable increase in menstrual flow, the mean blood loss per period after treatment being 157.7 ± 28.0 ml, or approximately double. The increase in blood loss following treatment was observed to be greatest in those women whose initial blood loss was above average. Jacobs and Butler (1965) concluded that in the majority of their cases the development of iron deficiency anaemia initiates a compensatory mechanism which tends to reduce the menstrual blood loss. In DUB with excessive blood loss the development of anaemia would appear to cause a relative reduction in the menstrual blood loss in the majority of cases.

Pathology

ENDOMETRIUM

DUB may be associated with almost any type of endometrium, even apparently normal endometrium. The endometrial findings in two series of DUB (Sutherland 1949, Kistner 1964a) are shown in Table 43.4.

The incidence of abnormal endometrial findings probably represents that found in routine gynaecological practice. It does not, however, necessarily indicate the true incidence of abnormalities of the endometrium as the incidence of abnormality will depend greatly upon the time when the endometrial biopsy was performed, both in relation to the cycle and to the episode of bleeding. The endometrial abnormalities in DUB are of three main types: 1 *Ovulatory* which may be (a) Irregular ripening of the endometrium, or (b) Irregular shedding of the endometrium; 2 *Anovulatory* with either (a) Proliferative endometrium, or (b) Endometrial hyperplasia; 3 *Atrophic*.

Ovulatory endometrium

Irregular ripening of the endometrium. This condition was first described by Traut and Kuder (1935) and an example is shown in Fig. 43.3. On histological examination of the endometrium obtained in the second half of the cycle there is a mixture of both proliferative and secretory phases with considerable areas that are definitely non-secretory and others which are as definitely secretory. Traut and Kuder (1935) stress that the changes must be found in the superficial zone of the endometrium as it is well recognized that the basal layers of the glands adjacent to the myometrium are almost completely unresponsive to the secretory stimulus of the ovary. They also stress that it is important to exclude myomata and polypi as the endometrium is frequently refractory in the vicinity of submucous fibroids and polyps. In a series of 100 cases of DUB Traut and Kuder (1935) found 21 cases of irregular ripening of the endometrium. Fourteen of the cases presented with bleeding commencing in the middle of the cycle. All responded to curettage without recurrence. It is suggested that there is either a functional defect of the corpus luteum or an irregular response of the endometrium to the normal hormonal influence.

Irregular shedding of the endometrium. Irregular shedding of the endometrium was first described by Driessen (1914) and was also discussed by Traut and Kuder (1935). They summarized their findings as follows: 'The history of the patient and the histological findings point definitely to maldeciduation of the endometrium with prolonged and exhausting secretory activity in the glandular elements of those fragments of the spongioma which remain attached to the basalis, while the stroma becomes shrunken and most often its cells have changed from large round nucleated forms to the spindle shape which is characteristic of the proliferative phase of the cycle' (Fig. 43.4). They found 11 cases in their series of 100 patients with DUB. The women all gave a history of having had normal menstrual periods until they came under observation because of a prolonged or profuse menses or of recurrent bleeding immediately following what was supposed to have been a normal menstrual period. The duration of the bleeding was from 10 to 43 days. Curettage, when performed, caused prompt cessation of the bleeding. McKelvey and Samuels (1947) describe 34 cases in which the endometrium had the same characteristics and was associated with prolonged and profuse menstrual bleeding. They emphasized that the endometrium

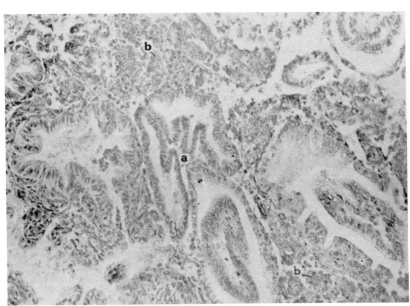

Fig. 43.3. Irregular ripening of endometrium. Glands and stroma in proliferative phase (a). Early secretory glands and stroma (b) (× 55) (Traut & Kuder 1935).

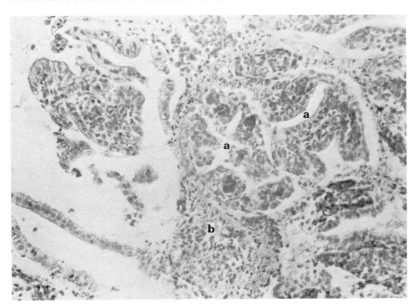

Fig. 43.4. Irregular shedding of endometrium. Collapsed 'star-shaped' glands with secretory epithelium (a). Shrunken, inactive endometrium (b) (× 55) (Traut & Kuder 1935).

must be taken on the fifth day of the bleeding or a day or two later. If the endometrium is taken earlier or at the end of the bleeding, accurate diagnosis is difficult. They also studied the pregnanediol excretion in 6 patients through 6 days of bleeding after which curettage was performed to establish the diagnosis. In 5 of the 6 cases pregnanediol was excreted throughout the periods. Holmstrom and McClennan (1947) showed that an identical microscopic picture to that of irregular shedding of the endometrium could be produced in normal patients by the administration of progesterone either immediately before or during menstruation. The reported incidence of irregular shedding in different series of cases of DUB varies from 3.7% to 25% (Sutherland 1949). Endometrial changes similar to irregular ripening and irregular shedding are seen following various steroidal contraceptives and the terms irregular secretory, suppressed or involuted endometrium and resting or inactive endometrium have been used (Maqueo 1980).

Anovulatory endometrium

Proliferative endometrium. Anovulatory cycles are common in adolescence and before the menopause. Though the mechanism is not known, the menstrual bleeding associated with the shedding of proliferative endometrium is frequently excessive and prolonged. The finding of proliferative endometrium in the second half of the cycle should always be regarded as abormal in DUB.

Endometrial hyperplasia. This is the classical and most common abnormality of the endometrium in DUB and is associated with metropathia haemorrhagica or completely acyclical bleeding. The hyperplasia varies from slight exaggeration of the proliferative phase to marked overgrowth, simulating adenocarcinoma of the endometrium. The overgrowth affects both the stroma and the glands, which increase in number and size, producing the typical 'Swiss cheese' endometrium. There is also abnormal vascularization with numerous large thick-walled blood vessels and markedly dilated veins or sinuses just under the endometrial surface (Fig. 43.5). Endometrial specimens obtained during bleeding, as Schroeder (1954) repeatedly emphasized, show infarction and thrombosis of the blood vessels with areas of necrosis and sloughing of the superficial layers of the endometrium. With the increased vascularity and the often grossly abnormal endometrium, it is not difficult to visualize that endometrial hyperplasia is often associated with bleeding, which may be very heavy. The incidence of endometrial hyperplasia in DUB has been quoted as high as 90%. Sutherland (1949), however, in an analysis of 4850 cases from 31 papers, found an incidence of 39.4% which is in reasonable agreement with the figure of 30.8% which he found in his own series. Discussion of the significance of endometrial hyperplasia, particularly in relation to the subsequent development of endometrial carcinoma, has occupied a large place in gynaecological literature. The subject has been reviewed by Kistner (1964b)

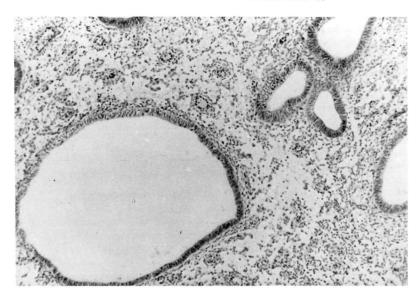

Fig. 43.5. Endometrial glandular hyperplasia showing dilated glands and 'Swiss cheese' appearance.

with particular reference to the effect of progestational agents.

Atrophy of the endometrium

There is considerable variation in the histological criteria for the diagnosis of this condition and in the incidence in different series, which ranges from 1.9 to 21.9 (Sutherland 1949). It is probably the least common abnormality in any age group though there seems little doubt that DUB can occur with a completely atrophic endometrium. Conclusions with regard to the incidence of atrophic endometrium may well change with the advent of hysteroscopy.

OVARY

The findings in the ovary in DUB vary with the age of the patient and the endometrial changes. In pubertal girls the ovaries may contain follicular cysts which may be up to 3 cm in diameter but there are usually no recent or old corpora lutea. In women of childbearing age with dysfunctional menorrhagia the ovaries usually appear normal though there may occasionally be a persistent corpus luteum or corpus luteum cyst. The ovaries of premenopausal women, in contrast, frequently contain multiple cysts of various types and these are particularly associated with endometrial hyperplasia.

ASSOCIATED FINDINGS

Organic disease of the genital tract is excluded by definition in DUB. It is nevertheless important to have some idea of the proportion of pathological conditions

which may be overlooked. The series of 861 cases of Sutherland (1949) was derived from 1000 cases of abnormal uterine bleeding in which careful pelvic examination under general anaesthesia failed to reveal any recognizable pathological lesion which might explain the haemorrhage. The pathological findings in the remaining 139 cases showed chronic endometritis in 11% and polyps, tuberculous endometritis and malignant disease in approximately 1% each of the total cases. Jacobs *et al.* (1957) reported 20 incorrect diagnoses in 112 cases of 'dysfunctional uterine bleeding', as follows: 6 pelvic inflammatory disease, 4 fibroids, 4 incomplete abortions, 3 threatened abortions and 1 polyp, 1 subinvolution and 1 case of precocious puberty.

Clinical presentation

Dysfunctional bleeding from the uterus may be abnormal in amount or duration, in regularity or frequency, and in its relation to menstruation. There is no specific pattern of bleeding which is characteristically dysfunctional and no specific pattern which is associated with organic disease. The incidence of pathological diseases and the prognosis varies both with age and the type of bleeding. In dealing with cases of abnormal uterine bleeding it is useful to consider the patients under three age groups and three types of bleeding: 1. *under 20 years*—adolescent uterine bleeding; *20–40 years*—uterine bleeding of adult reproductive years; *over 40 years*—perimenopausal bleeding.

Adolescent DUB

Uterine bleeding in adolescent girls (under the age of 20) is almost always dysfunctional in origin. In a group of 200 girls aged 20 or under, investigated by Sutherland (1953) there were no cases of malignancy but 8 cases of unsuspected tuberculous endometritis were found. It is estimated that as many as the first 30–40 cycles after menarche may be anovulatory. Distinction must be made between transitory oligomenorrhoea or some transitory irregularity of the cycles which may be regarded as physiological and a normal part of puberty, and persisting oligomenorrhoea and polymenorrhoea or excessive blood loss. Menorrhagia or metrorrhagia can be severe in adolescents and accounts for about 4% of cases of DUB. Southam and Rickart (1966) studied a series of 291 girls with dysfunctional bleeding and found that 40% had returned to normal in 2 years and 70% in 10 years (Fig. 43.6). The prognosis was better in patients whose abnormal bleeding started after a period of normal menstruation than those in whom it started at the menarche, though the overall prognosis for both groups was good.

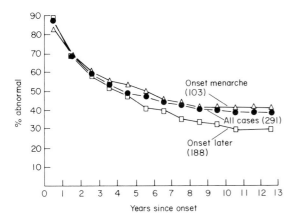

Fig. 43.6. Adolescent dysfunctional uterine bleeding. Rate of continued abnormality (Southan & Richart 1966).

Adult DUB

Abnormal uterine bleeding between the ages of 20 and 40 years is most commonly due to benign tumour, pelvic inflammatory disease or some complication of pregnancy. A diagnosis of DUB should therefore not be made until organic disease has been excluded. It is sometimes said that DUB is uncommon in this age group. This is, however, not borne out in the published series. Over 50% of Sutherland's (1949) patients were between the ages of 20 and 40 years. DUB is frequent in the puerperium and occurs in parous women more often than in nulliparae. The bleeding is most frequently ovulatory in type. Anovulatory bleeding and endometrial hyperplasia do, however, occur and were present in 21% of Sutherland's (1949) patients of childbearing age with dysfunctional bleeding. The prognosis in ovulatory DUB is good. Most of such cases either undergo spontaneous cure or remit after curettage or hormone therapy. The prognosis is, however, less favourable in patients with anovulatory bleeding and endometrial hyperplasia, which tends to recur.

Perimenopausal DUB

Abnormal uterine bleeding in women over 40 years is commonly due to organic disease. Carcinoma of the endometrium and of the cervix occurs with increasing frequency with increasing age and constitutes an important and serious cause of uterine bleeding in this age group. It is therefore essential to take every step to exclude carcinoma in all cases of perimenopausal bleeding. This period of life nevertheless has a high incidence of DUB associated with the alteration in ovarian pituitary function preceding the menopause. The bleeding tends to be acyclical and approximately 50% of cases are associated with endometrial hyperplasia.

Regular cyclical bleeding

Regular or cyclical uterine bleeding is frequently dysfunctional in origin and, if due to organic disease, is rarely associated with malignancy. Cyclical dysfunctional bleeding is most commonly ovulatory and the prognosis is good. Regular uterine bleeding is therefore usually considered relatively favourably, and uterine curettage or endometrial sampling may be deferred in younger women with menorrhagia of short duration in the absence of obvious organic disease.

Irregular or acyclical bleeding

Irregular or acyclical bleeding is more often associated with organic disease of the genital tract, including carcinoma of the cervix or endometrium. It is therefore regarded unfavourably and uterine curettage or endometrial sampling must be performed in every case.

Intermenstrual bleeding

Intermenstrual bleeding with normal regular periods falls into a separate category. If regular and occurring mid-cycle, it is often physiological and is due to the fall in oestrogen secretion following the oestrogen rise with ovulation. It usually lasts only 2–3 days but may occasionally linger until the next period. It is said to occur in 20% of women with 'mittelschmerz' (Diddle 1948) and in 60% of ovulatory women if the mid-cycle mucus is examined for erythrocytes (Kurzor *et al.* 1953). Intermenstrual bleeding is, however, common with endometrial polyps, submucus fibromyomata and cervical carcinoma. It is therefore essential to regard all cases of intermenstrual bleeding as abnormal until proved otherwise.

CLINICAL DIAGNOSIS

To establish a diagnosis of DUB it is necessary to take a full menstrual and medical history, to carry out an abdominal and pelvic examination and to perform dilatation and curettage or endometrial sampling of the uterus. In some cases other special investigations may be indicated.

The history should be detailed, with an assessment of the blood loss and the general condition of the patient. The presence or absence of associated menstrual symptoms and of symptoms of endocrine or other organic disease may provide a guide to the underlying dysfunction. The patient's background, home and marital circumstances and any history of emotional stress or psychiatric abnormality must also be elicited.

Pelvic examination should be performed in every patient complaining of any abnormality of menstruation. In adolescents with intact hymen pelvic examination may be deferred but, if the abnormality persists more than 3 months rectal and abdominal examination must be performed to exclude obvious uterine or ovarian pathology. The general condition of the patient must also be assessed and any overt endocrine or systemic disease excluded.

SPECIAL INVESTIGATIONS

Uterine curettage and endometrial biopsy

Curettage of the uterus is the first step in the management of patients with abnormal uterine bleeding. The objects of the curettage are: to exclude any lesion of the uterus, such as incomplete abortion, tubercu-lous endometritis or endometrial polyp or carcinoma; to obtain endometrium for histological examination in order to determine the functional state of the endometrium; for any possible therapeutic effect, particularly in cases of severe or persistent bleeding when bleeding may be arrested. Most gynaecologists are agreed that *in adolescence* curettage may be deferred unless the bleeding is severe or fails to respond to other measures; *in reproductive years* curettage should be performed but may be postponed for not more than 3 months, provided there is no abnormality on examination; *in the perimenopause* it is mandatory and must be performed without delay in every patient.

Curettage must be performed in the second half of the cycle and preferably 5–6 days before menstruation. Only at this stage can failure of ovulation, the response of the endometrium to progesterone and oestrogen, and tuberculous endometritis be diagnosed. Curettage *at the time of the bleeding* also has a place. Apart from arresting haemorrhage, it is of value diagnostically. 'Irregular shedding' of the endometrium in particular can be diagnosed only when curettage is performed on the 4th or 5th day of bleeding.

Formal dilatation and curettage and examination under general anaesthesia is desirable in all cases of abnormal uterine bleeding to enable a thorough examination to be carried out to exclude organic disease. Endometrial biopsy can be carried out as an office procedure and some gynaecologists feel this is adequate unless bleeding is recurrent or persistent.

Haematological investigations

All cases of DUB must have a haemoglobin estimation and appropriate investigation of anaemia if present. Patients with persistent and unexplained DUB should have a blood smear, platelet count, bleeding time and tourniquet test to exclude idiopathic thrombocytopenic purpura or other haemotological cause for the bleeding.

Gynaecological endocrine investigations

Gynaecological endocrine investigations have a limited use in DUB. Basal body temperature charts, vaginal smears and examination of the cervical mucus have all been advocated in the past but have been replaced by either endometrial biopsy or by the estimation of plasma progesterone on the 21st day of the cycle. These will indicate whether ovulation has occurred and whether there is corpus luteum insufficiency.

Other endocrine investigations

Tests of thyroid and adrenal function are indicated in all cases where there is clinical suspicion of associated endocrine disease. Tests of pituitary function and X-ray of the skull may be indicated in cases of DUB associated with oligomenorrhoea, particularly when this is of sudden onset and has occurred for no apparent reason.

Other gynaecological investigations: hysteroscopy, hystero-salpingogram, laparoscopy

It is sometimes difficult to exclude an organic gynae-cological lesion, particularly when it is not readily accessible to pelvic examination or uterine curettage. In all cases of presumed DUB which fail to resolve or to respond to treatment it is important to question the diagnosis, re-examine the patient and repeat the uterine curettage. Gynaecological procedures including hysteroscopy, hysterosalpingography and laparoscopy may then be of value in detecting diseases which otherwise might be missed. Hysterosalpingography and laparoscopy are alternative procedures when hysteroscopy is not available and may be of considerable value in the diagnosis of uterine polypi (particularly small single fibroid polyps) and malformations of the uterus, both of which may be easily overlooked on curettage. Laparoscopy is useful in the diagnosis of endometriosis, pelvic inflammation and unsuspected ovarian tumours and should be performed in all obscure cases of uterine bleeding, particularly when this is accompanied by pain.

Routine screening investigations

Routine screening investigations, such as blood pressure measurement, breast examination, cervical smear and urine testing should be performed in all women.

Management of dysfunctional uterine bleeding

Three principles should be borne in mind: it is essential to exclude organic disease, if necessary by repeated examination and special investigations; it is desirable to make a positive diagnosis of the likely functional defect underlying the dysfunctional bleeding; treatment should be individualized according to (a) age, parity, emotional and social background of patient, (b) the severity, pattern and duration of the bleeding and the general disturbance of the patient, (c) the nature of the underlying defect, the prognosis and the likelihood of organic disease.

The main measures available in the management of DUB are uterine curettage, conservative therapy including steroid hormones, prostaglandin synthetase inhibitors and antifibrinolytic agents, and radical therapy, which is now almost exclusively hysterectomy. A general strategy of management is set out in Table 43.5.

GENERAL MEASURES

Explanation of the situation and reassurance of the patient is one of the most important initial steps, particularly in adolescents. A useful measure if the exact nature and amount of the bleeding pattern is in doubt is to ask the patient to keep a detailed menstrual calendar with a precise record of the amount of menstrual or other blood loss for 2 or 3 months.

Age	Dilatation and curettage	Hormone and anti-fibrinolytic therapy	Hysterectomy
20 and under	*Only* if bleeding persists or is severe	*Whenever indicated*, e.g. excessive bleeding	*Never* (or almost never)
20–40	*Always*, but may be deferred (up to 3 months) if bleeding moderate, regular, and there is no suspicion of organic disease	*First resort* after dilatation and curettage	*Seldom*, only if bleeding is persistent or severe after dilatation and curettage and hormone therapy
40 and over	*Mandatory* in all cases	*Only after dilatation and curettage*, in absence of organic disease	*First resort* if bleeding is persistent after dilatation and curettage and hormone therapy

Table 43.5. Strategy of management of dysfunctional uterine bleeding.

Many episodes of DUB will resolve spontaneously and no specific treatment will be required. In those cases which persist, the menstrual calendar will provide a precise and accurate record on which to base treatment. On rare occasions the patient with DUB is exsanguinated and may require blood transfusion. If any generalized endocrine or systemic disease is suggested on clinical grounds this must be immediately investigated.

The possible therapeutic effect of uterine curettage in dysfunctional uterine bleeding has been much discussed. During episodes of profuse bleeding curettage may help to arrest the haemorrhage, probably by removing the necrotic areas of endometrium. Nillson and Rybo (1971) and Haynes *et al.* (1977) found that curettage reduces the amount of blood loss at the next menstrual period but has no effect on subsequent blood loss. Apart from these immediate benefits, it has no other therapeutic effect, and curettage should be regarded essentially as a diagnostic procedure.

CONSERVATIVE THERAPY

Hormone therapy
Oestrogens are rarely used by themselves except to arrest haemorrhage in cases of severe DUB. On discontinuing treatment they produce an oestrogen withdrawal bleeding which is itself often prolonged or excessive. They are however effective as an emergency measure in controlling severe bleeding by promoting regeneration of the endometrium but must be given in large doses e.g. conjugated equine oestrogens 25 mg i.v. This may be repeated but should be followed by cyclical oestrogen/progestogen preferably with an oestrogen dominant combination such as 'Lyndiol' (Organon).

The introduction of potent orally active *progestogens* has revolutionized the treatment of DUB. Unlike oestrogens, the different synthetic progestational agents have different effects. In particular, the 19 nortestosterone derivatives have an androgenic effect and appear to be more effective in controlling DUB. Most of the compounds are only available in formulations for oral contraception when they are combined with ethinyl oestradiol or mestranol.

Progestational agents are used in three ways in the treatment of DUB: *to arrest haemorrhage; cyclically throughout menstrual cycle* (5th to 25th day); *cyclically in second half of cycle* (20th to 25th day).
The use of progestogens to arrest haemorrhage. The most generally accepted regime for the arrest of haemorrhage is to give a 19-nortestosterone derivative such as norethisterone without added oestrogen (Norlutin A, Parke-Davis, Primolut-N, Schering) 20–30 mg daily for 3 days or until the bleeding stops, which it usually does within 24–48 hours.

The patient should be warned that a withdrawal bleeding will occur 2–4 days after cessation of treatment but this will stop of its own accord after 4 days or so. Kistner (1969a) recommended that cyclical progestogen therapy should be commenced on the 4th or 5th day of withdrawal flow. If endometrial biopsy has shown endometrium of a simple proliferative nature, cyclical progestogen therapy should be continued for at least 3 months. If the biopsy has shown endometrial hyperplasia or anaplasia, however, Kistner deems it advisable to continue cyclical therapy for 9 months to 1 year and then to perform uterine curettage. Other authors prefer to arrest the haemorrhage and then await events and to institute cyclical progestogen therapy only if there is further abnormal bleeding.

Cyclical progestogen therapy in dysfunctional uterine bleeding (5th to 25th day). In *ovulatory bleeding* with polymenorrhoea and menorrhagia, normal cycles may be produced by giving 19-nortestosterone derivatives with oestrogens from the 5th to the 25th day of the cycle, according to the usual regime adopted for contraception. This treatment is continued for 3 cycles. On discontinuing treatment normal menstruation resumes in the majority of cases due to the 'rebound phenomenon with restoration of a normally functioning pituitary-ovarian-endometrial axis'.

As many types of ovulatory bleeding were at one time thought to be due to a defective corpus luteum, it might be expected that cyclical progestogen therapy in the second half of the cycle would produce normal menstruation. Klopper (1962) and Kistner (1969b), however, found that if treatment is given only during the 7–10 days before the next expected period benefit is unlikely to occur. To control menstrual bleeding it is necessary to give progestogen from the 5th to the 25th day and to inhibit ovulation. According to Klopper (1962) the main action of the 19-nortestosterone derivatives is to suppress the pituitary and ovarian function and the endogenous production of ovarian steroids.

Anovulatory bleeding may be acyclical and is sometimes excessive, and measures such as dilatation and curettage or progestational therapy may be required to arrest the haemorrhage, as previously discussed. In adolescents and younger women of childbearing age every endeavour should be made to find the cause of anovulation and to institute appropriate treatment. If no cause is found the excessive bleeding may be controlled by cyclical progestogen therapy for 2–3 months. In cases of endometrial hyperplasia cyclical progestogen therapy should be continued for 9 months to 1 year, when repeat curettage should be performed.

Prolonged progestational therapy causes regression of benign cystic adenomatous and atypical endometrial hyperplasia and may obviate the need for hysterectomy, particularly in the younger patient. Many gynaecologists nevertheless prefer abdominal hysterectomy in such cases, particularly in the premenopausal patient, because of the very small risk of progression to invasive carcinoma.

Cyclical progestogen therapy in dysfunctional uterine bleeding in second half of cycle. Administration of progestogens in the second half of the cycle has found relatively little place in the treatment of DUB. One specific indication is of premenstrual staining which may be associated with 'irregular ripening' or 'progestationally immature' endometrium. In these cases 19-nortestosterone derivatives, with or without oestrogen, should be given from the 20th to the 25th day and repeated for three or more cycles. This treatment has the advantage or disadvantage of not suppressing ovulation.

Androgens and Danazol

Androgens have been used extensively in the treatment of DUB in the past and are an effective form of treatment. Because of the fear of masculinization most gynaecologists now prefer to use one of the new progestogens. Some gynaecologists, such as Israel (1967), have claimed there is still a place for androgens in the treatment of DUB, particularly in the premenopausal woman. Methyltestosterone is given 10 mg daily, either for 7 days preceding menstruation in cyclical menorrhagia or in 15-day courses with 10-day rest periods in acyclical bleeding.

Another agent in the treatment of DUB is the drug Danazol (Ladogar, Winthrop) which is an isoxazol derivative of 17-α-ethinyl-testosterone and has a pure progestogenic action. It is effective in reducing menstrual loss and has the advantage over oestrogen–progestogen of not producing any change in blood coagulation (Chimbira et al. 1979). Chimbira et al. (1980b) investigated various dosage regimes and found that the continuous administration of 200 mg daily for 12 weeks reduced the mean menstrual blood loss in 16 women from a pretreatment level of 183 ml to 38 ml in the first month and 26 ml in the second month. The majority of women had regular episodes of bleeding with no alteration in cycle length, but a reduction in the number of days of bleeding, and 14 patients had marked relief of dysmenorrhoea. Danazol had no effect when given cyclically in the early follicular and luteal phases of the cycle. The reduction of menstrual blood loss in this series appeared to be significantly greater than the 53% reduction achieved with the combined oestrogen and progestogen pill and the 74% reduction achieved by the antifibrinolytic agent epsilon aminocaproic acid. Danazol is, however, expensive and has side effects of weight gain, muscle cramp and skin rashes, though these were minimal with the dosage regime used. Danazol 200 mg daily continuously appears to be a useful agent for the treatment of DUB, particularly in patients in whom oestrogen and progestogen combinations are contraindicated or ineffective.

Prostaglandin synthetase inhibitors

New promising agents in the treatment of DUB are the prostaglandin synthetase inhibitors e.g. flufenamic acid and mefenamic acid (Ponstan, Parke-Davis). Anderson et al. (1976) originally showed, in 6 patients with menorrhagia, that mefenamic acid significantly reduced menstrual blood loss. Jakubowicz and Wood (1978) also showed that mefenamic acid significantly reduced the number of sanitary pads and tampons needed by women with menorrhagia. More recently, Haynes et al. (1980b) treated 22 women with unexplained heavy menstrual blood loss with mefenamic acid and showed a reduction in median loss from 137 ml before treatment to 76 ml after treatment. The reduction in menstrual loss varied from 2–78% in different patients and the women with the highest blood loss showed the greatest reduction on treatment. The fact that patients with the heaviest loss responded dramatically whereas others did not respond at all suggests that there was more than one mechanism responsible for the menorrhagia in the different patients. Prostaglandin synthetase inhibitors are clinically useful drugs particularly in patients in whom oestrogen and progestogen combinations are contraindicated or are ineffective.

Antifibrinolytic agents

The use of antifibrinolytic agents in the treatment of DUB appears to have been neglected. Nilsson and Rybo (1971) reported on a study of 215 menorrhagic women treated with curettage, a uterus-contracting agent (methylergobaseinmaleate), ovulation inhibi-

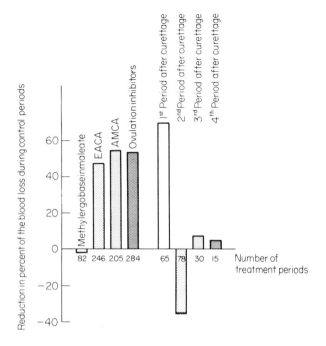

Fig. 43.7. The effect of various treatments of menorrhagia (Nilsson & Rybo 1971).

tors (combined contraceptive pills) and the antifibrinolytic agents, epsilonaminocaproic acid (EACA) and tranexamic acid (AMCA). They found that the percentage of patients whose menstrual blood loss was 'normalized' (not exceeding 80 ml) was about 50% with oral contraceptives, EACA and AMCA, whereas with methylergobaseinmaleate the blood loss was unchanged (Fig. 43.7).

After long term treatment with EACA for an average of 15 months, 3 out of 10 women had a blood loss of less than 80 ml per period. After long term treatment with oral contraceptives for an average of 22.5 months, 7 out of 21 women had a blood loss of less than 80 ml per period. On discontinuing treatment, however, the majority of women in both series showed no continuing benefit. The recommended dose of AMCA (Cyclokapron-Kambi) is 1 g four times daily for the first 4 days of the period, though Nilsson and Rybo (1971) used a slightly larger dose initially and continued treatment for up to 7 days.

Summary of conservative therapy
Antifibrinolytic agents EACA and AMCA and anti-prostaglandin agents such as mefenamic acid and flufenamic acid are an effective treatment for DUB and are as effective as the oestrogen–progestogen oral contraceptives. It is probable, however, that neither treatment cures the fundamental defect causing the bleeding, as the menorrhagia returns as soon as

treatment is discontinued, though a significant proportion of patients will undergo spontaneous cure.

The choice of agent is dependent upon several factors. *If contraception is desired* when combined oestrogen–progestogen oral contraceptives would be indicated; *if pregnancy is desired* when anti-prostaglandins and anti-fibrinolytics would be indicated. *If atrophic endometrium* is present then an oestrogen dominant oestrogen–progestogen combination is indicated; *if proliferation or hyperplastic endometrium* is present in 2nd half of cycle then a progestogen dominant oestrogen–progestogen combination is indicated; *if normal secretory endometrium is present* then a prostaglandin synthetase inhibitor or anti-fibrinolytic inhibitor is indicated.

As the primary endometrial defect in DUB in the absence of an ovulatory abnormality would appear to be an excessive formation of prostaglandin E2 and F2α and of thromboxane and prostacyclin, then an anti-prostaglandin agent such as mefenamic acid would appear to be the treatment of choice. This would particularly apply if there is associated primary dysmenorrhoea. Antifibrinolytic therapy such as AMCA is effective but relatively expensive and is perhaps best reserved as a second line drug to be given either with, or instead of, the prostaglandin synthetase inhibitors.

RADICAL THERAPY

Examination under anaesthesia, dilatation of the cervix and curettage of the uterus are essential to exclude both extra and intrauterine pelvic disease and to establish a diagnosis of DUB. Curettage is performed primarily to detect such conditions as endometrial polyps, hyperplasia or carcinoma. It also enables a sample of endometrium to be obtained for histological examination to determine the functional state of the endometrium (proliferative, secretory or hyperplastic) which may be of assistance in the management of DUB. Curettage however is essentially a blind procedure and has a number of drawbacks namely: some pathological conditions, including quite large polyps, may be missed even on repeat curettage; a patchy endometrial lesion may be missed; it is also not possible to make a positive diagnosis of conditions such as atrophic endometrium with dilated subendothelial venules or to identify the exact site of the bleeding in the uterus.

Hysteroscopy should obviate most of these difficulties. It is not a new procedure but progressive improvements in instrumentation have now made it a technique which is simple and easy to perform and a procedure in which every gynaecologist should be skilled. The advantage of hysteroscopy is that the whole endometrial cavity can be visualized in detail and any pathology including atrophic changes in the endometrium can be diagnosed. It is therefore advocated that all patients with abnormal uterine bleeding and on whom dilatation and curettage is indicated should also have hysteroscopy. This may be a 'policy of perfection' because of lack of instruments and suitably trained personnel but it nevertheless is a goal to be aimed at. It should be emphasized that hysteroscopy is a complementary procedure and does not substitute for histological examination of any material removed by curettage or endometrial biopsy.

Hysterectomy

The place of hysterectomy in the treatment of DUB depends upon the age and parity of the patient. *In younger women* of childbearing age it should be a last resort. The need to preserve reproductive function and to avoid a psychologically mutilating operation is paramount. The possibility of remission of symptoms for up to 10 years from the onset on the dysfunctional bleeding (Southam & Richart 1966) more than justifies an ultraconservative approach. *In women in their 'thirties'* it should be performed with reluctance and only after full investigation and failure of conservative therapy. It may however be considered in women who have completed their families and much will depend upon the wishes of the patient. *In 'older' women* hysterectomy should be considered in all cases of persistent or recurrent bleeding. In this age group the uterus is of less importance in psychological terms and hysterectomy is the treatment of choice in all cases where bleeding is persistent or severe. Though spontaneous cure may occur with the menopause, the possibility of a malignant or other organic lesion which may have been overlooked or may develop in the future fully justifies the operation in all cases of persistent DUB.

Radiotherapy

Radiotherapy has a small place in the treatment of DUB, primarily in women over 40 who are unfit for operation. Its advantages are that it is free of immediate risk, it causes little disturbance to the patient, and it is effective in producing amenorrhoea in 95–99% of cases. Its disadvantages are several. Operation is not completely avoided because it is essential to perform a D and C in all cases to exclude malignancy. The method is not without side effects and complications; Doll and Smith (1968) in the long term follow-up of 2068 patients with metropathia haemorrhagica and other benign gynaecological disease, treated by various forms of radiation over 20 years, found that there was a fourfold increase in leukaemia in these patients and an excess of cancer of the various organs in the heavily radiated areas. The procedure leaves a damaged organ which may develop haematometrà, pyometra or carcinoma. Corscaden *et al.* (1946) and Turnbull (1956) report an incidence of carcinoma of the cervix and endometrium of 1.5% in patients treated with radium or X-rays for benign uterine bleeding. It does not permit organic disease to be excluded with the same certainty as hysterectomy. Ovarian function is always suppressed and menopausal symptoms are common. In women under 40 years of age amenorrhoea may not be permanent and menstruation and ovulation may recommence after 1–2 years.

In most cases the disadvantages associated with radiotherapy heavily outweigh the advantages. Where radiotherapy is decided upon, external irradiation to the ovaries is now considered preferable to radium insertion because the dose of radiation to the various pelvic tissues can be more closely controlled and because of the lower incidence of serious side effects, such as radiation, cystitis and proctitis, and of complications such as radium burns.

Summary

DUB is not one disease but a category of diseases. The dysfunction underlying the abnormal bleeding is unknown, though it is widely believed to be due to a defect in ovulation and oestrogen and progesterone secretion. Recent work suggests that at least some, if not the majority, of cases are associated with some local endometrial dysfunction, possibly related to the excessive formation of prostaglandin E2, or prostacyclin. Diagnosis is by exclusion with curettage or endometrial sample and hysteroscopy to eliminate organic gynaecological disease. Anaemia and any obvious cause must be treated. Treatment of DUB in women of reproductive years is by observation to await spontaneous cure or combined oestrogen–progestogen, antiprostaglandin or antifibrinolytic therapy. Once a family is complete, hysterectomy with conservation of ovaries is indicated in persistent bleeding. Radiotherapy has a very small, if any, place in modern treatment.

REFERENCES

ANDERSON A.B.M., HAYNES P.J., GUILLEBAUD J. & TURNBULL A.C. (1976) Lancet, i, 774.

BELLER F.K. (1971) Amer. J. Obstet. Gynec., 111, 535.

BENSO R.C. & DAILEY M.E. (1955) Surg. Gynec. Obstet., 100, 19.

BOSHIER D.P. & LIGGINS G.C. (1974) Proceedings of the Fifth Asia Oceania Congress of Endocrinology, p. 18. The Endocrine Society of India, Clandrigah.

CHIMBIRA T.H., ANDERSON A.B.M. & TURNBULL A.C. (1980a) Brit. J. Obstet. Gynaec., 87, 610.

CHIMBIRA T.H., COPE E., ANDERSO A.B.M. & BOULTON F.G. (1979) Brit. J. Obstet. Gynaec., 86, 46.

CHIMBIRA T.H., ANDERSON A.B.M., NAISH C., COPE E. & TURNBULL A.C. (1980b) Brit. J. Obstet. Gynaec., 87, 1152.

CHRISTIAENS G.C.M.L., SIXMA J.J. & HASPELS A.A. (1982) Obstet. Gynecol. Surv., 37, 281.

CORSCADEN J.A., FERTIG J.W. & GUSBERG S.B. (1946) Amer. J. Obstet. Gynec., 51, 1.

DALLENBACH-HELLWEG G. (1980) In Endometrial Bleeding and Steroidal Contraception (Diczfalusy E., Fraser I.S. & Webb F.T.G. eds) p. 153. Pitman, London.

DICZFALUSY E., FRASER I.S. & WEBB F.T.G. (1980) Endometrial Bleeding and Steroidal Contraception. Pitman, London.

DIDDLE A.W. (1948) Amer. J. Obstet. Gynec., 56, 537.

DOLL R. & SMITH P.G. (1968) Brit. J. Radiol., 41, 362.

DRIESSEN L.F. (1914) Zbl. Gynäk., 38, 618.

FLOWER R.J. (1977) In The Fetus and Birth. Ciba Foundation Symposium n.s. No. 47. p. 297. Excerpta Medica, Elsevier, North Holland, Amsterdam.

FOWLER W.M. & BARER P.A. (1942) J. Amer. med. Ass., 118, 421.

GOLDSMITH R.E., STURGIS S.H., LERMAN J. & STANBURY J.B. (1952) J. clin. Endocrin., 12, 846.

GRANESTROM E., SWAHN M.-L. & LUNDSTROM V. (1983) Acta Obstet. Gynecol. Scand. Suppl., 113, 91.

GRAY R.H. (1980) In Endometrial Bleeding and Steroidal Contraception (Diczfalusy E., Fraser I.S. & Webb F.T.G. eds.) p. 14. Pitman, London.

GRIEVES S.A. & LIGGINS G.C. (1976) Prostaglandins, 112, 229.

GUILLEBAUD J. & BONAR J. (1978) Brit. J. Obstet. Gynaec., 85, 707.

GUILLEBAUD J., BONNAR J., MOREHEAD J. & MATTHEWS A. (1976) Lancet, i, 387.

GUILLEBAUD J., ANDERSON A.B.M. & TURNBULL A.C. (1978) Brit. J. Obstet. Gynaec., 85, 53.

HALLBERG L., HOGDAHL A., NILSSON L. & RYBO G. (1966) Acta. Obstet. Gynecol. Scand., 45, 320.

HAYNES P.J., ANDERSON A.B.M. & TURNBULL A.C. (1980a) Proceedings of 22nd British Congress of Obstetrics and Gynaecology. Royal College of Obstetricians and Gynaecologists, London.

HAYNES P.J., FLINT A.P.E., HODGSON H., ANDERSON A.B.M., DRAY F. & TURNBULL A.C. (1980b) Int. J. Obstet. Gynec., 17, 567.

HAYNES P.J., HODGSON H., ANDERSON A.B.M. & TURNBULL A.C. (1977) Brit. J. Obstet. Gynaec., 84, 763.

HENZL M.R., SMITH R.E., BOOST G. & TYLER E.T. (1972) J. clin. Endocriniol. Metab., 34, 860.

HOLMSTROM E.G. & McCLENNAN C.E. (1947) Amer. J. Obstet. Gynec., 53, 727.

ISRAEL S.L. (1967) Menstrual Disorders and Sterility, 5e., p. 388. Hoeber, New York.

JACOBS A. & BUTLER E.B. (1965) Lancet, ii, 407.

JACOBS W.M., LEAZER M.A. & LINDLEY J.E. (1957) Obstet. Gynec., N.Y., 10, 274.

JAKUBOWICZ D.L. & WOOD C. (1978) Aust. N.Z. J. Obstet. Gynec., 18, 135.

KISTNER R.W. (1964a) Gynecology, Principles and Practice, p. 238. Year Book Publishers, Chicago.

KISTNER R.W. (1964b) Gynecology, Principles and Practice, p. 278. Year Book Publishers, Chicago.

KISTNER R.W. (1969a) Progestins in Obstetrics and Gynecology, p. 44. Year Book Publishers, Chicago.

KISTNER R.W. (1969b) Progestins in Obstetrics and Gynecology, p. 45. Year Book Publishers, Chicago.

KLOPPER A. (1962) Proc. roy. Soc. Med., 55, 865.

KURZOR R., WILSON L. & BIRNBERG C.H. (1953) Fertil. Steril., 4, 479.

McKELVEY J.L. & SAMUELS L.T. (1947) Amer. J. Obstet. Gynec., 53, 627.

MARKEE J.E. (1950) In Progress in Gynecology (Meigs J.V. & Sturgis S.H. eds) Vol 2. Grune and Stratton, New York.

MAQUEO M. (1980) In Endometrial Bleeding and Steroidal Contraception, (Diczfalusy E., Fraser I.S. & Webb F.T.G. eds) p. 138. Pitman, London.

NEDOSS B.R. (1971) Amer. J. Obstet. Gnec., 109, 103.

Nilsson L. & Rybo G. (1971) *Amer. J. Obstet. Gynec.*, **110**, 713.

Novak E. R., Jones G. S. & Jones H. W. (1971) *Novak's Textbook of Gynecology*, 8th ed., p 319, Williams & Wilkins, Baltimore.

Ober W. B. (1966) *J. clin. Pathol.* **19**, 138.

Ober W. B. (1970) *Acta. Cytol. (Baltimore)*, **14**, 156.

Ober W. B. & Labay G. R. (1972) *Obstet. Gynecol. Ann.*, 373.

Quick A. J. (1966) *Obstet. Gynec., N.Y.*, **28**, 37.

Schroeder R. (1954) *Amer. J. Obstet. Gynec.*, **68**, 294.

Schultz F. M., Schwarz B. E., MacDonald P. C. & Johnston J. M. (1975) *Amer. J. Obstet. Gynec.*, **123**, 650.

Scott J. C. & Mussey E. (1964) *Amer. J. Obstet. Gynec.*, **90**, 161.

Simpson J. L. & Christakos A. C. (1969) *Obstet. Gynec. Surv.*, **24**, 580.

Smith S. K., Abel M. H., Kelly R. W. & Baird D. T. (1981) *Brit. J. Obstet. Gynaecol.*, **88**, 434.

Southam A. L. & Richart R. M. (1966) *Amer. J. Obstet. Gynec.*, **94**, 637.

Sutherland A. M. (1949) *Glasg. med. J.*, **30**, 303.

Sutherland A. M. (1953) *Glasg. med. J.*, **34**, 496.

Taymor M. L., Sturgis S. H. & Vonica C. (1964) *J. Amer. med. Ass.*, **187**, 323.

Traut H. F. & Kuder A. (1935) *Surg. Gynec. Obstet.*, **61**, 145.

Turnbull A. C. (1956) *J. Obstet. Gynaec. Brit. Emp.*, **63**, 179.

Vollman R. F. (1977) *Major Problems in Obstetrics and Gynecology*, Vol. 7. W. B. Saunders, Philadelphia.

Vorys N. & Neri A. S. (1968) In *Textbook of Gynecologic Endocrinology* (Gold J. J. ed.). Hoeber, New York.

Willman E. A., Collins W. P. & Clayton S. G. (1976) *Brit. J. Obstet. Gynaec.*, **83**, 337.

Zondek B. (1954) *Amer. J. Obstet. Gynec.*, **68**, 310.

CHAPTER 44
THE MENOPAUSE AND CLIMACTERIC

D. A. DAVEY

INTRODUCTION

The terms menopause, climacteric, pre-, peri- and postmenopause are often used interchangeably but strictly apply to different stages at the end of reproductive life in the human female. Menopause is derived from the Greek *men* 'month' and *pauo* 'to stop' and means the cessation of menstruation. The climacteric is derived from the Greek *klimakter*, 'rung of the ladder' meaning critical period of life. The climacteric is the equivalent of the perimenopause which may start 5–10 years before the menopause and continue up to 5 or 10 years afterwards. Pre-, peri- and postmenopause apply respectively to the periods immediately before, around and after the cessation of menstruation. This chapter deals with the whole period from the initial changes in ovarian-hypothalamic-pituitary function which precede the menopause to advanced age or postmenopause when the pathological and other consequences of the menopause may become manifest.

The human female is one of the few females of any species in whom reproduction ceases because of exhaustion of the oocytes in the ovary before the end of the natural life span. The only other species are certain strains of mice, designated CBA and DBA, who have also been shown to be non-reproductive for about half of their lives due to the depletion of the oocytes in their ovaries. With increasing age, virtually all animals have a decrease in fertility and a decrease in litter size but they remain in permanent low oestrus with continuing secretion of oestrogens to the end of their lives (Jones 1975). The decline in fertility in most animals is due to hypothalamic-pituitary dysfunction rather than to ovarian failure as occurs in CBA mice and in man. The menopause and postmenopause as seen in the human female is an almost unique biological phenomenon.

The number of women experiencing and living beyond the menopause has increased slowly over the centuries with the progressive increase in life expectancy. The average span of life in Roman times is believed to have been about 25 years. In the Elizabethan era the average life expectancy was 40 years and it has been estimated that at this time only 25% of women lived to experience the menopause. It was not until the present century that the average expectation of life reached about 50 years. Since 1900, however, the life expectancy has rapidly increased and is now approaching 75 years for females in developed countries. It may even reach 80 years by the year 2000 (Fig. 44.1). In contemporary developed countries approximately 95% of women live to experience the menopause, 50–60% achieve the age of 75 years and a third or more of all women are peri- or postmenopausal.

Contrary to beliefs that the age of the menopause is increasing, Amundsen and Diers (1973), who reviewed medieval records from the 6th to the 15th centuries, found that the average age of the menopause has remained remarkably constant at about 50 years. The median age of the menopause in a

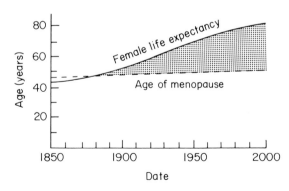

Fig. 44.1. Female life expectancy compared with age of menopause, 1850 to 2000 AD (from Beard 1975).

survey carried out in London in 1970 was 50.8 years (McKinley *et al.* 1972) and the figure of 50–51 years for the median or modal age is very similar in many different studies carried out at different periods and in different communities throughout the world (Frommer 1964). The age of the menopause does not appear to depend on socio-economic conditions, race, parity, height, weight or skinfold thickness (MacMahon, & Worcester 1966), though smokers may have an earlier natural menopause than non-smokers by on average 1–2 years (Jick *et al.* 1977). The constancy of the age of the menopause is in contrast to the age of the menarche, which is falling and is significantly affected by nutrition and socio-economic conditions (Flint 1976).

AETIOLOGY

The menopause and climacteric are primarily due to exhaustion of the stock of primordial follicles or oocytes in the ovary and the consequent fall in oestrogen and progesterone secretion. The ovaries of the human female at birth contain a maximum complement of primordial follicles which Hertig (1944) described as 'the ovarian capital' because the number of follicles is not added to or replaced during reproductive life. The menopause results from the progressive depletion of the follicles in the ovary starting at birth and continuing through prepubertal and reproductive life until the stock is eventually exhausted.

In a remarkable study, Bloch (1953) obtained ovaries postmortem from 150 females aged between 6 and 44 years who died a sudden death and had not been pregnant for up to one year beforehand (Table 44.1). He showed that the total number of primordial follicles in each pair of ovaries at birth is in the order of 750000 and that the number decreases to approximately 484000 in girls aged 6 to 9 years, to 155000 in those aged 18 to 24 years, to 74000 in

women between 32 and 38 years and to 8300 in women in their early forties. The two natural processes which reduce the number of oocytes are atresia and ovulation and, of these, ovulation *per se* accounts for a very small proportion of the loss. It has been calculated that for each single ovum shed an average of 1000 ovarian follicles commence development in each menstrual cycle and eventually become corpora atretica. In humans repeated pregnancy and suppression of ovulation by steroidal hormone contraceptives surprisingly have no obvious effect on the rate of decrease in oocyte number or on the age of the menopause. In mice the only known procedures which decrease the rate of oocyte decline are hypophysectomy and calorie restriction (Jones & Krohn 1961).

Endocrinology of the menopause and climacteric

Although ovarian follicular depletion is the primary cause of the menopause, the endocrine changes at the climacteric are not simply a matter of decreased or absent oestrogen secretion. Equally important is the decreased or absent secretion of progesterone and the compensatory hyperactivity of the hypothalamus and pituitary. After the menopause the ovarian stroma continues to secrete androgens, as does the adrenal cortex which also secretes other hormones which may be converted into oestrogens so that postmenopausal women are not necessarily oestrogen deficient. Changes in other ovarian, pituitary and hypothalamic hormones and neurotransmitters such as inhibin, prolactin and catecholoestrogens may also be involved in the endocrine changes at the climacteric though their role is poorly understood. The endocrine changes at the climacteric have been the subject of extensive investigations and have been reviewed by Asch and Greenblatt (1977), Mills and Mahesh (1977), Anderson (1979) and Utian (1980a). They may usefully be regarded as having three phases: (1)

		Number of primordial	
Number of females	Age in years	follicles	Range
5	6–9	484000	258000–755000
5	12–16	382000	85000–591000
7	18–24	155000	39000–290000
11	25–31	59000	8100–228000
8	32–38	74000	15000–208000
7	40–44	8300	350– 28000

Table 44.1. Influence on the number of primordial follicles in the human ovary (from Utian 1980, after Bloch 1952).

hypothalamic pituitary hyperactivity starting 5–10 years before and continuing after the menopause; (2) *ovulatory and corpus luteum failure* also starting 5–10 years before the menopause; (3) *ovarian follicular failure* starting at the menopause itself.

ENDOCRINE CHANGES BEFORE THE MENOPAUSE

The changes in ovarian function which result in the menopause in fact commence *in utero* as the number of oocytes in the fetal ovary is maximum at the 20th week of gestation. There is then a progressive depletion during the second half of intrauterine life, childhood and puberty and throughout the reproductive period. Not only does the total number of ovarian follicles decrease, however, but the oocytes that remain are those which are most resistant to stimulation by gonadotrophins. In the early reproductive years the normal feedback mechanisms of the hypothalamus and pituitary are usually more than suffi-

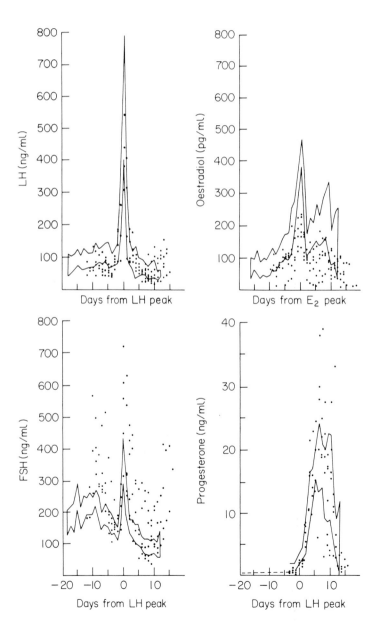

Fig. 44.2. Serum FSH, LH, oestradiol and progesterone in eight cycles in women 46–56 years old compared with mean ± 2 s.e.m. in ten cycles in women 18–30 years old (from Sherman *et al.* 1976).

cient to compensate for any increase in the resistance of the follicles to stimulation by gonadotrophins and to ensure regular ovulation, normal corpus luteum formation and a regular menstrual cycle. From about the age of 35 years onwards, however, follicular development tends to become progressively more deficient, and in the last 5–15 years of reproductive life the proportion of anovulatory cycles increases and the menstrual cycle may become irregular with unduly long or short cycles (Treloar et al. 1967). The incidence of anovulatory cycles as estimated from basal body temperature records by Doring (1969) increased from a range of 3–7% in women aged 26–40 years, to a range of 12–15% in those aged 41–50 years, and Sharman (1966) estimated the total incidence of anovulatory cycles in women over 40 years to be 25%. Doring (1969) further noted that the incidence of menstrual cycles with short luteal phases increased from 18% in women aged 40–45, to 36% in those aged 45–50. As a woman approaches the menopause one of the first changes in ovarian function is thus either a failure in ovulation or deficient corpus luteum formation, and the first hormone to become deficient or absent at the climacteric is progesterone.

In the years preceding the menopause the main oestrogen is oestradiol (E_2), which is secreted by the ovary, and is produced cyclically with low levels in the early follicular phase, a main peak in the late follicular phase, and a second peak in the luteal phase. Oestrone (E_1) is produced both cyclically by the ovary and continuously by the peripheral conversion of androstenedione. The early cross-sectional studies of plasma oestrogens and progestogens in menstruating women of different age groups did not show any change with increasing age or in women approaching the menopause (England et al. 1974), Reyes et al. 1977). Longitudinal studies, however, by Sherman and Korenman (1975) and Sherman et al. (1976), in which daily blood samples were taken from several premenopausal women aged 46–56 with regular menstrual cycles, showed that plasma oestradiol levels were lower and follicle stimulating hormone (FSH) levels higher than those in younger women at the same stage of the cycle (Fig. 44.2).

The reduction in plasma oestradiol in premenopausal women probably stimulates the negative feedback mechanism of the hypothalamus and pituitary (Sherman et al. 1976) causing the rise in FSH levels, which is the most characteristic feature of the endocrine changes at the climacteric and the first sign of approaching menopause. The rise in luteinizing hormone (LH) in general occurs later and is less marked than the rise in FSH, and LH levels are frequently normal in premenopausal women (Sherman et al. 1976). The rise in FSH levels may occur many years before the menopause and women of 34–39 years of age may have higher early follicular FSH levels than younger women (Fig. 44.3) (Reyes et al. 1977).

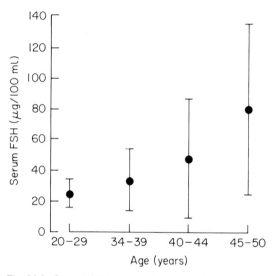

Fig. 44.3. Serum FSH concentrations (mean ± s.d.) during the early follicular phase of ovulatory menstrual cycles as a function of age (from Anderson 1979, after Reyes et al. 1977).

The same women may also have lower plasma progesterone levels in the luteal phase than the younger women (Fig. 44.4). The hyperactivity of the hypothalamic-pituitary axis initially compensates for the increasing resistance of the follicles to gonadotrophin stimulation and this first phase of the climacteric can be regarded as a state of compensated ovarian failure.

The second phase of the climacteric is the failure in ovulation or inadequate corpus luteum formation with absent or inadequate progesterone secretion. This results in unopposed oestrogen secretion (i.e. oestrogens unopposed by progestogens) which may give rise to dysfunctional uterine bleeding, endometrial hyperplasia and endometrial carcinima. As follicular development still occurs, even though ovulation and corpus luteum formation are defective, this second phase may be regarded as one of partial ovarian failure.

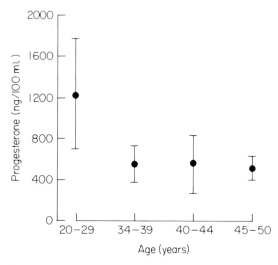

Fig. 44.4. Serum progesterone concentrations (mean ± s.d.) during the mid-luteal phase of ovulatory menstrual cycles as a function of age (from Anderson 1979, after Reyes *et al.* 1977).

ENDOCRINE CHANGES AT MENOPAUSE

The key change at the menopause itself is the failure of a sufficient number of ovarian follicles to develop and secrete enough oestrogens to produce endometrial growth with subsequent menstruation. This follicular failure may occur abruptly but, more commonly, it is a progressive process with fewer follicles developing, less oestrogen being secreted, less growth of the endometrium and decreased menstrual loss in succeeding menstrual cycles. Not infrequently follicular development and menstrual cycles become irregular with a prolonged follicular phase or shortened luteal

phase. A stage is however eventually reached in all women when in spite of the raised gonadotrophin levels and hypothalamic–pituitary hyperactivity too few ovarian follicles, which are sensitive to stimulation remain, and the menses then cease. Apart from the changes in levels of hormones, the cessation of menstruation, or menopause, also marks a change from cyclical to continuous hypothalamic, pituitary and ovarian function. The main steroid hormone changes at the menopause have been summarized by Utian (1980a) and are shown in Table 44.2.

ENDOCRINE CHANGES AFTER THE MENOPAUSE

Once a woman is postmenopausal the plasma oestradiol levels stay low although the plasma oestrone, androstenedione and testosterone remain unchanged, and may even increase. The extra-ovarian production of oestrone from androstenedione becomes the predominant source of oestrogens. Starting 5–10 years after the menopause, however, the plasma androstenedione and oestrone levels begin to fall, primarily due to a decrease in the ovarian secretion of androstenedione, so that postmenopausal women tend to become increasingly oestrogen deficient. At the same time plasma gonadotrophins begin to fall from their previous high levels and at this stage women may be regarded as truly postmenopausal.

Gonadotrophins
After the menopause the plasma levels of FSH and LH both rise, reaching a maximum in 2–3 years when the levels of FSH are increased approximately 13-fold and the levels of LH are increased 3-fold

Table 44.2. Serum sex steroid concentrations in μg/ml before and after spontaneous menopause and oophorectomy (from Utian 1980).

	Oestrone (E₁)	Oestradiol (E₂)	Oestriol (E₃)	Progesterone	Testosterone	Androstenedione
Premenopausal women						
Early follicular	25–50	25–75	7–8	100–500	200–400	1600–1750
Late follicular	150–200	200–600			300–800	1850–2000
Mid luteal	70–100	100–300	10–12		300–600	
Oophorectomy before menopause	20–40	15–25		50	75–150	600–1500
Postmenopausal women						
Spontaneous	20–40	9–15	6	100–200	200–300	600–900
Oophorectomy after menopause	20–40	9–15		100–200	100–150	500–800

above early proliferative phase premenopausal levels (Chakravarti *et al.* 1976). These levels are maintained for several years but, commencing 5–10 years after the menopause, also begin to decline and after 20–30 years may reach levels below those found in reproductive life (Fig. 44.5). The marked increase in

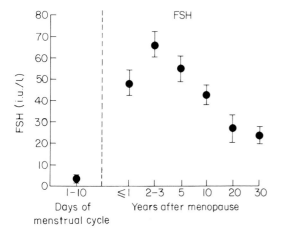

Fig. 44.5. Concentrations of plasma FSH (mean ± s.e.m.) as a function of age after the menopause compared with those in the first ten days of the menstrual cycle (from Chakavarti *et al.* 1976).

plasma levels in FSH and LH in the early postmenopause is not associated with any change in metabolic clearance of gonadotrophins so that the increase is directly due to increase in production rates by the pituitary (Saxena *et al.* 1969). Postmenopausally LH is released in pulses at the same frequency as in the follicular phase of the menstrual cycle (Anderson 1979). The amount of LH released with each pulse is, however, much greater than in the follicular phase and is similar to the amount released in the pulses occurring in the normal midcycle surge (Yen *et al.* 1972). The increased amount of LH released with each pulse was originally thought to be the result of an increased responsiveness of the pituitary. Seyler and Reichlin (1973), however, demonstrated an increase in luteinizing hormone releasing hormone (LHRH) activity in postmenopausal women and the increased LH and FSH secretion is almost certainly due to increased secretion of LHRH. With prolonged excessive secretion and with the course of time either the hypothalamus readjusts or the pituitary becomes exhausted so that commencing 5–10 years after the menopause the amount of gonadotrophin released progressively falls (Chakravarti *et al.* 1976).

Oestrogens

In postmenopausal women the average total urinary estrogen excretion is of the order of 5–6 µg/24 hr and is about one-half that of premenopausal women in the early follicular phase and one-tenth of that in the late follicular phase (Brown 1955). This level of excretion remains constant in the first 10 years of the postmenopause but later decreases markedly (Grattarola *et al.* 1975). In addition to the fall in the amount of oestrogen secreted there is an equally important change in the nature of the predominant circulating oestrogen from 17β-oestradiol premenopausally to oestrone postmenopausally. In the immediate postmenopausal period, plasma oestradiol levels are thus of the order of 10–15 µg/ml as compared with 25–75 µg/ml in the early follicular phase and 20–600 µg/ml in the late follicular phase in premenopausal women. Plasma oestrone levels in contrast are 25–50 µg/ml and are the same in postmenopausal women as in the early follicular phase, though less than in the late follicular phase when oestrone levels reach a peak of 150–200 µg/ml. The average production and clearance rates of steroid hormones have been summarized by Asch and Greenblatt (1977). In the case of oestrone the production rate is approximately 40 µg/24 hr after the menopause compared with 90–300 µg/24 hr before the menopause. The clearance of both hormones is decreased by about 25% after the menopause so that the plasma levels do not fall as much as the production rates. The ratio of plasma oestradiol/oestrone nevertheless shows a marked change from 0.67 during the follicular phase and 1.9 at ovulation to 0.42 postmenopausally. Oestrone is thus the predominant oestrogen in quantitative terms in postmenopausal women.

Following the pioneering work of MacDonald *et al.* (1967) many workers including Grodin *et al.* (1973) and Poortman *et al.* (1973) have shown that the major source of oestrogens in postmenopausal women is the peripheral conversion of androstenedione produced by the adrenal gland and by the ovary (Fig. 44.6). The aromatization of androstenedione to oestrone occurs in various peripheral extraglandular sites but mainly in adipose tissue and accounts for 98% of the total oestrone production in postmenopausal women. A small amount of oestradiol is produced by the peripheral conversion from testosterone, also mainly in body fat. Oestradiol may also be converted back into oestrone and oestrone sulphate, the latter being the major circulating oestrogen in postmenopausal women particularly after the oral ingestion of oestrogens (Anderson *et al.* 1978).

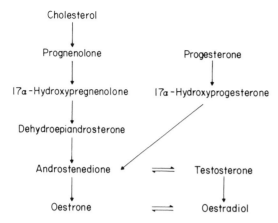

Fig. 44.6. Steroid biosynthetic pathways from androgen synthesis in the stroma of postmenopausal ovary (from Anderson 1979).

The average conversion rate of androstenedione to oestrone is 1.3%–2.5% which is sufficient to account for almost all of the total oestrone production rate of 40–50 μg/24 hr. The efficiency of conversion of androstenedione to oestrone, moreover, increases with increasing age and increasing obesity, the rate in women over 50 being 2–4 times greater than in women in their twenties (Hemsell *et al.* 1976, Rikzallah *et al.* 1975). In postmenopausal women the plasma levels of both oestrone and, to a lesser extent, oestradiol, correlate with body weight and excess body fat (Judd *et al.* 1976).

Although much work has been done on the changes in plasma levels of individual hormones at the climacteric, less attention has been paid to the overall hormonal status and end organ effects of these endocrine changes. Oestrone, which is the predominant oestrogen in postmenopausal women, has only one-tenth of the biological activity of oestradiol, both in terms of rat uterine weight gain (Velardo 1958) and of its affinity for oestrogen receptors in the pituitary and hypothalamus (Davies *et al.* 1975). In postmenopausal women the decrease in the oestrogenic biological activity is thus considerably greater than that suggested by the simple quantitative changes in plasma oestrogen levels and in total urinary oestrogen excretion. The examination of vaginal smears and of the various indices of maturation of the vaginal epithelium, such as the karyopynotic index, may provide some measure of the overall biological effect of oestrogens secreted. The use of vaginal smears in evaluating hormonal status in climacteric women has been studied by Wied and Bibbo (1975) and Ham-

mond (1977). In general there is a poor correlation between vaginal smear indices and the plasma and urinary oestrogen levels (Larsson-Cohn *et al.* 1978). Morse *et al.* (1979), however, have shown a highly significant correlation between the karyopynotic index and plasma oestradiol levels but no correlation with plasma oestrone levels. This ties in with a previous study by Hutton *et al.* (1978) in which it was found that postmenopausal women who complained of superficial dyspareunia had significantly lower plasma oestradiol levels but that the plasma oestrone levels were not significantly lower as compared with the levels in asymptomatic postmenopausal women. This suggests that in postmenopausal women the levels of oestradiol may be more important both biologically and clinically than the levels of plasma oestrone. The proportion of postmenopausal women with oestrogenic proliferative vaginal smears in different series varies from 9–50% which may depend upon the ages of the women in the groups studied. McLennan and McLennan (1971) thus found that the proportion of postmenopausal women with total absence of oestrogenic effect in vaginal smears increased from 14% under 50 years of age to 61% in patients over 75 years of age. It would appear that, at least in terms of the effect on the genital tract, the incidence of oestrogen deficiency is about 10–20% immediately postmenopausally and increases with increasing age and time after the menopause to at least 50–60%.

Androgens
After the menopause the ovary continues to secrete androgens, notably androstenedione, testosterone, dehydroepiandrosterone (DHA) and its sulphate (DHAS). In immediately postmenopausal women about 30% of the androstenedione is derived from the ovary and 70% from the adrenal, although the adrenal contribution tends to decrease with time. In the case of testosterone, 35% is derived from the ovary and 50% from the adrenal and a further 15% from the peripheral conversion of androstenedione (Fig. 44.7).

In postmenopausal women with intact ovaries the plasma levels of androstenedione and testosterone were moderately increased compared with younger premenopausal women in the follicular phase of the cycle (Longcope 1974). Following bilateral oophorectomy, the plasma androstenedione and plasma testosterone fall by about 50% in both pre- and postmenopausal women. The increased secretion of testosterone by the ovary combined with the de-

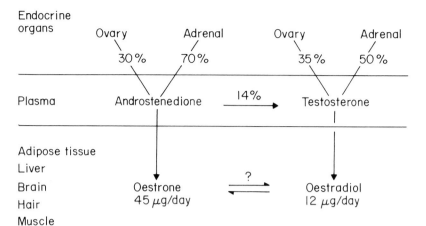

Fig. 44.7. Diagrammatic representation of the source of oestrogens in postmenopausal women (from Anderson 1979).

creased levels of oestrogens is thought to be responsible for the defeminization and hirsutism frequently seen in postmenopausal women (Sternberg 1949).

Progesterone

The plasma progesterone (P) and 17-hydroxyprogesterone (17 HOP) levels are considerably lower in postmenopausal women as compared with premenopausal women in the early follicular phase, falling from 31–19 μg/ml and from 400–240 μg/ml respectively (Vermeulen 1976, Abraham et al. 1971). The P and HOP in postmenopausal women are almost exclusively of adrenal origin, being completely suppressed by dexamethasone and increased 50% by ACTH (Vermeulen 1976). The levels are also unaffected by bilateral oophorectomy. The progesterone levels bear no relationship to vasomotor symptoms (Lauritzen 1973). It is noteworthy, however, that the mean value of pregnanediol excretion decreases from 1.5 μg/24 hr immediately after the menopause to 0.63 μg/24 hr in the late climacteric. It is important to remember that the climacteric is as much a progesterone deficiency as an oestrogen deficiency syndrome.

Prolactin

Prolactin levels fall after the menopause, probably due to the decrease in oestrogen secretion (Reyes et al. 1977). Prolactin increases the ratio of androgens to corticoids secreted by the adrenal cortex and Crilly et al. (1978) found that postmenopausal women with osteoporosis have a decreased androstenedione/cortisone ratio and postulated that the decreased androstenedione and increased cortisone might be due to the decreased prolactin secretion.

'Inhibin'

The increase in FSH at the climacteric generally precedes the increase in LH by many years and is also much greater in amount. The LH levels premenopausally may be in the normal range although there is usually some rise immediately preceding the menopause and a much greater rise thereafter (Faiman et al. 1976, Reyes et al. 1977). This differential increase in blood levels of FSH compared with LH has puzzled endocrinologists, and a number of different mechanisms have been invoked. These include differential secretion rates of FSH and LH by the pituitary (Coble et al. 1969), decreased clearance of FSH compared with LH (Yen et al. 1970), and differential response of the hypothalamus to changes in plasma oestradiol (Franchimont et al. 1975). Van Look et al. (1977) described four different patterns of abnormality in hypothalamic-pituitary and ovarian activity in premenopausal women with dysfunctional uterine bleeding, including a failure in the positive feedback effect of oestradiol and absence of the normal midcycle LH surge.

Other endocrinologists have been puzzled by the seeming lack of relationship between the plasma levels of sex hormones and the plasma levels of FSH and LH in both pre- and postmenopausal women, particularly as there is no apparent abnormality in hypothalamic-pituitary function on dynamic testing (Odell & Swerdloff 1968). This has led several investigators to speculate that the ovarian follicle produces a non-steroidal feedback factor, analogous to the peptide produced by the germinal tubule epithelium in the male, which inhibits FSH release, known as 'Inhibin' (Sherman & Korenman 1975) or 'FSH-release-inhibiting substance' (van Look et al. 1977). Inhibin exerts a specific negative feedback control on FSH secretion and has now been identified in both bovine and human ovarian follicular fluid (de Jong & Sharpe 1976, Chari *et al.* 1979). There is a close inverse correlation between the number of primordial follicles on ovarian biopsy and FSH levels (Goldenberg *et al.* 1973) and a decrease in inhibin would explain the disproportionate rise in FSH levels premenopausally. It could well be that a decrease in inhibin secretion is the main cause of the increase in gonadotrophins in both pre- and postmenopausal women (Lumpkin *et al.* 1984) and that lack of inhibin plays a much greater role in the endocrine changes at the menopause than currently thought.

SUMMARY OF ENDOCRINE CHANGES AT CLIMACTERIC

The endocrine changes at the climacteric can be summarized as follows:

1 Increased secretion of gonadotrophin with a disproportionate increase in FSH secretion commencing 10–15 years before the menopause;

2 anovulation or deficient corpus luteum formation with decreased or absent progesterone secretion commencing up to 10–15 years before the menopause;

3 failure in follicular development with a marked decrease in oestradiol secretion and cessation of menstruation at the menopause;

4 changes from cyclical to continuous secretion of sex hormones and gonadotrophins and a marked increase in gonadotrophin secretion reaching a maximum 2–3 years postmenopausally then slowly declining over next 20–30 years;

5 continued secretion of androstenedione and testosterone by the ovarian stroma, and continued secretion of androstenedione and other sex hormones by the adrenal cortex;

6 the peripheral conversion of the androstenedione derived from ovarian stroma and adrenal cortex to oestrone which is the predominant circulating oestrogen in postmenopausal women.

The endocrine changes at the climacteric may usefully be divided into three separate phases of development which frequently overlap but which have separate clinical and pathological connotations and consequences (Table 44.3).

Table 44.3. Phases of development and significance of endocrine changes at menopause.

Phase I   Hypothalamic–pituitary hyperactivity
(a) Starts 10–15 years before menopause.
(b) Compensatory for increased resistance of ovarian follicles and decreased follicular hormone secretion.
(c) Evidenced by raised FSH and, later, LH and associated with hot flushes—pituitary may become exhausted late postmenopause.

Phase II   Ovulation and corpus luteum failure
(a) Occurs in most women with increasing frequency as menopause approaches—anovulatory cycles or shortened luteal phase.
(b) Deficient progesterone and continued unopposed oestrogen secretion.
(c) Causes dysfunctional uterine bleeding, endometrial hyperplasia and carcinoma.

Phase III   Ovarian follicular failure
(a) Failure of follicular development causes fall in oestradiol secretion and cessation of menses.
(b) Ovarian stroma remains active; with adrenal cortex produces androstenedione and testosterone.
(c) Oestrone produced by extraglandular conversion of androgens; main postmenopausal oestrogen—only 10–50% postmenopausal women oestrogen deficient.

ANATOMICAL, PHYSIOLOGICAL AND PATHOLOGICAL CHANGES

CHANGES IN THE OVARY

As already discussed, ageing of the ovary with a progressive decrease in the number of ovarian follicles begins *in utero* (Hertig 1944) and continues in childhood during which time the ovary appears inactive both macroscopically and microscopically. At puberty the number of active follicles increases markedly and cyclical follicular activity commences and then continues throughout reproductive life. After the menopause the ovaries shrink, become wrinkled and white in appearance and have a fibrous consistency on palpation. There is a progressive thinning of the cortex of the ovary with a relative increase in the medulla where corpora albicanti can be found. The tunica albuginea thickens and sclerotic changes occur in the vessels of the cortex and medulla. Ultrastructural studies have shown however that the postmenopausal ovary is far from inactive (Costoff 1974). There is thus an abundance of stromal cells, some with well developed mitochondria, and an abundance of lipid droplets indicative of secretory activity, these cells being the likely site of steroid hormone synthesis of the postmenopausal ovary (Mattingly & Huang 1969).

Changes in the genital and urinary tracts

The changes in the genital and urinary tracts at the climacteric are partly related to the changes in sex hormones and partly to the normal ageing process. In general, the corpus of the uterus becomes smaller with a return to the 1/2 ratio of corpus/cervix found in childhood. The myometrium and endometrial stroma are partly replaced by fibrous tissue and the endometrium is thin and atrophic though cystic glands may persist for many years. In some women with high endogenous oestrogen production, however, the endometrium may become active and proliferative and even hyperplastic.

Changes in the vulva and vagina do not usually occur until some years after the menopause but as time goes by the vagina becomes narrower and less rugose and the vaginal epithelium becomes thin and more easily traumatized. The vulval and labial skin becomes shiny and atrophic, and the vulva and labia shrink and become flatter owing to loss of subcutaneous fat so that the introitus tends to gape. There may also be vaginal and uterine prolapse. Microscopically, the epithelium consists of only a few layers of cells, the cells lack glycogen and the stroma is infiltrated by lymphocytes and plasma cells. The lactobacilli disappear and the vagina becomes alkaline.

The bladder and urethra, which are lined by transitional epithelium, undergo similar changes to the vagina. The bladder epithelium also becomes thin and more prone to damage and infection resulting in recurrent urethritis and cystitis. There may also be bladder dysfunction with bladder irritability and stress incontinence.

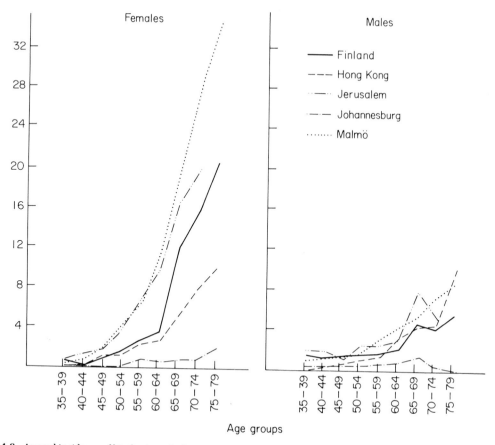

Fig. 44.8. Annual incidence of hip fractures in five centres (from Alhava & Puitinen 1973).

CHANGES IN OTHER ORGANS AND SYSTEMS

The postmenopausal female may show general body changes: greying of the hair, wrinkling and loss of elasticity of the skin, growth of facial hair, shrinking and laxity of the breasts and deposition of fat around the waist and shoulders. There may be loss of height and the development of kyphosis (Dowager's Hump) due to osteoporosis and crush fractures of the spine. She may develop cardiovascular disease, neoplasms and other medical disorders. There may also be mood, mental and personality changes. Many of these changes are part of the general ageing process but some are a direct result of changes in circulating sex hormones and it may be difficult to disentangle which changes are due to ageing *per se* and which changes are due to hormonal deficiencies.

Pathological changes

SKELETAL SYSTEM

The association between the menopause and osteoporosis was first described by Albright and his colleagues in 1941. They suggested that loss of ovarian oestrogens at the menopause leads to loss of bone and that administration of oestrogens can prevent bone loss. It has been known since ancient times that women lose bone to a greater degree than men (Perzigian 1973) and Sir Astley Cooper (1824) noted that in old age 'bones become thin in their shell and spongy in their texture'. Bruns (1882) noted that hip fractures occurred more commonly in women over 50 than in men but attributed this to women tripping over their long skirts. Current data show that after the age of 65 years hip, spine and wrist fractures are 8–10 times more frequent in women than in men of the same age (Alffram 1974, Alhava & Puittenen 1973—see Fig. 44.8). The increased incidence of forearm fractures occurs 10–15 years earlier than hip and spine fractures (Knowleden *et al.* 1964). In fact both men and women tend to lose bone after 40 years but the rate of mineral loss is on an average 3 times faster in women, with a 1% reduction in skeletal mass each year. Ultimately women lose on the average about 30% of their total bone mass whereas men, who start with a larger mass, lose on average only 20%. Osteoporosis has many causes: oestrogen deficiency; dietary deficiency or malabsorption of calcium and/or vitamin D; immobolization; excessive adrenocortical secretion; drug therapy—corticosteroids, cytotoxic drugs and heparin; other medical diseases

e.g. hyperthyroidism, hyperparathyroidism, chronic renal disease and rheumatoid arthritis.

The subject of the bone metabolism and the menopause is a large one and there have been a number of good reviews (Nordin *et al.* 1975, Aitken 1976, Gordon & Vaughan 1980, Utian 1980b) and only the main findings will be described here.

Effect of menopause and bilateral oophorectomy on calcium and phosphorus metabolism and mechanism of action of oestrogens

Following bilateral oophorectomy and following the menopause there is an increase in serum calcium and phosphorus, in urinary calcium and phosphorus, in serum alkaline phosphatase and in urinary hydroxyproline (Lindsay 1980) (Table 44.4) suggesting an increased resorption of calcium and phosphorus and a negative calcium and phosphorus balance (Gallagher & Nordin 1973 and 1975). These changes can be reversed by small doses of oestrogen with a restoration of the positive balance presumably due to inhibition of bone resorption (Recker *et al.* 1977). The exact mechanism of action of oestrogen on bone and calcium and phosphorus metabolism has not been determined. Bone is a dynamic structure and is being constantly remodelled with a fine homeostatic balance between bone formation and bone resorption. Oestrogens appear primarily to inhibit osteoclastic activity and bone resorption (Riggs & Jowsey 1969). Oestrogens may in addition have a beneficial effect on bone collagen as evidenced by the changes in hydroxyproline excretion. Heaney *et al.* (1978) have suggested that the primary action of oestrogen is to reduce the sensitivity of the bone to parathyroid hormone, but oestrogens also appear to have a direct inhibiting effect on bone resorption, possibly by increasing sensitivity of bone to calcitonin (Aitken 1976).

It is of interest that postmenopausal women with thin skins tend to have a high incidence of osteoporosis (83%) (McConkey *et al.* 1963) and that corticosteroid treated women often have reduced skin thickness and marked osteoporosis. This suggests that in postmenopausal women raised cortisol levels may have a significant inhibiting effect both on bone and on skin possibly due to changes in the amount of collagen or ground substance. Aitken *et al.* (1974), in a controlled trial of oestrogen therapy, showed that oestrogens increased cortisol secretion and that women with the increased urinary free cortisol had an increased rate of bone loss. Oestrogens may thus have a secondary indirect inhibitory effect on new

Table 44.4. Biochemical changes in postmenopausal women before and after oestrogen treatment (from Lindsay 1980).

	Premenopausal	Postmenopausal	Postmenopausal (oestrogen treated)
Serum calcium (mg/100 ml)	9.56 ± 0.08	9.84 ± 0.08	9.52 ± 0.04
Serum phosphate (mg/100 ml)	2.82 ± 0.09	3.32 ± 0.06	2.94 ± 0.06
Alkaline phosphatase (K.A. units)	7.06 ± 0.39	7.00 ± 0.42	7.00 ± 0.31
Urine Ca/Cr (mg/mg)	0.091 ± 0.007	0.114 ± 0.01	0.071 ± 0.006
Urine OHp5Cr (mg/mg)	0.015 ± 0.002	0.026 ± 0.003	0.011 ± 0.002
$\dfrac{TmPO_4}{GFR}$ (mg/100 ml)	2.90 ± 0.01	3.39 ± 0.09	2.87 ± 0.11

Ca Cr = Ratio of calcium to creatinine in urine after overnight fast

OHp Cr = Ratio of total hydroxyproline to creatinine in urine after overnight fast

$\dfrac{TmPO_4}{GFR}$ = Tabular maximum for phosphate reabsorption per unit glomerular filtration rate

bone formation by increasing cortisol secretion. The relationship between osteoporosis and oestrogen blood levels has been studied by Marshall *et al.* (1977). They compared plasma oestrone and androstenedione levels in normal and osteoporotic women (including a group on corticosteroid treatment for conditions such as asthma, rheumatoid arthritis). They found that the osteoporotic women had significantly lower oestrone and androstenedione levels. There was a significant curvilinear relationship between plasma androstenedione and oestrone levels suggesting that the reduced plasma oestrone was a the result of reduced plasma androstenedione levels. Lindsay (1980) showed that there was a significant relationship between bone loss and circulating androstenedione and circulating total oestrogen (oestrone plus oestradiol) and that women with the greatest bone loss also had the highest urinary free cortisol. Crilly *et al.* (1978) were unable to find any evidence of adrenal cortical or ACTH excess in osteoporotic women and suggested that the primary defect might be a change in the ratio of androstenedione and cortisol produced by the adrenal gland (Bassi *et al.* 1977). They postulated that as prolactin increases the androstenedione/cortisol production ratio, postmenopausal osteoporosis may in fact be due primarily to prolactin deficiency. Progestogen alone may also prevent bone loss (Lindsay *et al.* 1978a) apparently by increasing periosteal new bone formation without reducing bone resorption. Lindsay *et al.* (1978a) suggested that the ideal preparation for the prevention of bone loss may be a combination of oestrogen and progestogen which both inhibited bone resorption and stimulated new bone formation. Other factors such as physical activity and calcium intake have a major influence on bone formation. Nordin *et al.* (1975) have maintained that postmenopausal osteoporosis is due to a combination of oestrogen deficiency with malabsorption of calcium, and that supplementation of the diet with calcium (to about 1.5 g elemental calcium per day) is an important factor in the prevention of postmenopausal osteoporosis. Calcium administration however alone is not as effective as oestrogen therapy alone and both calcium and oestrogens may be necessary (Lindsay 1980, Riggs *et al.* 1982). Regular exercise may similarly be an important factor in maintaining normal bone structure as well as being beneficial to the general physical and psychological condition.

Decrease in bone density after the menopause: incidence of osteoporosis and fractures

Changes in bone density have been studied using X-ray metacarpal densitometry, X-ray grading of the trabecular pattern of the femoral neck (Singh index), radiogrammetry, photon absorptimetry and total-body neutron activation analysis. These studies have shown marked differences in total bone mass and the rate of bone loss between males and females and between different racial groups. While both sexes lose bone with increasing age, the loss is much more severe and occurs much earlier in women. Blacks, however, tend to have more bone and to lose it at a slower rate than whites, so that black women are less likely to develop osteoporosis or to sustain hip or other fractures (Goldsmith *et al.* 1977). Bone density has been shown to fall progressively in women who have had bilateral oophorectomy but to be maintained in women who have had hysterectomy with conservation of ovaries (Meema & Meema 1976). The prime candidate for the development of osteoporosis is the thin, elderly, white woman who smokes and has had an early menopause or bilateral oophorectomy (Daniel 1976). The true incidence of osteoporosis is difficult to estimate, depending upon the definition of osteoporosis followed, the methods of detection used and the precise population studied (Nordin *et al.* 1966). Using metacarpal bone densitometry, Smith *et al.* (1972) found that the prevalence of osteoporosis in Scottish females was 5%, 15%, 30%, 65% and 85% at the ages of 40, 50, 60, 70 and 80 years respectively. Barnes (1968) claimed that 25% of all postmenopausal women will experience some form of clinically disabling osteoporosis, and Marx (1978) estimated that 50% of all women over the age of 60 years in the USA will suffer some clinical consequence of osteoporosis.

The reported incidence of postmenopausal osteoporosis and of consequent fractures of the femur, vertebrae and radius and ulna varies in different series. Alffram and Bauer (1962), working in Sweden, found that the frequency of hip fractures doubles every five years in women over 65 years old, reaching the figure of 40% after the age of 80 years, and that 20% of Swedish women can expect to suffer one or more hip fractures during their lives. Barnes and Brown (1976) estimated that in England 1% of women over 65 years will sustain a hip fracture and that 34% of these women will die within 6 months of the accident. In both Britain and Sweden the incidence of forearm fractures in women over 40 progressively increases with age, becoming 10 times commoner than in men at the age of 60 years' so that by the age of 70 years over 10% of women will have sustained a Colles fracture at some time during their postmenopausal years (Alffram 1974, Knowleden *et al.* 1964, Alhava & Puittenen 1973). It has been calculated that in the Western world 25% of women will sustain a fracture of the femur, radius or vertebra some time in their lives (Horsman 1981).

One of the most characteristic features of postmenopausal osteoporosis is the vertebral crush fracture which causes the loss of height, the development of kyphosis and the typical short, hunchbacked appearance of older postmenopausal woman. In the USA it has been calculated that 50–70 in every 1000 postmenopausal women sustain a fresh vertebral crush fracture each year (Iskrant & Smith 1969) and it has been estimated that in general 25% of all white women over 60 years of age will develop spinal compression fractures due to oestoporosis.

The effect of oestrogens on bone loss, osteoprosis and occurrence of fractures

There is general agreement that oestrogen administration in the doses normally used for control of menopausal symptoms lowers urine calcium and prevents bone loss. Aitken *et al.* (1973) showed that bone loss was prevented by 20 μg mestranol/day but not by a placebo, and Lindsay *et al.* (1976) found that if oestrogen therapy is commenced within 3 years of bilateral oophorectomy the bone loss is not only prevented but the bone mass may be restored or increased (Fig. 44.9). There is a suggestion that when

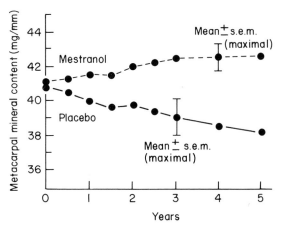

Fig. 44.9. Metacarpal mineral content during a 5-year follow-up of 120 patients who had been oophorectomized 3 years previously measured by photon absorptiometry. The women were divided into two groups and given either (a) mestranol 24.8 μg daily (dotted line) or (b) identical placebo (continuous line) (from Lindsay *et al.* 1976).

oestrogen therapy is stopped, a phase of accelerated bone loss may occur (Lindsay *et al.* 1978b) but it nevertheless seems that there is an overall benefit in prevention of bone loss which is proportional to the duration of oestrogen replacement. More recent work suggests a dose response relationship between the amount of oestrogen administered and the amount of bone loss. Using photon absorptiometry on the distal forearm Christiansen *et al.* (1982) found that bone mass was increased in women treated with high and medium dose micronized oestradiol (4 and 2 mg daily), was unchanged in the low dosage group (1 mg micronized oestradiol daily) and declined in the placebo group. Using radiographic morphometry of the metacarpals Horsman *et al.* (1983) found that bone mass increased in postmenopausal women treated with doses of 25 μg or more of ethinyloestradiol per day, was unchanged in doses between 15 and 25 μg/ day and decreased in women given 15 μg or less of ethinyloestradiol/day. This work suggests that in the prevention or treatment of osteoporosis a minimum dose of 2 mg oestradiol, or 20 μg ethinyloestradiol or their equivalent must be used.

Three case control studies have shown a marked and significant reduction in the risk of fractures in postmenopausal women treated with oestrogens, the risk ratio being 0.26–0.33 (Hutchinson *et al.* 1979); 0.38 (Weiss *et al.* 1980); (Paganini-Hill *et al.* 1981). Gordan and Vaughan (1980) in a retrospective study have shown a significant reduction in wrist and hip fractures in oestrogen treated postmenopausal women. More recently Riggs *et al.* (1982), in a study of rates of vertebral fractures in patients with post-menopausal osteoporosis, found a fracture rate of 35/ 1000 person years in women given oestrogens, fluoride and calcium as compared with 834/1000 person years in the untreated group, a reduction of almost 24-fold. It would thus appear that oestrogen replacement therapy, possibly in association with calcium and fluoride, can completely prevent, if not reverse, the occurrence of osteoporosis in postmenopausal women and can substantially reduce the risk of fractures of the wrist, hip and spine. As fractures are common and constitute a major source of disability, the prevention of osteoporosis and of fractures is one of the strongest arguments for prophylactic oestrogen replacement therapy.

It might be advocated that all postmenopausal women should be given hormone replacement to prevent osteoporosis. Not all postmenopausal women, however, are oestrogen deficient (at least in the early postmenopause), not all will develop osteoporosis and not all will sustain fractures. The cost and logistical difficulties of providing long term oestrogen replacement on a routine basis to large groups of women make such a policy of prophylactic therapy impractical both financially and medically. Experience has also shown, for example with antihypertensive therapy, that compliance is often poor and that patients give up such therapy after a few months or years particularly if they are asymptomatic and have no obvious disease. Attention is therefore now being focused on the identification of those menopausal women who have high rates of bone loss and who are at high risk of developing fractures: the 'fast bone losers'. It may be possible to detect such women by measurement of 24 hr urinary excretion of calcium or the urinary calcium/creatinine ratio. Such fast bone losers would have a specific medical indication

for long term prophylactic oestrogen replacement therapy, would probably be motivated to continue treatment and would justify the costs of the medical care involved (Christiansen and Rødbro 1983).

CARDIOVASCULAR LIPID AND COAGULATION CHANGES

Cardiovascular and cerebrovascular disease

It is widely believed that women are protected against coronary artery disease in their reproductive life as myocardial infarction is 5–6 times commoner in men than in women between the ages of 25 and 55 years (Ryan 1976). The incidence of cardiovascular disease, as shown in the Framingham study, is also 2–3 times greater in postmenopausal as compared with premenopausal women of the same age (Gordon *et al.* 1978). Several, but not all, workers have reported a greater increase in clinical coronary artery disease and in atherosclerosis in women following bilateral oophorectomy or premature menopause. Parrish *et al.* (1967) showed that on autopsy castrated patients had an excess of coronary atherosclerotic blockage and myocardial infarcts, and that this was related to the time interval from bilateral oophorectomy to time of death. It took on average 14 years after bilateral oophorectomy before excessive coronary artery disease became apparent, and women who undergo bilateral oophorectomy or premature menopause before the age of 40 years were found to have a significantly increased incidence of atherosclerosis and ischaemic cardiovascular disease.

The concept that women are protected premenopausally against coronary heart disease has been challenged by Heller and Jacobs (1978) who claim that, when the death rate due to coronary artery disease in England and Wales is analysed, the rate of increase with increasing age does not alter in women before and after the age of 50 years. Men, in contrast, do show a slower rise in death rate after the age of 50 years. The difference in the rate of increase of deaths due to coronary heart disease in males and females with age before and after the age of 50 years could be because: (1) women lose an endogenous protective factor which is present in the reproductive years, e.g. fall in oestrogen secretion; (2) men lose an endogenous risk factor at the age of 50 years, e.g. fall in testosterone secretion; (3) there are differences in environmental factors between males and females which change at the age of 50 years, e.g. work stress. Heller and Jacobs attributed the fall off in the rate of increase of death rate in men over 50 years to a reduction in a risk factor such as decreasing plasma testosterone level. Ryan (1976) has however pointed out that the decreased death rate in men could be due to a 'weeding out' of a 'coronary-prone' group in the younger men. It is also possible that women after the age of 50 years would show a similar falling off in the rate of increase to men if they did not become menopausal and if premenopausal oestrogen levels were maintained. The fact that women do not show a change in the increase in death rate with age after the age of 50 years, does not exclude a major effect of the menopause on ischaemic cardiovascular changes.

The effect of oestrogens on blood pressure and cardiovascular system in postmenopausal women
In premenopausal women the use of oestrogen containing oral contraceptives appears to be associated with an increased incidence of hypertension (MacKay *et al.* 1973). In postmenopausal women the situation is less clear. Von Eiff (1976) has shown that oestrogens decrease blood pressure. Pfeffer *et al.* (1979), using a variety of analytic techniques and controlling a large number of potentially confounding variables, found no association between oestrogens and hypertension. In the Boston Collaborative Drug Surveillance Program (1974) there was similarly no correlation between oestrogen therapy and the development of hypertension. Oestrogens may in fact decrease hypertension in postmenopausal women. Byrd *et al.* (1977), Hammond *et al.* (1979) and Lind *et al.* (1979) all found a statistically significant decrease in blood pressure in postmenopausal or hypo-oestrogenic women on oestrogen therapy. It would appear that in postmenopausal women administration of oestrogen is, if anything, associated with a fall rather than a rise in blood pressure, and that the presence of hypertension is no contraindication to hormone replacement therapy.

Effect of oestrogens on serum lipids and lipoproteins
Cholesterol, phospholipids and triglycerides exist in the plasma in association with specific proteins as lipoproteins. Under fasting conditions these form three groups: (1) high density alphalipoproteins (HDL) consisting of approximately half protein and containing more phospholipid than cholesterol and almost no triglyceride; (2) low density betalipoproteins (LDL), consisting of one-fifth protein and constituting most of the plasma cholesterol; (3) very low density prebetalipoproteins (VLDL) which consist mostly of triglycerides.

Premenopausal women differ from men in having higher serum HDL levels, lower VLDL levels, lower plasma cholesterol and lower cholesterol to phospholipid ratio. After the menopause the HDL level falls and LDL levels and cholesterol rise and the sex difference tends to disappear. Plasma cholesterol, phospholipids and triglycerides, moreover, all tend to increase with age. Cholesterol and phospholipid levels increase after the menopause but are not affected by dietary intake, whereas triglyceride levels do not appear to be related to the menopause but are related to body weight and diet (Oliver 1976). Increases in plasma cholesterol similarly occur in women following bilateral oophorectomy and following premature menopause (Oliver & Boyd 1959, Sznajderman & Oliver 1963), although Utian (1972c) was unable to detect any significant difference between different groups of premenopausal and oophorectomized women.

The effect of oestrogen and progestogen administered on lipid and lipoproteins in postmenopausal women appears to depend upon the type and dose of the oestrogen, the type and dose of progestogen, and the balance of effect of the two hormones. The administration of oestrogens alone causes a fall in plasma total cholesterol but a rise in HDL cholesterol levels (Fåhraeus & Larsson-Cohn 1982). The effect of oestrogens on triglycerides and VLDL and LDL lipoprotein fractions however is variable and appears to depend on the particular oestrogen administered. Oestradiol valerate thus causes a fall in triglyceride and VLDL and LDL phospholipid concentrations whereas ethinyloestradiol causes a rise in triglyceride and VLDL and LDL phospholipid (Silfverstolpe *et al.* 1982a, Samsioe *et al.* 1983).

The effect of oestrogens also depends on the route of administration; oestrogens administered percutaneously or vaginally have little effect on plasma lipid and lipoprotein levels, whereas the same dose administered orally has a marked effect (Fåhraeus & Larsson-Cohn 1982). High doses of oestrogens administered by implants however have a similar effect to lower doses given orally. It has been suggested that the effect of oral oestrogens is due to the high concentration of oestrogens in the hepatic portal circulation and to the 'first pass' effect on lipid and lipoprotein metabolism in the liver.

The effect of progestogens on lipid and lipoprotein metabolism in postmenopausal women depends on the particular progestogen administered. The 19 nor-testosterone (oestrane and gonane) type progestogen derivatives such as norethisterone or norgestrel appear to have marked effects, whereas 17 alpha-hydroxy-progesterone (pregnane) type derivatives have little or no effect on plasma lipids and lipoproteins (Silfverstolpe *et al.* 1982b). In general oestrane and gonane derivatives tend to decrease triglycerides, total cholesterol and HDL cholesterol levels and especially the important HDL2 fraction (Fåhraeus & Larsson-Cohn 1982, Silfverstolpe *et al.* 1982b). These progestogens also appear to reverse the beneficial effect of oestrogens on lipid and lipoproteins when oestrogen and progestogen are administered together. Little work has been done on the effect of combined oestrogen–progestogen preparation in postmenopausal women, although the combination of 2 mg of micronized oestradiol, 1 mg micronized oestriol and 1 mg norethisterone acetate leaves the plasma cholesterol, plasma triglyceride and plasma lipoproteins unchanged. In premenopausal women using a combined oestrogen–progestogen oral contraceptive pill Wahl *et al.* (1983) showed that, compared with non-pill users, low dose oestrogen with high dose progestogen pills caused higher LDL cholesterol and lower HDL cholesterol, while high dose oestrogen and low dose progestogen had higher HDL cholesterol levels. Wahl *et al.* (1983) concluded that the balance of oestrogen and progestogen in the pill determines the effect on LDL and HDL, and is an important factor affecting the incidence of stroke and myocardial infarction in women of childbearing age. The same considerations probably apply to the effect of combinations of oestrogen and progestogen on lipid and lipoprotein profiles in postmenopausal women. In order to prevent atherosclerosis and consequent cardiovascular disease in postmenopausal women any oestrogen–progestogen combination administered should have a significant positive beneficial effect on lipid and lipoprotein profiles. The preventive effects of oestrogens on atherosclerosis appear to be a major beneficial effect of hormone replacement and more information is urgently needed regarding the precise effect of different oestrogen–progestogen combinations on plasma cholesterol, triglycerides and lipoproteins. In the meantime it would appear to be advisable to use an effective dose of oestrogen, such as 2 mg oestradiol valerate or micronized oestradiol, and to combine this with the minimum dose of progestogen necessary to prevent the unwanted side effects and complications of endometrial hyperplasia and carcinoma.

The effect of oestrogens on blood coagulation and thromboembolic disease in postmenopausal women

Because the administration of oestrogens to premenopausal women in the form of the combined oestrogen–progestogen oral contraceptive pill is associated with coagulation changes and an increased incidence of thromboembolic disease it has been assumed that the same changes and risks are present to the same, if not greater, extent in postmenopausal women. In the case of premenopausal women on the pill however a potent oestrogen, usually ethinyloestradiol or mestranol, is given in high or 'supraphysiological' doses sufficient to inhibit ovulation in women who already have adequate oestrogen levels. In postmenopausal women, in contrast, a 'natural oestrogen' such as micronized oestradiol or conjugated equine oestrogen oestradiol valerate is given in small replacement doses to women who have abnormally low circulating levels of oestrogen with the aim of restoring these to normal premenopausal early follicular phase levels. It is therefore not valid to extrapolate any findings or conclusions regarding the effects of oral contraceptives in premenopausal women to postmenopausal women receiving oestrogen–progestogen replacement. Notelowitz *et al.* (1984) have shown that when either 1 or 2 mg 17-β oestradiol or 0.625 and 1.25 mg of conjugated equine oestrogens were administered to surgically menopausal women there were no abnormalities in intravascular coagulation or in dynamic tests of the coagulation cascade. They concluded that there were no adverse effects of oestrogens on the coagulation fibrinolysis system in postmenopausal women. In the Boston Collaborative Drug Surveillance Program (1974) there were 105 cases of thromboembolic disease but only 18 of these were idiopathic and in none of these was there any evidence of excess use of oestrogen. It is of interest that the overall incidence of idiopathic thromboembolic disease in the postmenopausal women was one-third to one-fifth of the incidence in premenopausal women on oral contraceptives. There is thus no evidence that the administration of oestrogens in replacement doses to postmenopausal or hypo-oestrogenic women is associated with any abnormalities in blood coagulation or any increase in thromboembolic disease. On the contrary, by their effect on lipid and lipoproteins the administration of oestrogens would appear to substantially reduce the incidence of ischaemic cardio-vascular disease and to have a major protective effect in postmenopausal women.

SKIN AND BREASTS

The skin shows marked changes at the time of the climacteric (Marks & Shahrad 1977). The dermis becomes thinner, less elastic and compressible, loses water and the total collagen may decrease. In the exposed areas, elastotic degeneration of the skin may occur causing the 'wrinkling' characteristic of advancing age. The epidermis also becomes thinner, the keratinocytes are smaller and the rate of re-epithelialization following injury decreases. Nail growth and sebaceous and sweat gland activity also decrease resulting in dry, scaly skin. How far these changes are due to ageing and how far to changes in circulating hormones has not been established. Oestrogens in general appear to cause thickening of the dermis but thinning of the epidermis, with a decrease in soluble collagen but an increase in insoluble collagen and in hyaluronic acid content (Henneman 1971). Ebling (1974) found that oestrogens had a biphasic effect on the skin with initial thinning and later thickening, supporting Punnonen (1972) who claimed that oestrogen caused proliferation and prevented atrophy of the epidermis. Oestrogens also increase skin pigmentation (Snell & Bischitz 1963) and inhibit the action of testosterone which normally stimulates sebaceous and sweat glands. Much of the work on oestrogens and skin has been done on mice and rats and it is of interest that when tritiated oestradiol was injected into women undergoing hysterectomy the labelled oestradiol was found in the endometrium and salpinges but could not be detected in muscle, subcutaneous fat or skin (Taylor 1974).

The breast volume in the normal menstrual cycle varies considerably, increasing by up to 100 ml in the luteal phase owing to glandular proliferation and water retention (Milligan et al. 1975). Following the menopause and after bilateral oophorectomy, the glandular tissue of the breasts becomes atrophic but the fat content may increase so that breasts may become large and pendulous. In thin women the breasts tend to become smaller and flat. Oestrogen administration in postmenopausal and postoophorectomized women however does not produce any significant change in breast size (Utian 1970) although oestrogen–progestogen combinations have been reported to do so (Dennerstein et al. 1979).

CLINICAL FEATURES OF THE MENOPAUSE AND CLIMACTERIC

A large number of symptoms and physical changes have been attributed to the menopause and it is often difficult to disentangle which symptoms are: (a) due to the climacteric; (b) due to contemporary unrelated diseases; (c) due to psychogenic causes originating from the patient's life circumstances, or some personality problem or psychiatric background.

As the climacteric is in large measure an oestrogen deficiency syndrome, a useful approach has been to determine which symptoms are relieved by oestrogen

Table 44.5. Menopausal symptoms and relation to oophorectomy and treatment with oestrogens and placebo. (From Utian 1972a.)

Group	Menopausal symptoms	Relation to oophorectomy, oestrogen and placebo treatment
1	Hot flushes and perspiration	Related to oophorectomy
	Atrophic vaginitis, dyspareunia and vaginal discharge	Relieved by oestrogens; not relieved by placebo
2	Agina pectoris	Related to oophorectomy
	Depression	Not relieved by oestrogens
	Insomnia	Relieved by placebo
3	Headache	Not related to oophorectomy
	Irritabilty	Possibly relieved by oestrogens; relieved by placebo
4	Backache	Not related to oophorectomy
	Reduced libido	Not relieved by oestrogens; not relieved by placebo

Table 44.6. Menopausal symptoms significantly improved by oestrogen therapy when compared with placebo in double-blind cross over trial. (From Campbell 1976b.)

2-month crossover study (64 patients)	6-month crossover study (56 patients)
1 Hot flushes	1 Hot flushes
2 Insomnia	2 Vaginal dryness
3 Vaginal dryness	3 Insomnia
4 Irritability	4 Urinary frequency
5 Poor memory*	5 Poor memory
6 Anxiety	
7 Worry about age*	
8 Headaches	
9 Worry about self*	
10 Urinary frequency	
11 Optimism	
12 Good spirits	

* Significant improvement in 20 patients without flushes

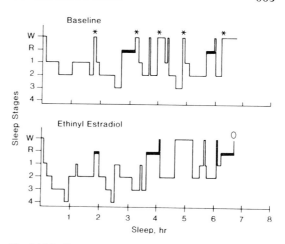

Fig. 44.10. Sleepgrams measured in a symptomatic patient before and after 30 days' administration of ethinyloestradiol, 50 µg four times daily.
* represents occurence of hot flush.
(From Erlik *et al.* 1981. With the permission of the *Journal of the American Medical Association.*)

replacement in either single-blind or double-blind trials (Greenblatt *et al.* 1950, Kupperman *et al.* 1953, Kaufman 1967, Utian 1972a, Lauritzen 1973, Campbell *et al.* 1976a). The conclusions from the trials are in surprisingly good agreement and the main findings of Utian (1972a) and Campbell (1976a) are shown in Tables 44.5 and 44.6

The symptoms and signs which are significantly relieved by oestrogens can be grouped under three headings: (1) vasomotor symptoms; (2) genital and urinary symptoms; (3) psychological symptoms.

VASOMOTOR SYMPTOMS

The most characteristic symptom of the climacteric is the 'hot flush', an uncomfortable and sometimes unbearable feeling of intense heat of sudden onset usually arising in the trunk, spreading upwards to the neck, face and forehead and sometimes over the whole body. The uncomfortable hot sensation characteristically lasts for only 1 to 2 min and is frequently associated with sweating, mostly of the forehead, face and upper trunk. It may be accompanied by palpitations and tachycardia which may be predominant features in some women. When the vasomotor attacks occur at night the patient is woken up and may be more aware of the sweating and complain of 'night sweats' which are frequently associated with dreaming and are probably related to episodes of REM sleep (Fig. 44.10) (Erlik *et al.* 1981).

Both hot flushes and night sweats may be exacerbated by hot weather, a hot room, woolly clothing or

bed clothes, spices, curries and alcohol. Though patients experiencing a hot flush may look 'hot and bothered', the change in appearance is often much less than might be expected from the patient's description. The endocrine and physiological mechanisms responsible for hot flushes are not fully understood but considerable new knowledge has been gained in recent years. Sturdee *et al.* (1978) showed that hot flushes were associated with an acute rise in skin temperature, with peripheral vasodilatation and a slight increase in heart rate suggestive of a sudden transient increase in sympathetic drive. Meldrum *et al.* (1979) recorded the changes in the skin temperature of the finger in postmenopausal women experiencing hot flushes and found a mean increase in skin temperature of 2.7°C which closely correlated with each hot flush. The subjective sensation, however, preceded the rise in temperature and lasted only 1—2 minutes whereas the rise in temperature lasted an average 30 minutes and recurred at intervals of 54 minutes (Fig. 44.14). Molnar (1979) continuously recorded the temperature of the vagina, cheek and toe in one postmenopausal woman for 5 days, during which time she experienced 63 hot flushes. During this period there were, in addition, 23 episodes of temperature increment not noted by the subject. Skin temperature rises of up to 6°C were recorded in the toes, and were higher than in the region where the hot flushes were experienced, such as the cheeks and forehead. In these areas however sweating occurred simultaneously with the hot flush and this may have limited the rise in skin temperature. The finding that the subjective sensation of hot flush precedes the rise in body temperature suggests that there is initially a change within the central nervous system which includes an acute resetting of the thermoregulatory centre. This gives rise to the acute discomfort, which is then followed by the generalized cutaneous vasodilatation causing the rise in skin temperature or flush. Studies on hot flushes occurring at night have shown that there is an increase in skin conductance, which is a measure of sweating, and that this may precede the rise in skin temperature and predominates over the flush (Fig. 44.11; Erlik *et al.* 1981). The initiation of sweating may result from an acute stimulation of cholinergic pathways, whereas the acute cutaneous vasodilatation probably results from acute stimulation of adrenergic pathways. The dissociation between sweating and vasodilatation, particularly at night, may provide an explanation for night sweats.

The physiological changes associated with hot flushes have been further elucidated by Kronenberg *et al.* (1984) who showed that they are accompanied by abrupt increases in plasma epinephrine (about 150%) and concomitant decreases in norepinephrine (about 40%). They confirmed that an aura precedes the onset of the hot flush by several seconds and that heart rate and finger blood flow also increases just before the flush, reaching peak levels of 10–20 beats/min and 30-fold respectively. Concurrent with the vasodilatation, the finger temperature increased an average of 3.9°C and oesophageal temperature fell 0.2 to 0°C. They further noted that, although hot flushes are usually discrete, self-limiting episodes lasting 3–6 min, prolonged hot flushes lasting up to 1 hr do occur and that the increase in LH, heart rate, sweating and heat sensation are then all raised parallel to each other. They also noted that the prolonged hot flushes occurred when the ambient temperature was raised 2°C above that found when discrete flushes were recorded, so that ambient temperatures may have an important effect on the duration of hot flushes. The observations of Kronenberg *et al.* (1984) are consistent with the hypothesis of a sudden resetting of the thermoregulating centre resulting in an adrenergic vasodilator discharge, followed by loss of body heat and a temporary lowering of body core temperature.

In view of the usual dramatic response of hot flushes to oestrogen therapy attempts have been made to relate the occurrence of hot flushes to oestrogen and gonadotrophin levels. Hutton *et al.* (1978), however, found no difference in oestrogen levels in postmenopausal women with and without flushes and Campbell (1976b), when he measured plasma oestrogens, LH, FSH, prolactin and growth hormone 2-hourly for 24 hours, also found no difference in women with and without flushes. Aksel and Schomber (1976) similarly could find no difference in luteal phase serum oestrogen, FSH and LH between a group of women who developed hot flushes and a group who did not following bilateral oophorectomy. More recently Erlik *et al.* (1982) studied two groups of women matched for age, years since menopause, and presence of ovaries. One group had never experienced hot flushes, the other had frequent hot flushes. The group with hot flushes had significantly lower plasma oestradiol, oestrone, non-steroid hormone binding globulin (non-SHBG) and total non-SHBG bound E_2. These workers also found that oestrogen levels and levels of SHBG correlated with body weight and suggested that thin, low mass women may have lower unbound oestrogen levels and may be more likely to experience hot flushes. Tataryn *et al.* (1979 and 1980) studied a series of 6 postmenopausal women having hot flushes, with continuous recording of the finger temperature and blood samples taken every 15 min for 8 hr and found that the pulses of LH release were closely correlated with the occurrence of hot flushes (Fig. 44.12). They con-

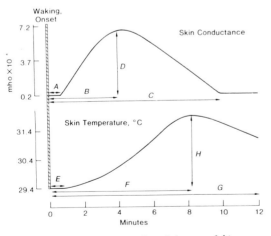

Fig. 44.11. Mean ± s.e. intervals and changes of skin conductance and temperature during 25 hot flushes that were associated with waking episodes (from Erlik *et al.* 1981. With permission from the *Journal of the American Medical Association*).

cluded that LH, or the factors that trigger its pulsatile release, are related to the mechanism responsible for the initiation of hot flushes.

The hot flush sensation coincides with the low point of pulsatile LH release when the rate of secretion of gonadotrophin releasing hormone (GnRH) is greatest, and it is suggested that the GnRH centre and the thermoregulatory centre stimulate and interact on each other or may be both simultaneously stimulated together from higher centres. Electrophysiological studies have shown that LHRH neurosecretory neurones can modify the thermoregulating

GENITAL AND URINARY TRACT SYMPTOMS

Symptoms which respond to oestrogen therapy but not to a placebo include vaginal dryness, dyspareunia and urinary frequency (Brown 1977). Atrophic vaginitis and atrophic changes as confirmed by vaginal cytology similarly show a rapid response to both local and systemic oestrogen therapy. In a group of 64 women between 54 and 56 years of age James et al. (1984) found that 55 (75%) were having regular intercourse, that 12 (20%) experienced some degree of dyspareunia which was severe in 5 (9%) of the

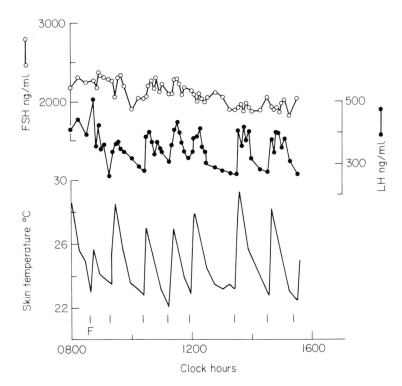

Fig. 44.12. Changes in cutaneous finger temperature and serum FSH and LH levels during an 8-hour study in a postmenopausal patient showing close temporal relationship between each subjective hot flush (indicated by vertical band), cutaneous skin temperature elevation and pulsatile LH release but not FSH levels (from Tataryn et al. 1979).

neurones (Lomax et al. 1979). It has further been shown that the rate of firing of the GnRH releasing neurones is increased in ovariectomized monkeys and is modulated by the level of circulating oestrogens (Kawakami & Sakuma 1974). The increased firing can also be reduced by alpha-adrenergic blocking agents such as phentolamine (Sawyer 1975) suggesting that alpha-adrenergic blocking agents may be of value in the treatment of hot flushes.

women. The 'urethral syndrome' of urgency, dysuria and recurrent urinary infections also responds to oestrogen therapy (Smith 1980). Oestrogens have further been shown to improve stress incontinence (Caine & Raz 1973, Walter et al. 1976).

PSYCHOLOGICAL CHANGES

Many patients of all ages experience anxiety, depression and a variety of psychological symptoms and when these occur at the climacteric they are often attributed to the menopause. Although there is very considerable improvement with placebo, it nevertheless appears from the work of Campbell (1976b) and others that a significant proportion of women given oestrogens do experience an improvement in mood over and above and distinct from the recognized placebo effect. There is thus a significantly greater reduction in anxiety, headaches, insomnia, irritability and worry about age and self, and significant improvements in good spirits, optimism and memory in women given oestrogens as compared with a placebo. The improvement occurred in women with and without vasomotor symptoms, although insomnia was improved only in those women who had hot flushes. Campbell (1976b) suggested that the improvement was in part a 'domino effect', i.e. due to relief from hot flushes and night sweats, patients felt better and slept better and were therefore less anxious and irritable. Other workers believed that oestrogens have a direct effect in improving mood and memory and reducing anxiety and have a genuine 'mental tonic effect' as originally suggested by Utian (1972b).

Apart from changes in mood and psychological symptoms directly related to endocrine changes, many women do experience psychological problems and symptoms at the climacteric which are the result of changes in their life situations. These symptoms include depression, tension, irritability, aggressiveness, nervous exhaustion, fluctuations in mood, sense of frustration and feelings of decreased energy and drive, reduced powers of concentration and feelings of inadequacy and loneliness. The modes of presentation of these symptoms at the climacteric have been reviewed by Christie-Brown and Christie-Brown (1976), Dominian (1977) and Dennerstein and Burrows (1978). It is now agreed that there is no specific psychological 'menopause syndrome' and the concept of a specific 'involutional melancholia' has been abandoned. The psychological disturbances that do arise in perimenopausal women result from the changes in life situation of the woman, which are common at the menopausal age, often combined with a previous personality problem or unhappy background. Changes in life situations and life stresses are very common in the climacteric years and include children growing up and leaving home ('the empty nest syndrome'), parents becoming ill or dying, husbands who show loss of affection, interest or sexual potency, widowhood, loneliness and social isolation. There is also the recognition that many of life's expectations in terms of money, marriage and position may never be fulfilled. Further stresses which may be very real are fears of loss of youth, femininity and beauty, fears of not being loved, needed or wanted and fears of old age, infirmity and even death. Sexual problems including dyspareunia or vaginal dryness in the female and loss of libido and of impotence in the male partner may also cause major disturbances between couples. The occurrence of psychological symptoms at the menopause is thus not surprising and is often a major part of the climacteric or critical age.

An important factor in determining the psychological response to the menopause and climacteric is the social and cultural background. In African tribes where women graduate from being 'bearers of children and drawers of water' to 'elders' and in India where women may end Purdah and stop wearing the veil, and also in Arab societies where women are no longer 'contaminated' by menstrual blood the menopause may indeed be welcomed. In Western society, however, with its current youth oriented culture and the emphasis on early achievement and success, physical attractiveness and prowess and sex, the menopause is regarded by many if not most women as something to be feared rather than a symbol of achievement and maturity.

Perimenopausal patients frequently present with a mixture of hormone-dependent and 'life-stress' symptoms. In the management of the perimenopausal patient, therefore, an assessment must be made not only of specific menopausal symptoms and conditions but of the patient's life and home circumstances, of her personality and disposition, and of any previous episodes of anxiety and/or depression. Such history taking, though time consuming, has considerable therapeutic benefit, and simple explanation and supportive psychotherapy, have a major place in the management of the climacteric.

COMPLICATIONS AND BENEFITS OF HORMONE REPLACEMENT

The use of oestrogens and hormones by climacteric women in the quest for eternal youth, or at least the prevention of ageing, and the complications that may arise, such as uterine cancer, has been the subject of much publicity in the medical and lay press and other media. Following the pioneer publication by Wilson and Wilson (1963) and of 'Feminine Forever' (Wilson 1966) oestrogens became widely, if not indiscriminately, used by many menopausal women, particularly in the USA. This treatment was popularized as 'oestrogen replacement' or 'hormone replacement therapy' (HRT). Some 10 years later Smith *et al.* (1975) and Ziel and Finkle (1975) claimed that oestrogen usage in postmenopausal women was associated with a significant increase in the incidence of endometrial carcinoma. Since 1975 there have been a large number of publications, mainly from the United States, claiming an association between oestrogen therapy and endometrial, breast and ovarian carcinoma and of other complications. These papers led at one stage to an almost complete abandomment or rejection of oestrogens and hormone replacement therapy in the management of the menopause and climacteric. More recently combined oestrogen–progestogen therapy has been introduced and shown to eliminate any increased risk and possibly even to reduce the 'natural' spontaneous incidence of endometrial hyperplasia and endometrial carcinoma.

ENDOMETRIAL CARCINOMA

The reported relative risk of carcinoma of the uterus due to unopposed oestrogen therapy varies in different series from 1.7–12.0%. Horwitz and Feinstein (1978) criticially reviewed these reports and concluded that, when important sources of surveillance and detection bias are allowed for, the 'true' mean unbiased relative risk is of the order of 2%. The most important factors influencing the risk of endometrial carcinoma are: (1) *Duration of use:* the risk of endometrial carcinoma is significantly increased after 3.5 years of use of unopposed oestrogens. There is a relatively long, 3–6-year, minimum latency period between the first administration of oestrogens and the development of endometrial carcinoma after which the relative risk progressively increases. A 2-year-free interval after stopping oestrogens is, however,

sufficient to significantly reduce the risk of endometrial carcinoma. (2) *Dosage of oestrogen:* in many patients the dose of oestrogen used may have been excessive and plasma oestrogen levels may have been well above premenopausal levels. (3) *Use of progestogens:* The use of progestogens in association with oestrogens when administered for a minimum of 10–14 days in any 28 days appears to eliminate any increase of endometrial carcinoma.

The endometrial carcinoma associated with unopposed oestrogen usage is usually Stage Ia clinically, Grade 1 histologically, and pathologically without any myometrial invasion and hence easily treated and of good prognosis.

There have been few studies of the incidence of endometrial carcinoma with combined oestrogen-progestogen therapy, principally because few patients have been on the combined therapy for long enough periods. Gambrell (1982), however, investigated the incidence of endometrial carcinoma in 3115 climacteric women who were treated with a variety of oestrogen and oestrogen–progestogen combinations and observed for a total of 13921 patient years (Table 44.7). The incidence of endometrial carcinoma in the oestrogen–progestogen users was approximately one quarter of that in both the oestrogen users and in the untreated women. It would thus appear that combined oestrogen–progestogen hormone replacement therapy in postmenopausal women not only prevents any increased risk but substantially reduces the incidence of endometrial carcinoma to approximately a quarter of the natural incidence. If this finding is substantiated the prevention of endometrial carcinoma may be one of the major benefits of hormone replacement therapy in pre- and postmenopausal women.

Table 44.7, Incidence of endometrial cancer in postmenopausal women 1975–1979 (Gambrell 1982).

Therapy group	Patient years of observation	Patients with cancer	Incidence per 100 000
I Oestrogen–progestogen users	7063	5	70.8*
II Oestrogen users	2302	10	434.4**
III Oestrogen vaginal cream users	7		
IV Progestogen or androgen users			
V Untreated women	2477	6	242.2
Total	13921	22	158.0**

*p 0.0001 difference between Groups I and II
**p 0.05 difference between Groups I and V

BREAST CANCER

Breast cancer is the commonest cancer in women, the death rate in the USA being approximately 23 per 100 000 women per year. It has been calculated that there are 10 times the number of deaths from breast carcinoma as there are from endometrial cancer (Gambrell 1980). The WHO Expert Committee reviewed a total of 15 studies of the association between oestrogens and breast carcinoma including 3 cohort studies and 12 case control studies. The Committee concluded that there was much circumstantial epidemiological evidence linking the occurrence of breast carcinoma to the hormonal status of different women including the age of the menarche, of the menopause and of the first pregnancy, and the effect of early bilateral oophorectomy which is strongly protective. In spite of this epidemiological evidence many of the early cohort and case control studies failed to demonstrate an association between breast carcinoma and oestrogen usage. However, 4 out of the 5 case control studies reported since 1980 (all of which were judged to be methodologically sound with adequate controls by the WHO Committee) found an increased relative risk ratio in breast carcinoma which varied from 0.7 in women who were taking oestrogens but had had bilateral oophorectomy to 2.5 in women taking high doses of oestrogen for long periods (Ross et al. 1980). There would appear to be a real small increased risk of breast carcinoma associated with the use of unopposed oestrogens in postmenopausal women, although the occurrence of

breast carcinoma and the degree of risk is affected by many factors. The duration of oestrogen treatment associated with increased risk of breast carcinoma is of the order of 10 or more years which is very much longer than that associated with an increase in risk of endometrial carcinoma. The relatively long exposure to unopposed oestrogens required to produce an increased risk of breast carcinoma may explain why earlier studies, where periods of exposure and observation were in general less than 10 years, failed to demonstrate an association between oestrogen usage and carcinoma of the breast.

It must be emphasized that all these studies have been based on the follow-up or analysis of women treated with oestrogens unopposed by progestogens. There have been very few studies of the risk of breast carcinoma in association with combined oestrogen–progestogen usage in postmenopausal women although there have been a number of studies of the relation between breast carcinoma and the combined oestrogen–progestogen oral contraceptives in premenopausal women. In premenopausal women taking oral contraceptives the situation is confused because two studies have reported an increased incidence of breast carcinoma after long use of oral contraceptives primarily on younger women. Other studies of women who have used oral contraceptives for 2 or more years have reported a decreased incidence of benign breast tumours, benign breast tumour being a major risk factor for subsequent breast carcinoma. In one study of postmenopausal women, half of whom were given Premarin 2.5 mg daily and 10 mg

Therapy group		Patient years of observation	Patients with cancer	Incidence per 100 000
I	Oestrogen–progestogen users	11.895	8	67.3*
II	Oestrogen users	15.6000	22	141.0**
III	Oestrogen vaginal cream users	3.130	3	95.8
IV	Progestogen or androgen users	1347	2	148.4
V	Untreated women	5258	18	342.3
	Total	37.236	53	142.3
NCI SEER (1980) Expected incidence age 55–59				229.2

* p 0.08 difference between Groups I and II
** p 0.01 differences between Groups I and V
     p 0.03   difference between Groups I and NCI SEER 1980
Reprinted with permission from the American College of Obstetricians and Gynecologists.

Table 44.8. Incidence of breast cancer in postmenopausal women 1975–1981 (Gambrell et al. 1983)

medroxyprogesterone acetate for 7 days each month, Nachtigall *et al.* (1979) reported a significant reduction in incidence of breast carcinoma. More recently Gambrell *et al.* (1983) in a study of 5563 postmenopausal women followed for 37 236 patient years of observation found 53 cases of breast carcinoma (Table 44.8). The incidence of breast carcinoma in untreated women, oestrogen users and oestrogen–progestogen users, was 342.3; 141.0 and 67.3 per 100 000 women respectively, so that in oestrogen–progestogen users the incidence of breast carcinoma was one-fifth of that in untreated women. There were no significant differences in intrinsic risk factors between the groups, and even in relation to expected incidence on the basis of national averages it would appear that oestrogen–progestogen usage significantly reduces the incidence of breast carcinoma in postmenopausal women to one-third or one-quarter of the 'natural' spontaneously occurring incidence. If this study is confirmed it will mean that combined oestrogen–progestogen replacement in postmenopausal women may in fact have a substantial protective effect against breast carcinoma and this may be one of the major benefits of hormone replacement therapy.

OVARIAN CARCINOMA

Ovarian carcinoma appears to be increasing in frequency and has become one of the commonest carcinomas and causes of death in women. Case control studies have not revealed any association between oestrogen usage and ovarian carcinoma, though one report had suggested an increased risk with stilboestrol (Hulka 1980). Oral contraceptives, however, have been shown to be associated with a low incidence of benign ovarian cysts (Ory 1974) and ovarian carcinoma (Newhouse *et al.* 1977). It has been postulated that the protective effect is due to suppression of gonadotrophin secretion which may be an aetiological factor in ovarian carcinoma. If this hypothesis is true, then it would be expected that the use of oestrogen and more particularly combined oestrogen–progestogen preparations which markedly reduce gonadotrophin levels in postmenopausal women would be associated with a reduction in the incidence of ovarian carcinoma.

CARDIOVASCULAR DISEASE

It is commonly asssumed that because long term oestrogen use in the form of the oral combined oestrogen–progestogen contraceptive is associated with

an increased risk of myocardial infarction and thromboembolic disease in premenopausal women, that oestrogen replacement therapy in postmenopausal women is also associated with an increased risk of myocardial infarction and thrombosis. As previously pointed out, however, the situation with regard to oestrogen use in pre- and postmenopausal women is entirely different. Premenopausal women have normal circulating levels of endogenous oestrogens to which potent synthetic oestrogens (usually in the form of ethinyloestradiol) are added in the relatively large doses sufficient to produce the 'high normal' or 'supraphysiological' levels of oestrogens required to suppress ovulation. Postmenopausal women in contrast have abnormally low levels of circulating oestrogens and natural oestrogens are given in hormone replacement doses to restore the levels of circulating oestrogens to the normal premenopausal level. Findings and conclusions on the risks of thromboembolic disease based on the use of oral contraceptives in premenopausal women are therefore not applicable to postmenopausal women.

One frequently quoted study on increased risk of myocardial infarction due to oestrogens was in fact carried out in men who had suffered a previous myocardial infarct (Coronary Drug Project Research Group 1973). The men were divided into two groups, one group being given 2.5 mg and the other 5 mg conjugated equine oestrogens daily. There was an increased recurrence of myocardial infarcts in both groups, but particularly in the group receiving 5 mg daily. The dosages of oestrogens however in both groups were excessive, so that quite apart from the fact that this study was carried out on men, it cannot be used as evidence of a deleterious effect of oestrogens when given in replacement doses to postmenopausal women.

Most other studies have shown a beneficial effect of oestrogen replacement on the incidence of ischaemic heart disease in postmenopausal women. Rosenberg *et al.* (1976) compared 336 postmenopausal women with myocardial infarction and 6730 normal control cases in the Boston Collaborative Drug Surveillance Program, and found a protective effect of oestrogen with a crude risk ratio of 0.39. Pfeffer *et al.* (1978) studied 220 newly diagnosed myocardial infarct cases in a Southern California retirement community and found a small but significant protective effect of oestrogens. Hammond *et al.* (1979) studied 309 hypo-oestrogenic women (e.g. Down's syndrome) who had had no treatment and a second similar group of 301 hypo-oestrogenic women who had had long term oestrogen replacement, and found a significant and substantially lowered rate of cardiovascular disease and hypertension as well as of osteoporosis and fractures, in the treated group. Ross *et al.* (1981), in a further follow up from the same Southern California retirement community, studied by Pfeffer found a significant beneficial effect of oestrogens and a reduction of deaths due to ischaemic heart disease, which could not be explained by any confounding factors such as hypertension, diabetes, smoking etc. The overall risk ratio (RR) was 0.43 so that the number of deaths in women taking oestrogens was more than halved. It is of interest that the effect of oestrogens in reducing the risk ratio also applied to women who smoke (RR 3.3 as compared with RR 0.58 non-smokers) and furthermore that women taking a lower dose of oestrogens (0.625 mg conjugated oestrogens daily) had a significantly lower RR of 0.39 as compared with 0.79 in women taking a higher dose of oestrogens (1.25 mg conjugated oestrogen daily).

Hulka in 1980 concluded that 'there is no firm epidemiological evidence of a detrimental effect of oestrogens in causing myocardial infarcts or thromboembolic events amongst postmenopausal women'. There would now appear to be sufficient evidence to believe that oestrogens in replacement dosages have a significant and important effect, probably by the prevention of atherosclerosis, in reducing the risk of ischaemic heart disease. Barrett-Connor *et al.* (1979) pointed out that risk of cardiovascular disease in women after the age of 55 years exceeds 10% as compared with 1% for endometrial carcinoma, and that even a small benefit in reducing deaths due to heart disease would outweigh any risks due to endometrial carcinoma.

The reported studies have all been on the effect of unopposed oestrogens and the effect of combined oestrogen–progestogen preparations on the incidence of ischaemic heart disease in postmenopausal women has yet to be investigated. The finding that with the current low dose oestrogen–progestogen oral contraceptive combinations in premenopausal women it is the progestogen component that is associated with increased risk of ischaemic heart disease (Bradley *et al.* 1978, Royal College of General Practitioners' Oral Contraception Study 1977, Meade *et al.* 1980) makes further investigation of the effect of progestogens in postmenopausal women a matter of urgency. In postmenopausal women some oestrogen–progestogen combinations would appear to have an overall deleterious effect on lipid and lipoprotein profiles, whereas in others the effects of the oestrogen–progestogen apparently balance each other out so that there is no detectable change in plasma lipids before and after therapy (Christiansen *et al.* 1984). The use of these latter 'balanced' preparations, which include oestradiol 2 mg or oestriol 1 mg combined with norethisterone acetate 1 mg, probably do not carry any increased risk of atherosclerosis, certainly in the short term (Christiansen *et al.* 1984). Because of the overwhelming importance of cardiovascular disease the WHO Scientific Group on Research in the Menopause has recommended that further studies on the effects of oestrogens and progestogens on lipids and lipoproteins and atherosclerosis should be given the highest priority.

It may be concluded that when oestrogens and progestogens are administered in physiologically balanced replacement doses these hormones not only do not carry any increased risk in terms of thromboembolic disease but in all probability have a substantial beneficial effect in preventing atherosclerosis and ischaemic cardiovascular disease. The effect of oestrogens in preventing atherosclerosis and its consequence may well prove to be one of the most important long term benefits of hormone replacement in postmenopausal women.

OSTEOPOROSIS AND FRACTURES

The benefits of oestrogens in preventing osteoporosis and fractures in postmenopausal women are real and substantial. It has been estimated that 20% of all women will suffer a hip fracture by the time they reach the age of 90 years; of these, 80% will be found to have pre-existing osteoporosis. Furthermore, as a result of complications stemming from hip fractures, 16% of the women will die within 3 months (Schiff & Ryan 1980). In addition, it has been estimated that 25% of all white women over 60 years old will develop spinal compression fractures due to osteoporosis. Riggs (1980), with reference to the situation in the USA, concluded that 'postmenopausal osteoporosis and senile osteoporosis are serious health problems, causing considerable morbidity because of fractures. The disease symptomatically affects about 4 million older Americans and causes an estimated 700 000 new fractures yearly. The incidence of fracture of the proximal femur in women doubles each decade after age 60 years. Based on currently available epidemiologic data, the economic cost of hip fractures in the United States can be estimated at approximately 1 billion annually'.

COST BENEFIT AND COST EFFECTIVENESS
ANALYSIS AND INDICATIONS FOR HORMONE
REPLACEMENT

The various attempts at cost benefit and cost effectiveness analysis of hormone replacement have been summarized by Utian (1980c). Aitken (1976) and Dewhurst (1976) estimated that in 1976 if conjugated oestrogens had been given to every postmenopausal woman, the total annual drug bill in the United Kingdom would have been approximately £90 000 000. In Britain, Dewhurst calculated that the bill for medical services would add a further £60 000 000, making a total of £150 000 000 per year. Aitken estimated that in the same population the cost of treating femoral neck and Colles fractures had amounted to roughly £10 000 000. This would not have allowed for the loss of earnings of the women or for the cost of the pain and disability, which are in many ways immeasurable. The prospects of achieving any scheme of long term prophylactic therapy to large populations are remote and cost benefit analyses, although of interest, are not really relevant in practical terms. Efforts need rather to be concentrated on the recognition and treatment of high risk subgroups of postmenopausal women such as women under 40 who have a premature menopause where benefit/cost ratios are unequivocal and treatment can be instituted effectively.

In the past the risks of oestrogen therapy have probably been overestimated and the benefits have been underestimated. With these considerations in mind, the following approach to hormone replacement may be advised:

1 Short term hormone replacement and appropriate therapy should be given for specific menopausal symptoms (hot flushes, atrophic vaginitis etc.) for as long as symptoms persist;
2 long term hormone replacement should be given in all women under the age of 40 who are hypo-oestrogenic or undergo a spontaneous premature menopause or induced premature menopause;
3 long term hormone replacement should be given to any informed patient who requests it provided there are no contraindications and adequate and continuing medical supervision is available. It is not ethically justifiable to withhold hormone replacement from fully informed patients who request it although all such patients must be assessed and managed on an individual basis.

MANAGEMENT OF THE MENOPAUSE AND CLIMACTERIC

Initial assessment: history

At the first visit the menopausal or climacteric woman requires assessment of her symptoms and direct enquiry into:
1 *Presenting complaints.*
2 *Specific menopausal symptoms*, including (a) vasomotor symptoms, hot flushes, night sweats, reaction to heat; (b) sleep pattern; (c) joint pains and arthritis; (d) menstruation; (e) sexual problems including dyspareunia and dry vagina; (f) mood and personality changes.
3 *Gynaecological history*, including: (a) last menstrual period and whether hysterectomy or bilateral oophorectomy has been performed; (b) menstrual history and amount of menstrual loss, and any postmenopausal bleeding; (c) patient's attitude to monthly withdrawal bleeding if postmenopausal.
4 *Previous medical and family history*, including: (a) thromboembolic disease; (b) liver disease; (c) hypertension/heart disease; (d) diabetes; (e) hyperlipidaemia; (f) other illness/operations.
5 *Previous treatment*, including: (a) oestrogens (type, dosage, duration); (b) other medical therapy; (c) psychotherapy.
6 Home/marital/social circumstances and background.

EXAMINATION

Examination must be performed in every case, including: (a) height, weight and obesity estimate; (b) urine for sugar and protein; (c) blood pressure; (d) breasts; (e) abdomen; (f) pelvis with assessment of oestrogen status.

SPECIAL INVESTIGATIONS

Special investigations which may be indicated include: (a) cervical smear and vaginal smear for hormonal assessment; (b) endometrial sample or dilatation and curettage; (c) FSH if diagnosis is in doubt; (d) plasma oestradiol and oestrone if measure of oestrogenicity required; (e) biochemical screen including plasma cholesterol and fasting blood sugar; (f) urinary calcium, calcium/creatinine ratio, urinary free cortisol and free cortisol/creatinine ratio.

At the conclusion of the initial examination a problem list and plan of management should be drawn up and discussed with the patient. The plan of management will depend upon the following factors.

Diagnosis and indications for oestrogen therapy

In most cases the occurrence of typical hot flushes is so characteristic as to be pathognomonic. Indications for treatment include: (a) vasomotor symptoms; (b) atrophic vaginitis; (c) recurrent urethritis cystitis; (d) Premature menopause; (e) osteoporosis; (f) type II: hyperlipoproteinaemia (Tikkanen *et al.* 1978).

Contraindications to oestrogen therapy

Some absolute or relative contraindications are: (a) previous thromboembolic disease particularly if associated with previous oestrogen or oral contraceptive usage; (b) chronic liver disease with impaired liver function; (c) porphyria; (d) hormone dependent carcinoma.

Diabetes and hypertension are not contraindications to oestrogen therapy but are indications for further investigations and treatment of these particular conditions.

Plan of management

The management of the climacteric patient consists of three equally important parts: (a) hormonal replacement therapy and other therapy for vasomotor symptoms; (b) medical therapy including antihypertensive therapy, weight reduction, etc.; (c) counselling and psychotherapy.

HORMONAL THERAPY

Strategies of management
In the present state of knowledge one of four alternative methods of treatment may be adopted: (a) cyclical oestrogen–progestogen therapy which will nearly always result in a monthly withdrawal bleeding in patients with intact uterus; (b) continuous unopposed oestrogen therapy, with 6-monthly or yearly endometrial sampling in patients with intact uterus; (c) continuous combined oestrogen–progestogen therapy in women who have had a hysterectomy or in women with intact uterus; (d) progestogens alone which are effective in relieving vasomotor symptoms in many women and may be given if oestrogens are contraindicated.

In the case of patients who have had a hysterectomy, or who are menstruating, the choice is fairly straightforward and there is a good case for cyclical oestrogen–progestogen therapy in both those groups of patients.

In postmenopausal women with intact uterus the choice is more difficult and depends upon whether the patient is prepared to accept withdrawal bleeding and whether or not the physician is prepared to undertake endometrial sampling. In general women under 60 years of age are usually prepared to accept monthly withdrawal bleeding when the reasons are explained to them, whereas women over 60 years are much more reluctant to accept a return of menstruation. Continuous combined oestrogen–progestogen therapy in women with intact uterus is still experimental as a significant proportion of women have irregular uterine bleeding which may prove unacceptable though this does decrease with time (Staland 1981). The bleeding results from an atrophic rather than a hyperplastic endometrium so that there is no risk of endometrial carcinoma and the problem is one of inconvenience. It is hoped that in time a balanced oestrogen–progestogen combination will be evolved which will not cause bleeding but will have all the therapeutic benefits of hormone replacement. At the present time the choice in women with intact uterus rests between monthly withdrawal bleeding with combined oestrogen–progestogen treatment or yearly endometrial sampling with oestrogen treatment alone. This choice is probably best left to the patient, though current evidence suggests that combined oestrogen–progestogen therapy is theoretically the treatment of choice.

In all hormonal replacement therapy certain principles should always be followed: (a) use the minimum dose of oestrogen and progestogen which will relieve symptoms and will provide effective hormone replacement in terms of prevention of osteoporosis, atherosclerosis and endometrial and breast carcinoma; (b) adjust the therapeutic regime to eliminate any side effects and achieve acceptable bleeding patterns, and wherever necessary to use appropriate additional treatment to obtain full relief of symptoms and to treat the general medical condition of the patient; (c) discontinue treatment when symptoms subside unless a definite decision has been made to carry out long term prophylactic hormone replacement therapy.

CHOICE OF HORMONE

(a) *Choice of oestrogen.* The ones most commonly used are: conjugated equine oestrogens (0.3–1.25 mg daily); oestradiol valerate (1–2 mg daily); ethinyl oestradiol (0.01–0.05 mg daily); oestriol succinate (2–4 mg daily); diethyl stilboestrol (0.25–0.5 mg daily); piperazine oestrone sulphate (3 mg daily).

It has been claimed that synthetic unconjugated steroids, e.g. ethinyl oestradiol, are associated with a relatively greater effect on liver metabolism as judged by effects on plasma proteins, than natural oestrogens in otherwise equipotent dosages and there is a trend away from the use of synthetic oestrogens in postmenopausal women. It has been shown however that, whereas ethinyloestradiol is absorbed and acts in its original form, most other preparations are metabolized in their passage through the gut and liver. Oestradiol valerate is thus metabolized in part to oestrone and oestrone sulphate in the gut and after oral administration of 2 and 4 mg micronized oestradiol valerate the oestrone sulphate levels were 2–50 times pretreatment levels. The levels of oestrone and oestradiol sulphate show a smaller increase of 4–10 and 2.5–5 times respectively, and the plasma oestradiol shows also a minor increase of 1.4–1.8 times. The levels of oestradiol moreover return to normal after 24 hr, whereas the levels of oestradiol sulphate, oestrone and particularly oestrone sulphate remain elevated for up to 72 hr so that on daily oral administration there will be a progressive build-up of oestrone sulphate (Dada et al. 1978). Conjugated equine oestrogens, which consist mainly of sodium oestrone, sulphate and sodium equiline sulphate similarly causes a predominant rise in oestrone and oestrone sulphate and causes only a small rise in plasma oestradiol levels in doses of 0.625 μg or greater (Utian et al. 1978). Anderson et al. (1978) have shown that, quantitatively, oestrone sulphate is the major circulating oestrogen after the oral administration of most oestrogens with the exception of ethinyloestradiol. In practice all oestrogen preparations appear to be equally effective in relieving symptoms and to have a similar incidence of side effects and complications when administered in equipotent dosages, and no oestrogen appears to have proven significant clinical advantages over any other. Advantages have been claimed for parenteral and intravaginal routes of administration in that oestrogens administered by these routes bypass the gut, produce relatively higher oestradiol/oestrone ratios and a more natural plasma oestrogen profile. Recent investigations however have shown that when oestrogens are administered by any route other than the gastrointestinal tract, the beneficial effect of the oestrogens on serum lipid and lipoproteins is lost. This may be an important consideration as presumably oestrogens so administered will fail to prevent atherosclerosis and ischaemic heart disease. The oral route is therefore the method of choice except under a few special circumstances such as in the treatment of atrophic vaginitis.

(b) *Choice of progestogen*. Unlike oestrogens, different progestogens do have significant differences in their actions, and 19-nortestosterone, pregnane and gonane derivatives in particular tend to have some androgenic effects. Many progestogens are available only in combinations with oestrogen in the form of the contraceptive pill. Those most commonly available not in combination with oestrogens are: medroxyprogesterone acetate (Provera Upjohn) Tab 5 mg; norethisterone (Primolut-N Schering AG) Tab 5 mg; medrogestone (Colpro Ayerst) Tab 5 mg.

The above progestogens may be given in combinations with any of the oestrogens. Norethisterone is 'more androgenic' and produces less withdrawal bleeding than the 17 alpha-hydroxyprogestogens but may tend to reverse possible 'beneficial' effects of oestrogens on plasma lipids and lipoproteins.

(c) *Choice of oestrogen–progestogen*. Several sequential oestrogen–progestogen combinations have been marketed for use in the treatment of climacteric women: Prem Pak (Ayerst)—21 tablets conjugated equine oestrogens 0.625 or 1.25 mg, and 10 tablets + Medrogestone 5 or 10 mg for last 10 days; Post-Oval (Wyeth) or Cyclo-Progynova (Schering)—11 tablets 2 mg oestradiol valerate, then 10 tablets 2 mg oestradiol valerate, then 10 tablets 2 mg oestradiol valerate plus 0.5 mg norgestrel; Trisequens (Novo)—12 tablets 2 mg oestradiol 1 mg oestriol, then 10 tablets 2 mg oestradiol 1 mg oestriol with 1 mg norethisterone acetate, then 6 tablets 1 mg oestradiol 0.5 mg oestriol.

These preparations have the advantage of convenience and ease of use. Their main disadvantage is that the dosages of oestrogen–progestogen are fixed and do not allow for adjustments in relative amounts of oestrogens and progestogens.

(d) *Other hormones*. Androgens have been largely abandoned in the management of the menopause because of the risk of virilization although some authors claim they are of benefit in women with decreased libido (Studd et al. 1977).

Route of administration

Oestrogens and progestogens may be administered orally and parenterally and in the case of oestrogens by local application to the skin and vagina. Injections and implants tend to give high peak dosages with uncertain duration of action and once administered the dose cannot be adjusted. They are popular with some gynaecologists and may be of particular value at the time of hysterectomy and bilateral salpingo-oophorectomy. The ability to adjust dosages according to response and to provide relatively constant day to day levels of hormone replacement, however, makes oral rather than parenteral administration the method of choice in most cases. Local application of oestrogens to the vagina in the form of creams and pessaries are very effective in the treatment of atrophic vaginitis. Such preparations are also well absorbed and have a general systemic effect. The oestrogens moreover are absorbed directly and not metabolized in the vagina so that relatively higher plasma oestradiol/oestrone ratios are obtained than when the same oestrogens are administered orally (Riggs *et al.* 1978). Oestrogen creams are similarly well absorbed when rubbed into the skin, and this percutaneous method of administration has been advocated in some countries such as France. In general however neither the vagina or percutaneous routes are as convenient for long term use as oral administration, and vaginal administration is probably best reserved for cases of atrophic vaginitis where a particular local effect is desired.

OTHER THERAPY FOR VASOMOTOR SYMPTOMS

The relief of vasomotor symptoms by oestrogens is usually so dramatic that oestrogens are sometimes regarded as a 'cure all' and it is assumed that all patients will be relieved by oestrogen. In most series (Utian 1972a, Lauritzen 1973, Campbell 1976a) however there is a 'hard core' of 5–10% of patients who, although they may be improved, are not completely relieved of their symptoms. In this group the vasomotor symptoms may have a different aetiological basis and may require additional therapy as well as oestrogens. It is important in these patients not to increase the dose of oestrogens to excessive levels but to use appropriate ancillary treatment depending upon the precise nature of the persisting symptoms. A number of other agents have been recommended for the treatment of hot flushes, including clonidine (Dixarit Boehringer Ingelheim), *β*-adrenergic blocking agents such as propanalol and tranqullizers, sedatives and antidepressants.

Clonidine is an imidazoline derivative which was introduced as an antimigraine drug and, in higher dose, as an antihypertensive and later for the prevention of hot flushes. It is believed to act as a central alpha-adrenergic stimulant. Some double blind cross-over trials of clonidine have shown no significant benefit over a placebo (Lindsay & Hart 1978). Other similar trials however have been reported as showing significant beneficial effects (Edington *et al.* 1980). It would appear, from personal experience, that clonidine is often effective in relieving hot flushes in women not responding, or only partially responding, to oestrogen replacement therapy. These women often respond to a combination of oestrogen and clinidine therapy. Clonidine may also be of considerable benefit when given at night to women troubled with night sweats or insomnia not relieved by oestrogens. It may in addition have a particular place as an antihypertensive agent in the treatment of hypertensive postmenopausal women with vasomotor symptoms. Some patients experience side effects to clonidine such as dizziness though these decrease with time and such patients may require progressive adjustment of dosage of clonidine to achieve optimum effect. Clonidine may have a particular place in the management of patients with vasomotor symptoms not responding to oestrogen replacement.

Beta-adrenergic blocking agents have also been used in the treatment of hot flushes and have been reported to be no better than placebos in double blind trials (Coope *et al.* 1978). Beta-blockers, however, may have a place in patients in whom palpitations, extrasystoles, tachycardia and anxiety symptoms predominate and are not relieved by oestrogens and by counselling. Beta-blockers also have an important place in the management of postmenopausal patients with hypertension. In some patients it may be necessary to use a combination of oestrogens, clonidine and beta-blockers.

Tranquillizers, sedatives and antidepressants, although widely used, probably have a small part to play in the management of the climacteric as such. Provided there is confirmatory evidence of hypothalamic pituitary hyperactivity (such as vasomotor symptoms or raised FSH) or of low oestrogen (as judged clinically by vaginal smears or plasma oestradiol) menopausal patients with anxiety, depression or mood changes should be given a therapeutic trial of oestrogen–progesterone therapy. At the same time, patients with home, marital or social problems should be treated by supportive explanation, reassurance and psychotherapy. Only when such measures have failed or where there is evidence of endogenous depression or anxiety should antidepressants or tranquillizers be used. Tranquillizers and sedatives may be of value on a short term for insomnia but habitual use of tranquillizers should be discouraged. In patients in whom oestrogens are contraindicated and where all else has failed, a combination of ergotamine tartrate (a sympathetic inhibitor), belladonna (a parasympathetic inhibitor) and phenobarbitone (Bellergal Sandoz) has been recommended though its effectiveness has not been tested in control trials.

OTHER MEDICAL THERAPY

Many women presenting at the menopause or postmenopause have other major medical problems such as obesity, osteoarthritis, hypertension and diabetes. In many instances the treatment of these medical conditions may be of as much importance and bring as much, if not greater, benefit to the patient than the treatment of the menopausal symptoms *per se*. In the past patients with hypertension and diabetes have often been refused oestrogen therapy for fear of causing an exacerbation of the hypertension, or of disturbing the blood sugar control in diabetes and in some instances hormone replacement has been discontinued. Such patients often experience considerable distress and disability from vasomotor symptoms. In these patients and in fact in all patients with medical conditions requiring treatment it is best to institute both appropriate medical therapy and menopausal treatment at the same time.

PSYCHOTHERAPY

The menopause means something to most women, whether it be departure of youth, loss of femininity or a sign of advancing years. The reality of middle age, with its grey hairs, wrinkles and spectacles, has to be faced and the menopause may symbolize the change. This realization, with other psychosocial problems which arise around the menopause, requires acceptance and adjustment on the part of most women. The climacteric is not without its compensations, with less anxiety over children and finance, more comfort and leisure and more opportunity and time for enjoyment. For the woman whom life has treated kindly, who adjusts easily and leads a full life, the menopause may present no problems. In such women the relief of any symptoms, simple explanations and reassurance may be all that is required. For the woman whom life has treated unkindly, who is maladjusted, unhappy or lonely more specific counselling and psychotherapy, and occasionally specialist psychiatric help, is often required. Adjustment and acceptance is not helped by the fact that the meno-

pause is often given a bad name with associations of failing powers, getting old and a wide variety of complaints. By attributing any unexplained symptom or condition in women over 40 years old to the 'change of life' many doctors are far from blameless. The menopause or climacteric should be regarded as what it is, no more and no less, that is the cessation of menstruation and of reproductive function. With this reassurance and the assurance that the end of menstruation is not the end of life but the beginning of a new phase to be lived and enjoyed, the doctor can enable most patients to make the necessary adjustments and live happily for the remaining third or more of their lives.

Role of menopause or mature women's clinic

Special clinics for the treatment of menopausal patients have been established in many centres. These have a number of advantages and have an important part to play in the management of climacteric patients. The advantage and purpose of such clinics are:

1   a considerable body of expertise, knowledge and skill is built by the personnel and a referral centre is provided both for routine treatment and for problems in management;

2   therapy can in general be more easily controlled and supervised under established regimes;

3   ancillary services such as dietetic and diagnostic screening facilities may be more readily available;

4   general health, education and fitness programmes can be introduced;

5   patients can and do share experiences, interests and problems providing a form of group therapy;

6   research can be carried out.

The aim of menopause clinics and indeed the aim of management of all menopausal or climacteric women should not just be the relief of menopausal symptoms and the prevention of complications such as fractures and myocardial infarcts but the broader, more positive aim of enabling and encouraging women to keep physically and mentally fit, and to maintain the confidence, interest and zest of life so as to be better able to enjoy a full and happy life into advanced age.

REFERENCES

ABRAHAM G.E., SWERDLOFF R.S., TULCHINSKY D., HOPPER K. & ODELL W.B. (1971) *J. clin. Endocr. Metab.*, **33**, 42.

AITEN J.M. (1976) In *The Menopause* (Beard R.J. ed.), p. 95. Lancaster MTP Press.

AITKEN J.M., HART D.M. & LINDSAY R. (1973) *Brit. med. J.*, **iii**, 515.

AITKEN J.M., HALL P.E., RAO L.G.S., HART D.M. & LINDSAY R. (1974) *Clin. Endocrinol.*, **3**, 167.

AKSEL S. & SCHOMBER D.W. (1975) *Amer. J. Obstet. Gynec.*, **126**, 165.

ALFFRAM P.A. (1974) *Acta Othop. Scand. (Suppl.)*, **65**, 9.

ALFFRAM P.A. & BAUER G.C.N. (1962) *J. Bone J. Surg. A.*, **44**, 105.

ALHAVA E.M. & PUITTINEN J. (1973) *Ann. clin. Res.*, **5**, 398.

AMUNDSEN D.W. & DIERS C.J. (1973) *Hum. Biol.*, **45**, 605.

ANDERSON A.B.M. (1979) In *Human Reproductive Physiology* (Shearman R.P. ed.), p. 445. Blackwell Scientific Publications, Oxford.

ANDERSON A.B.M., SKLOUSKY E., SAYERS L., STEELE P.A. & TURNBULL A.C. (1978) *Brit. med. J.*, **i**, 140.

ASCH R.H. & GREENBLATT R.B. (1977) *Clinics in Obstetrics and Gynaecology* (Greenblatt R.B. & Studd J.W. eds), **4**, 85. W.B. Saunders, London.

BARNES A.C. (1968) The long range problems of the post-menopausal woman. Ayerst Symposium.

BARNES R. & BROWN J.T. (1976) *J. Bone J. Surg. B.*, **58**, 2.

BARRETT-CONNOR E., BROWN W.U., TURNER J., AUSTIN M. & CRIQUI M.H. (1979) *J. Amer. med. Ass.*, **241**, 2167.

BASSI F., GIUSTI G., BORSI L., CATTANEO S., GIANNOTTI P., FORTI G., PAZZAGLI M., VIGIANI C. & SERIO M. (1977) *Clin. Endocrinol.*, **6**, 5.

BLOCH E. (1953) *Acta Anat.*, **17**, 201.

Boston Collaborative Drug Surveillance Program (1974) *New Engl. J. Med.*, **290**, 15.

BRADLEY D.D., WINGERD J., PETTITI D.B., KRAUSS R.M., RAMCHARAN S. (1978) *N. Engl. J. Med.*, **299**, 17.

BROWN J.B. (1955) *Lancet*, **i**, 320.

BRUNS P. (1882) *Dtsch. Chirug.*, **27**, 1.

BYRD B.F., BURCH J.C. & VAUGHAN W.K. (1977) *Ann. Surg.*, **185**, 574.

CAINE M. & RAZ S. (1973) *Abstracts of the International Society of Urology*, p. 30. Amsterdam.

CAMPBELL S. (1976a) *The Management of the Menopause and Post-Menopausal Years.* (Campbell S. ed.), p. 149. Lancaster MTP Press.

CAMPBELL S. (1976b) *The Management of the Menopause and Post-Menopausal Years.* (Campbell S. ed.), p. 63. Lancaster MTP Press.

CHAKRAVARTI S., COLLINS W.P., FORECAST J.D., NEWTON J.R., ORAM D.H. & STUDD J.W. (1976) *Brit. med. J.*, **ii**, 784.

CHARI S., HOPKINSON C.R.N., DAUME E. & STURM G. (1979) *Acta Endocrinol. (Kbh)*, **90**, 157.

CHRISTIE-BROWN J.R. & CHRISTIE-BROWN M.E. (1976) In *The Menopause.* (Beard R.J. ed.), p. 57. Lancaster MTP Press.

CHRISTIANSEN C., CHRISTENSEN M.S., LARSEN N.E. & TRANSBØL I.B. (1982) *J. clin. Endocrinol. Metab.*, **55**, 1124.

CHRISTIANSEN C., RØDBRO P. (1983) *Calcif. Tiss. Int.*, **35**, 720.

CHRISTIANSEN C., CHRISTENSEN M.S., GRANDE P. & TRANSBOL I. (1984) *Maturitas*, **5**, 193.

COBLE Y.D., KOHLER P.O., CARGILLE C.M. & ROSS G.T. (1969) *J. clin. Invest.*, **48**, 359.

COOPE J., WILLIAMS S. & PATTERSON J.S. (1978) *Brit. J. Obstet. Gynaecol.*, **85**, 472.

COOPER A. (1824) In *A Treatise on Dislocations and on Fractures of the Joints*, 3ed. Longman, London.

CRILLY R.G., HORSMAN A., MARSHALL D.H. & NORDIN B.E.C. (1978) *Front. Hormone Res.*, **5**, 53.

DADA O.A., LAUMAS V., LANDGREN B.M., CEKAN S.Z. & DICZFALUSY E. (1978) *Acta Endocrinol. (Kbh)*, **88**, 754.

DANIEL W.N. (1976) *Arch. int. Med.*, **136**, 288.

DAVIES I.J., NAFTOLIN F., RYAN K.J., FISHMAN J. & SIN J. (1975) *Endocrinology*, **97**, 554.

DE JONG F.H. & SHARPE R.M. (1976) *Nature*, **263**, 71.

DENNERSTEIN L., BURROWS G.D., HYMAN G.J. & SHARPE K. (1979) *Maturitas*, **2**, 19.

DENNERSTEIN L. & BURROWS G.D. (1978) *Maturitas*, **1**, 55.

DEWHURST C.J. (1976) In *The Menopause* (Beard R.J. ed.), p. 240. Lancaster MTP Press.

DOMINIAN J. (1977) In *The Menopause, Clinics in Obstetrics and Gynaecology* (Greenblatt R.B. & Studd J.W. eds.), **4**, 241. W.B. Saunders, London.

DORING G.K. (1969) *J. reprod. Fertil. Suppl.*, **6**, 77.

EBLING F.J. (1974) *J. invest. Dermatol.*, **62**, 161.

EDINGTON R.F., CHAGNON J.P. & STEINBERG W.M. (1980) *Can. med. Assoc. J.*, **123**, 1.

ENGLAND P.C., SKINNER L.G., COTTRELL K.M. & SELLWOOD R.A. (1974) *Brit. J. Cancer*, **29**, 469.

ERLIK Y., MELDRUM D.R. & JUDD H.L. (1982) *Obstet. Gynecol.*, **59**, 403.

ERLIK Y., TATARYN I.V., MELDRUM D.R., LOMAX P., BAJOREK J.G. & JUDD H.L. (1981) *J. Amer. med. Ass.*, **245**, 1741.

FAIMAN C., WINTER J.B. & REYES F. (1976) *Clin. Obstet. Gynaecol.*, **3**, 467.

FÅHRAEUS L. & LARSSON-COHN U. (1982) *Acta. Endocrinol. (Kbh)*, **101**, 592.

FLINT M. (1976) In *Consensus of Menopause Research* (Greenblatt R.B. & Albeaux-Fernet M. eds.), p. 78. Lancaster MTP Press.

FRANCHIMONT P., BECKER H., VALKE J.C., SCELLENS A.M.C.M., DERMOULIN A., THYS C., BOURGINGNON J.P. & LEGROS J.J. (1975) In *Reproductive Endocrinology* (Vokaer R. & Boch G. eds.), p. 185. Pergamon Press, Oxford.

FROMMER D.J. (1964) *Brit. med. J.*, **ii**, 349.

GALLAGHER J.C. & NORDIN B.E.C. (1973) *Front. Hormone Res.*, **2**, 98.

GALLAGHER J.C. & NORDIN B.E.C. (1975) *Front. Hormone Res.*, **3**, 150.

GAMBRELL R.D. (1980) In *The Menopause and Post-menopause* (Pasetto N., Paoletti R. & Ambrus J.C. eds.), p. 289. Lancaster MTP Press.

GAMBRELL R.D. (1982) *Acta Obstet. Gynecol. Scand. (Suppl.)*, **106**, 37.

GAMBRELL R.D., MAIER R.C. & SANDERS B.I. (1983) *Obstet. Gynecol.*, **62**, 435.

GOLDENBERG R.L., GRODIN J.M., RODBARD D. & ROSS G.T. (1973) *Amer. J. Obstet. Gynec.*, **116**, 1003.

GOLDSMITH N.F., JOHNSTON J.O., PICETTI G. & GARCIA C. (1977) *J. Bone J. Surg. A.*, **55**, 1276.

GORDAN G.S. & VAUGHAN C. (1980) In *The Menopause and Post-Menopause* (Pasetto N., Paoletti R. & Ambrus J.L., eds.), p. 179. Lancaster MTP Press.

GORDON T., KANNEL W.B., HJORTLAND M.C. & McNAMARA P.M. (1978) *Ann. intern. Med.*, **89**, 157.

GRATTAROLA R., SECRETO G. & RECCHIONE C. (1975) *Amer. J. Obstet. Gynec.*, **121**, 380.

GREENBLATT R.B., BARFIELD W.E., GARNER J.F., CALK G.L. & HARROD P.J. (1950) *J. clin. Endocrinol.*, **10**, 1547.

GRODIN J.M., SIITERI P.K. & MacDONALD P.C. (1973) *J. clin. Endocr. Metab.*, **36**, 207.

HAMMOND C.B., JELOUESK F.R., LEE K.L., CREASMAN W.T. & PARKER R.T. (1979) *Amer. J. Obstet. Gynec.*, **133**, 525.

HAMMOND D.O. (1977) In *Clinics in Obstetrics and Gynaecology. The Menopause* (Greenblatt R.B. & Studd J.W. eds.), **4**, 49. W.B. Saunders, London.

HEANEY R.R., RECKER R.R. & SAVILLE P.D. (1978) *J. lab. clin. Med.*, **92**, 964.

HELLER R.F. & JACOBS H.S. (1978) *Brit. med. J.*, **ii**, 472.

HEMSELL D.L., GRODIN J.M., BRENNER P.T., SIITERI P.K. & MacDONALD P.C. (1976) *J. clin. Endocr. Metab.*, **38**, 476.

HENNEMAN D.H. (1971) *Biochem. biophys. Res. Commun.*, **44**, 326.

HERTIG A.T. (1944) *J. clin. Endocrinol.*, **4**, 581.

HORSMAN A., (1981) In *Osteoporosis: Recent Advances in Pathogenesis and Treatment.* (De Luca H.F. ed.) p. 175. Baltimore University Park Press.

HORSMAN A., JONES M., FRANCIS R. & NORDIN C. (1983) *New Engl. J. Med.*, **309**, 1405.

HOWITZ R.I. & FEINSTEIN A.R. (1978) *New Engl. J. Med.*, **299**, 1089.

HUTCHINSON T.A., POLANSKY S.M. & FEINSTEIN A.R. (1979) *Lancet*, **ii**, 705.

HUTTON J.D., JACOBS H.S., MURRAY M.A.F. & JAMES V.H.T. (1978) *Lancet*, **i**, 678.

ISKRANT A.P. & SMITH R.W. (1969) *Publ. Hlth. Rep.*, **84**, 33.

JAMES C.E., BREESON A.J., KUVACS G., HILL J.G., GRANT C., ALLEN K.M., FRY D.E. & BAYLISS E.M. (1984) *Brit. J. Obstet. Gynaecol.*, **91**, 56.

JICK H., PORTER J. & MORRISON A.S. (1977) *Lancet*, **i**, 1354.

JONES E.C. & KROHN P.L. (1961) *J. Endocrinol.*, **21**, 497.

JUDD H.L., LUCAS W.E. & YEN S.C.C. (1976) *J. clin. Endocr. Metab.*, **43**, 272.

KAUFMAN S.A. (1967) *Obstet. Gynec., N.Y.*, **30**, 399.

KAWAKAMI M. & SAKUMA Y. (1974) *Neuroendocrinol.*, **15**, 290.

KNOWLEDEN J., BUHR A.J. & DUNBAR O. (1964) *Brit. J. prev. soc. Med.*, **18**, 130.

KRONENBERG F., COTE L.J., LINKIE D.M., DYRENFURTH I. & DOWNEY J.A. (1984) *Maturitas*, **6**, 31.

KUPPERMAN H.S., BLATT M.H.G., WIESBADEN J. & FILLER W. (1953) *J. clin. Endocrinol.*, **13**, 154.

LAURITZEN C. (1973) *Front Hormone Res.*, **2**, 2.

LIND T., CAMERON E.C., HUNTER W.M., LEON C., MORAN P.F.,

OXLEY A., GERRARD J. & LIND U.G.C. (1979) *Brit. J. Obstet. Gynaec.*, **86** (Suppl. 3), 1.

LINDSAY R. (1980) In *The Menopause and Post-Menopause* (Pasetto N. & Paoletti R. & Ambrus J.C. eds.), p. 163. Lancaster MTP Press.

LINDSAY R., AITKEN J., ANDERSON J.B., HART D.M., MacDONALD E.B. & CLARKE A.C. (1976) *Lancet*, **i**, 1038.

LINDSAY R. & HART D.M. (1978) *Maturitas*, **1**, 21.

LINDSAY R., HART D.M. & PURDIE D. (1978a) *Clin. Sci. Mol. Med.*, **54**, 193.

LINDSAY R., HART D.M., MacLEAN A., CLARK A.C., KRASKEWSKI A. & GARWOOD J. (1978b) *Lancet*, **i**, 1325.

LOMAX P., BAJOREK J.G., CHESAREK W. & TATARYN I.V. (1979) In *Thermoregulatory mechanisms and their therapeutic implications* (Cox B., Lomax P., Milton A.S. & Schonbaum E. eds), p. 208. Karger, Basle.

LONGCOPE C. (1974) In *The Menopausal Syndrome* (Greenblatt R.B., Makesh U.B. & McDorough P.G. eds.), p. 6. Medcom Press, New York.

LUMPKIN M.D., DEPAOLO L.V. & NEGRO-VILAR A. (1984) *Endocrinology*, **114**, 201.

MacDONALD P.C., ROMBATO R.P. & SIITERI P.K. (1967) *J. clin. Endocr. Metab.*, **27**, 1103.

MacKAY E.U., KHOO S.K. & SHAN N.A. (1973) *Obstet. Gynec. Surv.*, **28**, 155.

MacMAHON T. & WORCESTER J. (1966) *National Center for Health Statistics Series II.* Washington DC, 19.

MARKS R. & SHAHRAD P. (1977) *Clin. Obstet. Gynaecol.*, **4**, 207.

MARSHALL D.H., CRILLY R.G. & NORDIN B.E.C. (1977) *Brit. med. J.*, **ii**, 1177.

MARX S.J. (1978) *J. Amer. med. Ass.*, **240**, 1630.

MATTINGLY R.F. & HUANG W.Y. (1969) *Amer. J. Obstet. Gynec.*, **103**, 679.

McCONKEY B., FRASER G.M., BLIGH A.S. & WHITELEY H. (1963) *Lancet*, **i**, 693.

McKINLAY S., JEFFREYS M. & THOMPSON B. (1972) *J. Biosoc. Sci.*, **4**, 161.

McLENNAN M.J. & McLENNAN C.E. (1971) *Obstet. Gynecol.*, **37**, 325.

MEADE T.W., GREENBERG G. & THOMPSON S.G. (1980) *Brit. med. J.*, **i**, 1157.

MEEMA S. & MEEMA H.E. (1976) *Isr. J. med. Sci.*, **12**, 601.

MELDRUM D.R., SHAMONKI I.M., FRUMAR A.M., TATARYN I.V., CHANG R.F. & JUDD H.L. (1979) *Amer. J. Obstet. Gynec.*, **135**, 713.

MILLIGAN D., DRIFE J.O., & SHORT R.V. (1975) *Brit. med. J.*, **iv**, 494.

MILLS T.M. & MAHESH U.B. (1977) In *The Menopause, Clinics in Obstetrics and Gynaecology* (Greenblatt R.B. & Studd J.W. eds.), **4**, 71, W.B. Saunders, London.

MOLNAR G.W. (1979) *Amer. J. Physiol.*, **237 (5)**, 306.

MORSE R., HUTTON J.D., JACOBS H.S., MURRAY M.A.F. & JAMES U.H.T. (1979) *Brit. J. Obstet. Gynaec.*, **86**, 981.

NACHTIGALL L.E., NACHTIGALL R.H., NACHTIGALL R.D. & BECHMAN E.M. (1979) *Obstet. Gynec.*, **53**, 277.

NEWHOUSE M.L., PEARSON R.M., FULLERTON J.M., BOESEN

E.A.M. & SHANNON H.S. (1977) Brit. J. prev. soc. Med., 31, 148.

NORDIN B.E.C., GALLAGHER J.C., AARON J.E. & HORSMAN A. (1975) Front Hormone Res., 3, 131.

NORDIN B.E.C., MACGREGOR J. & SMITH D.A. (1966) Quart. J. Med., 35, 25.

NOTELOWITZ M., KITCHENS C.S. & WARE M.D. (1984) Obstet. Gynecol., 63, 621.

ODELL W.D. & SWERDLOFF R.S. (1968) Proc. N.Y. Acad. Sci., 61, 529.

OLIVER M.F. (1976) In The Management of the Menopause and Post-Menopausal Years (Campbell S. ed.), p. 175. Lancaster MTP Press.

OLIVER M.F. & BOYD G.S. (1959) Lancet, ii, 691.

ORY H. (1974) J. Amer. med. Ass., 228, 68.

PAGANINI-HILL A., ROSS R.K., GERKINS V.R., HENDERSON B.E., ARTHUR M. & MACK T.M. (1981) Ann. intern. Med., 95, 28.

PARRISH H.M., CARR C.A., HALL D.G. & KING T.M. (1967) Amer. J. Obstet. Gynec., 99, 155.

PERZIGIAN A.J. (1973) J. Amer. Geriatr. Soc., 21, 100.

PFEFFER R.I., KUROSAKI T.T. & CHARLTON S.K. (1979) Amer. J. Epidemiol., 110, 469.

PFEFFER R.I., WHIPPLE G.H., KUROSAKI T.T. & CHAPMAN J.M. (1978) Amer. J. Epidemiol., 107, 479.

POORTMAN J., THIJSSEN J.H.H. & SCHWARTZ F. (1973) J. Clin. Endocr. Metab., 37, 101.

PUNNONEN R. (1972) Acta Obstet. Gynec. Scand. (Suppl. 9), 9, 32.

RECKER R.P., SAVILLE P.D. & HEANEY R.P. (1977) Ann. intern. Med., 87, 649.

REYES F.I., WINTER J.S.D. & FAIMAN C. (1977) Amer. J. Obstet. Gynec., 129, 557.

RIKZALLAH T.H., TOVELL H.M.M. & KELLY W.G. (1975) J. clin. Endocr. Metab., 40, 1045.

RIGGS B.L. (1980) Obstet. Gynec. Surv., 35, 389.

RIGGS B.L. & JOWSEY J. (1969) J. clin. Invest., 48, 1065.

RIGGS B.L., SEEMAN E., HODGSON S.F., TAVES D.R. & O'FALLON W.M. (1982) New Engl. J. Med., 306, 446.

ROSENBERG L., ARMSTRONG B., PHIL D. & JICK H. (1976) New Engl. J. Med., 294, 1256.

ROYAL COLLEGE OF GENERAL PRACTITIONERS' ORAL CONTRACEPTION STUDY. (1977) Lancet, i, 624.

ROSS R.K., PAGANINI-HILL A., GERKINS V.R., MACK T.M., PFEFFER R., ARTHUR M. & HENDERSON B.E. (1980) J. Amer. med. Ass., 243, 1635.

ROSS R.K., PAGANINI-HILL A., MACK T.M., ARTHUR M. & HENDERSON B.E. (1981) Lancet, i, 858.

RYAN K.J. (1976) Clin. Obstet. Gynec., 19, 805.

SAMSIOE G., SKRYTEN A. & SILFVERSTOLPE G. (1983) Swed. Gynecol. Obstet. Invest., 15, 275.

SAWYER C.H. (1975) Neuroendocrinology, 17, 197.

SAXENA B.B., LEYENDECKER G., CHEN W., GANDY H.W. & PETERSON R.E. (1969) Diezfalusy Karolinska Symposium on Research Methods in Reproduction Endocrinology. 1st Symposium Immunoassay of Gonadotrophins, Stockholm.

SCHIFF I. & RYAN K.S. (1980) Obstet. Gynec. Surv. 35, 400.

SEYLER L.E. & REICHLIN S. (1973) J. clin. Endocr. Metab., 40, 413.

SHARMAN A. (1966) Reproductive physiology of the post-partum period, p. 73. Churchill Livingstone, Edinburgh & London.

SHERMAN B.M. & KORENMAN S.G. (1975) J. clin. Invest., 55, 699.

SHERMAN B.M., WEST J.H. & KORENMAN S.G. (1976) J. clin. Endocr. Metab., 42, 629.

SILFVERSTOLPE G., GUSTAFSON A., SAMSIOE G. & SVANBORG A. (1982a) Arch. Gynecol., 231, 279.

SILFVERSTOLPE G., GUSTAFSON A., SAMSIOE G. & SVANBORG A. (1982b) Maturitas, 4, 103.

SMITH D.A., AIKEN J.M., ANDERSON J., SHIMMINS J. & NORDIN B.E.C. (1972) The skeletal uptake of 855R in relation to age and bone loss in women. Presented at the Second International Conference on Strontium Metabolism, Glasgow, August 16–19.

SMITH D.C., PRENTICE R., THOMPSON D.J. & HERMANN W.L. (1975) New Engl. J. Med., 293, 1164.

SMITH P. (1980) In The Menopause and Post-Menopause (Pasetto N., Poletti R. & Ambrus J.C. eds.), p. 91. Lancaster MTP Press.

SNELL R.S. & BISCHITZ P.G. (1963) J. Anatom. (Lond.), 97, 361.

STERNBERG W.H. (1949) Amer. J. Path., 25, 493.

STUDD J., CHAKRAVARTI S. & ORAM D. (1977) Clin. Obstet. Gynaecol., 4, 3.

STURDEE D.W., WILSON K.A., PIPILI E. & CROCKER C.D. (1978) Brit. med. J., ii, 79.

SZNAJDERMAN M. & OLIVER M.F. (1963) Lancet, i, 962.

TATARYN I.V., LOMAX P., BAJOREK J.G., CHESAREK W., MELDRUM D.R. & JUDD J.L. (1980) Maturitas, 2, 101.

TATARYN I.V., MELDRUM D.R., LU K.N., FRUMAR A.M. & JUDD H.L. (1979) J. clin. Endocr. Metab., 49, 152.

TAYLOR R.W. (1974) J. Obstet. Gynaec. Brit. Cwlth., 81, 856.

THE CORONARY DRUG PROJECT RESEARCH GROUP (1973) J. Amer. med. Ass., 226, 652.

TIKKANEN M.J., NIKKALA E.A. & VARTIAINEN E. (1978) Lancet, ii, 490.

TRELOAR A.E., BOYNTON R.E., BENN B.G. & BROWN B.W. (1967) Int. J. Fertil., 12, 77.

UTIAN W.H. (1970) PhD Thesis, University of Cape Town.

UTIAN W.H. (1972a) 46, 732.

UTIAN W.H. (1972b) S. Afr. med. J., 46, 1079.

UTIAN W.H. (1972c) Int. J. Gynec. Ostet., 10, 95.

UTIAN W.H. (1980a) In Menopause in Modern Perspective, p. 26. Appleton-Century-Crofts, New York.

UTIAN W.H. (1980b) In Menopause in Modern Perspective, p. 63. Appleton-Century-Crofts, New York.

UTIAN W.H. (1980c) In Menopause in Modern Perspective, p. 121. Appleton-Century-Crofts, New York.

UTIAN W.H., KATZ M., DAVEY D.A. & CARR P.J. (1978) Amer. J. Obstet. Gynec., 132, 297.

VAN LOOK P.F.A., LOTHIAN H., HUNTER W.M., MICHIE E.A. & BAIRD D.T. (1977) Clin. Endocrinol., 7, 13.

VELARDO J.T. (1958) In The Endocrinology of Reproduction

(Velardo J.T. ed,), p. 148. Oxford University Press, New York.

VERMEULEN A. (1976) *J. clin. Endocr. Metab.*, **42**, 247.

VON EIFF A.W. (1976) *Front. Hormone Res.*, **3**, 177.

WAHL P., WALDEN C., KNOPP R., HOOVER J., WALLACE R., HEISS G. & RIFKIND B. (1983) *New Engl. J. Med.*, **308**, 862.

WALTER S., WALF H., BARLEBO H. & JENSEN K. (1976) *Abstracts of the International Continence Society*, Antwerp.

WIED G.L. & BIBBO M. (1975) In *Textbook of Gynecologic Endocrinology*, 2e (Gold J.J. ed.). Harper and Row, Hagerstown, Maryland.

WEISS N.S., URE C.L., BALLARD J.H., WILLIAMS A.R. & DALING J.R. (1980) *New Engl. J. Med.*, **303**, 1195.

WILSON R.A. (1966) *Feminine Forever*. Mayflower-Dell, New York.

WILSON R.A. & WILSON T.A. (1963) *J. Amer. geriatr. Soc.*, **11**, 347.

YEN S.S.C., LLERENA O., PEARSON O.H. & LITTEL A.S. (1970) *J. clin. Endocr. Metab.*, **30**, 325.

YEN S.S.C., TSAI C.C., NAFTOLIN F., VANDENBERG G. & AJABOR L. (1972) *J. clin. Endocr. Metab.*, **34**, 671.

ZIEL H.K. & FINKLE W.B. (1975) *New Engl. J. Med.*, **293**, 1167.

CHAPTER 45
PROLAPSE AND URINARY INCONTINENCE

D. W. WARRELL

Genital tract prolapse and urinary incontinence are closely linked by the important part played by pregnancy and childbirth in the aetiology of these two conditions.

Though uterine prolapse may occur in other circumstances such as in association with ectopia vesicae or in elderly spinsters; these are specialized and uncommon types of prolapse when compared with the general multiple organ involvement pattern of prolapse seen in multipara. The former represents a development failure of uterine supports while the latter is evidence of widespread damage sustained at childbirth.

Urinary incontinence has many causes; however, genuine stress incontinence is a disorder experienced mainly by multiparous women and is very much less common in nullipara. It is self-evident that reproduction initiates the damage which results in incontinence of urine and/or prolapse. However, an understanding of the relationship between prolapse and incontinence of urine has been slow to emerge, first of all because genuine stress incontinence has often been muddled with other types of incontinence, and secondly because techniques appropriate to study the problem are of recent evolution.

This chapter sets out to explore the link between these conditions and then goes on to describe the assessment and management of patients suffering from genital tract prolapse and those with incontinence of urine.

Pelvic floor and visceral sphincter damage is often widespread and many women suffering from genital prolapse suffer from urinary and faecal control problems. However the structure of specialist practice in the United Kingdom is so arranged that women with prolapse and urinary incontinence are usually looked after by gynaecologists while those suffering from anorectal problems are cared for by general or rectal surgeons. This arrangement carries the risk of each specialist being only aware of problems in his own field and being less aware of other pelvic damage. For

that reason emphasis is laid on the importance of a view of the pelvic floor as a whole structure both anatomically and functionally.

STRUCTURE AND FUNCTION OF THE PELVIC FLOOR AND THE VISCERAL SPHINCTERS

The major component of the pelvic floor is a pair of symmetrical striated muscle sheets usually termed the levator ani muscles or pelvic diaphragm. The muscle floor is defective in the midline where the urethra, vagina and bowel pass through it. The anterior attachment of the levator is linear and extends from the body of the pubis to the ischial spine. There is direct attachment to the bone of the body of the pubis lateral to the symphysis and to the ischial spine; in between the muscle arises from a condensation of the obturator fascia.

It is conventional to describe the levator in three parts, the most medial of which, the pubococcygeus, is further divided into two parts: a posterior flat muscle inserted into the tip of the coccyx and anococcygeal raphe and a thicker anterior part, the puborectalis, whose fibres swing medially and join those from the opposite side to mingle with the external anal sphincter.

The origin of the second part, the iliococcygeus, is contiguous with that of the pubococcygeus. It partly overlaps the latter to insert below it on the coccyx and the anococcygeal raphe. The third component, the coccygeus, is often rudimentary; it arises from the ischial spine and is inserted into the caudal part of the sacrum and upper coccygeal vertebrae.

The pelvic floor muscle has a double nerve supply, the pudendal nerve arising from the anterior primary rami of S2, S3 & S4, and direct branches from the motor roots of S3 and S4 to it's visceral surface. There is debate as to the precise parts of the pelvic floor supplied by these nerves. However, the weight of the evidence is that puborectalis is supplied by direct branches of the sacral nerves and that the rest of the pelvic floor is supplied via the pudendal nerve (Sato 1980, Percy *et al.* 1981).

The striated muscle of the pelvic floor is different from limb striated muscle in that it is in a state of continuous activity even during sleep (Floyd & Walls 1953). The heterogeneous mixture of slow and fast twitch fibres in the pelvic floor (Parks *et al.* 1977, Gosling *et al.* 1981) enables it to provide support for long periods with the capacity for increased activity and contraction when needed.

The urethra in the adult female is about 4 cm in length and runs from the bladder antero-inferiorly to the external meatus through the most anterior part of the gap between the origins of the pubococcygeus muscle. It is supported by the pubo-urethral ligaments (Zacharin 1962), and is intimately embedded in the vaginal fascia.

The urothelium is surrounded by smooth muscle whose fibres run both along and oblique to the long axis of the urethra. This smooth muscle layer is surrounded by a circular striated muscle sphincter whose fibres are mainly of the slow twitch type and

are thus able to maintain a closure force for long periods of time. There is conflicting evidence about the nerve supply of the striated urethral spincter. Last (1975) suggests that it is supplied by the perineal branch of the pudendal nerve, Gosling *et al.* (1981), from anatomical studies, suggest that it is supplied by a nerve from the pelvic plexus. However, Vodusek & Light (1983) demonstrated electrophysiologically that it is supplied by the pudendal nerve.

The anal sphincter consists of the internal sphincter which is smooth muscle, and the external sphincter which is striated muscle and into which the puborectalis muscle is partly inserted. The external anal sphincter is innervated via the pudendal nerve.

The pelvic floor fascia has a fundamental role in the integrity of the pelvic floor. It is attached to the pelvic brim and envelops pelvic floor muscle, thus providing a framework within the pelvis on which the pelvic floor can function. It is condensed in areas to provide strong supporting ligaments for the pelvic viscera. Thus, the uterus is supported by the utero-sacral, transverse cervical and round ligaments. The viscera passing through the gap between the medial muscle fibres of the pelvic floor rely on fascial

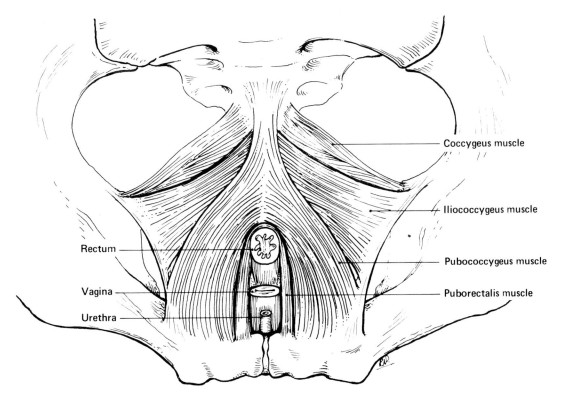

Fig. 45.1. Drawing of the pelvic floor as seen from the abdomen.

support. This gap between the two halves of the pelvic floor is filled by the urethra which is fixed anteriorly by the pubo-urethral ligament, and the bladder base which is supported by pubovesical fascia. Posterior to the uterus lies the musculofascial structure the perineal body, the anal canal and the post anal plate (Wendell-Smith 1967). The presacral fascia is condensed to form the suspensory ligaments of the rectum. Thus the pelvic floor consists of a sheet of muscle and fascia. The muscle depends on a fascial framework, the fascia also providing support for the midline gap in the floor and the viscera which traverse it (Fig. 45.1). The uterus relies on fascial support.

Urinary control

Genuine stress incontinence (GSI) is defined as the involuntary leakage of urine from the urethra when the intravesical pressure exceeds the maximum urethral pressure in the absence of detrusor activity (Bates *et al.* 1977).

The precise cause of GSI is as yet unknown but certain facts are agreed which are:—

1 Resting tone, i.e. the closure forces exerted by the urethral wall in women with GSI is considerably less than in women with normal control (Toews 1967, Brown & Wickham 1969, Edwards & Malvern 1974, Bunne & Obrink 1978, Hosker & Ward 1982). There is overlap in the values between the maximal urethral closure pressures of women with normal control and those suffering from GSI so that no single value of urethral closure forces at rest can be used to distinguish women with GSI from those with normal control.

2 More recently it has been shown that the striated muscle component of the sphincter mechanism is abnormal in many women with stress incontinence. Vereecken *et al.* (1981) reported electromyographic (EMG) abnormalities in the urethral striated muscle of 78% of women with stress incontinence. Snooks and Swash (1984) measured the conduction time of the nerve supply of the urethral striated sphincter and found it delayed in women with stress incontinence. This has been confirmed by Smith and Warrell (1985).

3 The transmission of increases in intra-abdominal pressure to the urethra is less in women with GSI than in women with normal control. In normal women an acute rise in intra-abdominal pressure is transmitted to the bladder as a opening force and simultaneously to the urethra as a closing force. If the urethra descends below the pelvic floor it no longer receives abdominal pressure transmission and continence depends on the urethral sphincter alone. These findings were clearly documented by Enhorning (1961) and have been confirmed by other workers since (Beck & Maugham 1964, Toews 1967, Heidler *et al.* 1979, Hilton & Stanton 1983).

4 Radiological studies have shown that descent of the bladder base and urethra together with loss of the angle normally seen between the bladder base and urethra is a common finding in women suffering from GSI. Like all other measurements there is overlap, and similar findings are sometimes seen in women with genital prolapse and normal control or with incontinence due to other causes. These findings have been documented by Jeffcoate & Roberts (1952), Hodgkinson (1953), Bailey (1963), Tenagho (1974) and Green (1975).

5 Lack of oestrogen lessens urinary control, and its administration helps to restore continence (Rud 1980).

The concept of urinary control that emerges from these facts is that in women with normal control urine is retained in the bladder by the occlusive forces generated by the urethral sphincter, and for this it is important that the urethral striated muscle is healthy. Increases in extra-abdominal pressure are transmitted to the urethra as closing forces. GSI is associated with weak intrinsic closure forces, partial denervation of the urethral striated muscle, descent of the bladder neck on strain, and loss of transmission of abdominal forces to the urethra. Urinary control is adversely affected by oestrogen loss.

Faecal control

Loss of faecal control is associated with loss of tone of the anal canal and EMG abnormalities in the anal sphincter. However, the major factor is descent of the perineum with loss of the anorectal angle. It seems that a healthy intact puborectalis muscle is essential for normal faecal control (Henry & Swash 1985).

There are similarities in urinary and faecal control. Both rely on a sphincter mechanism intrinsic in the wall of the exit channel of the viscus and also upon the transmission of abdominal forces to further close the exit tube. Continence is impaired if the sphincter becomes weak or if there is descent of the pelvic floor with loss of the urethrovesical or anorectal angle and a change in the transmission pattern of abdominal pressure changes.

FACTORS CONCERNED WITH GENITAL TRACT PROLAPSE

Much of the work in this field was reported long ago and it is a matter of regret there is comparatively little recent work in this area.

The factors concerned in genital tract prolapse are traditionally based on clinical observation. It is important that both pelvic floor muscle and pelvic fascia are healthy. Malpas (1955), in his book on genital tract prolapse, states that the fascia 'constitutes a fibrous framework upon whose integrity the effective action of the muscle depends'. He went on to state that in uterine prolapse the damage was more to the fascia, whereas in other visceral prolapse pelvic floor weakness is the dominant finding. Both Bonney (1934) and Mengert (1936) agreed that the lateral fascial attachments were the most important structures in the support of the uterus and lateral vaginal walls.

The clinical factors concerned in the aetiology of genital tract prolapse are well recognized to be the damage sustained in pregnancy and the weakening of the pelvic floor tissues seen at the menopause. Evidence is emerging that it is the act of childbirth which initiates the tissue damage. Measurement of urethral closure forces show a marked reduction after vaginal but not after abdominal delivery (Van Geelen 1981). EMG and histochemical studies in patients with the descending perineum syndrome and faecal incontinence has shown evidence of partial denervation of the pelvic floor and anal sphincter (Parks et al. 1977, Kiff & Swash 1984). Smith (1985), in a large study of women with genital tract prolapse, has shown by histochemical and EMG techniques that in these women the levator ani muscle is partly denervated. Finally Snooks et al. (1984) demonstrated, by an EMG study of the pelvic floor before and after delivery, that women who had undergone vaginal but not abdominal delivery suffered some degree of denervation to the pelvic floor.

All recent work points to the conclusion that parturition has the capacity to cause partial denervation of the pelvic floor and that this is a substantial fact in the aetiology of prolapse.

It is likely that damage to the fascia and ligaments also occurs at parturition and that this may be irreparable. Certainly the ligaments may undergo gross stretching, as for example when the cervix is seen at the vulva during the delivery of the placenta. Zacharin and Gleadell (1963) have emphasized the importance of damage and permanent elongation of the

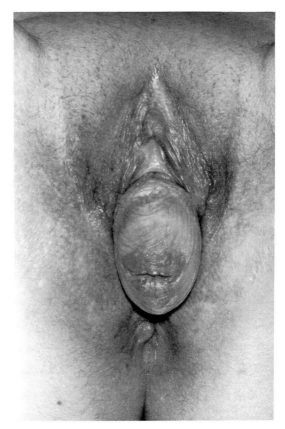

Fig. 45.2. An example of uterine prolapse without cystocele or rectocele.

pubo-urethral supporting ligaments in the aetiology of stress incontinence.

The concept that emerges is that parturition may cause damage to both the urethral and anal sphincters by partial denervation. Parturition may also cause partial denervation to the pelvic floor, and this damage to muscle together with fascial damage may lead to genital tract prolapse. If the latter occurs then the transmission of abdominal forces is changed so as to further impair both urinary and faecal control. Thus parturition has the capacity to cause damage which directly affects the visceral sphincters and also is a major factor in the aetiology of pelvic floor prolapse. If the latter ensues visceral control is further impaired.

Before proceeding to the care of the patient a brief outline will be given of the physiology of urinary control and the common causes of incontinence of urine, apart from fistulae.

PHYSIOLOGY OF URINARY CONTROL

There is an abundant and confusing literature in this field. Thus this short section contains only the core facts about which there is general agreement. The bladder and urethra should be considered as one unit with two main functions: (1) the storage and filling phase in which urine enters the bladder by ureteric peristaltic action and is retained at a low pressure until it is convenient to micturate; (2) the active phase, when, at a suitable time, the detrusor muscle contracts and the bladder empties. As the bladder fills the detrusor muscles fibres which constitute the bladder wall stretch so that intravesical pressure rises very little from empty to capacity which is usually at about 500–600 ml (Hodgkinson & Cobart 1960). This accommodation allows the ureter to pump urine into the bladder easily and also facilitates continence for the forces retaining urine need not be strong. As the erect position is assumed intravesical pressure rises due to the weight of the viscera. In a person of average build this rise is in order of 10–15 cm of water pressure. Activity causes further increases in intra-abdominal pressure which are transmitted to the bladder thus raising intravesical pressure.

The forces retaining urine are generated by the components of the urethra. These are striated and smooth muscle, elastic tissue and the turgor created by the venous plexus. In addition intra-abdominal pressure changes are transmitted to the upper urethra as forces occluding it. Also, closing forces can be generated by voluntary contraction of the pelvic floor.

As the bladder fills proprioceptive afferent impulses from receptors in the bladder pass to S2, S3 and S4 levels of the spinal cord via the parasympathetic nervous system, the nervi erigentes. In babies, when these afferent impulses reach a sufficient threshold, voiding takes place automatically because control is exerted at the level of the sacral reflex arc. With maturity, connections to higher inhibitory centres are established so that micturition comes under voluntary control, and the bladder usually holds 300–400 ml or more before the desire to micturate is perceived. Unconscious inhibition is mediated from the level of the basal ganglia. When the bladder is fairly full impulses reach the central cortex via the lateral spinothalamic tracts. Micturition is then consciously inhibited until it is convenient to void (Yeates 1972).

When an appropriate time for micturition has been selected the bladder changes from its passive to its active role.

Micturition is a complex process involving many higher centres (Boyarsky 1970). It is agreed that the detrusor muscle is innervated by parasympathetic nerves from the conus medullaris, mainly S3 as well as S2 and S4; their integrity is essential for detrusor activity.

The urethral smooth muscle is also under parasympathetic control. Both the bladder and urethra have a sympathetic innervation. In men its main function seems to be to prevent reflux of semen into the bladder at ejaculation. In women its role is unclear and division of the sympathetic presacral nerves does not usually have a discernable effect on bladder and urethral function. Micturition requires coordination of both striated and smooth muscle. Usually it is initiated by relaxation of the pelvic floor following which the bladder neck drops and funnels (Tenagho & Miller 1970). In sequence there is active relaxation of the striated and smooth muscle components of the urethra. In a few seconds the inhibitory influence of the higher centres on the sacral reflex arc is lifted. There is a rapid output of parasympathetic efferent impulses to the detrusor which contracts and pulls open the bladder neck. Intravesical pressure rises and micturition takes place. In some women the urethra opens and micturition occurs with a minimal rise in detrusor pressure. As the bladder empties intravesical pressure falls. At completion the pelvic floor and the striated muscle component of the urethral sphincter contract causing the mid-urethra to close. Urine in the proximal urethra is returned to the bladder. The inhibitory action of the higher centres is reapplied to the sacral reflex and the bladder enters its storage phase again.

URINARY INCONTINENCE

Incontinence of urine in women is a common problem. About 1 in 200 children suffers from troublesome incontinence. The incidence increases with age so that by the later reproductive years 5–10% of women suffer from incontinence, by the menopause 10–12%, and by old age 20%.

DEFINITION

It is difficult to decide the appropriate definition because what is barely a noticed degree of urinary incontinence in one woman may be a source of considerable embarassment to another and more fastidious patient. The International Continence Society defines incontinence as 'a condition in which involuntary loss of urine is a social or hygenic problem and is objectively demonstrable.' The author's own view is to accept the patient's description and to regard incontinence as troublesome and worth investigating if she finds it a social embarrassment limiting every day activity and forcing either the wearing of protective clothing or frequent changing of underwear. It is useful to try and quantify the amount of loss. This can be done by asking the patient to wear a pad and to take a substance which stains the urine such as pyridium so that over a twenty-four hour period a rough quantitative estimate can be made of the amount of urine lost. Alternatively she may be put through a set series of activities while wearing a pad; the pad is weighed and an estimate made of the volume of urine lost.

Urinary control depends on two main factors: firstly, the presence of a competent sphincter mechanism able to resist the changes in intra-abdominal pressure consequent on activity; secondly the capacity to inhibit a bladder contraction until it is convenient to micturate. It follows that incontinence may occur because of a loss of the normal inhibitory capacity, sphincter weakness or a combination of both factors. A third and much less common cause of incontinence is that of overflow incontinence where the failure of the bladder to empty is associated with intravesical pressure so high as to overcome the normal sphincter mechanism.

ABNORMALITIES OF BLADDER FUNCTION

As the bladder fills the walls stretch to accommodate the increased volume and pressure within it rises little, certainly less than 10–15 cm of water. This process does not reach conscious level until the bladder is fairly full. In people with normal control the capacity to inhibit a detrusor contraction is virtually 100% no matter the degree of provocation or discomfort. It seems that the capacity to inhibit a detrusor contraction, like all human affairs, has a physiological range and there are many individuals whose capacity to inhibit is less than adequate. A common example is found in the enuretic adult where tests of bladder function commonly reveal a basic or constitutional failure of inhibition.

As a female passes through the various stages of life she is likely to experience various trigger factors stimulating micturition. Incontinence will occur if her inhibitory capacity is exceeded by the particular trigger. These are inflammation and/or infection of the bladder and urethra and urethral atrophy. Inhibitory capacity may be impaired by emotional factors and by old age. The commonest cause of incontinence in the elderly is failure of inhibition. The other major cause of failure to inhibit is that of neurological disease of which multiple sclerosis is the best recognized example.

SPHINCTER WEAKNESS

The factors concerned in GSI have already been documented in the chapter.

EVALUATION OF THE PATIENT

Women presenting with incontinence of urine will often have symptoms due to genital tract prolapse and vice versa. If the presenting complaint is prolapse the purpose of the history and clinical examination is to decide if the symptoms can be accounted for by the type or extent of any prolapse found. If incontinence of urine is the main symptom the aim of clinical assessment is to decide what type of urinary incontinence is being described and to relate it to the physical findings. For clarity these two problems will be discussed separately.

History

Patients with incontinence of urine
It is essential to take a careful history and to listen to what the patient says for this alone may give the diagnosis. The aim of the history is to find out the circumstances under which urine is lost and to gain an impression of bladder behaviour. If the latter seems to be disturbed it is reasonable to ask leading questions to try and find the cause.

Patients with GSI have no reason to have disturbed bladder function, should have no frequency of micturition and should be able to restrain the desire to micturate for at least half an hour. Exceptions are those women with a cysto-urethrocele and a sphincter weakness who may have daytime frequency. The latter is due to mechanical stimulus of the stretch receptors in the trigone caused by descent of the prolapse.

A patient with GSI should give a history of incontinence by day but not by night. There should be no frequency of micturition by night. By day there should be no urgency, urine being lost only on

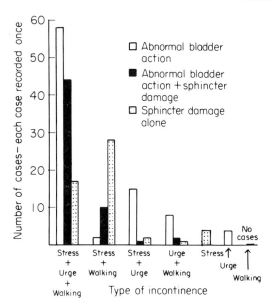

Fig. 45.3 The type of urinary incontinence, i.e. stress incontinence, urge incontinence and incontinence experienced on walking is related to a diagnosis made from the history.

exertion or raised intra-abdominal pressure. There should be no discomfort on holding or passing urine and patients should be able to inhibit a desire to micturate for at least half an hour.

Patients who are incontinent of urine due to a failure to inhibit will have a reduced functional bladder capacity and will have increased frequency of micturition by night and day. There is often a characteristic history of discomfort or pain on holding urine with urgency and incontinence if a lavatory cannot be quickly reached. Women with a history suggestive of a failure to inhibit often suffer from inflammatory lesions of the bladder or urethra.

In a patient with a urethral lesion the desire to micturate is felt low down or in the vagina and there may be difficulty or hesitation in initiating micturition.

Approximately 1 in 10 patients with incontinence will have difficult or hesitant micturition. Most commonly this is due to a subtle neurological abnormality of the sacral reflex arc. Less commonly it is due to a large cystocele kinking the urethra, or rarely a pelvic tumour lifting the trigone. It is easy to miss bladder emptying problems unless leading questions are asked. It is important to recognize the woman who has an impaired capacity to micturate for she is at risk of long term retention of urine if subjected to sphincter surgery.

Symptoms of genital prolapse

Gross prolapse may be present with minimal symptoms. On the other hand minor degrees may produce a surprising amount of discomfort. A possible explanation for this paradox is that the symptoms in the early stages of prolapse are due to stretch of the sensory afferent nerve supply from the uterus. As the prolapse progresses axonal damage takes place and the nerve ceases to conduct.

A sensation of an uncomfortable swelling at the introitus, often described as 'something coming down' is the classic and common symptom. This is often associated with a sense of suprapubic discomfort.

Sacral backache is common. However, backache is a common symptom with many causes and it is difficult to separate backache due to uterine descent from the many orthopaedic causes. The golden rule is to remember that symptoms due to genital tract prolapse are only experienced when the patient is on her feet. Symptoms present in bed are very unlikely indeed to be due to genital tract prolapse.

Examination

It is axiomatic that examination should be of the whole patient and not just the organ producing symptoms. Thus in women with symptoms suggestive of prolapse and urinary incontinence it is important to assess the factors which may increase intra-abdominal pressure such as chronic cough and obesity. Intravesical pressure in a thin woman examined supine is about 5 cm H_2O; standing causes little change. However, a fat woman who girdles her obesity with a corset may achieve an intravesical pressure of over 100 cm H_2O; clearly an important fact in the production of symptoms.

Pelvic examination

The aims of pelvic examination are: to assess the supports of the genital tract and the degree of descent; to assess the competence of the urethral sphincter mechanism; to recognize the type of prolapse which may hide genuine stress incontinence; to assess the health of the genital tract; to assess the health of the bladder and urethra; to make a formal assessment of the pelvic floor, perineal descent and the competence of the anal sphincter.

Abdominal examination is performed with the patient supine. The important points are palpation of the kidneys, to search for a pelvic tumour and the recognition of bladder tenderness. Palpation of the bladder should be carried out in every case. If palpation causes discomfort or produces a micturition desire it is likely that the bladder is inflamed and the capacity will be reduced.

Next the patient should abduct her legs so as to expose the introitus and be asked to strain. The presence or absence of stress incontinence, the support of the anterior and posterior vaginal walls and the degree of perineal descent should be noted. In a severe degree of perineal descent the degree of denervation is such as to resemble a cauda equina lesion. The most detailed assessment of genital tract prolapse is gained by the use of a Sims speculum. The speculum is passed with the patient in a Sims position and she is asked to strain. The support or descent of the different parts of the genital tract is documented. Descent of that part of the vagina overlying the urethra is conventionally described as a urethrocele (a term which urologists find confusing). Descent of the trigone of the bladder and that part of the anterior vaginal wall between the urethra and cervix is described as a cystocele or high cystocele; descent of the entire anterior vaginal wall is termed a cystourethrocele.

Uterine prolapse is often classified in grades. However, since the degree of descent is affected by the circumstances of the examination it is probably more accurate to simply describe the degree of prolapse and the position of the patient at the time of examination.

Next the uterus and anterior vaginal wall is restrained with sponge forceps or a similar instrument and the patient is asked to strain so as to demonstrate the presence or absence of a Pouch of Douglas hernia. Then the speculum is gradually withdrawn so as to demonstrate the presence or absence of a rectocele. Lastly, the patient is asked to contract the pelvic floor. Contraction should elevate the speculum and with it the anterior vaginal wall so demonstrating that the fascial attachments of the pubococcygeus to the vagina are intact.

It is important to recognize that two types of prolapse may compensate for or hide stress incontinence. If these are not recognized prior to operation their successful repair may uncover a pre-existing sphincter weakness and the patient may blame the operation for the loss of urinary control. A large rectocele can squash and close an incompetent urethra. Thus if a large rectocele is present it is important to ask the patient to cough forcefully while holding it back with a speculum. Another mechanism of urinary control which may conceal incontinence is that produced by a large cystocele without much descent of the urethra; straining or coughing by a patient who has

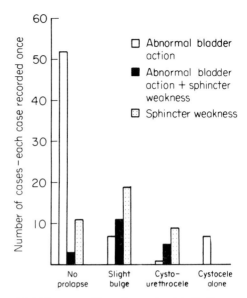

Fig. 45.4 The cause of incontinence is related to the degree of bladder base prolapse judged clinically. Note the preponderance of abnormal bladder action in women with no prolapse.

this defect causes descent of the cystocele and kinks the urethra. If this type of cystocele is present it should be elevated with the speculum blade and the woman asked to cough or strain.

Following the speculum examination a digital examination is made. First a bimanual examination is made for occasionally a pelvic tumour may present with urinary symptoms. The urethra is palpated against the back of the pubic symphysis. Normally it is barely palpable and the pressure of palpation causes no discomfort. Many women suffer urinary symptoms due to a chronic inflammatory lesion of the urethra and in these the urethra is often thickened; palpation causes discomfort and often reproduces the desire to micturate. The pelvic floor should be palpated at rest and during contraction, and assessments made of the degree of tissue damage or atrophy, the muscle bulk, the power of contraction of the pelvic floor and deficiencies due to an episiotomy or severe tear.

Lastly, the anal spincter is assessed. In health the anus will contract if the perineal skin is stimulated; this reflex is lost if the spinal reflex arc is damaged. Anal tone can be assessed by inserting a finger into the anus and pulling gently backwards, if anal tone is normal it is not possible to open the anus which continues to close around the finger.

Finally, the patient should be examined in the standing position. Prolapse causes symptoms only when the patient is erect and abnormalities may be present which can only be demonstrated with the patient erect. First the labia are parted, the external urethral meatus is visualized and the patient is asked to cough. This may be the only method of demonstrating the incontinence in women with mild GSI. It is useful to make a digital examination of the anterior vaginal wall and cervix while the patient strains for much greater degrees of descent will be found than when the patient is on the couch.

It is the author's experience that many women who have been thought not to have a cysto-urethrocele when examined supine can when examined erect be shown to have a substantial prolapse with the urethrovesical junction descending outside the introitus. The difference in the amount of prolapse between the two examination positions is so great as to render grading of a prolapse with patient supine inaccurate.

Investigation

At the conclusion of history taking and examination a working diagnosis will have been made, and the clinician will need to decide if this is sure enough for treatment to follow or if investigations are needed to strengthen or clarify the working diagnosis.

The following investigations have been found to be of help by demonstrating the mechanism of incontinence and throwing light on the cause.

Micturition volume chart

The simplest investigation is obtain a chart of a patient's voiding pattern and urinary control for a week. This is done by asking her to measure the volume of urine passed each time she micturates and the time it is voided. She should also note the time of each episode of incontinence. Women with normal control do not usually pass urine more than 6–8 times in 24 hours and are not normally woken from sleep by the need to micturate.

The voiding pattern in women with GSI should not be disturbed unless the patient initiates micturition before she is aware of a full bladder in an effort to keep dry. The normal voided volumes by day are in the order of 250–450 ml. The first volume voided after sleep is often the largest passed in the 24 hour period. If bladder behaviour is disturbed by a sensory disorder, e.g. the urethral syndrome, voided volumes will be smaller and more frequent, and nocturia is

usually present. Another use of the chart is to assess the degree of incontinence. It is not uncommon to find a marked discrepancy between the patient's description of incontinence as noted at the first consultation and what is recorded during a week's charting. This useful noninvasive assessment should be carried out by every woman who complains of incontinence before deciding treatment.

Microbiological investigation in a patient with urinary incontinence

Microbiological investigation is an important part of the assessment of the patient with urinary incontinence for urinary infection is a common association of the condition. There are two main reasons for investigation. Firstly, the patient with lower urinary tract symptoms may have upper renal tract infection which may be so serious as to risk her health and will certainly affect management. Secondly, infection of the bladder and/or urethra may cause inflammation of the urothelium and produce incontinence by increasing the stimulus to detrusor contractions. The investigator must be clear why he is looking for infection because the methods of investigation and the criteria by which infection is diagnosed are different for the upper and lower urinary tracts. The problem is further complicated because true infection may be asymptomatic while many women with lower tract symptoms suggestive of infection do not have significant number of bacteria in a fresh voided midstream urine (Gallagher et al. 1965). When greater than 10^5 bacteria per ml are found in fresh voided urine this is reliable evidence of bacteria multiplying in the urine, i.e. infection. This figure of 10^5 ml was introduced by Kass (1957) as being significant of upper urinary tract infection in women without lower urinary tract symptoms. In fact recent work has suggested that patients with fewer organisms may have genuine cystitis (Mond et al. 1965).

Approximately 50% of patients with greater than 10^5 bacteria per ml. do not have symptoms and on cystoscopy will be found to have a normal non-inflamed urothelium. Clearly, whether or not a patient with bacteria multiplying in her urine has lower urinary symptoms depends on if the urothelium of the bladder is inflamed.

The common bacteria causing infection are E. Coli, Proteus Miribilis and Staph. Epidermis which together account for 85% of urinary infections in domicillary practice. Other bacteria, e.g. Pseudomonas are generally a consequence of surgical intervention. There is also evidence that other organisms, e.g. My-

coplasma hominis (Stamm *et al.* 1982) and *Chlamydia trachomatis* may invade and infect the urethra causing lower urinary tract symptoms.

Urethral discomfort causing urge incontinence is common. However microbiological assessment is difficult. A midstream urine is an inappropriate specimen for any pathogen in the urethra will have been washed out and discarded with the first specimen. Examination of the first 2–3 ml of urine passed may reveal a pathogen. Alternatively a swab may be taken from the urethra, but special techniques are needed to avoid contamination (O'Neill 1981). Lastly it is of value to take an introital swab because the bacteria of the introitus and of the lower urethra are similar, and it is likely that a pathogen in the introitus will also be in the urethra.

The following schedule gives a practical guide to the detection of infection. A midstream specimen of urine is taken after the external meatus has been cleansed with sterile water. If less than 10^5 bacteria per ml is present then the patient is very unlikely to have an upper tract infection. If greater than 10^5 ml then the patient has an infection of the kidney or bladder.

If few bacteria are found it is worth both repeating the specimen and counting the pus cells. The presence of a persistent organism and more than 50 pus cells per ml suggests infection. If in doubt, a sample of bladder urine should be obtained by suprapubic aspiration or a catheter specimen. The presence of pus cells and lesser numbers of bacteria, say 10^3 per ml, is very suggestive of infection. If urethritis is suspected an introital swab and a urethral swab (via a fine catheter) should be taken. If these swabs are negative and the culture shows no pathogens fresh specimens should be obtained and cultured for Chlamydia.

Uroflowmetry

Measurement of the urinary flow rate gives information about both bladder and urethral function during micturition. A normal flow rate is pretty reliable evidence that detrusor contraction and urethral relaxation are normal.

If flow rate is poor this may be because the ability of the bladder to contract is impaired, or that the urethra is narrowed or fails to relax as the bladder contracts. Such a problem needs further study with measurement of bladder pressure during voiding. Uroflowmetry should be used as a screening test in all women with incontinence of urine, particularly those likely to undergo surgery for stress incontin-

ence. A proportion of women with GSI have impaired detrusor function. It is important to recognize this fact prior to operation.

Cystometric assessment

Even a simple cystometric examination, with the bladder filled by a drip set via a catheter and pressure measured intermittently with a manometer connected to the system by a T tube, is better than not performing the examination, for cystometric examination is the only method of objectively displaying bladder function.

Ideally intravesical pressure should be measured by a technique in which movement by the patient does not cause artifact. In practice this can only be done by introducing a gauge into the bladder capable of giving direct readings of intravesical pressure. Though such gauges are available commercially they are expensive and fragile when compared with external pressure gauges which are much more robust.

Usually intravesical pressure is recorded externally via a long fluid filled catheter. This system has the limitation of only being capable of measuring pressure relative to a base line. Conventionally, the zero reference for pressure is the level of the superior edge of the symphysis pubis. It also has the potential error that movement by the patient can cause fluid shifts in the catheter which may be mistaken for changes in intravesical pressure. Despite these limitations this system is in common use because it is robust and reasonably accurate. It is important to use similar apparatus to measure intrarectal pressure so that changes in intravesical pressure due to detrusor contraction can be distinguished from those secondary to abdominal pressure changes (which will affect both channels).

It is common for intrarectal pressure to be subtracted from intravesical pressure and the result called detrusor pressure i.e. a true measure of bladder function. This convention has errors e.g. rectal contractions, which are quite common, will appear on the subtracted line as a fall in intravesical pressure. Another limitations of subtracting intrarectal from intravesical pressure is that changes in intra-abdominal pressure, e.g. due to coughing, are not necessarily transmitted equally both to bladder and rectum. Therefore, although subtraction does separate out detrusor function from abdominal pressure changes, to avoid these pitfalls bladder and rectal recordings should be visualized as well as the subtracted pressure.

Bladder filling may be natural or retrograde via a

catheter. If via a catheter filling may be slow, e.g. 10 ml per minute, or rapid, over 100 ml per minute. Each technique has its own limitations and errors, so much so that the author believes cystometry is best thought of as a stress test and for a given set of apparatus the abnormal is compared with the normal, i.e. measurements are relative not absolute.

The aim of the investigation is to observe bladder function while as near as possible trying to reproduce the circumstances in which the patient is incontinent. The technique can be used to measure:

1 compliance, i.e. the relation between changes in volume and pressure, which is an indicator of both detruser tone and the physical state of the bladder wall;

2 sensation, which is important in the recognition of both the inflamed and the denervated bladder;

3 capacity, which is almost always determined by discomfort and is another measure of sensation;

4 detrusor control, which is a crucial assessment in making the fundamental distinction between GSI and incontinence due to failure to inhibit.

Normal values. With a filling rate between 50 and 100 ml per minute the first desire to void is usually experienced at between 200 and 250 ml and bladder capacity is between 500 and 600 ml. The pressure rise from empty to full is usually less than 10 cm H_2O (above 15 cm H_2O is abnormal). No detruser contractions should take place. On standing an increase in pressure is seen both in the bladder and rectum. Detrusor pressure does not change. Coughing and bouncing should not provoke contractions.

Evaluation of the sphincter mechanism
It would be ideal to be able to assess sphincter competence by measurement of the urethral occlusive forces at rest and the transmission of intra-abdominal pressure increases during activity. These are as yet research studies and in practice sphincter incompetence, i.e. GSI, is diagnosed by observing urethral dilatation either clinically or radiologically in the presence of normal bladder function.

Radiological assessment
Radiological assessment of bladder and urethral behaviour was the technique commonly used in the 1960s for the investigation of women with urinary incontinence. It is an excellent method of assessing urethral movement and dilatation in response to extra-abdominal pressure changes. However, it does not give information about bladder behaviour. It can-

not be used to distinguish patients with GSI from those with incontinence due to failure to inhibit. It is best used either following study of bladder behaviour with a filling cystogram or in combination with pressure measurements as a videocystogram.

Following cystometry it may be used to demonstrate the degree of bladder base and urethral descent as a guide to the choice of surgery. Usually the bladder is filled with a contrast material while the urethra is outlined with a bead chain or a soft pliable radio-opaque catheter. It is helpful to see vaginal movement with the aid of barium paste as contrast. The patient sits and a direct lateral view is obtained of the bladder base and urethra. Conventionally single shot radiographs are obtained at rest, during strain and during micturition.

Videocysto-urethrography
In this technique bladder function is assessed by a combination of intravesical pressure measurements and visualization by cineradiology. Urethral function is assessed visually. Intravesical, intrarectal and true detrusor pressure obtained by subtraction are recorded.

The bladder is filled by a contrast medium and the above pressures are recorded while the bladder shape is visualized radiologically. The first desire to void and bladder capacity are recorded. At capacity the filling catheter is removed and the X-ray table is raised so the patient has become erect. She is asked to cough and strain. The degree of movement and descent of the bladder base together with any urethral dilatation is seen. She is then asked to micturate while the flow rate and detrusor pressure are recorded.

The pressure together with the image of the bladder and urethra are seen on a video screen and recorded together with a sound commentary on a videotape. The technique has been documented by Bates *et al.* (1970). It has the advantage of assessing bladder and urethral function at the one investigation, so that in a case of stress incontinence the reaction of bladder function to filling can be assessed while any dilatation of the urethra in response to increased abdominal pressure can be seen. A major advantage of this technique is the ability to show that urethral dilatation is passive (i.e. secondary to abdominal pressure increases) or is due to a bladder contraction (i.e. an unstable bladder).

In summary the technique documents urethral competence, bladder neck mobility or the lack of it due to fibrosis, voiding problems, and incontinence due to inability to inhibit a bladder contraction. The apparatus is more complicated and more expensive than that needed for a simple X-ray cystogram, but it is a neat way of assessing malfunction of the lower urinary tract.

Cysto-urethroscopy

This examination is not indicated in every woman suffering from urinary incontinence. If bladder behaviour is normal, as assessed from the history and cystometric examination, then the chances of finding significant pathology are so small as to make it unnecessary. However, if abnormal cystometric values are found then cystoscopy is indicated.

The main reason for endoscopic examination of the bladder and urethra is to look for local lesions which may explain the abnormal behaviour, the most important but least common finding being that of a bladder tumour. Inflammatory lesions, particularly of the urethra, are common. Also, confirmation of a suspected neurological lesion may be found by the presence of trabeculation.

The examination can be performed without general anaesthesia, but the latter enables the sensation and compliance of the bladder to be compared with the cystometric findings in the conscious patient, thus enabling disturbed bladder function due to a pure sensory disorder to be distinguished from that due to a physical change in the bladder wall as in intercystial cystitis.

The investigations listed above are basic and readily available in the United Kingdom. For greater detail the reader may refer to *Urodynamics* edited by Munday A.R., Stephenson T.P. and Wein A.J. (Churchill Livingstone) and *Urodynamics* edited by Abrams P., Feneley R. and Torrens M. (Springer–Verlag).

CHOICE OF INVESTIGATION

At the conclusion of history taking and clinical examination patients will have been sorted out into three main groups. These are:—

1 Patients with symptoms due to a *genital tract prolapse and normal urinary control*. This group will contain the smallest number of women for it is uncommon for parturition to damage the pelvic floor and spare the urethral sphincter. In this group the clinician should be doubly sure that a rectocele is not hiding GSI. Providing the sphincter mechanism is satisfactory it is reasonable to advise treatment on the basis of clinical assessment.

2 Patients with a *genital tract prolapse and urinary incontinence* and who on the basis of history and ex-

amination are judged to have GSI. In this group it is important to be sure that the patient is not suffering from another type of incontinence. Another question to be decided is the relative importance of urethral sphincter weakness and bladder neck descent in the production of the stress incontinence for this judgement will influence the choice of operation. Lastly, the capacity of the bladder to contract needs to be assessed for if impaired detrusor function is overlooked the woman is at risk of postoperative retention.

The appropriate investigations in this group are as follows: (a) a micturition volume chart for a week, which tells more about the bladder function than any other test; voided volumes should be 300–400 ml with no daytime frequency or nocturia; (b) Uroflowmetry, which simple test is a satisfactory screening test of the ability of the bladder to contract; the flow of urine should be smooth and the maximum flow rate above 25 ml/sec; (c) filling cystometry, which should show normal bladder function (i.e. a capacity of between 500 and 600 ml with normal sensation, normal compliance and a normal capacity to inhibit despite provocation); (d) radiological demonstration of the degree of bladder neck prolapse; absence of prolapse will suggest that the urethral sphincter is very weak, conversely severe generalized prolapse points to gross pelvic floor damage.

At the conclusion of this set of tests the clinician should be confident of the diagnosis. When a diagnosis of sphincter weakness has been made it is important to have assessed the severity of the incontinence and the degree of prolapse for a decision has to be made to treat medically or surgically, and if surgically by the vaginal or abdominal approach.

3 A third group comprises patients with *incontinence of urine but who have no prolapse*, made up of women with GSI due to a severe sphincter weakness and women whose incontinence is due to abnormal bladder behaviour (usually a failure to inhibit bladder contractions). The important investigations are micturition volume chart, microbiological examination of the urine, uroflowmetry and cystometry. If clinical examination and the above tests point to GSI then radiological examination should be performed primarily to assess the response of the bladder base and urethra to increases in extra abdominal pressure. It is important to double check that there is no bladder neck prolapse.

If cystometry shows that incontinence is due to a failure to inhibit, cystoscopy is indicated to look for a local lesion which may be acting as an increased trigger to bladder contractions. If bladder behaviour is abnormal and cystometry is normal then it is likely that the problem is neurological. In most cases generalized pathology in the central nervous system cannot be recognized, and the problem is either a constitutional failure to inhibit or a local neurological fault in the pelvis.

TREATMENT OF GENITAL PROLAPSE AND GENUINE STRESS INCONTINENCE

The first decision to be made is whether to treat medically or surgically. Medical treatment should be considered if the symptoms and the degree of prolapse are mild, if surgery poses particular risks (for example in the very elderly), or as a preliminary measure prior to surgery, for example weight loss for the obese.

Medical treatment

Women with mild GSI associated with a small cysto-urethrocele should be encouraged to practise pelvic floor exercises. It is easy to advise this type of therapy; however, if advice alone is given the success rate is much less than if the patient is taken in hand by an enthusiastic physiotherapy department. Many patients have difficulty learning how to control the pelvic floor at will, indeed some strain down when asked to contract. It is likely that parturition causes sensory as well as motor nerve damage, and a patient with this pattern of response needs considerable help in learning how to contract and exercise the pelvic floor. There are several techniques available which may help. Pelvic floor faradism using a vaginal electrode stimulates the levator ani muscle group. This both exercises the muscle and helps the patient understand what muscle group should be exercised voluntarily. The patients need encouragement and support for they may not enjoy the benefits of this therapy until a month or so.

Other forms of electric stimulation have been tried, using either a perianal (Hopkinson & Lightwood 1967) or a vaginal electrode (Fall 1978. The author's experience with pelvic stimulation with a vaginal electrode is that although the device improves urinary control this benefit is outweighed by the discomfort and 'hassle' of wearing it. Recently Shepherd *et al.* (1985) reported a double blind trial, lasting six months, of an inflatable intravaginal electric stimulation pessary, but only 15 of 68 patients approached completed the trial. Another type of device used to help the patient exercise the pelvic floor was reported

by Kegel (1948). In essence this consists of a balloon attached to a pressure gauge visible to the patient. Successful pelvic floor contraction is evident to the patient who is thus encouraged to greater efforts! This device has not become popular. The choice of device is probably not important; what matters is that the patient is helped to become aware of pelvic floor contractions and is encouraged to exercise this muscle group long term.

At the other end of the age range are the patients in whom operation carries appreciable risks, either because of generalized disease or because of extreme age. Age in itself is not a contraindication to operation; indeed the rewards of repairing the prolapse of a very old but otherwise fit woman are considerable. She often experiences very little postoperative discomfort and soon returns to everyday activities.

Pessary treatment has a place in the management of those women in whom operation would carry special risks or problems, for example those with chronic respiratory disease. The pessaries available are ring pessaries constructed out of nontoxic polyvinal chloride and shelf pessaries. The disadvantage of pessaries is that they tend to produce vaginal infection and discharge which, if neglected, may lead to vaginal ulceration. Thus, if a satisfactory pessary is found which controls symptoms it will need to be changed every 3 or so months for the duration of its use. Patients need to have a reasonable pelvic floor in order to retain the pessary; women with severe obstetric tears or gross muscle denervation are unsuitable. Ring pessaries are best indicated to control rectocele and cystocele. Major degrees of uterine prolapse are best controlled with a shelf pessary.

At the initial fitting it is advisable to choose an oversmall rather than an overlarge pessary, for once the pessary is in place the vagina tends to shrink and an overlarge pessary may become very difficult to change.

In the postmenopausal patient the use of a pessary should be combined with the use of intravaginal oestrogen cream. In many cases the discomfort attributed to the prolapse is due to or at least exacerbated by the presence of atrophic vaginitis. Regular use of intravaginal oestrogen will minimize infection and add to the patient's comfort. It is a mistake to operate on the obese for the operative risks are increased compared to women of average weight and the long-term results are less satisfactory. Equally, patients with chronic chest disease pose operative risks and problems. It is difficult for a middle-aged person to change her lifestyle and to diet successfully, and sometimes the patient will try to persuade the surgeon to operate without preliminary weight loss. Experience has taught that this is bad practice.

Surgical treatment

The emphasis in this section is on general principles of management. Operative detail can be obtained by reference to current books of gynaecological surgical technique such as Shaw's Text Book of Operative Gynaecology (5th edition; Churchill Livingstone).

As a result of clinical evaluation the gynaecologist should have a clear concept of what damage is present in the genital tract, what symptoms are present and if the degree of damage is likely to be responsible for the patient's symptoms. Bearing in mind the degree of damage, it is important to know what surgical therapy can be expected to achieve and its limitations. It is also important to understand the patient's hopes, fears and aspirations. These days many patients have an expectation of cure which is unreal because problems produced by parturition damage and ageing are incurable. Before operating it is wise to have a thorough discussion, documenting what problems surgery may be expected to alleviate together with both the success and complication rate.

Preoperative evaluation

As in all surgical procedures the patient's general health should have been assessed and collaboration established with the anaesthetist. In each patient it is important to establish that both the urine and vagina are free from infection because the latter will add to the risk and may prejudice a satisfactory end result. If there is a history of recurrent urinary infection or if hypertension is present, renal function should be checked simply by estimating the urea and electrolyte levels in the blood. The patient should be questioned about coital function for this is an important constraint to keep in mind when planning the operation. The patient should be examined by the surgeon who is going to perform the operation a day or two before the event. The technique and scale of the surgery should be based on this preoperative evaluation. The operator should write a description of the prolapse and outline the operation he plans to carry out. It is not possible to satisfactorily assess prolapse under anaesthesia in the lithotomy position so to delay planning the scale of the operation until the patient is examined under anaesthesia is unsatisfactory.

PRINCIPLES OF REPAIR

In essence genital tract prolapse occurs because the pelvic floor and fascia becomes weakened by childbirth and ageing. The essence of all vaginal surgery is to adapt these weakened structures so as to retain the pelvic viscera in the anatomical position they occupied before parturition. Such a technique will only be satisfactory if the tissue damage is not great. If there is considerable descent and if the pelvic floor is very weak, consideration needs to be given to techniques of surgery in which parts of the genital tract are sutured to the fascia overlying the bony pelvis and the use of other tissues or material for support.

It is reasonable to consider vaginal surgery where there is moderate prolapse. Severe degrees of prolapse in young women are often due to gross pevic damage and muscle denervation and may be best treated by a combination of abdominal and vaginal surgery.

The vaginal approach should be used for almost all elderly women for, though the tissues are usually weak and atrophic, the stresses put on them are correspondingly less. Also it is usually possible to narrow the vagina. If this can be achieved, at worst the patient will be left with a degree of perineal descent due to poor pelvic floor tone. In the elderly this type of perineal descent causes little discomfort.

The choice of suture material is important. Since a fibroblast takes about four months to mature it is the author's view that catgut is inappropriate suture material to use to hold together the reconstructed genital tract supports. It seems odd that there has been a widespread swing to *Vicril* and *Dexon* for suture of the abdominal rectus sheath while catgut is used by the majority of gynaecologists for reconstructive vaginal surgery. *Vicril*, *Dexon* or non absorbable suture material should be used for the reconstructive deeper sutures. The use of catgut should be restricted to suture of the vaginal and perineal epithelium.

The aims of vaginal surgery are to excise redundant vaginal epithelium, to find the strongest and healthiest fascia available, which is usually out to the lateral side of the vagina, and to suture this together to support the viscera. In general the less complicated the suturing the better the long term results. Too many sutures will impair the blood supply of the healing tissues. Posteriorly, a decision has to be made to suture the fascia covering the levator muscles or the actual muscle. Major degrees of rectocele are most satisfactorily dealt with by formal dissection and suture of the pelvic floor. Faecal control can also be improved by bringing the medial fibres of the levator over the anal sphincter.

PARTICULAR PROBLEMS

A fundamental discussion point is whether to remove the uterus as part of a repair procedure. If the patient has menstrual problems or wishes sterilization then a repair and vaginal hysterectomy is the operation of choice. Apart from this clinical problem, there are points for and against vaginal hysterectomy.

An argument often advanced in favour of vaginal hysterectomy over a Manchester type of repair with cervical amputation is that better support is obtained. This is not the case; what matters is the efficiency with which the vaginal vault is supported by shortening the transverse cervical and uterosacral ligaments. Leaving aside the question of conserving the uterus for reproduction, the main advantage of a Manchester repair is that it is a simpler operation with less morbidity than a repair and vaginal hysterectomy. It's disadvantage is that, when used in women still menstruating, it may be followed by the appearance of menstrual problems. The author's own practice is to advise repair and vaginal hysterectomy in the menstruating woman who has completed her family and reserve the Manchester repair for the postmenopausal woman.

Prolapse in young women
Young women who present with prolapse may have suffered severe pelvic damage and should be assessed most carefully. Further childbirth will damage any pelvic floor repair so that every effort should be made to treat these women conservatively until their families are complete. However, if the prolapse is large this may not be practical.

A conventional Manchester repair operation with amputation of the cervix in contraindicated for this may leave the cervix incompetent. However, it is possible to remove just a sliver of cervix so as to expose the transverse cervical ligaments. These can be shortened in a conventional fashion with very satisfactory uterine support. There is debate regarding the place of posterior colporrhaphy in such women because the latter procedure may cause dyspareunia. Most young women with prolapse have suffered pelvic floor damage and in my view should undergo formal posterior repair with apposition of the medial borders of the levator muscles. Coital problems usually follow too wide a skin excision and can easily be avoided by appropriate surgical technique. It is possible to suture

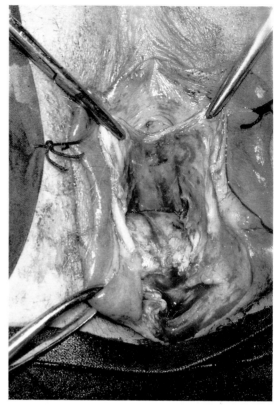

Fig. 45.5 Photograph taken during dissection for a posterior colporrhaphy illustrating the exposure of the rectum possible without removal of posterior vaginal wall epithelium.

the levators without removal of skin from the posterior vaginal wall (Fig. 45.5). The sutures should be placed far back near the rectum so as not to narrow the vagina. This type of posterior repair does not cause dyspareunia and helps support the whole genital tract.

Vault prolapse after hysterectomy
This is difficult to treat satisfactorily without disturbing coital function. In old women the bladder may be dissected off the transverse cervical ligaments, the enterocele opened and ligated at a high level. Then the transverse cervical ligaments are shortened and sutured together. Finally the vagina may be narrowed with generous skin excision and suture of the pelvic floor. In a younger woman this is not practical for normal vaginal dimensions need to be preserved. If the vaginal approach is used the vault can be sutured to the sacrospinous ligament (Richter & Albrich 1981). Satisfactory support can be obtained via an

abdominal approach by suture of the vaginal vault to the sacral fascia (Ridley 1976). It is important not to alter the axis of the vagina in relation to the rest of the pelvis.

Recurrent prolapse

Women who suffer from recurrent prolapse are in general those who have suffered the worst damage. They need the most careful assessment. In particular the quality, bulk and muscle tone of the pelvic floor should be documented. Sometimes the problem is simple in that an unoperated on part of the genital tract has descended, for example a rectocele in a patient who has not undergone posterior repair. This can be repaired in an orthodox fashion.

Enterocele is the commonest recurrence. It can usually be managed with high ligation via a vaginal approach. If this was part of the initial surgical procedure, then consideration should be given to an abdominal approach with obliteration of the peritonal sac and vault support.

In all cases of recurrent prolapse the surgeon should consider an abdominal approach combined with vaginal narrowing by suture of the levator muscles.

CHOICE OF OPERATION FOR GENUINE STRESS INCONTINENCE

Over the years there has been dissatisfaction with the results of vaginal surgery (Bailey 1954, Jeffcoate 1961, Low 1967) and because of poor results there has been a move towards suprapubic bladder neck suspension as a prime procedure. Though giving better success rates, these operations have brought their own special problems in the shape of detrusor instability and bladder emptying problems (Cardozo *et al.* 1979) (Fig 45.6). Current knowledge suggests that GSI is due to an intrinsic weakness of the urethral sphincter mechanism compounded by a loss of transmitted abdominal pressure as a closing force.

It is worth examining how surgery may restore urinary control so that treatment may be based on a rational basis. Vaginal surgery, if successful, will restore the bladder base and urethra to the position it was in before childbirth. The intrinsic urethral sphincter will still be weak, but transmitted abdominal pressure should now be restored as forces closing the urethra. Likewise suprapubic surgery restores the bladder neck to its normal position, but cannot change the power of the urethral sphincter. Suprapubic surgery differs from vaginal surgery in achiev-

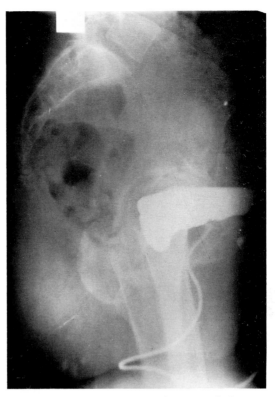

Fig. 45.6 Lateral X-ray cystogram of a patient who has voiding difficulties after a sling operation. Note the abnormally high position of the urethrovesical junction.

ing a greater and often more rigid bladder neck elevation and with this often a degree of outflow obstruction.

In summary, vaginal surgery achieves moderate bladder neck elevation but rarely creates urinary problems, while suprapubic surgery can achieve a greater and probably more permanent bladder neck elevation but carries the risk of producing bladder emptying problems.

It seems rational to select patients for either a vaginal or an abdominal approach according to the degree of damage. Green (1975) based his selection of patients on the alteration in relationship and the degree of descent of the bladder base and urethra. He reports a 90% cure rate by vaginal surgery in selected patients. Beck and McCormick (1982), using *Dexon* as suture material, report a 2 year cure rate of 80%. The cure rate for a suprapubic approach is in the order of 80% (Stanton 1984). However, this is achieved at the price of some patients having voiding problems. In our current state of knowledge, it would seem wise to operate vaginally on patients with moderate stress incontinence in association with prolapse, whose expelling forces are not increased and whose pelvic floor tissues have not been severely damaged. Patients unlikely to be cured by a vaginal technique are those who have already undergone a vaginal repair operation; those with a very weak urethral sphincter and minimal prolapse; and those with increased expelling forces (i.e. the obese): such patients should be considered for suprapubic surgery.

Urethroplasty

It is important to use either a nonabsorbable suture or a slowly absorbable suture material to restore the bladder neck to it's preparturition position. This may easily be achieved by plication of the pubocervical fascia as described by Kelly (1928). Pacey (1949) described suture of the medial border of the pubococcygeus muscles beneath the bladder neck; this is not always easy to achieve and can produce bands of scar in the anterior vaginal wall.

Figs. 45.7(a) and (b) show suture of the pubocervical fascia and the elevation that can be achieved.

Suprapubic surgery

Many suprapubic operations have been described and three most common in current use are: (a) sling operation; (b) Burch colposuspension and; (c) the Stamey Pereyra procedure.

The sling may be of the patient's own tissue, usually fascia from the abdominal wall, or inorganic material. The disadvantage of using the patient's own tissue is the degree of dissection needed to obtain the strip of fascia. Artificial material is readily available but has an appreciable incidence of infection and carries the risk of cutting through the urethra with formation of a fistula.

The Burch operation achieves elevation by suture of the vagina alongside the bladder neck to the ileopectineal ligament. The major long term complications are those of detrusor instability and voiding difficulties.

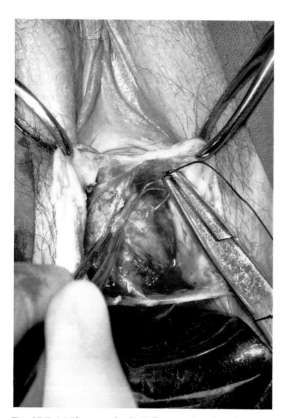

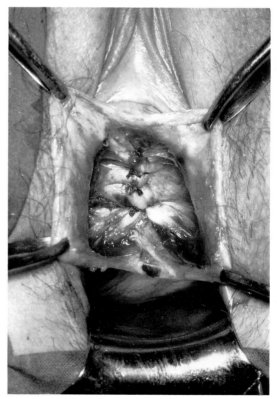

Fig. 45.7 (a) Photograph of a Kelly type of urethroplasty illustrating suture of the pubocervical fascia.

(b) Photograph of a completed Kelly type urethroplasty illustrating satisfactory support of the urethrovesical junction.

The Stamey Pereyra procedure is relatively simple and in essence the bladder neck is elevated by nylon sutures tied to the rectus sheath. A cure rate of 90% is reported (Stamey 1980). The disadvantages are of foreign body material which may in time cause infection or break. No one operation is clearly superior. It is important that the operator is comfortable with the technique and is able to achieve adequate elevation of the bladder neck without undue outflow obstruction. Postoperatively a suprapubic catheter should be used.

Many other operations have been described including the use of an artificial sphincter. The interested reader may consult books of surgical technique such as *Surgery of Female Incontinence*, edited by Stanton & Tenagho (Springer–Verlag).

Surgical restoration of urinary control is difficult. The best results will be achieved by the surgeon who assesses his patients objectively and selects the operation appropriate for the particular problem.

TREATMENT OF INCONTINENCE DUE TO FAILURE TO INHIBIT BLADDER CONTRACTIONS

This section is concerned with those women whose incontinence is due to a failure to inhibit a bladder contraction. The capacity to inhibit is the result of the relationship between the innate capacity to inhibit and any increased stimulus to micturition such as an inflammatory state in the urothelium of the bladder or urethra.

The innate capacity to inhibit varies so that an increased stimulus to micturition in one woman might result in frequency and urgency, and in another cause urge incontinence as well. The capacity to inhibit is innate but may be impaired by faulty habit, emotion, central nervous system disease and ageing. Thus un treatment a judgment has to be made as to which particular factor has allowed loss of inhibition to take place.

The common clinical entities are described below, but it is important to realize that more than one factor may be affecting the inhibitory capacity and to achieve success each needs to be treated.

Infection
Most chronic infections are in the urethra rather than the bladder. The aim of treatment is to isolate the organism responsible for the infection, to recognize what has gone wrong with the patient's defence mechanism to infection and if possible to correct it, and to treat the infection until the patient's natural defence to infection has been restored to normal.

In many cases of urethritis the organism will not be isolated and antibacterial therapy will be empirical. The drugs of choice are Trimethoprim and Furadantin, 100 mg daily for three months. The antibiotic should be combined with the following hygiene rules in order to promote a healthy vulval and hence urethral flora: wash the vulva once only per day with water only; no additives e.g. bubble bath or antiseptics to the bath water; stockings not tights and loose cotton pants; wash underwear with pure soap **not** detergents, avoid fabric softeners.

The urethra is often in spasm as judged by a reduced urine flow rate. If this does not improve urethral dilatation using a local anaesthetic gel or general anaesthesia should be performed. If there is urethral stenosis urethral dilatation should be performed under general anesthesia; a dilatation of 10–12 mm should be aimed for short of traumatizing the urethra; if restenosis takes place further dilatation should be performed. Urethrolysis has a place, but again stenosis may follow this procedure.

Atrophic urethritis
This condition responds well to oestrogen therapy. If it has been present for several years there may be secondary infection and stenosis which will require treatment in their own right. Initial treatment should be local with a weak oestrogen, for example dienoestral cream 0.01% w/w 5 ml inserted high into the vagina on alternate nights for 2 to 3 months, changes the cytology of the vagina and the lower urethra curing 80% of women with this condition, and it almost never causes endometrial growth. Patients who fail to respond should be given a small dose of oral oestrogen for three months, e.g. Ethinyl oestradiol 10 μg on alternate days. If a patient continues to suffer symptoms then it is likely some other factor is present.

Chronic abacterial inflammation of the bladder
This is an ill understood and incurable group of conditions. Treatment is empiric and at best can only alleviate the condition. The two treatments which may be of help are bladder dilatation, using general or epidural anaesthesia, and installations of silver nitrate solution into the bladder. If cystometric examination shows a reduced capacity with low compliance bladder it is worth distending it with normal saline. The installation pressure for a few minutes may be as

high as the patient's arterial pressure. If epidural anaesthesia is used the distention will be for 2 to 3 hours and the pressure should be released every half hour (Ramsden 1977).

Dilatation may achieve a considerable relief of symptoms for periods of up to a year. Many patients lead a tolerable life by means of bladder dilatation on a regular basis. The patient who has a vascular, irritable but more distensible bladder is best treated with silver nitrate bladder installations. After micturition 100 ml of 1/1000 silver nitrate is installed in the bladder via a catheter. This should be twice a day for 5 days. If there is no improvement the therapy should be abandoned, but if frequency of micturition diminishes it is worth continuing for a total of 10 days. Repeat cystocopy sometimes shows a surprising return to normality.

Patients with these conditions are a long term responsibility of the clinic and need help and support for many years.

Bladder training

In Britain, Jeffcoate and Roberts (1952), Frewen (1978), Mahady and Begg (1981), Cardozo et al. (1978) and Jarvis (1982) have all reported considerable success in the treatment of patients incontinent due to failure to inhibit bladder contractions and in whom there was no neurologic disease or local bladder pathology.

An 80% success rate is reported with up to a 4 year follow up (Mahady and Begg 1981). Different techniques have been used. Common to all is the need for the patients to be given an insight into the aetiology and mechanism of their disorder togethr with help to reinforce their capacity to inhibit. In essence, it is behaviour therapy aiding the patients to influence consciously their own autonomic functions.

DRUG THERAPY

Drug treatment of incontinence due to failure of inhibition is common, often expensive and rarely effective in the long term. The groups of drugs used are as follows:

1 *Anticholinergic drugs* Atropine-like drugs cause a competitive blockade of acetylcholine receptors primarily at post ganglionic receptor sites. *Propantheline bromide* (Probanthine) given intravenously produces a change in the cystometrogram and can abolish bladder contraction provoked by filling. However, when given orally in the dose range of 15–30 mg

every 4–6 hours side effects of dry mouth, mydriasis and constipation are common. The therapeutic benefits are small.

2 *Ganglion blockage. Emepronium bromide* is a quaternary ammonium compound said to possess both ganglion blocking and anticholinergic effects. Given systemically it can change intravesical pressure. However, it is poorly absorbed when given orally and may cause peptic ulceration. Administration of the drug produces only a marginal change in symptoms.

3 *Antispasmodics.* Other drugs are said to act directly on smooth muscle at a site distal to the cholinergic receptor mechanism. Of this group *flavoxate hydrochloride* (Urispas) is in most common use, in the dose range 100–200 g 3–4 times a day. It is expensive and has produced only minor relief of symptoms. Side effects are few. In general and in the dose range used, these drugs have little more than a placebo effect.

In order to produce an effect that can be recognized cystometrically the drugs have to be given systemically and in a dose producing unpleasant side effects.

PARTIAL DENERVATION OF THE BLADDER

This procedure, described by Ingleman-Sundberg (1959), has a place in the treatment of the unstable bladder when all other forms of conservative treatment has failed. In brief, the preganglia and autonomic fibres associated with the middle vesical artery are divided using a vaginal approach.

REFERENCES

BAILEY K.V. (1963) *J. Obstet. Gynaec. Brit. Emp.*, **70**, 947.
BAILEY K.V. (1954) *J. Obstet. Gynaec. Brit. Cwlth.*, **61**, 291.
BATES C.P., WHITESIDE C.G., & TURNER-WARWICK R. (1970), *Brit. J. Urol.* **42**, 714.
BATES P., BRADLEY E.W., GLENN E., GRIFFITHS E., MELCHIOR H., ROWAN D., STIRLING A., ZINNER N., & HALP T. (1977) *J. Urol.*, **9**, 237.
BECK R.P., & MAUGHAN C.B., (1964) *Amer. J. Obstet. Gynec.*, **89**, 746.
BECK P.R., & McCORMICK S. (1982) *J. Obstet. Gynaec.* **59**, 269.
BONNEY V. (1934) *J. Obstet. Gynaec. Brit. Emp.*, **41**, 669.
BOYARSKY S. (1970) In *Urology* 3rd Ed. (Campbell M.F. & Harrison J.H. Eds.). Saunders, Philadelphia.
BROWN M. & WICKHAM J.E.A. (1969) *Brit. J. Urol.*, **41**, 211.
BUNNE G. & OBRINK A. (1978) *Urol. Res.*, **6**, 127.

CARDOZO L.D., ABRAMS P.D., STANTON S.L. & FENELEY R. *Brit. J. Urol.,* (1978) **50**, 374.

CARDOZO L.D., STANTON S.L. & WILLIAMS J.E. (1979) *Brit. J. Urol.,* **51**, 204.

EDWARDS L. & MALVERN J. (1974) *Brit. J. Urol.,* **46**, 325.

ENHORNING G. (1961) *Act. Chir. Scand. suppl.,* **296**, 1.

FALL M. (1978) *Scand. J. Urol.,* **125**, 55.

FLOYD W.F. & WALLS E.W. (1953) *J. Physiol. London,* **28**, (3), 599.

FREWEN W.K. (1978) *Brit. J. Urol.,* **50**, 246.

GALLAGHER D.J.A., MONTGOMERIE J.Z. & NORTH K.D.K. (1965) *Brit. med. J.,* **1**, 622.

GOSLING J.A., DIXON J.S., CRITCHLEY H.O.D. & THOMPSON S.A. (1981) *Brit. J. Urol.,* **53**, 35.

GREEN T. Jr. (1975) *Amer. J. Obstet. Gynec.,* **122**, 368.

HEIDLER H., WOLK H. & JONAS U. (1979) *Eur. Urol.,* **5**, 110.

HENRY M.M. & SWASH M. (1985) *Colpoproctology and the Pelvic Floor,* p. 42. Butterworths, London.

HILTON P. & STANTON S.L. (1983) *Brit. J. Obstet. Gynaec.,* **90**, 919.

HODGKINSON C.P. (1953) *Amer. J. Obstet. Gynec.,* **1965**, 560.

HODGKINSON C.P. & COBART N. (1960) *Amer. J. Obstet. Gynec.,* **79**, 648.

HOPKINSON B.R. & LIGHTWOOD R. (1967) *Brit. J. Surg. Engl.,* **50**, 92.

HOSKER G. & WARD G. (1982) *Proc. I.C.S.,* **12**, 161.

INGLEMAN-SUNDBERG G.A. (1959) *Acta. Obstet. Gynecol. Scand.,* **38**, 487.

JARVIS G.J. (1982) *Brit. J. Urol.,* **54**, 374.

JEFFCOATE T.N.A. (1961) *J. roy. Coll. Surg. Edinb.,* **7**, 28.

JEFFCOATE T.N.A. & ROBERTS H. (1952) *J. Obstet. Gynaec. Brit. Emp.,* **1952**, 59, 685.

KASS E.H. (1957) *Arch. internal. Med.,* **100**, 709.

KEGEL A.H. 1948 *Amer. J. Obstet. Gynaec.,* **56**, 238.

KELLY H.A. (1928) *Gynaecology,* **26**, p. 823. D. Appelton, New York & London.

KIFF E. & SWASH M. (1984) *Brit. J. Surg.,* **71**, 614.

LAST R.J. (1975) *Anatomy Regional and Applied,* 5th Ed., p. 358. Churchill-Livingstone, Edinburgh.

LOW J.A. (1967) *Amer. J. Obstet. Gynec.,* **97**, 308.

MAHADY I.W. & BEGG B.M. (1981) *Brit. J. Obstet. Gynaec.,* **88**, 1038.

MALPAS P. (1955) *Genital Prolapse and Allied Conditions.* Grune & Stratton, New York.

MENGERT W.F. (1936) *Amer. J. Obstet. Gynec.,* **31**, 775.

MOND N.C., PERCIVAL A. & BRUMFITT W. (1965) *Lancet,* **1**, 514.

O'NEIL A.G.B. (1981) *Brit. J. Urol.,* **53**, 368.

PACEY K. (1949) *J. Obstet. Gynaec. Brit. Cwlth.,* **56**, 1.

PARKS A.G., SWASH M. & URICH H. (1977) *Gut,* **18**, 656.

PERCY J.P. NEILL M.E., SWASH M. & PARKS A.G. (1981) *Lancet,* **1**, 16.

RAMSDEN P.D. (1977) *Brit. J. Urol.,* **49**, 43.

RICHTER K. & ALBRICH W. (1981) *Amer. J. Obstet. Gynec.,* **141**, 811.

RIDLEY J.H. (1976) *Amer. J. Obstet. Gynec.,* **126**, 590.

RUD T. (1980) *Acta. Obstet. Gynaec. Scand.,* **59**, 265.

SATO K. (1980) *Acta. Anat. Nippon,* **55**, 220.

SHEPHERD A. BLANNIN J.P. & WINDER A. (1985) *Proc. I.C.S.,* **15**, 224.

SMITH A.R.B. & WARREL D.W. (1985) *Proc. I.C.S.,* **15**, 44.

SMITH A.R.B. (1985), M.D. Thesis on Pelvic Floor Denervation, submitted to the University of Manchester.

SNOOKS S.J. & SWASH M. (1984) *Brit. J. Urol.,* **56**, 401.

SNOOKS S.J., SETCHELL M., SWASH M. & HENRY M.M. (1984) *Lancet,* **2**, 546.

STAMEY T.A. (1980) *Surgery of Female Incontinence* (Ed. Stanton & Tenagho), p. 77. Springer-Verlag.

STAMM W.E., COUNTS G.W., RUNNING K.R., FIHN S., TURK M. & HOLMES K.K. (1982) *New Engl. J. Med.,* **307**, 463.

STANTON S.L. (1984) *Clinical Gynaecologic Urology,* p. 169. C.V. Mosby Co.

TENAGHO E.A. & MILLER E.R. (1970) *Brit. J. Urol.,* **42**, 175

TENAGHO E.A. (1974) *Brit. J. Urol.,* **46**, 295.

TOEWS H. (1967) *Obstet. Gynec.,* **29**, 613.

VAN GEELEN J. (1981) *Proc. I.C.S.,* **11**, 77.

VEREECKEN R.L., DEMEIRSMAN G. & PUERS B. (1981) *Advances in Diagnostic Urology,* p. 314. Springer.

VODUSEK D.B. & LIGHT J.K. (1983) *Proc. I.C.S.,* **13**, 108.

WENDELL-SMITH (1967) Studies in the Morphology of the Pelvic Floor, Ph.D. Thesis University of London, quoted in *Colpoproctology and the Pelvic Floor,* (Ed. Henry H.M. & Swash M. 1985) p. 5. Butterworths, London.

YEATES W.K. (1972) *Ann. roy. Coll. Surg. Engl.,* **50**, 335.

ZACHARIN R.F. (1962) *J. Anat.,* **97**, 183.

ZACHARIN R.F. & GLEADELL L.W. (1963) *Amer. J. Obstet. Gynec.,* **86**, 981.

CHAPTER 46
BENIGN DISEASE OF THE VAGINA AND VULVA*

J. S. SCOTT

VAGINA

The vaginal epithelial state changes greatly in different phases of life. In the newborn it is thick and contains abundant glycogen because of the influence of maternal oestrogens. It thins after a few weeks and the basal layer of cells is covered only by a thin cornified layer. With the menarche the epithelium regenerates but reversion to a form resembling the pre-pubertal occurs after the climacteric. In the reproductive phase there are minor changes with the menstrual cycle and relatively major ones with pregnancy when the basal layer shows increased mitotic activity; the intermediate layer thickens and the cells become packed with glycogen. Vascularity also increases. Changes in glycogen levels in the epithelium occur with the cellular change but there is not a close correlation with the amount of oestrogen stimulation (Langley 1973).

VAGINAL INFECTIONS

Vaginal infection of one type or another is responsible for a large proportion of gynaecological complaints. It may occur in childhood, presenting special problems (see Chapter 4, p. 421). Once reproductive life is reached vaginal infection is rare in virgins, the pH of 4.5 or less providing effective natural protection. Occasionally some obvious factor, like retention of a forgotten tampon, may precipitate an acute infection which settles quickly when the offending object is removed.

The commonest specific forms of vaginitis are trichomonas vaginitis and candidiasis which produce vulval pruritus as their main symptom. Spread of both conditions is usually by intercourse but they are so common that they do not carry any strong implication of extra-marital sexual activity and it is not usually regarded as appropriate to manage simple cases in special clinics as is done with the classic

venereal infections, syphilis and gonorrhoea. Both trichomonas and candidiasis can usually be simply diagnosed by direct microscopy on fresh specimens and culture is rarely necessary; there should be a high index of suspicion for the concomitant presence of another genital infection.

Trichomonas vaginalis infection

Trichomonas vaginalis is a flagellate organism about $20\,\mu$m long, similar in size to a leucocyte. Its appearance, four flagellae anteriorly and membranous stylus posteriorly, and typical movements make identification easy on microscopy of a saline preparation. It is not uncommon to find the organism present in asymptomatic women. Active trichomonad infection is associated with a shift in the bacterial flora of the vagina away from the normal predominance of lactobacilli. Symptoms are classically of discharge which causes pruritus on the vulva, sometimes with introital soreness. On examination the yellow-green frothy discharge is typical with punctate ('strawberry') injection of the vaginal epithelium. The pH is 5.0 or higher. However, it is only a minority of cases which show the classical discharge. Gardnerella vaginitis is the condition which is most frequently confused clinically.

Trichomonal infections require oral medication. Metronidazole has, over the last quarter of a century, established itself as an excellent drug for treating a condition which had previously caused a great deal of distress in the absence of effective therapy. Metronidazole rarely induces resistance in the organism and is also active against anaerobic bacteria.

Dosage for adults is a 200 mg tablet orally thrice daily for 7–10 days. Alternatively a single 2 gm dose may be given if there are reasons to doubt that the patient would take the full course. Gastrointestinal disturbance may occur and can be minimized by taking the tablets with food. Alcohol may give a reaction similar to that which it does with disulfiram ('Antabuse', C.P. Pharmaceuticals Ltd.) and its avoidance

---

* For prolapse please *see* Chapter 45 (p. 680).

should be recommended. Metronidazole administration should be avoided if possible in early pregnancy. Tinidazole is a similar drug with the sole advantage of a longer half-life, allowing less frequent administration. Nimorazole may also be given as a single oral dosage. Simultaneous treatment of sexual partners is wise and until cure is obtained the use of a contraceptive sheath should be advised at intercourse regardless of whether or not contraception is required.

Candida albicans vaginitis

Candida (monilia) *albicans* is a yeast-like fungus commonly affecting the vagina. In certain countries the closely related organism *C. glabrata* is commoner (Friedrich 1983). Direct microscopy shows the mycelial filaments or spores; a preparation in 10–20% potassium hydroxide helps to highlight the candida. Culture will confirm the diagnosis if necessary. *C. albicans* is frequently present in the vagina of asymptomatic women so its mere presence is not an indication for therapy. Candida is usually held in check by the normal flora of commensal organisms in the vagina. The appearances are of a light white discharge with curd-like patches adherent to the epithelium. The symptoms are of discharge with severe vulval pruritus and possibly introital soreness.

Predisposing factors are pregnancy, the use of anovulant contraceptives, the premenstrual phase, disturbed glucose tolerance, the taking of wide spectrum antibiotics and corticosteroid usage. Pregnancy is the strongest, 15–20% of women developing clinical infection near term (Gardner & Kaufman 1981).

Candidiasis, and some other forms of vaginitis, have in the past been treated by local antiseptic preparations such as gentian violet but these were messy and not very efficient. However nystatin, a polyene which became available as a by-product of streptomycin production in the 1950s, was soon established as the standard treatment of candidiasis. It is not prone to cause drug resistance. It is not absorbed from the gastrointestinal tract and is too toxic to give parenterally, so treatment is by pessaries or cream to the vagina and local application to the vulva if necessary.

More recently introduced imidazole anti-fungal preparations such as clotrimazole and miconazole have got few advantages except the need for less prolonged courses of treatment, which is possibly important when patient compliance is doubtful. Eliot *et al.* (1979) compared different regimes of nystatin, clotrimazole and miconazole and found no difference in the response rate though relapse rate varied. It is

important that the nystatin should be inserted high into the vagina, using a special tubular applicator nozzle for cream. Insertion *must* continue during the time of menstruation. One pessary (100 000 units of nystatin) nightly for up to six weeks is usually adequate dosage. In chronic cases longer periods of therapy are necessary (Gardner & Kaufman 1981). The use of a contraceptive sheath during treatment is wise, whether or not any treatment is being given to the consort.

Recurrence is common particularly if the full treatment course has not been completed, if steroids or antibiotics are being taken, if the patient is pregnant, if she has diabetes or an immune deficiency state, or there is another reservoir of infection e.g. in gut, nail-bed, bladder or umbilicus. Some women with recurrent candida have been found to have lymphocytes which fail to show mitogenic response to *candida albicans* (Witkin *et al.* 1983). While the exact immunological basis for candidiasis occurring and persisting in some individuals is not entirely clear, it is increasingly evident that the role of immunologic factors is a major one.

Whether it is necessary to treat simultaneously the partners of women with candida vaginitis is not agreed. Re-infection certainly occurs but a study in Denmark suggests that treatment of the partner does not influence the recurrence rate and that auto-infection from the large bowel is probably the important factor (Buch & Christensen 1982). The only rationale for oral treatment is to deal with such an intestinal reservoir of recurrent infection.

Gardnerella vaginalis vaginitis

Gardnerella (G.) *vaginalis* (previously known as *haemophilus vaginalis*) infection is reported with increasing frequency in asymptomatic patients who have had cervical smears taken. Lactobacilli are deficient and the cells may be heavily coated with the small bacteria involved, giving them a finely stippled or hazy appearance known as 'clue' cells (Fig. 46.1). The condition is related to sexual activity with non-barrier contraception.

When clinical disease is manifest there is usually a foul-smelling discharge and occasionally pruritus or a burning sensation. The appearances are similar to those of trichomonas infection but the colour is usually grey (Gardner & Kaufman 1981). The vaginal pH is above 4.5 and addition of KOH to the vaginal discharge leads to release of a fishy odour. Wet mount preparations show the 'clue' cells.

Whether or not it is necessary to treat the condi-

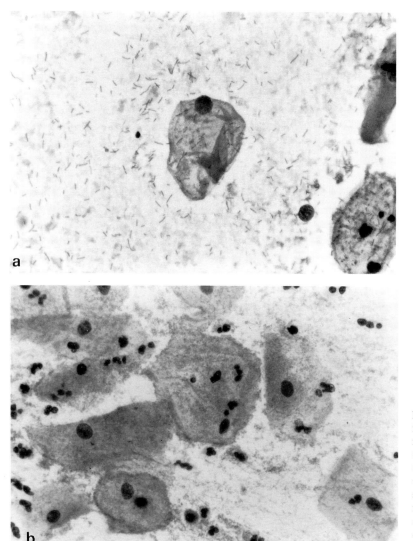

Fig. 46.1. (a) Cells and flora in normal smear with numerous Döderlein's bacilli (*lactobacilli*) evident. (b) Smear from patient with *G. vaginalis* infection showing 'clue' cells—the multiple, tiny bacilli adherent to cells give the characteristic hazy or very finely stippled appearance.

tion in the absence of symptomatology is not agreed. For therapy local sulphonamide cream may be given or metronidazole as a single 2 gm oral dose (Minkowski *et al.* 1983). More sophisticated antibiotics are also active but have no obvious benefit over these simpler drugs. Sheath contraception should be advised.

Non-specific vaginitis

As the name implies, the precise organism responsible is not defined in these cases. As with *G. vaginalis* infection a fishy odour is prominent and possibly an interaction between that organism and unidentified anaerobes causes the condition. Metronidazole therapy is usually effective.

Rarely a variety of pathogenic bacteria not usually associated with vaginitis may appear to be the cause of acute vaginitis but, before accepting that such a cultured organism is the cause of the pathology, every effort should be made to exclude the presence of one of the common pathogens.

POSTCLIMACTERIC VAGINAL PROBLEMS

Vaginal atrophy after the climacteric may cause coital difficulties. Bleeding may occur and discharge from secondary infection. Correction of these problems has for long been easily achieved by oestrogen applied locally. However the recent appreciation that there is a very close association between the action of oestrogens unopposed by a progestogen and the development of endometrial cancer demands review of this approach. Absorption of oestrogen applied locally is considerable especially from an atrophic vagina. If the uterus is still present it is probably safest to administer a low dose of oestrogen cyclically by mouth with a progestogen added in the second part of the cycle. One or two courses of treatment may be all that is necessary; they will restore vaginal acidity and cause regeneration of the epithelium.

Severe atrophy is common if there has been radiotherapy to the pelvis; in these cases particular difficulties may exist because if the tumour treated was possibly oestrogen dependent, the conventional therapy is contraindicated.

Atrophic vaginitis

This is *not* synonymous with postclimacteric vaginitis. Though the senile form is the commonest type a similar disorder may also occur in prepubertal children. In children foreign bodies must always be suspected as being the focus of the infection and can usually be demonstrated using a miniature Sims' speculum without need for anaesthesia. Faecal contamination may also sometimes be a factor in children, particularly if there is pinworm (*Enterobius vermicularis*) infestation.

In younger children therapy with gonadal steroids is best avoided and careful investigation and specific therapy will usually deal with the problem. Small applications of topical oestrogen cream to the introitus may, however, be used with care if specific relief is not possible.

EXCESSIVE VAGINAL DISCHARGE WITHOUT PATHOLOGY

In the past excessive discharge from the vagina without evident pathology was itself diagnosed as 'leuk(c)orrhoea'. This is no longer so but it is the case that women may complain of excessive discharge in the presence of an intrauterine device, with the use of an oral contraceptive (particularly one with a high oestrogen component), at the time of ovulation or in the presence of florid erosion or ectropion of the cervix. It is sometimes difficult to exclude an infection with confidence but if the pH is between 3.8 and 4.2, vaginitis is not present (Gardner & Kaufman 1981). Problems of interpreting vaginal flora may be overcome by using techniques of quantification (Onderdonk *et al.* 1977) and correlating the pH with the

bacterial flora (Langley 1973): Grade I only Döderlein's bacilli (lactobacilli) present pH 4.0–5.0; Grade II mixed flora including Döderlein's bacilli pH 4.5–5.5; Grade III mixed flora excluding Döderlein's bacilli pH 5.0–8.0.

TOXIC SHOCK SYNDROME AND VAGINAL TAMPONS

Forgotten vaginal tampons have long been recognized as a cause of vaginitis with acute offensive discharge the only symptom. The patient's embarrassment when the offending object was removed was often the major aspect of the condition. However in 1980 reports suddenly began to appear of women in the United States of America developing a strange and severe disease (Schrock 1980). The typical victim was a woman of reproductive age with high fever, vomiting and diarrhoea commencing at the time of menstruation. Hypotensive shock with dehydration was an early feature and death sometimes occurred. In surviving patients skin manifestations commonly appeared later. An association with use of vaginal tampons was a feature and certain aspects suggested that a toxin-producing *Staphylococcus aureus* infection might be involved. This was isolated from the cervix or vagina in most cases.

In a prompt piece of well coordinated sleuthing it was found that a particular new brand of tampon was most frequently involved: one which was designed to expand when in position. It seems that this may be associated with promotion of *S. aureus* colonization of the vagina and reflux of toxin-containing menstrual blood into the peritoneal cavity with resultant rapid absorption of toxin (Fuller *et al.* 1980). A similar *S. aureus* toxin syndrome occasionally occurs in other circumstances.

The tampons particularly implicated have been withdrawn but it is still a rare hazard with other brands. The management consists of urgent fluid replacement, all tampon fragments should be removed from the vagina and chemotherapy given. The chemotherapy will probably not affect the toxic state but by controlling the infection will prevent any recurrence.

VAGINAL INJURY

Vaginal injury is infrequent but for that of defloration and in association with parturition. Rape is a cause of injury to vulva or vagina, the significance being mainly psychological and medicolegal and this is dealt with in texts on that subject (*see also* Gardner & Kaufman 1981). In women of postclimacteric age, serious tears can occur as a consequence of consenting intercourse (Wilson & Swartz 1972) particularly if sexual activity is resumed after a prolonged gap, when the vagina has shrunk and lost its elasticity due to the lack of oestrogen and of regular coital stretching. The usual injury is a crescentic tear in the posterior fornix. The condition may seem a simple one with diagnosis and management self-evident. However, because of the circumstances in which the injury occurs, the patient often conceals the history. Furthermore when a vaginal speculum is passed, the blade pressing on the posterior vaginal wall may cover the tear, which is often not felt on palpation. The blood loss is often heavy and potentially life threatening. *Major postmenopausal bleeding not obviously coming from a cervical neoplasm should be suspected as being due to this cause.* If the lesion is not defined initially it should be found at examination under anaesthesia which gives the opportunity for curative suturing with absorbable material. Very occasionally such an injury can extend into the Pouch of Douglas.

Rarely rupture of a vaginal vault scar may occur with evisceration (Scott 1955, Powell 1973). It is liable to occur particularly when there has been prolapse of the vault after hysterectomy; then all intra-abdominal straining pressure comes directly on the scar. Bowel comes down through the vagina in a most alarming manner but restitution and repair is remarkably simple.

VAGINAL INTRA-EPITHELIAL NEOPLASIA

Local intra-epithelial carcinomatous lesions in the vagina present particular problems. The lesions are not confined to a small region like the squamo-columnar junction of the cervix; colposcopy is much less useful and excision biopsy of the whole area, as done with cone biopsy on the cervix, is rarely possible. Accordingly the locally acting anti-mitotic drug fluorouracil has been used. It is usually effective without serious side effects (Ballon *et al.* 1979) (*see* p. 715). Laser treatment may also be used (*see* Chapter 49, p. 761).

ADENOSIS VAGINAE

The appearance of adenomatous, columnar epithelium on the vagina has been recognized for over a century. More recently, however, the condition has sprung into prominence as the precursor of clear cell vaginal cancer in young women whose mothers had been treated with diethylstilboestrol in the course of the pregnancy resulting in the birth of the affected female (Chapter 49, p. 764).

ENDOMETRIOTIC CYSTS

Endometriotic cysts can form on the vagina giving pain, dyspareunia and post-coital bleeding (Fig. 46.2). Treatment is on an *ad hoc* basis as for endometriosis generally.

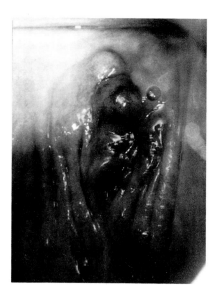
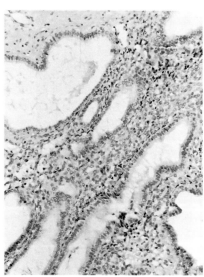

Fig. 46.2. Endometriosis of vaginal vault. There are dark nodules which were acutely tender. Histology shows the typical endometriotic pattern with glands and stroma.

MESONEPHRIC (GÄRTNER'S) AND PARAMESONEPHRIC DUCT CYSTS

Cysts of mesonephric origin may be found alongside the vagina lying laterally or antero-laterally. It has recently become appreciated that a higher proportion of paravaginal cystic lesions than was previously suspected have an origin in paramesonephric duct tissue (Gardner & Kaufman 1981). They may be at any level from the cervix to the urethra. The cysts are usually symptomless and are not tender so they may, if of low tension, be missed at vaginal examination or mistakenly diagnosed as representing a cystocele or bladder diverticulum (Fig. 46.3). They are lined

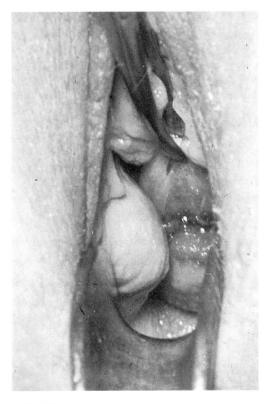

Fig. 46.3. Mesonephric cyst on lateral aspect of vaginal wall.

by cuboidal or flattened epithelium. Treatment is usually not necessary but, if large, marsupialization is often safer than attempts at excision which may lead the unwary operator into 'jungle' territory around ureter and uterine vessels.

VAGINAL FISTULAE

The anatomical situation of the vagina is such that fistulae may develop between it and both the gastrointestinal and urinary tracts. These may be congenital or acquired, either as a consequence of diseases such as tuberculosis, carcinoma or Crohn's, or as a complication of surgery. If a fistula follows surgery it may be after an operation done on the urinary or alimentary system but much more frequently it is a consequence of gynaecological surgery. This is not to be taken as implying a lower standard of gynaecological surgery, it is merely that surgery on the genital tract usually involves opening its surface and any leakage of faeces or urine will be likely to make its way through the suture line, creating a fistula.

CONDITIONS AFFECTING BOTH VULVA AND VAGINA

Many conditions described in the 'vaginal' and 'vulval' sections of this chapter frequently affect the other structure. However there are some conditions and circumstances in which both organs are usually affected together. For example, if the woman is suffering from a generalized deficiency state vulvovaginal candidiasis of chronic or recurrent nature is one of the commonest manifestations. Acute vulvovaginitis may develop due to infection with trichomonas, candida and *Neisseria gonorrhoeae* but the association of vulvovaginitis with other organisms which may be present in the vagina or on the vulva is not so precise. Osborne *et al.* (1982) studied 9 organisms in 253 patients and controls. They found that the presence of *Neisseria gonorrhoeae*, *trichomonas vaginalis*, *Gardnerella vaginalis* and herpes simplex showed a correlation with active infection. Childhood vulvovaginitis is a special problem (*see* p. 42).

VULVAL AND VAGINAL COLPOSCOPY

Colposcopy of the vagina is technically more difficult than colposcopy of the cervix because of problems with focusing on account of the tangential vision. Vault granulomas after hysterectomy have alarming vascular patterns. Pre-malignant lesions of the vaginal epithelium, seen mostly in women who have had similar cervical problems, show vessel pattern anomalies similar to those seen on the cervix.

The columnar epithelium of vaginal adenosis has the same appearance as columnar epithelium on the cervix. Typical grape-like structures can be seen after 3% acetic acid application. Conservatism is appropriate in management as squamous metaplasia will usually occur spontaneously.

Following the expansion and apparent success of colposcopy in the management of premalignant lesions of the cervix, the vulva seemed to offer scope for similar prophylactic care. However the colposcope is not very helpful on the keratinized vulval skin which has minimal translucency, though sometimes it is of use with lesions on the mucosal surface of the inner aspects of labia minora.

CONGENITAL ABNORMALITIES

Congenital abnormalities often affect vagina and vulva (*see* Chapter 1). In some cases they are manifestations of a profound disorder of sex differentiation and these conditions are considered in Chapter 3 (p. 25). In others, however, they occur in women who are otherwise normal.

Abnormalities of fusion of Müllerian ducts can lead to a variety of forms of duplication of the vagina. These range from total duplication to a small median band representing a region in which breaking down of the fused medial aspects of the Müllerian ducts has not occurred. When there is a complete duplication of the vagina it is remarkably easy for even the experienced examiner to fail to detect it; the speculum or finger may pass easily along one side of the septum and a single cervix is identified creating no suspicion of duplication. Once diagnosed no treatment may be necessary but in some cases division of the septum may be undertaken, which is usually a simple procedure.

Transverse septa are altogether different and treatment is usually necessary. These are commonly situated just above the hymen and are often mistakenly described as imperforate hymens. Presentation is often at puberty when amenorrhoea, pain, lower abdominal swelling and the evidence of the bulging dark blue membrane lead to the diagnosis of cryptomenorrhoea. Acute retention of urine may also be a feature. Haematocolpos may be combined with haematometra and haematosalpinx. Vaginal drainage is the appropriate treatment with precautions against the introduction of infection.

In other cases the obstruction is much more substantial; there may be no canalization of a large part of the lower vagina. In these circumstances much more complex surgery is required with either 'advancement' of the vagina (Jeffcoate 1969) or utilization of a segment of large bowel to construct a substitute for the missing section of vagina. This procedure may seem complex but to achieve satisfactory coital and reproductive function it has much to commend it (Goligher 1983).

Total absence of the vagina is usually associated with absence of the uterus, there having been no Müllerian duct development. Whether this represents a genetically controlled growth failure as occurs in relation to other organs from time to time, or there is an inappropriate production of the Müllerian inhibitory factor in an otherwise normal female, is unknown. Complex operations have been used in the past to deal with this problem but these operations have been superseded to a large extent by the simple Williams' 'marsupial' procedure. This merely involves creating a pouch from the labia minora which usually functions very well for purposes of coitus (Williams 1964). Feroze *et al.* (1975) in a review of the use of the Williams' operation as opposed to a complex grafting technique for cases of absence of the vagina found the results of the Williams' operation superior. The pouch created did *not* undergo contraction if intercourse did not take place.

In many cases, however, surgery is not necessary as regular use of graduated glass dilators will frequently result in the smallest of vaginal dimples enlarging to a depth and diameter adequate for intercourse which is satisfactory to both partners.

VULVA

The vulva being essentially an area of skin lying adjacent to the lower end of the vagina, it is not surprising that women with vulval diseases may attend a gynaecologist or a dermatologist; some may also attend a venereologist. Problems and confusions arise because of differing approaches, attitudes and terminologies of practitioners in these different specialties.

Skin conditions have different appearances, symptoms and implications when they present on the vulva and the response to local therapies can also be very different (Ridley 1983). Likewise there are great differences between the same disease affecting vulva and vagina. Most of the pathologies of the vulval skin do not respect anatomical limits and may extend to perianal, crural, upper thigh and lower abdominal skin.

Pruritus is an outstanding feature of vulval disorders. Skin conditions which are non-pruritic in other sites may be associated with intense pruritus when they occur on the vulva. As mentioned, trichomonas or candida vaginal infections produce no irritation in the vagina but cause intense vulval pruritus. Factors involved in this differential effect on the vulva include the special sensory innervation of the area (Ridley 1975) and the local climatic conditions. The importance of climatic factors is demonstrated by the evidence that vulval skin with lichen sclerosus transplanted to the thigh returned to normal, whereas thigh skin transferred to the vulva assumed the changes of lichen sclerosus (Whimster 1961). This local influence is also highlighted by Way's (1982) observation that 5.5% of patients he treated for cancer of the vulva by vulvectomy went on later to develop a fresh cancer in their new vulva: *re-occur*rence as opposed to recurrence.

Specialists involved with management of vulval lesions have been the subject of implied criticism for their hesitancy to do biopsies (Kolstad 1981). This view is a reflection of the current tendency to translate to the vulva the approach to problems of premalignancy which has developed in relation to the cervix. In the cervix, biopsy is very freely performed, particularly colposcopically directed punches or, less frequently, cone excision. However there are very important differences between cervix and vulva which make a direct translation of cervical management techniques to the vulva inappropriate (Friedrich 1983). When the vulva is biopsied a very sensitive area is left, usually sutured, and ultimately scarred. Furthermore the vulval equivalent of a cervical cone is a vulvectomy, a relatively major and unsatisfactory operation with considerable physical and psychological sequelae. Buckley *et al.* (1984) detail reasons from the pathologist's standpoint which make it inappropriate to draw a vulval/cervical analogy with regard to intra-epithelial neoplasia. This is far from saying that biopsy should *not* be done but merely that it can never be expected to be done with the same abandon as biopsy of the cervix.

CONDYLOMATA ACUMINATA*

Condylomata acuminata, venereal warts, though very common have long been regarded as benign condi-

---

* Previous editions have had the spelling 'accuminata'. The alternative spelling, now used, is 'acuminata' based on a derivation from the Latin 'acuminare' meaning 'tapering to a sharp point'. Although the lesions often seem far from being spear-like, they are pointed compared with the flat lesions of secondary syphilis, 'condylomata lata', and it was to distinguish these conditions that the terminology developed; 'Condyle', 'a knob', is the other part of the origin.

tions of no great importance (Fig. 46.4). However in recent years studies of the human papilloma viruses (HPVs), which apparently cause the lesions, have led to greatly increased interest in these warts and to consideration of their possible relationship to malignancy. There are currently a matter of 30 different types of HPV identified which share one common antigen (Editorial 1983); about a quarter produce genital tract lesions. HPV6 has a particular association with genital condylomata.

There has been a great increase in clinically obvious genital warts recently and it is thought that increased squamous cancer incidence may be a consequence of this (Singer *et al.* 1984). A synergism between herpes simplex virus and HPV has been suggested as being involved in the carcinogenetic mechanism (zur Hausen 1982). Smoking may also act as a cofactor or promoter in the presence of HPV infec-

Most of the attention to viral carcinogenesis in genital cancer has related to the cervix but interest is now developing in relation to the vulva. Intra-epithelial vulval neoplasia is becoming more commonly diagnosed and the evidence of an association between HPV lesions and vulval cancer is becoming increasingly strong (Singer *et al.* 1984). HPV genomes have been isolated from a number of vulval carcinomas. Condylomata acuminata have been recorded as being associated with intra-epithelial or invasive cancer of the vulva in as many as 20% cases (Crum *et al.* 1982). These authors reviewed 65 intra-epithelial lesions of vulva and distal vagina and defined criteria for differentiation of intra-epithelial neoplasia and condylomata. The histological features of condylomata are koilocytosis, parabasal hyperplasia, normal mitoses, minimal basal pleomorphism or nuclear enlargement and orderly epithelial maturation. Those of intra-epithelial neoplasia are disorderly maturation, abnormal mitoses, basal and parabasal pleomorphism with nuclear enlargement and hyperchromatism. Koilocytosis may also be present with intra-epithelial neoplasia but it is often focal and localized to the outer third of the epithelium.

Vaginal carcinoma has also been recorded as developing shortly after the presence of condylomata (Beck & Clayton 1984). It seems that the precise type of HPV is important. Type 16 apparently carries a high cervical cancer risk; type 2 has been reported with vulval cancer (Kàufman *et al.* 1981) but types 6 and 11 are found in benign vulval and cervical condylomata which tend to remain benign (Zoler 1983). The whole field is advancing rapidly and many further developments are likely.

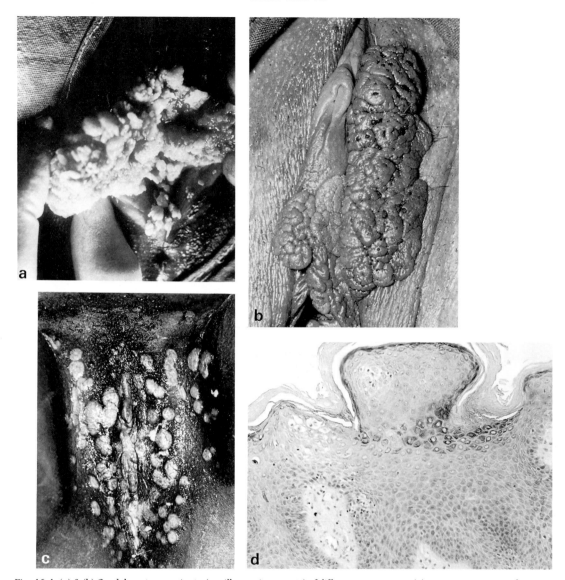

Fig. 46.4. (a) & (b) Condylomata acuminata (papilloma virus warts) of different appearance; (a) represents an acute form and (b) one of long-standing.
(c) Condylomata lata; secondary syphilis warts.
(d) Histology of a condyloma acuminatum shows parakeratosis and many vacuolated cells (koilocytes).

At one time topical application of the resin podophyllin, was the favoured local treatment of condylomata acuminata. Sometimes, however, it can cause excessive damage involving local healthy tissue. Central nervous system complications of local use of podophyllin have also been described and there have been occasional deaths of treated patients and of the fetus when treatment was given in pregnancy (Ridley

1975, Filley *et al.* 1982). However careful local applications to small warts in the non-pregnant probably carry little risk. Thermal cautery or laser treatment are usually more satisfactory if treatment appears indicated. Treatment may not prove necessary as spontaneous resolution sometimes occurs with surprising rapidity. A controlled trial of interferon therapy (Vesterinen *et al.* 1984) indicated that while colposcopic remission might be obtained, cells typical of condyloma persisted in all cases.

HERPES SIMPLEX INFECTION

Herpes simplex infection of the genital region is commonly due to the type 2 virus. At present the incidence appears to be increasing rapidly. It is commonest in young, unmarried women, frequently in association with the presence of other venereal diseases (Gardner & Kaufman 1981). Sexual contact is a major factor in transmission and incubation is less than a week. Vesicles appear which proceed to become ulcers and there is erythema with lymphadenopathy. Severe pain and tenderness are usual. Resolution takes place spontaneously but recurrence is common, representing a flare-up of latent infection. With type 2 virus infection recurrence is particularly common and the presence of antibodies makes this

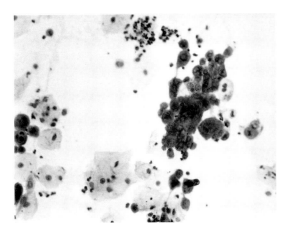

Fig. 46.5. Smear from patient infected with herpes genitalis showing characteristic multinucleated giant cells with intranuclear inclusions.

more likely. The antibodies are probably a marker for latent infection in the nerve ganglia. Recurrent lesions are usually much less severe than the primary variety unless secondary bacterial infection occurs.

A direct smear from the vagina shows characteristic multinucleated giant cells with intranuclear inclusions (Fig. 46.5). Direct viral culture of vesicular fluid and antibody studies on serum confirm the diagnosis. Local antiseptic treatment and antibiotics for secondary infection along with symptomatic measures have been the mainstay of treatment. Antiviral therapy both for local and systemic use (e.g. idoxuridine and acyclovir) is now available.

While this can reduce the time of virus-shedding and of resolution of lesions (Bryson *et al.* 1983, Mindel *et al.* 1982) there is not general agreement as to when it should be used beyond acceptance of its value for the immunocompromised individual. It has recently been reported (Mindel *et al.* 1984, Straus *et al.* 1984, Douglas *et al.* 1984) that acyclovir ('Zovirax', Wellcome Medical Division) will suppress recurrences but the effect does not persist when the drug is stopped.

It is not clear what the precise relationship is between vulval herpes infection, treated or untreated, and vulval carcinoma.

Neonatal infection with herpes is a risk for children born to women with active genital herpes (Nahmias *et al.* 1971, Ridley 1975). Caesarean section has been advocated for the delivery of such babies as they are suspected of acquiring the infection during passage through the infected birth canal but even with this precaution infection may still occur.

Syphilis
The primary chancre of syphilis may occur on the vulva. It starts as a small area of painless thickening, progressing to a round ulcer with raised borders. The floor is indurated and covered with grey slough; there is non-tender lymphadenopathy. Dark-ground microscopy reveals the spirochaete, *Treponema pallidum*.

Secondary syphilis occurs occasionally on the vulva in the form of condylomata lata which are to be differentiated from viral warts, condylomata acuminata. The syphilitic condylomata are coarse, flat topped, moist and necrotic (Fig. 46.4c) in contrast to the long, pointed fronds of condylomata acuminata (*see* footnote, p. 707).

Other venereal ulcers
Rarely exotic tropical venereal ulcerative conditions such as granuloma venereum (Donovanosis) or lymphogranuloma inguinale (venereum) may be encountered, the former due to a Rickettsial organism and the latter to a Chlamydia, presenting as vulval lesions. A high index of suspicion in patients likely to have had contacts in the tropics is necessary along with a co-operative diagnostic approach with a venereologist.

Chancroid (soft sore), said to be due to the Gram-negative streptobacillus *haemophilus ducreyi*, presents with tender ulcers associated with an injected circumference and lymphadenopathy.

VULVAL DYSTROPHY

For decades the terminology applied to conditions localized to the vulva which involved atrophy or hyperplasia has been a source of controversy and confusion amongst clinicans. Such terms as leukoplakia (hypertrophic and atrophic), kraurosis, lichen sclerosus (atrophic and otherwise) have been used with little discrimination; certainly there has been no reasonable anticipation that the reader would know to what the writer was referring. 'Leukoplakia' which merely means 'white patch', 'kraurosis' which means 'dry' and 'lichen' referring to a similarity to the growth found often on tree bark, are all terms of crude, macroscopic description bearing little or no relationship to the histo-pathological states. Jeffcoate and Woodcock (1961) in a classic paper put forward the view that most of the conditions were not specific entities. They regarded them all as different forms of dystrophy.

To create from such chaos a situation whereby a logical classification and common terminology can be accepted and understood between different doctors is not easy. Like the poor, outdated terminologies are always with us! However the International Society for the Study of Vulvar Diseases (Report of the Committee on Terminology, 1976) has made proposals to standardize diagnosis and nomenclature which go some way to rationalize matters. They are summarized in Table 46.1.

Vulval atypia as it is recognized may occur with or without dystrophy and may be mild, moderate or severe which can be equated with vulval intra-epithelial neoplasia (VIN) grades I, II or III. The grading is similar to that used for cervical intra-epithelial neoplasia, VIN III being equivalent to carcinoma-*in-situ*.

It is important to appreciate that, as with pathology in many organs, the disease state as defined by histology of a particular area at a specific time is neither representative of the total organ nor static. Change in the pathology can occur over months or years and an area not examined histologically may contain more sinister features from the point of view of malignancy than the area biopsied, actual or potential malignancy being the major concern of all involved.

Ia HYPERPLASTIC DYSTROPHY WITHOUT ATYPIA

This term covers lesions formerly labelled as lichen simplex and leukoplakia. The colour may range from dusky red, when hyperkeratosis is minimal, to white, when hyperkeratosis is severe; fissures and ulcers may develop. Scratching, rubbing, moisture and medications all affect the skin appearance.

Histologically there is hyperkeratosis, irregular thickening of the malpighian layer with elongation of epithelial folds (acanthosis) to give deep and distorted rete pegs. There is sometimes parakeratosis (retention of nuclear material in keratin layers) with a prominent granular layer. There is a variable dermal infiltration with lymphocytes and plasma cells but there is no epithelial cytological abnormality pointing to malignant potential (Fig. 46.6).

Ib HYPERPLASTIC DYSTROPHY WITH ATYPIA

(Dysplasia: atypical hyperplasia)

In this category there is an increased risk of malignancy and some in the past confined the use of the term leukoplakia to these cases. It comprises about 10% hyperplastic dystrophies.

Table 46.1

VULVAL DYSTROPHIES				
I	*Hyperplastic dystrophy*	(a) no atypia		
		(b) atypia	(i) mild	
			(ii) moderate	
			(iii) severe	
II	*Lichen sclerosus*			
III	*Mixed dystrophy*	(a) no atypia		
	(lichen sclerosus with foci	(b) atypia	(i) mild	
	of epithelial hyperplasia)		(ii) moderate	
			(iii) severe	
PAGET'S DISEASE OF THE VULVA				
SQUAMOUS CARCINOMA-IN-SITU				

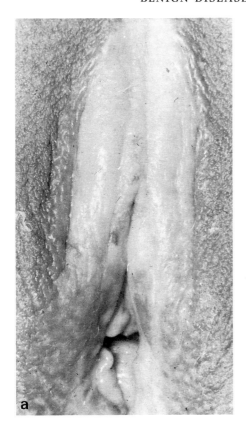

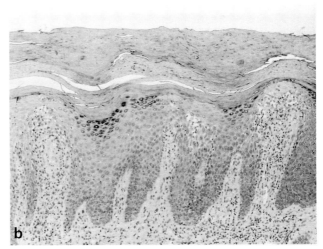

Fig. 46.6. (a) Vulva with hyperplastic dystrophy without atypia. (b) Histologically there is hyperkeratosis, elongated rete pegs and underlying chronic inflammation.

Macroscopically there are usually well delineated, slightly elevated, rough, white lesions evident. Microscopically the differentiating feature consists of variable nuclear size and shape in the deeper layers of the epidermis and rete pegs with hyperchromasia and scattered mitotic figures. There may be lack of the expected cellular maturation moving towards the surface of the epithelium. The more severe the condition the closer this abnormality approaches the surface. Pleomorphism and loss of polarity are other features and ultimately the picture is of carcinoma-in-situ (VIN III) (Fig. 46.7).

II LICHEN SCLEROSUS

Like leukoplakia this term has induced a lot of confusion particularly with kraurosis, primary atrophy and atrophic leukoplakia. Jeffcoate (1966) does not regard it as an entity but the International Society has accorded it this status, but without its common addendum 'et atrophicus'. Lichen sclerosus is a condition commonly associated with the post-climacteric era but it may occur in much younger, pre-menar-

chal females. In these cases it is usually relieved by the onset of the menarche. The deletion of 'et atrophicus' took place because several workers demonstrated that the epithelium was metabolically hyperactive rather than atrophic (Gardner & Kaufman 1981).

There is an association with morphoea (localized scleroderma) and possibly with vitiligo (Ridley 1983). It has recently been shown that, as in vitiligo, there is a relationship to autoimmune phenomena (Meyrick Thomas et al. 1982). Goolamali et al. (1974) found thyroid cytoplasmic antibodies in 40% of cases and antibodies to gastric parietal cells in 44% of cases; both figures increased highly significantly over age-matched controls. A familial pattern is sometimes evident (Friedrich & MacLaren 1984).

The primary lesion is a polygonal flat, pink, white or translucent macule. Confluent areas may be speckled or purpuric with telangiectasia and small blisters. Plugs resembling comedos may be evident along with surface depressions and oedema of the foreskin with phimosis (Gardner & Kaufman 1981). Lesions may be on the inner aspects of labia majora, labia

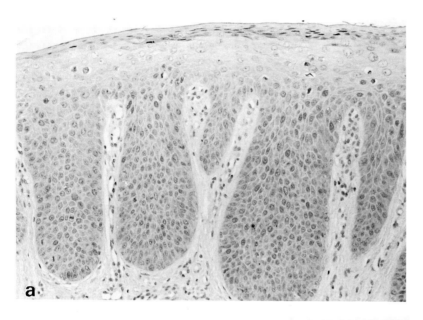

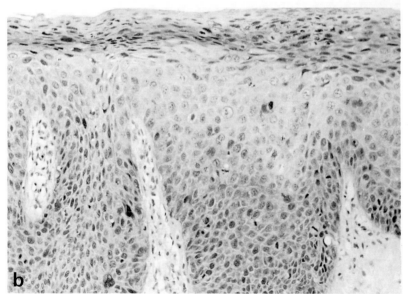

Fig. 46.7. (a) Histologcal
appearance of vulval intra-
epithelial neoplasia (VIN
grade II). The cellular
atypia is confined to the
lower two-thirds of the
epithelium.
(b) VIN grade III. There is
extensive cellular
hyperactivity, and frequent
mitoses and atypia
extending throughout the
thickness of the epithelium.

minora, clitoris, perianal regions and genito-crural folds. Lichenification often occurs. Ultimately a smooth waxen appearance develops with atrophy and the introitus can become constricted (Fig. 46.8). Sometimes there are median skin fissures. Coital difficulties become common. With the exception of the last feature, the childhood form is essentially similar (Fig. 46.9).

Microscopically there is hyperkeratosis, thin epithelium and flat rete pegs with cytoplasmic vacuoles and follicular plugging. The sub-epidermal region is relatively acellular with an homogeneous, pink-staining collagenous appearance, elastic fibres being absent. Below this region lies an infiltrate of chronic inflammatory cells. Ultrastructural studies show an absence of dopa-positive melanocytes and removal of degenerate dermal material into the epidermis with abnormal dermal collagen (Mann & Cowan 1973).

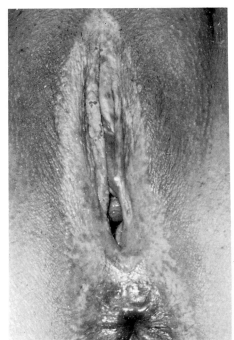 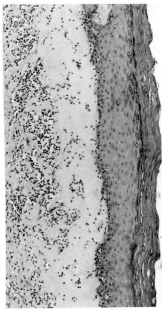

Fig. 46.8. Vulva with lichen sclerosus. Histologically there is hyperkeratosis, almost absent rete pegs and homogeneous subepidermal region with infiltrate of chronic inflammatory cells below this.

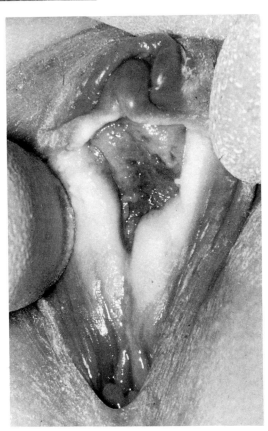

Fig. 46.9. Lichen sclerosus in a 5-year-old girl. The epithelial thickening has led to oedema of the clitoris and apparent enlargement. The child's original referral was as a case of masculinization.

III MIXED DYSTROHY

(Lichen sclerosus with foci of epithelial hyperplasia)

This confused term in itself encapsulates the nomen-clature problems! Lichen sclerosus in its ill-defined

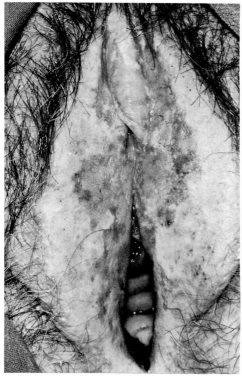

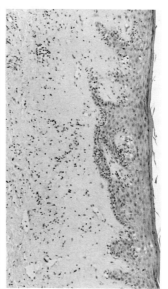

Fig. 46.10. Mixed vulval dystrophy (lichen sclerosus with foci of epithelial hyperplasia). There are a few somewhat elongated rete pegs and subepithelial homogeneity.

natural history may show hyperplastic or atrophic changes. Some of this may be reactive to scratching ('neurodermatitis*) around the atrophic area (Fig. 46.10). Other hyperplastic islands may be present in the midst of the atrophic lesion itself and show dysplasia.

Aetiology of vulval dystrophies

The precise mechanism of development of the range of dystrophic states which affect the vulva is unclear. It seems that a mixture of factors, traumatic, irritant, allergic, nutritional, infective, immunological, metabolic and, possibly, psychoneurotic, all play a part. Fungus infections and achlorhydria seem to have an

---

* The term 'neurodermatitis' is used in contradictory ways in the literature. Some writers use it to describe skin problems with a psychological basis, others to describe skin changes secondary to scratching.

important relationship (Jeffcoate 1966, Lavery *et al.* 1984) and may have a common immunologic basis.

A theory has been advanced that a normal balance of dermal stimuli to the epidermis and antimitotic chalones (inhibitory factors) within the epidermis is upset. Such inhibitory chemical substances have been recorded (Bullough *et al.* 1967). They are hormone-like proteins with a purely local action. In hyperplastic dystrophy the dermal stimuli would be highly active and the chalone production depressed. In lichen sclerosus of the pure type there may be a reverse situation with chalones dominant leading to low cellular activity and thinning of the epidermis.

Cancer risks and dystrophy

A major problem which has been hotly debated is the relationship of these dystrophic states to cancer. In the days when leukoplakia was an accepted diagnosis the quoted prevalence of it in patients with vulval cancer varied from 3% to 80%. It was also said that 50% of leukoplakias became cancerous (Gardner & Kaufman 1981). As the years passed the correlation became progressively less evident. It was noted that while most patients with vulval cancer had no history of dystrophy such changes were often found adjacent to the carcinoma. Woodruff and Baens (1963) estimated that 25% of hypertrophic vulval lesions became malignant. Jeffcoate (1966) put the risk of cancer with chronic vulval dystrophy at 5% based on a 3–25-year follow-up of 178 women but this was mainly related to the presence of atypical hyperplasia (dysplasia). More recently Buckley *et al.* (1984) have concluded that the risk of even VIN III proceeding to invasive cancer is very low and emphasize that spontaneous regression may occur. In one series only 4 of 106 women with VIN III proceeded to invasive cancer (Buscema *et al.* 1980).

There is general agreement that the cancer risk is low with lichen sclerosus (1–4%) but the two conditions may be found together. Some claim that it arises in the thinly keratinized mucosal aspects (Ridley 1983) while others believe it is the hypertrophic lesions which carry the risk (Wallace 1971). Hart *et al.* (1975) found it occurred in 5 out of 107 cases and when it did develop they noted that it seemed to be in an area uninvolved by the lichen sclerosus. Buscema *et al.* (1980) found changes of dystrophy in more than half of 98 cases of vulval squamous cancer; they regarded any long-standing itchy lesion as a predisposing factor.

Symptoms

Pruritus is the main symptom of most chronic dystrophies, being particularly severe in hyperplastic lesions. The itching produces a vicious circle, the scratching causing more skin damage. Soreness, pain, and dyspareunia or apareunia may also be present.

Management

Multiple punch biopsies are necessary at the outset before deciding on diagnosis and therapy (Fig. 46.11). Special attention should be paid to ulcerated and fissuring regions. An intense search for allergies, achlorhydria, infections, deficiency states, immunological and metabolic disorders, etc., is appropriate.

All possible contributory factors should be dealt with as far as possible. Bland local applications may give relief but failing this local corticosteroid applications such as betamethasone valerate cream 0.1% or 0.025%, applied sparingly 2–3 times per day, may help the cases of hyperplastic dystrophy without atypia. If a fungal infection is present a suitable inhibitor such as clioquinol should be added to the cream. With atrophic lesions such as lichen sclerosus, topical testosterone may be beneficial (Friedrich 1983). Testosterone cream is not available commercially but a preparation of 500 mg of testosterone propionate in 10 g of white petroleum jelly massaged into the vulva 2–3 times a day can be effective. Stimulation of libido is a frequent side effect which may or may not be a cause for complaint. Local progesterone application may also be effective (Friedrich 1983). If pruritus is very severe despite such therapy, local measures designed to relieve this distressing symptom are appropriate (*see* Pruritus vulvae, p. 717). Chloroquine has been used orally for lichen sclerosus (Janovski & Douglas 1972) but unless in unusual circumstances it is not the treatment of choice because of its side effects. Likewise vulvectomy is not a treatment to be recommended but it has been performed when there is persistent, progressive cellular atypia. The recurrence rate is extremely high as no matter how radical the excision new skin must

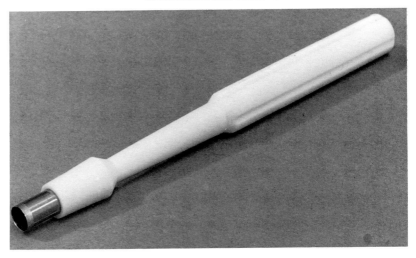

Fig. 46.11. Disposable skin biopsy punch suitable for use on vulva.

cover the external genital region again and be subject to the same environmental influences as the original vulva. Local therapy with fluorouracil is usually preferable to vulvectomy when progression to invasive cancer is feared. Fluorouracil, an antimitotic agent, blocks an enzyme essential for pyrimidine·synthesis and is used as a 5% cream applied topically twice daily for *a minimum of 6–8 weeks*. The area of excessive mitotic activity takes up the drug selectively and becomes fiery red and denudes, giving ulceration. Healing then occurs with normal epithelium. Treatment failures can often be attributed to the patient stopping treatment at an early stage, not appreciating that obtaining this reaction is an integral part of the regime. In-patient management can overcome this difficulty but is obviously expensive in terms of bed occupancy.

Regular follow up on a long term basis is required to detect any malignant development.

Treatment of children with lichen sclerosus is aimed at blocking the pruritus, usually best done with topical corticosteroid. The lesion can be expected to resolve in adolescence if not precisely at the time of puberty (Wallace 1971). The skin tends to be normal thereafter.

PAGET'S DISEASE OF THE VULVA

Vulval Paget's disease usually presents in the elderly. There is intense pruritus and a clearly demarcated injected, scaly area around the introitus. Such a presentation when there is no infection present to account for it should immediately arouse suspicion of Paget's disease and lead to biopsy.

The classic histological feature is the presence of unusual cells occurring singly or in clusters in the midst of the epithelium. They have irregular nuclei and plentiful pale, clear cytoplasm. With the periodic acid-Schiff reaction it can be shown that the cytoplasm contains large amounts of mucin (Fig. 46.12). As in the similar lesion in the nipple, it was originally thought to be secondary to an intraduct cancer in a sweat gland. However, often no such lesion is demonstrable. Willis (1967) has suggested that it may be due to a stimulus affecting tissues of common ectodermal origin causing them to proliferate in atypical ways, a metaplastic process.

Vulvectomy without gland dissection is usually adequate therapy. With recurrence, benefit may be obtained from fluorouracil applications (Gardner & Kaufman 1981).

Vulval intra-epithelial carcinoma (VIN) (Bowen's disease; carcinoma-*in-situ*).
This is considered in relation to vulval malignancy (Chapter 49) and vulval dystrophy (p. 714). There is no characteristic clinical feature and the diagnosis is a histological one based on the usual criteria for carcinoma-*in-situ*).

Senile and idiopathic vulval atrophy
In some post-climacteric women atrophy occurs to a degree greater than normal and this leads to clinical problems. There may be dyspareunia, and inflammatory change may develop secondary to trauma. The macroscopic and microscopic appearances are simply of atrophy. Also, vulval atrophy occurs occasionally before the climacteric without evident cause. In this

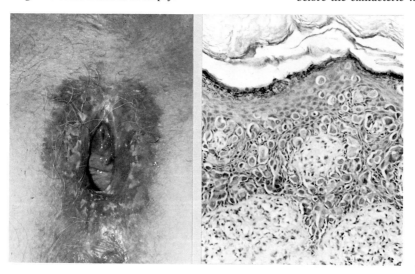

Fig. 46.12. Paget's disease of the vulva. There is a clearly demonstrated affected area. Typical Paget's cells are evident histologically.

idiopathic form there is no homogenization of the subepidermal collagenous tissue which is a feature of the atrophic form of lichen sclerosus (Janovski & Douglas 1972). Oestrogen administration in combination with progestogen is usually curative if there are symptoms.

PRURITUS VULVAE

Many conditions affecting the vulva and vagina have vulval pruritus as a leading symptom and the management is that of the underlying pathology. However there are a significant number of women who have itching in the vulval region as their main symptom and no cause is evident. In this circumstance the symptom becomes elevated to the status of a diagnosis. It may appear a trivial matter but it causes great distress and the patient who complains of it should be handled with sympathy and every effort made to alleviate it.

Intense localized scratching at a site of pruritus sometimes causes skin changes, formerly referred to as 'neurodermatitis'*. Vulval carcinoma often presents with pruritus as a leading symptom. However in many cases careful interrogation will reveal that the pruritus has long preceded any carcinomatous lesion. It is therefore more appropriate to think of prutitus in relation to the aetiology of the cancer rather than a consequence of it. Although evidence is now accumulating that various very specific types of genital virus infection carry a particular risk of cancer, in the vulva it seems that chronic irritation may, if associated with prolonged scratching, ultimately lead to development of a cancer (Buscema et al. 1980). Cancer prevention is therefore a further indication for a vigorous approach to pruritus vulvae as a clinical problem.

It is important to be sure that true pruritus, itching with a desire to scratch, is indeed the symptom. 'Irritation' of the vulva implies something quite different. Histamine, 5-hydroxytryptamine and plasma kinins have all been implicated in the induction of itching and it is probable that they are involved in vulval pruritus in some way.

The correct approach is to search with all diligence for any occult cause which, if detected, can be treated specifically. The investigations are often most efficiently conducted on an in-patient basis. If despite thorough and systematic search no cause is found then it becomes appropriate to seek relief with measures which are entirely symptomatic.

The commonest cause of vulval pruritus is trichomonas or candida vaginitis so at least three direct microscopic tests and cultures should be done on successive days from the vagina. A pipette may be used to instil into and then recover from the vagina a fluid culture medium.

Liver failure, uraemia, diabetes and lymphomatous pathologies all cause pruritus. The vulva is so sensitive that the itching may be present there long before any other aspect of the problem is evident. Blood analysis to exclude these conditions should be done even if there are no obvious features.

Pediculosis and local fungal infections other than vaginal candida may be responsible. Repeated vulval skin scrapings should be taken for examination for fungi. Infection should be looked for in the nailbeds, umbilicus, bowel, etc. Sarcoptes scabiei infection, threadworms and other intestinal parasites should also be sought.

Skin diseases present elsewhere but not causing pruritus there, may be relevant to the vulval problem.

Allergy to toilet preparations, the material of undergarments or contraceptive preparations may account for pruritus. Patch testing combined with systematic withdrawal of each possible factor one at a time should lead to the appropriate one being incriminated.

Some cases are associated with macrocytic anaemias, achlorhydria and vitamin B_{12} deficiency. In addition to the blood count, serum B_{12} estimation should be done. A pentagastrin stimulation test may reveal achlorhydria. The absence of acid appears to be part of an auto-immune disease state which also accounts for the pruritus. A search for antibodies, in addition to anti-intrinsic factor, is appropriate.

Retinol (vitamin A), riboflavine (vitamin B_2), folic acid and iron deficiencies have all been implicated. Iron deficiency is probably the commonest in this country and will usually be manifest as a microcytic hypochromic anaemia.

The relation between the mind and pruritus is a well known and close one. However it is entirely wrong to assume that a woman with vulval pruritus has a psychosomatic illness. *Chronic pruritus can lead to psychological disturbance* and this is probably commoner than the reverse mechanism. A psychological cause for the pruritus should be given consideration only when all possible physical mechanisms have been confidently excluded.

*See Footnote (p. 714).

Treatment

If a causal factor is found, treatment is that specific to the condition discovered. Otherwise symptomatic measures are the order and unfortunately they are often far from satisfactory. The use of loose fitting underwear to alter the local climate is advisable along with any other possible manoeuvre to keep the area well aerated. Sedatives to ensure sleep may be necessary. Local applications of cold cream may be helpful, as may washing with 1% sodium bicarbonate.

Corticosteroid applications as ointments or sprays may be tried and frequently produce relief. Local anaesthetic jellies, though disapproved of by some authorities (Jeffcoate 1975), may be beneficial. Nerve section and absolute alcohol injections have been used also. The alcohol temporarily destroys nerve endings. The technique must be meticulous otherwise skin sloughing may result (Sutherst 1979). Antihistamines and antifungicidal preparations may be worth trying empirically even when investigation fails to suggest these factors are specifically implicated.

If the epithelium is atrophic, oestrogen or testosterone applications may be beneficial. Vulvectomy is an irrational measure sometimes unwisely resorted to in intractable cases. The line of reasoning adopted is 'No vulva': no vulval pruritus'. The fallacy is that when the vulva is excised other skin is brought across or new skin develops to result in a new, albeit mutilated, vulva. This will be exposed to exactly the same climate as the excised vulva was and recurrence of the pruritus is to be expected.

URETHRAL CARUNCLE

Urethral caruncle is a well established clinical entity despite the fact that pathologists debate whether it exists. Patients affected have usually passed the climacteric. The external urethral meatus, usually the posterior aspect, shows a cherry-red pouting swelling which may bleed on touch and may be exquisitely tender (Fig. 46.13). Dyspareunia, dysuria and postcoital bleeding may be additional symptoms. It may be confused with urethral prolapse in which injected urethral mucosa bulges out around the whole circumference of the meatus.

Histologically there are different patterns, all benign. Commonly there is extreme granulation reaction, loss of surface epithelium and leucocyte infiltration; sometimes the picture is angiomatous and occasionally it points to a simple polypoid condition. The granulation variety causes most discomfort. The

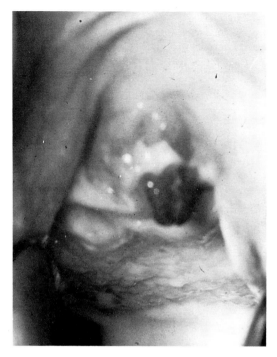

Fig. 46.13. Florid caruncle on posterior lip of urethral meatus.

angiomatous type shows stratified or squamous epithelium on the surface and deep crypts due to infolding and distended submucous capillaries, possibly representing a localized form of urethral prolapse.

A caruncle is often associated with infections such as trichomonas vaginitis. If this is treated the condition often resolves; if there is persistent infection other treatment is unlikely to be curative. If surgical treatment is felt necessary excision, with suturing of the base with fine atraumatic catgut, is preferable to cautery. Histological examination can then be done to exclude urethral carcinoma which in its early stages may have identical appearances. Even if any infection is treated, recurrence is not uncommon. Oestrogen/progestogen cyclic preparations may be helpful in cases in which postclimacteric atrophy appears to be a major factor.

SKENE'S DUCT CYSTS AND INFECTIONS

Skene's tubules (periurethral or paraurethral glands) lie on the floor of the urethra at its lower end. They are homologous to the prostate in the male and show along with that organ a tendency to chronic infection, and retention cysts may develop. Dysuria and frequency may be experienced and on compression pus may exude into the urethra. Excision of infected cysts is a possible treatment but opinions vary as to its necessity (Tancer 1965).

NOMA (ACUTE GANGRENOUS VULVITIS)

This was described in the old literature as occurring in severely debilitated individuals, being the vulval equivalent of cancrum oris. There is extensive tissue necrosis and labial fenestration may occur. It may not be a distinct entity from Behçet's syndrome.

TUBERCULOIS

Tuberculosis of the vulva was not common even when tuberculosis was rife but now it is an extreme rarity. However whenever an indolent ulcerative condition with irregular margins develops with no definite cause, it should be considered and excluded by histological, immunological and microbiological means.

DIABETIC VULVITIS

Patients with poorly controlled diabetes are particularly subject to vulvitis, the glycosuria being said to favour the growth of yeasts and other organisms (Janovski & Douglas 1972). *C. albicans* is frequently demonstrable. There is usually considerable irritation and the vulva is red and angry. Furuncle formation is common. The treatment consists of obtaining good diabetic control and dealing with the infection, usually by antifungal preparations.

LIPSCHUTZ ULCER

This term was applied to a non-venereal ulcer of unknown aetiology affecting the lower vagina or vulva. It is not clear if it is distinct from the ulcers which occur with Behçet's syndrome (Phillips & Scott 1955).

EPSTEIN–BARR VIRUS INFECTION

Attention has been drawn recently (Portnoy *et al.* 1984) to the occurrence of vulval ulceration as part of an attack of infectious mononucleosis ('glandular fever').

BARTHOLIN'S GLAND ABSCESSES AND CYSTS

Bartholin's glands are commonly involved in infection. Abscess formation usually occurs with pain,

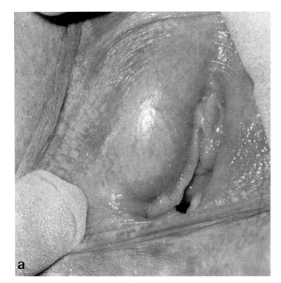

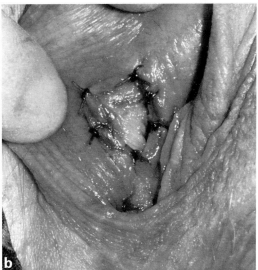

Fig. 46.14. (a) Abscess of Bartholin's gland before surgery. (b) After marsupialization. Sutures indicate the mouth of the pouch which has been created.

swelling and ultimately fluctuant 'pointing'. The pus discharges or is drained surgically. Recurrence is frequent in such circumstances. It is preferable to perform 'marsupialization' in which the abscess cavity is stitched open after incision, rather than a simple incision or excision. This leaves the ostium of the gland open, allowing free drainage and makes recurrent abscess or cyst formation less likely (Fig. 46.14). Antibiotics are given if necessary according to the

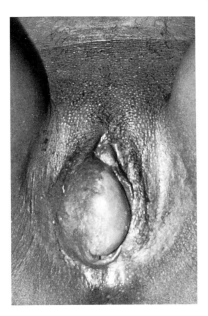

Fig. 46.15. Large, right-sided cyst of Bartholin's gland.

bacterium involved. Staphylococci, *E. coli* or gono-cocci are most common.

Cysts may form as a consequence of duct blockage following infections (Fig. 46.15). They may be dealt with by marsupialization in the same way as an abscess.

OTHER VULVAL CYSTS

Retention cysts of a variety of origins may occur in the vulva. Sebaceous gland, epidermoid, implantation dermoid, Gärtner's duct and clitoridal cysts all occur. Excision may be performed or, if they become in-fected, incision or marsupialization. Needle diathermy is sometimes preferred if there are multiple small se-baceous cysts. The canal of Nuck is the homologue of the inguinal canal in the male and occasionally a pouch of peritoneum is isolated and forms a cyst (hy-drocele) in the upper part of the labium majus (Woodcock 1973).

HIDRADENOMA

An adenoma may arise from a sweat gland in the vulva (hidradenoma), usually in the anterior part of the labium major. It has a size usually of up to one centimetre with a reddened surface. Malignancy is often suspected clinically and the complex adenoma-

tous pattern found histologically can be confused with malignancy but the condition is quite benign.

FIBROMA, LIPOMA, HAEMANGIOMA AND NEUROFIBROMA

Tumours of fibrous, adipose, vascular and neurofibro-matous tissue occasionally occur on the vulva. They are benign and unremarkable.

VULVAL VARICOSITIES

Vulval varicosities not infrequently develop in preg-nancy but rarely occur in the non-pregnant. The ease with which even the normal vulva can develop a massive haematoma on minor trauma inevitably causes apprehension at the appearance of such vari-cosities but they do not carry a high risk. If they produce symptoms such as aching on standing, sup-port pads and tights may be tried. If symptoms persist despite this, treatment is by injecting sclerosing fluids or high ligation of the long saphenous vein (Jeffcoate 1975).

PARTIAL ALBINISM, VITILIGO AND LEUKODERMA

Albinism is merely a congential lack of pigment on a localized section of skin. It has no clinical signific-cance. Vitiligo involves loss of pigment due to an auto-immune process destroying melanocytes. Various auto-immune diseases or antibodies may develop in patients with the condition so it should be regarded as a marker for likely systemic disorders. Leukoderma is acquired loss of pigment which may be secondary to local inflammatory or other injury. It is a marker of previous pathology.

VULVAL NAEVI, HAEMANGIOMATA AND TELANGIECTASIS

Coloured lesions of pigmented tissue of neural crest origin and vascular structures, both congenital and acquired, may occur on the vulva at various ages (Gardner & Kaufman 1981). Vascular lesions may be of capillary or cavernous type histologically. The pig-mented naevi carry a small risk of becoming malig-nant but otherwise the conditions have only minor significance. Granulomata may appear secondary to chronic infection.

ELEPHANTIASIS LYMPHANGIECTATICA

This gross enlargement of the vulva is a consequence of lymphatic obstruction, usually due to filariasis in countries where this is prevalent. Plastic surgery may be necessary but should be contemplated only when any infective element has been brought under control (Janovski & Douglas 1972).

DERMATOLOGICAL CONDITIONS OCCASIONALLY OCCURRING ON THE VULVA

Virtually any skin condition may occur on the vulva and present symptomatic problems. Psoriasis is an example being non-pruritic in most sites but capable of causing intense pruritis on the vulva. Eczema, impetigo, scabies, seborrhoeic dermatitis, pityriasis versicolour, reactive dermatitis, erythrasma, pemphigus or pemphigoid, tinea cruris, molluscum contagiosum, neurodermatitis and epidermolysis bullosa are all examples of dermatological conditions which sometimes occur on the vulva (Friedrich 1983).

FUSION OF LABIA MINORA

In young prepubertal girls, adhesions may form between the labia minora occluding the vaginal introitus partially or completely. They usually cause little symptomatology and can be separated easily under anaesthesia. Small doses of oestrogen locally have been advocated in the past. Jenkinson and Mackinnon (1984) have recently reported that such adhesions respond to completely conservative management. In all their cases they disappeared within 18 months without treatment. In the case shown in Fig. 46.16 the adhesions were so light that they separated as a consequence of a tremor of the hand holding the catheter, which is hardly a surgical procedure! Advice to the mother on thorough washing of the vulva seems all that is needed.

INTROITAL DYSPAREUNIA WITHOUT SPECIFIC CAUSE

Occasionally introital dyspareunia develops in a healthy woman who has previously had pain-free intercourse and is still in the reproductive era, but no specific pathological cause can be found. There may be the suggestion of a tiny fissure in the region of the fourchette where the tenderness is located; this seems similar to an anal fissure. Sometimes there is injection of the introitus but histology is non-specific. The suspicion exists that these are early forms of *lichen sclerosus* (Ridley 1983) and they may have an auto-immune basis.

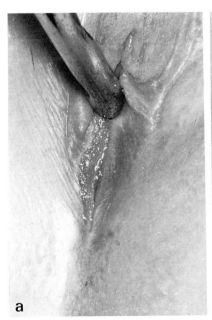
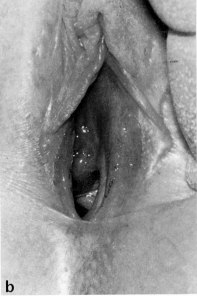

Fig. 46.16. Labial adhesions in a 3-year-old girl, originally referred as a case of absent vagina. In (a) a metal catheter marks the only opening over the urethra; (b) after a fine tremor movement of the catheter, the labia are separated and a vagina revealed.

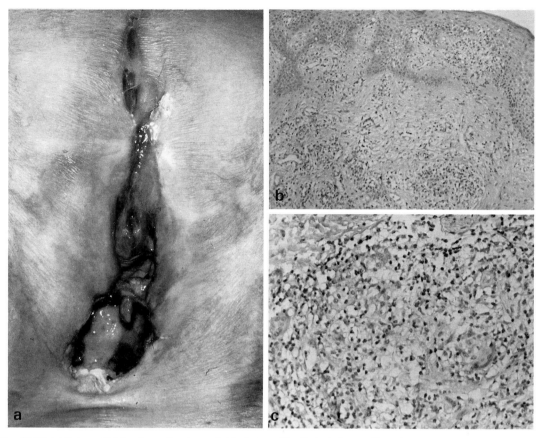

Fig. 46.17. (a) Vulva which has been almost completely destroyed by Crohn's disease. Extensive scarring represents areas in which healing of the disease has taken place.
(b) Low power histology of squamous epithelium and underlying dermis showing chronic inflammation with a poorly defined granuloma.
(c) High power showing giant cells as a cellular component of an epithelial granuloma.

CROHN'S DISEASE

There is increasing awareness that severe Crohn's disease (regional ileitis) may spread to the vulva causing serious tissue destruction (Parks *et al.* 1965, Kao *et al.* 1975, Prezyna & Kalyanaraman 1977). Fig. 46.17 shows the vulva of a patient who had suffered almost total destruction of it due to Crohn's disease. Only a small bridge of union is present anteriorly representing the remains of the perineum. This patient had previously had a total colectomy and ileostomy performed on the basis of an initial diagnosis of ulcerative colitis. There is a striking similarity between the gross destruction of vulval tissue produced by Crohn's disease on that site and the vulval lesions of severe Behçet's syndrome, and the pathologies may

be related. Tuberculosis must always be excluded in such cases as it can produce similar lesions.

Treatment of vulval Crohn's disease is difficult but a carefully timed complete excision of the affected tissue, when the bowel disease is quiescent, can be beneficial.

ACCESSORY BREAST TISSUE

The vulva lies along the 'milk line' and is rich in apocrine glands so rarely breast tissue develops in the site.

FOX–FORDYCE DISEASE

Fox–Fordyce disease is a condition similar to acne, involving blockage of apocrine sweat gland openings with formation of retention vesicles. It may affect other areas, especially the axilla. Intense pruritus is the main symptom, attributed to leakage of retained secretion into the surrounding tissue. Local or systemic oestrogen therapy is often beneficial (Friedrich 1983).

ENDOMETRIOSIS

Metaplastic or implantation endometriosis occasionally occurs in the vulva.

ACROCORDONS (SKIN TAGS)

Pedunculated skin polypi are often seen around the vulva or the internal aspect of the thigh. They are often, sensibly, referred to as skin tags but 'acrocordon' is the name preferred by some (Gardner & Kaufman 1981).

VULVAL INJURIES

Vulval injuries are, of course, common in association with vaginal tears due to various causes. Because of its vascularity the vulva has got a particular propensity to produce a massive haematoma when subjected to blunt trauma. Control by pressure should be attempted but often evacuation under general anaesthesia is required.

PATHOLOGIES WHICH ARE COMMON TO VULVA AND MOUTH

There are many climatic and other factors common to the vulval and oral regions. They are erogenous zones and the similarity extends to common pathologies. Syphilitic primary lesions are obvious examples. Trichomonas and candida albicans infections are common in both areas. 'Leukoplakia', though it is not an accepted vulval diagnosis today, has long been recognized as an oral pathology with a propensity to become malignant. Vitamin deficiency states such as riboflavine and vitamin B_{12} deficiency tend to have manifestations in mouth and vulva. Achlorhydria is associated with vulval dystrophy as it is with oral changes (Jeffcoate & Woodcock 1961, Lavery et al. 1984).

When there is serious diagnostic difficulty with a vulval condition it is worthwhile considering the matter in the light of recognized forms of oral pathology.

BEHÇET'S SYNDROME

Half a century ago a Turkish gynaecologist, Behçet, described a syndrome which has come to carry his name. It involved a triad of manifestations: ulceration of the external genitalia, ulceration of the mouth and inflammatory lesions of the anterior chamber of the eye, two of these constituting the criteria for diagnosis. It has since become the subject of increasing attention (Dewhurst 1955, Phillips & Scott 1955, Monacelli & Nazzaro 1966, Chamberlain 1977, O'Duffy 1978, Gardner & Kaufman 1981). It is now evident that it is not a clear-cut entity and overlaps with other conditions such as erythema multiforme, Stevens–Johnson and Reiter's syndromes. It affects males as well as females. In a study in the Yorkshire region, Chamberlain (1977) found an association with the antigens HLA B_5 and B_{27}, and an elevation of IgM level. HLA B_5 antiserum has been shown to identify at least two more specific antigens, Bw51 and 52. The association in most studies has been found to be with Bw51 (Barnes 1984). Erythema nodosum, acne and vasculitis were also all significantly associated.

Patient's with Behçet's syndrome are at serious risk of marital breakdown because of the effects of the long persisting ulcerative lesions of the vulva. There is also a high risk of suicidal attempts which gives an idea of the ghastliness of the persistent symptoms despite attempts at modifying the disease course by therapy (Chamberlain 1977). The aetiology has been debated at length and nutritional, hormonal, viral and immunologic factors have been advanced. Recently Behçet's syndrome seems to have established a place amongst the extensive group of multi-system immunological or collagen diseases (Bietti & Bruna 1966).

In a gynaecological context, the patient presents with ulceration of the vulva which may be indolent resembling the aphthous ulceration which is common in the mouth. There are often such ulcers present in the mouth or a history of them. On the other hand the ulcers may be actively destructive leading to fenestration of the labia reminiscent of cancrum oris. Ocular, neurological, arthritic, phlebitic, psychiatric and many other system involvements may occur and it can become a most serious and life threatening illness. Corticosteroid therapy may have a beneficial influence (Phillips & Scott 1955) as may ovarian steroid preparations (Friedrich 1983) and antibiotics will deal with any secondary infection. Vitamin supplements are appropriate if the oral lesions are preventing adequate dietetic intake.

REFERENCES

BALLON S.C., ROBERTS J.A. & LAGASSE L.D. (1979) *Obstet. and Gynec.* **54**, 163–6.

BARNES C.G. (1984) *J. roy. Soc. Med.*, **77**, 816.

BECK I. & CLAYTON J.K. (1984) *Brit. J. Obstet. Gynaec.*, **91**, 503–5.

BIETTI G.B. & BRUNA F. (1966) In *Behçet's Disease* (Monacelli M. & Nazzaro P. eds.), pp. 79–110. S. Karger and Basel, New York.

BRYSON Y.J., DILLON M., LOVETT M., ACUNA G., TAYLOR S., CHERRY J.D., JOHNSON L., WIESMEIER E., GROWDON W., CREAGH-KIRK T. & KEENEY R. (1983) *New Eng. J. Med.*, **308**, 916–21.

BUCH A. & CHRISTENSEN E.S. (1982) *Acta Obstet. Gynecol. Scand.*, **61**, 393–6.

BUCKLEY C.H., BUTLER E.B. & FOX H. (1984) *J. clin. Pathol.*, **37**, 1201.

BULLOUGH W.S., LAURENCE E.B., IVERSEN O.H. & ELGJO K. (1967) *Nature*, **214**, 578–80.

BUSCEMA J., STERN J. & WOODRUFF J.D. (1980) *Amer. J. Obstet. Gynec.*, **137**, 902–9.

CHAMBERLAIN M.A. (1977) *Ann. rheum. Dis.*, **36**, 491–9.

CRUM C.P., FU Y.S., LEVINE R.U., RICHART R.M., TOWNSEND D.E. & FENOGLIO C.M. (1982) *Amer. J. Obstet. Gynec.*, **144**, 77–83.

DEWHURST C.J. (1955) *J. Obstet. Gynaec. Brit. Emp.*, **62**, 562–6.

DOUGLAS J.M., CRICHLOW C., BENEDETTI J., MERTZ G.J., CONNOR J.D., HINTZ M.A., FAHNLANDER A., REMINGTON M., WINTER C. & COREY L. (1984) *New Engl. J. Med.*, **310**, 1551–6.

EDITORIAL (1983) *Lancet*, **ii**, 435–6.

ELIOT B.W., HOWAT R.C.L. & MACK A.E. (1979) *Brit. J. Obstet. Gynaec.*, **86**, 572–7.

FEROZE R.M., DEWHURST C.J. & WELPLY G. (1975) *Brit. J. Obstet. Gynaec.*, **82**, 536–40.

FILLEY C.M., GRAFF-RADFORD N.R., LACY J.R., HEITNER M.A. & EARNEST M.P. (1982) *Neurology (NY)*, **32**, 308–11.

FRIEDRICH E.G. JR. (1983) *Major Problems in Obstetrics and Gynaecology*, Vol. 9. W.B. Saunders Company, Philadelphia, London, Toronto, Mexico City, Rio de Janeiro, Sydney, Tokyo.

FRIEDRICH E.G. JR. & MACLAREN N.K. (1984) *Amer. J. Obstet. Gynec.*, **150**, 161.

FULLER A.F. JR., SWARTZ M.N., WOLFSON J.S. & SALZMAN R. (1980) *New Engl. J. Med.*, **303**, 881.

GARDNER H.L. & KAUFMAN R.H. (1981) Benign Diseases of the Vulva and Vagina (2nd ed). G.K. Hall Medical Publishers, Boston, Massachusetts.

GOLIGHER J.C. (1983) *Ann. roy. Coll. Surg. Engl.*, **65**, 353–5.

GOOLAMALI S.K., BARNES E.W., IRVINE W.J. & SHUSTER S. (1974) *Brit. med. J.*, **4**, 78–9.

HART W.R., NORRIS H.J. & HELWIG E.B. (1975) *Obstet. and Gynec.*, **45**, 369–77.

ZUR HAUSEN H. (1982) *Lancet*, **ii**, 1370–2.

International Society for the Study of Vulvar Diseases (1976) *Obstet. and Gynec.*, **47**, 122–4.

JANOVSKI N.A. & DOUGLAS C.P. (1972) *Diseases of the Vulva.* Harper & Row, Hagerstown, Maryland, New York, Evanston, San Francisco, London.

JEFFCOATE T.N.A. (1966) *Amer. J. Obstet. Gynec.*, **95**, 61–74.

JEFFCOATE T.N.A. (1969) *J. Obstet. Gynaec. Brit. Cwlth.*, **76**, 961–8.

JEFFCOATE SIR NORMAN (1975) *Principles of gynaecology* (4th edn.). Butterworths, London and Boston.

JEFFCOATE T.N.A. & WOODCOCK A.S. (1961) *Brit med. J.*, **2**, 127–34.

JENKINSON S.D. & MACKINNON A.E. (1984) *Brit. med. J.*, **289**, 160–1.

KAO M-S., PAULSON J.D. & ASKIN F.B. (1975) *Obstet. and Gynec.*, **46**, 329–33.

KAUFMAN R.H., DREESMAN G.R., BUREK J., KORHONEN M.O., MATSON D.O., MELNICK J.L., POWELL K.L., PURIFOY D.J.M., COURTNEY R.J. & ADAM E. (1981) *New Engl. J. Med.*, **305**, 483–8.

KOLSTAD P. (1981) In Coppleson M. (ed) *Gynecologic Oncology* Vol. 1, pp. 225–8. Churchill Livingstone, Edinburgh, London, Melbourne and New York.

LANGLEY F.A. (1973) In Fox H. & Langley F.A. (eds) *Postgraduate Obstetrical and Gynaecological Pathology*, pp. 71–93. Pergamon Press, Oxford, New York, Toronto, Sydney, Braunschweig.

LAVERY H.A., Pinkerton J.H.M. & MIDDLETON D. (1984) *Brit. J. Obstet. Gynaec.*, **91**, 694–6.

MANN P.R. & COWAN M.A. (1973) *Brit. J. Derm.*, **89**, 223–

MEYRICK THOMAS R.H., HOLMES R.C., ROWLAND PAYNE C.M.E., RIDLEY C.M., SHERWOOD F. & BLACK M.M. (1982) *Brit. J. Derm.*, **107**, Suppl. **22**, p. 29.

MINDEL A., ADLER M.W., SUTHERLAND S. & FIDDIAN A.P. (1982) *Lancet*, **i**, 697–700.

MINDEL A., WELLER I.V.D., FAHERTY A., SUTHERLAND S., HINDLEY D., FIDDIAN A.P. & ADLER M.W. (1984) *Lancet*, **ii**, 57–9.

MINKOWSKI W.L., BAKER C.J., ALLEYNE D., BAGHAI M., FRIEDLANDER, L. & SCHULTZ B. (1983) *J. Adolesc. Health Care*, **4**, 113.

MONACELLI M. & NAZZARO P. (1966) *Behçet's Disease.* S. Karger, Basel and New YORK.

NAHMIAS A.J., JOSEY W.E., NAIB Z.M., FREEMAN M.G., FERNANDEZ R.J. & WHEELER J.H. (1971) *Amer. J. Obstet. Gynec.*, **110**, 825–37.

O'DUFFY J.D. (1978) *J. Rheum.*, **5**, 229–33.

ONDERDONK A.B., POLK B.F., MOON N.E., GOREN B. & BARTLETT J.G. (1977) *Amer. J. Obstet., Gynec.*, **128**, 777—81.

OSBORNE N.G., GRUBIN L. & PRATSON L. (1982) *Amer. J. Obstet. Gynec.*, **142**, 962–7.

PARKS A.G., MORSON B.C. & PEGUM J.S. (1965) *Proc. roy. Soc. Med.*, **58**, 241–2.

PHILLIPS D.L. & SCOTT J.S. (1955) *Lancet*, **i**, 366–71.

PORTNOY J., AHRONHEIM G.A., GHIBU F., CLECNER B. & JONCAS J.H. (1984) *New Engl. J. Med.*, **311**, 966.

POWELL J.L. (1973) *Amer. J. Obstet. Gynec.*, **115**, 276–7.

PREZYNA A.P. & KALYANARAMAN U. (1977) *Amer. J. Obstet. Gynec.*, **128**, 914–6.

RIDLEY C.M. (1975) *Major Problems in Dermatology*, Vol. 5. W.B. Saunders Company Ltd., London, Philadelphia, Toronto.

RIDLEY C.M. (1983) *Brit. J. Hosp. Med.*, **30**, 158–66.

SCHROCK C.G. (1980) *J. Amer. med. Ass.*, **243**, p. 1231.

SCOTT J.S. (1955) *J. Obstet. Gynaec. Brit. Emp.*, **62**, 445–6.

SINGER A., WALKER P.G. & McCANCE D.J. (1984) *Brit. Med. J.*, **288**, 735–7.

STRAUS S.E., TAKIFF H.E., SEIDLIN M., BACHRACH S., LININGER L., DiGIOVANNA J.J., WESTERN K.A., SMITH H.A., LEHRMAN S.N., CREAGH-KIRK T. & ALLING D.W. (1984) *New Engl. J. Med.*, **310**, 1545–50.

SUTHERST J.R. (1979) *Brit. J. Obstet. Gynaec.*, **86**, 371–3.

TANCER M.L. (1965) *Clin. Obstet. Gynec.*, **8**, 982–96.

VESTERINEN E., MEYER B., CANTELL K. & PUROLA E. (1984) *Obstet. and Gynec.*, **64**, 535.

WALLACE H.J. (1971) *Trans. St. John's Hosp. derm. Soc. (Lond.)*, **57**, 9–30.

WAY S.A. (1982) Malignant disease of the vulva. Churchill Livingstone, Edinburgh.

WHIMSTER J.W. (1961) *J. Obstet. Gynaec. Brit. Cwlth.*, **69**, 889.

WILLIAMS E.A. (1964) *J. Obstet. Gynaec. Brit. Cwlth.*, **71**, 511.

WILLIS R.A. (1967) *Pathology of Tumours* (4th edn.). Butterworths, London.

WILSON F. & SWARTZ D.P. (1972) *Obstet. and Gynec.*, **39**, 182–4.

WITKIN S.S., YU I.R. & LEDGER W.J. (1983) *Amer. J. Obstet. Gynec.*, **147**, 809–11.

WOODCOCK A.S. (1973) In Fox H. & Langley F.A. (eds.) *Postgraduate Obstetrical and Gynaecological Pathology*, pp. 51–70. Pergamon Press, Oxford, New York, Toronto, Sydney, Braunschweig.

WOODRUFF J.D. & BAENS J.S. (1963) *Amer. J. Obstet. Gynec.*, **86**, 713–23.

ZOLER M.L. (1983) *J. Amer. med. Ass.*, **249**, 2997–9.

CHAPTER 47
BENIGN TUMOURS OF THE UTERUS

C.R. WHITFIELD

UTERINE POLYPS

Polyps are common tumours in the uterus, and may occur in either the endocervix or the corpus. They are of various types and are usually benign, apart from polypoidal masses found in carcinoma or sarcoma of the endometrium. Rarely, malignant change can occur in a benign polyp. The following are seen:

a) Corpus
> endometrial polyps
> fibroid polyps
> adenomyomatous polyps
> placental polyps

b) Endocervix
> mucous polyps
> fibro-epithelial polyps

Polyps arising in the uterine corpus

Endometrial polyps are the commonest in the uterine corpus, they are usually multiple and may form part of a hyperplastic endometrium. After the menopause they are single or only few in number. There is a tendency to recur, but sometimes this must be due to failure to remove them all at operation. A relationship with subsequent development of carcinoma of the endometrium has been noted by Armenia (1967), but in no sense are they to be regarded as premalignant.

PATHOLOGY

They are small, pale pink or red tumours projecting from the endometrial surface. Occasionally they have a long enough stalk to allow them to present through the cervix, or even at the vulva. Microscopically the polyp is composed of endometrial stroma and glands covered by a single layer of columnar epithelium. There is a variable response of the glands to the ovarian hormones. Progesterone-induced secretory change may be seen in the epithelium, but very often

there is no such response whether or not the rest of the endometrium is responsive. When one or more polyps are simply local exaggerations of hyperplasia extending throughout the endometrium their covering epithelium may show the typical metropathic 'Swiss cheese' histological appearance; and occasionally crowding of the glands produces an adenomatous appearance. Atypical changes and squamous metaplasia may cause difficulty in diagnosis from malignancy, but attention to the usual criteria for malignancy should avoid this. A malignant polyp is rare, and the histology will distinguish between adenocarcinoma *ab initio* and malignant change in an initially benign polyp; in the former there is adenocarcinoma throughout the entire polyp and usually also in the uterine tissue adjacent to its base, whereas in the latter there is malignancy in only parts of the polyp with none at its base. After the menopause endometrial polyps may have a fibrous stroma, and are sometimes then described as adenofibromata. Adenomyomatous polyps have smooth muscle and endometrial elements, they usually coexist with adenomyosis but are uncommon.

A submucous fibromyoma (fibroma) protrudes into the uterine cavity and may become polypoidal in shape. Such a polyp may then develop a pedicle that becomes long enough for the tumour to protrude into or through the cervical canal, occasionally even as far as the introitus. Circulatory changes caused by elongation and constriction of the pedicle may cause necrosis with sloughing of the covering epithelium.

Placental polyps are due to organization of small pieces of retained placental tissue. They are rare, they may cause severe haemorrhage on removal and they may resemble choriocarcinoma in appearance.

CLINICAL FEATURES

If polyps are part of an endometrial hyperplasia the symptoms are those associated with dysfunctional uterine bleeding, usually with increased menstrual loss. In particular, however, polyps are associated with intermenstrual bleeding, or with postmenopausal bleeding in the older woman. If extruded from the cervix, there may be discharge, intermenstrual bleeding or even postcoital bleeding, and sometimes the patient herself discovers the polyp in the vagina.

TREATMENT

Endometrial polyps are easily removed by small sponge forceps and by curettage; the former are the more useful and should always be introduced after dilatation of the cervix and before inserting the curette, because the latter on its own may miss the polyp. Careful histological examination of all polyps is necessary to exclude malignant change. Pedunculated submucous fibroids are usually easily avulsed by twisting the pedicle with sponge holders.

Polyps arising in the cervix

These are called mucosal polyps because of their histological appearance. They may be extruded distension cysts of the cervical racemose glands. Macroscopically they are single or multiple, small, cherry-red swellings appearing at the cervix and usually arising within the canal. Microscopically the polyp consists of cervical mucous glands, sometimes distended, in a vascular bed of fine fibrous tissue and covered usually by columnar, but sometimes squamous, epithelium. Inflammation and ulceration of the apex is common.

Their main symptom is mucoid discharge, which may be bloodstained. Intermenstrual bleeding and postcoital bleeding are also likely when the polyps are more vascular or if there is degeneration or inflammation of the apex. They may be the cause of bleeding in pregnancy, perhaps but not necessarily postcoital, when eversion of the cervix may expose a polyp within its canal. They are easily removed by avulsion, scissors or curettage; the canal should be dilated and explored for the presence of further unseen polyps and the stalk carefully removed and its base cauterized to prevent recurrence. Uterine curettage is also advisable, because there may be associated endometrial polyps. Larger polyps may have quite a large artery in the stalk. For these reasons it is wiser to remove cervical polyps under anaesthesia than in the out-patient department.

UTERINE FIBROIDS

Fibromyoma, more correctly termed leiomyoma and, by general usage, fibroid, is not only the commonest tumour found in the uterus, or even in the genital tract, but in the human body. It is estimated that 20% of all women have one or more present in the uterus at death; the vast majority of these have been symptomless and often are very small. The aetiology is unknown, but inevitably the female sex hormones have been incriminated, particularly stimulation by oestrogen unbalanced by progesterone as a result of persistent anovulation. Myomata in women receiving hormone treatment (usually oral contraceptives) have sometimes enlarged quite rapidly. Experimental production of myomata in humans has, however, been conspicuously unsuccessful, and the tumours produced by oestrogen stimulation do not persist when the hormone is withdrawn, they tend to be more fibrous than myomatous, and do not occur solely in the uterus. The theory that the tumours arise from smooth muscle cells rather than fibrous tissue is supported by the tissue culture experiments of Miller and Ludovici (1955). While these tumours are commonest in women who have not borne children, this is by no means always the case. There is an obvious racial factor in women of negro origin, many of whom develop myomata when young and despite having had children. The association with nulliparity is common to endometriosis and carcinoma of the corpus uteri, in association with either of which myomata may also be found. In European women fibroids tend to cause symptoms around the age of 30 years and are then more frequently observed towards the menopause, after which they cease to cause trouble because they no longer grow but, instead, undergo atrophy. This is most probably related to the cessation of ovarian function, but is as likely to be due to the associated reduced blood supply and general gradual atrophy of the uterine muscle as to any direct effect of oestrogen withdrawal on the tumours. Jeffcoate (1962), however, stated that fibroids do sometimes grow after the menopause.

PATHOLOGY

Macroscopically the appearance is of a firm, round tumour in the uterine wall, which itself may be thickened and hypertrophied. Fibroids within the wall of the uterus are described as being intramural, if projecting from the peritoneal surface of the uterus as subserous, if between the layers of the broad ligaments as intraligamentary, and if projecting into the cavity as submucous. Subserous fibroids may become pedunculated and submucous ones polypoidal. Pedunculated fibroids may become adherent to other structures, particularly the omentum, gain a secondary blood supply, and lose their uterine attachment; they are then termed parasitic.

The tumours usually arise in the body of the uterus or, less commonly, in the cervix; infrequently, they spring from the round ligaments. They may be single or multiple, and very large numbers have been reported. Their size varies from microscopic to large enough for a single tumour to fill the whole abdomen. Characteristically, they are firm in consistency, but as a result of degeneration may be soft and cystic, or rock-hard due to calcification. A single fibroid can cause symmetrical enlargement of the uterus, whereas multiple fibroids transform the organ into an irregular mass. On cutting into a uterus containing fibroids it is immediately apparent that the tumour is enclosed in a false capsule of compressed uterine muscle, thus allowing it to be easily enucleated; this is in contradistinction to an adenomyoma. The tumour itself is white with a characteristic whorled appearance. On microscopical examination the tumours when small are mainly composed of smooth muscle cells, but as they become larger fibrous tissue is more abundant and degenerative changes become more frequent. The muscle cells are arranged in bundles in the classically whorled pattern. The proportion of muscle cells to fibrous tissue is very variable; a preponderance of the former gives a superficial resemblance to sarcoma, and of the latter to fibroma. The blood supply enters from the periphery and the tumours are relatively avascular.

Degenerative changes

The very poor vascularity of fibroids encourages the degenerative changes that are common in all but the smaller tumours. The various degenerative changes which may occur are as follow.

Hyaline degeneration. This is present to some degree in most tumours, leading to the loss of the usual whorled appearance of the cut surface. There is a tendency to liquefaction of larger areas of hyaline change and this leads on to cystic degeneration.

Cystic degeneration. Usually this occurs irregularly with the formation of multiple small cystic spaces, giving a sponge-like appearance and soft consistency

to the tumour. Less commonly, a single cystic cavity may almost replace the fibroid.

Calcification. This is seen most often in pedunculated subserous fibroids with poor blood supply, or in women well beyond the menopause also as a result of devascularization. The fibroid becomes rock-hard, shows up on X-ray and represents what used to be called a 'wombstone'.

Necrosis. This may occur in any tumour, particularly following other degenerations and may be either microscopical or macroscopical; in the latter a putty-like area is seen, usually in the centre of the tumour.

Necrobiosis or red degeneration. This occurs most often in pregnancy or near the menopause, but can occur at any time. The general experience seems to be that it is much less common than some of the literature, particularly from Britain, would suggest. It is similar to the process of infarction. Necrosis is either diffuse or focal; there is thrombosis of the peripheral vessels, loss of the fibromyomatous pattern with absence of nuclei, and distended thin-walled vessels are engorged with red blood cells. Central necrosis and cyst formation may occur. If the fibroid is freshly sectioned, its colour is the appearance of raw beef, but it soon turns to a dull red on exposure; later, the colour may turn a greenish yellow. The mechanism underlying this form of degeneration remains uncertain.

Sarcomatous degeneration. This is a very infrequent occurrence. Novak and Woodruff (1974) considered the incidence to be less than 0.5%, although about two-thirds of uterine sarcomas do arise in fibromyomas. Typically there is a soft homogeneous area in the fibroid, and this may extend into the adjacent myometrium at one part on the circumference. In a gross case diagnosis is easy, but real difficulty may be encountered with what are known as cellular myomata, in which there is lack of distinctive fibrous tissue and a preponderance of muscle cells. It was once customary to classify these sarcomas into different histological types, for example round, spindle, mixed or 'giant' cell types, but this is a subjective interpretation and serves no useful practical purpose.

Infection

Infection occurs in minor degree when fibroids become adherent to bowel or pyosalpinges. Suppuration and abscess formation is uncommon but may occur, particularly in submucous fibroids or in fibroid polyps during the puerperium. Sometimes a fibroid polyp sloughs off as a result of infection.

Rare complications

Certain rare conditions are reported in relation to fibroids. Benign metastasizing fibroleiomyoma has been described with benign metastases in the omentum or lung (Barnes & Richardson 1973). Secondary parasitic attachment of fibroids to other structures in the abdomen, giving them an alternative blood supply with subsequent detachment from the parent organ, rarely occurs. An association with polycythaemia has been described (Payne *et al.* 1969).

CLINICAL FEATURES

The clinical presentation is very variable and often fibroids are symptomless, especially when small but also sometimes even when of considerable size. They may become apparent for the first time on palpation during pregnancy, or they may be an unexpected finding when the woman has a pelvic examination or laparotomy for a reason unrelated to them. It is extremely rare for fibroids to cause symptoms after the menopause, as they usually undergo atrophy along with the uterus. Such atrophy occasionally allows an abdominal mass to drop back into the pelvis and cause increased frequency of micturition or acute retention of urine, but these occurrences are very rare and it is most unwise to diagnose as being a fibroid a tumour which causes symptoms after the menopause. Abdominal swelling is a common presentation and may be noticed by the patient herself or by her doctor at a routine examination. The swelling is due to the mass itself appearing in the abdomen, but a slow increase in growth is often ignored as attributable to menopausal obesity.

Pressure effects may be produced on the pelvic veins or on the inferior vena cava. Oedema and varicose veins in the leg will result, and may be unilateral or bilateral depending on which vessel is subjected to pressure. Haemorrhoids may similarly occur or be exacerbated. A large tumour filling the abdomen may cause dyspnoea. Pressure on the bladder may cause increased frequency of micturition, and may sometimes cause stress incontinence of urine or accentuate it if it is already present. Cervical fibroids or fundal fibroids in a retroverted uterus occasionally displace the cervix so as to cause retention of urine in the same manner as does an impacted retro-

verted gravid uterus. Constipation is not caused by fibroids.

Increased menstrual loss is very common and the reason is not always obvious unless the uterine cavity is enlarged by submucous fibroids. Often, however, quite large tumours may be present without any increase in size of the cavity, and if heavy periods occur in these women it may be due to the generally increased vascularity of the uterus. But in cases where heavy periods are associated with only small fibroids it is presumed that the condition is one of dysfunctional uterine bleeding, either coincidental or associated in that some unspecified hormonal disturbance is responsible for both. Indeed, a hormonal mechanism is likely to be the explanation, or at least an important contributing factor, when fibroids are associated with anovulatory cycles and endometrial hyperplasia.

Intermenstrual bleeding may occur as a result of a fibroid polyp undergoing necrotic ulceration. This may take the form of a bloodstained discharge if such a fibroid has become infected, or there may also be postcoital bleeding when a pedunculated fibroid has been extruded through the cervical canal.

There is a well recognized, but far from invariable, association between fibroids and infertility. This resembles the relationship between infertility and endometriosis in that there is often no obvious explanation for the association, and some patients with sizeable fibroids or with more than mild endometriosis may be fertile; sometimes the three conditions (fibroids, endometriosis and infertility) coexist. Infertility, either voluntary or involuntary, is likely to be followed in time by the development of uterine fibroids, and on the other hand once fibroids have developed fertility is likely to be decreased or in abeyance. Whilst uterine distortion or mechanical obstruction of the Fallopian tubes by fibroids is an understandable cause for infertility, this may also be present when the uterine cavity and Fallopian tubes are apparently normal and undisturbed by the tumours, yet occasionally pregnancy occurs in a uterus grossly distorted by fibroids. At operation some patients with uterine fibroids are found to have associated hydrosalpinges, which may precede and predispose to the formation of fibromyomas by producing infertility. Once pregnancy has occurred then abortion may follow, and this is probably more likely if implantation occurs in relation to a submucous fibroid. Most pregnancies, however, continue undisturbed. During pregnancy, fibroids may increase in size as the uterus enlarges, but not to any great extent. Usually, due to marked oedema in the connective tissue, they soften and flatten out and may actually become more difficult to distinguish on palpation. During the puerperium they undergo involution and may become smaller than they were before the pregnancy.

Pain may result from the presence of uterine fibroids. This may be a simple congestive dysmenorrhoea resulting from the increased vascularity in the pelvis; or a more constant dull backache may be complained of when the fibroids are of moderate size in a retroverted uterus, although persistence of this pain after removal of such a uterus is a common enough experience in practice. Torsion of a pedunculated fibroid will result in acute or subacute pain demanding fairly urgent treatment. Generally less severe, but still unpleasant, pain is associated with red degeneration; occasionally, especially during pregnancy, the pain and general upset caused by this complication may mimic an acute abdominal emergency. A fibroid polyp may be associated with some degree of uterine colic as the uterus contracts to expel it through the cervix; this may at first be chronic and intermittent, usually coinciding with the menses, but is likely to become an acutely painful episode. Infection and sarcomatous degeneration also cause pain but are rare complications.

The physical signs associated with uterine fibroids are also extremely variable and can simulate conditions as dissimilar as pregnancy and malignant disease. Much depends on the size, number, situation and type and, later on, the presence of degenerative changes. Fibroids are so common that they may occur coincidentally with other pelvic pathology, and they may thus obscure a more important lesion such as an ovarian tumour or carcinoma of the endometrium.

Differential diagnosis
This must include all other pelvic tumours and those conditions which might be mistaken for one. Fortunately, in the majority of cases the diagnosis is relatively simple, and perhaps the most distinctive feature is that of consistency: 'fibroids feel like fibroids'. The tumours are rounded, smooth swellings of characteristic firm consistency. Mostly intramural, they distort the shape of the uterus, but a single fibroid can cause symmetrical enlargement. If it can be certain that fibroids are situated in the uterus there is little difficulty, unless there is cystic degeneration of a single fibroid, which can then simulate pregnancy; the reverse mistake is more important to avoid, as a lap-

arotomy for presumed fibroids which reveals a pregnant uterus is an unfortunate error. Pedunculated fibroids may be thought to be ovarian tumours, either cystic or solid, and if calcified may be mistaken for ovarian fibromas; occasionally, it is possible to feel the pedicle of attachment and to recognize that the mobility of the tumour is restricted by its being tethered to the uterus. Sometimes a fibroid polyp is seen to have been extruded through the cervical canal, but occasionally extrusion may be intermittent and only during menstruation.

The difference between myoma and adenomyoma may not be appreciated until attempted removal reveals the lack of capsule, but in general the latter are firmer tumours and there is severe dysmenorrhea.

The main differential diagnosis is from ovarian tumours when, as a rule, the uterus can be detected as separate from the swelling and menstrual disorders are not so common. But if the ovarian tumour is adherent to the uterus difficulty arises, and it is not unusual for the correct diagnosis to be reached only at laparotomy. Ascites is uncommon, but occasionally may result from peritoneal irritation by a freely mobile, firm, pedunculated tumour.

TREATMENT

Conservative treatment undoubtedly has a place in the management of uterine fibroids. When the tumours are small, the diagnosis is certain and there are no symptoms, patients may be reassured but must be kept under regular supervision to detect any subsequent enlargement. Near the menopause, larger symptomless fibroids may also be left untreated, in the anticipation of atrophy after cessation of the menstruation, but the patient must be kept under regular supervision. The advent of symptoms or an increase in size of the tumours demands surgical intervention in case the diagnosis is incorrect or malignant degeneration has supervened.

In cases where, apart from the finding of a few small fibroids, the diagnosis would be dysfunctional uterine bleeding, then a diagnostic curettage may be all that is required. If the abnormal bleeding persists, hormone therapy with progestogens may be instituted, but the fibroids must be carefully observed in case they enlarge, in which case surgery is called for.

When fibroids are causing symptoms, when the diagnosis is in doubt, or when they are larger than a size corresponding to a 12-week pregnancy, then surgical treatment is indicated.

Two main forms of operation are possible: myomectomy or hysterectomy. Both are usually performed abdominally but occasionally the vaginal route is preferred. Hysterectomy is usually the better procedure because the fibroids cannot recur and the symptoms can be relieved with certainty. This operation is generally easier to perform, there is less blood loss, and less postoperative morbidity. Obviously it is indicated when the age and parity of the patient make further pregnancy unlikely or undesirable. For younger patients myomectomy is indicated, because it is possible for successful pregnancy to occur after this operation. Loeffler and Noble (1970) reviewed 180 patients subjected to myomectomy, about 1 in 3 of whom subsequently conceived; over one-third of pregnancies subsequently aborted, and of the 41 viable infants 25% were delivered by Caesarian section. It must always be understood, of course, that recurrence of the fibroids is a distinct possibility, either from seedling fibroids overlooked at the time of operation or because the stimulus to regrowth is maintained. Loeffler and Noble found that 27% of their cases came to hysterectomy and two others had repeat myomectomies. In performing myomectomy the surgeon must be careful to avoid damaging the Fallopian tubes in their course through the myometrium. Incisions on the posterior uterine wall are to be avoided as far as possible because of the increased risk of adhesions involving the intestines. The 'hood' operation devised by Victor Bonney is a useful method for removing posterior intramural fibroids and advancing the uterine incision anteriorly over the fundus so as to avoid this complication. His treatise on the minutiae of myomectomy and ovarian cystectomy (Bonney 1946) remains a classic textbook to this day, and should be read by those interested in the techniques of myomectomy. Myomectomy is often followed by a slightly stormy convalescence associated with abdominal pain and raised temperature; this is seldom due to infection and usually results from oozing of blood into either the myomectomy cavity in the uterus or into the peritoneal cavity. Intestinal obstruction is the most serious complication, resulting from the small bowel becoming adherent to the uterine scar. Rupture of a myometcomy scar in a subsequent pregnancy or labour is very rare, but has been described. The uterus, which is often still quite enlarged after the operation, tends to shrink to normal size within 2–3 months.

In some black races removal of the uterus is considered a serious mutilation and permission for hysterectomy is not often granted, even where multiple fibroids are associated with gross pelvic sepsis and where there is no possible hope of subsequent pregnancy. A modified subtotal hysterectomy which leaves a modicum of functioning endometrium may then be the most acceptable procedure.

Fibroids and pregnancy

During pregnancy myomata often enlarge but, because they also tend to become soft as a result of interstitial oedema, they flatten out and may become indistinct. Subserous tumours, on the other hand, may be readily palpated as the uterus enlarges, and on occasion may be mistaken for fetal parts.

Certain accidents and degenerations are more common in fibroids during pregnancy, and of these red degeneration and torsion of pedunculated fibroids are the most important. When red degeneration occurs there is subacute abdominal pain which may be severe enough to require opiates for relief, tenderness over the fibroid and, at times, signs of peritoneal irritation with rigidity and guarding in the area. Constitutional effects are not severe, but there may be initial vomiting and both temperature and pulse rate are raised slightly. There is an associated leucocytosis, but in pregnancy this does not signify in view of the physiological leucocytosis that is present. The differential diagnosis from acute appendicitis may be difficult if the fibroid is situated in the right iliac fossa, but usually in appendicitis there is a rapid thready pulse raised out of proportion to the body temperature which is only slightly raised or may even be subnormal. Pyelonephritis may also have to be considered in the diagnosis, but here the temperature is high, and usually there is also symptomatic and bacteriological evidence of urinary tract infection. The treatment of red degeneration in fibroids is conservative; bedrest, reassurance and analgesics to relieve pain will be followed by subsidence of symptoms and signs within about ten days.

Torsion of pedunculated fibroids may occur antepartum, but is more likely to occur early in the puerperium when there is rapid uterine involution and laxity of the abdominal wall results in increased mobility of the intra-abdominal contents. Symptoms and signs of an acute or subacute abdomen follow, but guarding and rigidity are usually absent due to the lax abdominal muscles. Diagnosis is seldom difficult if a fibroid is already known to be present; but if not, an accident to an ovarian cyst is likely to be diagnosed, and intestinal volvulus, appendicitis and ureteric colic should be considered, as should the possibility of a rectus muscle haematoma. Laparotomy is required if torsion of either a pedunculated fibroid or an ovarian cyst (or an acute 'surgical abdomen') is diagnosed. The offending fibroid should be removed, but the temptation to deal with any other coexistent myomas must be resisted.

Infection in fibroids may also occur postpartum or, more commonly, after an abortion; fibroid polypi and submucous fibroids are the most likely to be infected, and the former may be cured spontaneously by sloughing and passage *per vaginam*.

Fibroids may influence the course of pregnancy and labour. The uterine size may seem greater than would be consistent with the period of gestation. In early pregnancy abortion may result, and is probably more likely if implantation occurs over a submucous fibroid. Later on, cervical fibroids, or those situated in the lower half of the corpus, may prevent engagement of the fetal head, and cause instability of the fetal lie, or alternatively a persistent abnormal lie or presentation. During labour, fibroids seldom interfere with uterine action, although there is a widely held but unsubstantiated view that they predispose to postpartum haemorrhage. A cervical fibroid will result in obstructed labour unless it is very well taken up into the lower uterine segment as this develops during late pregnancy, and becomes further stretched over the presenting fetal part during labour. If the tumour is in the lower segment early in pregnancy it is even more likely to be pulled up and out of the way in this manner, and fortunately pregnancy in association with a cervical fibroid is a rare occurrence.

Obstructed labour must be relieved by Caesarean section, but the temptation to undertake Caesarean myomectomy should be resisted unless the fibroid is actually in the line of the incision; uncontrollable haemorrhage may be the reward of such interven-tion. Caesarean hysterectomy is a safer procedure if it is deemed that removal of the uterus is both desirable and inevitable. Postpartum haemorrhage may occur, perhaps because the presence of the fibroids may interfere with proper contraction and retraction of the uterus. In the puerperium, retarded involution may occur or may be simulated. The ultimate effect of pregnancy on fibroids is variable, they may become much smaller or they may remain unchanged, but they do not increase in size.

RARE TUMOURS

Rare benign tumours are lipomas, lymphangioma, haemangioma and haemangio-perictyoma, although the latter has been reported as having a low-grade malignancy in some cases.

REFERENCES

ARMENIA C.S. (1967) *Obstet. Gynaec. NY*, **30**, 524.
BARNES H.M. & RICHARDSON P.J. (1973) *J. Obstet. Gynaec. Brit. Cwlth.*, **80**, 569
BONNEY V. (1946) *The Technical Minutiae of Extended Myomectomy and Ovarian Cystectomy*. Cassell, London.
JEFFCOATE T.N.A. (1962) *Principles of Gynaecology*. Butterworths, London.
LOEFFLER F.E. & NOBLE A.D. (1970) *J. Obstet. Gynaec. Brit. Cwlth.*, **77**, 167.
MILLER N.F. & LUDOVICI P.P. (1955) *Amer. J. Obstet. Gynec.*, **70**, 720.
NOVAK E.R. & WOODRUFF J.D. (1974) *Novak's Gynecologic and Obstetric Pathology*. W.B. Saunders, Philadelphia.
PAYNE P., WOODS H.F. & WRIGLEY P.F.M. (1969) *J. Obstet. Gynec.*, **76**, 854.

CHAPTER 48
BENIGN AND MALIGNANT TUMOURS
OF THE OVARY

K. R. PEEL

Introduction

The ovary gives rise to a wider variety of tumours than any other organ in the body which present to the clinician, often not a gynaecologist, in a number of different ways. Symptoms may or may not be associated with the lesion. The enlargement may be such as to produce a pelvic swelling or, if larger, a tumour which can be felt in the abdomen. The tumours may be solid, cystic or a mixture of both, and may be benign, malignant or in a borderline state. The diagnostic problems associated with smaller cysts are increased by the development of so-called functional cysts (sometimes called cystic ovaries) due to alterations in the follicular system. Ovarian enlargement can be due to infection, endometriosis or to an ovarian pregnancy though these latter conditions are discussed elsewhere.

Ovarian malignancy accounts for almost 25% of gynaecological cancer and, more important, 50% of all deaths from cancer of the female genital tract. No satisfactory screening test is available and the disease has often spread widely when first found. We are better informed about the spread of the disease as a result of better surgical staging, but in spite of radical surgery coupled with the introduction of many new cytotoxic drugs, which together have on occasions produced significant remissions, the overall five-year survival rate has changed little in recent years and remains at around 25–30%. Ovarian cancer, without doubt, presents the greatest challenge to the gynaecological oncologist.

FUNCTIONAL CYSTS

Derangements of the pituitary ovarian cycle can alter the physiological ovarian changes associated with ovulation leading to ovarian enlargement which rarely exceeds a diameter of 5 cm. Cysts arising in the follicular phase do so when the Graafian follicle fails to rupture at the expected time though the resultant

follicular cyst may do so at a later stage. Follicular cysts may arise as a consequence of excessive ovarian stimulation with drugs such as Clomiphene or with human chorionic gonadotrophin. When follicular cysts develop in early normal pregnancy, they will normally disappear in the second or third month of the pregnancy.

OVARIAN TUMOURS

The variety of ovarian tumours is such that a classification is essential so as to facilitate communication between clinicians of different disciplines and to provide a basis for the orderly study of tumour pathology and behaviour. Over the years various classifications based on morphological characteristics, histogenetic features or clinical behaviour have been tried. The one favoured is that recommended by the World Health Organization (Serov *et al.* 1973) which depends on the microscopic appearances of the various cell types and arrangements and which is set out in detail in Table 48.1.

In broad terms tumours are classified as being
1   of epithelial origin (sometimes referred to as serosal tumours),
2   sex cord stromal tumours,
3   germ cell tumours,
4   miscellaneous primary tumours,
5   metastatic tumours,
6   tumour-like conditions referred to earlier.

Approximately 50% of ovarian tumours are benign epithelial tumours. Of the malignant tumours 90% are epithelial in origin whilst the remaining 10% include those arising in ovarian stroma, cells of sex cord or germ cell origin, or those which are the result of metastases from primary tumours elsewhere in the body.

'Tumours of borderline malignancy' is the term currently used in the WHO classification of ovarian tumours to describe a group of tumours which are intermediate in both behaviour and histological

Table 48.1. Histological classification of ovarian tumours

I COMMON 'EPITHELIAL' TUMOURS

A *Serous Tumours*

   1 Benign
      (a) cystadenoma and papillary cystadenoma
      (b) surface papilloma
      (c) adenofibroma and cystadenofibroma

   2 Of borderline malignancy (carcinomas of low
      malignant potential)
      (a) cystadenoma and papillary cystadenoma
      (b) surface papilloma
      (c) adenofibroma and cystadenofibroma

   3 Malignant
      (a) adenocarcinoma, papillary adenocarcinoma,
      and papillary cystadenocarcinoma
      (b) surface papillary carcinoma
      (c) malignant adenofibroma and
      cystadenofibroma

B *Mucinous Tumours*

   1 Benign
      (a) cystadenoma
      (b) adenofibroma and cystadenofibroma

   2 Of borderline malignancy (carcinomas of low
      malignant potential)
      (a) cystadenoma
      (b) adenofibroma and cystadenofibroma

   3 Malignant
      (a) adenocarcinoma and cystadenocarcinoma
      (b) malignant adenofibroma and
      cystadenofibroma

C *Endometrioid Tumours*

   1 Benign
      (a) adenoma and cystadenoma
      (b) adenfibroma and cystadenofibroma

   2 Of borderline malignancy (carcinomas of low
      malignant potential)
      (a) adenoma and cystadenoma
      (b) adenofibroma and cystadenofibroma

   3 Malignant
      (a) carcinoma
         (i) adenocarcinoma
         (ii) adenoacanthoma
         (iii) malignant adenofibroma and
         cystadenofibroma
      (b) endometrioid stromal sarcomas
      (c) mesodermal (Müllerian) mixed tumours,
      homologous and heterologous

D *Clear Cell (Mesonephroid) Tumours*
   1 Benign: adenofibroma
   2 Of borderline malignancy (carcinomas of low
      malignant potential)
   3 Malignant: carcinoma and adenocarcinoma

E *Brenner Tumours*

   1 Benign

   2 Of borderline malignancy (proliferating)

F *Mixed Epithelial Tumours*

   1 Benign

   2 Of borderline malignancy

   3 Malignant

G *Undifferentiated Carcinoma*

H *Unclassified Epithelial Tumours*

II SEX CORD STROMAL TUMOURS

A *Granulosa–Stromal Cell Tumours*

   1 Granulosa cell tumour

   2 Tumours in the thecoma-fibroma group
      (a) thecoma
      (b) fibroma
      (c) unclassified

B *Androblastomas: Sertoli–Leydig Cell Tumours*

   1 Well differentiated

      (a) tubular androblastoma; Sertoli cell tumour
      (tubular adenoma of Pick)
      (b) tubular androblastoma with lipid storage;
      Sertoli cell tumour with lipid storage
      (folliculome lipidique of Lecène)
      (c) Sertoli–Leydig cell tumour (tubular adenoma
      with Leydig cells)
      (d) Leydig cell tumour; hilus cell tumour

   2 Of intermediate differentiation
   3 Poorly differentiated (sarcomatoid)
   4 With heterologous elements

C *Gynandroblastoma*

D *Unclassified*

III LIPID (LIPOID) CELL TUMOURS

IV GERM CELL TUMOURS

A *Dysgerminoma*

B *Endodermal Sinus Tumour*

C *Embryonal Carcinoma*

D *Polyembryoma*

E *Choriocarcinoma*

F *Teratomas*

    1 Immature

    2 Mature
       (a) solid
       (b) cystic
           (i) dermoid cyst (mature cystic teratoma)
           (ii) dermoid cyst with malignant transformation

    3 Monodermal and highly specialized
       (a) struma ovarii
       (b) carcinoid
       (c) struma ovarii and carcinoid
       (d) others

G *Mixed Forms*

V GONADOBLASTOMA

A *Pure*

B *Mixed with Dysgerminoma or other form of Germ Cell Tumour*

VI SOFT TISSUE TUMOURS NOT SPECIFIC TO OVARY

VII UNCLASSIFIED TUMOURS

VIII SECONDARY (METASTATIC) TUMOURS

IX TUMOUR-LIKE CONDITIONS

A Pregnancy Luteoma

B Hyperplasia of Ovarian Stroma and Hyperthecosis

C Massive Oedema

D Solitary Follicle Cyst and Corpus Lutem Cyst

E Multiple Follicle Cysts (Polycystic Ovaries)

F Multiple Luteinized Follicle Cysts and/or Corpora Lutea

G Endometriosis

H Surface-epithelial Inclusion Cysts (Germinal Inclusion Cysts)

I Simple Cysts

J Inflammatory Lesions

K Parovarian Cysts

---

features between benign tumours and those obviously malignant. Such a tumour is defined as one 'that has some, but not all, of the morphological features of malignancy: those present include, in varying combinations, stratification of epithelial cells, apparent detachment of cellular clusters from their sites of origin and mitotic figures and nuclear abnormalities intermediate between those of clearly benign and unquestionably malignant tumours of similar cell type: on the other hand obvious invasion of the stroma is lacking'. It is this lack of ovarian stromal involvement that is paramount. Extra-ovarian spread can occur with implantation of peritoneal surfaces and local invasion. Lymph node metastases are sometimes seen, but even so survival is often prolonged.

Other terms for the same condition have been used. Taylor (1929) reported a hyperplastic variety of papillary cystadenoma which behaved in this fashion and called it a 'semi-malignant tumour'. The International Federation of Gynaecologists and Obstetricians in its classification (FIGO 1971) adopted the term 'tumours of low malignant potential'. It would seem that borderline malignancy is the term most commonly used.

The prognosis is dependent not only on the tumour type but also on the extent of spread. It is the pathologist who determines the nature of the tumour, examining histologically many samples when the tumour is large, and who, when the degree of differentiation is important, analyses carefully the cytological detail of the specimen. It is the lot of the surgeon to assess the extent of spread when the laparotomy is performed. As with other malignant diseases staging, in this disease surgical staging, is of paramount importance. Two systems are in use, the one according to FIGO (1982) which is shown in Table 48.2, and the other, the TNM (Tumours, Nodes, Metastases) system which is shown in Table 48.3. It is the FIGO system which is more commonly used.

OVARIAN CANCER

Epidemiology

During the last fifty years the death rate from ovarian cancer has doubled (OPCS 1981). Whereas it is possible the frequency of diagnosis has increased, it is more likely the result of an increase in incidence. Ovarian cancer, long the commonest killer of the

Table 48.2. Carcinoma of ovary: staging according to FIGO.

STAGE I Growth limited to the ovaries.

    Stage Ia Growth limited to *one* ovary; no ascites.
        (i)   No tumour on the external surface; capsule intact.
        (ii) Tumour present on the external surface and/or capsule ruptured.

    Stage Ib Growth limited to *both* ovaries; no ascites.
        (i)   No tumour on the external surface; capsule intact.
        (ii) Tumour present on the external surface and/or capsule(s) ruptured.

    Stage Ic Tumour either Stage Ia or Stage Ib, but with ascites* present or positive peritoneal washings.

STAGE II Growth involving one or both ovaries with pelvic extension.

    Stage IIa Extension and/or metastases to the uterus and/or tubes.

    Stage IIb Extension to other pelvic tissues including peritoneum and the uterus.

Stage IIc Tumour either Stage IIa or Stage IIb, but with ascites* present or positive peritoneal washings.

STAGE III Growth involving one or both ovaries with intraperitoneal metastases outside the pelvis and/or positive retroperitoneal nodes.

    Tumour limited to the true pelvis with histologically proven malignant extension to small bowel or omentum.

STAGE IV Growth involving one or both ovaries with distant metastases.

    If pleural effusion is present there must be positive cytology to allot a case to Stage IV.

    Parenchymal liver metastases equals Stage IV.

SPECIAL CATEGORY Cases which are thought to be ovarian carcinoma, but where it has been impossible to tell the origin of the tumour.

* Ascites is peritoneal effusion which in the opinion of the surgeon is pathological and/or clearly exceeds normal amounts.

Table 48.3. Carcinoma of ovary: staging according to TNM.

TP1 The tumour involves one ovary which remains mobile.

TP2 The tumour involves both ovaries, each remaining mobile.

TP3 The tumour extends into the uterus or Fallopian tubes.

TP4 The tumour extends to other surrounding structures.

N Regional lymph nodes
    NX− lymph nodes not involved.
    NX+ lymph nodes involved.
    NX lymph node involvement not known.

M Distant metastases.

MO No distant metastases.

M1 Implantation or metastases present:
    M1a In the true pelvis only.
    M1b Within the peritoneal cavity.
    M1c Outside the peritoneal cavity.

female pelvic malignancies, has now become the commonest pelvic cancer amongst women resident in England and Wales (Fig. 48.1). The rate of increase has not been uniform for all age groups. Although there is an increasing incidence with age up to the sixth decade (Fig. 48.2) a downward trend in mortality has been noted for some age groups, and Beral *et al.* (1978) describe a cohort effect demonstrating that women born between 1900 and 1910 had an especially high risk of developing ovarian cancer and this they attributed to their smaller family size as compared with predecessors or successors and the result of having their childbearing years at the time of the depression in the 1930s which occurred in both the United Kingdom and the United States.

The disease is seen more often in industrialized societies and particularly in the Western World. It has its highest incidence in Sweden, followed by Norway, the United States of America, Germany and the United Kingdom. Japan has one of the lowest incidences. A study of immigration trends suggests the variation is more likely accounted for by environmental or behavioural reasons than by racial or genetic variation e.g. second generation Japanese women living in the United States show an incidence of ovarian

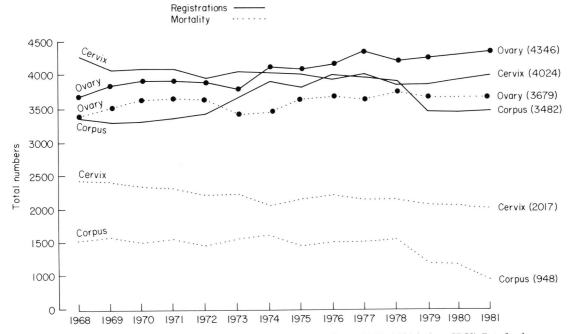

Fig. 48.1. England and Wales cancer registrations and mortality, by site and year 1968–1981 (source OPCS). Data for the ovary are marked with solid dots.

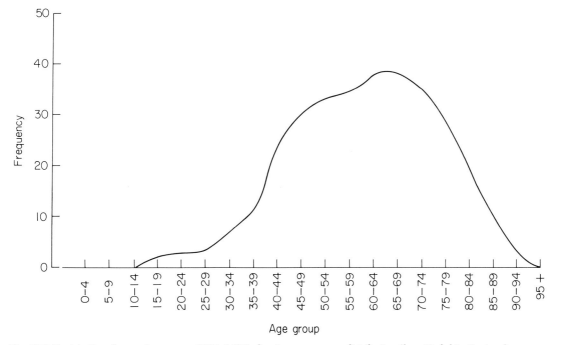

Fig. 48.2. Registrations for ovarian cancer, 1981–1983, showing average age distribution (from Yorkshire Regional Cancer Organization).

cancer equivalent to that of their American neighbours.

No direct relationship has been established between either industrial pollution or cigarette smoking and ovarian cancer, but asbestos and talc have both been suspected of being relevant to ovarian cancer aetiology. Keal (1960) first suggested a link between asbestosis and ovarian cancer. Newhouse *et al.* (1972) reported high rates of ovarian cancer among women working with asbestos, a finding later confirmed by Acheson *et al.* (1982). Talc particles are similar to asbestos and until recently most talc powders contained asbestos. Henderson *et al.* (1971) found a high proportion of ovarian tumours contained talc particles within them. Talc is found in soap powders and deodorants, and is used in the packaging of condoms and contraceptive diaphragms. All are possible sources of talc on the perineum or in the vagina which might then migrate via the uterus and tubes to the ovaries. Cramer *et al.* (1982) report that women with ovarian cancer were three times as likely to use talc on the perineal area. Some workers have cast doubt on the association between asbestosis and ovarian cancer on the grounds that sometimes mesotheliomata have been wrongly diagnosed as ovarian cancer.

An increased risk of pelvic cancer, including ovarian cancer, in women previously treated with pelvic irradiation for benign gynaecological diseases such as metropathia haemorrhagica was reported by Smith (1977).

The influence of hormones, reproduction and ovulation on the incidence of ovarian cancer has been studied and reported by Beral *et al.* (1978). They point out that ovarian cancer is less common in women of high parity and that pregnancy would seem to be protective whether ending in an abortion or at term. La Vecchia *et al.* (1983) have shown an early age of first pregnancy confers a greater protection against ovarian cancer than high parity. Breast feeding can also be protective (Risch *et al.* 1983). An early menarche and a late menopause are associated with an increased risk. Newhouse *et al.* (1977) first described the protective effect of oral contraception and they believe that the longer the pill is used the less the likelihood of subsequent ovarian cancer. All these facts point to ovarian cancer being more common in those women who ovulate often. Fathalla (1971) has used the term 'incessant ovulation' to highlight these facts. Casagrande *et al.* (1979) introduced the term 'ovulatory age' i.e. the number of years a women spends menstruating less those years

pregnant or having ovulation suppressed. They found this to be a high predictive index for the risk of ovarian cancer when the figure is high.

Both nutrition and infection have also been considered as possible aetiological factors. The high incidence in western societies has been assoiated with a high animal fat intake but this was not confirmed by Byers *et al.* (1983). They found no association between ovarian cancer and a high intake of fat, protein, vitamin C or alcohol, but noted a relationship between the disease and those ingesting a high quantity of fibre or vitamin A in their diet.

Infective agents have not been incriminated, but it has been suggested that suffering from mumps oophoritis may be protective perhaps by a diminution of future ovulation (West 1966) yet a check on the levels of neutralizing antibodies (Golan *et al.* 1979) failed to confirm such a view.

Women whose mothers or sisters had ovarian cancer run a twenty-fold risk of developing the disease (Hildreth *et al.* 1981) and, whereas inheritance would seem to be mainly via the maternal line, paternal inheritance has been described by Matheson *et al.* (1981). It would be remembered however that the cause may be an environmental factor to which all the family are exposed.

Significant ovarian function after the menopause is unlikely so oophorectomy to prevent subsequent malignancy is indicated whenever an abdominal hysterectomy for benign disease is done in the postmenopausal woman. When such a woman is premenopausal the risk of subsequent ovarian cancer, variously reported as 0–0.2%, must be weighed against the advantages of less coronary artery disease and less osteoporosis which result from ovarian conservation. Annegers *et al.* (1979) produced data which suggest that hysterectomy, even with preservation of one or both ovaries, may reduce the risk of subsequent ovarian cancer.

EPITHELIAL TUMOURS

Pathological features

Benign serous cystadenomata occur slightly more often than benign mucinous tumours, but in the malignant form serous cystadenocarcinomata are three to four times more common than mucinous cystadenocarcinomata. Serous and mucinous borderline tumours are seen but other types of epithelial tumours of borderline malignancy, such as the variants of Brenner and endometrioid tumours, are rare. When borderline tumours occur they are most often seen in women aged between twenty and forty years.

Serous tumours

Forty per cent of ovarian tumours are serous in origin and 50–70% of these are benign serous cystadenomata. They are usually smaller cysts than the mucinous variety and bilateral in approximately 50% of cases. The cyst is most often unilocular, with a smooth outer surface which rarely exhibits exophytic lesions, and a lining which nearly always contains papilliferous processes. The fluid content is a thin serous fluid. The papillae may be few in number and just cause a localized roughened area or fill the whole cyst so that it appears solid. As described earlier the papillae may sprout through the capsule in which case ascites is commonly found and, though this is very suggestive of malignancy, such tumours may be histologically benign. The lining cells are cuboid or columnar and may be ciliated, often resembling the epithelium of the Fallopian tube. Serous tumours may contain cells which secrete abundant mucin, though in contrast to true mucinous tumours (the cells of which contain mucin within the upper part of their substance) the mucin in serous tumours is secreted from the surface of the cells. The papillae of borderline tumours tend to be finer and softer than in their malignant counterparts. Serous cystadenocarcinomata, the commonest malignant primary ovarian tumour, may be predominantly cystic or predominantly solid with fine papillae which are irregular, often with slit-like glandular lumens and associated with the presence of small deposits of calcium in the stroma known as psammoma bodies. These latter lesions do however occur in a variety of other benign and malignant ovarian neoplasms.

Mucinous tumours

Mucinous cystadenomata tend to be large, unilateral cysts, sometimes reaching enormous proportions and yet still remaining benign. Shaw (1932) reported a number of benign tumours weighing more than 200lb, the heaviest being a case described by Spohn of Texas which weighed 328lb. This latter tumour extended from the patient's chin to midway between the knees and feet; thirty gallons of fluid were drained by tapping one week prior to removal of the tumour, and the patient survived the operation. Atlee of Pennsylvania, between 1861 and 1900, tapped a cyst 269 times, removing nearly 17 000 pints of fluid. They are multilocular with smooth outer and inner sur-

faces. The fluid content is mucinous, of variable consistency but characteristically jelly-like, and can be discoloured with blood or pus. The loculi, lined by a single layer of tall mucus secreting columnar cells with dark staining nuclei, are of variable size. It is unusual for papillary processes to be present, but when they are they are suggestive of malignancy. Malignant change in mucinous cystadenomata is thought to occur in 5–10% of cases. Unlike serous tumours, the mucinous variety may have benign, borderline and malignant elements in the same tumour, and it is therefore important that extensive sampling is undertaken by the pathologist when examining the tumour. Mucinous cystadenocarcinomata tend to be predominantly solid.

Pseudomyxoma peritonei is a rare complication of mucinous tumours which occurs when spontaneous perforation of the cyst leads to implantation of cells of low malignancy on the peritoneum. These cells form cysts or pockets of mucin surrounded by dense connective tissue. Mucocele of the appendix may also be a cause of the condition and may coexist with a mucinous tumour of the ovary. The patient usually dies from malignant cachexia after several laparotomies to remove the collected mucin. Unfortunately, treatment seems to be of little avail as regards ultimate survival though Long et al. (1969) report a 45% five year survival from the condition with death occurring from between four months and twenty-four years after diagnosis.

Endometrioid tumours

Ovarian tumours which contain tubular glands with the appearance of those within proliferative endometrium are called endometrioid tumours. Also included in this group of tumours are endometrioid adenofibromas, which if they contain areas of squamous metaplasia are known as adenoacanthofibromas. Benign endometrioid tumours are rare. Endometrioid tumours of borderline malignancy do occur in which the glandular epithelium appears malignant but does not invade the stroma.

Endometrioid carcinomas account for between 16 and 30% of all ovarian carcinomas. The term is used whenever the primary ovarian carcinoma has microscopic features resembling carcinoma of the endometrium whether or not an origin from endometriosis is found. The tumours average 10–20 cm in diameter and are less cystic than serous or mucinous carcinomas. The solid areas tend to be yellow to dark red in colour and, within the cystic areas, dark haemorrhagic fluid is often found. Intracystic papillary projections occur in some. Grading varies as with uterine adenocarcinomas. Such tumours are often found in association with carcinoma of the uterine corpus and it is believed that the lesions are independent primary growths in both organs. Mixed epithelial and stromal tumours of the endometrioid type are also included in this group of tumours. Malignant mesodermal mixed tumours, which are entirely derived from mesoderm and almost always occur in postmenopausal and menopausal women, must be differentiated from immature teratomas which contain tissue from all three germ cell layers and tend to occur in women under fifty years of age.

Clear cell tumours

Clear cell carcinoma is regarded as being of Müllerian origin and is closely related to endometrioid carcinomas and endometriosis. They are more frequently associated with ovarian and pelvic endometriosis than any other ovarian tumour. Tumours with an identical histological appearance can also arise in the cervix, vagina, endometrium or broad ligament. The vaginal variants are usually seen in young females who, whilst *in utero*, were exposed to diethylstilboestrol. The ovarian tumours are often in excess of 15 cm in diameter, partly solid and partly cystic and uncommonly bilateral. The cells are arranged in solid sheets or lined glandular spaces and are, as expected, clear cells or so-called hobnail cells, i.e. cells having scanty cytoplasm draped around a prominent protruding nucleus. The prognosis for clear cell carcinoma is said to be worse for its endometrioid counterpart.

Clear cell carcinomas were once considered mesonephric in origin and called mesonephric or mesonephroid carcinoma. Now that clear cell carcinoma is thought to be of Müllerian nature, there is doubt as to whether the mesonephroma is a distinct entity.

Brenner tumours

The Brenner tumours are a relatively frequent variety of epithelial tumour being composed of nests of benign transitional epithelium resembling that found in the urinary bladder, surrounded by dense fibrous tissue. Areas of mucinous cells are found in up to 25% of Brenner tumours. These tumours are usually benign, often quite small (less than 5 cm in diameter) and as a result are often found incidentally during pelvic surgery or during the pathological examination of an operative specimen. Borderline and malignant variants do occur but uncommonly. Malignant Brenner tumours (transitional cell carci-

nomas) may be predominantly solid or predominantly cystic and have no distinctive gross features Mucinous elements should be found on microscopic examination.

Undifferentiated carcinomas

Undifferentiated carcinoma accounts for 10% of ovarian carcinomas. The term is used to describe primary ovarian carcinomas with minimal or no differentiation. Most are probably undifferentiated serous or endometrioid carcinoma, more than 50% are bilateral, and the tumour which is nearly always solid has often spread widely at the time of diagnosis. The prognosis for such patients is very poor indeed.

Mixed epithelial tumours

Whenever examination of a tumour shows a significant component of a second or third cell type the tumour can be designated a mixed epithelial tumour. One exception is the Brenner tumour which so often contains mucinous or serous elements that it is excluded from this category.

Clinical features

Ovarian tumours may be cystic or solid and of such a size as to remain within the pelvis or, if larger, to become apparent on abdominal examination. Not uncommonly ovarian tumours are symptomless in their early stages. They may be found during the course of a pelvic examination done as part of antenatal care and therefore usually in early pregnancy, during a routine examination to obtain a cervical smear, or during an examination done for insurance purposes or some similar reason. Postmenopausal patients undergoing hormone replacement therapy may be found to have a palpable ovary and such patients require further investigation. In recent years an ultrasonic scan may have revealed a previously unsuspected ovarian swelling.

When symptoms do occur they commonly take the form of either dyspareunia or dysmenorrhoea. When the ovarian tumour has reached such a size as to be found in the abdomen the patient may complain of abdominal discomfort, an increase in abdominal girth, an increase in weight, or a failure to lose weight from the abdomen as a result of dieting.

If an ovarian cyst undergoes torsion, rupture, haemorrhage or infection, acute or subacute abdominal symptoms may occur.

It is usually benign cysts of moderate size on long pedicles which undergo torsion. Acute or subacute pain in one or other side of the lower abdomen will occur, and will often be associated with nausea or vomiting. The patient may have an elevated pulse rate. Tenderness, guarding or rigidity of the lower abdomen may be apparent, and on pelvic examination an acutely tender swelling might be found in one or other adnexal region. In such circumstances laparotomy is indicated. As a result of the torsion, infarction of the ovary and its related tube may be found and only rarely will it be possible to conserve ovarian tissue. Invariably the tumour mass requires excision.

When an ovarian cyst or a loculus of a larger ovarian cyst ruptures, the acuteness of the symptoms will depend on the amount and character of the cyst contents released into the peritoneal cavity. The contents of dermoid cysts are extremely irritant as is, to a lesser extent, the chocolate material released from endometriotic cysts. The contents of a simple serous cyst are significantly less irritant and may be associated with only minimal symptoms. In this latter group of patients mild tenderness may be noted, whereas rupture of an endometriotic or demoid cyst will usually lead to severe pain often in association with collapse and the signs of an acute abdomen.

Haemorrhage can occur from the torn edge of a ruptured cyst or the bleeding may be into the cavity of the cyst. The amount of associated pain varies but can be severe.

Whenever infection is a complication of an ovarian tumour, constitutional signs by way of pyrexia and an elevated pulse rate may be associated with localizing signs due to peritoneal irritation, such as tenderness, rigidity and guarding of the abdomen. If an infected cyst ruptures and disgorges its contents into the abdominal cavity, pelvic or general peritonitis will follow.

Even though malignant change may occur a tumour may remain symptomless. It is said that 15% of patients with malignant ovarian tumours are asymptomatic at the time of diagnosis (Piver et al. 1976), and more than 50% of patients with ovarian malignancy have widespread disease at the time of laparotomy.

When symptoms do develop abdominal distension with a noticeable increase in abdominal girth occurs, soon followed by abdominal pain. Non-specific digestive upset is common. The patient may complain of pelvic discomfort, vaginal bleeding, or of a palpable tumour. As the disease progresses the patient may be aware of a loss in weight. Dypsnoea may occur if the ovarian tumour causes pressure on the diaphragm or is associated with a pleural effusion. Other pressure effects include unilateral or bilateral lower limb oedema or varicosities and haemorrhoids. Deep venous thrombosis may be the presenting sign. Pressure on the bladder may give rise to frequency or urgency of micturition. If the tumour is of such a size that it can become impacted in the pelvis, then acute retention of urine may occur. Extrinsic pressure from tumour masses on the small bowel not uncommonly leads to intestinal obstruction causing abdominal colic and vomiting. In the terminal stages of malignant ovarian disease cachexia is common, but cachexia is not always the result of malignant disease since sometimes large tumours interfere with absorption and digestion. Very large tumours are commonly benign since had they been malignant they would have destroyed the patient before reaching such a size. One exception is the patient whose benign tumour undergoes malignant change late in its natural history.

Ascites is a common accompaniment of ovarian malignancy but, as has been mentioned earlier, it can arise in association with benign or malignant tumours. Meigs' syndrome (Meigs & Cass 1937) is of ascites associated with a benign ovarian fibroma and a right-sided hydrothorax.

Hormone producing tumours may be associated with specific symptoms. Masculinizing tumours such as the androblastoma at first lead to a loss of feminization with amenorrhoea and atrophy of the breasts, and then later to masculinizing effects such as acne, hirsutism, deepening of the voice and enlargement of the clitoris. The symptoms caused by feminizing tumours, such as the granulosa cell tumour, vary according to the age of the patient. In the prepubertal child precocious puberty occurs, whereas postmenopausal bleeding may be apparent after the menopause due to oestrogen stimulation of the atrophic endometrium. Postmenopausal bleeding can also be due to ovarian tumours other than those which are obvious feminizing. During menstrual life feminizing tumours may induce cystic glandular hyperplasia of the endometrium with a clinical story such as occurs with metrophathia haemorrhagica. Gonadal dysgenesis may be present in association with dysgerminoma. Although rare, if stroma ovarii (a teratoma containing thyroid tissue) is present symptoms of thyrotoxicosis occur.

Intrapelvic benign tumours, when mobile, can usually be recognized readily as adnexal swellings distinct from the uterus. Endometriomata however, are not uncommonly confused with fibroids as a result of being tense and fixed to the uterus. Tubo-ovarian or tubal inflammatory lesions are more likely to be bilateral, tender and fixed, and have associated symptoms suggestive of infection. Broad ligament cysts are usually unilateral, fixed, and push the uterus to one or other side of the pelvis. Pedunculated fibroids may be confused with ovarian fibromata. Diagnostic difficulties arise in the differentiation of follicular cysts and early neoplasms, and can usually be resolved in the young patient by observation over a short period of time, but if there is any suspicion of malignant disease, laparoscopy, and immediate precise diagnosis, is necessary.

Ovarian cysts which are palpable in the abdomen are usually discrete with a smooth surface and associated with limited mobility. Dullness to percussion will be apparent over the cyst with resonance over the displaced bowel. On pelvic examination the lower pole of the tumour may be felt and the uterus defined separately from the tumour. Confusion may arise if abdominal distension due to flatus is present, if gross constipation has resulted in an abdominal mass, or if ascites due to some other cause is present. The clinician should always be aware of the possibility of a full bladder which must be emptied by spontaneous voiding or catheterization prior to further examination. Fibroids undergoing degenerative or cystic change may, particularly when subserous, confuse the clinician. Less common conditions which should be considered in the differential diagnosis of ovarian tumours include accessory lobes of the liver, an enlarged spleen, hydronephrosis, mesenteric cyst, pancreatic or pseudopancreatic cyst, pseudocysts formed by adhesions due to drug therapy such as practolol, large hydrosalpinges particularly if of tuberculous origin, and lesions of the pelvic colon such as diverticulitis, endometriomata or much less commonly carcinoma. Other conditions which can cause confusion on pelvic examination include a pelvic kidney or a mobile and dependent pelvic caecum. Obesity invariably makes the examination more difficult and less precise, and if doubt occurs it should be resolved by ultrasonic examination or by examination under anaesthesia. These latter steps will also exclude pseudocyesis and the apparent tumour of a patient whose distended abdomen is due to a failure of abdominal muscle relaxation. Pregnancy deserves special mention and should always be considered in a woman of childbearing age who has either a pelvic or lower abdominal swelling. Errors may occur if a false history is given by the patient or if scanty bleeding occurs in an irregular way during early pregnancy. The clinician who always thinks of pregnancy

as a possibility is much less likely to make errors, and the ready availability of ultrasound in recent years has meant an inappropriate laparotomy is much less commonly done.

Specific physical signs may point to malignancy. Malignant tumours are more likely to be solid than cystic and many undergo rapid growth. Ascites is common and fixity is usual, often associated with irregular masses felt in the Pouch of Douglas. Bilateral tumours are much more likely to be malignant. When ovarian tumours are the result of metastases, signs or symptoms referrable to the primary disease in the breast, stomach or large bowel may be apparent.

Ancillary investigations

Malignant cells of ovarian origin may be seen in a Papanicolaou smear (usually when the disease is far advanced) or as a result of aspiration of fluid via the posterior fornix of the vagina. Neither method is suitable for use as a screening procedure, nor are they normally used as part of the investigation of a patient with an ovarian tumour.

Radiological studies of the upper and lower gastrointestinal tract are necessary if the ovarian tumour is thought to be metastatic, and X-rays of the chest should be taken to exclude metastases to the lungs or diaphragm. Intravenous pyelography is indicated to check on renal function and confirm renal tract anatomy. Lymphography, which has no place in the FIGO staging for ovarian cancer, is said to have 100% predictive value when the nodes are positive but only 87% predictive value when they are negative (Musumeci *et al.* 1977) but the technique does not displace or facilitate surgical intervention and is therefore not indicated.

Ultrasound can be useful in establishing the size and situation of tumours and in determining consistency, but it will not differentiate the benign from the malignant cyst nor demonstrate tumour deposits of less than 2 cm in diameter. Computer Assisted Tomography (CAT) scanning is being used much more often than was previously the case but has little to offer at this stage in the management of ovarian tumours. Early reports (Mamtora & Isherwood 1982, Solomon *et al.* 1983) of retrospective studies failed to demonstrate a clear benefit resulting from CAT scanning. Involved para-aortic nodes are often recognized but Sheils *et al.* (1984), in a prospective study of CAT in the staging of ovarian cancer, demonstrated its failure to differentiate benign disease from Stage I disease and whether adhesions and distant lesions were due to malignancy or unrelated pathology.

Laparoscopy can be useful if the exclusion of ovarian cancer means a laparotomy can be avoided. One such example is the postmenopausal woman with a small pelvic swelling which is most likely a subserous fibroid but which could be an ovarian cancer. Although laparoscopic diagnosis might seem attractive, needle biopsy to confirm a diagnosis might lead to the dissemination of malignant cells and is almost never indicated. Invariably the final diagnosis will be made at laparotomy.

Treatment

Surgery for an ovarian tumour is best done through a vertical lower abdominal incision, preferably paramedian, which can be extended above the level of the umbilicus so that adequate and safe surgery can be undertaken and any possible error in diagnosis overcome. It might however be reasonable to deal with a small ovarian cyst in the pelvis of a young woman, through a low transverse incision when the diagnosis has been confirmed by ultrasound.

BENIGN DISEASE

Whenever benign disease is confirmed, there is an opportunity to consider conservative treatment. Simple cysts may be enucleated from an ovary and the ovarian tissue reconstituted, though on occasions large cysts so involve an ovary that conservation of ovarian tissue on that side is impractical. If there is a solid component associated with the ovarian tumour then oophorectomy or salpingo-oophorectomy is to be preferred. In women over 45 years of age it is customary to remove both ovaries and the uterus, in the belief that further ovarian pathology will be avoided and secondly lest an unsuspected carcinoma be found in the single ovary removed which would have necessitated a second laparotomy.

The management of endometriosis presents particular problems and has been dealt with in Chapter 42 (p. 616).

MALIGNANT DISEASE

Current thinking on the surgical treatment of ovarian cancer demands that at the primary operation the surgeon should have the opportunity of confirming the diagnosis, staging the extent of the disease and then either undertaking a curative operation or, al-

ternatively, removing as much malignant tissue as is possible, a so-called debulking operation, so that the chance of success with subsequent chemotherapy or radiotherapy is improved. Staging of ovarian cancer is a surgical procedure and is done according to the FIGO recommendations in Table 48.2. It is clear therefore that the surgical incision must be such that the whole abdominal cavity can be explored and the tumour removed intact whenever possible.

Bloody ascitic fluid, bilateral tumours, irregularities of the cyst capsule, rupture of the cyst, or tumours which are partly solid and partly cystic, are all pointers to malignancy. Palpable lymph nodes or metastatic implants on viscera or the peritoneum are more significant signs. The extent of spread must be recorded carefully.

Ascitic fluid, if present, should be sent for cytological examination, otherwise 100 ml of normal saline should be instilled into the Pouch of Douglas and into each of the paracolic gutters in turn and then withdrawn for subsequent but immediate cytological evaluation. The liver and diaphragm should be inspected carefully and diaphragmatic nodules biopsied using laparoscopic biopsy forceps. Any enlarged para-aortic lymph nodes should also be removed for histological examination. A careful search of the peritoneal surfaces and of the large and small bowel should be undertaken and tissue removed for biopsy when appropriate. The omentum should be inspected and then removed, whether or not metastases are apparent to naked eye examination.

The careful and extensive evaluation of ovarian cancer, described above, has become necessary to explain the previously reported poor survival rates in women with apparent Stage I disease. Bagley et al. (1972) had attributed treatment failure to the subclinical metastases which were present outside the normal treatment field. Pemberton (1940) had much earlier recommended removal of the omentum during an operation for ovarian cancer so as to deal with gross or microscopic metastases and avoid a source of subsequent recurrence. Keettel and Elkins (1956) used peritoneal washings to demonstrate malignant cells in the peritoneal cavity in association with early disease, and Knapp and Friedman (1974) reported a prospective study dealing with the incidence of subclinical metastases in apparently normal omenta in State I disease. Data regarding diaphragmatic metastases were reported by Bagley et al (1973) and subsequently by Rosenhoff et al. (1975). Current data suggest that in apparent Stage I and Stage II disease cytological washings will be positive in 10–50% of cases, positive para-aortic nodes will be found in up to 20% of cases, omental secondaries will be present in 0–4.7% of patients, and diaphragmatic metastases will be confirmed in 0–44% of cases. All this would seem to explain the previous high mortality associated with early ovarian cancer.

The latest collected world data (FIGO 1982) on the distribution of patients in the different stages show 25% in Stage I, 18% in Stage II, 40% in Stage III and 18% in Stage IV, but since the patients were treated between 1973 and 1975 it is unlikely that the work referred to above would have been taken into account. The reader should be careful not to be misled by the apparent improvement in results of treatment of both early and late disease that might appear in future literature which is simply a consequence of modern staging and mathematical manipulation.

Initial treatment of Stage I and Stage II disease
The standard surgical treatment of apparent Stage I disease is to perform a total hysterectomy, bilateral salpingo-oophorectomy and omentectomy. The surgical treatment of Stage II disease is more complicated due to the fixity of the ovarian growth to other pelvic tissues. Hudson (1968, 1981) has advocated an extrapelvic approach which mobilizes the pelvic peritoneum with the pelvic tumour and allows removal of the tumour within a false capsule. Such a procedure, for success, is dependent on the fact that ovarian tumours, although involving serosal surfaces, rarely invade deeply.

This policy might be modified in a young woman whose fertility is to be protected. In such cases the tumour should be unilateral, encapsulated, free of adhesions, and well differentiated (i.e. borderline or grade 1); metastases should have been excluded and the contralateral apparently normal ovary examined carefully and biopsied. Frozen section facilities are needed if this management is to be undertaken safely. Endometrial curettage is needed if an endometrial primary is to be excluded. Whenever conservative surgery has been undertaken it is recommended that the patient is sterilized by removing the uterus and residual ovary when her family is complete (Williams *et al.* (1973)).

Further treatment of patients with Stage I and Stage II ovarian carcinoma
Adjuvant therapy is used to deal with subclinical metastases and the choices available to the clinician include the use of intraperitoneal radioactive substances, whole abdominal irradiation and systemic chemotherapy. There is no good evidence to suggest that adjuvant therapy, whether it be chemical or radiological, is of benefit to patients with borderline tumours.

Experience with intraperitoneal radioactive isotopes comes mainly from the American literature. Radioactive chromic phosphate (P32) and radioactive gold (Au198), have both been used and a retrospective analysis reported by Rosenshein *et al.* (1979). Ninety per cent cure rates can be expected, which is a significant improvement over surgery alone. Chromic phosphate is easier to use by virtue of its longer half-life and its higher beta energy which allows greater penetration of tissues. No isolation of the patient is necessary and the patient can be discharged from hospital the day following treatment. The one significant complication, intestinal obstruction, occurs rarely (1.2%), but if multiple adhesions are present in the peritoneal cavity, which would prevent an even distribution of the chemical, its use is best avoided.

Stage I disease. Retrospective data on the treatment of Stage I disease by surgery and adjuvant intraperitoneal P32 suggest an improved survival as compared with surgery alone. Hester and White (1969) gave a figure of 89%, Clark *et al.* (1973) 92.5% and Piver *et al.* (1972) 94%. These figures can be compared with five year survival figures quoted by Bagley *et al.* (1972) of 67% and Tobias and Griffiths (1976) of 70% for Stage I disease treated by surgery alone. A well controlled, prospective clinical trial on the use of P32 is necessary to judge accurately its efficacy and to establish if it is better than surgery alone.

Various studies have been undertaken to assess whether postoperative radiotherapy is necessary for all patients with Stage I disease, what form such therapy should take, and what benefits such therapy might confer on the patients to whom it is given. Dembo and Bush (1983) reported a clinical trial at the Princess Margaret Hospital, Toronto, in which no treatment was compared with pelvic irradiation after surgery. No curative benefit from pelvic irradiation was demonstrated, but those patients who had pelvic irradiation were less likely to develop pelvic recurrence. It became clear that, when irradiation was given, it should be directed at the whole peritoneal cavity and the study was therefore abandoned. Information was available from the trial which indicated that relapse occurred in patients with poorly or moderately differentiated tumour, and that postoperative X-ray therapy is not necessary if the tumour is well differentiated in its worst differentiated parts. It was also clear that the assessment of rupture of the cyst, ascites and capsule penetration were of dubious prognostic value.

In the United States the Gynecology Oncology Group (Hreshchyshyn et al. 1980), using more than twenty institutions, compared postoperative therapy using melphalan with postoperative pelvic irradiation. Neither method of postoperative therapy, when compared independently with no therapy, produced a significantly greater prevention of relapse, but it was noted that there were significantly fewer relapses in the melphalan treated patients than among those who received pelvic irradiation. This study has however been criticized because 49% of patients entered in it were removed from the analysis, and it is thought that the treatment aims thereafter may have been unequally matched with respect to the distribution of prognostic variables.

It would seem therefore that there are no data available which indicate that additional therapy improves the survival of patients with Stage I disease. Investigations continue and whilst they do it is the current practice in the Princess Margaret Hospital to give postoperative irradiation to the abdomen and pelvis to those Stage I patients at increased risk, i.e. those with poorly differentiated tumours.

Stage II disease. The number of patients presenting with Stage II disease is relatively few. It is thought (Fuks 1977) that surgery and irradiation offers a better prognosis than surgery alone. (The average five-year survival for surgery alone being 21% as compared with 32% five-year survival for surgery plus irradiation.) Smith and Rutledge (1975), reporting work from the M. D. Anderson Hospital and Tumour Institute, demonstrated that irradiation to the abdomen and pelvis was better than irradiation given to either the abdomen or pelvis alone or when radio-isotopes were used.

Treatment of Stage III and IV ovarian epithelial cancer
Since the first report of an objective response using melphalan (L-phenylalanine mustard) to treat advanced ovarian cancer alkylating agents have become the accepted single agent for cytoxic therapy in ovarian cancer. A partial response with the reduction in tumour size occurred in 54.8% of patients (Burns et al. 1963). As a result of second look laparotomy, Rutledge and Burns (1966) showed that inoperable tumour had disappeared following treatment with melphalan and that, after the drug had been discontinued, subsequent initial progress was satisfactory in

eleven out of thirteen patients. Later reports were less reassuring so that, latterly, complete response (that is a complete disappearance of all clinical and X-ray evidence of malignancy for a minimum of one month) has been observed in only 70% of patients.

Other available alkylating agents such as chlorambucil, cyclophosphamide and triethylenethyophosphoramide have been used with similar results (Smith & Rutledge 1970). Only those patients achieving a complete response showed a significant prolongation of survival, and even then the median survival was only nineteen months.

Other drugs have also been used. 5-fluorouracil and methotrexate have been shown to be active against ovarian adenocarcinoma as has cis-diaminodichloroplatinum. Wiltshaw and Kroner (1976), using this latter drug, demonstrated a 26% response rate when it was used as second line chemotherapy in patients whose initial treatment with an alkylating agent had failed. The efficacy of adriamycin was demonstrated by Bonadonna et al. (1975) and of hexamethylmelamine by Wharton et al. (1979). Chemotherapeutic agents used singly have been shown to achieve a complete response in 10–20% of patients, although this has never been adequate to demonstrate a long term improvement in survival.

Once it had been shown that cytotoxic drugs having differing modes of action were equally effective, oncologists, not surprisingly, investigated their use in combination so that the drugs could be used to interfere with different stages of the mitotic process in the malignant cells. Combination therapy was shown to achieve a higher response rate and, perhaps more importantly, a higher complete response rate than did treatment with melphalan alone. A combination of hexamethylmelamine, cyclophosphamide, methotrexate and 5-fluorouracil (HEXACAF) was shown by Young et al. (1978) to produce a 75% overall response rate, as compared with one of 54% for melphalan. The comparable complete response rates were 33% as compared with 16%. This work by Young and his colleagues has not been substantiated by other workers, and further investigations are necessary if the superiority of a multiple drug regimen with acceptable toxicity is to be demonstrated.

In the United Kingdom, a Medical Research Council Study on Advanced Ovarian Cancer (1981) compared the use of continuous oral cyclophosphamide with pulsed combination therapy using cyclophosphamide, hexamethylmelamine and methotrexate. The mortality attributed to cancer was somewhat less in those patients on combination therapy but such therapy was associated with a greater toxicity. The conclusion was that there was little evidence of greater clinical benefit using the triple regimen.

Wiltshaw and Kroner's work on cisplatinum as second line chemotherapy was followed by a report from Vogl et al. (1979) who used hexamethylmelamine in combination with adriamycin and cisplatinum as second line chemotherapy with a response rate of 67%. The same workers later added cyclophosphamide to the regimen and used the four drugs as primary chemotherapy, reporting a response rate of 90.4% in 21 patients with previously untreated ovarian adenocarcinoma, of which 46.7% of the patients had a complete response. Ehrlich et al. (1979) reported similar results (an overall response rate of 68.5% with a complete response rate of 37%) using a combination of cisplatinum, adriamycin and cyclophosphamide as primary therapy.

One other highly active combination has been described by Barlow et al. (1980), in which high dose methotrexate with citrovorum factor rescue and cyclophosphamide were used for primary therapy, with an overall response rate of 68% and a complete response rate of 48%.

The development of second generation platinum analogues has shown a number of them to be less toxic than cisplatinum in pre-clinical testing and several clinical trials using these drugs are in progress.

Chemotherapy regimes in current use are reviewed by Richardson et al. (1985) and it would seem that one which includes cisplatinum gives the Stage III or IV patient with residual disease the best chance of an identifiable response to therapy, but it should be remembered that evidence is not available which demonstrates an improved chance of survival.

Stem cell assay of chemotherapeutic agents
Human tumour cells can be grown in tissue culture media and then used to test the potency of cytotoxic drugs, so-called stem cell assay. Previously it was often the case that drug sensitivities did not correlate with the response *in vivo*, but recently better results have been achieved by Welander et al. (1983) who have shown 100% correlation when a negative response has been predicted and 53% when the response was positive. All patients under investigation had not received prior chemotherapy.

Cytotoxic drugs are expensive, and if unnecessary therapy can be avoided it will not only be of benefit to the patient but will also save valuable financial resources.

SECOND LOOK LAPAROTOMY AND LAPAROSCOPY

Wangensteen introduced the concept of second look laparotomy in 1949 to evaluate the progress of patients suffering from carcinoma of the colon (Wangensteen et al. 1951). At that time the purpose of the operation was to see whether further surgery for subclinical recurrence of the disease was required.

With the development of cytotoxic drugs second look surgery has been used in the management of ovarian cancer. Initially, patients whose disease at the time of the original operation had been too extensive or fixed to allow radical surgery were subsequently treated with melphalan, and then subjected to a second laparotomy to determine whether effective surgery had become possible (Rutledge & Burns 1966). More recently second look procedures have also been performed to see if cytotoxic therapy can be discontinued after a full course of treatment. Schwartz and Smith (1980) using melphalan found an increased satisfactory outcome when the number of treatments was increased from ten to twelve, and thus second look surgery was normally undertaken twelve months after the initial operation. Indefinite treatment with alkylating agents may lead to the development of acute nonlymphocytic leukaemia, and many of the newer cytotoxic agents have toxic side effects which do not allow treatment for longer than is absolutely necessary.

If at a second look operation subclinical residual disease is found, resection of the persisting or recurrent disease should be attempted prior to the use of an alternative cytotoxic agent though the prognosis in such patients is poor.

Were it not for the fact that most patients will have recurrent disease at second look laparotomy the alternative would be to discontinue treatment without confirmation of the true state of the disease, but unfortunately if the patient is left until there are clinical signs of recurrence further effective treatment is rarely possible.

Second look laparotomy should not be confused with delayed primary surgery, i.e. a second operation done for a patient whose first operation had been incomplete by virtue of the inadequate experience of the surgeon, nor with the case in which a laparotomy proves to be necessary to deal with a late complication of the disease such as intestinal obstruction.

Procedure
Prior to a second look procedure, preliminary investigation should include a chest X-ray and an intra-

venous pyelogram. A formal preoperative bowel preparation should be undertaken. A vertical incision such as is used in a staging laparotomy is performed. Peritoneal fluid is sent for cytological assessment or, if none is present, fluid is instilled into each of the paracolic gutters and into the Pouch of Douglas and then recovered for cytological examination. The peritoneal cavity is explored by inspection and palpation, and then multiple biopsies are taken from suspicious areas and from sites known to be at risk such as the peritoneal surfaces, the serosa of the colon, and the inferior surface of the diaphragm. The omentum, if still present, should be removed. Any retroperitoneal nodules should be removed along with a sample of the paraaortic lymph nodes.

Patients developing recurrent disease after a negative second look laparotomy will normally do so within six to twenty-eighth months (Schwartz & Smith 1980).

Second look laparoscopy
Laparoscopy is inadequate as a method of excluding persisting disease since all possible areas of persistent or recurrent disease cannot be seen with the laparoscope, but can be helpful in monitoring patients with known diseases who are undergoing chemotherapy. It may, for example, be a satisfactory alternative to laparotomy when information is needed to allow a decision on the need to change a chemotherapeutic agent.

IMMUNOTHERAPY

Immunotherapy is still in its infancy, as yet of unproven value, and should be regarded as experimental. An impaired immune status has been demonstrated in patients with malignant disease, and in patients with ovarian cancer it has been suggested that there is a relationship between the immunological status of the patient and the progress of the disease. Laboratory work has identified tumour-associated antigens and antibodies with antitumour activity but all the tests lack specificity.

Immunotherapy can be non-specific or specific. Corynebacterium Parvum (C. Parvum) and Bacillus-Calmette-Guerin (BCG) are two of the best known non-specific stimulators of cell mediated immunity. Alberts *et al.* (1979) demonstrated an unproved response and survival using BCG with adriamycin and cyclophosphamide in the treatment of patients with Stage III, Stage IV and recurrent ovarian cancer.

Creaseman *et al.* (1979) showed similar benefits, although this was in a trial without randomization, using C. Parvum with melphalan, as compared with melphalan alone. C. Parvum, given intraperitoneally, has been used with some degree of success by Mantovani *et al.* (1981) to reduce the amount of ascitic fluid associated with ovarian cancer, whilst Miller *et al.* (1979) have shown intrapleural C. Parvum to be more effective than nitrogen mustard in controlling pleural effusions associated with malignancy.

Specific immunotherapy implies the use of tumour associated antigens. Hudson *et al.* (1979) used allogeneic irradiated tumour cells (and BCG), given by intradermal inoculation to patients with advanced or recurrent cancer. Improved survival in the short term was seen but there were no long term survivors. Similar work has been done elsewhere.

Interferons, proteins secreted by virus treated cells which can then absorb onto other cells and give them resistance to virus infection, have been used as a possible agent against human cancers. Animal work had previously shown an effect against tumours thought to be produced by oncogenic viruses. Human leucocyte interferon was given by Einhorn *et al.* (1982) to a small number of patients with ovarian cancer with some benefit, and at least one prospective study evaluating interferon is in progress. Other such studies are necessary to determine the place of immunotherapy in cancer management.

TUMOUR MARKERS

Tumour markers are proteins, selectively produced by tumour cells, which upon release into the circulation can be measured in peripheral blood. Immunological methods are usually employed. To be an ideal marker the specific protein would be produced by the tumour in its earliest stage so allowing a rapid diagnosis. The concentration of the tumour marker would fall following treatment but rise again should a recurrence occur. Of the available markers few have the specificity to be of value in clinical work. Ovarian tumour markers fall into four groups:

Carcinoplacental antigens include placental alkaline phosphatases, which are elevated in a substantial number of patients with ovarian cancer but also with other cancers, and placental hormones such as human chorionic gonadotrophin (HCG). Beta-HCG is elevated in over 90% of patients with specific germ cell tumours (embryonal carcinoma and ovarian choriocarcinoma) and measurement of this marker can be of value in the management of patients with such tumours.

Carcinoembryonic antigen (CEA), alphafetoprotein (AFP), beta-oncofetoprotein (BOFA) and fetal ferritin are all *fetal proteins*. They are found in a variety of tumours and in normal tissue. CEA is produced not only by many ovarian epithelial tumours but also by cervical and endometrial cancers amongs others. Its lack of specificity means it is not helpful in differentiating the various types of tumour. AFP however is a specific marker for endodermal sinus tumour of the ovary, embryonal cancer of the ovary and ovarian teratomata which contain either of these elements.

Tumour associated antigens are glycoproteins present on the surface of ovarian cancer cells. They are usually recognized in peripheral blood by immunoassay. Ovarian tumour antigen (OCA) and ovarian cystadenocarcinoma associated antigen (OCAA) levels are elevated in more than 70% of patients with ovarian tumour and ovarian cystadenocarcinoma respectively, but in neither case is the specificity sufficient to make them of established clinical value.

Miscellaneous tumour markers, the fourth group, include fibrin degradation products (FDP), galactosyl transferase and alpha-L-fucosidase. Alpha-L-fucosidase is present in diminished levels in patients with ovarian cancer and may prove to be of value in the early diagnosis of ovarian cancer (Bhattachanja & Barlow 1979).

There are also other potential uses for tumour markers. If, for example, radio-labelled antibodies raised against specific tumour associated antigens will accumulate in tumour tissue they might be used to identify primary or metastatic tumour with the aid of a gamma scintillation camera. If antibodies can be coupled with chemotherapeutic agents or radiotherapeutic sources, then there is the potential for concentrating the agent in the tumour, assuming that the antibody reacts with the tumour specific antigens.

RESULTS OF TREATMENT

The results of the treatment of ovarian cancer vary considerably depending on histological type, stage and grade. In general those patients having the longest tumour-free interval will have the best prognosis. If all cases of ovarian cancer are considered together (i.e. both epithelial and special tumours) five-year survival figures as shown in Table 48.4 have been achieved world wide. It should be remembered that five-year survival figures relating to the more recently introduced aggressive chemotherapy are not yet available. Data for obvious malignancy published in 1985 differ very little (FIGO 1985).

SPECIAL OVARIAN TUMORS

Sex cord stromal tumours
Gonadal mesenchymal stroma gives rise to ovarian stromal cells and their theca and luteal derivatives. The cells within the developing gonads that have been called sex cords give rise to the granulosa cells of the ovary. All tumours which include these various cell types, singly or in combination, are called sex cord stromal tumours. Some of these tumours produce steroid hormones, giving rise to oestrogenic or androgenic changes, and the tumours have in the past frequently been referred to as feminizing tumours (granulosa and theca cell tumours) and masculinizing tumours (androblastoma, previously known as arrhenoblastoma). It should be emphasized that it is current practice to classify such varieties of tumour on a morphological basis and not according to their possible hormonal effect.

Table 48.4. Results of treatment of ovarian cancer: percentage 5 year survival.

Stage	Ia	Ib	Ic	IIa	IIb/c	III	IV
Obvious malignancy							
(5268 patients)	69.7	63.9	50.3	51.8	42.4	13.3	4.1
Borderline malignancy							
(304 patients)	87.4	82.6	—	—	77.8	33.3	—

Data taken from Clinical Report on the results of treatment in gynaecological cancer. International Federation of Obstetrics and Gynecology, 1982.

Data based on 5268 patients with obvious malignancy and 304 patients with borderline malignancy treated between 1973–1975 in seventy-six institutions.

Where no figure is given the number of patients is too small for significant analysis.

Granulosa cell tumours

Granulosa cell tumours are said to account for about 2% of ovarian tumours and less than 10% ovarian cancers. They occur in any age group, are usually unilateral and vary in size from an impalpable small nodule to a large tumour. The tumours are often lobulated and vary in consistency, being mainly solid but partly cystic. The colour may be yellow or, if cysts containing bloodstained fluid are present, red or blue. The gross appearances are of such variation as to mimic almost any other type of ovarian neoplasm. The granulosa cells appear in sheets, sometimes taking on a microfollicular pattern (so-called Call-Exner bodies), and are separated by fibroblasts or theca cells of ovarian stromal origin. The granulosa cells are characteristically round, ovoid or angular with an eosinophilic cytoplasm and indistinct cell boundaries. Luteinization of the cells is sometimes seen.

Associated endometrial abnormalities are common. Cystic hyperplasia of the endometrium is seen quite commonly and less often atypical endometrial hyperplasia. It is believed that there is an association between granulosa cell tumours and endometrial adenocarcinoma, and Fox and Langley (1976) report a prevalence of endometrial adenocarcinoma in 6.6% of their cases which fits quite closely with a figure of 6% reported by Diddle (1952) from a series of over a thousand cases of granulosa cell tumours.

Theca cell tumours

It is only an arbitrary line which distinguishes fibromas which consist entirely of fibroblast like-cells producing collagen from thecomas which contain predominantly lipid-rich theca-like cells.

Fibromas

Fibromas are large, hard, mobile, lobulated tumours with a white glistening surface and are bilateral in about 10% of cases. They are often associated with ascites; and in a small proportion ascites and hydrothorax, usually right sided, are found in association with a benign fibroma. Meigs, whose name is given to the syndrome, drew attention to the benign and curable nature of the condition. Both the ascites and the hydrothorax should resolve after removal of the tumour.

Thecomas

Thecomas have the appearances, to a varying degree, of theca interna cells of the Graafian follicle containing fibroblast type cells and rounded cells which contain lipid. When this is present in moderate to large amounts, the tumour is sometimes described as a luteinized thecoma. Oestrogenic changes are sometimes seen in association with thecomas, and morphological changes in the endometrium occur similar to those seen in association with granulosa cell tumours. It is unusual for fibromas and thecomas to be malignant. Fibrosarcomas, when they occur, firstly spread within the pelvis, later to the peritoneum of the abdominal cavity, and at a later date disseminate via the lymphatics to distant organs such as the lung, liver and bones.

Germ cell tumours

These tumours, derived from multipotential germ cells, occur most commonly in the second or third decade of life. Unilateral disease occurs in two-thirds of patients. Teilum (1965) described their potential to develop as dysgerminoma or as embryonal carcinomas. These latter tumours can be either embryonic, i.e. teratomata or extra embryonic tumours such as endodermal sinus tumour, or choriocarcinoma of the ovary.

Dysgerminomas

These tumours are often found as a large lobulated mass, pale yellow or cream in colour with a consistency that varies from soft to firm. They are surrounded by a fibrous capsule. Histological examination shows them to consist of rounded polyhedral cells which contain abundant clear cytoplasm rich in glycogen. The nuclei are central and the nucleoli are often prominent. Lymphocytes are sometimes seen in the connective tissue. Rarely, cells with the appearance of syncytiotrophoblast may be present and, if they are, chorionic gonadotrophin is secreted. Oestrogenic and androgenic manifestations may be seen.

The tumours usually present in the second or third decades of life, and are bilateral in 10–20% of cases. They are sometimes found in patients with subnormal gonadal development or pseudohermaphroditism. Patients often present with abdominal swelling or pain, and on occasions as an acute abdominal emergency due to some accident to the tumour, most commonly torsion.

Malignant metastases, when they occur, often do so late in the disease process. The best guide to the prognosis is the extent of the spread found at operation.

If, at laparotomy, the disease appears unilateral then it is worth doing a biopsy on the contralateral ovary for frozen section and taking biopsies of any palpable pelvic or paraaortic nodes. If there is no evidence of spread and the patient is young and wanting children, conservative treatment with a unilateral salpingo-oophorectomy is reasonable. In such a patient it would be important to follow her progress with careful clinical examinations and chest X-rays, and many would argue in favour of a second look laparotomy some nine months after primary surgery.

If the disease has already spread at the time of operation or the patient is not wanting children, then a total abdominal hysterectomy, bilateral salpingo-oophorectomy and omentectomy should be followed by external irradiation (the tumour is radiosensitive) to the abdomen and pelvis, and to the paraaortic areas if paraaortic node biopsies are positive.

Should recurrence occur cytoreductive surgery followed by further external irradiation is indicated if tissue tolerance allows but, if not, chemotherapy using vincristine, actinomycin D and cyclophosphamide (VAC) is worthwhile.

Five year survival rates for pure dysgerminoma are around 90–95%.

If a young patient has been treated in a conservative way, there is good reason for doing a total hysterectomy and unilateral salpingo-oophorectomy when she has completed her family, and following this by external irradiation if there is any suggestion of recurrence having occurred.

Endodermal sinus tumours

These highly malignant germ cell tumours were once known as Mesonephromas Ovarii or as Yolk Sac Tumours. The gross appearance is of encapsulated smooth but nodular tumours, grey or yellow in colour, which by virtue of underlying haemorrhage, degeneration and necrosis, become friable and undergo rupture.

They grow rapidly, usually presenting with an obvious abdominal or pelvic mass, abdominal pain and sometimes the effects of rupture. Serum AFP is usually raised and can be used as a tumour marker but the serum HCG level is not elevated.

As with other germ cell tumours if the patient is young and the other ovary normal unilateral oophorectomy should be performed, if not radical cytoreductive surgery is indicated. Postoperative chemotherapy using VAC has resulted in an improved prognosis (68% alive at two years or more) whereas previously a 95% mortality within two years would have been expected.

Embryonal carcinomas

Kurman and Norris (1976) described these germ cell tumours resembling embryonal carcinoma of testis, which could be distinguished from endodermal sinus tumour by histological and histochemical means. Embryonal carcinomas are solid but soft tumours, subject to haemorrhage and necrosis. Presentation is usually as a result of pain and a pelvic mass, but in young individuals precocious puberty may be seen.

Elevated serum levels of both AFP and HCG are found and can be used as tumour markers following surgery and chemotherapy (normally VAC). The prognosis is somewhat better than that expected for endodermal sinus tumour.

Choriocarcinomas

Ovarian choriocarcinomas are rare tumours. When they occur, they are most commonly nongestational and often mixed with other germ cell elements. If gestational, they are more likely to be uterine metastases than primary ovarian tumours. Progress is monitored using serum beta-HCG levels as a tumour marker. Chemotherapy, after prior surgery, most usually involves the agents methotrexate, actinomycin D and chlorambucil.

Teratomas

Germ cell tumours differentiating along embryonic lines can result in benign cystic teratomas, benign cystic teratomas with malignant change or solid teratomas.

Monophyletic teratomas containing only one tissue are rare and include such tumours as carcinoid tumour of the ovary, struma ovarii, strumal carcinoid and primary malignant melanoma of the ovary.

Benign cystic teratomas, often called ovarian dermoids, account for 97% of ovarian teratomata and 10–20% of ovarian neoplasms. The fully differentiated tissue is most commonly squamous, but mesodermal and endodermal elements are often seen. Ten to seventeen per cent are bilateral. They are usually around 5–15 cm in diameter, often heavy for their size and frequently on a long pedicle. These latter features account for a ready liability to torsion. The cysts have a wrinkled outer surface, are variable in colour, are fluctuant until cool when they feel 'doughy', and they contain a brownish-grey greasy material with the features of sebum. Hair with any of a wide variety of characteristics is frequently found in the cyst, along with teeth in one-third of cases. Osseus tissue is less commonly found.

The cysts can occur at any age, but 90% occur in

women of reproductive age so it is not surprising that they are the commonest ovarian cyst to be found in pregnancy.

They present as a swelling, perhaps with pain, dyspareunia, backache or urinary symptoms. Symptoms may be due to complications such as torsion, rupture or infection. Rupture can occur into the bladder, causing pilomicturition, or less commonly into the rectum.

Removal of the tumour is indicated to deal with symptoms and avoid complications. Conservation of ovarian tissue on the affected side is acceptable but bisection of the contralateral ovary is indicated to exclude bilateral disease.

In 1–2% of cases benign cystic teratomata undergo malignant change. Squamous carcinomata is the result in 85%, but many other varieties of tumour are found such as adenocarcinoma, carcinoids, sarcomas or melanomas.

Treatment is such as would be recommended for epithelial ovarian tumours. The prognosis is poor.

Solid teratomas
Although called solid, these tumours often have microcystic areas. They tend to be large unilateral tumours with a white, brown or yellow surface and though encapsulated the surface is irregular. Underlying haemorrhage and necrosis makes them friable. Benign (mature) variants are rare but immature malignant teratomata constitute the third commonest germ cell tumour. They contain a wide variety of tissues from 2 to 3 germ layers.

They spread by direct extension and implantation. Lymphatic spread is uncommon as are metastases. When seen, metastases are usually to brain or lung.

It is thought important to grade carefully the tumour (Norris & Adams 1981) the incidence of recurrence being related to the tumour grading.

As with other germ cell tumours, young people are affected with a mean age presentation of around 16 years for immature teratomata. The presenting symptoms are usually due to the pelvic or abdominal mass which is invariably present. Neither AFP nor beta-HCG levels will be elevated.

When possible unilateral surgery is first performed. Patients with Grade 0 and Grade 1 tumours are then kept under observation, but those with Grade 2 or 3 tumours are given chemotherapy using VAC. Regimens using platinum derivatives are being tried but experience is limited. Radiotherapy seems ineffective for these highly malignant tumours. Prior to modern chemotherapy patients with Grade 3 tumours would

not survive, and the rate of survival of those with lesser gradings was 40–50%.

Androblastomas (Sertoli–Leydig tumours)
Androblastomas is a term for tumours, previously called arrhenoblastomas, which are sex cord tumours containing Sertoli and Leydig cells with an indifferent stroma. Morris and Scully (1958) prefer the term Sertoli–Leydig tumours because only 80% of them are masculinizing, some being feminizing or inert. Testosterone levels will be elevated in those with viri.-lization.

Subclassification is according to the degree of differentiation. All have well differentiated Leydig cells as seen in the male testis. Well differentiated tumours have hollow tubules separated by Leydig cells, whilst the intermediate variety have more primitive Sertoli cells arranged in cords as in the immature testis. Poorly differentiated tumours are sarcomatoid, containing cells resembling spindle cell sarcoma. This last group includes those tumours which contain heterologous elements such as argentaffin cells, cartilage, skeletal muscle or mucus secreting epithelium.

The tumours have a gross appearance similar to granulosa cell tumours and only 1–3% are bilateral. Because patients are most often in the 2nd or 3rd decades of life this allows conservative surgery when there is a need to maintain fertility, otherwise a total hysterectomy and bilateral salpingo-oophorectomy is indicated. One may expect 94% of patients to survive the disease with surgery alone, but when poorly differentiated sarcomatoid lesions are found postoperative radiotherapy should be considered but it is of unproven value. Recurrences warrant therapy with VAC.

Lipid cell tumours
Lipid cell and lipoid cell are terms applied to ovarian tumours containing cells with the appearance of steroid hormone producing cells, e.g. lutein cells, adrenocortical cells and Leydig cells. They may or may not have a high lipid content, but when they do they are yellow or orange in colour and reddish-brown when the lipid content is low. Virilization occurs in 75% of patients and symptoms of hyperoestrogenism are found in 25%. The tumours are almost always unilateral and therefore salpingo-oophorectomy is normally sufficient for the young patient.

Hilus cell tumours are found both in the ovarian hilus and elsewhere in the ovary. The cells contain lipid and are benign.

Gonadoblastomas

These rare tumours almost always occur in the gonads of intersexual patients. The patients are usually phenotypically female with hypoplastic uteri and tubes and streak gonads. Primary amenorrhoea is usual and sex chromatin is negative. The degree of malignancy is dependent on the germ cell content of the tumour.

Because the patients are infertile both gonads should be removed whether or not the tumour is unilateral.

OVARIAN METASTASES

Eight to ten per cent of ovarian tumours presenting clinically with an adnexal mass are metastatic, most commonly from primary disease in the gastrointestinal tract. Secondary spread from breast carcinoma is very common (more than 25% of ovaries removed therapeutically from patients with breast cancer contain metastases) though may be subclinical.

Of gynaecological tumours 8–10% of endometrial lesions spread to the ovary. Spread from primary disease in the tube is seen, but direct spread from the vulva, vagina or cervix is extremely rare.

Krukenberg tumours, the best known metastatic tumours, result from primary tumours with mucus secreting cells, i.e. usually from stomach or colon. In such cells the nucleus is peripheral and the cells have a signet ring appearance. The tumours are usually bilateral, solid, often reniform in shape and have a smooth surface with a soapy feel.

Metastatic tumours should be removed whenever possible, as would be the case with primary ovarian disease, but long term survival in such patients is unusual.

OVARIAN SARCOMAS

Primary ovarian sarcomas account for less than 1% of malignant ovarian tumours. They usually occur in postmenopausal women of low parity. Adenosarcomas, carcinosarcomas, mixed mesodermal sarcomas and fibrosarcomas are all seen, but rarely. The tumours, with the exception of adenosarcomas, are characterized by rapid growth and wide spread and a high mortality. Treatment is by way of radical surgery, and although additional radiotherapy and multiple agent chemotherapy has been tried little has been achieved.

OVARIAN TUMOURS IN PREGNANCY

Ovarian tumours are found in 1 in 1000 pregnancies. Corpus luteum cysts account for 10%, and 5% are malignant. The remainder are most often benign epithelial tumours, germ cell tumours or gonadal stromal tumours.

If a smooth, mobile unilateral ovarian tumour is found in early pregnancy observation until the second trimester will reduce the risk of abortion resulting from premature intervention.

Ultrasound scanning can be used to detect any change in size and to recognize features such as consistency or septa.

If the tumour persists laparotomy is indicated. Unilateral intervention is adequate for benign disease. Malignant disease is treated as in the non-pregnant patient, remembering that the pregnancy will not affect the cancer nor will the cancer affect the pregnancy.

In the third trimester the tumour will be dealt with by elective Caesarean section and the appropriate surgical management. Timing will depend on whether the tumour is malignant or not, the viability of the fetus and the wishes of the patient.

Unrecognized ovarian cysts are liable to torsion in the early puerperium, though this probably occurs less often than was previously the case by virtue of routine ultrasound investigations in pregnancy.

Inspection of the tubes and ovaries at the time of any Caesarean section should be routine practice.

REFERENCES

ACHESON E.D., GARDNER M.J., PIPPARD E.C. & GRIME L.P. (1982) *Brit. J. industr. Med.*, **39**, 344.

ANNEGERS J.F., STROM H., DECKER D.G., DOCKERTY M.B. & O'FALLON W.M. (1979) *Cancer*, **43**, 723.

ALBERTS D.S., MOON T.E., STEPHENS R.A., WILSON H., OISHI N., HILGERS R.D., O'TOOLE R. & THIGPEN J.T. (1979) *Cancer Treat. Rep.*, **63**, 325.

BAGLEY C.M. JR., YOUNG R.C., CANELLOS G.P. & DEVITA T. (1972) *New Engl. J. Med.*, **287**, 856.

BAGLEY C.M. JR., YOUNG R.C., SCHEIN P.S., CHABNER B.A. & DEVITA V.T. (1973) *Amer. J. Obstet. Gynec.*, **116**, 397.

BARLOW J.J., PIVER M.S. & LELE S.B. (1980) *Cancer*, **46**, 1333.

BERAL V., FRAZER P. & CHILVERS C. (1978) *Lancet*, **i**, 1083.

BHATTACHARYA M. & BARLOW J.J. (1979) *Int. Advances surg. Oncol.*, **2**, 155.

BONADONNA G., BERRETTA G., TANCINI G. *et al.* (1975) *Cancer Chemotherapy Reports*, **6 (2)**, 231.

Burns B.C., Rutledge F. & Gallagher H.S. (1963) *Obstet. and Gynec.*, **22**, 30.

Byers T., Marshall J., Graham S., Mettlin C. & Swanson M. (1983) *J. nat. Cancer Inst.*, **71**, 681.

Casagrande J.T., Louie E.W., Pike M.C., Roy S., Ross R.K. & Henderson B.E. (1979) *Lancet*, **ii**, 170.

Clark D.G.C., Hilaria B., Roussis C. & Brunschwig A. (1973) *Clinical Cancer*, vol. 5, p. 227. Grune & Stratton, New York.

Cramer D.W., Welch W.R., Scully R.E. & Wajciechowski C.A. (1982) *Cancer*, **50**, 372.

Creasman W.T., Gall S.A., Blessing J.A., Schmidt H.J., Abu-Ghazaleh S., Whisnant J.K. & Disaia P.J. (1979) *Cancer Treat. Rep.*, **63**, 319.

Dembo A.J. & Bush R.S. (1983) In *Gynecologic Oncology* (Griffiths C.T. & Fuller A.F. eds.). p. 263. Nijhoff, Boston.

Diddle A.W. (1952) *Cancer*, **5**, 215.

Ehrlich C.E., Einhorn L., William S.D. & Morgan J. (1979) *Cancer Treat. Rep.*, **63**, 281.

Einhorn N., Cantell K., Einhorn S. & Strander H. (1982) *Amer. J. clin. Oncol.*, **5**, 167.

Fathalla M.F. (1971) *Lancet*, **ii**, 163.

FIGO (1971) *Acta obstet. gynec. scand.*, **50**, 1.

FIGO (1982) Annual report on the results of treatment in gynecological cancer. Statements of results obtained in 1973 to 1975 inclusive. Edited by H.L. Kottmeier, p. 20.

FIGO (1985) Annual report on results of treatment in gynaecological cancer. Statements of results obtained in 1976–1978. Edited by F. Pettersson.

Fox H. & Langley F.A. (1976) *Tumours of the Ovary*. Heinemann, London.

Fuks Z. (1977) *Israel J. med. Sci.*, **13**, 815.

Golan A., Joosting A.C.S. & Orchard M.E. (1979) *Sth. Afr. med. J.*, **56**, 18.

Henderson W.J., Joslin C.A.F., Turnbull A.C. & Griffiths K. (1971) *J. Obstet. Gynaec. Brit. Cwlth.*, **78**, 266.

Hester L.L. & White L. (1969) *Amer. J. Obstet. Gynec.*, **103**, 911.

Hildreth N.G., Kelsey J.L., Livolsi V.A., Fischer D.B., Holford T.R., Mostow E.D., Swartz P.E. & White C. (1981) *Amer. J. Epidemiol.*, **114**, 398.

Hreshchyshyn M.M., Park R.C., Blessing J.A., Norris H.J., Levy D., Lagasse L.D. & Creasman W.T. (1980) *Amer. J. Obstet. Gynec.*, **138**, 139.

Hudson C.N., Crowther M. & Levin L. (1979) *Recent results in Ca research* (Mathe G. ed).

Hudson C.N. (1968) *J. Obstet. Gynaec. Brit. Cwlth.*, **75**, 1155.

Hudson C.N. (1979) *Brit. J. Obstet. Gynaec.*, **86**, 154.

Hudson C.N. (1981) *Ann. roy. Coll. Surg. Engl.*, **63**, 118.

Keal E.E. (1960) *Lancet*, **ii**, 1211.

Keettel W.C. & Elkins H.B. (1956) *Amer. J. Obstet. Gynec.*, **71**, 553.

Knapp R.C. & Friedman E.A. (1974) *Amer. J. Obstet. Gynec.*, **119**, 1013.

Kurman R.J. & Norris H.J. (1976) *Cancer*, **38**, 2420.

La Vecchia C., Franceschi S., Gallus G., De Carli A.,

Liberati A. & Tognoni G. (1983) *Int. J. Epidemiol.*, **12**, 161.

Long R.T., Spratt J.S. Jr. & Dowling E. (1969) *Amer. J. Surg.*, **117**, 162.

Mamtora H. & Isherwood I. (1982) *Clin. Radiol.*, **33**, 165.

Mantovani A., Sessa C., Peri G., Allavena P., Introna M., Polentarutti N. & Mangioni C. (1981) *Brit. J. Cancer*, **27**, 437.

Masson J.C. & Ochsenhirt N.C. (1929) *Surg. Gynec. Obstet.*, **48**, 702.

Matheson J.A.B., Matheson H. & Anderson S.A. (1981) *J. roy. Coll. gen. Practit.*, **31**, 743.

Medical Research Council, Working Party of Ovarian Cancer (1981) *Brit. J. Obstet. Gynaec.*, **88**, 1174.

Meigs J.V. & Cass J.W. (1937) *Amer. J. Obstet. Gynec.*, **33**, 249.

Miller J.W., Hunter A. & Horne N.W. (1979) *Thorax*, **35**, 856.

Morris J.M. & Scully R.E. (1958) *Endocrine pathology of the ovary*, p. 89l Mosby, St. Louis.

Musumeci R., Banfi A., Bolis G., Candani G.B., De Palo G., Di Re F., Lucina L., Lattuada A., Mangioni C., Mattioli G. & Natale N. (1977) *Cancer*, **40**, 1444.

Newhouse M.L., Berry G., Wagner J.C. & Thurok M.E. (1972) *Brit. J. industr. Med.*, **29**, 134.

Newhouse M.L., Pearson R.M., Fullerton J.M., Boeson E.A. & Shannon H.S. (1977) *Brit. J. prev. soc. Med.*, **31**, 148.

Norris H.J. & Adam A.E. (1981) In *Gynecologic Oncology* (Coppleson M. ed.) Vol 2, p. 680. Churchill Livingstone, Edinburgh.

Office of Population Censuses and Surveys (1981) Cancer Statistics: incidence, survival and mortality in England and Wales, **34**, 76.

Pemberton F.A. (1940) *Amer. J. Obstet. Gynec.*, **40**, 751.

Piver M.S. (1972) *Obstet. and Gynecol.*, **40**, 42.

Piver M.S., Lele S. & Barlow J.J. (1976) *Obstet. and Gynecol.*, **48**, 312.

Piver M.S., Barlow J.J. & Lele S.B. (1978) *Obstet. and Gynec.*, **52**, 100.

Richardson G.S., Scully, R.E., Nikrui N. & Nelson J.H. (1985) *New Engl. J. Med.*, **312**, 415.

Risch H.A., Weiss N.S., Lyon J.L., Daling J.R. & Liff J.M. (1983) *Amer. J. Epidemiol.*, **117**, 128.

Rosenhoff S.H., DeVita V.T. Jr., Hubbard S. & Young R.C. (1975) *Sem. Oncol.*, **2**, 223.

Rosenshein N.B., Leichner P.K. & Vogelsang G. (1979) *Obstet. gynec. Surv.*, **34**, 708.

Rutledge F. & Burns B.C. (1966) *Amer. J. Obstet. Gynec.*, **96**, 761.

Schwartz P.E. & Smith J.P. (1980) *Amer. J. Obstet. Gynec.*, **138**, 1124.

Serov S.F., Scully R.E. & Sobin L.H. (1973) International Histological Classification of Tumours No. 9: Geneva Histological Typing of Ovarian Tumours, World Health Organization.

Shaw W.F. (1932) *J. Obstet. Gynaec. Brit. Emp.*, **39**, 234.

SHIELS R., PEEL K.R., MACDONALD H.N., THOROGOOD J. & ROBINSON P.J. (1984) *Brit. J. Obstet. Gynaec.*, **92**, 407.

SMITH J.P. & RUTLEDGE F. (1970) *Amer. J. Obstet. Gynec.*, **107**, 691.

SMITH J.P. & RUTLEDGE F. (1975) In *Progress in Gynecology* (Taymor M.L. & Green T.H. eds.) Vol. 6, p. 627. Grune & Stratton, New York.

SMITH P.G. (1977) *Cancer*, **53** (Suppl), 1901.

SOLOMON A., BRENNER H.J., RUBINSTEIN Z., CHAITCHIK S. & MORAG B. (1983) *Gynec. Oncol.*, **15**, 48.

TAYLOR H.C. (1929) *Surg. Gynecol. Obstet.*, **48**, 204.

TEILUM G. (1965) *Acta path. microbiol. scand.*, **64**, 407.

TOBIAS J.S. & GRIFFITHS C.T. (1976) *New Engl. J. Med.*, **294**, 818.

VOGL S.E., BERENZWEIG M., KAPLAN B., MOUKHTAR M. & BULKIN W. (1979) *Cancer Treat. Rep.*, **63**, 311.

WANGENSTEEN O.H., LEWIS F.J. & TONGEN L.A. (1951) *J-Lancet.*, **71**, 303.

WELANDER C.E., HOMESLEY H.D. & JOBSON V.W. (1983) *Amer. J. Obstet. Gynec.*, **147**, 188.

WEST R.O. (1966) *Cancer*, **19**, 1001.

WHARTON J.T., RUTLEDGE F., SMITH J.P., HERSON J. & HODGE M.P. (1979) *Amer. J. Obstet. Gynec.*, **133**, 833.

WILLIAMS T.J., SYMMONDS R.E. & LITWAK O. (1973) *Gynec. Oncol.*, **1**, 143.

WILTSHAW E. & KRONER T. (1976) *Cancer Treat. Rep.*, **160**, 55.

YOUNG R.C., CHABNER B.A., HUBBARD S.P., FISHER R.I., BENDER R.A., ANDERSON T., SIMON R.M., CANELLOS G.P. & DeVITA V.T. Jr. (1978) *New Engl. J. Med.*, **299**, 1261.

CHAPTER 49
MALIGNANT DISEASE OF THE VULVA AND VAGINA

K. R. PEEL

VULVAL CARCINOMA

Carcinoma of the vulva is a rare condition seen by the average British gynaecologist only once or twice per year. For informed opinion, the gynaecologist is reliant on the work of individuals who have attracted and treated large numbers of patients with the disease such as Rothschild (1912), Taussig (1941), Way (1954, 1982), Green et al. (1958), Green (1978) and Franklin and Rutledge (1971).

The clinical work of Taussig was based on earlier descriptions of surgical and post-mortem material in Basset's MD thesis of 1912. It was he who described the lymph drainage upon which modern radical vulvar surgery is based. More recent work on lymphatic drainage by Way (1948), Green et al. (1958), Parry-Jones (1960) and Reiffenstuhl (1964) has led to more conservative surgery being undertaken in some instances.

AETIOLOGY

The aetiology of vulval carcinoma is unknown but it has long been realized that women at higher risk are menopausal or postmenopausal with a history of chronic vulvitis. Krupp (1981) reports 18% of his cases of vulval carcinoma were preceded by vulvar granulomatous venereal disease and 14% by hypertrophic leukoplakia. One per cent of cases were the result of malignant change in condylomata acuminata. Carcinoma of the vulva in the majority of cases is a disease of older women. Way (1982) described 28.5% of patients aged over 70 years at presentation, 38.5% in the age group 60–70 years and only 1.8% in women under 30 years. In his experience when the disease occurs in women under 20 years, it is invariably a sarcoma.

Marital status and parity are not of significance but the disease is more common in women in social classes III, IV and V. The vulval skin is analogous to scrotal skin, and 'mule spinner's cancer' is seen in both the male as scrotal carcinoma and the female as vulval carcinoma. Premalignant changes in vulval skin have been discussed in detail in Chapter 46.

PATHOLOGY

Vulval carcinomas are frequently painful ulcers but hypertrophic lesions are seen and flat non-ulcerative lesions are seen infrequently. These latter lesions are hard on palpation, painful and often associated with 'peau d'orange'.

The tumours are usually seen in the anterior part of the vulva affecting mainly the skin of the labia majora. Involvement of the clitoris is common, but this is rarely the site of origin of the tumour. So-called 'kissing ulcers', i.e. small ulcers arising in opposite labia yet in apposition are probably of multifocal origin though possibly due to contralateral implantation of malignant cells.

Direct spread occurs in 25% of cases with involvement of the urethra, vagina or rectum and in 2% of cases the pelvic bone. Spread via the lymphatics is more usual and has occurred in more than 50% of patients by the time they present to a clinician. The lymphatic vessels of the vulva are numerous and interconnecting, running as they do upwards and laterally to the superficial and deep nodes of the groin. It is important to note that the lymphatic vessels do not cross the labial crural fold. The nodes themselves are arranged in five groups in each groin being situated in either a superficial or deep layer. The superficial nodes include the medial and lateral inguinal nodes and the medial and lateral femoral nodes and the deep nodes the inguinal, femoral and external iliac nodes. The superficial inguinal nodes are arranged in a lateral chain on a line below the inguinal ligament and a medial group lying inferior to the superficial inguinal ring. The deep inguinal nodes, when present, lie in the inguinal canal. The superficial femoral nodes are clustered in two groups on either side of the saphenous vein as it enters the femoral vein at the fossa ovalis. The deep femoral nodes lie in the femoral canal, on the medial aspect of the femoral vein, and are often represented by a single node only, the node of Cloquet, which lies more on the abdominal side of the opening with only its lower pole in the proximal part of the femoral canal. The external iliac nodes are disposed in three groups, the most important lying medial and inferior to the external iliac vein, another situated lateral to the artery and the anterior group when present, is in the sulcus between the artery and the vein.

The lymphatics from the perineum, however, may travel in the fold alongside the vulva as do those from the skin lateral to the vulva. These vessels travel through the mons veneris to reach their destination, and those from the clitoris and urethra run upwards and medially to enter the pelvic cavity between the origins of the rectus abdominis muscles and then turn laterally on the superior ramus of the pubic bone, on the inner surface of which may be found an intermediary lymph node which interconnects with the node of Cloquet. The superficial and deep nodes intercommunicate and all drain into the node of Cloquet which thus assumes great importance as being the recipient of all lymphatic drainage of the vulva. The flow is then upwards through the external iliac, common iliac and paraaortic nodes finally reaching the thoracic duct. When pelvic nodes are removed some internal iliac nodes and the obturator nodes are invariably removed with the external iliac nodes.

Usually, left sided lesions will spread to the left groin and a right sided lesion to the right groin, but bilateral node involvement is seen in 13.8% of cases (Way 1982) and contralateral node involvement without ipsilateral disease in 5% of cases. Way never found pelvic nodes to be involved in the absence of inguinal node metastases. The clinical diagnosis of node involvement is unreliable with a 25% error as regards both false positive and false negative findings.

Ninety per cent of lesions are of squamous origin with 3.5% being melanoma, 1% basal cell carcinoma and 1% originating in Bartholin's gland. Vulval melanomas, which account for 9% of body melanoma, have a high incidence of node involvement and a a negligible 5 year survival. Sarcoma and adenocarcinoma each contribute less than 1% of cases. Size is not necessarily indicative of prognosis. The large tumour might be a well differentiated lesion and slow growing, and the smaller tumour be a rapidly growing poorly differentiated lesion.

Sarcomas are rare. In children they are usually of mixed mesodermal or round cell origin and in adults due to spindle cell tumours. Tumours arising in Bartholin's gland are adenocarcinomata though squamous carcinomas are seen if the tumour arises from the duct.

Secondary carcinoma is on occasion found in the vulva. One or more firm nodular homogeneous masses present within or beneath the epidermis of the labia majora or clitoris. Most commonly the primary lesion is in the cervix or endometrium, though less often it may be found in a variety of sites including the vagina, ovary, urethra, kidney, rectum or lung. Deposits secondary to choriocarcinoma and melanoma elsewhere are also rarely seen.

CLINICAL FEATURES

Patients with vulval cancer often fail to seek advice until the disease is quite advanced. This is surprising when one takes into account the fact that the lesion is frequently preceded by pruritus, often associated with discomfort or pain, and frequently there is an obvious lesion that the patient can see. Other symptoms which might occur include a bloodstained discharge or a palpable swelling in the groin. Dysuria may be present if the lesion is close to the urethral meatus and is the result of urine flowing over an ulcerated tumour. The lesion may be discovered on routine pelvic examination when no symptoms are present or when the patient is examined by virtue of her complaint of pruritus.

DIAGNOSIS

The diagnosis of vulval cancer may be obvious but should be confirmed by biopsy. Early invasive and intraepithelial lesions may present more difficulty. When a small ulcer is visible, the biopsies should be taken in such a way that the growing edge of the ulcer is included in the specimen. Small tumours and naevi should be dealt with by excision biopsy. All white lesions should be biopsied. The use of a colposcope may help to identify abnormal areas by the recognition of atypical blood vessel patterns as may the use of Collin's test. One per cent toluidine blue (a nuclear stain) is applied to the vulval skin and then washed off with 1% acetic acid. The affected areas retain the blue dye and are submitted to biopsy and histological analysis.

Staging
Staging should be undertaken prior to treatment and it is recommended that it should be done according

to the method favoured by FIGO (Table 49.1). This takes into account the primary tumour (T), the regional lymph nodes (N), and the possible presence of distant metastases (M). It has however serious shortcomings in that it fails to recognize intraepithelial cancer, it depends on an arbitrary lesion size of smaller or larger than 2 cm in diameter, and lastly it is known that the diagnosis of lymph node metastases by palpation is unreliable.

The staging can be made more meaningful if the cytological or histological findings on lymph node analysis reveals malignant cells. The symbol + (plus) should be added to N if malignant cells are found, and if such examinations do not reveal malignant cells, the symbol − (minus) should be added to N.

TREATMENT

It should be made clear at the outset that in assessing a patient's suitability for treatment, not only should the staging be taken into account but the patient's general health and suitability for what might be extensive surgery must be assessed carefully. The options available include surgery, radiotherapy and chemotherapy, but of these only surgery seems to be of significant value.

Surgery involving a wide excision of the primary tumour and an *en bloc* dissection of the nodal areas is the first choice. A review of the literature would suggest that an operability rate of 80–90% can be achieved with an operative mortality of the order of 2–5%.

Limited surgery such as simple vulvectomy leads to poor results. Way (1951) quoting 8 cases reported a 5 year survival of only 24%, a survival rate borne out by Green's series of 78 cases described in 1958 (Green *et al.* 1958).

Radiotherapy has led to similar poor results. Paterson *et al.* (1950) quoting 100 cases reported a 24% 5 year survival, and Helgason *et al.* (1972) describe a similar success. Any radiotherapeutic technique must take into account the need to irradiate regional lymph nodes. Complications which might follow radiotherapy include severe vulvitis, tissue necrosis, fistulae formation, urethral obstruction and possible mortality. It should also be remembered that verrucous carcinoma of the vulva, a variant of squamous carcinoma which is normally locally invasive and indolent, can be made to become rapidly invasive as a result of radiotherapy.

Chemotherapy has proved uniformly unsuccessful in the treatment of vulval carcinoma. Bleomycin and

Table 49.1. Carcinoma of vulva, FIGO method of staging (TNM classification).

T *Primary tumour*

T1   Tumour confined to the vulva, 2 cm or less in larger diameter.

T2   Tumour confined to the vulva, more than 2 cm in diameter.

T3   Tumour of any size with adjacent spread to the urethra and/or vagina and/or perineum and/or to the anus.

T4   Tumour of any size infiltrating the bladder mucosa and/or the rectal mucosa or both, including the upper part of the urethral mucosa and/or fixed to the bone.

N *Regional lymph nodes*

N0   No nodes palpable.

N1   Nodes palpable in either groin, not enlarged, mobile (not clinically suspicious of neoplasm).

N2   Nodes palpable in either one or both groins, enlarged, firm and mobile (clinically suspicious of neoplasm).

N3   Fixed or ulcerated nodes.

M *Distant metastases*

M0   No clinical metastases.

M1a   Palpable deep pelvic lymph nodes.

M1b   Other distant metastases.

Definitions of the different clinical stages in carcinoma of the vulva (FIGO)

Stage I

T1 N0 M0   Tumour confined to the vulva, 2 cm or less in the larger diameter. Nodes are not palpable, or are palpable in either groin, not enlarged, mobile (not clinically suspicious of neoplasm).

Stage II

T2 N0 M0   Tumour confined to the vulva, more than 2 cm in diameter. Nodes are not palpable, or are palpable in either groin, not enlarged, mobile (not clinically suspicious of neoplasm).

Stage III

T3 N0 M0   Tumour of any size with (1) adjacent spread
T3 N1 M0   to the lower urethra and/or the vagina, the
T3 N2 M0   perineum, and the anus, and/or (2) nodes
T1 N2 M0   palpaple in either one or both groins,
T2 N2 M0   enlarged, firm and mobile, not fixed (but clinically suspicious of neoplasm).

Stage IV

T4 N0 M0   Tumour of any size (1) infiltrating the bladder
T4 N1 M0   mucosa, or the rectal mucosa, or both,
T4 N2 M0   including the upper part of the urethral
T1 N3 M0   mucosa, and/or (2) fixed to the bone or other
T2 N3 M0   distant metastases. Fixed or ulcerated nodes in
T3 N3 M0   either one or both groins.
T4 N3 M0

All other conditions containing M1a or M1b

methotrexate have been used and, whereas a response to treatment has been achieved, this has been without cure (Deppe *et al.* 1979).

SURGICAL TREATMENT

The standard radical vulvectomy used in the treatment of vulval carcinoma should include a wide excision of the primary growth, which is not only wide in extent but also deep, and an appropriate bilateral lymphadenectomy. The excision should extend laterally to the genitocrural folds, posteriorly to include three-quarters of the perineum and anteriorly some 3–4 cm above the clitoris. The groin incisions are extended in each thigh to the apex of the femoral triangle so that the superficial and deep femoral nodes can be removed *en bloc* along with the superficial and deep inguinal nodes. In suitable patients, the operation can be extended by way of dividing the inguinal ligament so that extraperitoneal access to the pelvic nodes is possible in order that a suitable pelvic lymphadenectomy be performed. Many surgeons would remove only the pelvic nodes if there was evidence of metastases to inguinal nodes as judged by intra-operative frozen section examination of nodal tissue. An alternative technique, which allows a more comprehensive histological examination of excised nodes rather than frozen section nodal sampling, is to leave the pelvic lymphadenectomy, should it be necessary, to a second stage abdominal procedure done after the full histological report on the operative specimen is available.

Surgical treatment such as is described briefly above and amplified in descriptions by Way (1982) and Stenning (1980) is appropriate in the management of fit patients with Stage I, II or III disease.

In certain circumstances more conservative surgery might be appropriate. Kolstad (1981) reports the results of a more limited operation done in Oslo for Stage I squamous carcinoma of the vulva. It is performed only after an excision biopsy of a tumour less than 2 cm in diameter has been examined histologically with the exclusion of lymph vessel or blood vessel invasion by tumour. In such circumstances a hemivulvectomy is performed with an ipsilateral lymphadenectomy. Conservation of the clitoris is practised if the lesion is perineal or on the labia majora or minora on one side. The clitoris is removed if an anterior lesion is present. A bilateral lymphadenectomy is undertaken if the clitorial or perineal region is involved. With this technique, the mutilation of a more radical operation is avoided and the incidence

of groin skin necrosis and lymph oedema of the leg reduced. Less interference with sexual activity is reported. These advantages have not been at the expense of cure.

Multifocal microinvasive lesions may require a wide local excision but with only a superficial groin gland dissection.

When Stage IV disease exists, urinary or faecal diversion may be necessary. It has been found that the lower third of the urethra may be removed without urinary incontinence occurring but, when more than a third needs to be removed, an ileal conduit will be necessary. If the tumour has spread to the anus then a preliminary defunctioning sigmoid colostomy will be required, and also time for the colostomy to heal, before the radical vulval procedure is undertaken. Some surgeons would recommend a temporary transverse colostomy, with a later permanent left iliac fossa sigmoid colostomy, so as to allow the colostomy bag to be kept further away from the groin incisions in the hope that, as a result of reduced contamination, improved healing will occur.

Complications

The breakdown of groin wounds as a result of tissue necrosis is probably the commonest complication of radical surgery and the cause of the prolonged in-patient stay needed by such patients. The incidence of breakdown can be reduced by attention to surgical detail. The use of preoperative antiseptic baths (using either povidone-iodine or Hibitane) to reduce the skin bacterial colonization is beneficial. Prophylactic antibiotic therapy, using cephradine 500 mg intravenously six hourly and metronidazole 500 mg intravenously eight hourly over a period of 48 hours, is worthwhile as is the use of a postoperative povidone-iodine wound spray. As important is to use suction drainage to each groin. Quarter-inch-diameter polythene drains should be employed, each brought out through a stab wound towards the posterior aspect of the perineum. Drainage should be continuous until negligible amounts of fluid are obtained and this often may take as long as 10 days. Sedlacek *et al.* (1976) have reported a reduction in incidence of wound breakdown from 73–20% with a corresponding reduction of average in-patient stay from 37 to 18 days by the use of oral zinc (220 micrograms t.i.d.) to improve wound healing.

If breakdown does occur then Eusol packs on a twice daily basis are necessary. Such nursing care is frequently painful and the patient's comfort improved by the use of analgesia such as sublingual buprenorphine, 200 micrograms sucked 20 minutes prior to nursing care. Once the granulation tissue has been freed of its secondary infection, epithelialization of the wounds will occur.

Haemorrhage may be primary and results either from oozing which, with drainage as recommended, can be measured and this normally responds to pressure, or as a result of a vessel which requires religature. Secondary haemorrhage is invariably due to sepsis and can be serious, and sometimes fatal, if major blood vessels are involved and are the site of necrosis. Transplantation of the sartorius muscles to cover the femoral vessels would seem to avoid this possible complication.

Osteitis may present with local pain and tenderness and an associated swinging temperature, some days after the surgery has been performed and will require excision of necrotic bone. The incidence of deep venous thrombosis following surgery can be reduced by teaching patients leg exercises prior to surgery, using anti-emboli stockings, giving subcutaneous heparin prior to and following surgery and by encouraging postoperative leg exercises. If suspected the diagnosis should be confirmed by phlebography. Pulmonary embolism may follow and accounts for a 1% operative mortality. Urinary tract infection after surgery is common unless a urinary antiseptic such as trimethoprim is given whilst an indwelling Foley catheter is in use (normally for around seven days). The catheter should be strapped to one or other leg on alternate days so as to keep the urethra straight whilst healing occurs. The incidence of postoperative femoral and inguinal herniae can be reduced by closing routinely the hernial orifices with a nonabsorbable suture material. Care should be exercised in closing the femoral canals lest constriction of the femoral vessels is produced which may predispose to venous thrombosis. A careful reconstruction of the perineal body will avoid the development of a rectocele. Lymphoedema affecting both legs is a not uncommon consequence of the operation. It is associated with discomfort, a loss of mobility and a deleterious cosmetic effect. Secondary infection with a streptococcus may occur and lead to erysipelas. Symptomatic treatment by way of support stockings is indicated but it is recognized that antidiuretics are of no value.

Results of treatment
Way (1982) reporting on 642 patients treated between 1939 and 1975 had a 49% absolute five year survival. During the overall period of surveillance 31.7% of patients developed recurrence and died from

the disease and, of those patients, 93% had developed their recurrence within three years of surgery. Thirty-four per cent of patients died from intercurrent disease. Stenning (1981), quoting a series of 204 patients with an operability rate of 96% and an operative mortality of 1%, achieved a 62% absolute five year survival. Franklin & Rutledge (1972) in a series of 164 patients achieved a similar figure of 55.7%.

Way (1960) demonstrated the improved survival in those patients with negative nodes (70–80% five year survival as compared with 45–50% when the nodes were involved). Even better survival figures for patients with negative nodes were reported by Morley (1976). Ninety per cent of his patients (corrected mortality) and all of the 53 patients described by Rutledge *et al.* (1970) remained free of recurrence.

The treatment of recurrence is often unrewarding, more so for the patient than the surgeon. Palliation by way of surgical excision or alternatively diathermy excision may have some benefit but rarely do patients live long after such procedures.

As with many carcinomas the best chance of cure is that associated with the initial operation, and there would seem to be evidence to suggest that the experience gained by surgeons working in oncological centres to which patients are referred is of benefit to the patient.

RARE MALIGNANT TUMOURS OF THE VULVA

BASAL CELL CARCINOMA

Basal cell carcinoma has the typical appearance of a rodent ulcer and accounts for between 2 and 4% of all vulval malignancies. As would be expected, a nodule appears and then breaks down leaving an ulcer with a rolled beaded edge. The lesion is locally invasive but invasion takes place slowly. If the clinical diagnosis is confirmed by a careful histological examination of a biopsy specimen and co-existent invasive squamous carcinoma is excluded, wide local excision may prove sufficient treatment. The lesion is radiosensitive but on balance surgical treatment is preferred.

MELANOMA OF THE VULVA

This lesion presents as a soft fungating protuberant mass of black or purple colour. Early lesions are small and nodular but metastases occur early. Spread is to the regional lymph nodes and by the blood stream. Radical surgery on early cases is the only hope of cure, and invariably it will be necessary to remove the deep pelvic nodes as well as performing a radical vulvectomy and bilateral groin lymphadenectomy. The quoted five year survival ranges from 25% (Karlen *et al.* 1975) to 50% (Morrow & Rutledge 1972), but the average five year survival is of the order of 34%.

CARCINOMA OF BARTHOLIN'S GLAND

This is a rare unilateral vulval tumour, and is an adenocarcinoma in most cases although squamous carcinoma can arise from the duct of Bartholin's gland. The appearances are similar to other vulval tumours but the lesion might well be suspected from its situation. Treatment is as for carcinoma of the vulva. The prognosis may be less favourable than with squamous carcinoma of the vulva by virtue of the fact that the lesion develops deep in the vulva and diagnosis may be delayed.

CARCINOMA OF THE URETHRA

Urethral malignancy occurs uncommonly. Whereas it is normally squamous in origin, adenocarcinoma may arise in the paraurethral glands. Cases of sarcoma and melanoma are also reported. Tumours of the distal end of the urethra drain to vulval lymphatics, but in addition lymphatics of the remaining portion of the urethra follow those of the vagina deep into the pelvis. Apart from the swelling, the patient may notice haematuria and dysuria. Biopsies should be taken whenever the diagnosis is suspected.

By virtue of its rarity, there is no agreed standard therapy. Radiotherapy when used usually takes the form of radium needles inserted in and around the urethra in combination with external irradiation. Surgical treatment can vary from local excision of the tumour to a radical vulvectomy which might or might not be in combination with an anterior exenteration necessitating diversion of the urinary flow. Grabstadd (1973) quotes a 27% 5 year survival rate of 96 collected cases.

SARCOMA OF THE VULVA

These rare lesions can be one of four types, i.e. leiomyosarcoma, rhabdomyosarcoma, neurofibrosarcoma or fibrosarcoma. The leiomyosarcoma appears most commonly, whilst the rhabdomyosarcoma occurs at the earliest age. The mean age of presentation of vulval sarcoma is around 42 years. Spread is as with other vulval tumours, though in addition the sarcoma tends to be associated with early haematogenous spread.

Surgical treatment is recommended when the lesion is restricted to the vulva and regional lymphatics, but if blood-borne metastases are known to have occurred additional systemic cytotoxic therapy will be necessary.

With this disease long term survival is unusual.

VAGINAL INTRAEPITHELIAL NEOPLASIA

Vaginal intraepithelial neoplasia is seen coexisting with cervical intraepithelial neoplasia in 1–3% of such patients. Hummer *et al.* (1970) examining a series of 66 patients with vaginal intraepithelial neoplasia showed that one-third had developed within two years of a previous cervical lesion being treated and that the longest time interval between cervical and vaginal intraepithelial neoplasia was 17 years. The patients' ages ranged from 24–75 years with a mean age of 52 years.

The aetiology of vaginal intraepithelial neoplasia is not known. Radiotherapy for carcinoma of the cervix some 10–15 years prior to the development of vaginal intraepithelial neoplasia has been noted, and it is thought by some that a sublethal dose of radiation is of more harm than a lethal dose and that radiation of the vagina may be relevant. No relationship between vaginal intraepithelial neoplasia and herpes simplex virus has as yet been found, but the possibility of human papilloma virus being an aetiological factor is under suspicion. A higher incidence of vaginal intraepithelial neoplasia than normal has been noted in patients on chemotherapy and immunosuppressive therapy.

PATHOLOGY

As with cervical disease, vaginal intraepithelial neoplasia Grade I is equated with mild dysplasia, Grade II with moderate dysplasia and Grade III with severe dysplasia or carcinoma-*in-situ*. The disease is normally recognized as the result of abnormal cytology seen on a vaginal smear specimen. Townsend (1981) recommends that vaginal smears are done on patients having previously had a hysterectomy on a three-yearly basis if the hysterectomy was done for benign disease, or annually if the hysterectomy was done for cervical intraepithelial neoplasia. Colposcopic assessment of patients with abnormal smears is indicated. Five per cent acetic acid will show up aceto-white areas from which biopsies should be taken and the abnormal area can frequently be delineated by using a half-strength Lugol's iodine solution which will stain suspect lesions light yellow. Punctation may be apparent in more than 50% of cases. Vaginal biopsies can usually be taken without anaesthesia for subsequent histological examination, and if bleeding occurs haemostasis can be achieved using Monsell's solution (ferric sub-sulphate). Not uncommonly atrophic changes in the vagina lead to difficulties in diagnosis and a preliminary course of oestrogen cream to correct the oestrogen deficiency is often needed. Oestrogen deficiency changes should always be corrected before treatment is initiated.

Natural history

No adequate study on the progression of vaginal intraepithelial neoplasia to invasive disease has been reported. There is uncertainty as to whether the pattern of progression equates with cervical intraepithelial neoplasia. Vaginal vault lesions may be residual, resulting from adjacent cervical intraepithelial neoplasia already removed, or if distant from the vault, the result of a multifocal origin.

TREATMENT

There are and have been a wide variety of treatments available. The smallest lesions can be removed by biopsy excision or if the lesions are more extensive treatment with either 5-fluorouracil cream or with the laser undertaken.

Provided the lesion is not hyperkeratotic the application of 5-fluorouracil cream, as introduced by Woodruff *et al.* (1975), has advantage in that widely scattered lesions can be treated effectively. The cream, a cytotoxic metabolite, is used *per vaginam* as a test dose using 5 grams of a 5% preparation. The patient is re-evaluated colposcopically four days later and if a satisfactory response has occurred, 5 grams of cream are used *per vaginam* on a nightly basis for five days. Further colposcopic assessment is undertaken at six and then twelve weeks after treatment and, if any residual lesion is found, a further five-day course recommended. If this fails, laser therapy may be necessary.

Whereas in the past cryotherapy and thermal cautery have been used to deal with vaginal intraepithelial neoplasia, treatment with a carbon dioxide laser would seem to have significant advantage in that general anaesthesia is rarely required and the treatment can be repeated as necessary. It is possible for the surgeon to control both the area and depth of tissue destruction.

A third alternative is local excision of the lesion. If the lesion is at the vault and there is danger of vaginal narrowing, the vaginal vault should be left open. A vaginal pack is used and subsequently changed on a regular basis, and then vaginal dilators used by the patient until re-epithelialization without constriction has occurred which normally needs an interval of six weeks.

Total vaginectomy is used but rarely. Radiotherapy is an alternative for the post-menopausal woman who is no longer sexually active.

VAGINAL CARCINOMA

Vaginal carcinomas may be primary or secondary. Primary carcinoma of the vagina is most commonly of squamous origin but can be an adenocarcinoma. Squamous carcinomas most commonly present in the sixth and seventh decades of life but the range is from the third to the ninth decade. Adenocarcinoma, in contrast, can occur at any age. In young women it is normally of the clear cell (mesonephric) variety, and some but by no means all of such patients are the daughters of women who took diethylstilboestrol in early pregnancy. Papillary or tubal cell adenocarcinomata have been described and these varieties usually present in the older age group.

Rarely, melanoma of the vagina is seen. Sarcomas are also rare. Sarcoma botryoides and endodermal sinus tumours are diseases which normally occur in infancy or childhood.

Secondary disease can arise as a result of direct extension of carcinoma from the cervix, as a result of an endometrial lesion spreading onto the cervix and then to the vagina, from the vulva, or from the rectum, anus or rectovaginal septum. Distal metastases may be the result of a primary carcinoma in the breast or gastrointestinal tract.

CLINICAL FEATURES

As might be expected from the age at presentation, postmenopausal bleeding is one of the commonest symptoms. Vaginal discharge is another which, if it be the result of tissue necrosis, is foul smelling. If the lesion is on the anterior wall of the vagina there may be urinary symptoms. If the posterior wall is affected, rectal symptoms and pain may be the result of infiltration resulting in either visceral involvement or being associated with secondary infection.

Examination normally shows the lesions to be exophitic or ulcerative, but they can be of the infiltrative variety. More than 50% of lesions occur in the upper vagina, with 30% occurring in the lower third of the vagina, and approximately 19% in the middle third (Pentyl & Friedman 1971). Posterior vaginal lesions are said to be more common than anterior lesions which in turn are more common than lateral vaginal lesions.

Spread is by way of direct extension and by the involvement of lymphatic pathways. If the disease arises in the upper vagina it tends to spread as does cervical disease, whereas if it is in the lower third of the vagina it spreads as does a vulval carcinoma. If the bladder or rectum are involved, spread is more extensive and via the appropriate lymphatic pathways. Information on the incidence of nodal involvement is deficient but, as a result of Pentyl & Friedman's study (1971) on postmortem and surgical material, the incidence of nodal involvement is said to be around 21%.

DIAGNOSIS

Diagnosis is the result of a histological examination of biopsy material obtained after an appropriate clinical examination. A Papanicolaou smear is unreliable as a diagnostic indicator unless taken specifically from the vaginal lesion. Vaginal carcinoma is said to be often missed by the clinician as a result of the gynaecologist's cursory examination of the vagina. The use of a bivalve vaginal speculum does not help and a much better view of the vagina is obtained using the Sims' position for examination and a speculum of the Sims' type.

Investigation

A vaginal biopsy can normally be obtained in the outpatient clinic without the need for anaesthesia, but examination under anaesthesia is indicated to establish whether the lesion be of primary or secondary origin, to establish the extent of the lesion and so that cystoscopy and sigmoidoscopy can be undertaken. Associated investigations should include an X-ray of the chest, X-rays of the renal tract and a barium enema and, if the lesion is thought to be an adenocarcinoma, X-rays of the gastrointestinal tract. More special investigations by way of ultrasound,

computerized axial tomography and lymphography are occasionally of value.

Staging should be according to the recommendations of FIGO and the details of staging are seen in Table 49.2. It should be remembered that if the carcinoma involves both the vagina and the cervix, vulva or urethra, then the carcinoma should be designated as arising in the tissue other than the vagina.

Table 49.2. Carcinoma of the vagina. FIGO method of staging.

Pre-invasive carcinoma	
Stage 0	Carcinoma-*in-situ*, intraepithelial carcinoma.
Invasive carcinoma	
Stage I	The carcinoma is limited to the vaginal wall.
Stage II	The carcinoma has involved the subvaginal tissue, but has not extended on to the pelvic wall.
Stage III	The carcinoma has extended on to the pelvic wall.
Stage IV	The carcinoma has extended beyond the true pelvis or has involved the mucosa of the bladder or rectum.
Stage IVa	Spread of the growth to adjacent organs.
Stage IVb	Spread to distant organs.

TREATMENT

There is no consensus view as to the optimum treatment for carcinoma of the vagina. The disease occurs but rarely and a variety of treatments involving the use of surgery, radiotherapy or a combination of surgery and radiotherapy in either order have been tried. Patients themselves are of a wide age range, vary in their degree of fitness for radical surgery, and the lesions themselves are associated with a variable spread of disease. Even so, the majority would favour using radiotherapy as primary treatment for vaginal carcinoma.

In determining the success of radiotherapy the tumour size and the extent of spread are more important than the cell type. Radiotherapists will invariably use external irradiation to first reduce the size of the tumour mass, and they will follow this by local irradiation using a colpostat for delivery or, alternatively and particularly when the lesion is in the lower vagina, by using radium needles. Some would use hollow needles which are 'after-loaded' with Irridium 192 wires.

Complications following radiotherapy are not uncommon. Vaginal necrosis is not infrequently seen.

Cystitis, urethritis and proctosigmoiditis are not unusual, and sometimes followed by either a vesicovaginal or rectovaginal fistula. Urethral necrosis can occur. The small or large bowel can be affected by mucosal ulceration, perforation, stenosis or obstruction. Postirradiation fibrosis may lead to subsequent dyspareunia and to the clinician having difficulty in recognizing recurrent tumour.

When the disease is in the upper third of the vagina, then treatment by way of a radical hysterectomy with partial vaginectomy and pelvic lymphadenectomy is recommended by some (Frick *et al.* 1968, Herbst *et al.* 1970, Underwood & Smith 1971). Disease affecting the middle third of the vagina, if treated surgically, invariably needs an exenterative procedure, though very superficial disease has been treated by total vaginectomy alone, often with unfavourable results. If surgery is used to treat disease affecting the lower third of the vagina then the extent of the operation must include a radical vulvectomy with an appropriate lymphadenectomy. Palumbo *et al.* (1969) describe their results.

Results of treatment

Pentyl and Friedman (1971) reviewing world literature suggested that there has been an improvement during the previous 40 years. They found an 11.5% 5 year survival rate prior to 1940, with a 24% 5 year survival in the subsequent two decades and a 31% 5 year survival between 1961 and 1968. Other more recent papers suggest that the 5 year survival is now nearer 40%. In particular, results quoted from the M. D. Anderson Hospital (Wharton *et al.* 1981) relating to a series of 114 patients, of which 89 were treated by radiotherapy alone with the remainder treated by radiotherapy and surgery, indicated a 50% 5 year survival.

Diethystilboestrol and related diseases

Diethylstilboestrol (DES) has been used from the late 1940s for the treatment of recurrent abortion and unexplained fetal loss late in pregnancy, predominantly in the United States of America where it is estimated that two million women were so treated, and also in Canada, Mexico, Western Australia and Western Europe.

Herbst and Scully (1970) reported seven cases of clear cell adenocarcinoma of the vagina seen and treated in the Massachusetts General Hospital, Boston, in young women aged between 14 and 22 years. A retrospective study by them the following year linked these carcinomata with the intrauterine exposure of the patients to diethylstilboestrol (DES) given to their mothers during pregnancy. A more extensive survey (Herbst *et al.* 1979) looked at 346 cases of clear cell adenocarcinoma of the cervix and vagina. In 317 patients the maternal history was available, and it was found that two-thirds of the patients had been exposed *in utero* to DES or a similar non-steroid oestrogen given to the mothers during pregnancy. In a further 10%, drugs of doubtful origin were given, but in 25% no history of maternal hormone therapy could be obtained.

They found that the age incidence for clear cell adenocarcinoma of the vagina in young women begins at age 14, peaks at 19 years and then subsequently undergoes a rapid decline. They estimated the probable risk of development of clear cell carcinoma in women exposed to DES *in utero* to be 0.14–1.4 per thousand.

Clear cell vaginal carcinomas were normally found in the upper third of the anterior vaginal wall or on the portio of the cervix. They ranged in size from 0.3–10 cm in diameter and were polypoid or nodular, less commonly being flat and ulcerated. Hobnail cells are often present and were described by Scully *et al.* (1974). Abnormal vaginal smears were identified in 80% of cases. Early spread to lymph nodes was seen (16% in Stage I and 50% in Stage II or more) but was thought to be absent if the lesion was less than 1 cm in diameter or had invaded to a depth of less than 3 mm.

Treatment for Stage I disease was normally surgical taking the form of a radical hysterectomy, partial (or complete) vaginectomy and pelvic lymphadenectomy with a split thickness skin graft being done at the same time so as to create an artificial vagina. The ovaries were normally conserved. With this regime, 87% of patients with Stage I vaginal disease will survive 5 years and 91% of patients with Stage I cervical disease will survive 5 years. Similar results are achieved after radiotherapy used in combination with pretreatment node biopsy to exclude metastases. Radiotherapy is limited and does not deal with nodal areas. Stage II disease is normally treated by irradiation, with 5 year survival figures of 76% for Stage II vaginal disease and 77% for Stage IIA cervical disease. The 5 year survival of patients with Stage IIB cervical disease is 60% falling to 30% for Stage III disease.

Overall there is a 78% 5 year survival for patients with clear cell carcinoma of the vagina (Herbst *et al.* 1979).

NON-MALIGNANT CHANGES

Vaginal adenosis is often seen in combination with cervical ectropion or eversion. The patients often have a ridge between the vaginal and cervical tissue often referred to as a collar, a rim or 'a cock's-comb cervix'. Such appearances tend to occur in approximately 25% of patients. The adenosis can affect the anterior and posterior vaginal walls and lateral vaginal fornices but is usually restricted to the upper third of the vagina.

Squamous metaplasia is common in the transformation zone of DES affected patients. Confusion with malignant change is not uncommon. Fu *et al.* (1978) have used a microspectrophotomimetic method to establish nuclear DNA in an effort to differentiate aneuploid (neoplastic) from euploid (metaplastic) cells.

Women who are known to have been exposed to DES *in utero* should be screened from the age of 14 years with both cytological and colposcopic examination. It should be realized that the saline method of colposcopic examination can be misleading in that punctation and mosaic changes are often seen in an extended transformation zone. The acetic acid technique combined with the use of half-strength Lugol's iodine is usually sufficient to indicate abnormal areas, and it is important that biopsies are taken from such areas for histological evaluation.

SQUAMOUS CELL LESIONS

There is no evidence that there is an increased incidence of squamous cell neoplasia in DES exposed females. It has been postulated that, by virtue of the increased transformation zone, there may be an increased risk of cervical intraepithelial neoplasia, though workers vary in their assessment of the degree of risk. It is thought that the risk of an exposed patient developing cervical intraepithelial neoplasia exceeds the risk of developing clear cell adenocarcinoma of the vagina, though there is as yet no statistical evidence that there is a significant difference in the frequency of squamous cell carcinoma in DES exposed and unexposed women.

VAGINAL SARCOMA

The commonest vaginal sarcoma is a leiomyosarcoma which grows locally yet only spreads via lymphatics and the blood stream late in its natural history. It is surrounded by a pseudocapsule which too

is malignant and which should be removed with the tumour. Wide local excision is often sufficient treatment.

Rhabdomyosarcoma on the other hand spreads via the lymphatics and blood-stream early. It is normally recommended that adjuvant radiotherapy or chemotherapy be used with surgery.

Sarcoma botryoides may occur in the vagina of children as part of multicentric disease affecting the vagina, cervix, uterus and bladder. The treatment of sarcoma botryoides is discussed in Chapter 51 (p. 794).

VAGINAL MELANOMA

Melanoma of the vagina, which is rare, normally presents as a slightly elevated pigmented lesion, commonly in the lower third of the vagina. Spread can be direct, via lymphatics or via the blood stream. Treatment is surgical, often radical and frequently unsuccessful.

REFERENCES

BASSETT A. (1912) *L'epithelioma primitif du clitoris: son retentissment ganglionaire et son traitment operatoire.* G. Stenheil, Paris.

COLLINS D. (1965) *Amer. J. Obstet. Gynec.,* **91**, 818.

DEPPE G., COHEN C.J. & BRUCKNER H.W. (1979) *Gynec. Oncol.,* **7**, 345.

FRANKLIN E.W. & RUTLEDGE F.N. (1971) *Obstet. and Gynec.,* **37**, 892.

FRANKLIN E.W. III & RUTLEDGE F.D. (1972) *Obstet. and Gynec.,* **39**, 165.

FRICK H.C., JACOX H.W. & TAYLOR H.C. JR. (1968) *Amer. J. Obstet. Gynec.,* **101**, 695.

FU Y., ROBBOY S.J. & PRAT J. (1978) *Obstet. and Gynec.,* **52**, 129.

GRABSTADD H. (1973) *Cancer,* **32**, 1236.

GREEN T.H. JR. (1978) *Obstet. Gynec.* **52**, 462.

GREEN T.H. JR., ULFELDER H. & MEIGS J.V. (1958) *Amer. J. Obstet. Gynec.,* **75**, 848.

HELGASON N.M., HASS A.C. & LATOURETTE H.B. (1972) *Cancer,* **30**, 997.

HERBST A.L. & SCULLY R.E. (1970) *Cancer,* **25**, 745.

HERBST A.L., GREEN T.H. JR. & ULFELDER H. (1970) *Amer. J. Obstet. Gynec.,* **106**, 210.

HERBST A.L., NORVSIS M.J., ROSENOW P.J., WELCH W.R. & SCULLY R.E. (1979) *Gynecol. Oncol.,* **7**, 111.

HUMMER W.K., MUSSEY E., DECKER D.G. & DOCKERTY M.B. (1970) *Amer. J. Obstet. Gynec.,* **108**, 1109.

KARLEN J.R., PIVER M.S. & BARLOW J.J. (1975) *Obstet. and Gynec.,* **45**, 181.

KOLSTAD P. (1981) In *Gynecologic Oncology* (Ed. Coppleson, M.), p. 838. Churchill Livingstone, Edinburgh.

KRUPP P.J. (1981) In *Gynecologic Ocology* (Ed. Coppleson M.) p. 329. Churchill Livingstone, Edinburgh.

MOLEY G.W. (1976) *Amer. J. Obstet. Gynec.*, **24**, 874.

MORROW C.P. & RUTLEDGE F.N. (1972) *Ostet. and Gynec.*, **39**, 745.

PALUMBO L. JR., SHINGLETON H.M., RISHBURN J.I. JR., PEPPER F.D. JR. & KOCH G.G. (1969) *Sth. Med. J.*, **62**, 1048.

PARRY-JONES E. (1960) *J. Obstet. Gynaec. Brit. Cwlth.*, **67**, 919.

PATERSON R., TOD M. & RUSSELL M. (1950) *The Results of Radium and X-Ray Therapy in Malignant Disease.* E. & S. Livingstone, Edinburgh.

PENTYL A.A. & FRIEDMAN E.A. (1971) *Lymphatics of the Female Genitalia.* W.B. Saunders, Philadelphia.

REIFFENSTUHL G. (1964) *The Lymphatics of the Female Genital Organs.* Lippincott, Philadelphia.

ROTHSCHILD F. (1912) Inaugural dissertation. *Freiburg* (quoted by F.J. Taussig 1931. Diseases of the Vulva p. 142). Appleton & Co. New York.

RUTLEDGE F., SMITH J.P. & FRANKLIN E.W. III (1970) *Amer. J. Obstet. Gynec.*, **106**, 1117.

SCULLY R.E., ROBBOY S.J. & HERBST A.L. (1974) *Ann. clin. lab. sci.*, **4**, 222.

SEDLACEK T.V., MANGAN C.E., GUINTOLI R.L. & MUKUTA N.J. (1976) *Gynec. Oncol.*, **4**, 324.

STENNING M. (1980) *Cancer and Related Lesions of Vulva.* Adis Press, Sydney, New York.

STENNING M. (1981) In *Gynecologic Oncology* (Ed. Coppleson M.) Churchill Livingstone, Edinburgh.

TAUSSIG F.J. (1941) *Amer. J. Roentgenol.*, **45**, 813.

TOWNSEND D.E. (1981) In *Gynecologic Oncology* (Ed. Coppleson M.) Churchill Livingstone, Edinburgh.

UNDERWOOD P.B. & SMITH R.T. (1971) *J. Amer. med. Ass.*, **217**, 46.

WAY S. (1948) *Ann roy. Coll. Surg.*, **3**, 187.

WAY S. (1951) *Malignant Disease of the Female Genital Tract*, p. 20. J. & A. Churchill, London.

WAY S. (1954) *J. Obstet. Gynaec. Brit. Emp.*, **61**, 1.

WAY S. (1960) *Amer. J. Obstet. Gynec.*, **79**, 692.

WAY S. (1982) *Malignant Disease of the Vulva.* Churchill Livingstone, Edinburgh, London, Melbourne & New York.

WHARTON J.T., FLETCHER G.P. & DELCLOS L. (1981) In *Gynaecologic Oncology* (Ed. Coppleson M.). Churchill Living stone, Edinburgh.

WOODRUFF J.D., PARMLEY T.H. & JULIAN C.G. (1975) *Gynecol. Oncol.*, **3**, 124.

CHAPTER 50
PREMALIGNANT AND MALIGNANT DISEASE OF THE CERVIX

K. R. PEEL

Cancer of the cervix, a disease with a fascinating aetiology, is that which most women think of as cancer of the womb. By virtue of its accessibility it can be readily diagnosed even in its pre-invasive state, and if treated in its early stages the patient can be very often cured of the disease. Papanicolaou, who gives his name to the 'Pap' smear, laid the foundation for preventive medicine at its best. Regrettably in some poorer countries, where the disease is common, the resources for such measures are not available though hopefully this situation will change with time.

PATHOLOGY

Carcinoma of the cervix may develop in either the squamous epithelium or the glandular epithelium of the endocervix, approximately 90% of the growths being squamous carcinoma and the remaining 10% adenocarcinoma; proportions of 95 and 5% used to be quoted but there seems to be an increasing incidence of adenocarcinoma.

Pre-invasive lesions. The existence of a pre-invasive stage in the development of squamous carcinoma has been known since Sir John Williams in the Harveian lecture for 1886 presented a case of symptomless carcinoma of the cervix which is now thought to have been a case of carcinoma-*in-situ*. Rubin (1910), along with others, described non-invasive change at the margins of invasive carcinomas and it was he who introduced the term 'carcinoma-*in-situ*'. The concept of dysplasia, that is, a stage in the pre-invasive process prior to carcinoma-*in-situ* was put forward by Walters and Reagan (1956).

Cervical intra-epithelial neoplasia has, during the last decade, gradually replaced the older terms of dysplasia (mild, moderate and severe) and carcinoma-*in-situ*, previously used to describe the various stages of cellular atypia seen in abnormal cervical epithelium. The World Health Organization (WHO) recommendations (Poulsen & Taylor 1975) set out the

pathological features of the various stages of the disease. Although these features remain the same mild dysplasia is regarded as Grade I cervical intra-epithelial neoplasia, moderate dysplasia as Grade II cervical intra-epithelial neoplasia, and severe dysplasia and carcinoma-*in-situ* as Grade III cervical intra-epithelial neoplasia.

The newer terminology is intended to emphasize that the disease is a continuum, yet its degree of severity, i.e. grading, reflects the prognostic differences in the untreated lesion. If the lesion is removed, then the recurrence rate should be the same, irrespective of grading. A transition stage between carcinoma-*in-situ* and invasive carcinoma is recognized and is called microinvasion which can be further subdivided into early stromal invasion and microcarcinoma. In early stromal invasion small finger-like processes break through the basement membrane and extend into the stroma. If these finger like processes become confluent, then the lesion is termed microcarcinoma and attempts are made to measure the volume of invasive tumour, although there are varying opinions as to the maximum acceptable depth that should be regarded as microinvasion. The pathologist should also report whether or not vascular invasion has occurred. The most commonly held opinion is that for microinvasion the invasion should not extend beyond a depth of 5 mm from the basement membrane, and for a microcarcinoma the volume of tumour should not exceed 500 mm³. In the United States the Society of Gynecological Oncology in 1973 took the view that for microinvasion to exist invasion must not go beyond 3 mm nor should involvement of lymphatics be seen. Burghardt (1984) believes that in early stromal invasion the presence of vascular involvement is not significant, but that when vascular invasion occurs in association with microcarcinoma there is a significant risk of metastases, and that this should be taken into account in planning treatment.

Invasive lesions. When the extent of invasion exceeds the limits described above, though a clinical lesion is not yet apparent, the tumour is described as an occult invasive carcinoma. The Fédération Internationale de Gynécologie et Obstétriques (FIGO) staging recommendations (Kottmeier 1982) take into account the higher risk of lymph node metastases with occult invasive carcinoma as will be seen in the staging (Table 50.1) in which microinvasion (Stage IA) is separated from occult invasive disease (Stage IB occult).

Table 50.1. FIGO staging of carcinoma of the uterine cervix.

Pre-invasive carcinoma

Stage 0	Carcinoma-*in-situ*, intraepithelial carcinoma. Stage 0 should not be included in any therapeutic statistics for invasive carcinoma.

Invasive carcinoma

Stage I	Carcinoma strictly confined to the cervix. Extension to the corpus should be disregarded.
Stage Ia	Microinvasive carcinoma (early stromal invasion).
Stage Ib	All other cases of Stage I. Occult cancer should be marked 'occ'.
Stage II	The carcinoma extends beyond the cervix but has not extended onto the pelvic wall. The carcinoma involves the vagina, but not the lower third.
Stage IIa	No obvious parametrial involvement.
Stage IIb	Obvious parametrial involvement.
Stage III	The carcinoma has extended onto the pelvic wall. On rectal examination, there is no cancer-free space between the tumour and the pelvic wall. The tumour involves the lower third of the vagina. All cases with hydronephrosis or non-functioning kidney.
Stage IIIa	No extension onto the pelvic wall.
Stage IIIb	Extension onto the pelvic wall and/or hydronephrosis or kidney.
Stage IV	The carcinoma has extended beyond the true pelvis or has clinically involved the mucosa of the bladder or rectum. A bullous oedema as such does not permit a case to be allotted to Stage IV.
Stage IVa	Spread of the growth to adjacent organs.
Stage IVb	Spread to distant organs.

Clinical cervical cancers appear in a variety of forms and may be exophytic, endophytic, ulcerative or polypoid. Adenocarcinomas do not differ markedly in clinical presentation, though tend to be more often endophytic and polypoid than the squamous varie-

ties, yet even so the commonest adenocarcinoma is an exophytic lesion.

Spread can be by extension into the endometrium which is difficult to recognize clinically, laterally into the parametrium, or less commonly anteriorly into the bladder, or posteriorly into the rectum. As a result of parametric spread, ureteric obstruction may occur and renal failure follow. Direct extension into the vaginal fornices is seen, and less commonly extension into the lower third of the vagina.

Lymphatic spread may occur early in the disease so that the obturator, internal iliac and external iliac nodes are not uncommonly involved, with less frequent involvement of the sacral, inguinal and para-aortic nodes. Rarely dissemination may occur to the periadrenal, peribronchial or supraclavicular nodes. Haematogenous spread to the lungs, liver and bones is seen. The commonest causes of death include uraemia and pyelonephritis, infection and haemorrhage.

Langley and Fox (1981) reviewed the much rarer variants of cervical carcinoma which are beyond the scope of this text.

EPIDEMIOLOGY

One of the first recognized epidemiologidal studies on cancer of the cervix was done by Rigoni-Stern in 1842. Using the death records for Verona between the years 1760 and 1839 he noted a higher prevalence of uterine cancer in married than in unmarried women and that the disease was extremely rare in nuns. Nearly all early reports of uterine cancer invariably referred to cancer of the cervix.

Since that time many other epidemiological studies on the aetiology of cervical cancer have been done and excellent reviews on the subject are available by Coppleson (1969) and Rotkin (1973). Evidence suggests an association of the disease with sexual behaviour and, although the age of first pregnancy, parity and promiscuity all seem to be relevant aetiological factors, it is likely that an early age of first intercourse is the most important factor (Rotkin 1973, Terris *et al.* 1967). Harris *et al.* (1980) however found that the most important factor was the number of sexual partners, and that this appeared to be the case quite independent of the age of first intercourse. They also reported a higher risk for women who smoke. Vineberg (1919) noted a twenty-fold difference in the incidence of cervical cancer in non-Jewish as compared with Jewish women in New York city. Other later observations confirm this finding. It was initially thought that the Jewess might be protected by the fact that the male partner had been circumcised and that there was a diminished risk of exposure to smegma, although there has never been laboratory evidence to suggest that smegma is carcinogenic. Abou-Daoud (1966) found no difference in incidence of the disease between Lebanese Christians and Muslims despite their different circumcision status. Other reasons put forward for the low incidence of the disease in Jewesses were a hereditary factor, the avoidance of intercourse around the time of menstruation, during pregnancy and in the postpartum period, and the strong ethnic ties to solidarity of family life. More recently, Pridan and Lilienfeld (1971) have suggested that the increasingly liberal sexual behaviour of Jewish males may be a factor in the development of cervical cancer in Jewesses, and to substantiate this they reported that 80% of Jewish males whose wives have developed a cervical carcinoma (as compared with 44% in a matched control group) had more than 9 sexual partners.

In the British Isles carcinoma of the cervix has the steepest social class gradient of any cancer. There is also evidence from elsewhere, primarily from Third World countries where it is a major cause of death, that the disease is associated with poverty. Stamler (1967) has shown that in the United States the disease is most likely to kill Puerto Ricans, blacks and poor whites. United Kingdom social class data indicate that the wives of manual workers are at greater risk than those married to non-manual workers, and that this is even true when social class 3 is separated into non-manual and skilled manual workers. Not surprisingly, the husband's occupation has therefore been examined as a possible risk factor. The women at greatest risk are those married to fishermen, barge and boatmen, long-distance lorry drivers and hotel and lodging house keepers (Beral 1974, Wakefield et al. 1973), with the implication that such occupations offer more than the usual opportunity for extramarital sexual relationships and an excess of sexual partners. The wives of commercial travellers whose husbands have similar opportunities do not fall into such a high risk group as would be expected. Possible exposure of the male to carcinogens such as tar or diesel oils might therefore be significant. Whatever the reason, the wives of men who have had more than 18 partners outside marriage have a 7.8-fold risk of developing cervical cancer (Buckley et al. 1981). Still with the male, Swan and Brown (1979) have reported a reduced risk in women married to vasectomized men. Is this accounted for by some alteration to the semen?

A high incidence of carcinoma of the cervix in prostitutes, women attending venereal disease clinics and women in prison has been observed. Moghissi et al. (1968) showed carcinoma of the cervix to be four times as common in a group of female prisoners, one-third of whom were prostitutes, as in a control group, and Singer (1973) studied a group of 768 women in a London prison and found a histologically proven rate for cervical intra-epithelial neoplasia of 92 per 1000 with a rate of 60 per 1000 in women under 21 years old. Because of the importance of sexual behaviour in the aetiology of cervical cancer, sexually transmitted infectious agents have been studied as possible aetiologic factors. In recent years most work has been centred on herpes simplex virus type II (HSV II) and human papilloma virus, but even spermatozoa have been considered.

Herpes Simplex Virus II

HSV II virus is responsible for a highly infectious disease primarily transmitted by venereal means. Antibodies are produced in the host and have been measured quantitively, early results indicating a high titre in women with cervical cancer or with premalignant stages of the disease. Conflicting reports are also available and the explanation may in part be that the antibody tests are not yet sufficiently specific. It is postulated that the nucleus of the virus becomes integrated into the host cell genome, the so-called oncogene theory. Laboratory tests have shown the virus to have oncogenic potential as judged by the transformation of cells *in vitro*. Other venereal diseases, such as syphilis and trichomoniasis, often present along with HSV II infection, have been excluded as causal factors.

Human Papilloma Virus (Wart Virus)

A large number of women with asymptomic intra-epithelial neoplasia are also found to have changes recognized by cytology, colposcopy and on histological examination of biopsy specimens which are consistent with wart virus infection. No satisfactory antibody tests are available, such as is the case with HSV II, but a similar causal mechanism is suggested. One-third of men with carcinoma of the penis have had penile warts (Cocks et al. 1982) and a common aetiology for carcinoma of the penis and cervix, e.g. human papilloma virus, was postulated by Cocks et al. (1980). The subject has recently been reviewed by Singer and McCance (1985) and the question posed 'a casual or causal association?'

Spermatozoa

Reid (1964) has put forward the view that the nucleic acid in the sperm head may be integrated into the epithelial cell genome in a similar way to that described for viruses, and that this may modify the metabolism of the host cell so as to cause uncontrolled growth.

As with many other cancers, the aetiology may well be multifactorial, in this case involving not only the host female but the male and the environment. Further research is necessary before conclusions can be drawn which will allow effective protective policies to be developed.

CERVICAL CYTOLOGY

Papanicolaou and Traut (1941) claimed that the examination of vaginal smears would allow pre-invasive carcinoma of the cervix to be recognized in a symptomless population, and that treatment of the disease at this stage would prevent the onset of cervical cancer and later reduce the incidence of mortality from the disease. It was some years before national screening programmes developed.

Cytological methods have since been used to recognize pre-invasive and preclinical invasive disease of the cervix. Ayre (1951) improved the precision of the test by designing a wooden spatula, specially shaped so as to collect cells from the squamocolumnar junction of the cervix. The preparation is immediately spread on to a glass slide and fixed with 95% ethyl alcohol, or with an aerosol alternative, and subsequently examined after staining with haematoxylin and eosin or the Papanicolaou staining method. The cytologist's report is usually presented on the basis of a classification which uses 5 sub-groups. A smear may be normal or be one showing cells with inflammatory changes but no evidence of malignancy. Together such smears may be reported as 'negative'. Some smears include cells suggesting dysplasia or lead the cytologist to report the smears as 'doubtful'. Positive smears are those which include cells suggestive of severe dysplasia or carcinoma-*in-situ* or cells suggestive of invasion.

It should be remembered that this classification is only a pointer to the likely pathology and in no way represents a definitive diagnosis. The technique carries with it a false negative rate which has been variously reported as being between 1% and 28%. Yule (1973) in Manchester, as a result of re-examining a cohort of women at regular intervals, found a 12.7% false negative rate.

False negative reports may arise as a result of: a sampling error, i.e., that, because the lesion was small or inaccessible, insufficient cells had been exfoliated to be available in the specimen; a technical error as a result of the smear being badly taken so that the preparation was too thick or thin or contaminated by an excess of red cells; or because the staining technique was incorrect; or lastly a professional error arising as a result of inexperience, inadequate training, or fatigue by the personnel involved in reading the smears.

It has been suggested that all women should have a second smear a year after the first in the hope of reducing the false negative rate.

False positive smears can be the result of errors in interpretation as a result of acute inflammation, be it bacterial, viral or the result of monilial or trichomonad infection. Atrophic conditions of the epithelium due to oestrogen deficiency may lead to a similar difficulty in interpretation.

SCREENING FOR CERVICAL CANCER

A screening programme, to be deemed effective, should reduce both the incidence of the clinical lesion and the mortality from the disease. Evaluation of such a programme may be made more difficult by virtue of changes in predisposing factors leading to changes in the incidence of the disease. The Walton Report (1976) concludes that in Canada it was not possible to confirm that screening had reduced the incidence of cervical cancer but, on the other hand, reports from both Finland (Hakama 1978) and Iceland (Johannson *et al.* 1978), where intensive screening programmes are in being, suggest that observed falls in incidence are likely to be due to screening. Mortality, the most important criterion, has been shown to fall in Canada, Finland and Iceland. Screening in the United Kingdom by comparison has been unsatisfactory and a relative failure due to poor implementation of the programme. Its shortcomings have been attributed (Draper 1982) to the lack of a national call system, an unsatisfactory recall system and the inadequate handling of data. One particular observation of this Working Group was the high number of smears done in women under 35 years old (55% smears taken for 5% of cervical cancer deaths) as compared with the smaller number taken from women over 35 years who are at a greater risk of dying from the disease. MacGregor and Teper (1978) report more favourably from Scotland. In one Scottish region where screening was intensive, mortality from the disease was seen to fall. Hakama's study (1982) of data from Nordic countries led him to believe that the changes in incidence corresponded with the level of screening, being most pronounced in Iceland, which has the most effective screening programme, followed by Finland and Sweden. A smaller effect was observed in Denmark where only 40% of women are screened. In Norway where organized screening is done on only 5% of the population, there was an increasing incidence during the period under review.

It is possible that the presumed changes in sexual practices, leading to a high incidence of cervical intra-epithelial neoplasia in young women, might have resulted in a higher mortality from carcinoma of the cervix had it not been for screening. Yule (1978), reporting on United Kingdom data, highlighted a doubling in mortality from cervical cancer in women under 35 years old between 1970 and 1976 in spite of screening, though admittedly the absolute numbers were small.

The possible effect of total hysterectomy done for benign disease was considered (Walton 1976) but it was concluded that such treatment had played no significant part in the reduction of mortality in British Columbia.

High and low risk groups
It has been apparent for many years that women in the lower socio-economic groups, though at greatest risk, are the ones least likely to avail themselves of screening facilities. The United Kingdom experience has been that only 45% of smears done are on women over 35 years, yet in this age group 95% of the deaths occur. Those women embarking on sexual activity early in life should be screened at the first opportunity which is usually at a Family Planning Clinic. Women who attend venereal disease clinics or routine gynaecological outpatient clinics should also have smears. Those women at greatest risk are quite likely to be found in female prisons (Singer 1973).

The Canadian Task Force (Walton 1976) identified those at low risk who need not be included in a programme as women who had never had sexual activity, women who have had a hysterectomy for benign disease, and women who, having had negative smears throughout life, reach the age of 60 years.

Age and frequency
The recommendations for screening in any health programme invariably are influenced by the cost of the service. If only one smear can be done then a smear at around age 35–40 years seems to offer a considerable degree of protection.

Knox (1976) using a mathematical model, claims ten tests on a woman between the ages of 35 and 80 years should, in England and Wales, save 77% of all deaths from cervical cancer in women screened, a yield of 0.67 deaths saved per 1000 tests performed. Both Canadian and United Kingdom experience suggests that there are diminishing returns with increasing frequency of screening in a given cohort of women. It is better to spend money on increasing the number of women being screened for the first time than to increase the frequency of screening in women previously screened, and it is primarily cost that has determined the 5-yearly recall interval recommended in England and Wales. It is also believed that screening programmes are best organized on a National Health Service District basis and that it is as important to improve the quality and sensitivity of screening programmes as it is to increase the frequency of screening.

The most recent Walton Report (1982) recommends that for women who have had sexual intercourse, screening tests be done on an annual basis between the ages of 18 and 35 years and that thereafter women should be screened every five years. Women over 35 years, who are thought at high risk by virtue of their contact with venereal disease clinics, penal institutions or by their own judgement, should not be discouraged from having smears done more than once every five years if they request them.

In the United Kingdom, on the advice of the Committee of Gynaecological Cytology, the Department of Health and Social Security (1984) advise screening for any woman who is or has been sexually active at her first presentation for contraceptive advice or whenever she first requests screening. Screening should be repeated after that first occasion at the ages of 20, 25, 30 and 35 years and thereafter every five years. In addition every woman should be screened early in the course of care for each pregnancy. A statement from the Imperial Cancer Research Fund Co-ordinating Committee on Cervical Screening (1984) sets out in detail how such a scheme can be organized.

Management of the patient with the abnormal cervical smear

If smear changes resulting from infection are recognized, then the specific infection should be treated, and a further smear taken from the patient once the infection has been eradicated. Patients with atrophic smears should be treated with oestrogen and the smear test repeated when the epithelium has returned to normal. All other patients with abnormal smears should have a colposcopic examination of the cervix unless there is an obvious clinical lesion from which a biopsy can be taken without doubt or difficulty. The English-speaking nations have been slow to recognize the advantages of colposcopy, which was first described by Hinselmann (1925) but, as a result of numerous reports in the English literature, it should now be readily available to all gynaecologists.

COLPOSCOPY

The patient is examined in the modified lithotomy position so as to allow easy exposure of the cervix using a bivalve speculum. Alternative speculae should be available in order to get the best view of the vagina. The colposcope itself is a binocular microscope which is used to view the cervix telescopically at magnifications ranging from 6–40 times. Once the cervix has been exposed, the mucus is cleared away using a cotton wool swab soaked with normal saline and then the vascular patterns of the subepithelial capillaries are examined. These blood vessels are more easily seen when a green filter is used so that the vessels appear black, a technique made popular by Koller (1963). With experience the nature and extent of the cervial epithelial lesion can be determined. When the green filter is removed, and 5% acetic acid applied gently to the cervix, the atypical epithelium becomes more readily visible as the acetic acid coagulates the proteins of the epithelial lesion which then takes on a white appearance. Biopsies should be taken from such areas.

Schiller (1929) had observed that squamous carcinomas of the cervix were lacking in glycogen and as a result failed to take up an iodine solution (Lugol's iodine containing iodine 2 g, potassium iodide 4 g and distilled water to 300 ml) applied to the cervix and upper vagina. Normal epithelium, however, being rich in glycogen stains dark brown. Schiller recommended that biopsies be taken from all non-staining areas, but most colposcopists now believe that it adds little to the acetic acid test which is currently the most used method of determining those areas of the cervix which require biopsy. Schiller's test can be of value, if there is a good correlation between the acetic acid and Schiller's tests, to a surgeon who is going to undertake a cone

biopsy on another occasion, enabling him to know exactly the extent to which the cone need go without resorting to a second colposcopic examination. More detailed accounts of colposcopic techniques can be found by consulting Coppleson et al. (1971), Kolstad and Stafl (1982), Jordan and Singer (1976) and Cartier (1984).

It is important that during a colposcopic examination of the cervix, the squamocolumnar junction is seen in its entirety. Special instruments, such as a Kogan endocervical speculum, are available to facilitate this procedure. If the squamocolumnar junction is not seen, then the colposcopist cannot be sure that the full extent of the lesion has been recognized, and under such circumstances a cone biopsy is obligatory. At the end of a satisfactory colposcopic examination, the colposcopist should have decided on the nature and extent of the lesion and have taken biopsy specimens from the worst affected areas for subsequent histological examination. When the histological report becomes available treatment can be planned. A suggested scheme of management is shown in Fig. 50.1.

TREATMENT OF PRE-INVASIVE LESIONS

If the examination has been incomplete, if microinvasion or invasion is suspected, or if the colposcopic examination revealed no abnormality in spite of further positive smears being obtained, then a cone biopsy should be performed. The size of the cone biopsy can be kept to a minimum, being tailored to the colposcopic findings. By keeping the cone biopsy as small as is necessary, the incidence of the complications which can follow cone biopsy can be reduced or avoided. Once the dimensions of the cone have been determined it is cut using a knife with an angled Beaver blade. The dilatation and curettage should then be performed. Haemostasis can be achieved using Dexon sutures in the 3 and 9 o'clock positions or sutures of the Sturmdorf type in the anterior and posterior aspects of the cervix, supplemented by sutures at each lateral angle. It is important that the squamocolumnar junction remains visible for subsequent assessment, and with this in mind Krebs (1984) describes a circumferential suturing technique which seems to have much to offer.

Prior to the use of colposcopy, cone biopsy was followed by a primary or secondary haemorrhage rate approaching 10%. Less commonly perforation of the uterus may precede local infection or peritonitis. Scarring may lead to cervical stenosis with conse-

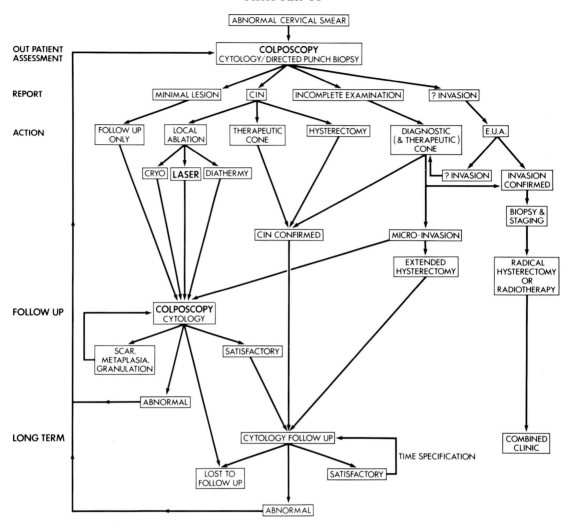

Fig. 50.1. Flow diagram depicting management of cervical epithelial abnormality by colposcopy.

quent cryptomenorrhoea. Subsequent fertility can be impaired by virtue of cervical scarring or the loss of cervical mucus, and pregnancy, should it occur, may be complicated by an increased incidence of abortion, premature labour or cervical dystocia in labour.

It is essential that after a cone biopsy has been performed, the patient is examined on a regular basis and that a cytological smear is submitted for examination at each visit. An acceptable regime would be to see the patient at 4 monthly intervals during the first year, at 6 monthly intervals during the second year, and thereafter at yearly intervals provided the cervical smears remain negative. It is extremely rare for invasive cancer to develop after cone biopsy (0.9% according to Kolstad & Klem 1976).

Treatment by total hysterectomy does not give significantly better results but should be considered when residual lesions persist after treatment by conization, if the lesion extends on to the upper vagina (as judged by colposcopy), or if there is a co-existing indication for hysterectomy, such as menorrhagia due to benign disease or prolapse.

Treatment by local destruction
Many women we see with cervical intra-epithelial neoplasia are young, often unmarried and frequently wanting children in the future.

In an effort to avoid the complications which sometimes follow cone biopsy, premalignant disease of the cervix has been treated by local destruction using one of a variety of methods. It is now generally accepted that before such methods are used, the patient should be seen and assessed by an expert colposcopist who has satisfied himself that he can see all the lesion, is confident that he can exclude invasive carcinoma as a result of his colposcopic examination and subsequenthistological examination of the colposcopically directed biopsies, and that he himself carries out the ablative procedures. It is also important that the patient is available for regular cytological and if necessary colposcopic surveillance after treatment.

Cryocautery, electrocautery, electrodiathermy, cold coagulation and the carbon dioxide laser have all been used in recent years and the results of treatment reported.

Cryocautery, which destroys the tissue by freezing is an outpatient procedure associated with little discomfort but which has the disadvantage of not destroying tissue to a depth greater than 3–4 mm. There are those (Richart *et al.* 1980) who believe that the new regenerating epithelium may cover residual disease so that it may not become apparent prior to it becoming invasive.

Electrocautery done on an outpatient basis without anaesthesia will not achieve a satisfactory depth of tissue destruction without causing too much pain, though if electrodiathermy is done under general anaesthesia a satisfactory depth of destruction can be achieved but with the risk of subsequent cervical stenosis. Duncan (1983) reported on the use of a SEMM 'cold' coagulator used on an outpatient basis, without anaesthesia, and he claims that although most patients experienced pelvic cramp-like pains lasting for the duration of the treatment, on no occasion did treatment need to be abandoned. Post-treatment complications were few.

Bellina (1977) and Jordan (1979) have advocated the use of a carbon dioxide laser and this equipment is now used in many centres to treat pre-invasive disease on an outpatient basis. *LASER* is an acronym from the first letters of the words *Light Amplification by the Stimulated Emission of Radiation*. Within the laser tube carbon dioxide is converted into radiant energy of a special kind. Laser light has three qualities: it is coherent (all the waves are exactly in phase with each other in space and time), it is collimated (the rays are parallel to each other) and it is monochromic (all the rays are of exactly the same wavelength). The laser beam is directed and manipulated through the colposcope and aimed precisely at abnormal tissue. The tissue is destroyed by vaporizing the intracellular fluid so that the cells burst. Smoke

is removed by suction. The depth of tissue destruction is dependent on two factors, time and the power density which is measured in watts/cm². The power and the time for which it is used are adjusted on the console and the laser is then controlled by a protected foot switch. Although claims are made that almost all patients can be treated without any form of analgesia or anaesthesia, this is not our experience and we currently use paracervical blocks with 2% lignocaine for all patients. It is essential that the depth of destruction must reach 5–7 mm so that all involved glands are treated, and with such a technique cure rates in the region of 94% for selected patients can be expected (Jordan & Mylotte 1980). Healing is quick and post-treatment complications, such as bleeding or infection, are few. Cervical function is retained after treatment. It is our practice to see the patient four months after treatment for colposcopic examination and for cervical cytology, and then if these findings are satisfactory to review her as after cone biopsy.

CLINICAL FEATURES AND PRETREATMENT ASSESSMENT

Early invasive cancers of the cervix produce few symptoms. In the premenopausal woman, irregular bleeding is usually noticed as intermenstrual bleeding which commonly follows intercourse. After the menopause, the postmenopausal bleeding that occurs can be either postcoital or spontaneous. If tissue necrosis is present, an offensive vaginal discharge becomes apparent, characteristically thin and watery, but sometimes brown in appearance. It is only when the growth reaches the pelvic side walls that nerves become involved and severe pain occurs. Pain may also be the result of metastatic deposits in bone. Lower limb oedema may follow the neoplastic involvement of the lymphatic channels in the pelvis. In the later stages of the disease, ureteric involvement may lead to symptoms due to uraemia, and progressive bleeding may cause anaemia. Should the tumour invade the bladder or bowel a fistula may occur which leads to obvious urinary or bowel incontinence, but a urinary fistula may be preceded by frequency and urgency of micturition, dysuria and haematuria and a bowel fistula by tenesmus, diarrhoea and rectal bleeding.

Any patient with such suggestive symptoms should have a careful, general and pelvic examination and the latter must include a speculum examination, so that the cervix can be examined and a smear taken from it for cytological assessment, and both digital vaginal and rectal examinations. When necrosis is associated with superficial ulceration and infection, the cervical smear may be negative and in such circumstances the smear report should be ignored.

To confirm the diagnosis, a histological examination of biopsy material is undertaken, the specimen being obtained either in the outpatient clinic or under anaesthesia. Primary carcinoma of the cervix can sometimes be confused with other malignant lesions involving the cervix. The cervix is rarely a site for metastatic carcinoma, but can nevertheless be involved with lymphomas in the pelvis, or as a result of direct extension of carcinomata from adjacent organs, i.e. spread from an endometrial or a vaginal lesion. Benign lesions may cause confusion at the time of the clinical examination but are readily excluded by cytology and an appropriate biopsy. Tuberculosis of the cervix can result in a friable lesion and the shedding of giant cells can confuse the cytologist.

Staging is used to determine the extent of spread prior to treatment, and for cancer of the cervix it should, by convention, take into account the findings under anaesthesia. Pre-operative evaluation of the patient will include a detailed past medical and past surgical history. A general examination to include a search for possible lymph nodes in the supraclavicular fossae or inguinal regions, and an abdominal examination with particular reference to the renal areas, the liver, and to exclude swellings arising out of the pelvis, are necessary. Laboratory tests will include a full blood count, as well as estimates of liver and renal function. Simple radiographic studies including X-rays of the chest and renal tract are essential and included in the staging process, but the results of more sophisticated investigations, such as lymphography and computerized axial tomography, if performed, must not affect staging.

Lymphography has frequently been used to look for nodal metastases prior to surgical treatment or pre-treatment staging laparotomy. Leman et al. (1975) quote a 94% accuracy and Piver and Barlow (1973) 95% for early disease, but Averette et al. (1969) reported 79% for pelvic nodes. Lagasse et al. (1979) investigating more extensive disease found unrecognized common iliac or paraaortic nodes in 19% of patients and concluded that it was unwise to plan any treatment on the basis of lymphography findings. It is probable that the technique offers a high predictive value when nodes are negative but is of low predictive value when nodes are positive (Ashraf et al. 1982).

The worth of lymphography increases when it is used with intraoperative lymphograms done to ensure nodal clearance during surgery (Kolbenstvedt & Kolstad 1974). It can also be used with some value in the investigation of recurrent disease.

Computerized axial tomography has not yet been shown to be of value in the pre-operative assessment of the disease. Grumbine et al. (1981), recorded only 58% accuracy in the assessment of parametric spread, and nodal metastases were frequently missed.

It is generally agreed that the current staging system recommended by FIGO (Table 50.1) is preferable to other staging systems, such as the TNM (tumour, node, metastases) classification. When the patient is examined under anaesthesia to determine the extent of spread, a cystoscopy is undertaken to check the bladder and, if appropriate biopsies have not been obtained earlier, biopsy specimens from the cervix and curettings from the corpus are sent for histological examination.

TREATMENT OF INVASIVE DISEASE

Historical review

Towards the end of the 19th century simple hysterectomy and removal of the growth was shown to be inadequate treatment for invasive cancer of the cervix. In 1898 in Vienna, Wertheim first treated the disease by performing a radical hysterectomy which included wide excision of the parametrium and removal of all the pelvic lymph nodes. He later modified his lymphadenectomy technique to one of a selective removal of enlarged suspicious nodes in the hope of reducing the high mortality and the incidence of ureteric complications. He reported on his results (Wertheim 1905, 1911) but the high incidence of complications did little to popularize the operation. Also in Vienna, Schauta (1904) favoured a radical vaginal hysterectomy which allowed the removal of the uterus and adnexae with, if anything, a more radical excision of the paracervical tissues than the Wertheim's procedure, but without removal of the pelvic lymph nodes. The Curies' discovery of radium in 1898 (Roentgen having previously discovered X-rays in 1825) meant that an alternative method of treatment for carcinoma of the cervix became available with well known techniques being developed in Manchester, Paris and Stockholm. Rivalry between surgeons and radiotherapists became commonplace. In this country Victor Bonney (1935) reported a personal series of 483 Wertheim's procedures performed as treatment for cervical and endometrial cancer between 1907 and 1935. His operative mortality for the first 100 patients was 20% but had fallen to 9.5% for the last 200. With improvements in anaesthesia, antisepsis and resuscitation, gynaecologists world-wide have reduced progressively the operative mortality and morbidity resulting from radical surgery. Currie (1971) and Stallworthy and Wiernik (1976) have reported big series in which radiotherapy was combined with radical surgery with improved results and lowered mortality. Wertheim's operation has been used extensively in Japanese clinics since its introduction, and modified there so as to allow a more extensive anatomical dissection and excision of the parametrium (Okabayashi 1921, Natsume 1973).

Schauta's operation was further developed by Amreich (1941), Bastiaanse (1955) and Navratil (1954) and by Mitra (1954) who combined the radical vaginal operation with an abdominal extraperitoneal lymphadenectomy.

Although the cooperation between surgeon and radiotherapist has improved as years have gone by there is still a considerable geographical variation in the way carcinoma of the cervix is treated. The review of world data by Kottmeier (1982) indicates that in general terms the results of surgery and radiotherapy, used singly or in combination, differ little. Treatment should therefore be selected on an individual basis for each patient, bearing in mind the advantages and disadvantages which each has to offer.

RADIOTHERAPY

Radiotherapy can be used, with few exceptions, to treat carcinoma of the cervix irrespective of the extent to which the disease has spread. The uterus and vagina allow ready access for the placement of sources and the cervix tolerates high doses of irradiation. The dose given is normally quoted for point A, an arbitrary point defined in Manchester as being 2 cm lateral to the centre of the uterine canal and 2 cm up from the vaginal skin of the lateral fornix in the plane of the uterus. Seven thousand to eight thousand rads at this point are given over a time varying from 50–100 hours as a single or multiple application. In Stockholm, Forsell (1917) used uterine sources in tandem and vaginal sources in boxes. Heyman (1947) individualized the treatment regimes. In Paris, Regaud (1926) used a protracted low dose rate employing a colpostat. Tod and Meredith (1938) working in Manchester developed a system using a uterine tube and rubber ovoids employed with a spacer. The ovoids were of variable size to cope with differing vaginal dimensions and the dose of the source was modified according to the size of the ovoid to keep the dose of irradiation affecting the tissues constant.

Caesium has superseded radium as a source, being of lower energy and having a short half life, thus reducing the radiation hazard to the staff who handle it.

The methods described above all use radiation sources which are introduced into the patient under general anaesthesia. Packs are used to maintain the sources in position and normally the position of the sources will be checked by radiographic means. After-loading systems have more recently been developed (Joslin 1971) which allow empty tubes to be placed within the patient and then, after the position of the tubes has been checked radiologically, radioactive sources can be introduced along catheters from machines in which the sources are stored. A high dose after-loading system using Cobalt 60 as a source is shown in Fig. 50.2. With such a system the insertion time lasts for only a few minutes. The necessary protection for staff is achieved by inserting the applicators in a protected operating theatre, by checking the position of the applicators by X-ray and then by introducing the sources by remote control outside the operating theatre. The patient is kept under observation using television.

A low dose system using Caesium 137 requires a longer insertion time and is used in a somewhat different way. The blank sources are introduced into the patient in the operating theatre and then after the position of the sources has been checked radiologically, the patient is transferred to a protected room (Fig. 50.3). The equipment is designed so that the nurse can, having left the room, introduce the radioactive sources into the patient and subsequently withdraw those sources prior to re-entering the room for any nursing procedure. The accumulative time that the sources are in the patient is recorded. To date, it is thought that the tumour response with these higher-dose-rate treatments is very similar to that achieved with conventional radium treatments.

Intracavitary treatment is likely to be adequate to deal with the central tumour, but if tumour or enlarged lymph nodes on the pelvic wall are present additional therapy in the form of external irradiation is necessary. On occasions a central lead block or wedge is employed to minimize the effect of the external therapy on the bladder and rectum. The radio-

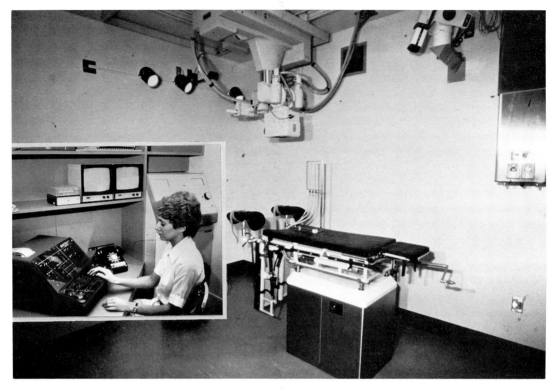

Fig. 50.2. A high dose after-loading system using Cobalt 60 designed by Nucletron. Inset, the operator working outside the protected room.

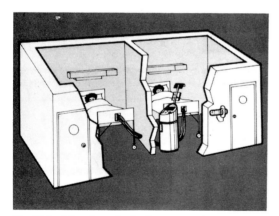

Fig. 50.3. A low dose after-loading system showing equipment used for two patients in adjacent rooms, by Nucletron.

therapist will vary the way in which he combines intracavitary and external irradiation according to the particular features of any patient's disease. For example, if extensive tumour is present or if a barrel lesion exists, external therapy is used initially to shrink the tumour mass prior to the employment of intracavitary sources.

Various attempts have been made to assess the degree of radiocurability that can be expected. Glucksman and Spear (1945) looked for a correlation between cellular differentiation and a favourable prognosis, but Atkin (1971) found the prognosis more closely linked to chromosome variability independent of histological grading. Dixon and Stead (1977) have used sequential biopsies during treatment to allow a qualitative assessment of the proliferative parts of the tumour to predict the likely results of treatment.

Complications of radiotherapy

Symptoms observed during treatment may herald long term complications so, in addition to dealing with the immediate problem, further irradiation may need to be delayed. Proctitis is one such symptom and can normally be managed by giving the patient a kaolin and morphine mixture along with Predsol enemas. Cramp-like abdominal pain may be a warning that small bowel complications might appear later. If the patient develops frequency of micturition, urgency of micturition or dysuria, she should be encouraged to take a high intake of fluid and infection, if present, should be treated. Patients with pyometra should have the uterus drained and be given antibiotics prior to any radiotherapy being undertaken. Skin reactions such as erythema or pigmentation may occur towards the end of external therapy, but severe burns can be avoided by using multiple ports of entry and high voltage radiotherapy.

Dyspareunia, the result of vaginal adhesions or fibrosis, may be minimized by the use of vaginal dilators, and is said to be less when shorter treatment times in combination with high dose sources are used. Subdermal fibrosis is unsightly, uncomfortable and unresponsive to remedial action. If the small bowel is damaged by irradiation, malabsorption, obstruction, perforation or peritonitis may follow and bowel resection may be necessary. Rectal bleeding and pain can occur and be followed by the development of a recto-vaginal fistula which may require a defunctioning colostomy to provide symptomatic relief. The colostomy is often permanent. Haematuria is the most common urinary complication, usually being due to telangiectasia which is apparent on cystoscopy, but contraction of the bladder, a radiation ulcer, or the development of a vesico-vaginal fistula can occur making a urinary diversion necessary, usually achieved by the creation of an ileal conduit.

Representative results of treatment of carcinoma of the cervix by radiotherapy are shown in Table 50.2.

Table 50.2. Results of radiotherapy for carcinoma cervix.

| Institution | Cases | Percentage 5 year survival by Stage | | | |
		I	II	III	IV
Toronto, Canada	600	74	68	37	14
Tokyo, Japan	367	92	70	50	19
Oslo, Norway	700	82	59	32	13
Stockholm, Sweden	377	88	55	17	0
Manchester, U.K.	1074	78	51	36	7
Minneapolis, U.S.A.	108	91	64	36	0

Table constructed from data published in the *Eighteenth Annual Report on Results of Treatment in Gynecological Cancer for the period 1973–1975*, FIGO.

SURGICAL TREATMENT

Surgical treatment confers considerable advantages for the patient when the disease being treated is still restricted in its spread. Most surgeons would operate only on patients whose disease was within the FIGO staging IA, IB and IIA. When the disease has spread into the parametrium, radiotherapy is more suitable.

Surgical treatment is of the greatest advantage to the younger woman. It can offer the preservation of ovarian function if pre-operative radiotherapy is omitted. There is evidence that carcinoma of the cervix is more common in younger women than it was previously (Fig. 50.4) and it has been suggested that the disease may be more aggressive in these younger women. Dyspareunia is less common, whether or not pre-operative radiotherapy is used. Technical problems for the radiotherapist, i.e. infected adnexae, the big uterus and pregnancy, can all be avoided by using surgical treatment. Irradiation of normal tissue need not take place and radiotherapy complications can be avoided. Local recurrence in the uterus is not possible and pelvic recurrence after treatment is uncommon. The possibility of radioresistance can be avoided. From the educational point of view the clinician's pre-operative staging can be confirmed, though of course not altered as a result of his surgical findings. Bonney (1935) drew the comparison 'between what one man sees and another man thinks he feels'. A histological report of adenocarcinoma should not dissuade the surgeon. Such a histological diagnosis, like the poorly differentiated squamous carcinoma, carries a worse prognosis but Kottmeier's analysis (1982) reveals that patients do better when surgery is used alone or in combination with radiotherapy than when radiotherapy is used alone.

Attitudes vary as to the way in which microinvasive disease (Stage IA) should be treated. Nelson *et al.* (1975) recommend radical surgery when the depth of invasion exceeds 1 mm, but Coppleson (1976), in an excellent review, draws attention to the overtreatment of microinvasion and points out that microinvasive carcinoma can frequently be treated with surgical procedures which fall short of a radical hysterectomy and lymphadenectomy. Minimal lesions with only stromal invasion can be dealt with by cone biopsy but when the microinvasive lesion is associated with lymph channel involvement a more radical procedure is indicated. This should take the form of an extended hysterectomy. Lymph node sampling is often wise but a wide dissection of the parametrium is unnecessary.

Occult Stage IB lesions (including those described as microcarcinoma) along with those clinical lesions staged as IB and IIA require a formal radical hysterectomy combined with an appropriate lymphadenectomy.

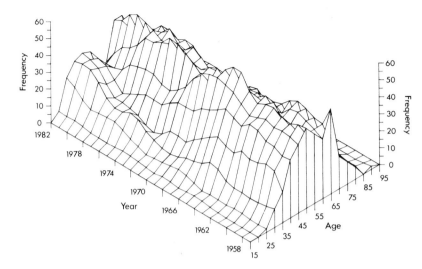

Fig. 50.4. Yorkshire Regional Cancer Registry data shown in three-dimensional form. From Paterson *et al.* (1984) with permission from the *British Medical Journal*.

The reader should consult operative surgery texts, e.g. Shaw (1983), Nelson (1976), Coppleson (1981) for details of surgical technique, but it is appropriate to mention here some relevant points.

Adequate exposure is essential for safe surgery and this can be achieved by using either an extended lower oblique incision (preferred) or a transverse incision which employs a rectus muscle cutting technique. Careful exploration of the abdominal contents is important, and there is advantage in sampling para-aortic lymph nodes so that if metastatic tumour is found by frozen section the surgical procedure can be abandoned and radiotherapy used, thus avoiding undue morbidity in a situation which is associated with a reduced survival rate.

The ovaries need not be sacrificed if apparently healthy. Surgeons differ as to the thoroughness of the lymphadenectomy. When pre-operative lymphography has been used there is the opportunity to take intra-operative films after lymphadenectomy so as to check that all the pelvic lymph nodes have been removed (Kolbenstvedt & Kolstad 1976). It is thought however that there is a higher incidence of postoperative lymphocysts and lower extremity oedema after a more extensive pelvic node dissection.

The essential feature of a Wertheim's operation is the lateral displacement of the ureters and forward displacement of the bladder so as to allow a wide excision of the parametria and upper vagina when the total hysterectomy is undertaken. This means that the uterine artery is divided at its origin from the anterior division of the internal iliac artery and brought medially so that the tunnel surrounding the terminal ureter can be opened and the ureter dis-

placed safely. Such a dissection creates a risk of postoperative ureteric fistula, a risk increased when surgery is combined with radiotherapy. Other aspects of technique will be considered during the discussion of postoperative complications.

POSTOPERATIVE COMPLICATIONS

Bleeding during the operation most commonly occurs whilst the bladder and terminal ureter are being dissected, but there is also a risk of haemorrhage if an abnormal obturator vein is not recognized or when removing lymph nodes from adjacent blood vessels. This can be particularly troublesome if there is a fixed node where the common iliac vein is formed. With adequate blood replacement postoperative shock should be uncommon. Postoperative pyrexia is frequently observed. Pulmonary atelectasis with subsequent infection is one possible cause but this readily responds to physiotherapy and antibiotics. The incidence of pelvic infection due to cellulitis or abscess is reduced when suction drainage is employed and haematomas are avoided. Various measures to reduce the incidence of infection including wound infection are taken. Pre-operative infection should be identified and treated. Pre-operative Betadine vaginal douches are used to reduce the bacterial flora in the vagina. Prophylactic antibiotics (a combination of metronidazole and cephradine) are given intravenously immediately prior to surgery and for 48 hours afterwards. Urinary tract infection is the commonest postoperative infection observed as patients need an indwelling urinary catheter in the postoperative period.

Pulmonary embolism is the complication most

likely to lead to the death of the patient. Preceding deep vein thrombosis may or may not have been recognized. It is of vital importance that the patient is handled carefully both on and off the operating table. Whenever the Trendelenburg position is used, attention must be paid to the proper placing of the patient's knee joints in relation to the angulation of the table. Early postoperative mobilization is important. Many surgeons use prophylactic subcutaneous heparin, given in a dose of 5000 i.u. 2 hours pre-operatively and 8 hourly thereafter for 7 days or until the patient is ambulant whichever is the shorter. Therapeutic doses of anticoagulants will be required if a presumptive diagnosis of deep vein thrombosis is confirmed by phlebography.

The incidence of ureteric fistula has been reduced significantly and different surgeons attribute their success (Table 50.3) to different intra-operative or

Table 50.3. Changing incidence of uretero-vaginal fistula after radical hysterectomy.

		No. of cases	% of fistula
Green *et al.*	(1962)	623	8.5
Green	(1966)	65	1.5
Novak (1947–54)	(1963)	246	11.4
Novak (1954–63)	(1963)	850	2.8
Symmonds	(1966)	72	0

postoperative regimes. Stallworthy (1964) emphasized the need to maintain a mesentery running along the inferior surface of the ureter, whilst Green (1966) employed a technique of suspending the ureter to the obliterated hypogastric artery at the end of the operation. Novak (1963) thought it important to leave the ureter intraperitoneally on completion of the pelvic part of the operation, whilst Symmonds and Pratt (1961) like many others attribute their success to routine postoperative bladder drainage. Their normal practice is to drain the bladder for two weeks after surgery or for six weeks if pre-operative radiotherapy has been employed. Surgeons differ in their choice of either suprapubic catheterization or the use of a Foley catheter.

Interference with bladder denervation (Smith *et al.* 1969) seems to be responsible for the voiding difficulties experienced by patients after operation. Episodes of overdistension of the bladder (often due to inappropriate catheter management) may make the situation worse. Bladder drainage is therefore necessary until normal function has been restored. This may rarely mean that long term catheter drainage is

necessary or a technique of self-catheterization by the patient is required. Urinary tract infection must be avoided and prophylactic urinary antiseptics are given so long as the patient is experiencing difficulty in emptying the bladder.

The incidence of pelvic lymphocyst following pelvic surgery is of the order of 5%. Ligature of afferent lymphatics may help to reduce the incidence of this complication. When they occur, simple aspiration (more safely employed with ultrasound control) may be curative but, if not, operative transperitoneal marsupialization of the lymphocyst may be required.

Infrequently damage to pelvic nerves can occur. The obturator nerve may be divided during the dissection of lymphatic channels in the region of the common iliac bifurcation but with resuture a restoration of function normally occurs. Numbness on the anterior aspect of the thigh may follow the division of femoral branches of the genitofemoral nerve.

Postoperative dyspareunia resulting from shortening of the vagina can be avoided by using a technique described by Symmonds and Pratt (1961) in which the peritoneum on the front of the rectum and the base of the bladder is used to extend the vagina. The vaginal extension becomes covered spontaneously by vaginal squamous epithelium over a matter of some weeks. An alternative is to use Williams' operation to achieve lengthening of the vagina.

Wound dehiscence can be prevented by careful surgical technique and the avoidance of abdominal distension. In this respect the use of nasogastric aspiration following the operation is helpful.

The incidence of psychological problems can be reduced by careful counselling.

COMBINED THERAPY USING IRRADIATION AND SURGERY

Local irradiation prior to radical surgery has been much more commonly used in England than in America. Stallworthy's technique involved an intracavitary regime with a dose of 5000 rads at point A six weeks prior to the patient having radical surgery, and Currie used a similar regime but with a lower dose. Both had excellent results from treatment. More recently Rampone *et al.* (1973) have used a modified radical Wertheim's hysterectomy 6–8 weeks after intracavitary radium (5000 rads at point A), believing that central irradiation reduced the need for extensive parametrial dissection, undue stripping of the lower ureter and the removal of a vaginal cuff. The 5 year cure rate of 88.3% for Stage IB compares favourably with those clinics using surgery alone. The incidences of 0.7% for urological complications reported by Stallworthy & Wiernik (1976) and of 1.4% by Currie (1971) are no worse than in many series employing surgery alone.

In spite of the theoretical advantage of pre-operative local radiotherapy, i.e. that it destroys visible tumour cells around the cervix which may implant into the vaginal wall during operation, and that it also shrinks the primary tumour making surgery easier and less haemorrhagic, there are few controlled trials which justify its use. Surwit et al. (1976) quoted a 5 year survival rate of 89.7% in patients receiving pre-operative irradiation, as compared with 75.1% in matched controls treated by primary surgery. Hansen (1981) found no such advantage. On balance, it would seem that pre-operative irradiation is indicated except in those young women with a well differentiated lesion in early stage disease whose ovaries it is intended to conserve.

Many surgeons believe that the patients with the bulky, usually barrel-shaped, endocervical lesions are at increased risk. These patients in particular benefit from pre-operative irradiation, normally megavoltage external irradiation which has the effect of shrinking the disease at the outset of treatment. Such therapy is then followed by either intracavitary irradiation or an extrafascial hysterectomy (Nelson et al. 1975).

There is a similar lack of information as to the value of postoperative irradiation given to women whose pelvic nodes contain metastatic disease. Controlled trials are underway in the United States, but until such information becomes available it would seem reasonable to continue to treat patients with positive nodes by giving postoperative megavoltage therapy.

RESULTS OF TREATMENT

When Stage IB carcinoma of the cervix is treated by primary surgery in specialist centres the 5 year survival varies from 85–89% (Morley & Seski 1976, Webb & Symmonds 1979). The figure for Stage IIA disease is somewhat lower at 70–75%. When pelvic lymph nodes are affected by tumour the 5 year cure rate falls to 50–60%. Hsu et al. (1972) report a worse prognosis when more than 4 pelvic nodes are affected (19% as compared with 48.5% 5 year survival). Some workers (Pilleron et al, 1974. Hsu et al. 1972) report a worse prognosis when pelvic nodes in both sides of the pelvis are affected, but this is not the experience reported by Webb and Symmonds (1979).

Perez et al. (1980) reported a randomized study of patients with Stage IB and IIA disease and demonstrated that patients treated by combined intracavitary irradiation followed by radical hysterectomy, as compared with conventional irradiation, did not have an improved 5 year survival.

In summary, similar cures can be achieved with either primary radical surgery or irradiation. Although the morbidity from surgery and irradiation is similar, the complications of surgery are more easily remedied and primary surgery is to be preferred for the early carcinoma, particularly in young women where ovarian conservation is practised.

Carcinoma of the cervix in special circumstances

CARCINOMA OF THE CERVIX IN PREGNANCY

The incidence of carcinoma of the cervix in pregnancy is variously quoted at 1 in 2000 to 1 in 5000 pregnancies. A speculum examination of the cervix, during which a smear is taken for cervical cytology, done at the first antenatal visit is regarded as good antenatal practice so it is not surprising that 80% of cervical cancers in pregnancy are discovered during the first two trimesters. The availability of colposcopy allows investigation of the patient with an abnormal smear without undue interference in the pregnancy. A colposcopically directed punch biopsy for histological assessment is often sufficient to exclude invasion; if so, continued colposcopic assessment of the cervix at intervals of 8–10 weeks throughout the pregnancy would thereafter be indicated and a more formal revaluation of the cervix will be done at the time of the postnatal examination.

If an obvious carcinoma is present a punch biopsy is often sufficient for diagnosis but if occult disease is suspected then a cone biopsy will be necessary even though the patient be pregnant. If microinvasion is found and the lesion is totally within the cone biopsy specimen, conservative management is reasonable with revaluation at the time of the postnatal examination and such management is likely to prove acceptable to the patient.

Whenever invasion is found, the patient must be informed of the diagnosis, of the dangers and of the need for treatment. If the patient agrees that treatment be undertaken, then in early disease (Stage IB, Stage IIA) there is a choice between using radical surgery or radiotherapy and, as in the non-pregnant patients, the results of treatment are essentially similar. It is likely that patients who are pregnant will be young and surgery seems therefore the best option in the first trimester and in the third trimester, when a Caesarean section will be combined with a radical hysterectomy and pelvic lymphadenectomy. Surgery in pregnancy is no more difficult than in the non-pregnant patient. The tissue planes dissect easily and the uterus is mobile and is easily brought up into the abdominal cavity. Ovarian conservation is possible. It is in the second trimester of pregnancy that the ethical problems are greatest and the selection of treatment more difficult. With recent advances in neonatal care, it would seem reasonable to await viability of the fetus and then do a classical Caesarean section followed immediately by a radical hysterectomy and pelvic lymph node dissection, but as an alternative, the patient can be treated by external irradiation as primary treatment and then when the fetus has died and abortion takes place, intracavitary irradiation given.

Cancer of the cervix found later in pregnancy carries a worse prognosis, but when staging is taken into account Creasman *et al.* (1970) found no difference in survival throughout the three trimesters.

CANCERS OF THE CERVICAL STUMP

It is becoming unusual to see a patient with cancer of the cervical stump now that an abdominal hysterectomy is almost invariably total. Surgical treatment is appropriate if the disease is restricted to the cervix or vaginal vault. When radiotherapy is used it may not be possible to use an intracervical source. Instead, reliance is placed on a vaginal applicator. When the disease is advanced then external irradiation will be given initially followed by intracavitary irradiation.

Results of treatment of the cervical stump equate with those for the intact uterus.

UNSUSPECTED INVASIVE CARCINOMA OF THE CERVIX

On occasions a routine histological examination of a vaginal or abdominal hysterectomy specimen will show unsuspected invasive carcinoma of the cervix. Shingleton and Orr (1983) favour re-operation in such circumstances so as to remove the residual parametrium and pelvic lymph nodes. This view is supported by Green and Morse (1969) and Barber *et al.* (1968). On the other hand, Andras *et al.* (1973) and Davy *et al.* (1977) have reported good results when high energy radiation treatment is used soon after the diagnosis has been reported by the pathologist.

RECURRENT DISEASE

After primary treatment for cervical cancer, careful observation of the patient is necessary. Forty-six per cent of patients who develop recurrence will have done so within the first year, 73% by the end of the second year, and overall, 93% by the end of the fifth year. Patients should be seen on a 3 monthly basis during the first year and a careful examination undertaken so as to exclude new physical signs appearing in the supraclavicular regions, in the abdomen (where paraaortic swellings or hepatomegaly might be observed) or in the pelvis. It is recommended that X-rays of the chest and renal tract are done in alternate years and that frequent observations on renal and liver function are undertaken. It is important to differentiate between persistent disease and recurrence. Persistent disease after irradiation therapy or surgery is further tumour appearing within a period of 3 months, whereas recurrent disease is tumour appearing after a period of complete clinical remission.

Recurrence or persistence of tumour will be suspected when the patient suffers a loss of appetite, often associated with a loss in weight. Oedema of the legs associated with pelvic pain which radiates either to the buttock posteriorly or into the upper thighs invariably has sinister implications. Pulmonary metastases are relatively uncommon but may present with chest pain, haemoptysis or a cough.

It is always necessary to get histological confirmation of recurrence before further therapy is contemplated. On occasions, lymph node needle biopsy can be helpful. Ewing *et al.* (1982) describe one such technique using monoplanar fluoroscopy. Having got a histological diagnosis, further specific investigations by way of computerized axial tomography, ultrasonic scanning or lymphography may be undertaken, although all have their limitations.

Treatment
When previous surgery has been undertaken and an isolated pelvic recurrence found, irradiation treatment may be appropriate. Re-irradiation of previously treated areas is rarely of value unless the primary course of radiotherapy has been suboptimal. Chemotherapy for recurrent disease has proved disappointing and, if the patient with recurrent disease after irradiation therapy is to be cured, ultraradical surgery, normally of the exenterative type, becomes necessary.

There is a place for removal of a small central

recurrent tumour by a radical hysterectomy, provided the fascial planes between both the bladder and the rectum and the genital tract can be divided without causing an unacceptably high risk of fistula formation. The more usual situation is that a central recurrence is spreading to either the bladder or bowel, even if not clinically evident, and that a total exenteration, which involves removing the bladder, urethra, cervix, uterus and adnexae, vagina and rectum is required. Rarely when the spread is only in a forward direction an anterior exenteration (removal of the bladder, urethra, uterus, adnexae, cervix and vagina) is possible, or if the spread is limited to the posterior aspect a posterior exenteration (removal of the rectum, uterus, adnexae, cervix and vagina) may suffice. Earlier reports on partial exenteration (anterior or posterior) indicated a poor survival and such operations went out of favour, but more recent literature suggests that these procedures can be performed successfully.

Pre-operative discussion with the patient and appropriate close members of their family is important, and during such discussion the magnitude of the procedure must be indicated and the need for a prolonged rehabilitation period emphasizes. Shingleton and Orr (1983) emphasize the importance of regarding extrapelvic disease, the triad of unilateral leg oedema, sciatica and ureteral obstruction, tumour related pelvic side wall fixation and bilateral ureteral obstruction, which is secondary to a recurrence, as absolute contraindications to an exenteration. They also point out the need to avoid such surgery in patients with severe life limiting medical illnesses or psychoses, patients with religious objections to blood transfusion, and if medical staff or hospital facilities such as are required for successful surgery are unavailable. They regard patients over 70 years old and those with a large tumour volume, unilateral ureteral obstruction or metastases to the distal vagina as relative contraindications.

From this, it becomes clear that the final decision to go ahead with an exenterative procedure will be taken during the operation when negative frozen section histology reports become available on tissue taken from the limits of the pelvic tumour and from paraaortic lymph nodes. Extrapelvic disease, malignant ascites, multiple positive pelvic nodes, tumour invasion of major vessels or bowel serosal involvement all provide intra-operative contraindications to proceeding. Symmonds and Webb (1981) and Nelson (1976) provide excellent accounts of the surgical technique required for successful surgery and should

be consulted by the reader. Traditionally a urinary conduit was, and often is, fashioned from a length of ileum, but one alternative described by Nelson is to use part of the transverse colon which will not have been subjected to the same amount of irradiation. More recently surgeons have used a length of sigmoid colon taken from that part of the bowel immediately proximal to the resected area. End to end anastomosis between the residual sigmoid and the anal canal, using a stapling technique, has avoided the need for a permanent colostomy.

Survival was adversely affected when metastases in lymph nodes were demonstrated, and significantly improved when a urinary conduit was used as a method of diversion as compared with the diversion of ureters directly into the faecal stream. No significant difference could be demonstrated between adenocarcinoma and squamous cell carcinoma as far as survival was concerned. Between 1950 and 1971, 198 pelvic exenterations were performed at the Mayo Clinic (Symmonds et al. 1975). The operation was done as a primary treatment for 37 patients and for recurrence in the remaining 161. Total exenteration had been performed in 34% of the patients, anterior exenteration in 57% and the remaining 9% had posterior exenteration. The overall mortality was 8.1% (16 patients dying within 60 days of their surgery), but during latter years the operative mortality was only 3% in 102 patients. This was attributed to better techniques of urinary diversion, improved fluid balance management and to the availability of newer and better antibiotics. The overall 5 year survival was 32% in the series. Other similar results have been reported.

Chemotherapy

There is no evidence that chemotherapy has been successful in treating recurrent carcinoma of the cervix, and since approximately half the patients with cancer of the cervix will die of the disease, in spite of modern management with surgery and radiotherapy, the need for another mode of treatment is apparent. Barker (1983) drew attention to a number of reasons as to why chemotherapy has been unsuccessful. Fibrosis commonly exists as a result of previous surgery or radiotherapy and, as a result, the blood stream to the tumour is impaired, making it difficult for the chemotherapeutic agent to reach its target organ. The tumour itself is commonly of squamous origin and few agents have been shown to be efficacious against this type of tumour. Apart from fibrosis, bone marrow function may have been impaired by previous radiotherapy and if renal failure occurs, as a result of late disease, chemotherapy regimes are compromised. The lack of a reliable tumour marker and the inaccuracies of ultrasound and computerized axial tomography, make it difficult to assess response. To date, cervical tumours have not appeared sensitive to hormone manipulation, though trials are in progress to see whether or not the use of oestrogens in combination with radiotherapy leads to improved results.

Chemotherapy has been used as primary treatment for advanced disease. Trussel and Mitford-Barberton (1961) used a pelvic infusion of methotrexate via cannulated internal iliac arteries when no radiotherapy facilities were available in East Africa. Tumour regression was reported in all 14 patients treated, with complete regression in one of the 14. Wertheim's hysterectomy became possible in another three of the 14 patients.

Morrow et al. (1977) reported on a multi-centre study using continuous pelvic arterial infusion of bleomycin for recurrent squamous cell carcinoma after irradiation therapy and concluded that the technique was not helpful. Guthrie and Way (1978) used Adriamycin and methotrexate for advanced disease and showed an improved survival time in those patients whose tumour responded to treatment. Cis-diamminedichloroplatinum (cisplatinum) has been used with Adriamycin in a trial under the auspices of the Gynecologic Oncology Group in the United States of America with a near 50% response rate.

More recently pilot studies aimed at primary treatment using cisplatinum, vinblastine and bleomycin (Friedlander et al. 1984) and cisplatinum and bleomycin (Wertheim et al. 1985) have been reported for the treatment of patients with locally advanced tumours and high risk early tumours respectively, with results sufficiently encouraging to warrant further investigation.

TERMINAL CARE

When treatment for cure is no longer appropriate, and instead only palliative measures are indicated, the management of the patient is often referred to as terminal care. Death may be imminent though not necessarily so.

Invariably patients who have had treatment for cancer of the cervix will know the diagnosis. Anxiety and depression may occur, presenting problems in communication for both relatives and staff alike. Time to talk or, perhaps more important, time to listen is essential. Help from appropriately trained social workers and churchmen can be invaluable.

Many patients will want to die in their own home but unfavourable circumstances such as relatives unable to cope by virtue of emotional problems or financial inadequacy may prevent this. It may be that the nursing care will be beyond the relatives in spite of help from the domiciliary services of the local hospice or local authority.

When admission is required the hospital in which the patient has received most of her care, i.e. the gynaecological unit, should be prepared to accept the responsibility for further care. This will usually present no problem in the short term, but if care is prolonged a hospice will be the better alternative where staff can ensure comfort and the relief of pain in a caring environment.

Symptoms requiring control may well include soreness of the mouth, anorexia, nausea or vomiting and constipation or diarrhoea. Cancer of the cervix is often associated with anaemia which may need correction, and uraemia which can lead to fits and the need for anticonvulsive therapy.

Pain is commonly the most significant problem and an accurate diagnosis of the cause should precede treatment. Regular therapy is essential and further treatment should precede the recurrence of pain. The dosage and time interval should be varied as necessary. Simple analgesics may be sufficient but narcotics such as diamorphine may be needed for visceral pain. Pain resulting from the involvement of bone may respond to an antiprostoglandin. When pelvic nerves are infiltrated corticosteroid, to reduce perineural oedema, may be combined with psychotropic drugs and anticonvulsants. Neurosurgical procedures such as nerve blocks, intrathecal injections or even a cordotomy may need to be considered in special circumstances. With thoughtful care the relief of pain can be achieved. Patients can invariably be helped towards a positive outlook if they accept reality and if they have confidence and trust in their medical and nursing advisers.

REFERENCES

Abou-Daod K.T. (1966) Cancer, 19, 1293.

Amreich A.I. (1941) Zbl. Gynäk., 65, 457.

Andras E.J., Fletcher G.H. & Rutledge F. (1973) Amer. J. Obstet. Gynec., 115, 647.

Ashraf M., Elyaderani M.K., Gabriele O.F. & Krall J.M. (1982) Gynec. Ocol., 14, 96.

Atkin N.B. (1971). In Gynaecological Cancer (Ed. T.J. Deeley), p. 138. Butterworth, London.

AVERETTE H.E., LEMAIRE W.J. & LEPAGE J.R. (1969) *Clin. Obstet. Gynec.*, **12**, 372.

AYRE J.E. (1952) *Amer. J. Obstet. Gynec.*, **55**, 609.

BARBER H.R.K., PECE G.V. & BRUNSCHWIG A. (1968) *Amer. J. Obstet. Gynec.*, **101**, 959.

BARKER G.H. (1983) *Chemotherapy of Gynaecological Malignancies*, p. 107. Castle House Publications, Ltd., Guildford.

BASTIAANSE M.A. VAN B. (1955) *J. Obstet. Gynaec. Brit. Emp.*, **62**, 761.

BELLINA J.H. (1977) *Ann. Obstet. Gynec.*, **6**, 371.

BERAL V. (1974) *Lancet*, i, 1037.

BONNEY V. (1935) *Amer. J. Obstet. Gynec.*, **30**, 815.

BUCKLEY J.D., HARRIS R.W.C., ROLL R., VESSEY M.P. & WILLIAMS P.T. (1981) *Lancet*, ii, 1010.

BURGHARDT E. (1984) *Clin. Obstet. Gynaec.*, **11**, 239.

CARTIER R. (1984) *Practical Colposcopy.* Gustav Fischer Verlag. Stuttgart, New York.

COCKS P.S., ADIB R.S. & HUNT K.M. (1982) *Brit. J. Obstet. Gynaec.*, **89**, 408.

COCKS P.S., PEEL K.R., CARTWRIGHT R.A. & ADIB R. (1980) *Lancet*, ii, 855.

COPPLESON M. (1969) *Brit. J. hosp. Med.*, **2**, 961.

COPPLESON M., PIXLEY E.C. & REID B.L. (1971) *Colposcopy: A Scientific and Practical Approach to the Cervix in Health and Disease.* Charles C. Thomas, Springfield, Illinois.

COPPLESON M. (1976) (Jordan J.A. & Singer A., eds.) *The Cervix.* W.B Saunders. London, p. 453.

COPPLESON M. (1981) Ed. *Gynecologic Oncology*, Vol. 2, Churchill Livingstone, Edinburgh and London.

CREASMAN W.T., RUTLEDGE F.N. & FLETCHER G.H. (1970) *Obstet. Gynecol.* **36**, 495.

CURRIE D.W. (1971) *J. Obstet. Gynaec. Brit. Cwlth.*, **78**, 385.

DAVY M., BENTZEN H. & JAHREN R. (1977): *Acta Obstet. Gynec. Scand.*, **56**, 105.

Department of Health and Social Security (1984) *Hosp. Circ.*, **84**, 17.

DIXON B. & STEAD R.H. (1977) *J. clin. Path.*, **30**, 907.

DRAPER G.J. (1982) *Health Trends*, **14**, 37.

DUNCAN I. (1983) In *Progress in Cancer Research and Therapy.* Recent Developments in Gynecological Oncology. (Ed. Morrow C.P.) Vol. 24, p. 15. Raven Press, New York.

EWING T.L., BUCHLER D.A., HOOGERLAND P.L., SONEK M.G. & WIRTANEN G.W. (1982) *Amer. J. Obstet. Gynec.*, **143**, 824.

FORSELL G. (1917) *Fortschr. Röntgenstr.*, **25**, 142.

FRIEDLANDER M.L., ATKINSON K., COPPLESON J.V.M., ELLIOT P., GREEN D., HOUGHTON R., SOLOMON H.J., RUSSELL P. & TATTERSALL M.H.N. (1984) *Gynecol. Oncol.*, **19**, 1.

GLUCKSMANN A. & SPEAR F.G. (1945) *Brit. J. Radiol.*, **18**, 313.

GREEN T.H. JR. (1966) *Obstet. Gynec.*, **28**, 1.

GREEN T.H. JR., MEIGS J.V., ULFELDER H. & CURTIN R.R. (1962): *Obstet Gynec.*, **20**, 293.

GREEN T.H. & MORSE W.J. JR. (1969) *Obstet. Gynec.*, **33**, 763.

GRUMBINE F.C., ROSENSHEIN N.B., ZERHOUNI E.A. & SIEGELMAN S.S. (1981) *Gynec. Oncol.*, **12**, 286.

GUTHRIE D. & WAY S. (1978) *Obstet. Gynecol.*, **52**, 349.

HAKAMA M. (1978) In *Screening in Cancer* (Ed. Miller A.B.) *U.I.C.C. Technical Report Series*, **40**, 93.

HAKAMA M. (1982) In *Trends in Cancer incidence. Causes and practical implications* (Ed. Magnu K.). Hemisphere Publishing Corporation, Washington D.C.

HANSEN M.K. (1981) *Gynecol. Oncol.*, **11**, 275.

HARRIS R.W., BRINTON L.A., COWDELL R.H., SKEGG D.C., SMITH P.G., VESSEY M. & DOLL R. (1980) *Brit. J. Cancer*, **42**, 359.

HEYMAN J. (1947) *J. Amer. med. Assoc.*, **135**, 412.

HINSELMANN (1925) *Münch. med. Wschr.*, **77**, 1733.

HSU C.-T., CHENG Y.-S. & SU S.-C. (1972) *Amer. J. Obstet. Gynec.*, **114**, 954.

Imperial Cancer Research Fund Co-ordinating Committee on Cervical Screening (1984) *Brit. med. J.*, **289**, 894.

JOHANNESSON G., GEIRSSON G. & DAY N. (1978) *Int. J. Cancer*, **21**, 418.

JORDAN J.A. (1979) *Obstet. Gynec. Surv.*, **34**, 831.

JORDAN J.A. & MYLOTTE M.J. (1980) In *Gynecologic Laser Surgery* (Ed. Bellina J.) p. 245. Plenum Press, New York.

JORDAN J.A. & SINGER A. (1976) Eds. The Cervix, W.B. Saunders Company Ltd, New York.

JOSLIN C.A.F. (1971) In *Modern Radiotherapy-Gynaecological Cancer* (ed. T.J. Deeley) p. 71. Butterworths, London.

KNOX E.G. (1976) *Brit. J. Cancer*, **34**, 444.

KOLBENSTVEDT A. & KOLSTAD P. (1974) *Gynec. Oncol.*, **2**, 39.

KOLBENSTVEDT A. & KOLSTAD P. (1976) *Gynec. Oncol.*, **115**, 597.

KOLLER O. (1963) A colpophotographic study of *The vasculature patterns of the uterine cervix.* Universitetsforlaget Oslo.

KOLSTAD P. & KLEM V. (1976) *Obstet. Gynecol.*, **48**, 125.

KOLSTAD P. & STAAFL A. (1972) *Atlas of Colposcopy.* Universitetsforlaget, Oslo. Churchill Livingstone, London.

KOTTMEIER H.L. (1982) Ed. in Annual Report of the Results of Treatment in Gynecological Cancer. FIGO, 1973–1975, **XVIII**.

KREBS H.B. (1984) *Obstet. and Gynec.*, **63**, 430.

KREBS L.D., BALLAN S.C., BERMAN M.L. & WATRING W.G. (1979) *Amer. J. Obstet. Gynec.*, **134**, 219.

LAGASSE L.D., BALLAN S.C., BERMAN M.L. & WATRING W.G. (1979) *Amer. J. Obstet. Gynec.*, **134**, 219.

LANGLEY F.A. & FOX H. (1981) In *Gynecologic Oncology* (Coppleson, Ed), **1**, 465. Churchill Livingstone. Edinburgh.

LEMAN M.H., PARK R.C., BARHAM E.D.D., CHISM S.E., PETTY W.M. & PATOW W.E. (19975) *Gynec. Oncol.*, **3**, 354.

MacGREGOR J. & TEEPER S. (1978) *Lancet*, ii, 774.

MILLER A.B., VISENTIN T. & HOWE G.R. (1981) *Int. J. Cancer*, **27**, 651.

MITRA S. (1954) In *Surgical Treatment of Carcinoma of the Cervix* (Meigs, J.V. ed.) p. 267. Grune & Stratton, New York.

MIYAMOTO T., TAKABE Y., WATANABE, M. & TERASIMA T. (1978) *Cancer*, **41**, 403.

MOGHISSI K.S., MACK H.C. & PORZAK J.P. (1968) *Amer. J. Obstet. Gynec.*, **100**, 607.

MORLEY G.W. & SESKI J.C. (1976) *Amer. J. Obstet. Gynec.*, **126**, 785.

MORROW C.P., DI SAIA P.J., MANGAN C.F. & LAGASSE L.D. (1977) *Cancer Treat. Rep.*, **61**, 1403.

NATSUME M. (1973) *Systematic Radical Surgery for Carcinoma of Uterine Cervix*, Nankodo, Tokyo.

NAVRATIL E. (1954) In *Surgical Treatment of Carcinoma of the Cervix*. (Ed. Meigs J.V.) p. 218. Grune & Stratton, New York.

NELSON A.J., FLETCHER G.H. & WHARTON J.T. (1975) *Amer. J. Roentgenol.*, **23**, 91.

NELSON J.H. JR. (1976) *Atlas of Radical Pelvic Surgery*. Appleton-Century-Crofts, New York.

NELSON J.H., AVERETTE H.E. & RICHART R.M. (1975) *Dysplasia and Early Cervical Cancer*. Professional Education Publication, American Cancer Society, New York.

NOVAK F. (1963) In *Progress in Gynecology*, Vol. 4 (Ed. Meigs J.V. & Sturgis S.) p. 495. Grune & Stratton, New York.

OKABAYASHI S. (1921 *Surg. Gynecol. Obstet.*, **33**, 335.

PAPANICOLAOU G.N. & TRAUT H.F. (1941) *Amer. J. Obstet. Gynec.*, **42**, 193.

PATERSON M.E.L., PEEL K.R. & JOSLIN C.A.F. (1984) *Brit. med. J.*, **289**, 896.

PEREZ C.A., CAMEL H.M., KAO M.S. & ASKIM F. (1980) *Cancer*, **45**, 2759.

PILLERON J.P., DURAND J.C. & HAMELIN J.P. (1974) *Amer. J. Obstet. Gynec.*, **119**, 458.

PIVER M.S. & BARLOW J.J. (1973) *Cancer*, **32**, 367.

PIVER M.S., BARLOW J.J. & XYNOS F.P. (1978) *Amer. J. Obstet. Gynec.*, **131**, 311.

POULSEN H.E. & TAYLOR C.W. (1975) *International histological classification of tumours*. WHO, Geneva.

PRIDAN H. & LILIENFELD A.M. (1971) *Israel J. med. Sci.*, Vol. 7, **12**, 1465.

RAMPONE J.F., KLEM V. & KOLSTAD P. (1973) *Obstet. Gynecol.*, **41**, 163.

REGAND C.L. (1926) *Rapp. Vlle Cong. Soc. Int., Chirurg.*, **1**, 35.

REID B.L. (1964) *Lancet*, **i**, 21.

RICHART R.M., TOWNSEND D.E., CRISP W., DE PETRILLO A., FERENCZY A., JOHNSON G., LICKRISH G., ROY M. & VILLA SANTA U. (1980) *Amer. J. Obstet. Gynec.*, **137**, 823.

RIGONI-STERN (1842) *G. sevire Progr. pathol. terrap. Ser.*, **2**, 507.

ROTKIN I.D. (1973) *Cancer Res.*, **33**, 1353.

RUBIN I.C. (1910) *Amer. J. Obstet.*, **62**, 668.

SCHAUTA F. (1904) *Mschr. Geburtsh. Gynäk.*, **19**, 475.

SCHILLER W. (1929) *Zlb. Gynäk.*, **53**, 1056.

SHAW'S *Textbook of Operative Gynaecology* (1983) (Eds. Howkins J. & Hudson C.N.), Churchill Livingstone, Edinburgh and London.

SHINGLETON H.M. & ORR J.W. (1983) Eds. *Cancer of the Cervix*. Churchill Livingstone, Edinburgh and London.

SINGER A. (1976) In *The Cervix* (Eds. Jordan J. & Singer A.) Vol **8**, p. 87. W.B. Saunders, London.

SINGER A. & McCANCE D. (1985 *Brit. J. Obstet. Gynec.*, **92**, 1083.

SMITH P.H., TURNBULL G.A., CURRIE D.W. & PEEL K.R. (1969) *Brit. J. Urol.*, **41**, 685.

STALLWORTHY J.S. (1964) *Ann. roy. Coll. Surg. Eng.*, **34**, 161.

STALLWORTHY J. & WIERNIK G. (1976) In *The Cervix*. (Eds. Jordan J.A. and Singer A.) p. 474. Saunders, London.

STAMLER J., FIELDS C. & ANDELMAN S.L. (1967) *Amer. J. publ. Hlth.*, **57**, 791.

SURWIT E., FOWLER W.C. JR., PALUMBO L., KOCH G. & GJERTSEN W. (1976) *Obstet. and Gynecol.*, **48**, 130.

SWAN S.H. & BROWN W.L. (1979) *New Engl. J. Med.*, **46**, 301.

SYMMONDS R.E. (1966) *Amer. J. Obstet. Gynec.*, **94**, 663.

SYMMONDS R.E. & PRATT J.H. (1961) *Obstet. and Gynec.*, **17**, 57.

SYMMONDS R.E., PRATT J.H. & WEBB M.J. (1975) *Amer. J. Obstet. Gynec.*, **121**, 907.

SYMMONDS R.E. & WEBB M.J. (1981) In *Gynecologic Oncology*. (Ed. Coppleson M.). Vol 2, p. 896. Churchill Livingstone, Edinburgh.

TERRIS M., WILSON F., SMITH H., SPRUNG E. & NELSON J.J. (1967) *Amer. J. Publ. Hlth.*, **57**, 840.

TOD M.C. & MEREDITH W.J. (1938) *Brit. J. Radiol.*, **11**, 809.

TRUSSEL R.T., MITFORD-BARBERTON G. DE B. (1961) *Lancet*, **i**, 971.

VINEBERG H.N. (1919) In *Contributions of medical and biological research* (ed. Osler Sir William)., Vol 2, p. 217. Hoeber, New York.

WAKEFIELD J., YULE R., SMITH A. & ADELSTEIN A.M. (1973) *Brit. med. J.*, **ii**, 142.

WALTERS W.D. & REAGAN J.W. (1956) *Amer. J. clin. Path.*, **26**, 1314.

WALTON R.J. (1976) *Can. med. Assn. J.*, **114**, 981.

WALTON R.J. (1982) *Can. med. Assn. J.*, **127**, 953.

WEBB M.J. & SYMMONDS R.E. (1979) *Obstet. & Gynec.*, **54**, 140.

WERTHEIM E. (1905) *Brit. med. J.*, **ii**, 689.

WERTHEIM E. (1911) *Die erweitert abdominale Operation bei Carcinoma Colti Uteri* (Auf Grund Voon 500 Fallon) Urban, Berlin.

WERTHEIM M.S., HAKES T.B., DAGHESTANI A.N., NORI D., SMITH D.H. & LEWIS J.L. (1985) *J. clin. Oncol.*, **3**, 7, 912.

WILLIAMS Sir JOHN (1888) *Harveian Lecture for 1886*, Lewis, London.

YULE R. (1973) In *Cancer of the Uterine Cervix*. (Ed. Easson, E.C.) p. 11. W.B. Saunders Co. Ltd.

YULE R. (1978) *Lancet*, **i**, 1031.

CHAPTER 51
MALIGNANT DISEASE OF THE UTERINE BODY

K. R. PEEL

The commonest of the primary tumours encountered in the uterine body is adenocarcinoma. Squamous carcinoma is rare but when it occurs it develops in a glandular epithelium which has undergone squamous metaplasia. Sarcomas occur much less frequently than adenocarcinomas and include leiomyosarcoma which can develop within the myometrium or within a leiomyofibroma and the rarer sarcomas developing from endometrial stroma. For convenience, cancer of the Fallopian tube is described in this chapter, but gestational tumours, which also occur in the uterus, are described elsewhere (Chapter 37).

CARCINOMA OF THE CORPUS UTERI

Corpus cancer accounts for 4% of cancer in females, being in England and Wales the ninth commonest female cancer, with carcinoma of the ovary the sixth commonest and cervix the eighth commonest (Office of Population Census and Surveys 1983). In the United States of America, however, it is the commonest female pelvic malignancy occurring twice as commonly as cancer of the cervix or ovary (Cancer Statistics 1979). The increased incidence noted in America has been associated with a slight fall in the death rate from endometrial cancer. A detailed analysis of the aetiological factors would suggest that endometrial cancer is hormone dependent. The changed incidence in America is thought to be due to a number of factors including an increased incidence of occult endometrial cancer in association with the use of continuous oestrogen therapy for postmenopausal patients, without either regular endometrial sampling or its combination with progesterone. The misdiagnosis of hyperplasia is another possible reason. Other factors may be relevant, however, because an increased incidence has also been observed in Norway and Czechoslovakia even though oestrogens have been used rarely in those countries or have not been available.

Aetiology

The disease most commonly occurs in postmenopausal women who have had a long menstrual life and few pregnancies if any. Three-quarters of women presenting are over 50 years old, with few under 40 and a peak incidence around 61 years. Nullipara, accounting for 24–31% of patients with endometrial cancer, run twice the risk of developing the disease as women with one child and three times the risk of women with five children or more (McMahon 1974).

Roberts (1961) reported that 73% of patients with endometrial carcinoma ceased menstruation between the ages of 51 and 55 years and a similar increased risk in association with the late menopause has been reported by others. The frequency of anovulatory cycles has been thought relevant by Fox and Sen (1970).

Novak and Yui (1936) first described the association between endometrial cancer and the so-called feminizing tumours, such as granulosa cell or theca cell tumours. Wide-ranging estimates for the development of endometrial hyperplasia (22–56%) and adenocarcinoma (9–23%) in such patients are reported by Evans et al. (1980). Interesting though these tumours are, they account for only a small proportion of cases in young women.

Unopposed endogenous oestrogen is produced in patients with polycystic ovary syndrome, though accurate estimates of their current risk of developing endometrial cancer should be lower than Jackson and Docherty (1957) reported (37.2% of 43 patients) by virtue of the presently recommended practice of treating the failure of ovulation that occurs in this condition.

Obese women have an increased risk of developing endometrial cancer varying from 3 times normal when 21–50 lb overweight to 10 times when the excess of weight is greater than 50 lb (Wynder et al. 1966). Macdonald et al. (1977) suggest the large fat mass allows an increased conversion of androstenedione to oestrone with a subsequently high plasma level thought by them to be crucial to the development of endometrial cancer. Excess oestrogen stimulation may cause endometrial hyperplasia but the malignant potential of hyperplasia varies significantly according to its type. Cystic hyperplasia progresses to malignancy in less than 1% of cases (Schroeder 1954, McBride 1959). Adenomatous hyperplasia carries a greater risk estimated as 14% by Gusberg and Paplan (1963) and also by Chamilion and Taylor (1970).

Atypical hyperplasia is the most dangerous precursor, and according to whether it be mild, moderate or severe it may go on to endometrial cancer in 15, 24 and 45% of cases respectively (Campbell & Baxter 1961). Even higher rates are quoted by Wentz (1974) and Sherman (1978). In spite of the known association, the use of unopposed oestrogens as hormone replacement therapy continued until Smith et al. (1975) first suggested that oestrogen therapy might cause endometrial cancer. This study was later criticized for using patients with other gynaecological malignancies, often showing diametrically opposite aetiological factors, as controls. They reported a 4.5 times greater risk of endometrial cancer in women on oestrogen therapy as compared with the controls. Ziel and Finkle (1975) in the same year suggested risk ratios of 5.6 when therapy had been continued for 1–5 years, rising to 13.9 when more than 7 years' exposure to oestrogen had occurred. Weiss (1978) came to a similar conclusion after studying trends in mortality from uterine cancer. Mack et al. (1976) estimated a risk ratio for any oestrogen use of 8 times, with a risk ratio of 5.6 times for conjugated oestrogens, and they concluded that the risk is dose related with respect to the length of exposure and the magnitude of the dose. Antunes et al. (1979) also showed as much risk with conjugated oestrogens as with diethylstilboestrol and no difference between cyclical and continuous treatment. It was first thought that endometrial cancer so induced was easy to cure but, when grading is taken into account, the results of treatment are no better for drug induced disease than for naturally occurring cancer (Robboy & Bradley 1979).

It is believed by Whitehead et al. (1977) that the risk of endometrial hyperplasia and presumably cancer can be reduced by combining progesterone with oestrogen when hormone replacement therapy is used. Sturdee et al. (1978) suggested that the longer the duration of progesterone use the less is the incidence of hyperplasia. It is therefore now recommended that, whenever oestrogens are prescribed for more than 6 months to the woman with a uterus, oestrogen should be given cyclically and progesterone added for at least 5 and possibly as long as 14 days in the second half of the cycle. Sturdee et al. (1978) warn that regular bleeding does not necessarily imply the absence of an underlying carcinoma and endometrial sampling, with a histological examination of the specimen, should be undertaken regularly.

Whilst Lyon (1975) and Silverberg and Makowski (1975) linked endometrial cancer with sequential oral contraceptives, Weiss and Sayvetz (1980) demonstrated that, whereas the use of Oracon (a preparation contaning 100 μg of ethinyloestradiol which was used by a majority of the patients reported in the earlier papers) carried more than 7-fold the normal risk, the users of oral contraceptives in general had only a 50% incidence of endometrial cancer as compared with non-users.

Because patients with ovarian dysgenesis (Turner's syndrome) require long term oestrogen therapy, it would seem sensible to use a combined oestrogen and progesterone preparation such as would be used for the postmenopausal patient, but a number of authors comment on the rarity of endometrial carcinoma developing in such patients.

Evidence as to the risk in diabetic patients is conflicting. Those with access to large diabetic populations deny a high incidence of endometrial cancer (Kessler 1970, Feroze 1981) yet Wynder et al. (1966) reported an increased risk after correcting for height and weight.

Whereas hypertension is prevalent in the age group in which endometrial cancer is most commonly found, hypertensive patients do not seem to be at increased risk.

An excess of observed over expected cases of endometrial cancer in patients who received pelvic irradiation (McMahon 1974) may be due to the underlying condition for which they were irradiated rather than to the effect of the irradiation.

PATHOLOGY

It is thought that most invasive cancer must evolve through an *in situ* stage and the association between endometrial hyperplasia and adenocarcinoma of the uterus is well recognized. Terminology has in the past been confused, but the classification based on glandular pattern, cell structure and the relationship to the basement membrane as described by Vellios (1972) is generally accepted and shown in Table

Table 51.1. Precursor lesions of invasive endometrial carcinoma.

Cystic hyperplasia
Adenomatous hyperplasia
Atypical hyperplasia
Carcinoma-*in-situ*

From Vellios (1972)

51.1. There are those who dislike the concept of carcinoma-*in-situ* and prefer to classify such cases with atypical hyperplasia (Haines & Taylor 1962). For detailed information on the histological features, the reader is referred to the paper by Vellios (1972) and one by Welch and Scully (1977). Wentz (1974), using the criteria of Vellios, presented data (Table 51.2) on patients with adenomatous hyperplasia, atypical hyperplasia and carcinoma-*in-situ*, who within the subsequent 2–8 years developed invasive endometrial carcinoma. Similar, though less striking, figures, also seen in Table 51.2, were presented by Sherman (1978). It is extremely rare (less than 0.4% according to McBride (1959)) for cystic hyperplasia to progress to carcinoma.

Table 51.2. The risk of carcinoma developing in endometrium previously the site of hyperplasia.

	Percentage patients developing carcinoma according to	
	Wentz (1974)	Sherman (1978)
Adenomatous hyperplasia	26.7	19.8
Atypical hyperplasia	81.8	57.1
Adenocarcinoma-*in-situ*	100.0	57.1

When invasive cancer exists the tumour is nearly always an adenocarcinoma of polypoid or nodular type which spreads around the endometrium or projects into the cavity. The lesion may be diffuse or localized and in the latter case may be in the form of a single, large polyp. In the early stages the growth is usually confined to the fundus, but as it spreads it may come to involve the whole endometrium and then extend into the cervical canal. The uterine wall may become very thin and friable, and this more so if pyometra, due to cervical stenosis, is present, the latter being usually the result of infection rather than obstruction by the tumour itself. Associated lesions are fibroids, commonly, and granulosa cell ovarian tumours rarely. The uterus will, at operation, be found to be enlarged in just over half the cases, but

such enlargement may not easily be detected on clinical examination prior to surgery.

Spread of the tumour is direct in the endometrium itself and, to a lesser degree into the myometrium; the latter, in contradistinction to the cervix and paracervical tissues, is fairly resistant to the invasion by tumour, presumably because of the close interlacing network of muscle fibres, so that penetration to the serosa is unusual. Ovarian involvement is usually the result of direct spread but the ovaries may also be involved (as may the peritoneum or the Pouch of Douglas) by transtubal embolism. Ovarian secondaries are found in about 5 to 7% of cases.

Lymphatic spread occurs along three pathways. The lymphatics draining the upper uterus follow the ovarian vessels and drain into the paraaortic nodes and, in view of the results obtained by treatment which makes no attempt to include them in the surgical resection, their secondary involvement would appear to be uncommon. Lymphatics from the fundus itself pass via the round ligament to the superficial and deep inguinal nodes. When the lower or midportion of the uterus is involved, the lymphatic spread is as for cervical cancer, i.e. to the paracervical, obturator, internal iliac, external iliac and parametrial lymph nodes and less commonly to the sacral, common iliac, inguinal and paraaortic nodes. In order to assess the extent of the surgical procedure required for cure, a number of authors have reported on the incidence of involved lymph nodes (Table 51.3) which ranges from 6.7–28% of cases.

Table 51.3. Frequency of involvement of lymph nodes in endometrial carcinoma.

Authors	No. of cases	(%) Nodes involved
Javert (1952)	50	28
Schwartz & Brunschwig (1957)	96	13
Liu & Meigs (1955)	47	23
Lees (1969)	76	17
Lewis *et al.* (1970)	129	13.2
Milton & Metters (1972)	30	6.7
Winterton (1954)	85	7.1
Rickford (1967)	50	10

The pathologist has the opportunity to assess factors which have a significant bearing on the prognosis, being primarily the extent of spread and also the degree of differentiation of the neoplasm, namely whether the lesion be well differentiated (Grade I), moderately differentiated (Grade II) or undifferentiated (Grade III).

The Cancer Committee of the Fédération Internationale de Gynécologie et Obsetriques (FIGO 1982) recommends that when uterine corporeal carcinoma is staged the staging be based on the findings obtained by inspection and palpation, including examination under anaesthesia, and that one may take into account the information derived from a fractional curettage, cystoscopy or proctoscopy, and the results of radiological studies of the chest, skeleton and urinary tract.

In recent years the hysterscope has been used to assess the extent of tumour spread within the uterus by direct vision. It will be seen that although the FIGO staging (Table 51.4) takes into account only the spread as judged by clinical methods and the histological grading as reported by the pathologist, the additional information made available to the clinician by the pathologist regarding the depth and extent of myometrial involvement is of great value in planning further treatment.

Table 51.4. Definitions of the clinical stages in carcinoma of the corpus uteri (FIGO 1982).

Stage O. Carcinoma-*in-situ*. Histological findings suspicious of malignancy. Cases of Stage O should not be included in any therapeutic statistics.

Stage I The carcinoma is confined to the corpus.
Stage Ia: The length of the uterine cavity is 8 cm or less.
Stage Ib: The length of the uterine cavity is more than 8 cm.
The Stage I cases should be sub-grouped with regard to the histological type of adenocarcinoma as follows:
G1: highly differentiated adenomatous carcinoma
G2: differentiated adenomatous carcinoma with partly solid areas
G3: predominantly solid or entirely undifferentiated carcinoma

Stage II The carcinoma has involved the corpus and the cervix.

Stage III The carcinoma has extended outside the uterus but not outside the true pelvis.

Stage IV The carcinoma has extended outside the true pelvis or has obviously involved the mucosa of the bladder or rectum.
A bullous oedema as such does not permit a case to be allotted to Stage IV.

CLINICAL FEATURES

The commonest presenting symptom in patients suffering from endometrial carcinoma is abnormal uterine bleeding. It is most commonly postmenopausal and the bleeding can be scanty with irregular and sometimes quite long intervals between episodes of bleeding. It should be remembered that 20–25% of cases of corpus cancer present before the menopause and in such patients the bleeding is usually intermenstrual but may be prolonged or heavy menstruation. On occasions the patient may complain of a watery or purulent vaginal discharge. Nearly always symptoms due to local disease will precede those due to metastatic spread to the lungs, spine or long bones.

A full general and pelvic examination is indicated, though frequently abnormal physical signs are not found. The postmenopausal woman can be expected to have a small, atrophic uterus and if in such a patient the uterus is found to be soft and enlarged, having many of the characteristics of a pregnant uterus, an endometrial tumour possibly in association with a pyometra should be suspected. A speculum examination may reveal blood coming through the cervical os or that small, red or plum coloured swellings are present at the lower end of the vagina, alongside the urethra which are due to secondary metastes. Rarely enlarged inguinal lymph nodes are palpable.

Other common causes of postmenopausal bleeding which enter the differential diagnosis are a history of oestrogen therapy, and cervical polypi or atrophic vaginitis which might be seen on examination. Such causes should be discounted until endometrial carcinoma has been excluded by diagnostic curettage.

Attempts have been made to find a screening technique, analogous to cervical smears, which might help in the diagnosis of endometrial cancer. Smears or aspirates taken from the posterior vaginal fornix too often give false negative findings to be regarded as a reliable method of diagnosis. Various mechanical devices for obtaining cytological samples from the endometrial cavity, such as uterine sounds, endometrial brushes or irrigation instruments have been tried with a diagnostic accuracy of cytological preparations ranging from 57–92%. Creasman and Weed (1976) found no single method proved entirely satisfactory. The use of a vacuum curettage does yield specimens which lead to as high a detection rate as a conventional curettage, but this can mean that the opportunity for an associated examination under anaesthesia is missed. Examination under anaesthesia and a fractional curettage therefore remains the diagnostic method of choice. The advantage of a fractional curettage, (i.e. when the surgeon curettes first the endocervical canal, subsequently dilating the cervix prior to using the curette to get specimens from the uterine fundus and then from the lower uterine walls) is that Stage II disease can be recognized. The dilatation and curettage must always be performed with extreme care because the uterine wall may be soft and thin and easily perforated, and this is particularly so when pyometra is present. If pus is found, then the uterus should be drained with a rubber tube left in the cervical os for 2–3 days and the curettage left in abeyance. Antibiotic therapy will be required and it will be necessary to do a further curettage once the infective condition has resolved, if endometrial cancer is not to be missed. Hysterography is used by Continental gynaecologists to delineate the extent of an endometrial tumour. This method has not found favour in Britain because of the theoretical fear of disseminating the growth. Hysteroscopy (Sugimoto 1975) has been recommended to locate small early tumours missed by dilatation and curettage. It can also be used to outline the extent of endometrial carcinoma which could well help in planning appropriate therapy. Provided the procedure is carried out correctly and with scrupulous care, the possible side effects of uterine massive haemorrhage, with dissemination of cancer cells into the abdominal cavity and pelvic infection can be avoided. Additional investigations (cystoscopy, chest X-ray, electrocardiogram, glucose tolerance test and estimation of liver and renal function, blood urea and serum electrolytes) may be required to assess the patient's general physical state before making a decision as regards the best treatment.

TREATMENT OF STAGE I AND STAGE II DISEASE

Whenever possible surgical treatment should be the first and main line of attack. The operation most frequently used for Stage I disease is an abdominal total hysterectomy and bilateral salpingo-oophorectomy. There has been, and is, much discussion as to whether more radical surgery is required to deal with lymph nodes and prevent vaginal vault recurrence, and to a much lesser extent as to the place of vaginal surgery.

The commonest site for recurrence of endometrial cancer is the vaginal vault. The incidence of vault recurrence can be reduced by either removing a cuff of vagina with the uterus or by using pre-operative local irradiation or postoperative vault irradiation, in combination with an abdominal total hysterectomy and bilateral salpingo-oophorectomy. It will be seen from the paragraphs which follow that when irradiation is used postoperative vault irradiation is preferred. Other techniques used to try to avoid recurrence have aimed at preventing vault recurrence resulting from tumour spill during surgery. Simple suture closure of the cervix has been recommended commonly whilst others have tried suturing a flap of vagina over the cervix created from the upper anterior and posterior vaginal walls. Spratt (1960) has described a metal screw which can be used to occlude the cervix. Although these ideas seem attractive, most studies have not shown that any of these techniques result in a reduced rate of vaginal recurrence or an improved 5 year survival (Coperhaver & Barsamian 1967). When the partial vaginectomy is performed to avoid vault recurrence it must be done in a radical way if it is to remove subvaginal lymphatics. Nelson (1977) recommends and describes the 'modified radical hysterectomy' which essentially involves dividing the uterine arteries at their origins from the internal iliac vessels so that the ureters can be dissected free and displaced laterally whilst the bladder is separated from the anterior vagina, so allowing clamps to be applied safely to the parametric tissues and allowing the upper third of the vagina to be removed with the uterus. The modified radical hysterectomy is valuable for treating the patient with Stage I Grade 1 disease so that radiotherapy can be avoided. Patients with carcinoma of the body of the uterus are frequently old, hypertensive and obese and as a result not all patients present an ideal operative risk. Routine radical hysterectomy with pelvic lymphadenectomy in patients with endometrial carcinoma is associated with a higher morbidity than when the operation is performed for cervical cancer, and at the sime time it does not offer the patient a better prospect of cure than when simpler procedures are performed in combination with radiotherapy. Jones (1975) reviewed the results of radical surgery in reported series, which included the Lees' series (1969) from Sheffield and the Oxford series reported by Lewis et al. (1970). The overall 5 year survival rate as 77%, but of those patients who had positive nodes only 24% survived 5 years. From the Oxford series it would appear that most node positive patients already have extrapelvic disease at the time of their original operation and hence even radical surgery cannot be curative.

Although such radical surgery is not recommended as a routine procedure, it is indicated in the treatment of the patient who has Stage II disease (that is, extension of tumour on to the cervix) and who presents no increase in operative risk. Pre-operative intracavity radiotherapy 4–6 weeks prior to surgery is indicated for such patients.

Surgery via the vagina is a poor route to deal with endometrial cancer which has spread to the ovaries, but in the very obese patient with disease restricted to the uterus vaginal hysterectomy may be the operation of choice.

THE PLACE OF RADIOTHERAPY

Postoperative intravaginal radiotherapy offers the same degree of control over vaginal vault recurrence as does pre-operative radiotherapy and is preferred. This procedure however would not adequately treat lymph node disease, so when lymph node metastases are suspected, a combination of intravaginal radiotherapy and external beam therapy should be used. Dobbie (1953) recommended a simple vaginal obturator which, when loaded with the appropriate dose of radium and used over a period of 96 hours, would deliver a dose of 6000 rads to the tissues 0.5 cms beneath the surface from the vaginal vault to the vaginal introitus. This technique reduced the incidence of vaginal vault recurrence to less than 1% but was associated with rectal complications. Joslin (1971) recommended a simple modification to the obturator along with the use of Cobalt 60 sources, resulting in a high activity after loading technique. Treatment is on a daily basis over 5 days with 600–700 rads being delivered throughout the vaginal length to tissues 0.5 cm from the surface of the obturator. A 5 year vaginal vault recurrence rate of about 1% was reported (Joslin 1978). When the risk of lymph node metastases is high (i.e. when the tumour is poorly differentiated, or when myometrial invasion has occurred), then external pelvic irradiation is also indicated. This is normally given in 15 fractions over a period of 21 days with a dose varying from 3000 rads to 3500 rads. When external irradiation is used, the dose of intravaginal irradiation is reduced, normally by giving only 4 daily fractions instead of the usual 5.

In certain circumstances endometrial carcinoma may be treated by radiotherapy alone and this is normally the case with patients considered unfit for surgery. Intracavitary treatment using Heyman's capsules, the Manchester system (which uses a straight intrauterine tube in combination with vaginal ovoids) or the Strickland system which employs a horseshoe shaped source within the uterine cavity, result in 5 year survival figures or around 55–60%.

TREATMENT OF STAGE III AND STAGE IV DISEASE

The treatment of late disease is mainly by radiotherapy with the prime objective being to achieve bulk reduction of the primary tumour by external beam therapy. Once this has been achieved, then a decision can be made as to whether or not the tumour has become operable or whether intracavitary treatment is required. If treatment does not have the required result, then hormone therapy using progestational agents should be added.

Whenever Stage IV disease is associated with spread beyond the pelvis, the aim of radiotherapy should be to control local symptoms which might take the form of bleeding from the uterus, pain in association with bone metastases or occasionally discomfort due to enlarged inguinal or supraclavicular nodes. Progestational agents are indicated just as with Stage III disease.

RECURRENT DISEASE

Recurrent disease may occur: at the vault of the vagina; in the lower third of the vagina; as a mass within the pelvic cavity usually on the side wall and probably arising from lymph node involvement; as distant metastases in lungs or bone.

When previous treatment has been by surgery alone, vaginal or external radiotherapy is indicated to deal with vault recurrence, radium needles for low vaginal lesions and external irradiation for pelvic wall recurrence. Solitary lesions may be suitable for surgical removal. If primary treatment has included radiotherapy and no tissue tolerance remains, the use of progestational agents or cytotoxic drugs should be considered. Metastases in the lungs, spine or long bones can be dealt with by radiotherapy but in some cases they may respond dramatically to hormone therapy.

THE USE OF PROGESTATIONAL AGENTS

Kistner (1959) reported on the favourable effect of synthetic progestogens on endometrial hyperplasia or carcinoma-in-situ of the endometrium, so much so that complete regression was often observed. As a consequence progestogens were used in the treatment of advanced endometrial carcinoma, and Kelly and Baker (1961) first reported significant regression in 6 of their 21 patients in whom 5 had multiple pulmonary metastases which decreased in size or disappeared. It has been reported that pulmonary and skeletal lesions respond better than visceral ones, and that in some cases there is a considerable delay before a favourable therapeutic response is achieved. Kistner and Griffiths (1968) favoured a high loading dose to shorten this time interval. Reifenstein (1974) reported similar objective responses with the use of hydroxyprogesterone hexanoate at a dose of 1 g weekly by intramuscular injection for advanced endometrial carcinoma which had not responded to surgery and the radiotherapy. Of 314 women in the series, regression was noted in 30% of the patients and arrest in a further 7%. The average survival of responding patients was 4 times that of non-responders with an average survival time of 27 months. It appeared that slow growing tumours were more likely to respond, a view supported by the work of Rozier & Underwood (1974) who also noted that the response was likely to be better when the tumour had recurred or when metastases had presented many years after the initial treatment had been undertaken. The most commonly used preparation was medroxyprogesterone acetate (Depo-provera) given at a dose of 200 mg weekly by intramuscular injection. Of their patients, 8 of 13 with lung metastases, 10 of 15 with abdominal lesions and 8 of 17 with pelvic recurrence responded to treatment, Bonte (1983) analysed the remission rate in 3700 patients collected from 84 reports on the use of 11 different pregestogens on patients with advanced or recurrent uterine cancer. By calculating the mean objective remission rate for each individual report, he found a difference in response to the various progestogens, noting a 47% response rate for medroxyprogesterone acetate compared with a 28% response when 17-α hydroxyprogesterone was used.

Ehrlich et al. (1978) looked at the relationship between the rate of response of advanced endometrial adenocarcinoma to progestogens and the presence or absence of progesterone receptors in the corresponding endometrium. In 70 patients accumulated from 4 series, progesterone receptors were found in 88% of those responding and in only 6% of those failing to show a response to treatment.

The place of progestogen therapy in the treatment of persistent or recurrent disease is well established, particularly as the therapy does not give rise to unpleasant side effects, indeed patients frequently report an increased sense of well-being, but the place of progestogen therapy in early disease is far from clear.

Bonte et al. (1978) have claimed that adjuvant hormone therapy using medroxyprogesterone acetate prior to and following treatment with surgery and radiotherapy led to enhanced survival of patients with Stage I disease and believed the improvement is due to the radiosensitizing effect of the hormone. John et al. (1974) observed tumour regression in those patients given gesteronol hexamoate (Depostat) between the diagnostic curettage and the subsequent hysterectomy whilst Boyd et al. (1973) used hydroxyprogesterone hexanoate (Primolut Depot) before pre-operative irradiation was given and up to the time of the hysterectomy in 38 patients. The subsequent recurrence rate was half that in a control group.

On the other hand, following an American multicentred trial, Lewis et al. (1974) reported no significant difference in survival between 2 groups of patients, the first (285 patients) received medroxyprogesterone acetate and the second (287) received a placebo. The 4 year survival figures were 93% for those treated by surgery and radiotherapy and placebo, and 87% for those treated with a progestogen in association with hysterectomy whether or not they had also had associated intracavitary radium. The shortcoming of this trial is that the medroxyprogesterone acetate therapy was given over a period of only 3 months.

Taylor (1983) presented data of a series of 130 patients with carcinoma of the body of the uterus who in addition to having an abdominal hysterectomy and bilateral salpingo-oophorectomy, with or without pre- or postoperative radiotherapy, were also given medroxyprogesterone acetate orally in a dose of 300 mg per day from the time of the first diagnostic curettage, either for 6 weeks when there was no evidence of pelvic spread at laparotomy or indefinitely if such spread was discovered. The death rate was compared with the expected death rate calculated from an earlier study from St. Thomas's Hospital. There were 28 deaths from intercurrent disease in patients who were thought to be free of recurrent carcinoma, but in only 4 of those patients was recurrence formally excluded by postmortem examination. There were no known deaths from recurrent carcinoma when medroxyprogesterone acetate was used, though 8 deaths would have been 'expected' on the basis of their earlier series. Further controlled clinical trials on the use of progestational agents are in progress in Italy, Norway and under the aegis of the Yorkshire Regional Cancer Organization.

CYTOTOXIC THERAPY

Non-hormonal chemotherapy has proved disappointing in the treatment of endometrial cancer. Both Donovan (1974), and Carbone and Carter (1974) reviewed collected reports on treatment with single agents with response rates as follows: 5 fluorouracil 20–25%, cyclophosphamide 25–28% and Adriamycin 38%. Carbone and Carter in their series found no response to treatment with Chlorambucil and Mercaptopurine. It is thought that combination therapy will produce better results and, on the basis of initial reports by Lloyd et al. (1975), and Bruckner and Deppe (1977), the American Gynecologic Oncology Group have initiated a study to establish the efficacy and tolerance of adjunctive cytotoxic therapy. Their results are awaited.

Non-steroid anti-oestrogens such as tamoxifen and aminogluthemide have been tried in patients who have failed to respond to progesterone therapy. Only small numbers of patients were reported by Quinn et al. (1981) but the results were sufficiently encouraging to make further trials worthwhile. The lack of side effects with both of these drugs favours their use in elderly patients who are less likely to tolerate cytotoxic chemotherapy. Anti-oestrogens block the oestrogen receptor system and induce progesterone receptor synthesis. Bonte (1983) has used tamoxifen and medroxyprogesterone acetate in various combinations so as to achieve better results.

OVERALL RESULTS OF TREATMENT

Data available from FIGO(1982) about 7656 patients treated between 1973 and 1975 indicate an overall 5 year survival of 66.6%, with 3.4% lost to follow up and 6.3% dying of intercurrent disease. Survival by stage and the effect of grade is shown in Fig. 51.1 (ungraded patients are not included).

Sarcoma of the uterus

Sarcoma of the uterus, a mesodermal tumour, is rare, accounting for only 1% of female genital tract tumours, yet it is the most malignant of all uterine tumours. It can occur in a variety of forms (see Table 51.5) but the three most common variants are leiomyosarcoma, endometrial stromal sarcoma and malignant Müllerian mixed tumours. Clement and Scully (1981) have provided an excellent review of the pathological features of these lesions. The disease spreads into the myometrium, into pelvic blood ves-

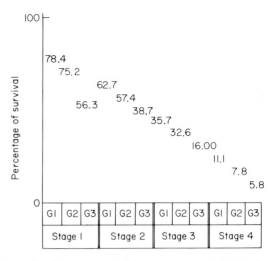

Fig. 51.1. Five year survival data on 7656 patients treated world-wide between 1973 and 1975 (FIGO 1982).

sels and lymphatics, and into adjacent pelvic structures. Distant metastases to the lungs occur not infrequently. The disease is staged using the FIGO staging for endometrial carcinoma.

Little is known about their aetiology but an increased incidence of uterine sarcomas following pelvic irradiation therapy, e.g. for the treatment of carcinoma cervix, has been observed. Piver and Lurain (1981), quoting 8 publications, indicated previous radiotherapy in between 5 and 37% of patients with a figure of 8.3% overall. Such cases occur on average 10–20 years after treatment, are usually malignant Müllerian mixed tumours and carry a worse prognosis

Table 51.5. Types of uterine sarcoma.

Leiomyosarcoma
  (1) Arising in leiomyofibroma
  (2) Arising in myometrium
Endometrial sarcoma
  (1) Stromal sarcoma, to include some or all cases of stromal endometriosis
  (2) Mixed mesodermal-cell tumour, to include:
      sarcoma botryoides
      osteosarcoma
      chondrocarcoma
      rhabdomyosarcoma
      fibromyosarcoma
      carcinosarcoma
Vascular
      Angiosarcoma
      haemangiopericytoma: some cases
Lymphosarcoma

than when sarcomas develop without preceding radiotherapy.

Leiomyosarcoma

The risk of malignant change in a fibroid is difficult to establish yet has been variously quoted as ranging from 1–8 per thousand. The median age at presentation varied from 43 to 56 years in different series, and no relationship with parity has been demonstrated. Both Gudgeon (1978) and Silverberg (1971) have reported a better prognosis for the premenopausal patient.

Clinical features. The symptoms are not specific for the disease and are usually of recent origin. Vaginal bleeding is the commonest presenting complaint and this is often associated with pelvic pain, pressure or discomfort. The patient may be aware of an abdominal mass. Other symptoms include weakness, lethargy, weight loss and fever, and rarely the presenting symptoms may be due to metastatic disease. The usual physical sign is a pelvic mass which may extend into the abdomen. Sarcoma should be suspected if rapid growth in a previously diagnosed fibroid occurs and particularly if the patient is postmenopausal.

Treatment. Dilatation and curettage is not often helpful in establishing the diagnosis, but on the other hand if the sarcoma is protruding through the cervical os, a biopsy may prove conclusive. The mass is nearly always of such a size that a laparotomy is indicated and the normal surgical treatment is an abdominal total hysterectomy and bilateral salpingo-oophorectomy.

Five year survival rates of from 20–63% have been quoted and attempts have been made to use mitotic counts as a prognostic indicator, but probably the best prognostic feature is the extent of the disease at the time of laparotomy.

Oddities include pelvic sarcomas occurring after the removal of apparently benign fibroids by hysterectomy, and the co-called intravenous leiomyomatosis where cords of tumour spread through the uterus and into the vessels of the broad ligament. Such intravenous extensions, it is postulated, originate in the muscle wall of the vein. Pulmonary metastases have also been recorded in some of these cases.

Endometrial stromal tumours

Endometrial stromal tumours are rare. Classification is on the basis of the appearances of the margin of the tumour and the mitotic rate of the central cells. They can take the form of either an endometrial stromal nodule, usually considered benign; endolymphatic stromal myosis, which is characterized by myometrial infiltration (by virtue of vascular and lymphatic invasion spread beyond the uterus both locally and by metastases is common); or endometrial stromal sarcoma which is usually diagnosed on the basis of excessive mitotic activity. This latter tumour is aggressive and carries the worst prognosis.

Stromal tumours occur in the perimenopausal age group, though one-third of patients are postmenopausal. No relationship with parity has been observed, nor is the disease characteristically associated with other diseases. Prior pelvic radiotherapy is not a feature of the disease. Whereas abdominal pain may lead to the palpation of an abdominal mass, it is normally only on pelvic examination that a regular or irregular enlarged uterus is found, often with associated parametrial induration. At operation the uterus is found to be filled with soft brain-like tissue, often showing signs of haemorrhage and necrosis and worm-like extensions into adjacent tissue. Primary treatment is by way of an abdominal total hysterectomy and bilateral salpingo-oophorectomy.

Malignant Müllerian mixed tumours

These tumours can be a mixture of sarcoma and carcinoma. When the sarcomatous element resembles normal endometrial stroma, it would be regarded as homologous, but if tissues foreign to the uterus, such as cartilage, bone or striped muscle are present, it would be called heterologous.

It is usual for these tumours to occur after the menopause and there are often associated clinical conditions such as is seen with endometrial carcinoma, i.e. obesity, diabetes mellitus and hypertension. It is not uncommon for there to be a history of previous pelvic irradiation for carcinoma of the cervix or benign disease of the uterus. Abdominal bleeding is the commonest symptom, though vaginal discharge can occur, occasionally in association with the passage of tissue through the vagina. Pain in either the abdomen or pelvis may be noticed by the patient as may weight loss.

In most patients the uterus is enlarged and often there is a polypoid mass appearing through the cervical os. The grape-like appearance of such polypoid tumours has led to the term, sarcoma botryoides. It is this variety of tumour which affects the cervix and vagina in young children usually in the first decade of life. As with other sarcomas, treatment in the adult is total hysterectomy and bilateral salpingo-oophorectomy.

Whereas sarcoma botryoides in the child was once treated by radical surgery, often to the extent of exenteration, chemotherapy (a triple regime using vincristine, actinomycin D and cyclophosphamide) is now preferred as initial treatment, followed by pelvic radiotherapy and frequently thereafter by an extended hysterectomy and vaginectomy with lymph node dissection. When possible, exenteration is now avoided.

Adjunct radiotherapy and chemotherapy. Evidence is accumulating that radiotherapy may be of some benefit to the patient with either malignant Müllerian mixed tumours or endometrial stromal sarcomas, if confined to the pelvis, by improving the degree of pelvic control and increasing the disease-free interval. There is little to suggest that the overall survival is significantly improved. Leiomyosarcoma seems to be resistant to radiotherapy.

Although, in general, adult sarcomas do not respond to chemotherapy as well as do childhood rhabdomyosarcomas, a number of trials in America have been undertaken using triple therapy (vincristine, adriamycin and diclophosphamide) and, more recently, two other agents, adriamycin and dimethyl-triazeno-imidazole carboxamide, have been used and found active against sarcomas. The drugs have been used in various combinations. Whereas Gottleib *et al.* (1975) and Azizi *et al.* (1979) reported favourably, workers at the Mayo Clinic were unable to come to the same conclusion. Further work is in progress and the situation may change for the better as years go by.

Carcinoma of the Fallopian tube

Carcinoma of the Fallopian tube is often a chance finding when other pelvic pathology had been suspected. Primary carcinoma of the tube is exceedingly rare, accounting for 0.3% of genital tract cancer, but secondary disease, often from adjacent ovarian cancer, is more common. It most commonly occurs in women between 40 and 60 years old, with a peak incidence at about 55 years. Approximately 50% of the patients are nulliparous.

Pathology
The tumour varies in size but often has become palpable by the time it is diagnosed. It is usually unilateral, but 20% of cases are bilateral. The lesion is a papillary adenocarcinoma which tends to occur more often in the lateral part of the tube. In its early stages

it is a purplish fusiform swelling, but if the tumour breaks through the serosal surface of the tube, then papillary growths are apparent and spread to adjacent structures occurs.

Clinical features
It is unusual for the disease to be diagnosed preoperatively, being most commonly mistaken for an ovarian tumour. Unexplained postmenopausal bleeding, a watery vaginal discharge or intermittent unexplained cervical smears showing adenocarcinoma cells should all make the gynaecologist think of a possible tubal carcinoma. In practice only 50% of patients have bleeding or discharge, 30% abdominal pain and 12% a palpable mass.

Treatment
No official FIGO staging exists for carcinoma of the tube, but, as with other tumours, the prospect of cure is dependent upon the stage at which the disease is discovered. The normal treatment is total hysterectomy and bilateral salpingo-oophorectomy. During the operation a careful search of the upper abdominal cavity should be undertaken and biopsies taken from the areas suspected of being the site of secondary carcinoma. The place of omentectomy is not yet established. Postoperative radiotherapy or chemotherapy has been tried, but the relative worth of either remains controversial. Benedet and White (1981) quoting collected series, give 5 year survival figures ranging from 60% for early disease to 15% for late disease.

REFERENCES

ANTUNES C.M.F., STOLLEY P.D., ROSENHEIM N.G., DAVIES J.L., TANASCIA J.A., BROWN C., BURNETT L., RUTLEDGE A., POKEMPNER M. & GARCIA R. (1979) *New Engl. J. Med.,* **300,** 9.

AZIZI F., BITRAN J., JAREHARI G. & HERBST A.L. (1979) *Amer. J. Obstet. Gynec.,* **133,** 379.

BENEDET J.L. & WHITE G.W. (1981) In *Gynecologic Oncology* (Ed. Coppleson M.) **48,** 621. Churchill Livingstone, Edinburgh and London.

BONTE J. (1983) Role of Medroxyprogesterone in Endocrine related tumours. Vol 2 (Eds. Campio L. Robustelli Della Cuna G. & Taylor R.W.), 141. Raven Press, New York.

BONTE J., DECOSTER J.M., IDE P. & BILLIET G. (1978) *Gynec. Oncol.* **6,** 60.

BOYD I.E., POLLARD W. & BLAIKLEY J.B. (1973) *J. Obstet. Gynaecol. Brit. Cwlth.* **80,** 360.

BRÜCKNER H.W. & DEPPE G. (1977) *Obstet. and Gynec.,* **50,** 10.

CAMPBELL P.E. & BAXTER R.A. (1961) *J. Obstet. Gynaec. Brit. Cwlth.,* **68,** 668.

Cancer Statistics (1979) *Ca—A Cancer Journal for Clinicians,* **29,** 6.

CARBONE P.P. & CARTER S.K. (1974) *Gynecol. Oncol.,* **2,** 348.

CHAMILION D.L. & TAYLOR H.B. (1970) *Obstet. and Gynec.,* **36,** 659.

CLEMENT P.B. & SCULLY R.E. In *Gynecologic Oncology* (Ed. Coppleson M.) **46,** 591. Churchill Livingstone Edinburgh and London.

COPERHAVER E.H. & BARSAMIAN M. (1967) *Amer. J. Obstet. Gynec.,* **99,** 864.

CREASMAN W.T. & WEED J.C. JR. (1976) *Cancer,* **38,** 436.

DOBBIE B.M.W. (1953) *J. Obstet. Gynaecol. Brit. Cwlth.,* **60,** 702.

DOOVAN J.F. (1974) *Cancer,* **34,** 1587.

EHRLICH C.E., CLEARY R.E. & YOUNG P.C.M. (1978) *Endometrial Cancer* (Eds. Brush, King & Taylor), **28,** p. 258. Ballière-Tindall, London.

EVANS A.T., GAFFEY T.A., MALKASIAN G.D. & ANNEGERS J.F. (1980) *Ostet. and Gynec.,* **55,** 231.

FEROZE R.M. (1981). In *Integrated Obstetrics and Gynaecology for Postgraduates* (Ed. Dewhurst J.) p. 731. Blackwell Scientific Publications, Oxford.

FIGO (1982) Annual Report on the Results of Treatment in Gynaecological Cancer. Eighteenth volume. Radiumhemmet, Stockholm.

FO H. & SEN D.K. (1970) *Brit. J. Cancer,* **24,** 30.

GOTTLIEB J.A., BAKER L.H., O'BRYAN R.M. et al. (1975) *Cancer Chemother. Rep.,* Part 3, **6,** 271.

GUDGEON D.H. (1978 *Obstet. and Gynec.,* **32,** 96.

GUSBERG S.B. & PAPLAN A.L. (1963) *Amer. J. Ostet. Gynec.,* **87,** 662.

HAINES M. & TAYLOR C.W. (1962) *Gynaecological Pathology.* Churchill, London.

JACKSON R.L. & DOCHERTY M.B. (1957) *Amer. J. Obstet. Gynec.,* **73,** 161.

JAVERT C.T. (1952) *Amer. J. Obstet. Gynec.,* **64,** 780.

JOHN A.H., JACKSON J.W. & BYE P. (1974) *J. Obstet. Gynaec. Brit. Cwlth.,* **81,** 786.

JONES H.W. III (1975) *Obstet. Gyn. Survey* Vol. 30, No. 3.

JOSLIN C.A. (1971) *Modern Radiology in Gynaeccological Cancer* (Ed. T.J. Deeley) p. 71. Butterworths, London.

JOSLIN C.A. (1978) *Endometrial Cancer* (Eds. Brush, King and Taylor) p. 158–62. Ballière-Tindall, London.

KELLY R. & BAKER W. (1961) *New Engl. J. Med.,* **246,** 216.

KESSLER I.I. (1970) *J. natl. Cancer Inst.,* **44,** 673.

KISTNER R.W. (1959) *Cancer,* **12,** 1106.

KISTNER R.W. & GRIFFITHS C.T. (1968) *Clin. Obstet. Gynecol.,* **11,** 439.

LEES D.H. (1969b) *J. Obstet. Gynaec. Brit Cwlth.,* **76,** 615.

LEWIS B.V., STALLWORTHY J.A. & COWDELL R. (1970) *J. Obstet. Gynasec. Brit. Cwlth.,* **77,** 343.

LEWIS G.C. JR., SLACK N.H., MORTEL R. & BROSS I.D.J. (1974) *Gynecol. Oncol.,* **2,** 368.

LIU W. & MEIGS J.V. (1955) *Amer. J. Obstet. Gynec.,* **69,** 1.

LLOYD R.E., JONES S.E. & SALMON S.E. (1975) *Proc. Amer. Assn. Cancer Res.,* **16,** 265.

LYON F.A. (1975) *Amer. J. Obstet. Gynec.,* **123,** 299.

MACK T.M., PIKE M.C., HENDERSON B.E., PFEFFER R.I., GERKINS V.R., ARTHUR M. & BROWN S.E. (1976) *New Engl. J. Med.,* **294,** 1262.

McBRIDE J.M. (1959) *J. Obstet. Gynaec. Brit. Emp.,* **66,** 288.

MACDONALD J.W., ANNEGERS J.F., O'FALLON W.M., DOCHERTY M.B., MALKASIAN G.D. JR. & KIRKLAND J.T. (1977) *Amer. J. Obstet. Gynec.,* **127,** 572.

McMAHON B. (1974) *Gynecol. Oncol.,* **2,** 122.

MILTON P.J.D. & METTERS J.S. (1972) *J. Obstet. Gynaec. Brit. Cwlth.,* **79,** 455.

NELSON J.H. (1977). In *Atlas of Radical Pelvic Surgery,* 2e. Appleton-Century-Crofts, New York.

NOVAK E. & YUI E. (1936) *Amer. J. Obstet. Gynec.,* **32,** 674.

Oce of Population Census and Surveys (1983) *Cancer Statistics,* HMSO, London.

PIVER & LURAIN (1981) In *Gynecologic Oncology* (Ed. Coppleson M.) **47,** p. 608. Churchill Livingstone, Edinburgh and London.

QUINN M.A., CAMPBELL J.J., MURRAY R., PEPPERELL R.J. (1981) *Aust. N.Z. J. Ostet. Gynaecol.,* **21,** 226.

REIFENSTEIN E.C. JR. (1974) *Gynecol. Oncol.,* **2,** 377.

RICKFOD R.B.K. (1967) *Fifth World Congress of Gynaecology and Obstetrics.* Butterworth, Sydney.

ROBBOY S.J. & BRADLEY R. (1979) *Obstet. and Gynec.,* **54,** 269.

ROERTS D.W.T. (1961) *J. Obstet. Gynaec. Brit. Cwlth.,* **68,** 132.

ROIER J.C. & UNDERWOOD P.B. (1974) *Amer. J. Obstet. Gynec.,* **44,** 60.

SCHROEDER R. (1954) *Amer. J. Obstet. Gynec.,* **68,** 294.

SCHWARTZ A.E. & BRUNSCHWIG A. (1957) *Surg. Gynec. Obstet.,* **105,** 697.

SHERMAN A.I. (1978) *Israel J. Med. Sci.,* **14,** 370.

SILVERBERG S.G. (1971) *Obstet. and Gynecol.,* **38,** 613.

SILVERBERG S.G. & MAKOWSKI E.L. (1975) *Obstet. and Gynaec.,* **46,** 503.

SMITH D.C., PRENTICE R., THOMPSON D.J. & HERRMAN W.L. (1975) *New Engl. J. Med.,* **293,** 1164.

SPRATT D. (1960) *Obstet. and Gynecol.,* **15,** 526.

STURDEE D.W., WADE-EVANS T., PATERSON M.E.L., THO M.H. & STUDD J.W.W. (1978) *Brit. med. J.,* **1,** 1575.

SUGIMOTO O. (1975) *Amer. J. Obstet. Gynec.,* **21,** 105.

TAYLO R.W. (1983) In *Role of Medroxyprogesterone in Endocrine Related Tumours.* Vol. 2, p. 157. (Eds. Campio L. Rubustelli Della Cuna G. & Taylor R.W.) Raven Press, New York.

VELLIOS F. (1972) *Pathol. Annu.,* **7,** 201.

WEISS N.S. (1978) *J. Chronic Dis.,* **31,** 705.

WEISS N.S. & SAYVETZ T.A. (1980) *New Engl. J. Med.,* **302,** 551.

WELCH W.R. & SCULLY R.E. (1977) *Human Pathol.,* **8,** 503.

WENTZ W.B. (1974) *Gynecol. Oncol.,* **2,** 362.

WHITEHEAD M.I., McQUEEN J., BEARD R.J., MINARDI J. & CAMPBELL S. (1977) *Acta Obstet. Gynecol. Second Suppl.*, **65**, 91.

WINTERTON W.R. (1954) *Proc. roy. Soc. Med.*, **47**, 895.

WYNDER E.L., ESCHER G.C. & MANTEL N. (1966) *Cancer*, **19**, 489.

ZIEL H.K. && FINKLE W.D. (1975) *New Engl. J. Med.*, **293**, 1167.

INDEX